Reconstructive Surgery of the Rectum, Anus and Perineum
直肠、肛管与会阴重建手术学

注 意

医学知识和临床实践在不断进步。随着新的研究成果展现、临床经验的积累，临床实践、治疗和药物也应有相应的变化。建议读者宜仔细检查展示的操作方法、制造商所提供最新的信息，以核对所推荐药品的剂量或剂型、给药方法和时间、禁忌证。医生有责任根据自己的经验和患者的资料做出诊断，确定每一个患者最佳的剂量和最佳的治疗方法，并采取各种安全预防措施。在法律的最大范围内，出版社和编辑均不承担由于应用本书中的内容或与本书内容相关的对患者造成的损伤或损害的责任。

出版者

Reconstructive Surgery of the Rectum, Anus and Perineum
直肠、肛管与会阴重建手术学

原　著　Andrew P. Zbar
　　　　Robert D. Madoff
　　　　Steven D. Wexner

主　审　李　宁

主　译　王西墨　姜　军　王荫龙

北京大学医学出版社
Peking University Medical Press

ZHICHANG GANGGUAN YU HUIYIN CHONGJIAN SHOUSHUXUE

图书在版编目（CIP）数据

直肠、肛管与会阴重建手术学 /（以）巴（Zbar, A.P.）,（美）玛多弗（Madoff, R.D.）,（美）维克斯纳（Wexner, S.D.）著；王西墨，姜军，王荫龙译 . —北京：北京大学医学出版社，2014.8

书名原文：Reconstructive surgery of the rectum, anus and perineum

ISBN 978-7-5659-0822-4

Ⅰ . ①直… Ⅱ . ①巴… ②玛… ③维… ④王… ⑤姜… ⑥王… Ⅲ . ①直肠疾病－外科手术②肛门疾病－外科手术③会阴－外科手术Ⅳ . ① R657.1 ② R713.2

中国版本图书馆CIP数据核字（2014）第 061167 号

北京市版权局著作权合同登记号：图字：01-2014-4137

Translation from English language edition:
Reconstructive Surgery of the Rectum, Anus and Perineum
by Andrew P. Zbar, Robert D. Madoff and Steven D. Wexner
Copyright © 2013 Springer London
Springer London is a part of Springer Science+Business Media
All Rights Reserved

Simplified Chinese translation copyright © 2014 by Peking University Medical Press.
All rights reserved. Except for use in a review, the reproduction or utilization of this work in any form or by any electronic, mechanical, or other means, now known or hereafter invented, including xerography, photocopying, and recording, and in any information storage and retrieval system, is forbidden without the written permission of the publisher.

版权所有，除以评论为目的外，未经出版者书面许可，禁止以任何形式使用原著，不论是电子的、机械的还是其他形式，不论是现在已知的，还是将来可能出现的使用方式，包括复印、影印、录音，或用于其他形式的信息储存或检索系统。

直肠、肛管与会阴重建手术学

主　　译：	王西墨　姜　军　王荫龙
出版发行：	北京大学医学出版社
地　　址：	（100191）北京市海淀区学院路38号　北京大学医学部院内
电　　话：	发行部：010-82802230；图书邮购：010-82802495
网　　址：	http://www.pumpress.com.cn
E-mail：	booksale@bjmu.edu.cn
印　　刷：	北京圣彩虹制版印刷技术有限公司
经　　销：	新华书店
责任编辑：	罗德刚　金美娜　　责任校对：金彤文　　责任印制：张京生
开　　本：	889mm×1194mm　1/16　印张：34.5　字数：1029千字
版　　次：	2014年8月第1版　2014年8月第1次印刷
书　　号：	ISBN 978-7-5659-0822-4
定　　价：	320.00元

版权所有，违者必究

（凡属质量问题请与本社发行部联系退换）

译校者名单

主　审：李　宁

主　译：王西墨　姜　军　王荫龙

副主译：龚剑峰　李国逊

译　者：（按姓氏笔画排序）

天津市南开医院

于向阳　王西墨　邹常林　陈建军　邵　伟　崔志刚

南京军区南京总医院　全军普通外科研究所

丁威威　王　刚　王绪林　韦　瑶　冯啸波　刘建磊
江志伟　李　宁　李　民　李　毅　汪志明　陈启仪
范朝刚　赵　坤　胡雄辉　姜　军　倪　玲　龚剑锋
管　群

天津市人民医院暨南开大学人民医院　天津市大肠肛门病研究所

王荫龙　王树森　尹注增　石　洋　许　晨　李　超
李　鹏　李国逊　李淑媛　杨　东　张　帅　张　林
张　昭　张巨东　张明庆　张春泽　陈　硕　郑　阳
徐　彬　徐　靖　曹　磊

秘　书：冯啸波　陈建军

统　筹：王云亭

策　划：黄大海

主审简介

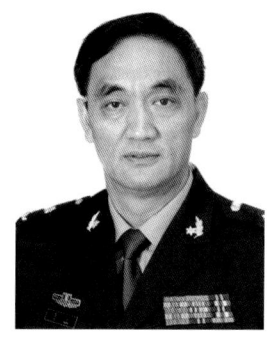

李宁，1952年生，医学硕士，南京军区南京总医院、全军普通外科研究所主任，主任医师，博士后联系导师，博士研究生导师，硕士研究生导师。南京大学医学院教授，第二军医大学教授。全军普通外科专业委员会主任委员；中华医学会外科学分会常务委员、营养支持学组组长；中华医学会肠外肠内营养学分会主任委员；南京军区普通外科专业委员会主任委员；江苏省医学会常务理事、省外科学会副主任委员；南京医学会常务理事、普通外科专业委员会副主任委员；国家食品药品监督管理局药品评审专家；国家基本药物目录遴选与调整专家；国家自然科学基金评审专家。

主译简介

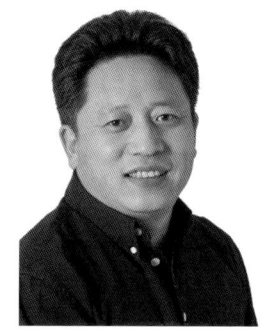

王西墨，1966年生，外科学博士，主任医师。天津市南开医院院长，天津市大肠肛门病研究所所长。南开大学医学院外科学教授。天津中医药大学中西医结合外科学博士研究生导师组成员，天津医科大学硕士研究生导师，南开大学医学院硕士研究生导师。加拿大西安大略大学多器官移植中心博士后。美国哈佛大学医学院、美国匹兹堡大学医学院、美国明尼苏达大学胰岛移植与糖尿病治疗中心访问学者。中国中西医结合学会理事，中国中西医结合学会大肠肛门专业委员会副主任委员，中华医学会外科学分会委员，中华医学会外科学分会结直肠外科学组委员，中华医学会消化内镜分会内镜外科学组委员，天津市医学会外科学分会副主任委员，天津中西医结合学会常务理事，天津市中西医结合研究院副理事长，天津中西医结合研究院学术委员会副主任委员，《中华肝胆外科杂志》编委，《天津医药》编委。

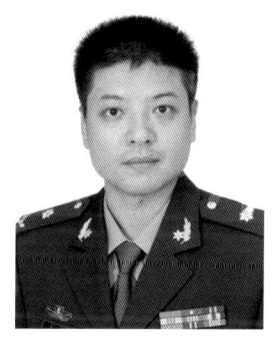

姜军，1969年生，外科学博士，南京军区南京总医院普通外科副主任医师，南京大学医学院副教授，硕士研究生导师。中华医学会外科学分会中青年委员，中华医学会外科学分会结直肠肛门外科学组委员；全军结直肠病学专业委员会常务委员，胃肠功能性疾病学组副组长；全军普通外科专业委员会结直肠外科专业学组委员；全军中医药学会肛肠专业委员会常务委员。

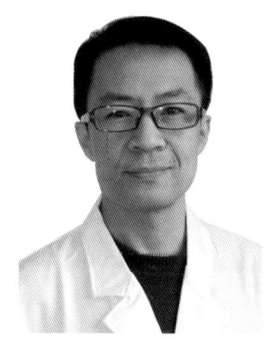

王荫龙，1964年生，副主任医师，医学硕士，毕业于天津中医药大学。自1987年开始从事普通外科的临床和科研工作。2004年起任天津市人民医院疝和腹壁外科主任，曾主持"天津市腹股沟疝流行病调查"。现任中国医师协会普通外科分会疝和腹壁外科委员会委员，天津市医学会外科分会疝和腹壁外科学组副主任委员，《中华疝和腹壁外科杂志》编委。

副主译简介

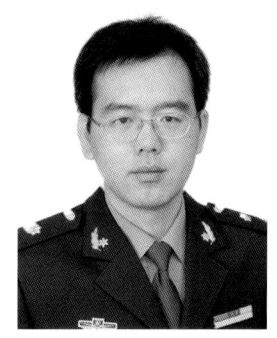

龚剑峰，南京军区南京总医院普通外科主任助理，副主任医师，副教授。2005年获南京大学外科学博士学位。现任南京大学医学院及南方医科大学硕士生导师，中华医学会肠内肠外营养分会青年委员会副主任委员。主要研究方向：炎症性肠病的外科治疗、复杂胃肠疾病的外科治疗、临床营养支持。获国家自然科学基金面上项目2项，江苏省自然科学基金项目1项。发表SCI论文5篇，中文核心期刊论文20余篇。

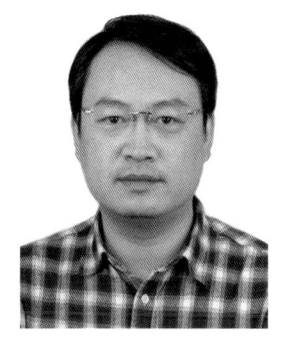

李国逊，医学博士，副主任医师。南开大学硕士生导师，天津市人民医院普通外科副主任和营养科主任。中华医学会外科学分会感染与危重症学组委员，天津市医学会外科学分会感染与危重症学组副组长，天津中西医结合学会普通外科专业委员会委员，《中国临床药理学杂志》青年编委。2010年到2011年在美国和英国做访问学者，在美国匹兹堡大学医学中心重点研修胃肠外科腹腔镜治疗方法及小肠移植的实施，在英国圣马克医院医院则重点研修结直肠外科中良性疾病的诊治。目前在国内外核心专业期刊发表学术文章20余篇，参编学术专著6部，参译学术专著1部。

译者序言

2013年，我们这个译者团队合作翻译了美国结直肠外科医师学会（ASCRS）的教科书《美国结直肠外科医师学会结直肠外科学》，出版后反响较好。在该书的翻译过程中，主审李宁教授就向我提及并积极推荐翻译《直肠、肛管与会阴重建手术学》一书；机缘巧合的是，这本书的中文版权恰好就在北京大学医学出版社，在与相关人员接洽后，我们这个团队很荣幸再次承接了这本书的翻译任务。

本书的主要译者们是一群极富活力的年轻外科医生，他们绝大部分时间都在忙于临床繁琐的日常工作，书稿的翻译都是他们挤出少得可怜的业余时间完成的；虽然辛苦，但这两本书的翻译工作让他们获益匪浅。如果说《美国结直肠外科医师学会结直肠外科学》是系统的理论讲述的话，那么《直肠、肛管与会阴重建手术学》则是非常贴近临床实战的经验交流汇总，两本书相互呼应、相得益彰。正是由于原著作者们丰富的临床经验和深厚的学术造诣，才保证了本书拥有极高的学术价值，所以我要在这里对原著作者们表示由衷的敬佩和衷心的感谢！

正如先前所说，本书的主要译者们都是年轻的外科医生，翻译对于他们来说都停留在业余水平上，距离傅雷先生对翻译要求的"信、达、雅"还相差很大一段距离。同时由于时间仓促，尽管已尽极大的努力，但错误肯定在所难免，还请阅读本书的各位专家同道批评指正；若有可能，我们还是建议大家阅读原汁原味的原版著作。

在本书的翻译过程中，编译秘书陈建军医生和冯啸波医生居中协调，统稿联络；同时还承担绝大部分稿件的文字校对工作，为本书的顺利成稿和出版付出了大量的心血。中华国际医学交流基金会的黄大海老师从本书的筹备到最后出版的全过程都给予了我们巨大的帮助；本书能顺利付梓，还包含了出版社其他老师在幕后的大力支持，在此一并表示衷心的感谢！

王西墨
2014年4月

原著序言

《直肠、肛管与会阴重建手术学》这本专业教材由来自五大洲的国际知名专家组参与编写，Andrew Zbar、Robert Madoff 和 Steven Wexner 共同主编完成，包括 54 章，共 600 多页。本书重点论述了如何处理直肠、肛管和会阴疾病先前治疗失败所导致的病例，包括良、恶性疾病或并发症导致的治疗失败，如吻合口瘘。这些问题在结直肠外科中很常见，本书详细介绍了处理这些问题的措施，包括通过挽救性治疗（通常是手术治疗）来处理某些重要的问题，如癌症复发、贮袋失败；同时，本书对其他结直肠疾病进行了十分深入的阐述。本书是一本高级教科书，主要读者是三级医学中心的外科医师和渴望完成三级临床实践的实习医生，其他结直肠外科书籍都未能达到此高度。

本书分为 8 篇，包括前期检查、决策制订、炎性肠病的再手术方案、便秘和排便梗阻、大便失禁、肛门重建技术、造口和其他专题。每一篇均以专家引言作为开始。

本书文字讲解清晰，各章都很易懂。每章内容都涵盖了最新研究资料，并且包含了极好的细节。参考书目来源广泛，是非常有用的资源。参考文献在文中很容易找到，在基本不干扰阅读的同时能很容易地查询。文中的彩图都是高质量的，在手术治疗盆腔复发的章节尤为突出，包含了很多信息。线条图都很清晰，并且很容易理解；书中还有很多高质量的临床照片，表格设计也很合理且容易阅读。

本书不仅涵盖了整个大肠肛门病学范畴内较常见的疾病，还介绍了一些罕见疾病的治疗方法。部分章节介绍了较新的技术，如腹腔镜、机器人手术和 STARR，并阐述了可能发生的问题及解决方法。另外，介绍肛管和会阴部重建方法的章节也非常有用。本书最后一章介绍了医疗法律方面的内容，对临床实践也十分有益。

作为一本权威著作，本书满足了结直肠外科医师和实习医师在临床实践中的更高需求，可以说是一座知识宝库，对相关医生来说具有很高价值。

Emeritus Consultant Surgeon,
St Mark's Hospital, London
Professor of Colorectal Surgery,
Imperial College, London

John Nicholls
MA (Cantab), M.Chir, FRCS (Eng),
EBSQ (Coloproctology), hon FRCP (Lond),
hon FACS, hon FRCSE,
hon FRCS (Glasg), hon ASCRS,
hon ACPGBI, hon ESCP, hon BSG

原著前言

很少有文献提出直肠、肛管和会阴良恶性疾病重建手术的治疗原则，然而，结直肠专家经常要面对因复杂疾病而多次治疗失败的患者，如高位复杂性肛瘘或难治性肛周克罗恩病，面对这种情况，我们就必须熟悉各种新的手术方法及辅助技术。虽然良性肛门直肠病学并没有从大肠肛门病学中发展成为一个独立的附属学科，但随着更多的结直肠医生在这个领域获得显著声誉，这个学科会变得越来越专业化。随着复杂修复技术和骶神经调节技术成为新的亚学科，对排泄功能障碍的患者的治疗和影像检查也被归入这个方向。目前，并没有面向大肠肛门病学员的认证规范，来指导他们对于常规影像学检查或是其他放射学技术如磁共振或排粪造影的理解。

本书第一篇介绍了不同的影像学检查对于需要行重建手术或再次手术的患者的作用。论述了在这些复杂病例中，传统 X 线平片、排粪造影、腔内超声、磁共振和内镜检查的适应证，如何选择、如何解读及其局限性。此部分还评估了肛门直肠测压、向量容积测压、阻抗面积测量法、电子恒压器检测、神经生理学检测用于再手术病例的生理原则。

第二篇介绍了推荐用于改进超低位吻合的技术，超低位吻合通常会伴有明显的术后功能紊乱，尤其是在新辅助放射治疗后或出现吻合口瘘后。这部分介绍了新直肠贮袋及其修正手术，还同时介绍了用于放射损伤性直肠的特定手术。进行广泛癌肿切除和盆腔脏器廓清患者的手术细节是由世界上不同区域的两个主要的手术团队来确定的，他们描述了进行广泛 R0 切除的方法。还讨论了进行高难度腹腔镜手术和机器人结直肠手术的机械原理，并同时介绍了肛管癌及其瘤前综合征的治疗原则，以及在直肠根治性切除后进行完全肛门直肠重建的结局。

第三篇概述了炎性肠病的手术方式，并讨论了结肠炎患者肠上皮增生的临床重要性、回肠贮袋肛管吻合后的重复手术、再手术原则、结肠克罗恩病和溃疡性结肠炎的结局、不同方法治疗复杂和反复肛周克罗恩病的效果。

第四篇探讨了失功性肠病的再手术，并讨论了如何处理手术失败的严重便秘、巨直肠和修补失败的直肠前突，以及如何处理肛内吻合器手术效果不太满意的病例；还总结了妇科医生对于原发性盆底疾病、会阴部软组织及盆腔间隔问题的看法。

第五篇确定了与反复大便失禁患者有关的已知数据，评估了重复括约肌成形术的作用，同时评估了失败的股薄肌成形术、仍存有疑问的人工括约肌植入术和骶神经刺激术，以及括约肌功能加强治疗的效果。

第六篇分析了肛管和会阴部的表面修复的手术方法和替代治疗，特别关注了难治性反复或顽固的肛裂，以及复杂性肛瘘、困难的直肠阴道瘘重复手术及直肠前列腺瘘的治疗。

第七篇讨论了造口修复手术，包括造口移位及局部修复，以及最近成功的腹腔镜造口旁疝修补术、Hartmann 反转术的手术方法、儿科造口的修复。

第八篇概述了一些需要进行修复手术的混杂性结直肠和肛门直肠病变的治疗方法。讨论了对于这些患者麻醉管理的新方法，治疗复杂憩室炎的新方法，以及吻合口裂开的治疗方法。重温了骶前肿瘤及其手术方法，以及直肠脱垂手术治疗失败后的处理方法。评估棘手的反复藏毛窦疾病及结肠直肠子宫内膜异位的再手术治疗。最后还提及了需要再手术或重建手术患者的医疗法律方案，其中着重介绍了在再手术后功能预后处于危险状态的患者。

正是由于癌症的多学科综合治疗需要专业化的

知识，成功治疗直肠、肛门及会阴复杂疾病需要在一个类似的领域里拥有复杂的专业知识，最好由可以与其他学科专家合作并对记录前瞻性功能预后数据有兴趣的人来进行。这本新书为治疗复杂病例提供了协同方法的依据。

感谢所有章节的作者，感谢他们付出的时间、专业知识和创造力，这些对这本新书来说是必需的。我们还要进一步感谢 Springer 的 Mlissa Morton 推动本书被 Springer-Verlag 和 Maureen Pierce 收录；还要感谢我们孜孜不倦的编辑，使这本书成功出版。

Andrew P. Zbar
Robert D. Madoff
Steven D. Wexner

原著者名单

Herand Abcarian, M.D. Division of Colon and Rectal Surgery, Stroger Hospital of Cook County, Chicago, IL, USA

Division of Colon and Rectal Surgery, University of Illinois at Chicago, Chicago, IL, USA

Donato F. Altomare, M.D. Department of Emergency and Organ Transplantation, University Aldo Moro of Bari, Bari, Italy

Corrado R. Asteria, M.D. Department of Surgery and Orthopaedics, General Surgery Unit, Carlo Poma, Mantua, Italy

Kirk Austin, B.Sc., MBBCh, BAO, LRCP & SI, AFRCSI, FRACS Department of Colorectal Surgery, Royal Prince Alfred Hospital, Camperdown, NSW, Australia

C.G.M.I. Baeten, M.D., Ph.D. Department of Surgery AZM, University Hospital Maastricht, Maastricht, The Netherlands

Goran I. Barišić, M.D., Ph.D. Clinical Center of Serbia, First Surgical Clinic, Belgrade, Serbia

Medical School, University of Belgrade, Belgrade, Serbia

Rosilma Gorete Lima Barreto, M.D., Ph.D. School of Medicine, Clinic Hospital, Federal University of Maranhão, Fortaleza, Brazil

David C.C. Bartolo, M.S. (Lond), FRCS Department of Surgery, Western General Hospital, Edinburgh, Scotland, UK

Geerard L. Beets, M.D., Ph.D. Department of Surgery, Maastricht University Medical Centre, Maastricht, The Netherlands

Regina G.H. Beets-Tan, M.D., Ph.D. Department of Radiology, Maastricht University Medical Centre, Maastricht, Limburg, The Netherlands

Sergio Bellarosa, M.D. Department of Radiology, Carlo Poma, Mantua, Italy

Roberto Bergamaschi, M.D., Ph.D., FRCS, FASCRS, FACS Division of Colon and Rectal Surgery, State University of New York, Stony Brook, NY, USA

Mitchell Bernstein, M.D., FACS, FASCRS Division of Colon & Rectal Surgery, NYU Langone Medical Center, New York, NY, USA

John Beynon, B.Sc., M.B.B.S., M.S., FRCS (ENG.) Department of Colorectal Surgery, Singleton Hospital, Sketty Lane, Swansea, UK

Andrea Bischoff, M.D. Colorectal Centre for Children, Cincinnati, OH, USA

Department of Pediatric Surgery, Cincinnati Children's Hospital Medical Center, University of Cincinnati, Cincinnati, OH, USA

Ronald Bleday, M.D., FACS, FASCRS Department of Surgery, Brigham and Women's Hospital, Harvard Medical School, Boston, MA, USA

Jennifer Blumetti, M.D. Division of Colon and Rectal Surgery, Stroger Hospital of Cook County, Chicago, IL, USA

Division of Colon and Rectal Surgery, University of Illinois at Chicago, Chicago, IL, USA

Edward C. Borrazzo, M.D., FACS Department of Surgery, University of Vermont College of Medicine, Burlington, VT, USA

Stepahnie O. Breukink, M.D., Ph.D. Department of Surgery AZM, University Hospital Maastricht, Maastricht, The Netherlands

Valérie Bridoux, M.D. Digestive Surgery Unit, Rouen University Hospital, Rouen, France

Luigi Brusciano, M.D., Ph.D. XI Division of General and Obesity Surgery, Second University of Naples, Aversa, Italy

Federica Cadeddu, M.D. Department of General Surgery, University Hospital Tor Vergata, Rome, Italy

Hester Y.S. Cheung, FRACS, FHKAM (Surgery) Department of Surgery, Pamela Youde Nethersole Eastern Hospital, Chai Wan, Hong Kong, China

Peter Christensen, M.D., Ph.D., DmSci Department of Surgery P, Aarhus University Hospital, Aarhus, Denmark

Cliff C.C. Chung, FRCSEd, FHKAM (Surgery) Department of Surgery, Pamela Youde Nethersole Eastern Hospital, Chai Wan, Hong Kong, China

Fernando de la Portilla, M.D., Ph.D., MAECP, EBSQ-C Coloproctology Section, Department of Surgery, Virgen del Rocio University Hospital, Seville, Spain

A. Del Genio, M.D. XI Division of General and Obesity Surgery, Second University of Naples, Aversa, Italy

J. Manuel Devesa, M.D., EBSQC Department of Surgery, University of Alcalá de Henares, Madrid, Spain

Colorectal Unit, Hospital Universitario Ramón y Cajal, Madrid, Spain

Colorectal Unit, Hospital Ruber Internacional, Madrid, Spain

C. Di Stazio, M.D. XI Division of General and Obesity Surgery, Second University of Naples, Aversa, Italy

Javier Die, M.D. Colorectal Unit, Hospital Universitario Ramón y Cajal, Madrid, Spain

Hans Peter Dietz, M.D., Ph.D. Discipline of Obstetrics, Gynaecology and Neonatology, Sydney Medical School Nepean, Nepean Hospital, Penrith, NSW, Australia

Eric J. Dozois, M.D., FACS, FACRS Division of Colon and Rectal Surgery, Mayo Clinic, Rochester, MN, USA

Adam Janusz Dziki, M.D., Ph.D. Department of General and Colorectal Surgery, Medical University of Lodz, Lodz, Poland

Łukasz A. Dziki, Ph.D. Department of Clinical Nutrition, Medical University of Lodz, Lodz, Poland

Department of General and Colorectal Surgery, Medical University of Lodz, Lodz, Poland

Yair Edden, M.D. Department of Colorectal Surgery, Cleveland Clinic Florida, Weston, FL, USA

C. Neal Ellis, M.D., FACS, FASCRS, FACG Chief of Surgery, VA Gulf Coast Veterans Health Care System, Biloxi, MS, USA

Sanne M.E. Engelen, M.D., Ph.D. Department of Surgery, Catharina Hospital, Eindhoven, The Netherlands

David A. Etzioni, M.D., MSHS Department of Surgery, Mayo Clinic, Phoenix, AZ, USA

Martyn D. Evans, B.M., M.Phil., FRCS (Gen Surg) Department of Colorectal Surgery, Singleton Hospital, Sketty Lane, Swansea, UK

Przemysław Galbfach, Ph.D. Department of Surgery Second Division, Wojewodzki Szpital Zespolony, Plock, Poland

Marc A. Gladman, M.B.B.S., DRCOG, DFFP, Ph.D., MRCOG, FRCS (Gen Surg) FRACS Academic Colorectal Unit, Concord Hospital, University of Sydney, Sydney, NSW, Australia

Brooke H. Gurland, M.D., FASCRS, FACS Department of Colorectal Surgery A30, Cleveland Clinic, Cleveland, OH, USA

Najib Y. Haboubi, MBChB, FRCS, FRCPath, FRCP, DPTH Department of Cellular Pathology, University Hospital of South Manchester, Manchester, UK

Olof Hallböök, M.D., Ph.D. Department of Surgery, University Hospital, Linköping, Sweden

James Hill, MBChB, FRCS, ChM Department of Surgery, Manchester Royal Infirmary, Oxford Rd, Manchester, UK

Kok Sun Ho, M.B.B.S., FRCSED, FAMS, MMED (Surg) Department of Colorectal Surgery, Singapore General Hospital, Outram Road, Singapore, Singapore

Tracy L. Hull, M.D. Department of Colorectal Surgery, The Cleveland Clinic Foundation, Cleveland, OH, USA

Neil Hyman, M.D. Department of Surgery, University of Vermont College of Medicine, Burlington, VT, USA

Division of General Surgery, Digestive Disease Center, Burlington, VT, USA

Joshua R. Karas, M.D. Division of Colon and Rectal Surgery, State University of New York, Stony Brook, NY, USA

Urban Karlbom, M.D., Ph.D. Department of Surgical Sciences, University Hospital, Uppsala, Sweden

Hasan T. Kirat, M.D. Department of Colorectal Surgery, Cleveland Clinic Foundation, Cleveland, OH, USA

Zoran Krivokapić, M.D., FRCS, Ph.D. Clinical Center of Serbia, First Surgical Clinic, Belgrade, Serbia

Medical School, University of Belgrade, Belgrade, Serbia

Mary R. Kwaan, M.D. Division of Colon and Rectal Surgery, Department of Surgery, University of Minnesota Medical School, Minneapolis, MN, USA

Mariano Laporte, M.D. Colorectal Surgery Section, General Surgery Department, Hospital Aleman de Buenos Aires, Buenos Aires, Argentina

Søren Laurberg, M.D., DmSci Department of Surgery P, Aarhus University Hospital, Aarhus, Denmark

Peter Jun Myung Lee, M.B.B.S., B.Sc. (Med), FRACS Colorectal Department, Royal Prince Alfred Hospital (Sydney), Newtown, NSW, Australia

Anne-Marie Leroi, M.D. Service de Physiologie Digestive, Hôpital Charles Nicolle, Rouen, France

Physiology Unit, Rouen University Hospital, Rouen, France

Marc A. Levitt, M.D. Colorectal Centre for Children, Cincinnati, OH, USA

Department of Pediatric Surgery, Cincinnati Children's Hospital Medical Center, University of Cincinnati, Cincinnati, OH, USA

Bruce F. Levy, MBChB (Hons), M.Sc., FRCS, M.D. Department of Surgery, Minimal Access Therapy Training Unit, Guildford, Surrey, UK

Michael K.W. Li, FRCS (Eng), FRCSEd, FHKAM (Surgery) Department of Surgery, Pamela Youde Nethersole Eastern Hospital, Chai Wan, Hong Kong, China

Walter E. Longo, M.D., M.B.A. Colon and Rectal Surgery, Department of Gastrointestinal Surgery, Yale University School of Medicine, New Haven, CT, USA

F. Lucido, M.D. XI Division of General and Obesity Surgery, Second University of Naples, Aversa, Italy

Jonathan N. Lund, BMedSci (Hons), BMBS, DM, FRCS (Gen) Division of Surgery, School of Graduate Entry Medicine and Health, Royal Derby Hospital, University of Nottingham, Derby, UK

Robert D. Madoff, M.D. Division of Colon and Rectal Surgery, Department of Surgery, University of Minnesota Medical School, Minneapolis, MN, USA

Yasuko Maeda, MRCS, M.Phil. Sir Alan Parks Physiology Unit, St Mark's Hospital, Harrow, Middlesex, UK

David J. Maron, M.D., M.B.A. Department of Colorectal Surgery, Cleveland Clinic Florida, Weston, FL, USA

Klaus E. Matzel, M.D. Department of Surgery, University Erlangen, Erlangen, Germany

Francis Michot, M.D., Ph.D. Digestive Surgery Unit, Rouen University Hospital, Rouen, France

Giovanni Milito, M.D. Department of General Surgery, University Hospital Tor Vergata, Rome, Italy

Litza Mitalas, M.D., Ph.D. Department of Surgery, Reinier de Graaf Gasthuis, Delft, The Netherlands

Sthela Maria Murad-Regadas, M.D., Ph.D. Department of Surgery, School of Medicine of the Federal University of Ceara, Fortaleza, Brazil

Juan J. Nogueras, M.D., FACS, FASCRS Department of Colorectal Surgery, Cleveland Clinic Florida, Weston, FL, USA

Lars Påhlman, M.D., Ph.D. Department of Surgical Sciences, University Hospital, Uppsala, Sweden

Joel Palefsky, M.D., FRCP(C) Department of Infectious Diseases, University of California, San Francisco, CA, USA

Alberto Peña, M.D. Colorectal Centre for Children, Cincinnati, OH, USA

Department of Pediatric Surgery, Cincinnati Children's Hospital Medical Center, University of Cincinnati, Cincinnati, OH, USA

Mario Pescatori, M.D., FRCS, EBSQ Department of Coloproctology Unit, Ars Medica Hospital and La Sapienza University, Rome, Italy

Johann Pfeifer, M.D. Department of General Surgery, Medical University of Graz, Graz, Austria

Vittorio Luigi Piloni, M.D. SICCR Imaging Section,
Diagnostic Imaging Center "N. Aliotta", Villa Silvia Clinic, Senigallia (AN), Italy

Filippo Pucciani, M.D. Department of Medical and Surgical Critical Care,
University of Florence, Florence, Italy

Micha Rabau, M.D. Proctology Unit, Department of Surgery B, Tel Aviv Sourasky Medical Center, Sackler School of Medicine, Tel-Aviv University, Tel-Aviv, Israel

Vikram Reddy, M.D., Ph.D. Colon and Rectal Surgery, Department of Gastrointestinal Surgery, Yale University School of Medicine, New Haven, CT, USA

F. Sergio P. Regadas, M.D., Ph.D. Department of Surgery, School of Medicine of the Federal University of Ceara, Fortaleza, Brazil

Feza H. Remzi, M.D., FACS, FASCRS, FTSS (Hon) Department of Colorectal Surgery, Cleveland Clinic Foundation, Cleveland, OH, USA

Patricia L. Roberts, M.D. Department of Colon and Rectal Surgery, Lahey Clinic, Burlington, MA, USA

Timothy A. Rockall, M.B.B.S., FRCS, M.D. Department of Surgery,
Royal Surrey County Hospital, Guildford, Surrey, UK

Jack W. Rostas III M.D. Department of Surgery, University of South Alabama College of Medicine, Mobile, AL, USA

Nicolás A. Rotholtz, M.D. Vice Director, Colorectal Surgery Program,
University of Buenos Aires, Buenos Aires, Argentina

Chief of Colorectal Surgery Division, Hospital Aleman de Buenos Aires, Buenos Aires, Argentina

Emil N. Salmo, FRCPath Department of Histopathology, Royal Bolton NHS Foundation Trust, Bolton, UK

William Samson, M.D. Department of Plastic Surgery, St Luke's – Roosevelt Hospital, Colombia University, New York, NY, USA

Dana R. Sands, M.D., FACS, FASCRS Department of Colon and Rectal Surgery, Cleveland Clinic Florida, Weston, FL, USA

Mandeep S. Saund, M.B.B.S., M.S., FACS, FRCS(G) Department of Surgery,
Brigham and Women's Hospital, Harvard Medical School, Boston, MA, USA

W. Rudolph Schouten, M.D., Ph.D. Department of Colorectal Surgery,
Erasmus Medical Centre, Rotterdam, The Netherlands

Jamie Schwartz, M.D. Department of Surgery, St Luke's – Roosevelt Hospital, Colombia University, New York, NY, USA

M.J.P Scott, M.B.B.S., FRCA Department of Anaesthesia, Royal Surrey County Hospital, Guildford, Surrey, UK

Asha Senapati, Ph.D., M.B.B.S., FRCS Department of Colorectal Surgery,
Queen Alexandra Hospital, Portsmouth, UK

Francis Seow-Choen, M.B.B.S., FRCSED, FAMS, FRES Department of Colorectal Surgery, Seow-Choen Colorectal Centre, Mt. Elizabeth Hospital, Singapore, Singapore

Ali A. Shafik, M.D. Department of Surgery and Experimental Research, Faculty of Medicine, Cairo University, Cairo, Egypt

Michael John Solomon, MBBCh, BAO, M.Sc., FRACS Department of Colorectal Surgery, Royal Prince Alfred Hospital, Missenden Road, Camperdown, NSW, Australia

Michael J. Stamos, M.D. Department of Surgery, University of California, Irvine, CA, USA

Patrick S. Sullivan, M.D. Colon and Rectal Surgery, Division of Surgical Oncology, Emory University Midtown Hospital, Atlanta, GA, USA

Division of Colon and Rectal Surgery, Mayo Clinic, Rochester, MN, USA

Ursula M. Szmulowicz, M.D., B.S., AB Department of Colorectal Surgery, The Cleveland Clinic Foundation, Cleveland, OH, USA

Hagit Tulchinsky, M.D. Department of Surgery, Tel Aviv Sourasky Medical Center, Tel-Aviv, Israel

Proctology Unit, Department of Surgery B, Tel Aviv Sourasky Medical Center, Sackler School of Medicine, Tel-Aviv University, Tel-Aviv, Israel

Selman Uraneus, M.D., FACS Clinical Division of General Surgery, Department of Surgery, Medical University of Graz, Graz, Austria

Rosana Vicente, M.D. Colorectal Unit, Hospital Ruber Internacional, Madrid, Spain

Nir Wasserberg, M.D. Department of Surgery B, Beilinson Campus, Rabin Medical Center, Tel Aviv, Israel

Sackler School of Medicine, Tel Aviv University, Tel Aviv, Israel

Eric G. Weiss, M.D., FACS, FASCRS, FACG Department of Colorectal Surgery, Cleveland Clinic Florida, Weston, FL, USA

Steven D. Wexner, M.D., Ph.D. (Hon), FACS, FRCS, FRCS (Ed.) Professor & Chair, Department of Colorectal Surgery

Emeritus Chief of Staff Cleveland Clinic

Associate Dean for Academic Affairs, Florida Atlantic University College of Medicine

Affiliate Dean for Clinical Education, Florida International University College of Medicine, Florida, USA

Malcolm Wilson, FRCS Colorectal Surgeon, Christie Hospital, Manchester, UK

Norman S. Williams, M.B.B.S., LRCP, M.S., PRCS, FMed Sci. FDGP (Hon) Academic Surgical Unit, Centre for Digestive Diseases, Blizard Institute of Cell and Molecular Science, Barts and The London School of Medicine and Dentistry, Queen Mary, University of London, The Royal London Hospital, London, UK

Andrew P. Zbar, M.D. (Lond), M.B.B.S., FRCS (Ed.), FRACS Department of Surgery and Transplantation, Chaim Sheba Medical Center, Ramat Gan, Israel

Sackler School of Medicine, Tel Aviv University, Tel Aviv, Israel

David D.E. Zimmerman, M.D., Ph.D., F.E.B.S. (Coloproctology) Department of Surgery, Twee Steden Ziekenhuis and St. Elisabeth Ziekenhuis, Tilburg, The Netherlands

Oded Zmora, M.D. Department of Surgery and Transplantation, Sheba Medical Center, Tel Hashomer, Israel

Sackler School of Medicine, Tel Aviv University, Tel Aviv, Israel

Massarat Zutshi, M.D., FACS Department of Colorectal Surgery A30, Cleveland Clinic, Cleveland, OH, USA

目 录

第一篇 重建手术的成像技术和生理机制

- 第1章 常规放射影像学检查 ····· 3
- 第2章 排粪造影 ····· 12
- 第3章 腔内超声检查（包括三维超声） ····· 20
- 第4章 直肠肛管疾病的磁共振成像 ····· 33
- 第5章 结肠直肠再手术前内镜评估 ····· 43
- 第6章 直肠肛门疾病再次手术的压力测定、直肠肛管抑制反射和顺应性评估 ····· 48
- 第7章 再手术病例中向量测压和神经生理评估时的建议 ····· 73

第二篇 肛门直肠重建手术的决策制定

- 第8章 外科直肠重建：超低位吻合术的术式选择 ····· 85
- 第9章 新直肠贮袋及其修正手术 ····· 94
- 第10章 放射性损伤直肠的重建 ····· 101
- 第11章 复发性直肠癌的手术切除 ····· 110
- 第12章 廓清术及重建 ····· 124
- 第13章 首次腹腔镜手术后再手术 ····· 139
- 第14章 探讨困难性腹腔镜手术的解决途径 ····· 146
- 第15章 机器人手术的思考 ····· 153
- 第16章 完全肛门重建 ····· 159
- 第17章 肛管上皮内瘤样变的医疗对策 ····· 171
- 第18章 肛管癌复发后挽救性切除 ····· 180

第三篇 炎性肠病的再次手术策略

- 第19章 炎性肠病异型增生 ····· 193
- 第20章 再次手术行贮袋肛管吻合术的手术注意事项 ····· 204
- 第21章 结肠克罗恩病的再手术 ····· 215
- 第22章 肛周克罗恩病的治疗 ····· 223

第四篇 功能性便秘和排便困难的再次手术

- 第23章 慢性便秘行回肠/盲肠直肠吻合失败后再手术 ····· 243
- 第24章 Malone治疗方法及其衍生治疗方式 ····· 247
- 第25章 巨直肠的处理 ····· 256

第26章	直肠前突修补失败的处理	268
第27章	STARR术式的利与弊	274
第28章	直肠前突与直肠疝：妇科医生的处理方式	282

第五篇　大便失禁的再手术

第29章	重复括约肌成形术	295
第30章	电刺激股薄肌成形术失败后治疗策略	302
第31章	人工肛门括约肌植入术后并发症的处理	306
第32章	肛门括约肌重建的手术方式	313
第33章	肛门内括约肌增强方法	318
第34章	自体新建括约肌和排便控制的新技术	329
第35章	尚有争议的骶神经调节	334

第六篇　肛门会阴重建手术的相关技术

第36章	复发性复杂肛瘘的再手术治疗	341
第37章	成人肛管前移畸形与肛管前庭瘘的治疗	356
第38章	直肠阴道瘘的重复手术治疗	362
第39章	直肠尿道瘘的处理	374
第40章	复发性肛裂的个体化治疗	385
第41章	肛管狭窄的肛管皮肤填补术	390
第42章	会阴皮肤填补与重建	399

第七篇　改良式造瘘术

第43章	造口重造、移位和关闭	407
第44章	造口旁疝的治疗	418
第45章	哈特曼手术后重建的相关问题	424
第46章	儿童肠造口并发症的再手术治疗	433

第八篇　肛肠再手术学的特殊论题

第47章	结直肠及肛门再次手术的麻醉相关问题——快速康复外科的作用	441
第48章	憩室病并发症的再手术治疗	448
第49章	肠吻合口瘘的外科问题	455
第50章	直肠后肿瘤	461
第51章	直肠脱垂手术失败后的治疗方法	491
第52章	藏毛窦疾病复发的治疗	498
第53章	结直肠子宫内膜异位症的外科治疗	506
第54章	结直肠肛门外科再手术的医疗法律问题	514

第一篇
重建手术的成像技术和生理机制

引 言

Andrew P. Zbar

本部分主要明确了放射学、内镜和生理学检测方法在评估行再次手术和重建手术患者中的作用。虽然这些章节由一些专家编写，但其中仍有很多争议。如何选择肛肠疾病的影像检查方法经常让人感到迷惑，在选择时，临床医师首先要回答一个问题：这些检查是否会影响患者的治疗？对于良性肛门直肠疾病，我们可以看到在反复发作的复杂性肛瘘中，增强磁共振检查比手术能提供更好的金标准（尤其对于多次复发患者），静态经会阴超声可以作为补充诊断。但是某些特殊情况下，如病变位置超出了内镜超声探头的聚焦范围，或肛提肌以上发生实质病变，却只配有经肛探头时，超声和磁共振检查都不是最佳选择。

有很多患者为了治疗局部顽固性肛裂进行手术，在这种情况下，虽然在术中想象肛门内括约肌的解剖结构受到很大限制，但在分离肛门内括约肌时应仔细地考虑是否安全。在这方面，虽然没有影像指导的前瞻性数据帮助我们决定是否采取保留括约肌手术，但在很多病例中，可直观地使用术前影像学检查来决定是否做括约肌切开术。

我们很难处理一些存在形态学异常却有功能的患者，而且我不完全相信动态经会阴或三维经直肠超声排粪造影用来指导手术的准确性，无论是单独使用一种检查方法还是联合使用。对于这些患者，我们支持使用动态MRI直肠排粪造影或更广泛更传统的排粪造影。

在恶性疾病中，虽然治疗意向上仍有一些偏见，但术前高分辨率MRI检查指导我们在低位直肠癌患者中使用短期放疗还是正式的新辅助治疗，在全直肠系膜切除术中保证环切缘阴性。这些患者的随访十分困难，如果可行，必须依靠PET/CT。同样的方法还推荐用于在活检后使用放化疗能完全缓解的直肠小病变。对于接受放化疗的肛管癌患者，随访应联合使用PET/CT，因为其他方法不够准确，随访应不早于初始治疗后的3个月，因为3个月内检查的假阳性率比较高。

对于接受过腹腔镜切除的患者行内镜评估，需要进行病变染色。对于放置结肠支架，已经有确定位置（但仍未证实）。非随机试验显示，在治疗低位直肠吻合口瘘中定制的封闭式负压引流技术有一定作用，在很多病例中，避免了重复开腹手术，但这种治疗的功能预后仍需得到确认。

实话实说，再次手术患者的肛门直肠测压和生理学测试结果比他们初次诊疗时的结果更加让人难懂，我们只把它作为辅助手段，用在将要进行括约肌修复或骶神经调节治疗的患者，从而使某些患者避免进行广泛的经肛手术、直肠肛管直接端端吻合和直肠乙状结肠切除术。虽然文献中很少有客观证据来支持这一观点，但是对于肛门直肠测压可能有更好的使用方法；对接受广泛肛肠手术的患者，通过确定的压力指数来预测是否存在功能不良。

目前，对于结直肠实习医生是否应花时间去放射科学习超声并被认证，或学习肛肠 MR 检查中的细微差别，还没有达到共识。只有当他们需要更复杂的肛肠影像解读和转诊技术时，才需要进行这些方面的训练。

第 1 章 常规放射影像学检查

Johann Pfeifer

胡雄辉 译 姜 军 审校

摘 要

各种术前准确的影像学检查极大促进了肿瘤患者新辅助治疗策略的发展。这些影像学检查有助于实现更准确的肿瘤分期和病例筛选，促进治疗方案的个体化运用、提高保肛率、R0 切除率和肿瘤复发再切除成功率及多脏器切除成功率。常规行计算机断层扫描（CT）能更好发现术后感染性并发症，有助于复杂憩室病手术方式的制订。本章主要介绍结直肠手术患者术后常用的影像学检查方法，包括 X 线平片、CT 扫描、放射核素显像和正电子发射断层扫描。

关键词

X 线平片；计算机断层扫描（CT）；正电子发射断层扫描（PET）；放射核素显像

引 言

新兴的影像成像及重建技术可使癌症患者获得更新、更好的综合治理方案，包括帮助制订术中辅助治疗方案、选择重建方式（详见本书相关章节）和术后疗效评价。这些影像检查使得术前获得更准确的肿瘤分期、更好的病例筛选，制订更适宜的个体化治疗方案成为可能，降低发病率和死亡率，帮助提高 R0 切除率，提高晚期癌症多脏器切除成功率及复发再切除成功率。计算机断层扫描（CT）的普及使用使结直肠术后并发症（特别是感染性并发症）的诊断变得更容易而准确，改变了吻合口瘘诊断及治疗的"传统方案"。CT 结肠成像逐渐成为继电子结肠镜检查之外的另一检查手段，而正电子发射断层扫描（PET）也越来越多地应用于判断盆腔肿瘤的复发、转移，以及是否适合再切除的评价方面。本章概述了结直肠癌术后患者各种放射学检查的使用原则，包括 X 线平片、CT、PET 和放射性核素显像等。关于磁共振成像（MRI）及直肠腔内超声在准备再手术和重建患者中的应用，本书将另行讨论。

X 线平片

X 线平片依然是有腹部不适症状患者的一项快速而有力的检查方法。原则上有 3 种不同体位的摄片：①平卧位，能获得腹腔各组织结构最好的细节及对比度显示，及腹腔游离气体的显示；②立位或侧卧位，用于显示腹部气体的分部状态；③立位胸部摄片，专门用于显示膈下游离气体。腹部 X 线平片能显示 4 种不同组织密度：软组织、脂肪、气体及金属密度。气体可作为一个"阴性"对照。因粪便在结肠中的缓慢传输，其内可有气体存在，因此可在结肠的各个部位查见气体密度。

消化道内正常气体分布

一名受过良好训练的观片者可迅速识别正常的气体分部形态。气液平面最多见于胃，少量的气液平面也可见于小肠，而大多数气体聚集于结肠。肠管内气体分部还取决于患者体位：直立位，气体聚集于肠道弯曲处；俯卧位，气体多聚集于直肠；仰卧位，气体可广泛分部于肠管各处。正常小肠直径应不超过 2.5cm，横结肠最大直径应不超过 6~8cm[1]。

气 腹

立位胸部摄片是显示膈下游离气体最敏感的摄片方式。左侧卧位可用于有残疾不能站立或不能搬动患者，但摄片前需保持该体位 10~15min，以便气体聚集[2]。在 32% 的气腹患者中，可出现气体同时聚集于肠壁两侧，称"双壁征"[3]。虽然肠腔外游离气体多提示有空腔脏器穿孔，但近期有腹部手术史也可在腹腔查见少量游离气体。到术后第 6 天，无论是否保留腹腔引流管，80% 的患者在立位胸部摄片中已看不见膈下游离气体[4-5]。

肠梗阻

小肠梗阻

腹部 X 线平片的一个最大作用之一就是鉴别小肠梗阻与结肠梗阻、机械性肠梗阻与功能性肠梗阻。但需指出的是影像学诊断必须与临床表现相结合。影像学表现主要取决于症状持续时间、反复呕吐、是否应用胃肠减压及梗阻程度。异常的腹部气体形态表现为气体聚集于一处或多处扩张的小肠腔内（肠腔直径 >2.5cm），且气体形态多变。气液平面是小肠梗阻（SBO）的特异性影像学征象。完全性 SBO 患者结肠中多无气体影。另外，扩张显影的肠袢越多，梗阻部位越低（图 1.1）。腹部 X 线平片对机械性肠梗阻诊断的敏感性约为 52%，特异性约 71%[6]。

大肠梗阻

结肠梗阻与小肠梗阻具有相似的影像学征象，但是结肠有环绕肠壁全周的皱襞形成的结肠袋，因此呈现出特征性的深入结肠腔但又未达对侧肠壁的

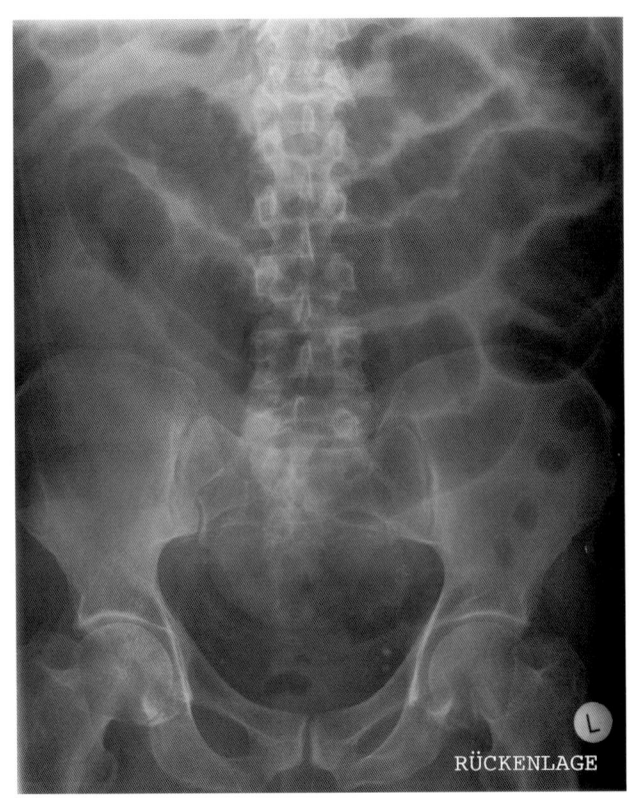

图 1.1 腹部 X 线平片：小肠梗阻。扩张显影肠袢越多，梗阻部位越低

结肠袋影。引起小肠梗阻的原因包括粘连、嵌顿疝、克罗恩病及肿瘤；引起大肠梗阻最常见的原因是恶性肿瘤、肠扭转、假性结肠梗阻（Ogilvie's syndrome）及粪石梗阻，其次是克罗恩病、结肠憩室、结肠缺血性疾病、吻合口狭窄及子宫内膜异位症[7]。

恶性肿瘤

典型表现是结肠癌近端肠管扩张，远端肠管萎陷，肠腔内无气体影。当回盲瓣功能良好，横结肠直径大于 12cm 时将有结肠穿孔危险；若回盲瓣关闭不完全，结肠将不会如此扩张，继而出现小肠梗阻假象。

假性结肠梗阻

假性结肠梗阻又称 Ogilvie 综合征，表现为结肠重度扩张但又无机械性梗阻因素。影像学上，右半结肠多呈重度扩张表现，少数患者累及左半结肠。在侧卧位片上，直肠积气扩张是功能性结肠梗阻与机械性低位大肠梗阻的鉴别点[8]。

肠扭转

乙状结肠扭转表现为扩张的结肠袢的结肠袋消失，且呈倒"U"形。必要时，泛影葡胺灌肠造影可用于鉴别结肠假性梗阻、肿瘤性梗阻和结肠扭转。肠扭转的典型表现是在扭转部位出现尖端平行于肠腔的造影剂聚集，为肠壁扭曲尖端，又称"鸟嘴征"[9-11]。盲肠扭转在腹部X线平片上的典型表现为扩张盲肠内单一的液平面，可出现于腹部任何部位，取决于盲肠位置、扭转部位及扭转程度，而它多出现在左上腹。在泛影葡胺灌肠造影中，典型的"咖啡豆"样或"泪滴"样表现仅在50%的病例中出现[12]。总之，腹部X线平片对乙状结肠扭转和盲肠扭转的诊断率可高达75%[7]。

结肠炎

因炎症、感染或缺血导致的暴发性结肠炎将导致肠管松弛和结肠扩张。当全结肠有扩张而横结肠直径达到6.5cm时，可定义为中毒性巨结肠。因为有肠穿孔危险，中毒性巨结肠被视为结肠造影的禁忌证。

缺血性结肠炎可因全身低灌注（非闭塞性肠系膜缺血）或肠系膜血栓栓塞导致。在腹部X线平片上，非特异性肠壁增厚和"拇纹征"是肠壁水肿或黏膜下出血的特征性表现。有时，位于髂嵴上的粪石和升结肠不规则结肠袋影提示有阑尾炎的可能。若存在阑尾穿孔，可同时出现腹膜后气体影[13]。

其 他

在某些特殊情况下，腹部X线平片还可用于检查骨性结构改变（如骨盆骨折、尾骨痛）或检查人工肛门括约肌是否在位、有无移位或液体渗漏；同样还可用于检查骶神经调节装置位置的损坏或移位，如骶神经刺激（SNS）电极放置、电极位置及人工肛门括约肌（ABS）系统可能的液体渗漏（图1.2）。

结 论

在术后怀疑有肠梗阻或肠麻痹、气腹及有发展为中毒性巨结肠可能的患者中，腹部X线平片是一

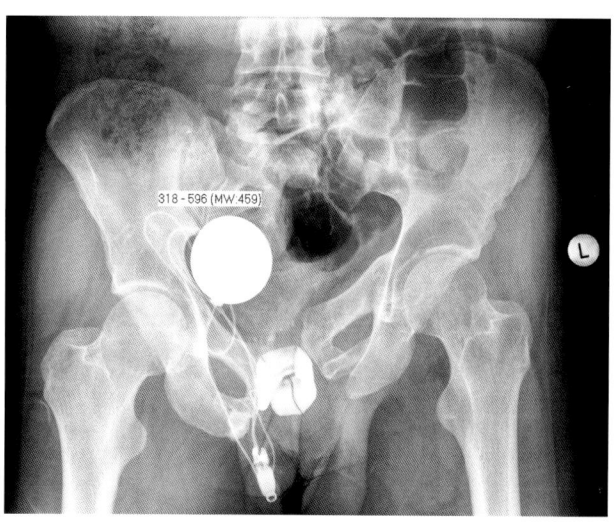

图1.2 一例35岁摩托车事故男性患者人工肛门装置植入后的腹部X线平片。可以看到位于肛门附件的袖带、阴囊内的泵及右下方装满不透射线液体的球囊，同时还可以看到耻骨联合分离

种简便、快捷、射线量小且有很高诊断价值的检查方法，同时还可用于肾绞痛及体内异物检查[14]。对于ICU内的危重患者，特别是机械通气等转运风险很大的患者，床旁摄片因无需将患者转运至放射科而具有极大优势[15]。

造影检查

技 术

造影检查用于显示结肠黏膜的细微改变已有几十年历史，基本可分为应用钡剂的单对比造影、气钡双重造影和应用水溶性造影剂造影两种。为了克服单对比造影只有在病变足够大时才能显影的不足，20世纪60年代开始应用的双重造影用气体作为第二种对比剂，通过在肠黏膜涂布一层薄约0.2mm的钡剂，可良好显示肠道病变。无论采用哪种检查技术，良好的肠道准备十分必要。与传统的结肠气钡双重造影（DCBE）相比，数字技术的应用明显减少了射线剂量[16]。

结肠气钡双重造影

很多研究认为，结肠气钡双重造影因为诊断依靠间接征象而非直接影像，在早期结肠炎、<1cm

息肉及结直肠癌诊断的准确性方面不及结肠镜检查；另一方面，结肠气钡双重造影为纯诊断性检查，无法行可疑病变组织活检及治疗（如息肉切除）。但结肠气钡双重造影仍是一个简单、安全、廉价的排除明显病变的方法，同时它几乎总能完成全结肠检查，因此，仍是那些行结肠镜检查存在技术难度的患者所需检查的一个重要补充。例如，结肠镜检查经常出现的因乙状结肠曲度过大，很难通过或肠镜无法成功到达盲肠等情况[18]。未行肠道准备而直接行钡剂灌肠仍可显示结肠炎的程度和范围，但不能在中毒性巨结肠或怀疑有肠穿孔患者中应用[17]。

水溶性造影剂造影检查

如果有肠穿孔的可能风险，应避免使用硫酸钡作为对比剂，而采用水溶性造影剂如胃影葡胺（gastrografin®）、泛影葡胺（urografin®）。因造影剂有黏膜刺激性，口服造影剂可用于部分麻痹性肠梗阻、不全性肠梗阻[19]。水溶性造影剂黏滞度低，可用于显示小肠瘘[20]。虽然部分患者可通过肛瘘外口行瘘管造影，但传统的肛瘘瘘管造影已较少应用，更多应用超声内镜和MRI[21, 22]。另外，水溶性造影剂还用于在回肠肛管贮袋吻合术后近端回肠造口还纳前行贮袋造影[17, 20]，或直肠癌结肠肛管吻合后检查吻合口的完整性[23]。水溶性造影剂应用的适应证还包括怀疑有膀胱阴道瘘或结肠/直肠阴道瘘时[24-25]，以及在回肠造口或结肠造口还纳时怀疑有远端肠管梗阻或瘘[26]。

小肠摄影和小肠灌肠

虽然小肠约占整个消化道长度的75%，但小肠疾病发病率却明显低于胃和结直肠。小肠造影的适应证包括不明原因消化道出血、原发性小肠梗阻、小肠肿瘤、克罗恩病和营养吸收不良[17]。小肠造影包括两种检查方式：①小肠摄影：由患者口服大量稀释钡剂或水溶性造影剂；②小肠灌肠：先经鼻放置导管，跨过幽门，再经导管注入对比剂加甲基纤维素，可获得更好的肠管扩张度和显影，但不足是需放置经鼻导管。造影检查过程将持续90～120min，最佳适应证是腹部大手术术后不全性小肠梗阻[27]及多节段性小肠克罗恩病[28]。

肠套叠

肠套叠发生于一段近端肠管全层套入远端肠管中时，多发生于3岁及3岁以下儿童；也可出现于成人[29-30]，特别是接受过胃旁路手术的患者[31]。肠套叠可分为原发性和继发性，最常见的套叠部位是回盲部，小肠和结肠也可发生。依据套入病变肠管的性质，可分为良性和恶性。在儿童患者，透视监视下的液体造影剂或气体灌肠常可使套叠肠管成功复位[1]。肿瘤性病变所致儿童及成人术后早期的肠套叠发生率很低，且在成人患者更多见，儿童与成人在临床表现、影像学特点及病因方面有很多不同表现[32]。

结论：造影检查

随着检查技术的不断发展，结肠气钡双重造影已逐渐被超声内镜、CT、MRI取代，但水溶性造影剂造影检查仍然是常规检查中不可缺少的一部分，特别是在术后治疗麻痹性肠梗阻、检查有无手术并发症（如吻合口瘘）及某些疾病（如瘘和疾病进展）的诊断方面有重要价值。

减影技术

减影技术现广泛用于获取经血管增强后强化不明显组织的图像。在普通扫描后再经血管注入造影剂获取增强图像，两次图像叠加相减后获得只有被造影剂强化的组织图像。动脉造影检查是一种需股动脉经皮穿刺的侵入性检查方法，其并发症除最常见的造影剂过敏外，还包括血肿、假性动脉瘤、动静脉瘘及穿刺部位血栓形成，其总体死亡率约为1/4万[7]。动脉造影技术的一大优势是在诊断明确后可马上采取治疗措施。例如消化道出血患者，一种止血方式是在肠系膜上动脉或肠系膜下动脉主干注射血管加压素[33]，或经动脉超选后弹簧栓栓塞出血动脉，其成功率在50%～90%，而缺血性并发症小于5%[34]。虽然血管造影不是下消化道出血的一线诊断方法，但在多次肠镜检查阴性的复发性隐匿性消化道出血患者有重要价值，在0.5ml/min以上出血时可获得阳性结果，比核素扫描所需的0.1～0.2ml/min略高[7]。

计算机断层扫描（CT）

技 术

CT机通过扫描获取大量不同方向扫描图像，经计算机软件重建后获取横断面图像，可识别组织密度的细微差异，重建后可获得二维图像。常规CT扫描以1cm层厚环绕人体进行旋转扫描。新型的更快速的螺旋CT通过对人体进行螺旋形扫描生成连续的图像。通过消化道增强或血管增强方法可获得更准确的组织分辨能力。静脉增强在扫描时造影剂经弹丸式注入血管。造影剂除了可导致过敏外，还不能应用于肾衰竭患者[35]。CT扫描在检查腹部病变、评估憩室炎严重程度及结直肠癌分期等方面有重要作用；在某些情况下，还是诊断一些术后并发症的金标准；另外，CT还可引导细针穿刺活检或脓肿穿刺引流。

憩室炎

当怀疑有憩室炎时，CT是首选检查方法[36]。通过腹部CT（最好是增强CT）检查可诊断憩室炎的范围、严重程度及可能存在的憩室穿孔或脓肿形成。与过去常用的结肠气钡双重造影相比，CT能够诊断早期的憩室炎，且能依据CT表现制订个体化治疗方案[37]，可使大多数患有急性局限性脓毒性憩室炎并发症的患者接受非手术治疗[38]。

克罗恩病

克罗恩病可使小肠和（或）结肠肠壁及肠周组织受累，CT表现包括典型的肠壁增厚伴或不伴靶形征、跳跃性病变、脂肪增生肥大（爬行脂肪）和（或）纤维性脂肪增生、增大淋巴结、瘘及窦道伴或不伴脓肿形成[39]。有结肠壁增厚、肠周脓肿形成不伴纤维脂肪性增生的患者，CT不能区分憩室炎伴脓肿形成、克罗恩病及结肠癌伴穿孔[1]。与MR肠道显像相比，CT肠道显像可能更少产生诊断误差[40]。CT肠道显像能显示肠壁增厚（包括双层黏膜增强、多层肠壁改变）及治疗后肝静脉期肠壁的增强或强化减弱[41]。

其他类型结肠炎

溃疡性结肠炎肠壁增厚不如克罗恩病，且肠周没有增生脂肪，较少形成肠瘘。CT在回肠肛管贮袋吻合术后并发症的诊断方面有重要价值[42]。感染性改变可分为仅侵犯结肠和炎症侵犯结肠及末端回肠两种。散在的或局限性肠壁增厚作为结肠炎的一个典型表现，可出现典型的"拇纹征"表现（如伪膜性肠炎、巨细胞病毒性结肠炎）。若出现"拇纹征"和肠壁内气体，伴或不伴门静脉内气体影，则考虑缺血性肠炎的可能性大。CT对缺血性结肠炎的诊断敏感性为83%，特异性为93%，阳性预测值为79%，阴性预测值为95%[43]。

小肠梗阻

小肠梗阻的首选检查方法是腹部X线平片检查，其准确率为50%~92%[44]，CT因其准确率较高，越来越多地应用于小肠梗阻的诊断。CT除了能判断有无肠梗阻存在，还能判断肠梗阻的部位、梗阻原因及有无血管源性病因存在。通常在扩张肠管与塌陷肠管之间存在一个过渡区，但当此过渡区不明显时，鉴别机械性肠梗阻与小肠炎症所致动力性肠梗阻将存在困难[7]。CT还有助于查找肠梗阻的病因，如疝、肠套叠、克罗恩病或小肠肿瘤。

结直肠癌

虽然结直肠癌最佳的检查方法是结肠镜，但CT在肠壁内及肠腔外肿瘤诊断方面有较大优势。结直肠癌分期包括：①有无肝转移；②区域淋巴结受累情况；③腹膜内有无转移。增强CT图像常包括两个时相：肝动脉期及门静脉期。依据在不同象病灶强化的不同表现，增强CT可诊断1cm以上的肝转移灶[45]。CT不仅可用于术前诊断，还可用于结直肠癌术后复查。但常见的肠壁增厚和肠周包块表现并不只在恶性肿瘤中出现，憩室炎或结肠炎也可能有类似表现。不良的肠道准备也会降低CT诊断的特异性，其对肿瘤原发灶及淋巴结转移的总体敏感性分别为53%~77%和22%~73%[46]。

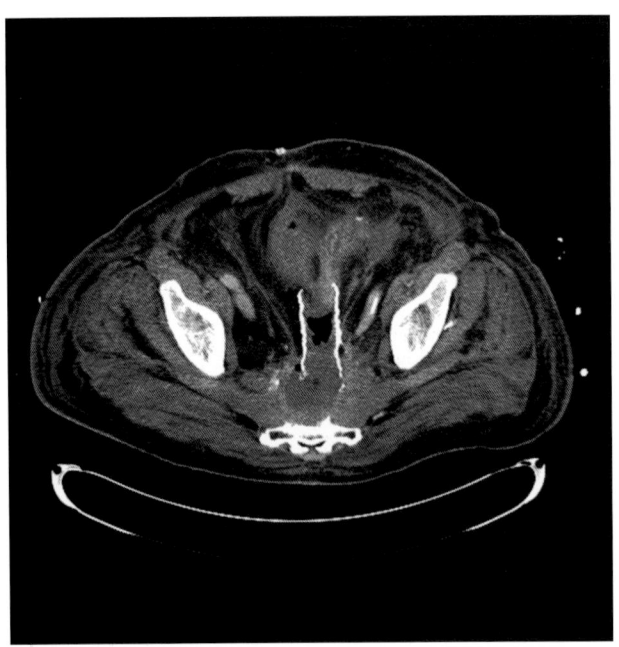

图1.3 CT图像示一例患者低位直肠前切除术后吻合口狭窄,直肠支架置入后直肠穿孔伴脓肿形成(支架周围气泡影)

术后评价

当术后患者有炎性指标(如白细胞计数、C反应蛋白)升高、发热、持续存在的肠梗阻或无法解释的腹痛出现时,CT是最重要的一种检查方法。值得注意的是,当临床上怀疑患者有特别问题存在时,如是否有腹腔脓肿或吻合口漏,CT是最有效的检查方法(图1.3)[47]。

CT 仿真肠镜

目前,CT仿真肠镜(CTC)尚不是结直肠肿瘤的一线检查方法。但是CTC有很多特有的优势,包括准确性高、针对所有患者的全结肠检查、无创、安全、舒适、可发现肠外病灶及效价比高[48]。不足之处是需要像肠镜一样行肠道准备;另一个缺点是需要暴露在电离辐射之下,但现在已采用低辐射剂量的检查技术,其辐射剂量相当于或仅略高于正常人群每年接受的辐射量。有间接证据显示辐射暴露不会导致额外的肿瘤发生[49]。另外,采用显影葡胺"粪便标签技术"特别是在老年患者中优势更明显[50-51],可作为除结肠镜之外的另一选择[52]。

结论:CT

CT是临床常用的良好的检查方法之一,主要的应用适应证包括憩室炎、结直肠癌分期及术后并发症的评估。虽然新的CT检查技术使检查更快捷,但不足仍然是有电离辐射,特别是对于那些有术后并发症需经常行CT检查的患者。

核素显像

核素显像(核素闪烁扫描)通过特殊的探测器(伽马探测器)来显示放射性核素在器官和机体中的不同分布。核素显像主要用于评价组织器官功能,而很少用于检查解剖学异常。最常用的放射性核素是锝99(^{99m}Tc),因为它只发射γ射线,有唯一的能量峰,易于制备,半衰期为6h且适用于多器官功能检查(如骨、甲状腺、肾)。在消化道检查中,核素显像的主要应用是将^{99m}Tc标记的红细胞注入人体,用于显示隐匿性下消化道出血的出血部位。常用^{99m}Tc标记的红细胞显像寻找幼儿和青少年异位的胃黏膜出血(Meckel扫描)[53]。

正电子发射断层扫描

正电子发射断层扫描(PET)用于代谢活跃组织的显像。在PET检查中,通过将低剂量放射性核素标记的葡萄糖注入血管,探测器于体外螺旋扫描记录葡萄糖中放射性原子发射的射线。因恶性肿瘤组织较正常组织摄取更多的葡萄糖而被动态成像。应用18F-FDG行PET/CT显像,现已在肿瘤患者肿瘤分期、术后评估及治疗后疗效评价方面广泛应用。结直肠癌患者行PET/CT检查的适应证包括:术前评估远处转移病灶(图1.4),监测有无肿瘤复发,鉴别可疑肿块,对肿瘤标志物异常增高患者寻找原发灶及查找卫星病灶[54]。

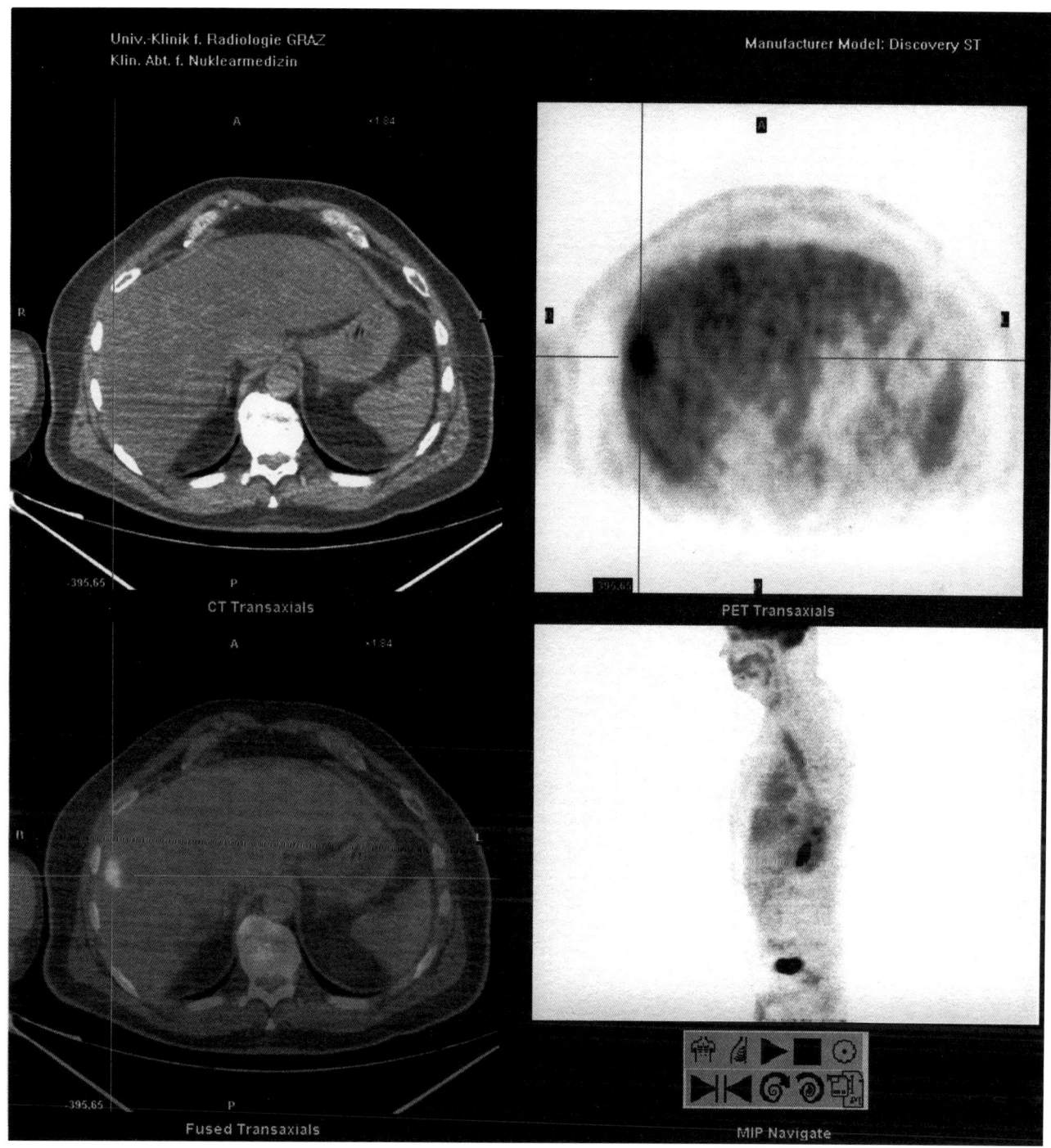

图 1.4 一例 56 岁男性直肠癌患者 PET/CT 图像，显示直肠病灶及肝第Ⅷ段单发转移灶。左上图：CT 图像；右上图：PET 图像；左下图：PET 图像与 CT 图像整合后高亮显示肝单发转移灶

结　论

CT 在评估结肠炎性、肿瘤性疾病，以及结直肠癌术后并发症检查方面的作用已十分明确，同时 CT 仿真肠镜（CTC）的临床应用也迅速发展。在目前的临床工作中，虽然 PET/CT 的适应证主要是肿瘤性疾病患者，但它在结直肠炎性疾病的诊断方面也有巨大潜力，应用也逐渐增加。其他影像学检查方法，如常规放射学及结肠气钡双重造影，现主要满足结直肠重建手术前后的检查需要[55]。

参考文献

1. Thoeni RF, Thornton R. Radiology of the colon. In: Wexner SD, Stollman N, editors. Diseases of the colon. New York: Informa Healthcare; 2007. p. 163–210.
2. Miller RE, Becker GJ, Slabaugh RA. Detection of pneumoperitoneum: optimum body position and respiratory phase. AJR Am J Roentgenol. 1980;135:487–90.
3. Levine MS, Scheiner JD, Rubesin SE, Laufer I, Herlinger H. Diagnosis of pneumoperitoneum on supine abdominal radiographs. AJR Am J Roentgenol. 1991;156:731–5.
4. Miller RE. The radiological evaluation of intraperitoneal gas (pneumoperitoneum). CRC Crit Rev Clin Radiol Nucl Med. 1973;4:61–85.
5. Tang CL, Yeong KY, Nyam DC, Eu KW, Ho YH, Leong AF, et al. Postoperative intra-abdominal free gas after open colorectal resection. Dis Colon Rectum. 2000;43:1116–20.
6. Harlow CL, Stears RL, Zeligman BE, Archer PG. Diagnosis of bowel obstruction on plain abdominal radiographs: significance of air-fluid levels at different heights in the same loop of bowel. AJR Am J Roentgenol. 1993;161:291–5.
7. Mutch MG, Birnbaum EH, Menias CO. Diagnostic evaluations – radiology, nuclear scans, PET, CT-colography. In: Wolff BC, Fleshman JW, Beck DE, Pemberton JH, Wexner SD, editors. The ASCRS textbook of colon and rectal surgery. New York: Springer; 2007. p. 69–100.
8. Low VH. Colonic pseudo-obstruction: value of prone lateral view of the rectum. Abdom Imaging. 1995;20:531–3.
9. Ballantyne GH. Volvulus of the colon. In: Fazio VW, editor. Current therapy in colon and rectal surgery. Philadelphia: BC Decker; 1990. p. 254–65.
10. Bubrick MP. Volvulus of the colon. In: Gordon PH, Nivatvongs S, editors. Principles and practice of surgery for the colon, rectum and anus. St. Louis: Quality Medical Publishing Inc.; 1992. p. 799–816.
11. Pfeifer J, Hammer H. Volvulus. In: Wexner SD, Stollmann N, editors. Diseases of the colon. New York: Informa Healthcare; 2006. p. 463–75.
12. Kerry RL, Lee F, Ransom HK. Roentgenologic examination in the diagnosis and treatment of colonic volvulus. AJR Am J Roentgenol. 1971;113:343–8.
13. Karkhanis S, Medcalf J. Plain abdomen radiographs: the right view? Eur J Emerg Med. 2009;16:267–70.
14. Smith JE, Hall EJ. The use of plain abdominal x-rays in the emergency department. Emerg Med J. 2009;26:160–9.
15. Löw M, Jaschinski U. Intrahospital transport of critically ill patients. Anaesthesist. 2009;58:95–107.
16. Martin CJ, Hunter S. Reduction of patient doses from barium meal and barium enema examinations through changes in equipment factors. Br J Radiol. 1994;67:1196–205.
17. Bartram CI, Halligan S. Imaging. In: Nicholls JR, Dozois RR, editors. Surgery of the colon and rectum. New York: Churchill Livingstone; 1997. p. 85–113.
18. Morini S, Zullo A, Hassan C, Lorenzetti R, Campo SM. Endoscopic management of failed colonoscopy in clinical practice: to change endoscopist, instrument, or both? Int J Colorectal Dis. 2011;26:103–8.
19. Branco BC, Barmparas G, Schnüriger B, Inaba K, Chan LS, Demetriades D. Systematic review and meta-analysis of the diagnostic and therapeutic role of water-soluble contrast agent in adhesive small bowel obstruction. Br J Surg. 2010;97:470–8.
20. Kalady MF, Mantyh CR, Petrofski J, Ludwig KA. Routine contrast imaging of low pelvic anastomosis prior to closure of defunctioning ileostomy: is it necessary? J Gastrointest Surg. 2008;12:1227–31.
21. Zbar AP, Armitage NC. Complex perirectal sepsis: clinical classification and imaging. Tech Coloproctol. 2006;10:83–93.
22. McIntyre PB, Ritchie JK, Hawley PR, Bartram CI, Lennard-Jones JE. Management of enterocutaneous fistulas: a review of 132 cases. Br J Surg. 1984;71:293–6.
23. Severini A, Civelli EM, Uslenghi E, Cozzi G, Salvetti M, Milella M, et al. Diagnostic and interventional radiology in the postoperative period and follow-up of patients after rectal resection with coloanal anastomosis. Eur Radiol. 2000;10:1101–5.
24. Casadesus D, Villasana L, Sanchez IM, Diaz H, Chavez M, Diaz A. Treatment of rectovaginal fistula: a 5-year review. Aust N Z J Obstet Gynaecol. 2006;46:49–51.
25. Biewenga P, Mutsaerts MA, Stalpers LJ, Buist MR, Schilthuis MS, van der Velden J. Can we predict vesicovaginal or rectovaginal fistula formation in patients with stage IVA cervical cancer? Int J Gynecol Cancer. 2010;20:471–5.
26. Karsten BJ, King JB, Kumar RR. Role of water-soluble enema before takedown of diverting ileostomy for low pelvic anastomosis. Am Surg. 2009;75:941–4.
27. Ohmiya N, Arakawa D, Nakamura M, Honda W, Shirai O, Taguchi A, et al. Small-bowel obstruction: diagnostic comparison between double-balloon endoscopy and fluoroscopic enteroclysis, and the outcome of enteroscopic treatment. Gastrointest Endosc. 2009;69:84–93.
28. Jensen MD, Kjeldsen J, Nathan T, Rafaelsen SR. Diagnostic imaging and endoscopic methods in Crohn's disease of the small intestine. Ugeskr Laeger. 2009;171:2383–8.
29. Rea JD, Lockhart ME, Yarbrough DE, Leeth RR, Bledsoe SE, Clements RH. Approach to management of intussusception in adults: a new paradigm in the computed tomography era. Am Surg. 2007;73:1098–105.
30. Guillén Paredes MP, Campillo Soto A, Martín Lorenzo JG, Torralba Martínez JA, Mengual Ballester M, Cases Baldó MJ, et al. Adult intussusception – 14 case reports and their outcomes. Rev Esp Enferm Dig. 2010;102:32–40.
31. Simper SC, Erzinger JM, McKinlay RD, Smith SC. Retrograde (reverse) jejunal intussusception might not be such a rare problem: a single group's experience of 23 cases. Surg Obes Relat Dis. 2008;4:77–83.
32. Zbar AP, Murphy F, Krishna SM. Adult postoperative intussusceptions: a rare cause of small bowel obstruction. South Med J. 2007;100:1042–4.
33. Walker TG. Acute gastrointestinal hemorrhage. Tech Vasc Interv Radiol. 2009;12:80–91.
34. van Delden OM, Rauws EA, Gouma DJ, Lamèris JS. Increasing role for angiographic embolisation in the treatment of gastrointestinal haemorrhage. Ned Tijdschr Geneeskd. 2006;150:956–61.
35. Katzberg RW, Newhouse JH. Intravenous contrast medium-induced nephrotoxicity: is the medical risk really as great as we have come to believe? Radiology. 2010;256:21–8.
36. Destigter KK, Keating DP. Imaging update: acute colonic diverticulitis. Clin Colon Rectal Surg. 2009;22:147–55.
37. Hansen O, Stock W. Prophylaktische Operation bei Divertikelerkrankung des Kolons – Stufenkonzept durch exakte Stadieneinteilung. Langenbecks Arch Chir. 1999;(Suppl II);1257–60.
38. Dharmarajan S, Hunt SR, Birnbaum EH, Fleshman JW, Mutch MG. The efficacy of nonoperative management of acute complicated diverticulitis. Dis Colon Rectum. 2011;54:663–71.
39. Gore RM, Marn CS, Kirby DF, Vogelzang RL, Neiman HL. CT findings in ulcerative, granulomatous, and indeterminate colitis. AJR Am J Roentgenol. 1984;143:279–84.
40. Jensen MD, Ormstrup T, Vagn-Hansen C, Ostergaard L, Rafaelsen SR. Interobserver and intermodality agreement for detection of small bowel Crohn's disease with MR enterography and CT enterography. Inflamm Bowel Dis. 2011;17:1081–8.
41. Wu YW, Tang YH, Hao NX, Tang CY, Miao F. Crohn's disease: CT enterography manifestations before and after treatment. Eur J Radiol. 2012;81:52–9.
42. Hoeffel C, Marcus C, Arrivé L, Bouché O, Tubiana J. Postoperative imaging after colorectal surgery. J Radiol. 2009;90(7–8 Pt 2):954–68.
43. Balthazar EJ, Yen BC, Gordon RB. Ischemic colitis: CT evaluation

of 54 cases. Radiology. 1999;211:381–8.
44. Kidmas AT, Ekedigwe JE, Sule AZ, Pam SD. A review of the radiological diagnosis of small bowel obstruction using various imaging modalities. Niger Postgrad Med J. 2005;12:33–6.
45. Inaba Y, Arai Y, Kanematsu M, Takeuchi Y, Matsueda K, Yasui K, et al. Revealing hepatic metastases from colorectal cancer: value of combined helical CT during arterial portography and CT hepatic arteriography with a unified CT and angiography system. AJR Am J Roentgenol. 2000;174:955–61.
46. Stevens WR, Johnson CD. Computed tomography and magnetic resonance imaging. In: Nicholls RJ, Dozois RR, editors. Surgery of the colon and rectum. New York: Churchill Livingstone; 1997. p. 114–34.
47. Danse E, Goncette L, Kartheuser A. Optimal diagnosis of anastomotic colorectal leak by combination of conventional colonic enema and CT. JBR-BTR. 2007;90:526–7.
48. Veerappan GR, Ally MR, Choi JH, Pak JS, Maydonovitch C, Wong RK. Extracolonic findings on CT colonography increases yield of colorectal cancer screening. AJR Am J Roentgenol. 2010;195:677–86.
49. Laghi A, Iafrate F, Rengo M, Hassan C. Colorectal cancer screening: the role of CT colonography. World J Gastroenterol. 2010;16:3987–94.
50. Faccioli N, Foti G, Barillari M, Zaccarella A, Camera L, Biasiutti C, et al. A simplified approach to virtual colonoscopy using different intestinal preparations: preliminary experience with regard to quality, accuracy and patient acceptability. Radiol Med. 2011;116:749–58.
51. Liedenbaum MH, Denters MJ, Zijta FM, van Ravesteijn VF, Bipat S, Vos FM, et al. Reducing the oral contrast dose in CT colonography: evaluation of faecal tagging quality and patient acceptance. Clin Radiol. 2011;66:30–7.
52. Keeling AN, Slattery MM, Leong S, McCarthy E, Susanto M, Lee MJ, et al. Limited-preparation CT colonography in frail elderly patients: a feasibility study. AJR Am J Roentgenol. 2010;194:1279–87.
53. Yang JG, Yin CH, Li CL, Zou LF. Meckel's diverticulum and intestinal duplication detected by Tc-99m pertechnetate scintigraphy. Clin Nucl Med. 2010;35:275–6.
54. Chowdhury FU, Shah N, Scarsbrook AF, Bradley KM. [18F]FDG PET/CT imaging of colorectal cancer: a pictorial review. Postgrad Med J. 2010;86:174–82.
55. Mirnezami AH, Sagar PM, Kavanagh D, Witherspoon P, Lee P, Winter D. Clinical algorithms for the surgical management of locally recurrent rectal cancer. Dis Colon Rectum. 2010;53:1248–57.

第 2 章 排粪造影

Vittorio Luigi Piloni · Corrado R. Asteria · Sergio Bellarosa
胡雄辉 译 姜 军 审校

摘 要

传统的排粪造影检查是一些结直肠术后标准的解剖学检查方法，如回肠-肛管贮袋吻合术后、结肠-肛管吻合术后或新近发展的经肛门吻合器切除术后 [如经肛门吻合器下直肠切除术（STARR）及其改良手术]。排粪造影除了能显示出术后最常见的并发症（如吻合口裂开、窦道形成），还能显示出导致术后功能障碍的潜在可能病因，如吻合口狭窄、排便延迟所致直肠扩张和对比剂残留、不对称肠壁膨出、直肠异常脱垂至吻合口位置。本章重点阐述此类有术后排便功能障碍的复杂患者的放射学表现，为制订再手术治疗方案提供参考。

关键词

X 线排粪造影；STARR 手术；结肠-肛管吻合；直肠癌；回肠-肛管贮袋；溃疡性结肠炎；排便障碍综合征

引 言

虽然 X 线排粪造影在检查方法及结果方面的不足早已人所共知，如射线暴露、检查的个体差异性、无法显示周围软组织等，但它仍是各种良、恶性疾病的直肠肛门部术后检查和评价的极为重要的方法。这些手术包括：①溃疡性结肠炎和家族性息肉病的回肠-肛管贮袋吻合重建手术；②低位直肠肿瘤切除术后结肠-肛管吻合；③针对排便障碍综合征的 STARR 手术。要求放射科医师完成以下两方面主要任务：①显示新吻合口形态；②评价重建后直肠排粪能力。其检查目的是排除任何可能导致功能障碍和（或）原有症状复发的解剖学异常，因为以上状况是否存在将帮助结直肠科医师决定手术方式。

虽然为治疗不同的病理改变设计了许多不同的手术方式，但放射科医师要认识到不同手术方式后直肠肛门部解剖学改变仍有很多共同点，包括任何吻合口都会有吻合线贯穿吻合口近远端。正常状况与手术并发症出现都会有其特有的影像学表现和解释，对结直肠科医师有巨大帮助。

回肠-肛管贮袋吻合

在部分经严格选择的溃疡性结肠炎和家族性息肉病患者行全结肠切除、直肠黏膜切除联合直肠内回肠肛管吻合术有以下一些优点：①全病变黏膜切除；②避免永久性腹壁造口；③保持经肛门排便。近端暂时性转流性回肠造口通常在 6～8 周后还纳，可使吻合口充分愈合并最大限度保留储便功能。关于贮袋设计,文献中提到3种方法[4-5],其中两种临床中较常用。第1种S形贮袋是将3段末端回肠顺蠕动制作成一球形贮袋后,输出段与肛管吻合;第2种是小一些的J形贮袋,用两段肠管制成贮袋后,因无输出袢而直接与肛管吻合;第3种是更大的4段肠管制成的W形贮袋,但此种方式因造成过多的粪便潴留而基本被弃用。

第一次的X线排粪造影检查可在术后1周进行,用于排除吻合口瘘[6]。吻合口瘘可源于制作贮袋的小肠管间吻合,也可源于贮袋与肛管吻合。在射线监视下经柔软的橡胶导管注入造影剂(稀释的泛影葡胺或稀钡),可使贮袋适当地充盈扩张,为了避免损伤回肠-肛管吻合口,需注意给气囊导管球囊充气应不超过3ml。在可能情况下,造影剂最好通过近端造口注入(图2.1)。在拔除导管后,应摄取贮袋充盈状态下的前后位及侧位影像,用于显示贮袋的完整形态。S形贮袋呈带有明显的输出袢的球形,而J形贮袋显示为两条明显的指向吻合口的吻合线,没有明显的输出袢。需注意勿将不透射线的输入袢误认为是吻合口瘘,有聚集在吻合口周围肠腔外的造影剂显示,可诊断有吻合口瘘和(或)吻合口破裂。另外,需仔细观察侧位片上有无因骶前积液所致贮袋移位等征象。

Thoeni等[7]报道各种不同检查方式中并发症诊断方面的总体敏感性如下:贮袋造影60%,CT 70%,核素标记的白细胞显像79%[8]。据这些学者报道,3种检查方法最易漏诊的是瘘,而仅CT能准确诊断所有的脓肿形成。目前,MRI逐渐成为可选甚至首选的检查,若MRI检查阴性,则应行核素闪烁扫描。在没有任何并发症出现的条件下,术后6～8周可经近端造口快速注入200ml稀钡(图2.2),使输入端贮袋充盈,即所谓的"液体超载试验"。X线排粪造影检查可为评价贮袋功能提供基本依据,在检查中加压状态下出现肛门失禁患者可预测在消化道重建后可能在临床上出现大便失禁。因此,若检查显示患者肛门控便功能不良,回肠造口还纳需延迟至盆底康复治疗,直至控便功能良好以后。

虽然很多因素可影响术后贮袋功能,如贮袋容量、储存能力、小肠动力、肠道激素水平、脓毒血症和细菌过度繁殖,但X线排粪造影检查可以提供更多关于贮袋排空功能方面的诊断信息,在术后3个月进行,应用特制的坐便器取侧位摄片[9-10]。检查时,将约200ml硫酸钡混悬液通过肛门注入,然后记录以下信息:

1. 重建后直肠或贮袋的几何形态和大小,它取决于贮袋的设计方式;

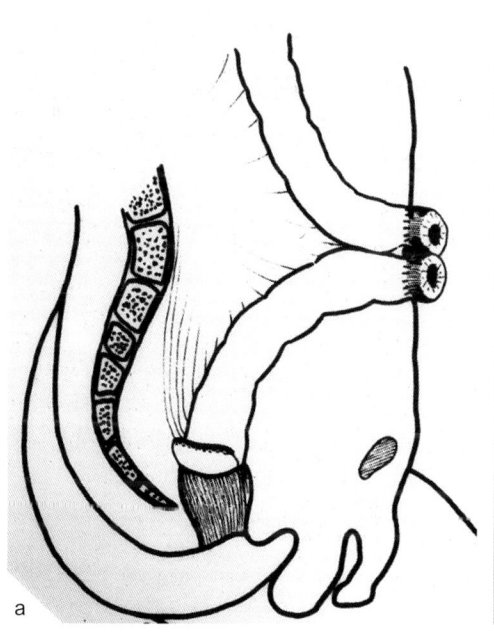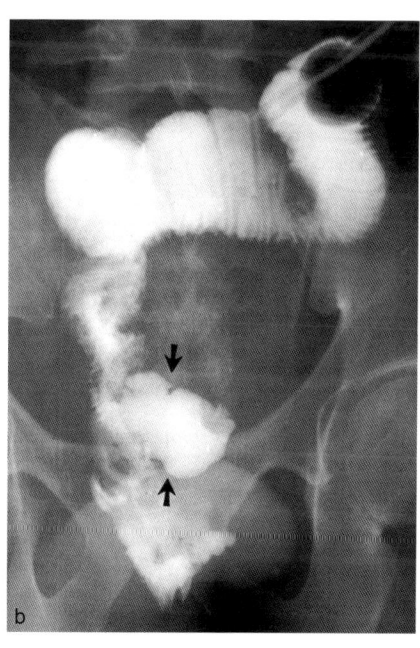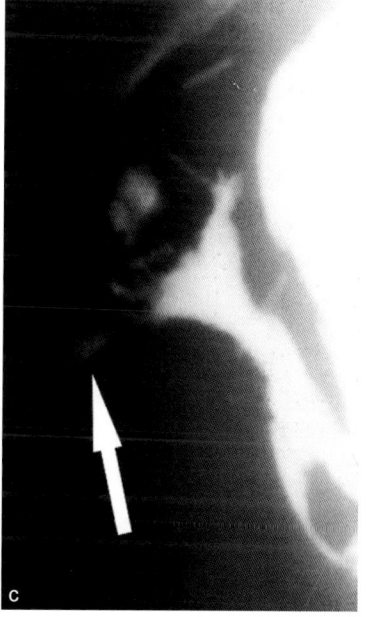

图2.1 回肠肛管J形贮袋吻合术后早期并发症。(a)示意图;(b)经暂时性回肠造口注入造影剂,可见因吻合线不完整所致造影剂聚集于吻合口周围肠腔外(箭头所指);(c)造影剂由输出袢肠段漏出至骶前,酷似窦道形成表现

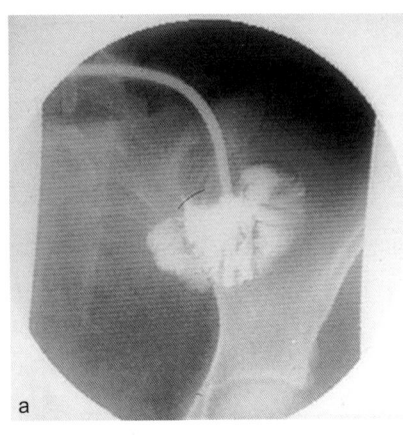 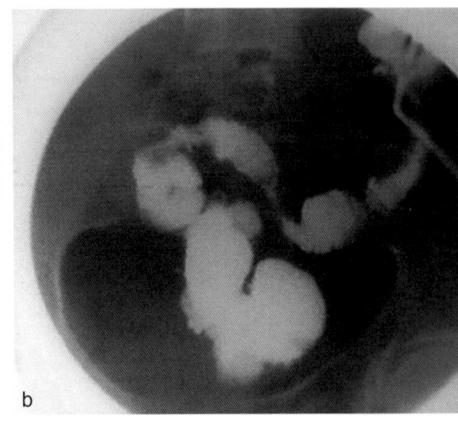 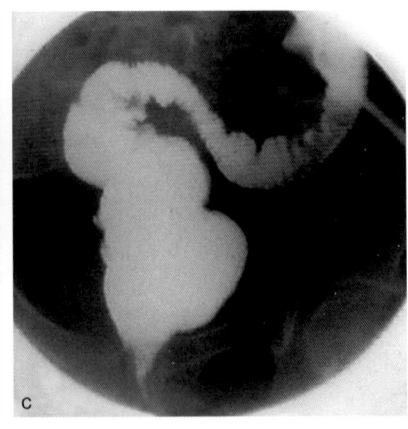

图 2.2　回肠造口还纳恢复肠道连续性前行液体超载试验：将 200ml 稀钡于 2min 内经回肠造口注入，分别于 15s 后（a）、60s 后（b）、90s 后（c）摄片，检查贮袋蠕动功能及其容量和完整性

2. 盆底贮袋的位置以贮袋 - 肛管结合部到耻尾线的垂直距离来描述，Pescatori 等[11]定义贮袋与肛缘之间肠管为远端肠道；

3. 沿重建后直肠或贮袋后壁作一条直线，肛管 - 贮袋角定义为肛管轴线与该直线所成的夹角。该直线被 Kmiot 等[8]所推崇，而非经直肠或贮袋中心所做的所谓"中心线"。他认为"中心线"更易受贮袋设计方式及贮袋充盈程度影响。肛管 - 贮袋角需在静息、提肛、力排及黏膜相测量并记录其大小；

4. 不论患者做 1 次或多次排便动作，都应在患者用力排出尽可能多的对比剂不少于 3min 以后再记录贮袋的黏膜形态；

5. 对比剂残留的量以注入对比剂量的分数表示，如 1/3、2/3 或更多。

直肠肛门功能良好时（例如每天排便次数不多于 3～4 次、无气体或固体粪便漏出的肛门失禁），排粪造影表现包括：重建后直肠或贮袋最大直径不大于 5～6cm；肛管内无造影剂残留；提肛和力排相时肛管 - 贮袋结合部上移或下降幅度均不超过 3cm；60s 内做出排便动作不多于 2～3 次；直肠内剩余 2/3 造影剂时，直肠直径明显缩小；排便结束后造影剂残留不超过 1/3。直肠肛门功能不良表现包括：肛管狭窄；吻合口环形狭窄；吻合口至肛门口距离增长；伴有排空困难和钡剂残留的贮袋不对称性扩张（图 2.3）。

据报道，术后贮袋炎的最好的诊断方法是核素闪烁扫描（敏感性 80%），其次是 CT（71%）和贮袋造影（53%）[7]。贮袋炎相对比较常见，发生率在 9%～34%，可严重影响贮袋功能，造成排便

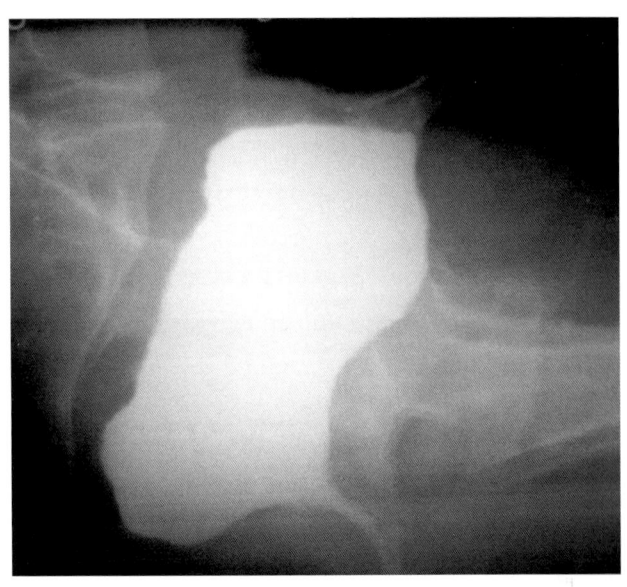

图 2.3　W 形回肠 - 肛管贮袋吻合术后力排后侧位片，显示大量钡剂残留于贮袋内

次数增加、便时疼痛、便急、肛门刺激和大便失禁。据报道，贮袋炎可能的病因包括贮袋动力异常导致蠕动停滞、细菌过度繁殖、缺血 - 再灌注损伤和隐匿性克罗恩病[12-13]，组织学和内镜学因素包括白细胞增多、肠外风湿性疾病、病变起始于结肠脾曲、发病年龄、类固醇使用史等。术中造成贮袋炎的高危因素包括 S 形贮袋、多期手术、围术期输血等提示手术操作复杂的情况[14]。克利夫兰诊所的 Lipman 等[14]最近的研究显示发生贮袋炎的患者临床预后较无贮袋炎的患者差，包括吻合口狭窄、小肠梗阻和瘘发生率高，生活质量较差。仅在组织活

检中偶然发现的无临床症状的组织学层面贮袋炎不影响临床结局。

结肠 – 肛管吻合

2/3 的低位直肠肿瘤患者行结肠 – 肛管吻合的保肛手术，该术式虽然存在主要因重建后新"直肠"容积减小导致排便次数增加和便急等不足，但在世界范围内已被广泛接受。为了改善术后功能，Lazorthes 等[15]在吻合口近端添加结肠 J 形贮袋，Parc 等[16]介绍行直肠全切除、结肠 – 肛管吻合术。虽然很多学者报道 J 形贮袋吻合在术后 2 年内较单纯结肠 – 肛管吻合有很多优点[17]，但至今仍没有一种检查方法能够很充分地预测某一种手术方式优于其他手术方式。动态的放射学检查（如排粪造影）可为临床医生评价术后直肠肛门功能提供客观依据[18-19]。检查中，患者取左侧卧位，在重建的直肠肛管内充盈标准量的硫酸钡混悬液（200ml 浓度为 70% 混悬液，Bracco Spa 公司）。直肠内充盈的造影剂量需考虑患者排便阈值，同时还需考虑不同贮袋吻合方式后贮袋的最大承受容积。造影剂注入完成后，将检查床直立，患者取侧位坐于特制的坐便器上(Bipot 125, Platinum, Giordanoshop, Naples, Italy)，透视下将重建的吻合口置于视野中央，应用电视记录设备记录所需图像，该记录设备需拥有重播及慢放功能，同时将计时器设置至 1/100s。

患者侧坐位于坐便器上，记录以下时相：充盈相、静息相、提肛相、力排相、强忍相及排空后黏膜相。另外，需记录患者突然控制停止排便的能力，称为"暂停试验（stop test）"，结果可记录为正常（0）、功能减退（−1）和功能缺失（−2）。必要时可摄取前后位及斜位片。在矢状位上，放射学医师需识别和画出某些基线，记录以下变量的距离和角度：

- 排便前后记录新"直肠"的前后径最大值；
- 耻尾线：耻骨联合至尾骨尖的连线，代表盆底的位置水平；
- 记录直肠 – 肛管结合部在静息、强忍、力排和排空时的不同位置；
- 肛直角，定义为肛管轴线与直肠或贮袋轴线的夹角，直肠或贮袋轴线为沿直肠或贮袋后壁所做的直线。

造成放射科医师计算肛直角困难的因素包括直肠壶腹前有肠管遮挡、直肠形态不规则、直肠后壁界限不清、耻骨直肠肌压迹形态多变。检查中所见任何导致贮袋排空障碍的因素均应被记录，包括肛管狭窄和（或）异常成角、贮袋至吻合口间肠管长度增长（图 2.4）以及肛门失禁。

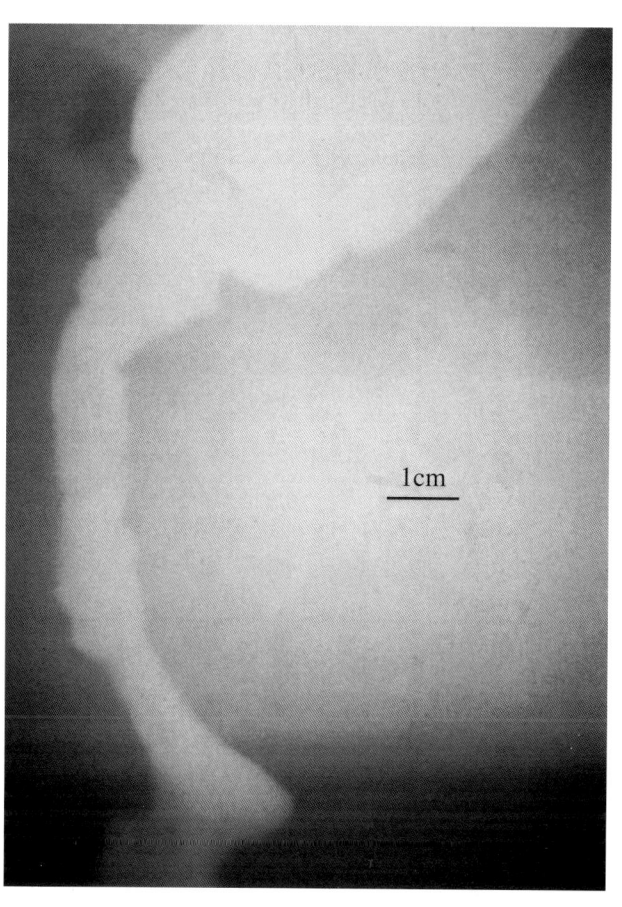

图 2.4 一例 54 岁男性患者直肠肿瘤切除、结肠肛管吻合术后 1 年行排粪造影检查，同时存在排便困难和肛门失禁，贮袋至吻合线距离增长至 7cm 以上，伴有此段肠管动力减退

吻合器下经肛门直肠切除术（STARR）

STARR 手术最早由 Longo[20]在 20 世纪 90 年代报道，用于治疗痔疮脱垂，此后逐渐被用于因直肠内套叠、直肠前突、直肠黏膜脱垂所致排便障碍综合征（ODS）经内科及康复治疗失败的患者。该手术通过两个环状吻合装置(PPH-01, Ethicon Endo-Surgery, Cincinnati, OH) 或改进的 STARR/trans-STARR 吻合器分别于直肠前壁和后壁行直肠切除术，客观上重建相对正常的直肠结构[21-22]。直肠前

壁切除用于减轻内套叠和直肠前突，同时纠正直肠前壁肌肉功能不良，直肠后壁切除用于纠正直肠内套叠。该手术可切除3~10cm直肠全层，纠正直肠的解剖异常。在女性患者，直肠前壁切除后需检查阴道后壁，排除直肠阴道隔损伤及因盆底疝导致的偶然的小肠损伤。但直肠后壁切除后因耻骨直肠肌影响而无法行类似检查，因此在闭合吻合器时有可能误伤耻骨直肠肌，可导致术后肛门部剧烈疼痛[23]。

手术需在齿状线上2cm及5cm分别行荷包缝合，包括黏膜层、黏膜下层及部分肌层。吻合器击发后常会在吻合线部位出现出血点，需可吸收线缝合止血，在使用新型的PPH-03型吻合器行直肠脱垂或混合痔手术后，这种需缝合止血的出血点已明显减少。因前壁和后壁两个吻合线常不是严格的圆环形，在两个吻合线交界的部位可形成黏膜隆起，又称为"狗耳朵"，必要时可将此处黏膜切除。最近，发展出了一种称为凯图Transtar（Contour Transtar）的新型的弧形切割吻合器，可提供更标准化的、全层环形切除，且使手术者可在直视下切除足够多的组织量。尽管如此，STARR术后仍有一些严重并发症报道，如直肠阴道瘘、肛门失禁、吻合口裂开等[24]，这些并发症还需一些特殊的放射学检查帮助诊断。

STARR手术在外科医生中很快被接受并流行开来，特别是在欧洲及意大利，其原因很多，包括缩短手术时间（平均25min）、减少肛门损伤、缩短住院时间、减少术后疼痛、早期恢复正常生活。另外，很多治疗团队[25-27]的短期研究得出高达91%的患者临床效果很好，但同时，STARR手术的快速推广应用导致在缺乏足够随机对照研究及明确的指南规定适应证和禁忌证的情况下，它的适应证被扩大至治疗排便障碍综合征（ODS）。此外，对STARR术后出现的生理学及形态学改变还缺乏足够的认识[26, 28]。这些因素也许可以解释STARR术后新出现的一些临床症状，及时有发生的危及生命的并发症，如顽固性难治性盆底痛、直肠肛门狭窄、需行转流性造口的直肠穿孔伴盆底脓毒症[29]。很多症状持续甚至需再次手术，最常见的是重度的肛门痛和肛门失禁，且这类患者多可查见有精神心理障碍存在[30]。

最近，另外一些研究[31-33]报道有44%的患者术后症状持续存在，术后随访20个月，有35%症状改善不明显，9%因术后并发症需再次干预，11%患者复发。现在，STARR手术已逐渐从某种程度上的滥用回归到对其手术疗效的现实性理性认识上来，这已被写入《专家共识》中[34]，并列出了STARR的禁忌证包括：会阴部感染、炎性肠病、肛门狭窄伴或不伴肛门失禁、盆底疝、肛门痉挛、直肠周围有补片置入、盆底结构异常[35]。另外，有盆底疝的患者也可在腹腔镜引导下行STARR手术以避免小肠损伤[36]。现在更平衡的观点认为STARR可作为结直肠医生在某些特殊病例中的可供选择的治疗方法，特别是在一些排便障碍综合征伴直肠前突和直肠内套叠患者中可获益；但需注意，18个月内它仍有高达19%的因术后并发症或复发需再次治疗的比例。另外，就算是专家手术，也有手术失败可能，且术后可能有持续的难治性的不适症状，如便急、排便次数增加、慢性肛门痛等。表2.1列出了常见的和不常见的STARR术后不良事件。

联合小肠和阴道增强的X线排粪造影检查是在检查前2h口服400ml稀钡，同时在检查时阴道注入3~4ml硫酸钡混悬液。术前行此检查十分必要，因为它不仅可以在某种程度上决定治疗方案，还在术前病例筛选（图2.5）、术后预测疗效方面发

表2.1 导致STARR手术失败的原因

异常表现	可能原因
顽固性疼痛	吻合口距齿状线过近，吻合钉钉合部瘢痕组织
直肠囊袋及憩室形成	荷包缝合不当
吻合口狭窄	吻合口慢性出血，吻合口处纤维瘢痕增生，吻合钉残留，吻合口过度加强缝合
直肠阴道瘘	吻合口感染，吻合器误伤阴道壁
便急和便频	直肠容积或直肠顺应性降低
大便失禁	括约肌损伤，扩肛过度
盆底感染、坏死性筋膜炎	吻合线裂开，术中误伤小肠或致小肠穿孔
直肠前突持续存在	直肠前壁组织切除量不足
肛直角开大受限	术前对肛门痉挛预计不足

Sources: See Refs. [23, 29, 31-33]

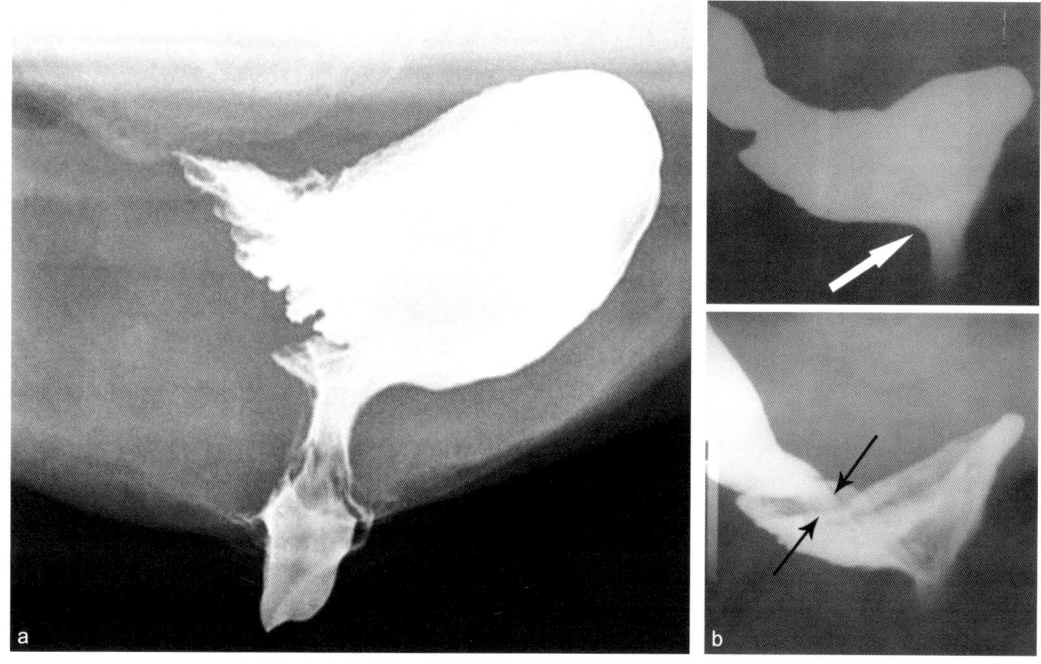

图 2.5 STARR 手术的纳入（a）及排除（b）。（a）直肠前突深度 >2cm，排便后钡剂残留；（b）直肠前突（上图）、直肠内套叠（下图黑色箭头）伴有耻骨直肠肌痉挛所致耻骨直肠肌压迹（白色箭头）

挥重要作用。排除慢传输型便秘的排便障碍综合征（ODS）患者术前完善排粪造影检查，STARR 手术的具体纳入标准如下：

- 无盆底疝及耻骨直肠肌痉挛的临床证据；
- Bartram 法[9]测量直肠前突深度 >2.5cm；
- 直肠内套叠或肛管内套叠；
- 肠腔内黏膜冗长所致直肠黏膜脱垂长度 >1cm；
- 直肠扩张 >7cm，排便时间延长，排便完成后肠腔内钡剂残留。

术后 3~6 个月行 X 线排粪造影或 MRI 排粪造影[37]用于评价解剖学改变及功能状况，但需注意，形态学与症状学相关性较差，可能解剖学异常已被纠正，但症状学改善不明显。STARR 术后一个重要的预期结果是那些导致患者接受手术的解剖学异常消失或在程度上得到明显纠正，如直肠前突、直肠内套叠、无粪便或造影剂排出障碍的直肠扩张。手术成功后最常见的排粪造影表现包括：①吻合线水平直肠平均直径为 5cm（4~8cm）；②吻合环形态规则，仅有极小程度缩小（图 2.6）；③吻合线至直肠肛管结合部或肛门内口平均距离为 5cm，（3.8~11.6cm）；④强忍和力排时直肠肛管结合部移动度为 1~4cm；⑤偶尔可见不透射线的吻合钉影。相反，STARR 手术失败的表现有吻合线不对称、吻合口狭窄、直肠囊袋形成（图 2.7）、持续存在的直肠内套叠伴或不伴直肠前突深度 >2cm、排便不完全、直肠内钡剂异常聚集、静息时钡剂渗漏入周围组织或窦道形成、肛门失禁。

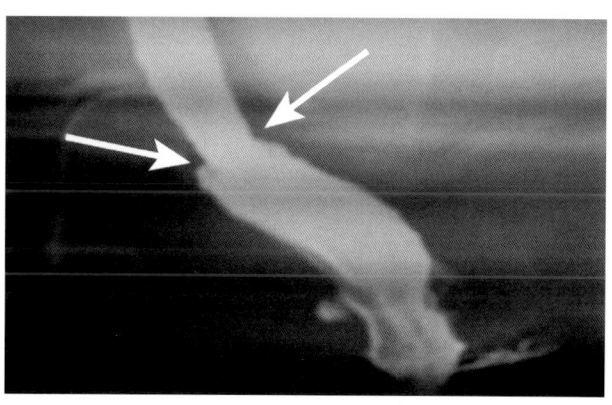

图 2.6 STARR 术后排粪造影的常见表现，可见吻合环位置对称、规则的轻微缩窄（箭头所指）

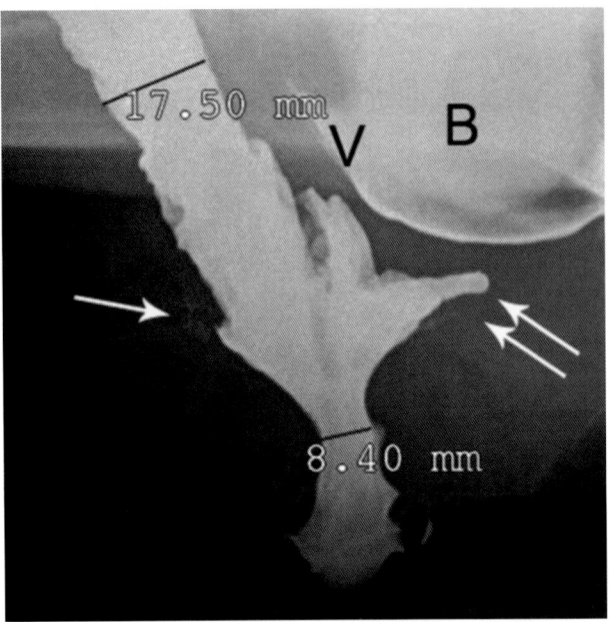

图 2.7　55 岁女性 STARR 术后 2 年持续存在排便障碍及疼痛，行四重排粪造影检查可见吻合线对侧不对称狭窄（单箭头所指）及直肠囊袋形成（双箭头所指）。B：膀胱；V：阴道

结　论

常规（X 线）排粪造影检查是针对盆底功能评价的一项极其重要的传统检查方法，特别是在贮袋 - 肛管吻合及经肛门吻合器手术病例筛选及术后疗效评价方面作用巨大。在日常临床工作中，它常用于准确描绘术后盆底解剖结构及诊断常见并发症，例如吻合口裂开、窦道形成、吻合口狭窄、吻合口溃疡、排空障碍、造影剂残留及直肠囊袋形成。

参考文献

1. Utsunomiya J, Iwama T, Imago M, Matsuo S, Sawai S, Yaegashi K, et al. Total colectomy, mucosal proctectomy and ileo-anal anastomosis. Dis Colon Rectum. 1980;23:459–66.
2. Parks AG, Nicholls RJ, Belliveau P. Proctocolectomy with ileal reservoir and anal anastomosis. Br J Surg. 1980;67:533–8.
3. Dozois RR, Goldberg SM, Rothemberger DA, Utsunomiya J, Nicholls RJ, Cohen Z, et al. Restorative proctocolectomy with ileal reservoir. Int J Colorectal Dis. 1986;1:2–19.
4. Nicholls RJ, Pezim ME. Restorative proctocolectomy with ileal reservoir for ulcerative colitis and familial adenomatous polyposis: a comparison of three reservoir design. Br J Surg. 1985;72:470–4.
5. Thayer ML, Madoff RD, Jacobs DM, Bubrick M. Comparative intrinsic and extrinsic compliance characteristic of S, J and W ileoanal pouches. Dis Colon Rectum. 1992;35:547–51.
6. Kremers PW, Scholz FJ, Schoetz DJ, Veidenheimer MC, Coller JA. Radiology of the ileoanal reservoir. AJR Am J Roentgenol. 1985;145:559–67.
7. Thoeni RF, Fell SC, Engelstad B, Schrock TB. Ileoanal pouches: comparison of CT, scintigraphy and contrast enemas for diagnosing postsurgical complications. AJR Am J Roentgenol. 1990;154:73–8.
8. Kmiot WA, Yoshioka K, Pinho M, Keighley MR. Videoproctographic assessment after restorative proctocolectomy. Dis Colon Rectum. 1990;33:566–72.
9. Bartram CI, Turnbull GK, Lennard-Jones JE. Evacuation proctography: an investigation of rectal expulsion in 20 subjects without defecatory disturbance. Gastrointest Radiol. 1988;13(1):1372–80.
10. Turnbull GK, Bartram CI, Lennard-Jones JE. Radiological studies of rectal evacuation in adults with idiopathic constipation. Dis Colon Rectum. 1988;31:190–7.
11. Pescatori M, Manhire A, Bartram CI. Evacuation pouchography in the evaluation of ileoanal reservoir function. Dis Colon Rectum. 1983;26:365–8.
12. Ascanelli S, Bartolo DCC. Functional outcome after restorative proctocolectomy. Tech Coloproctol. 1999;3:145–51.
13. Yu ED, Shao Z, Shen B. Pouchitis. World J Gastroenterol. 2007;13:5598–604.
14. Lipman JM, Kiran RP, Shen B, Remzi F, Fazio VW. Perioperative factors during ileal pouch-anal anastomosis predict pouchitis. Dis Colon Rectum. 2011;54:311–7.
15. Lazorthes F, Fages P, Chiotasso P. Resection of the rectum with construction of a colonic reservoir and colo-anal anastomosis for carcinoma of the rectum. Br J Surg. 1986;73:136–8.
16. Parc R, Tiret E, Frileux P, Moszkowski E, Loygue J. Resection and coloanal anastomosis with colonic reservoir for rectal carcinoma. Br J Surg. 1986;73:139–41.
17. Nicholls RJ, Lubowski DZ, Donaldson DR. Comparison of colonic reservoir and straight colo-anal reconstruction after rectal excision. Br J Surg. 1988;75:318–20.
18. Landi E, Marmorale C, Piloni V, et al. Functional assessment of coloanal anastomosis with and without reservoir. Coloproctology. 1993;6:359–62.
19. Piloni V, Pieri L, Pomerri F, Pittarello F, Salvetti M, Leo E, et al. The 3rd National workshop on defecography: functional radiology of the (neo)rectum (ileal pouch, colo-anal-anastomosis, continent perineal colostomy) [in Italian]. Radiol Med. 1996;91:66–72.
20. Longo A. Treatment of haemorrhoidal disease by reduction of mucosal and haemorrhoidal prolapse with a circular-suturing device: a new procedure. In: Proceedings of the sixth world congress of endoscopic surgery. Rome: Monduzzi Editori; 1998. p. 777–84.
21. Schwandner O, Stuto A, Jayne D, Lenisa L, Pigot F, Tuech J-J, et al. Decision-making algorithm for the STARR procedure in obstructed defecation syndrome: position statement of the group of STARR pioneers. Surg Innov. 2008;15:105–9.
22. Boccasanta P, Venturi M, Roviaro G. What is the benefit of a new stapler device in the surgical treatment of obstructed defecation? Three-year outcomes from a randomized controlled trial. Dis Colon Rectum. 2011;54:77–84.
23. De Nardi P, Bottini C, Faticanti Scucchi L, Palazzi A, Pescatori M. Proctalgia in a patient with staples retained in the puborectalis muscle after STARR operation. Tech Coloproctol. 2007;11:353–6.
24. Jacopo M, Pasquale T, Alfonso C. Early complications after STARR with Contour Transtar. Int J Colorectal Dis. 2010;20:83–85. [Epub ahead of print].
25. Boccasanta P, Venturi M, Stuto A, Bottini C, Caviglia A, Carriero A. Stapled transanal rectal resection for outlet obstruction: a prospective, multicenter trial. Dis Colon Rectum. 2004;47:1285–96.
26. Dindo D, Weishaupt D, Lehmann K, Hetzer HFH, Clavien PA, Hahnloser D. Clinical and morphological correlation after stapled transanal rectal resection for obstructed defecation. Dis Colon

27. Stuto A, Renzi A, Carriero A, Gabrielli F, Gianfreda V, Villani RD, et al. Stapled trans-anal rectal resection (STARR) in the surgical treatment of the obstructed defecation syndrome: results of STARR Italian Registry. Surg Innov. 2011;18:248–253.
28. Boenicke L, Jayne DG, Kim M, Reibetanz J, Bolte R, Kenn W, et al. What happens in stapled transanal rectum resection? Dis Colon Rectum. 2011;54:593–600.
29. Dodi G, Pietroletti R, Milito G, Binda G, Pescatori M. Bleeding, incontinence, pain and constipation after STARR transanal double stapling rectotomy for obstructed defecation. Tech Coloproctol. 2003;7:148–53.
30. Pescatori M, Zbar A. Reinterventions after complicated or failed STARR procedure. Int J Colorectal Dis. 2009;24:87–95.
31. Pescatori M, Dodi G, Salafia C, Zbar AP. Rectovaginal fistula after double-stapled transanal rectotomy (STARR) for obstructed defecation. Int J Colorectal Dis. 2005;20:83–5.
32. Sciaudone G, Di Stazio C, Guadagni I, Selvaggi F. Rectal diverticulum: a new complication of STARR procedure for obstructed defecation. Tech Coloproctol. 2008;12:61–3.
33. Pescatori M, Gagliardi G. Post operative complications after procedure for prolapsed hemorrhoids (PPH) and stapled transanal rectal resection(STARR) procedures. Tech Coloproctol. 2008;12:7–19.
34. Corman ML, Carriero A, Hager T, Herold A, Jayne DG, Lehur PA, et al. Consensus conference on the stapled transanal rectal resection (STARR) for disorders defaecation. Colorectal Dis. 2006;8:98–101.
35. Stuto A, Schwander O, Jayne D. Assessing safety of the STARR procedure for ODS: preliminary results of the European STARR registry. Dis Colon Rectum. 2007;50:724.
36. Carriero A, Picchio M, Martellucci J, Talento P, Palimento D, Spaziani E. Laparoscopic correction of enterocele associated to stapled transanal rectal resection for obstructed defecation syndrome. Int J Colorectal Dis. 2010;25:381–7.
37. Grassi R, Romano S, Micera O, Fioroni C, Boller B. Radiographic findings of postoperative double stapled trans-anal rectal resection (STARR) in patients with obstructed defecation syndrome (ODS). Eur J Radiol. 2005;53:410–6.

第3章 腔内超声检查（包括三维超声）

Martyn D. Evans · John Beynon

汪志明 译 李 宁 审校

摘 要

直肠和肛门腔内超声检查技术的发展彻底改变了直肠肛门肿瘤、肛门失禁和肛周复杂脓肿的治疗策略。近几十年来，腔内超声已经从相对原始的 4-MHz 超声探头，发展成最新的三维超声，分辨率极大提高，肛肠疾病的图像显示更为清晰。本章主要介绍腔内超声技术的临床应用，及其在盆腔和会阴重建手术中的作用。

关键词

直肠内超声（ERUS）；肛门内超声；腔内超声；三维（3D）ERUS

引 言

近 30 年来，直肠和肛门腔内超声检查技术的发展改变了结直肠疾病的治疗。腔内超声已经从相对原始的 4-MHz 超声探头，发展成最新的三维（3D）超声，极大地改善了图像分辨率，对复杂肛肠疾病显示更为清晰。本章主要介绍腔内超声技术的临床应用，及其在盆腔和会阴重建手术中的作用。

直肠内超声的历史和发展

1956 年，Wild 和 Reid 首先建立了直肠内超声（ERUS）技术[1-3]。Wild 和 Foderick 于 1978 年改进了该项技术[1-3]，发明了"腔内超声探头"（echoendo probe）。该探头为手提式，手柄柔韧可屈，声源为椭圆型体含压电结晶、驱动柄和马达。传感器外被充水气囊，所产生的声束与其长轴成角。虽然最初的探头从未应用于临床，但与目前临床应用的装置极其相似，手柄更坚硬，使其可通过乙状结肠镜进入直肠，通过在肠道内旋转探头获得图像。这种早期的设备制作了第一张肠壁的分层图像，之后又得到第一张直肠癌的原始照片。由于受技术条件的限制，在近 30 年中，该技术更多保持了理论优势，而非临床实际应用，直到 Dragsted 和 Gammelgaard[4] 报道了应用 8901 型 Bruel & Kjaer 超声扫描仪和装备 4.5-MHz 传感器的硬质探头（最初设计用于前列腺图像采集）诊断 13 例直肠肿瘤的经验，对比了术前 ERUS 结果与术后组织病理结果，结果有 11 例准确预测了肿瘤浸润。

在 Dragsted 和 Gammelgaard 后，ERUS 有了技术改进，提高了准确度。目前既能横断面扫描也能纵切面扫描，有些探头还能两个切面同时扫描。径向扫描的图像与手术中所见更为接近，故更容易理解。只有自动旋转探头才能 360° 成像，并需要充水气囊。水囊的作用：①形成声学介质；②可扩张直肠，防止肠腔内折。此方法要求肿瘤（如能被扫描到）尚未引起肠腔狭窄影响探头放置，并且肿瘤的位置不超出探头范围。

在目前已发表 ERUS 相关文章中多数采用 Bruel & Kjaer（丹麦，1850 探头）超声仪和 5.5-MHz 或 7-MHz 探头，近期多为 10-MHz 探头。最近大多数的系列研究多采用 7-MHz 探头（焦距 2～5 cm）。为保证图像质量，应清洁灌肠清除粪便。检查通常采用左侧卧位，探头通过直肠镜或盲插入直肠，当病变位置较高或狭窄性病变时以前种方式更佳，可发现位置更高或导致狭窄的病变。在插入探头后，球囊充水，打开超声机。当探头达到预定部位时，通过调整探头位置和气囊充水量，以获得最佳图像。

要明白 ERUS 的作用，必须先理解经直肠成像的原理。通常情况下，直肠结构分为 5 层，其中 3 层为强回声，间隔 2 层为低回声（如图 3.1 所示）：

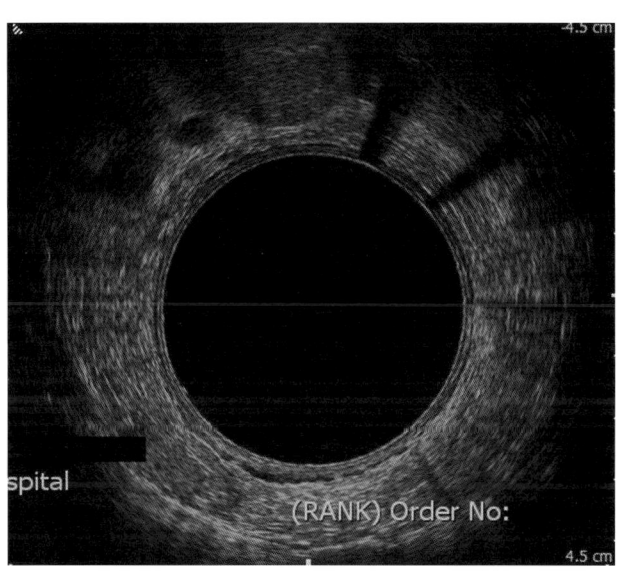

图 3.1　正常直肠的前面观。直肠内超声可见，正常直肠分为 5 层结构（如文中所述）；前列腺位于前方。在某些区域，可见 7 层结构，为环行和纵行直肠肌

- 第 1 强回声层：水 / 气囊与黏膜表面层的界面
- 第 2 低回声层：黏膜和黏膜肌层的混合图像
- 第 3 强回声层：黏膜下层
- 第 4 低回声层：固有肌层
- 第 5 强回声层：固有肌层与直肠周围脂肪，或浆膜层的界面

ERUS 还能识别直肠外器官如子宫、阴道、前列腺和精囊的解剖结构，判断直肠与上述器官间的筋膜是否完整。

三维超声

在最近 10 年中，3D ERUS 的应用逐年增加，主要与二维（2D）超声对三维结构成像存在很大缺陷有关，也是传统 ERUS 的缺陷。以直肠肿瘤为例，2D 超声不能提供肿瘤纵深径及其空间定位，操作者必须进行连续横断面扫描，才能集成真实的解剖意象图[5]。

三维（3D）图像需要大量平行的横断面 2D 图像来合成[6]。只有少数配套有 3D 软件超声设备才能实现此功能[7]。2D 图像的分辨率以像素来衡量（每个像素都有一个 x 平面和 y 平面）。3D 超声的像素被转化为小的 3D 图像元素称为体素。体素的深度对于 3D 图像的分辨率尤为重要：高分辨率的 3D 超声通常要求在 z 平面上每毫米成像 4～5 帧[7]。成像的原理有以下 3 种[6-7]：

1. 基于表面的成像技术：操作者或系统通过识别结构的边缘来创建一个有框架的图像。如果不能探及该结构边缘，则不能通过该技术成像，比如分辨肛管精细的分层结构。

2. 多平面成像技术：通过 3 个垂直正交平面（纵轴、横轴和长轴）同时成像，并通过操作者的移动或旋转从不同角度观察病变。

3. 体积渲染模式：通过光线铸件技术将 3D 图像投射到一个 2D 平片上，每条光线分割体素值可以与各种因素累加，以产生不同的效果，如厚度、滤光、亮度和透明度等。

最近 10 年，3D ERUS 技术已用于许多疾病的诊断（包括直肠肿瘤分期[8-9]，识别直肠癌的复发[10]、肛瘘[11]，以及评价大便失禁患者的括约肌功能等[12]），而以往通常采用传统的 2D ERUS 技术。已经发表的文献证实了 3D 成像技术的可行性及优于 2D 技术之处，但其真正的优势仍有待研究[13]。

直肠腔内超声和直肠肿瘤

历史上，直肠肿瘤的手术切除通常采用钝性盲视分离法，导致术后肿瘤复发的概率很高。近 30 年来，随着手术技术的发展，术前新辅助疗法的应用以及分期放疗技术的发展，极大地丰富了直肠肿瘤的治疗手段。对于进展期肿瘤患者可采用完全直

表 3.1 美国肿瘤 T 分期联合委员会对直肠癌的分期[15]

TNM T 分期	组织病理学	超声特征
Tx	原发肿瘤无法评价	难以确定肿瘤的深度
T0	无原发肿瘤证据	未见肿瘤
Tis	原位癌（局限于黏膜层）	突破第一低回声层，第二强回声层完整
T1	肿瘤侵犯黏膜下层但未达固有肌层	肿瘤未突破中间强回声层
T2	肿瘤侵犯固有肌层	肿瘤局限于固有肌层所在强回声层，未影响脂肪层
T3	肿瘤累及肛周脂肪/浆膜层	最外强回声层被突破，肿瘤边缘不规则通常呈锯齿状
T4	肿瘤累及邻近器官/腹腔	肿瘤转移至邻近器官

肠系膜切除术（total mesorectal excision，TME），保留或不保留肛门括约肌；早期肿瘤患者可采用经肛门内镜下微创手术切除（transanal endoscopic microsurger，TEMS），这些手术方式已成为临床常规。新辅助治疗已成为局部进展期肿瘤的治疗常规，术前通过 ERUS 和磁共振成像（MRI）对肿瘤进行分期，也显著提高局部肿瘤分期的精确度。现今诊断为直肠肿瘤的患者通常可以接受个体化的、有循证医学证据的疾病分期和治疗方案。制订治疗方案时，必需解决以下关键问题：肿瘤是否局限于黏膜和黏膜下层？如果肿瘤局限，则肿瘤能否通过非 TME 的方式成功根除？如果肿瘤已侵犯固有肌层，则患者在 TME 术前是否具备新辅助治疗的指征？患者是否需要切除多个器官？肿瘤对新辅助治疗是否有反应，是否需要修改手术方式或完全避免手术？MRI 和 ERUS 对于这些问题的回答起到了关键作用。本章重点介绍 ERUS 的作用。

在 ERUS 下，直肠肿瘤通常表现为低回声，当肿瘤侵犯直肠壁深层时，直肠正常的超声解剖影像被破坏。通过比较肿瘤引起的变化和正常超声影像，即可进行肿瘤 T 分期（以字母 u 表示）（表 3.1）[15]。直肠肿瘤的 T1～T4 期如图 3.2 所示。

ERUS 在早期直肠肿瘤的应用

早期黏膜内病变不伴有淋巴结转移者可考虑行经肛门肿瘤切除术或 TEMS。对 16 年中发表文献的多因素分析表明，ERUS 诊断累及固有肌层肿瘤的敏感性和特异性分别为 94% 和 86%[16]。比较研究发现，ERUS 和 MRI 诊断的敏感性相似，而前者的特异性更佳（86% vs 69%）[16]。本书重点介绍盆腔手术重建和会阴手术再造，后文将深入探讨 ERUS 在早期直肠肿瘤诊断中的作用。

ERUS 在晚期直肠肿瘤的应用

多数直肠肿瘤患者在确诊时已穿入或穿透固有肌层（>T2 期），通常认为这些患者可受益于新辅助放射治疗或放化疗（CRT）。其治疗目标是减少进展期原发肿瘤灶的大小或降低分期，以加强对原发病灶的控制。此外，一些作者认为新辅助治疗可有助于改变手术方式，部分肿瘤可以改为局部切除而非既往实施的 TME/腹会阴联合切除术[17-19]。部分原来不能手术的患者也可以手术切除[20-21]。此外，可使一些低位直肠肿瘤缩小得以保留肛门括约肌[22]。约 25% 的患者通过 CRT 可获得完成缓解，部分学者甚至主张坐等策略（watch-and-wait policy），而不建议立即手术根治[23]。

ERUS 在 T4 期判断局部病灶进展和邻近器官受侵中的作用

直肠肿瘤 <T3 期和 ≥T3 期的治疗和预后显著不同，淋巴结阴性的 T3 和 T4 期患者生存率低于淋巴结阳性的 T1 和 T2 期患者[24]，≥T3 期的患者通常都要接受新辅助治疗。在术前评估时明确原发肿瘤是否影响到邻近的器官尤为关键，特别是膀胱、阴道、前列腺或精囊，必要时应行多脏器切除术，以提高患者治愈的机会[25-26]。

文献中已广泛介绍了 ERUS 和 MRI 在区分直肠周围组织侵犯（T3）以及邻近器官受累中所起的重要作用，对 16 年内研究的荟萃分析结果表明，ERUS 确定直肠周围受侵的敏感性优于 MRI（表 3.2）[16]，两种方法的准确性相似，在判断邻近器官是否受累时都具有高度特异性。

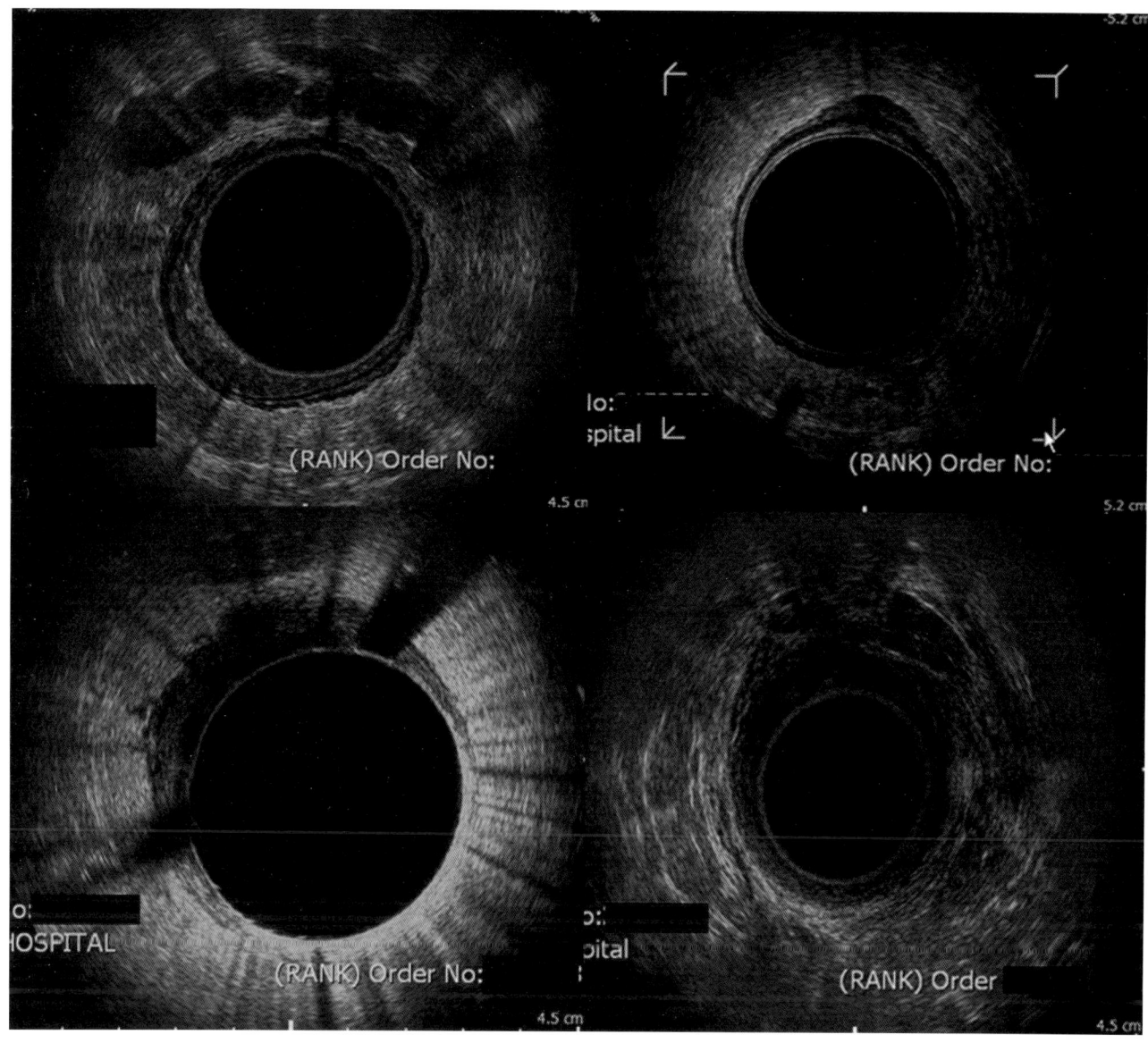

图 3.2 T1~T4 期直肠肿瘤的 ERUS 影像。T1 期（上左图）：直肠肿瘤前部可见精囊；T2 期（上右图）：直肠肿瘤侵入固有肌层，黏膜下层有少量缺失；T3 期（下左图）：外强回声层断裂，表明肿瘤穿透固有肌层进入直肠周围脂肪中；T4 期（下右图）：患者为男性患者，伴前列腺转移，表现为 Denovillier 筋膜断裂

表 3.2 EURS 和 MRI 对直肠肿瘤分期的敏感性和特异性比较汇总[16]

分 期	检查方式	敏感性（95% 可信区间）	特异性（95% 可信区间）
直肠周围组织受侵	ERUS	90%（88~92）	75%（69~81）
	MRI	82%（74~87）[a]	76%（65~84）
邻近器官受侵	ERUS	70%（62~77）	97%（96~98）
	MRI	74%（64~79）	96%（95~97）
累及淋巴结	ERUS	67%（60~73）	78%（71~84）
	MRI	66%（54~76）	76%（59~87）

a：显著低于 ERUS

ERUS 与淋巴结侵犯

是否出现淋巴结转移是预测直肠肿瘤患者生存率和局部病灶控制是否失败的最重要的因素之一，因而在手术前影像学诊断有淋巴结转移的患者通常先给予 CRT，以便于术中淋巴结清扫。临床应当利用 ERUS 的特点，对局部病灶和淋巴结进行分期。"正常"情况下直肠周围淋巴结在超声下通常不可见，但"异常"的恶性淋巴结通常可被发现（图 3.3）[27]。转移的"恶性淋巴结"的超声表现通常为直径较大（>3 mm）、回声较低、不均一、形状较圆、边界较清楚；而炎症性淋巴结通常回声较强、呈卵圆形、边界不清楚，两者的超声特征有所不同。尽管如此，在手术前通过 ERUS 或 MRI 对淋巴结分期都有一定的误诊率，结节的大小对于预测病变的性质尤其不可靠[28]，因为在一些小结节中可能隐藏着小的恶性病灶，而一些大的结节也可能只是炎症。在对 16 年文献的荟萃分析发现，ERUS 诊断淋巴结病变的敏感性和特异性分别为 67% 和 78%，MRI 的敏感性和特异性分别为 66% 和 76%（表 3.2）[16]。因此，ERUS 和 MRI 在鉴别淋巴结性质方面均有一定的局限性，但这些是现有最佳的诊断方法。最初曾有学者寄希望于正电子发射断层扫描（positron emission tomography scanning，PET/CT）技术，但最终发现 PET/CT 不能区分氟代脱氧葡萄糖（FDG）代谢活跃的原发肿瘤和与之性质相似的淋巴结[29]。

ERUS 的不足之处

虽然 ERUS 可用于早期和局部进展期直肠肿瘤的分期，但该技术仍有一些局限性。在一些研究单位发现的完美结果，在其他单位不能复制，使得 ERUS 的准确性波动于 54% ~ 92%[14, 30]。准确性不一致的原因之一是该技术高度依赖操作者的技术[31]，有一个公认的学习过程，特别是对淋巴结病变的评估[32-33]。发表文章的偏倚可能导致对 ERUS 准确性的高估[34]。常见的分期错误是高估患者分期而非低估[31, 33]，可能与操作者的谨慎态度有关，害怕低估了病变程度导致严重后果。此外，传统的 2D ERUS 通常不能确定 TME 的平面，也就不能确定直肠肿瘤的系膜环周切缘（CRM）是否受侵犯和是否需要新辅助治疗，而 MRI 在此方面具有更多的优势。最近的研究表明，3D ERUS 可在术前评估 CRM[35]，但迄今为止对该项技术的推广经验有限。同样，ERUS 不能显示所有的直肠周围和肠系膜下动脉根部淋巴结，而 MRI 对此更具优势。在一些在超声检查前做过活检，形成血肿，从而导致解剖结构不完整的患者，ERUS 结果也是不准确的，或息肉切除术后证实为恶性的患者，需要进行影像学检查，进行正式的肿瘤分期。

新辅助治疗可显著影响正常的超声影像解剖结构，可能导致对 CRT 后正常组织反应和肿瘤进展的鉴别困难。ERUS 对于 CRT 后患者的作用及困难将随后进行讨论。

ERUS 在直肠肿瘤化放疗后的应用

新辅助治疗在直肠肿瘤的应用越来越广泛。如前文所述，一些研究者认为降低肿瘤的分期可能会使某些患者免于手术[23]，或从 TME 术式改为局部切除术式[17-19]，而其中一项挑战是明确哪些患者采取这种方法是安全的。CRT 可导致照射部位炎症反应和纤维化，为临床医师在治疗后重新评估肿瘤分期带来困难，特别是在坐等疗效时，因为在炎症性病变中可能隐藏一些本应当手术切除的难以确认的微小恶性病灶。要想精确诊断这些病灶或精确分期有赖于临床检查与影像学检查（如 ERUS）相结合。

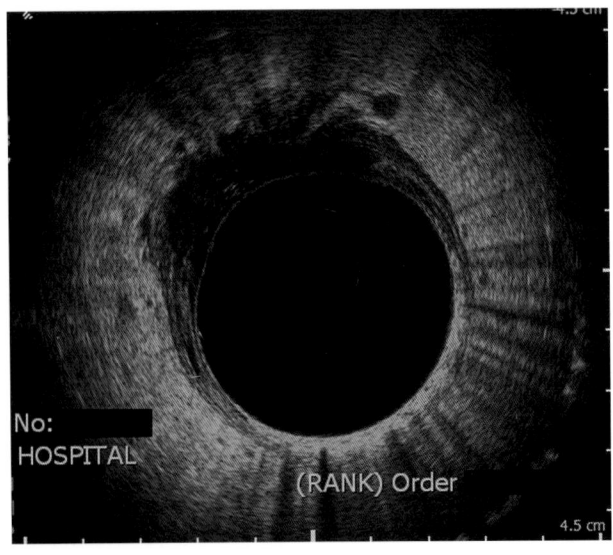

图 3.3 T4 期直肠肿瘤伴直肠周围淋巴结肿大。T4 期肿瘤已侵犯前列腺前部，在直肠前部 9 点钟方向可见肿大的淋巴结

一些研究者报道了在 CRT 后,多种手段(ERUS、MRI 或 CT)对原发病灶进行分期的准确性明显下降,因为炎症和瘢痕性病变与恶性病灶很难区分。Maretto 等[36] 研究了 46 例中下段直肠肿瘤患者 CRT 后采用 ERUS、MRI 和 CT 分期的结果,发现 ERUS 预测 T 期肿瘤的准确性为 64%,N 期为 61%,与 MRI 和 CT 的准确度相似。Huh 等[37] 观察了 ERUS(60 例)和 CT(80 例)在 CRT 后的应用情况,发现 T 期肿瘤 ERUS 和 CT 的准确性分别为 38% 和 46%,对淋巴结病变分期的准确性分别为 73% 和 70%。有趣的是,在该研究中治疗后达到完全缓解的 11 例患者,无 1 例通过上述两种方法准确分期。在 Radovanovic 等[38] 的另一项研究中,44 例 CRT 后患者采用 ERUS 进行评估,对 T 期和 N 期肿瘤分期的准确率分别为 75% 和 68%,该研究中 5 例完全缓解的患者中仅 1 例在术前通过 ERUS 确认。Pomerri 等[39] 采用 ERUS、MRI 和 CT 对连续 90 例 CRT 患者进行评估,发现三种方法的准确性都不高,T 期的准确性分别为 ERUS 27%、MRI 34%、CT 37%;N 期的准确性分别为 ERUS 65%、MRI 68%、CT 68%;该研究证实对于 ≤T3 和 T4 期的患者,ERUS 对于肠壁病变分期的准确性较高,敏感性和特异性分别为 92% 和 95%,但该组研究中只有 7 例 T4 期患者。

因此,在临床上存在的最主要问题是在 CRT 后根据临床和影像检查结果制订合适的手术方案,但在手术切除病灶、病理结果出来之前,难以预测 CRT 的疗效。因此,本书作者认为手术方式的裁定更多依据 CRT 前的影像检查结果,而非 CRT 后的结果。

局部复发的诊断

尽管局部根治手术的成功率较高,但直肠肿瘤术后局部复发率高达 12%[40]。位于直肠下 1/3 段的肿瘤以及肿瘤体积大、已发生局部转移和淋巴结转移的病灶复发率更高。在术后复查超声时应当谨记手术之后的盆腔解剖结构已发生变化,尤其是在术后近期复查时的变化多为明显,因此建议在手术后 3 个月再复查超声。通常称为"吻合口复发"病灶多来源于盆腔内局部病灶复发,在穿过吻合口并在此处复发。

ERUS 在直肠肿瘤术前分期的准确性高,但其在诊断和评估术后局部肿瘤复发中的临床价值如何?由于检查相对价廉、易行、耗时较短的优点,ERUS 应该同临床检查及乙状结肠镜作为临床术后随访检查的常规方法。进行恢复性切除或腹会阴联合切除的女性患者也可行经阴道超声检查。在直肠肿瘤术后,ERUS 下仍能清楚区分 5 层结构的患者,ERUS 评估复发的临床意义不亚于术前分期的意义,结直肠吻合钉在超声下表现为小而明亮的强回声,但不伴后声影,并不影响图像质量。手术后盆腔的解剖结构发生了变化,复查超声的时间宜在术后 3 个月时,要谨慎地理解所见影像。

手术后通过指诊或乙状结肠镜确诊的复发性肿瘤的特点与原发肿瘤极为相似,内镜超声下均表现为低回声影。其浸润程度的评估也与原发病灶相同,表现为超声下肠壁结构完整性的破坏。直肠外的局部复发病灶早期即可被发现,通常表现为吻合口旁局限性低回声病灶,但有时单凭 ERUS 难以早期诊断肿瘤复发。

在这种情况通常采用以下两种策略(图 3.4):①在 1 个月或 6 周后重复超声检查,如发现病灶体积增大,通常可以确诊为肿瘤复发;②经皮经会阴进行细针穿刺活检术。

已有少数中心报道了 ERUS 在随访中的作用,Hildebrandt 等[41] 报道了 22 例复发患者,其中仅 6

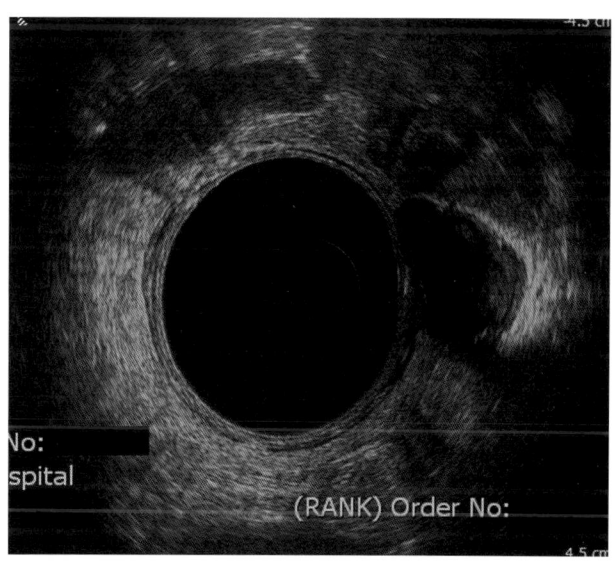

图 3.4 可疑的复发病灶。一例男性患者在直肠前壁切除术后 6 个月复查,ERUS 在 3 点钟位置见一混合超声强度团块,建议 3 个月后复查,或行经会阴穿刺活检检查

例单凭 ERUS 作出了诊断，3 例患者同时有癌胚抗原水平升高，10 例患者在癌胚抗原升高的同时，也有其他影像或内镜学改变。Romano 等[42] 报道了随访的 42 例患者中有 8 例复发，2 例患者通过经皮超声引导下穿刺活检确诊为纤维化，证实超声检查结果为假阳性。Beynon 等[43] 观察的 85 例患者中有 22 例复发，只有 3 例单纯依赖 ERUS 明确诊断，其他的病例都能通过指诊或乙状结肠镜发现病灶。在另一项意大利的研究中，Mascagni 等[44] 随访的 120 例患者中 17 例复发，7 例无症状，12 例通过直肠内超声确诊，5 例使用了经阴道超声，总准确率高达 97%，敏感性和特异性分别为 94% 和 98%，其中有 6 例患者经过指诊和单纯内窥镜检查也可发现病灶。Morken 等[45] 报道了 525 例局部或根治性术后直肠肿瘤患者采用 ERUS 随访的经验，任何提示局部复发的病灶都应行 ERUS 引导下活检术。其中 39 例在随访中证实局部复发，其中 5 例（13%）只有 ERUS 检查发现了异常，82% 患者在 ERUS 后明确了诊断。Doornebosch 等[46] 报道了一组患者 TEMS 治疗后 T1 期肿瘤患者的预后，18 例复发，其中 6 例只在 ERUS 下发现异常。

因此，小的直肠外复发性肿瘤可通过 ERUS 早于腔道复发而诊断，并可行 ERUS 引导下穿刺活检术。在直肠肿瘤术后常规使用 ERUS 来评估盆腔病变，这在以前只能通过昂贵的 CT 或 MRI 检查才能实现。在 TEMS 和 TME 后，ERUS 都能发挥早期诊断肿瘤复发的作用，从而有可能通过再次手术达到根治的目的。

小　结

目前已经发表的有关直肠肿瘤局部分期和手术后随访的文献都在试图回答一个问题，即 ERUS 或 MRI 是更精确的检查手段吗？事实上，两种方法各有优点（表 3.3），临床医生可联合使用两种检查方法以达到最佳的结果（图 3.5）。因此本书作者的观点是，所有的直肠肿瘤患者都应常规行这两种检查。

表 3.3　ERUS 和 MRI 诊断直肠肿瘤优劣的比较

	ERUS	MRI
发现早期黏膜病变	更好	较差
区分 <T3 和 >T3 病灶	更好	较差
邻近器官侵犯	相仿	相仿
淋巴结侵犯	较差	更好
判断潜在系膜环周切缘	较差	更好

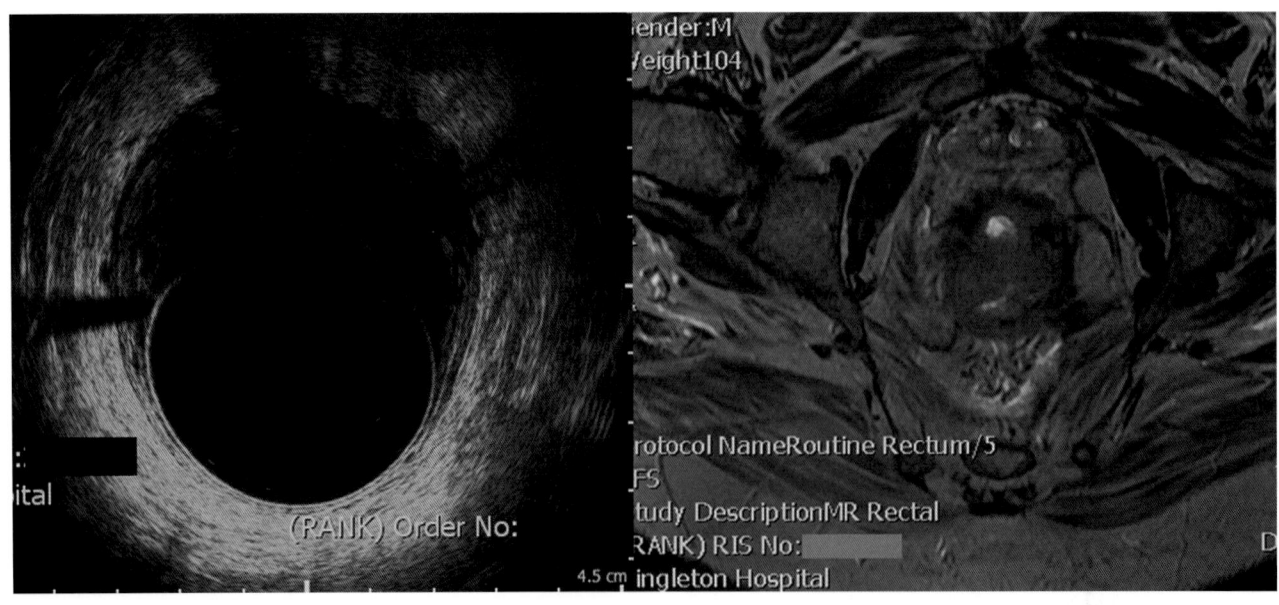

图 3.5　一例 T4 期直肠肿瘤前列腺转移患者 ERUS（左图）与 MRI（右图）结果的对照。MRI 提示前列腺转移的可能，ERUS 证实前列腺回声不均均匀，从而显示了两种检查方法相结合的优势

肛门内超声

肛门内超声（EAUS）是一种微创、简便、可提供肛门细微解剖结构的检查手段。结肠直肠吻合重建术后行EAUS检查的适应证包括肛门肿瘤行CRT术前和术后，严重的肛瘘性疾病和肛门失禁。最终希望获得360°横断面图像。该技术需要一个能自动旋转的探头，外面包被着经除气处理的塑料囊，避免气泡产生的假象。整个装置被置于一个避孕套中，两面均涂有凝胶做为声耦合剂。患者取俯卧位，以保持会阴部处于对称位置，从患者的脚部往上看时保持图像的前面在上。肛管检查是个动态过程，分别获得浅层、中层和深层图像。EAUS获得的肛管各层结构通常描述如下（图3.6 a-c）：

1. 黏膜表层——强回声层
2. 黏膜层——低回声层（但不一定可见）
3. 上皮下层——强回声层
4. 内括约肌层——混合回声层
5. 纵行肌层——强回声层
6. 外括约肌层——混合回声层

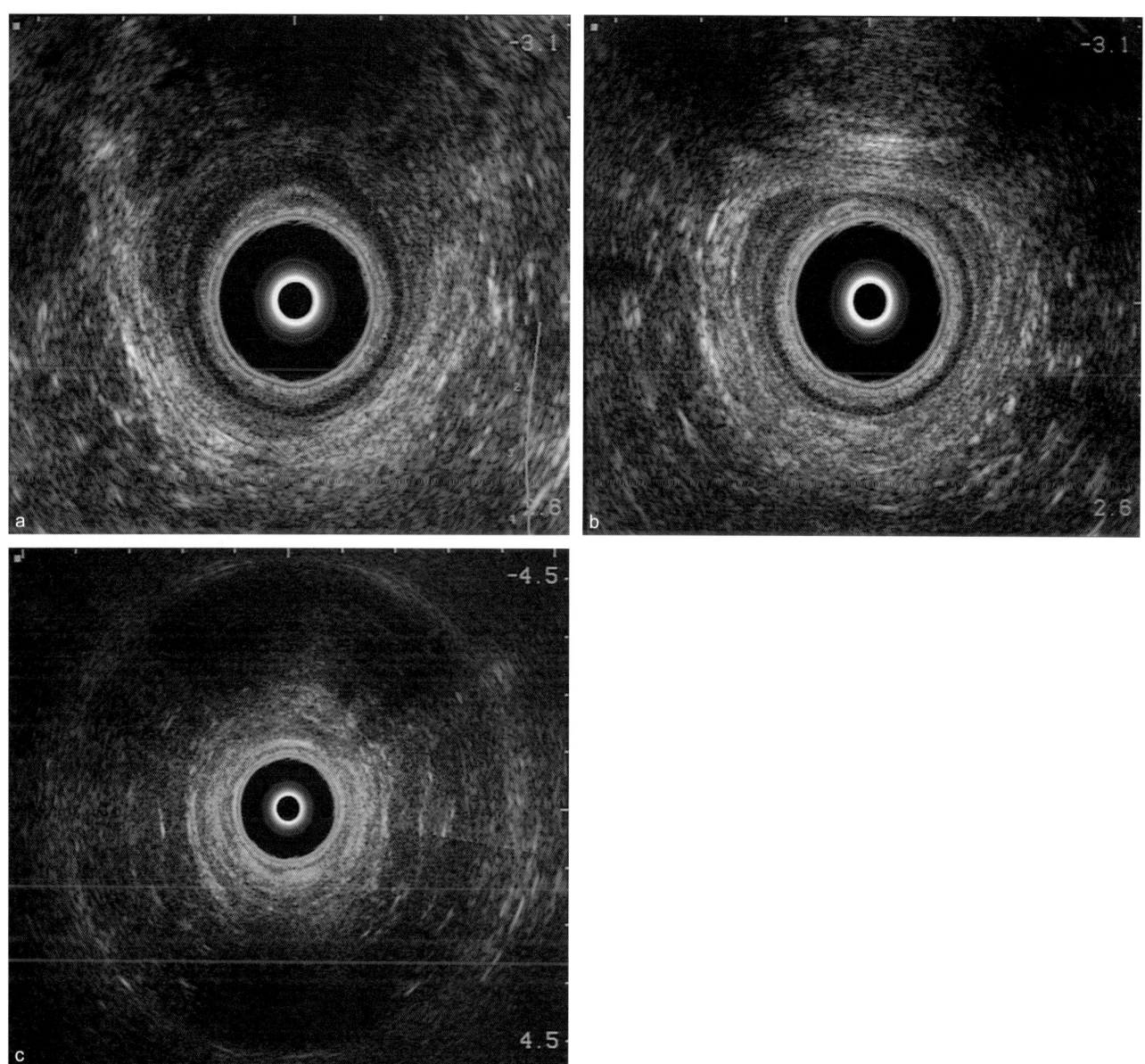

图3.6 正常直肠内超声显示的肛管上段（a）、中段（b）和下段（c）影像，可见低回声的肛门内括约肌和混合回声的肛门外括约肌，在肛管上段（a），可见逐渐分开的耻骨直肠肌

男性和女性的肛管解剖结构存在明显差异，尤其是肛门外括约肌层的结构。不同年龄者肛门括约肌的形态也有所不同，在解释 EAUS 检查结果时应考虑到这些正常的差异。

在无症状的未经产女性中，肛管上段和中段内括约肌层的厚度与年龄正相关[45]，而上段、中段和下段外括约肌的厚度与年龄负相关。肛门外括约肌结构复杂，通常分为深层、浅层和皮下层3层，退出探头时可见到呈强回声的 U 形耻骨直肠肌。在退出探头的过程中肛门外括约肌逐渐向前会聚形成肛环。女性的前部肛门外括约肌较为薄弱，男性的肛门外括约肌更为对称，在各个平面都为环型结构，在外部有一段回声环。女性肛管的各层回声较为均匀，通常难以分层，在肛管前部深层肌肉自然缺如[47]。随着数字图像时代的来临，3D EAUS 成像已成为可能，可通过大量的平行轴面 2D 图像重建 3D 图像，与前文所述的直肠内超声方法相似。

EAUS 和肛门肿瘤

肛门肿瘤历来是一种需要通过手术切除根治的疾病，但是随着 Nigro 技术的发展[48]，非手术性 CRT 根治疗法已替代手术成为首选的治疗方法。

EAUS 和肛门肿瘤分期

（同时参见第 18 章，作者 James Hill）

目前尚无国际统一的肛门肿瘤分期体系，目前最常使用的是美国癌症联合委员会 TNM 分期系统。在该系统中 T 期是直肠指诊、CT 和 MRI 等检查确定的肿瘤大小（表 3.4），该系统潜在的问题是（T4 期除外）对肿瘤侵犯的深度没有明确规定。使用 EAUS 技术之后，根据肿瘤侵犯的深度，T 期肿瘤的分期方法发生了变革，与普遍使用的小肠肿瘤的 T 分期方法更为相似（表 3.4 和图 3.7）[49]。

不管初始分期如何，多数肛门肿瘤患者都采用根治性 CRT 治疗，唯独小的 T1 期肿瘤除外，可考虑做局部切除。因此影像检查对于抗肿瘤治疗最有意义在于其随访阶段。但 EAUS 在随访中的作用饱受争议[50-51]。其中最困难的问题之一是区分治疗引起的瘢痕和恶性病灶（图 3.8）。支持在随访过程中进行系列 EAUS 检查者，认为可以早期发现治疗后

表 3.4 美国癌症联合委员会（AJCC）的分期系统与 Goldman 等[49] 提出的超声分期系统的比较

AJCC 分期系统	超声分期系统[49]
T1 直径 <2cm	局限于上皮下
T2 2～5cm	局限于括约肌内
T3 >5cm	穿透外括约肌
T4 侵犯邻近器官如阴道、前列腺、子宫、膀胱（不包括侵犯括约肌）	侵犯邻近器官

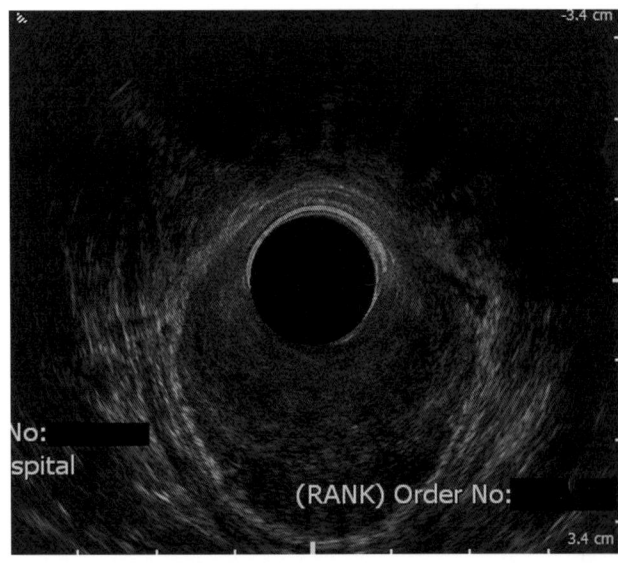

图 3.7 一例肛门鳞癌患者化放疗前直肠内超声所见，病灶位于肛管后部，侵犯内、外括约肌，根据 Goldman 分期（表 3.4）定义为 T3 期

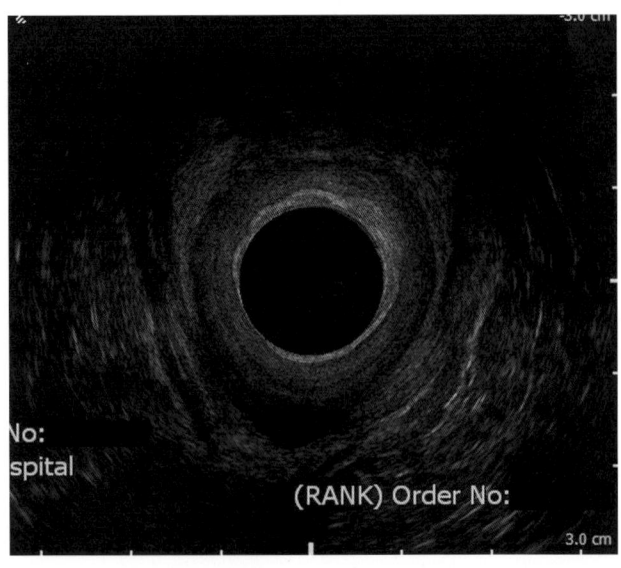

图 3.8 一例肛门癌患者在化放疗后行直肠内超声所见。肛管后部持续可见一低回声影像结节，经穿刺证实为瘢痕，表明在 CRT 后鉴别良性病变和恶性病灶较为困难

的变化[52]，而且可以在 EAUS 指引下行细针穿刺活检术[53]，彩色多普勒显示的彩色信号可提示疾病复发，增加了对肿瘤复发诊断的可靠性[54]。但 Lund 等[51]认为，EAUS 在现有常规的指诊和可视检查的基础上添效甚微：在他们报道的 14 例复发中，无一例不是因为临床的原因而确诊的。

在放疗后进行 EAUS 检查的时机也颇为关键，有研究认为在治疗后 45 天之内检查太早，由于照射导致的水肿增加了图像理解的难度，而穿刺也有导致医源性瘘管的风险[55]。此外，通常认为放疗的效果在停止治疗后仍可持续一段时间，过早检查可能导致对治疗结果的误判。最佳的随访方案仍不得而知，但有研究者建议，在术后行 EAUS 和临床检查的频率为第 1 年每 3 月一次，第 2 年和第 3 年每 6 个月一次，以后每年一次[55]，并建议由手术的医生或放疗医师进行检查，采用动态记录的 3D 影像结果可有助于动态比较检查结果的变化，而非单一的照片之间的比较[55]。

EAUS 和肛瘘及肛周脓肿

肛周脓肿是一种常见的症状，通常表现为急性脓肿或慢性肛瘘。虽然简单的肛瘘通常不需要放射性检查，但一些患者通过麻醉下检查（EUA）不能明确窦道的解剖特点，必需联合放射性检查。在这种情况下，EAUS 和盆腔 MRI，与 EUA 联合使用可增加对瘘管评估的精确性[56]。

在 EAUS 下，脓肿表现为不均质的低回声区，中间偶见强回声光点；肛瘘表现为低回声的腔道，有时可穿透括约肌（图 3.9）。文献报道 EAUS 诊断原发性窦道的准确性为 50%～91.7%，继发性窦道的准确性为 60%～68%[57-59]。目前已有大量研究对比传统 EAUS 和 MRI，研究结果仍存在争论。EAUS 的确是评估肛瘘的有效手段，不仅可在手术室使用还可当成一种 EUA 进行；而多数一线研究者多首选 MRI，可能与 EAUS 的某些局限性有关，如观察范围有限，对超出括约肌的脓肿和窦道评估困难，在既往手术史的患者，其脓肿和瘢痕性病变的区分较困难，并且其准确度受操作者影响较多，特别是反复发作的复杂肛瘘[60]。

通过窦道外口注射 H_2O_2 可增加 EAUS 诊断肛瘘的准确性[61]。注入的 H_2O_2 可显著增强窦道的回声，从低回声变为强回声，在需要区分窦道和瘢痕时该

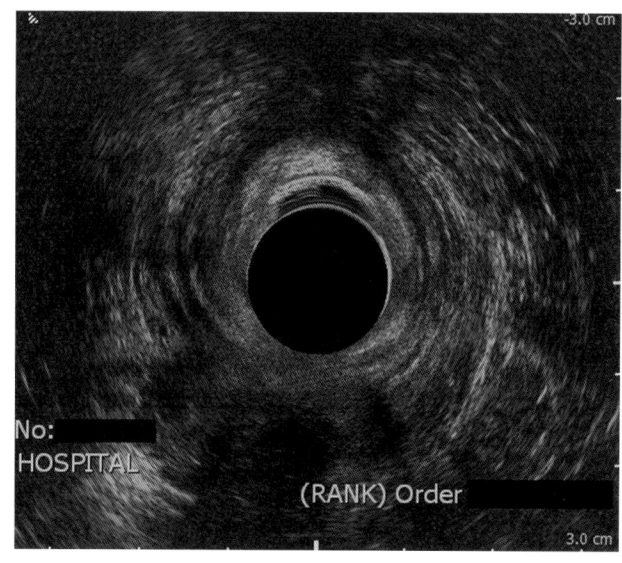

图 3.9　一例男性患者克罗恩病患者直肠超声见肛周瘘道形成，肛管后部可见一低回声、不均一的脓肿，7 点钟位置见一穿透括约肌的瘘管

技术尤为有效[7]，与 3D EAUS 联合使用时可明显提高诊断的准确率[62]。

EAUS 与肛周克罗恩病

克罗恩病是各种导致肛瘘的原因之一，但它应被单独提出讨论，因为它可能会导致严重的后果，重症患者甚至需要行直肠切除和会阴重建。

在处理直肠和肛门克罗恩病时，EAUS 很多情形都可发挥作用。传统上 EUA 是治疗肛周克罗恩病的金标准，Schwarz 等[56]的前瞻性研究发现，单用 EUA 的准确性为 90%，而联合使用 EAUS 或 MRI 时，准确度可高达 100%。内镜超声还被成功地用于诊断和辅助引流深部盆腔感染[63]。在复杂瘘管的患者中，与单纯 EUA 相比，联合 EAUS 能更容易地发现原发和继发瘘管。

EAUS 还可用于评价药物治疗的效果，特别是抗肿瘤坏死因子单抗（英夫利昔单抗）。有人评估了 EAUS 在预测抗肿瘤坏死因子单抗治疗疗效中的作用，研究包括了 30 例合并有直肠阴道瘘或肛瘘的克罗恩病患者[64]，在纳入研究时、治疗 10 周以及每 6 个月时均行 EAUS 检查，结果发现 EAUS 显示瘘管闭锁消失的患者要比虽然瘘管闭锁而内镜超声仍提示存在瘘管的患者的复发率低。

EAUS 和肛门失禁

EAUS 技术极大地帮助了我们理解复杂性括约肌损伤如何引起肛门失禁[65]。许多研究指出 EAUS 可准确反映括约肌缺陷，将其与特发性大便失禁相鉴别，确定哪些患者需要行括约肌修补术，并在修补术后评估括约肌功能。

采用 EAUS 评估括约肌功能时，操作者应考虑以下因素：病变是累及 1 种括约肌还是都累及了；累及数量、部位，纵向缺失还是横向缺失，缺失的径向角方向，括约肌的超声特性和厚度。多数肛门内括约肌（IAS）的损伤比较容易确定，通常表现为正常低回声的括约肌环上出现强回声的缺口[7]，肛门外括约肌（EAS）的缺失表现为外围混合强回声带上出现缺口（图 3.10 所示为 IAS 和 EAS 损伤）[7]。在诊断大便失禁时，了解不同性别 IAS 的生理差别极为重要，不论男女，EAS 的后外侧在各个层面都应当是完整的；但在女性中，肛管较深水平的前方，EAS 存在生理缺失[66]。

有报道称，在诊断大便失禁患者时，3D EAUS 显著优于 2D 图像[67-69]，但也有学者认为 EAUS 图像虽有改善，但与临床病情并不相符[70]。Gold 等[67] 认为 3D EAUS 在显示括约肌的纵向和放射状撕裂时较为有效，可用于评价手术治疗的有效性。Christensen 等[69] 证实，3D EAUS 能提高诊断的可信度，增加不同研究者在诊断括约肌缺陷时的一致性。

结 论

近 30 年来 ERUS 和 EAUS 的应用逐渐增多，技术设备越来越完善，应用范围越来越广泛。两种技术在诊断恶性肛门直肠疾病和肛瘘中都有重要地位，在评价大便失禁患者的括约肌形态学中发挥了重要作用。大多数文献都侧重于比较 ERUS、EAUS 与 MRI 诊断效能，但不同技术各有优劣之处。本书作者认为，在大多数临床情况下，特别是在恶性疾病患者，ERUS 和 EAUS 都应当成为各种互补检查手段之一（包括指诊），使患者接受到最合理的治疗。

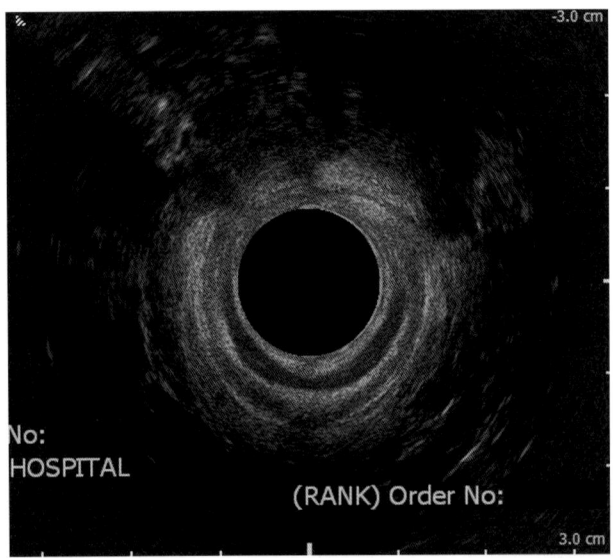

图 3.10 一例产科括约肌损伤患者在损伤 3 个月后行直肠内超声见肛管前部内、外括约肌均发生撕裂

参考文献

1. Wild JJ, Reid JM. Diagnostic use of ultrasound. Br J Phys Med. 1956;19:248–57.
2. Wild JJ, Foderick JW. The feasibility of echometric detection of cancer in the lower gastrointestinal tract. Part II. Am J Proctol Gastroenterol Colon Rectal Surg. 1978;29(2):11–3. 5–6, 18–20.
3. Wild JJ, Foderick JW. The feasibility of echometric detection of cancer in the lower gastrointestinal tract. Part I. Am J Proctol Gastroenterol Colon Rectal Surg. 1978;29(2):16–25.
4. Dragsted J, Gammelgaard J. Endoluminal ultrasonic scanning in the evaluation of rectal cancer: a preliminary report of 13 cases. Gastrointest Radiol. 1983;8:367–9.
5. Hunerbein M. Endorectal ultrasound in rectal cancer. Colorectal Dis. 2003;5:402–5.
6. Giovannini M, Ardizzone S. Anorectal ultrasound for neoplastic and inflammatory lesions. Best Pract Res Clin Gastroenterol. 2006;20:113–35.
7. Santoro GA, Fortling B. The advantages of volume rendering in three-dimensional endosonography of the anorectum. Dis Colon Rectum. 2007;50:359–68.
8. Hunerbein M, Below C, Schlag PM. Three-dimensional endorectal ultrasonography for staging of obstructing rectal cancer. Dis Colon Rectum. 1996;39:636–42.
9. Kim JC, Cho YK, Kim SY, Park SK, Lee MG. Comparative study of three-dimensional and conventional endorectal ultrasonography used in rectal cancer staging. Surg Endosc. 2002;16:1280–5.
10. Hunerbein M, Dohmoto M, Haensch W, Schlag PM. Evaluation and biopsy of recurrent rectal cancer using three-dimensional endosonography. Dis Colon Rectum. 1996;39:1373–8.
11. Buchanan GN, Bartram CI, Williams AB, Halligan S, Cohen CR. Value of hydrogen peroxide enhancement of three-dimensional endoanal ultrasound in fistula-in-ano. Dis Colon Rectum. 2005;48:141–7.
12. West RL, Felt-Bersma RJ, Hansen BE, Schouten WR, Kuipers EJ. Volume measurements of the anal sphincter complex in healthy controls and fecal-incontinent patients with a three-dimensional reconstruction of endoanal ultrasonography images. Dis Colon Rectum. 2005;48:540–8.
13. Gravante G, Giordano P. The role of three-dimensional endolumi-

nal ultrasound imaging in the evaluation of anorectal diseases: a review. Surg Endosc. 2008;22:1570–8.
14. Hildebrandt U, Feifel G. Preoperative staging of rectal cancer by intrarectal ultrasound. Dis Colon Rectum. 1985;28:42–6.
15. Sobin LH, Wittekind C. UICC TNM classification of malignant tumors. 6th ed. New York: Wiley-Liss; 2002.
16. Bipat S, Glas AS, Slors FJ, Zwinderman AH, Bossuyt PM, Stoker J. Rectal cancer: local staging and assessment of lymph node involvement with endoluminal US, CT, and MR imaging – a meta-analysis. Radiology. 2004;232:773–83.
17. Schell SR, Zlotecki RA, Mendenhall WM, Marsh RW, Vauthey JN, Copeland 3rd EM. Transanal excision of locally advanced rectal cancers downstaged using neoadjuvant chemoradiotherapy. J Am Coll Surg. 2002;194:584–91.
18. Bonnen M, Crane C, Vauthey JN, Skibber J, Delclos ME, Rodriguez-Bigas M, et al. Long-term results using local excision after preoperative chemoradiation among selected T3 rectal cancer patients. Int J Radiat Oncol Biol Phys. 2004;60:1098–105.
19. Callender GG, Das P, Rodriguez-Bigas MA, Skibber JM, Crane CH, Krishnan S, et al. Local excision after preoperative chemoradiation results in an equivalent outcome to total mesorectal excision in selected patients with T3 rectal cancer. Ann Surg Oncol. 2010;17:441–7.
20. Glimelius B, Gronberg H, Jarhult J, Wallgren A, Cavallin-Stahl E. A systematic overview of radiation therapy effects in rectal cancer. Acta Oncol. 2003;42:476–92.
21. Braendengen M, Tveit KM, Berglund A, Birkemeyer E, Frykholm G, Påhlman L, et al. Randomized phase III study comparing preoperative radiotherapy with chemoradiotherapy in nonresectable rectal cancer. J Clin Oncol. 2008;26:3687–94.
22. Habr-Gama A, Perez RO, Kiss DR, Rawet V, Scanavini A, Santinho PM. Preoperative chemoradiation therapy for low rectal cancer. Impact on downstaging and sphincter-saving operations. Hepatogastroenterology. 2004;51:1703–7.
23. Habr-Gama A, Perez RO, Nadalin W, Sabbaga J, Ribeiro Jr U, Silva e Sousa Jr AH. Operative versus nonoperative treatment for stage 0 distal rectal cancer following chemoradiation therapy: long-term results. Ann Surg. 2004;240:711–8.
24. Kozak KR, Moody JS. The impact of T and N stage on long-term survival of rectal cancer patients in the community. J Surg Oncol. 2008;98:161–6.
25. Moriya Y, Akasu T, Fujita S, Yamamoto S. Aggressive surgical treatment for patients with T4 rectal cancer. Colorectal Dis. 2003;5:427–31.
26. Nguyen DQ, McGregor AD, Freites O, Carr ND, Beynon J, El-Sharkawi AM, et al. Exenterative pelvic surgery – eleven year experience of the Swansea Pelvic Oncology Group. Eur J Surg Oncol. 2005;31:1180–4.
27. Beynon J, Mortensen NJ, Foy DM, Channer JL, Rigby H, Virjee J. Preoperative assessment of mesorectal lymph node involvement in rectal cancer. Br J Surg. 1989;76:276–9.
28. Monig SP, Baldus SE, Zirbes TK, Schroder W, Lindemann DG, Dienes HP, et al. Lymph node size and metastatic infiltration in colon cancer. Ann Surg Oncol. 1999;6:579–81.
29. Abdel-Nabi H, Doerr RJ, Lamonica DM, Cronin VR, Galantowicz PJ, Carbone GM, et al. Staging of primary colorectal carcinomas with fluorine-18 fluorodeoxyglucose whole-body PET: correlation with histopathologic and CT findings. Radiology. 1998;206:755–60.
30. Konishi F, Muto T, Takahashi H, Itoh K, Kanazawa K, Morioka Y. Transrectal ultrasonography for the assessment of invasion of rectal carcinoma. Dis Colon Rectum. 1985;28:889–94.
31. Garcia-Aguilar J, Pollack J, Lee SH, de Hernandez Anda E, Mellgren A, Wong WD. Accuracy of endorectal ultrasonography in preoperative staging of rectal tumors. Dis Colon Rectum. 2002;45:10–5.
32. Badger SA, Devlin PB, Neilly PJ, Gilliland R. Preoperative staging of rectal carcinoma by endorectal ultrasound: is there a learning curve? Int J Colorectal Dis. 2007;22:1261–8.
33. Li JC, Liu SY, Lo AW, Hon SS, Ng SS, Lee JF, et al. The learning curve for endorectal ultrasonography in rectal cancer staging. Surg Endosc. 2010;24(12):3054–9.
34. Harewood GC. Assessment of publication bias in the reporting of EUS performance in staging rectal cancer. Am J Gastroenterol. 2005;100:808–16.
35. Giovannini M, Bories E, Pesenti C, Moutardier V, Lelong B, Delpero JR. Three-dimensional endorectal ultrasound using a new freehand software program: results in 35 patients with rectal cancer. Endoscopy. 2006;38:339–43.
36. Maretto I, Pomerri F, Pucciarelli S, Mescoli C, Belluco E, Burzi S, et al. The potential of restaging in the prediction of pathologic response after preoperative chemoradiotherapy for rectal cancer. Ann Surg Oncol. 2007;14:455–61.
37. Huh JW, Park YA, Jung EJ, Lee KY, Sohn SK. Accuracy of endorectal ultrasonography and computed tomography for restaging rectal cancer after preoperative chemoradiation. J Am Coll Surg. 2008;207:7–12.
38. Radovanovic Z, Breberina M, Petrovic T, Golubovic A, Radovanovic D. Accuracy of endorectal ultrasonography in staging locally advanced rectal cancer after preoperative chemoradiation. Surg Endosc. 2008;22:2412–5.
39. Pomerri F, Pucciarelli S, Maretto I, Zandona M, Del Bianco P, Amadio L, et al. Prospective assessment of imaging after preoperative chemoradiotherapy for rectal cancer. Surgery. 2011;149:56–64.
40. Sebag-Montefiore D, Stephens RJ, Steele R, Monson J, Grieve R, Khanna S, et al. Preoperative radiotherapy versus selective postoperative chemoradiotherapy in patients with rectal cancer (MRC CR07 and NCIC-CTG C016): a multicentre, randomised trial. Lancet. 2009;373(9666):811–20.
41. Hidebrandt U, Fiefel G, Schwarz HP, Scherr O. Endorectal ultrasound: instrumentation and clinical aspects. Int J Colorectal Dis. 1986;1:203–7.
42. Romano G, de Rosa P, Vallone G, Rotondo A, Grassi R, Santangelo ML. Intrarectal ultrasound and computed tomography in the pre- and postoperative assessment of patients with rectal cancer. Br J Surg. 1985;72(Suppl):S117–9.
43. Beynon J, Mortensen NJ, Foy DM, Channer JL, Rigby H, Virjee J. The detection and evaluation of locally recurrent rectal cancer with rectal endosonography. Dis Colon Rectum. 1989;32:509–17.
44. Mascagni D, Corbellini L, Urciuoli P, Di Matteo G. Endoluminal ultrasound for early detection of local recurrence of rectal cancer. Br J Surg. 1989;76:1176–80.
45. Morken JJ, Baxter NN, Madoff RD, Finne 3rd CO. Endorectal ultrasound-directed biopsy: a useful technique to detect local recurrence of rectal cancer. Int J Colorectal Dis. 2006;21:258–64.
46. Doornebosch PG, Ferenschild FT, de Wilt JH, Dawson I, Tetteroo GW, de Graaf EJ. Treatment of recurrence after transanal endoscopic microsurgery (TEM) for T1 rectal cancer. Dis Colon Rectum. 2010;53:1234–9.
47. Frudinger A, Halligan S, Bartram CI, Price AB, Kamm MA, Winter R. Female anal sphincter: age-related differences in asymptomatic volunteers with high-frequency endoanal US. Radiology. 2002;224:417–23.
48. Nigro ND, Vaitkevicius VK, Considine Jr B. Combined therapy for cancer of the anal canal: a preliminary report. Dis Colon Rectum. 1974;17:354–6.
49. Goldman S, Norming U, Svensson C, Glimelius B. Transanorectal ultrasonography in the staging of anal epidermoid carcinoma. Int J Colorectal Dis. 1991;6:152–7.
50. Giovannini M, Bardou VJ, Barclay R, Palazzo L, Roseau G, Helbert T. Anal carcinoma: prognostic value of endorectal ultrasound (ERUS). Results of a prospective multicenter study. Endoscopy. 2001;33:231–6.
51. Lund JA, Sundstrom SH, Haaverstad R, Wibe A, Svinsaas M, Myrvold HE. Endoanal ultrasound is of little value in follow-up of anal carcinomas. Dis Colon Rectum. 2004;47:839–42.
52. Martellucci J, Naldini G, Colosimo C, Cionini L, Rossi M. Accuracy of endoanal ultrasound in the follow-up assessment for squamous cell carcinoma of the anal canal treated with radiochemotherapy. Surg Endosc. 2009;23:1054–7.

53. Magdeburg B, Fried M, Meyenberger C. Endoscopic ultrasonography in the diagnosis, staging, and follow-up of anal carcinomas. Endoscopy. 1999;31:359–64.
54. Drudi FM, Giovagnorio F, Raffetto N, Ricci P, Cascone F, Santarelli M, et al. Transrectal ultrasound color Doppler in the evaluation of recurrence of anal canal cancer. Eur J Radiol. 2003;47:142–8.
55. Martellucci J. Endoanal ultrasound for anal cancer follow up. Int J Colorectal Dis. 2011;26:679–80.
56. Schwartz DA, Wiersema MJ, Dudiak KM, Fletcher JG, Clain JE, Tremaine WJ, et al. A comparison of endoscopic ultrasound, magnetic resonance imaging, and exam under anesthesia for evaluation of Crohn's perianal fistulas. Gastroenterology. 2001;121:1064–72.
57. Law PJ, Talbot RW, Bartram CI, Northover JM. Anal endosonography in the evaluation of perianal sepsis and fistula in ano. Br J Surg. 1989;76:752–5.
58. Cataldo PA, Senagore A, Luchtefeld MA. Intrarectal ultrasound in the evaluation of perirectal abscesses. Dis Colon Rectum. 1993;36:554–8.
59. Lindsey I, Humphreys MM, George BD, Mortensen NJ. The role of anal ultrasound in the management of anal fistulas. Colorectal Dis. 2002;4:118–22.
60. Halligan S, Stoker J. Imaging of fistula in ano. Radiology. 2006;239:18–33.
61. Kruskal JB, Kane RA, Morrin MM. Peroxide-enhanced anal endosonography: technique, image interpretation, and clinical applications. Radiographics. 2001;21:S173–89.
62. West RL, Dwarkasing S, Felt-Bersma RJ, Schouten WR, Hop WC, Hussain SM, et al. Hydrogen peroxide-enhanced three-dimensional endoanal ultrasonography and endoanal magnetic resonance imaging in evaluating perianal fistulas: agreement and patient preference. Eur J Gastroenterol Hepatol. 2004;16:1319–24.
63. Giovannini M, Bories E, Moutardier V, Pesenti C, Guillemin A, Lelong B, et al. Drainage of deep pelvic abscesses using therapeutic echo endoscopy. Endoscopy. 2003;35:511–4.
64. Ardizzone S, Maconi G, Colombo E, Manzionna G, Bollani S, Bianchi Porro G. Perianal fistulae following infliximab treatment: clinical and endosonographic outcome. Inflamm Bowel Dis. 2004;10:91–6.
65. Law PJ, Bartram CI. Anal endosonography: technique and normal anatomy. Gastrointest Radiol. 1989;14:349–53.
66. Bartram CI. Anal endosonography. In: Freeney PC, Stevenson GW, editors. Alimentary tract radiology. St Louis: Mosby-Year Book; 1994.
67. Gold DM, Bartram CI, Halligan S, Humphries KN, Kamm MA, Kmiot WA. Three-dimensional endoanal sonography in assessing anal canal injury. Br J Surg. 1999;86:365–70.
68. Williams AB, Spencer JA, Bartram CI. Assessment of third degree tears using three-dimensional anal endosonography with combined anal manometry: a novel technique. BJOG. 2002;109:833–5.
69. Christensen AF, Nyhuus B, Nielsen MB, Christensen H. Three-dimensional anal endosonography may improve diagnostic confidence of detecting damage to the anal sphincter complex. Br J Radiol. 2005;78:308–11.
70. Wasserberg N, Mazaheri A, Petrone P, Tulchinsky H, Kaufman HS. 3D Endoanal ultrasonography of external anal sphincter defects in patients with faecal incontinence: correlation with symptoms and manometry. Colorectal Dis. 2011;13:449–53.

第4章 直肠肛管疾病的磁共振成像

Sanne M.E. Engelen · Geerard L. Beets · Regina G.H. Beets-Tan
刘建磊 译　姜　军 审校

摘　要

磁共振成像技术（MRI）对软组织有较高的分辨率，有助于肿瘤及复杂肛瘘的诊治，有助于深入了解直肠肛管解剖及盆底和会阴在排便、提肛、力排过程中的相互作用，有助于直肠癌患者进行新辅助治疗的效果随访。对复杂性肛瘘及克罗恩病的肛周表现，MRI 有助于某些新手术方法的开展，如括约肌间瘘管挂线术（LIFT）、瘘管塞和纤维蛋白胶等，同时有助于筛选适宜行肛门成形术或肠道转流术的患者。本章阐述了直肠肛管正常解剖的 MRI 表现、直肠癌和肛瘘的分级，以及确定需重建或再次手术的病例。

关键词

直肠肛管疾病；磁共振成像技术（MRI）；肛瘘；直肠癌

引　言

磁共振成像技术（MRI）有助于指导直肠肛管疾病，尤其是直肠癌和肛瘘的治疗。近年研究显示直肠肛管 MRI 有利于直肠癌的最佳治疗方案选择，通过 MRI 进行局部分级，评估直肠癌的复发概率，依据其制订治疗方案，及治疗过程出现的相关并发症来评估方案的优劣，从而选择最佳的个体化方案。肛瘘治疗的研究发现，MRI 在复杂性及复发性肛瘘最佳治疗方案筛选方面优于其他检查方法，还可探查复杂性肛瘘的所有瘘管及潜在的脓肿，指导术中探查，从而降低瘘管或脓肿残留概率及复发率。本章主要介绍直肠肛管的正常 MRI 表现、MRI 对直肠癌及肛瘘的分级，以及 MRI 为复杂肛瘘的初次或再次手术治疗提供影像学指导。

解　剖

直肠肛管与盆腔临近器官

直肠是从直肠肛管交界向上至直乙交界，长度12～15cm，与测量的基准线不同有关，如以肛缘、齿状线或直肠肛管交界为基线。直乙交界位于第3骶椎水平，肛管位于直肠尾端，直肠肛管交界处向后显著弯曲（图4.1）。直肠肛管位于盆腔的后半部，在骶骨和尾骨前方，在其前方女性为阴道和子宫，男性为前列腺和精囊腺（图4.2）。

直肠系膜腔

是由直肠系膜筋膜（图4.3）围绕而成，内有直肠及直肠系膜，后者内包含血管、淋巴结及淋巴管。

MRI 的 T2 加权像上正常的直肠是双层结构：外侧低信号层是直肠固有肌层，内侧高信号层是黏膜层。当直肠出现炎症，如炎性肠病或放疗后，MRI 显示在直肠内外层之间出现另一高信号层（图 4.4）。

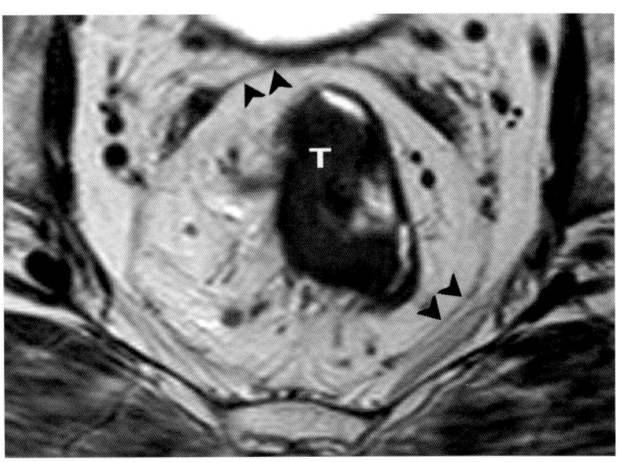

图 4.3　骨盆的横断面图像，T2 加权，快速自旋回波（TR/TE 为 342/150ms），直肠肿瘤及周围的直肠系膜脂肪被低信号的直肠系膜筋膜包绕（黑色箭头）

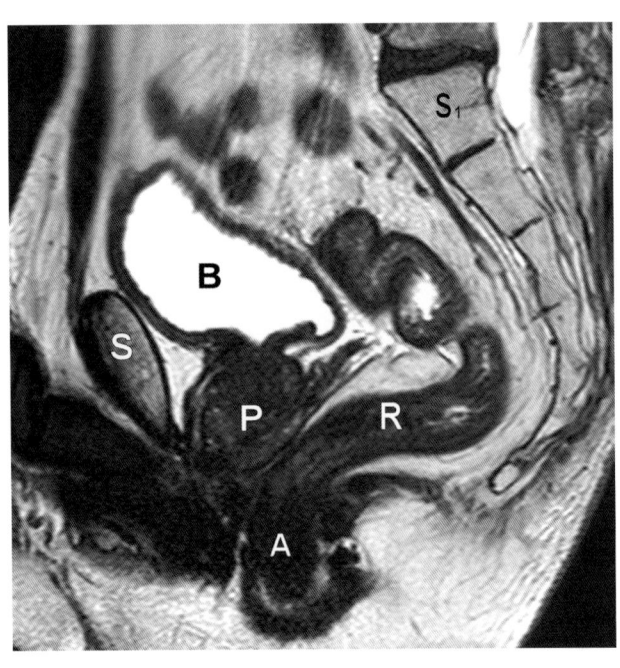

图 4.1　盆腔 T2 加权矢状位成像（TR/TE 为 342/150ms），显示直肠（R）、肛管（A）、前列腺（P）、膀胱（B）。S：耻骨联合；S_1：第 1 骶骨

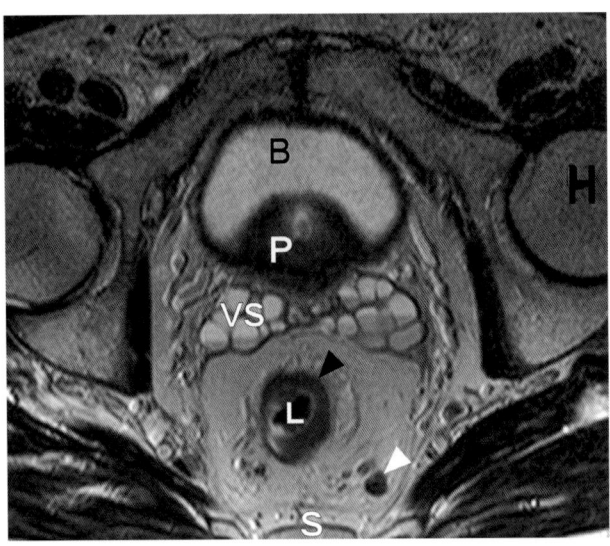

图 4.2　男性骨盆的横断面图像，T2 加权，快速自旋回波（TR/TE 为 342/150ms），显示盆腔内各器官的关系：后面是骶骨（S），两侧是股骨头（H），直肠腔（L）是低信号区。直肠壁上有一环形等信号肿瘤（黑色箭头）。直肠前是直肠周围脂肪组织、精囊腺（VS）、前列腺（P）和膀胱（B）。此例直肠癌患者的直肠系膜内可见一淋巴结（白色箭头）

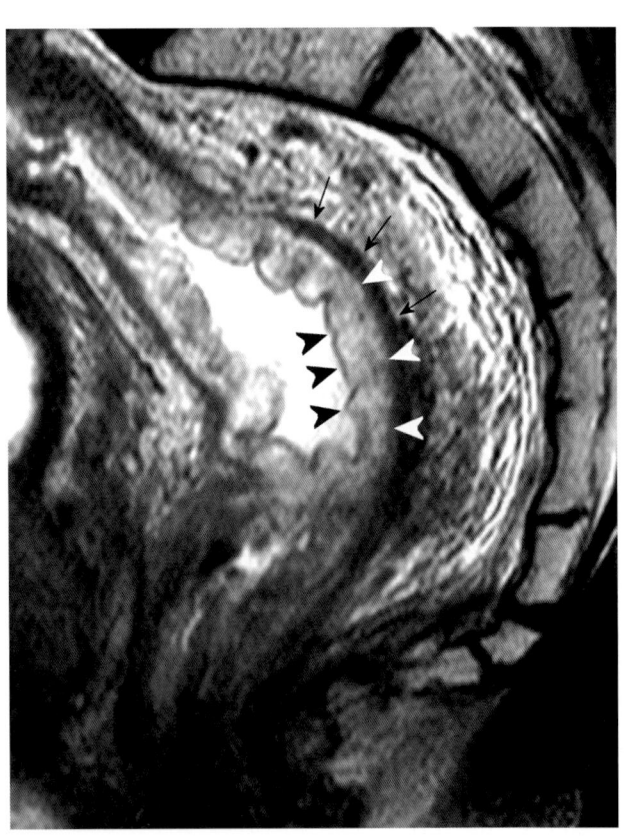

图 4.4　男性直肠癌患者骨盆的 MR 矢状位图像，T2 加权，快速自旋回波（TR/TE 为 3427/150ms），高信号区（白色箭头）提示黏膜下水肿，内侧为黏膜层（黑色箭头），外侧为直肠固有肌层（黑色箭头）（Reprinted with permission from Lahaye et al.[1]）

在 MRI 的 T2 加权像上，直肠系膜脂肪是一个高信号结构，环绕直肠，但纵行及环行密度不均，在直肠前壁稍厚，因此前壁信号与生殖腺信号相似（男性的精囊腺、前列腺，女性的阴道、子宫颈）。直肠前壁与邻近器官关系紧密，且直肠下段系膜脂肪变薄，直肠癌易侵犯前壁邻近器官及盆壁（图 4.5）。

在 MRI 的 T2 加权像上，直肠系膜筋膜是包绕直肠系膜脂肪的低信号细线（图 4.3）[2]。在直肠前方分隔直肠周围脂肪与精囊腺或阴道，此处直肠系膜筋膜增厚，被称为 Denonvilliers 筋膜；直肠后方低信号的骶前筋膜-Waldeyer 筋膜位于直肠系膜筋膜与骶骨之间，手术切除直肠时，应沿上述两层筋膜之间的层面分离。直肠上 2/3 的前壁被腹膜包绕，前壁的腹膜在精囊腺（男性）或子宫颈/阴道后壁处反折形成直肠膀胱陷凹或直肠子宫陷凹，即 Douglas 窝。

肛门括约肌

肛门肌肉是由肛门内、外括约肌及两层间的纵行肌肉层组成。括约肌复合体近端为肛提肌复合体，是盆底肌肉的重要组成部分（图 4.6）。肛提肌复合体及肛门外括约肌（EAS）是受阴部神经支配，而肛门内括约肌（IAS）是受 $S_2 \sim S_4$ 的副交感神经支配。

血 供

直肠血供主要来自直肠上动脉，起源于肠系膜下动脉。直肠上动脉分为左右两支，供应直肠两侧，直肠上静脉在直肠背侧与动脉伴行，在 MRI 的 T2 加权像上，直肠上动脉是低信号的（图 4.7）。直肠远端也接受来自髂内动脉的直肠中动脉供应。

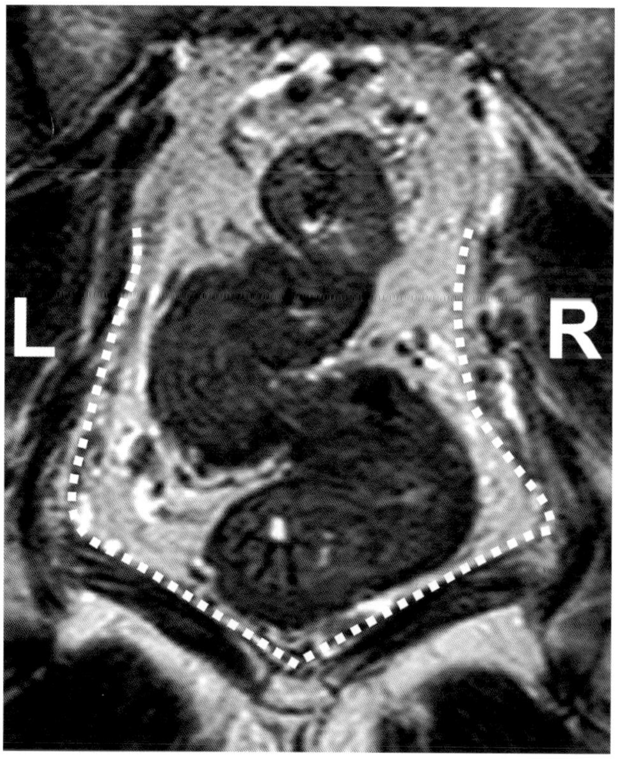

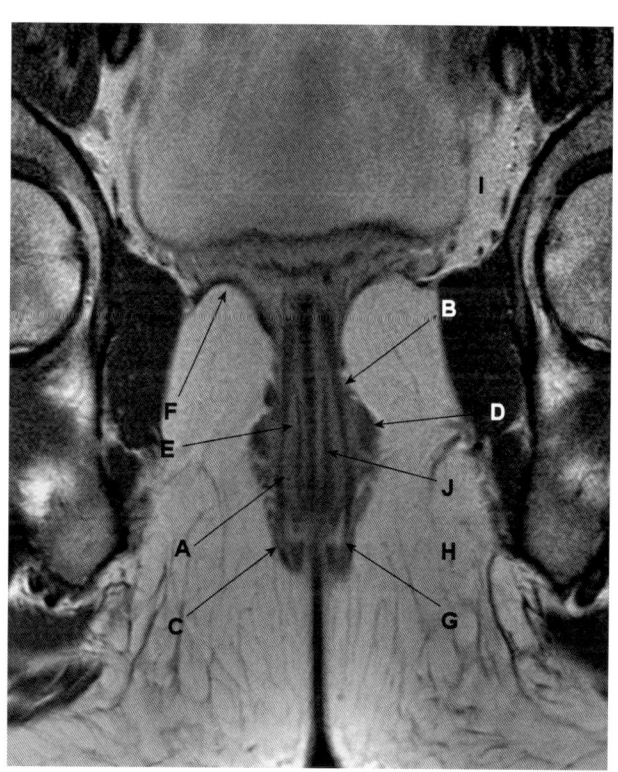

图 4.5 直肠肿瘤患者骨盆的 MRI 冠状位图像，T2 加权，快速自旋回波（TR/TE 为 3427/150ms），显示直肠系膜远端逐渐变细，且与直肠壁及盆底肌肉关系密切（白色虚线）（Reprinted with permission from Lahaye et al.[1]）

图 4.6 MRI 快速自旋回波，T1 加权，钆剂增强，可以显示肛门的肌肉组织。A. 肛门内括约肌；B. 纵行肌层；C. 肛门外括约肌；D. 耻骨直肠肌；E. 肛门黏膜下肌肉；F. 肛提肌；G. 括约肌间隙；H. 坐骨肛管/直肠间隙；I. 肛提肌上间隙；J. 位于黏膜下层的薄肌肉层

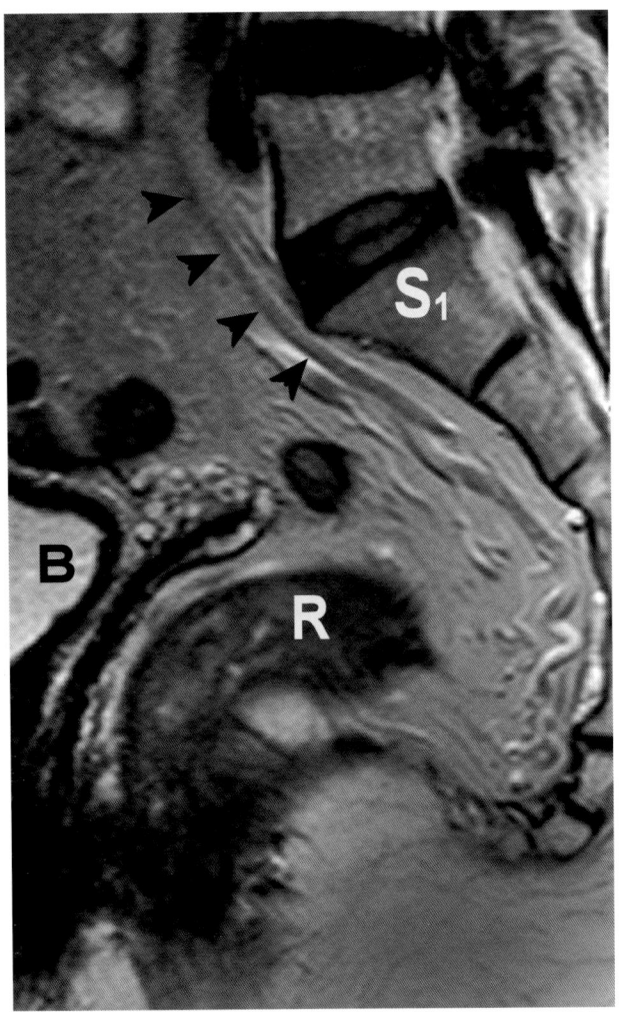

图 4.7 盆腔 MRI 矢状位图，T2 加权，快速自旋回波（TR/TE 3427/150ms），直肠上动脉是低信号区（黑色箭头表示），可见直肠（R）、膀胱（B）和第 1 骶骨（S_1）

髂内动静脉位于盆腔侧壁，直肠下动脉来自于阴部动脉，后者是髂内动脉的一个分支。骶前静脉丛位于 Waldeyer 筋膜后，对外科医师来说，该静脉丛非常重要，如不慎损伤，可导致大出血，且止血困难。

淋巴回流

直肠的淋巴回流管路主要与直肠上静脉、肠系膜下静脉伴行，汇入主动脉旁淋巴。直肠系膜淋巴结主要位于直肠的侧方和后方[3]。直肠下段的淋巴回流是沿着直肠中血管，即所谓的骨盆侧壁淋巴结，肿瘤转移往往发生于这些淋巴结，尤其是低位肿瘤，直肠系膜淋巴结最常受累（图 4.8）[4-5]。

神经分布

支配直肠肛管、泌尿系统和性功能的神经位于盆腔，交感和副交感神经均沿骨盆侧壁走形，汇入直肠系膜，因此增大了肿瘤侵犯及手术损伤神经的可能性[6-7]。下腹上神经位于骶岬水平，在直肠的背面分为左右两支，沿着盆壁绕过直肠，支配膀胱和性器官。在 $S_2 \sim S_5$ 水平，这些神经与副交感神经纤维伴行，经相同的途径到达膀胱和性器官。交感和副交感神经纤维共同形成左、右下腹下神经丛，MRI 不能显示该神经丛。

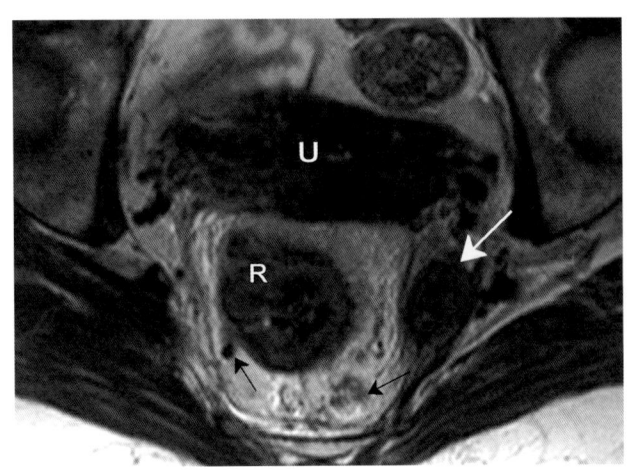

图 4.8 MRI 横断面，T2 加权，快速自旋回波（TR/TE 3427/150ms）。有一个巨大的淋巴结在直肠系膜外（白色箭头），位于直肠中动脉水平，考虑为转移淋巴结，直肠系膜内也有肿大淋巴结（黑色箭头），左侧的淋巴结边界清楚、信号均匀，因此可能为良性的反应性增生；右侧的淋巴结边界不清、信号强度不均匀，考虑为肿瘤转移。同时可见直肠肿瘤（R）、子宫（U）

直肠肿瘤

直肠癌

2006 年欧洲共有约 30 万人患结直肠癌，结直肠癌已成为第 3 大常见肿瘤，在肿瘤相关性死亡原因中占第 2 位[8-9]。结直肠肿瘤中约 30% 为直肠癌，直肠癌除可直接导致死亡外，其局部复发率高，因此直肠癌的治疗聚焦于局部及远期控制，近年来直肠癌的治疗进展主要是手术方式和新辅助疗法。肿瘤细胞可沿着直肠周围脂肪组织播散，全直肠系膜切除（TME）是沿着直肠系膜外锐性分离直肠系膜腔，将直肠周围脂肪组织、淋巴结和血管一并切除，可显著降低局部复发率[10]。TME 的源头来自于肿瘤距离环形切缘（CRM）的距离，病理学家认为该距离是决定局部复发率的一个重要因素[11]。与此同时，斯堪的纳维亚研究证实传统手术方式术前放射治疗在降低肿瘤局部复发率方面优于术后放射治疗，荷兰的 TME 研究[12]和 MRC CR07 研究[13]表明，在 TME 术前辅助 5×5Gy 的短期放疗，可显著降低局部复发率，因此在荷兰和斯堪的纳维亚，TME 术前进行 5×5Gy 的放射治疗成为所有直肠癌的标准治疗方案。荷兰的 TME 亚组研究同时发现术前放疗（5×5Gy）没有提高Ⅰ期肿瘤（T1-2N0）的治疗效果，可能与Ⅰ期肿瘤本身预后较好相关[12]，因该结论是亚组研究结果，且术前根据淋巴结进行肿瘤分期存在困难，因此临床医师并没有停止对此类患者进行术前放射治疗。另外，进展期肿瘤（尤其是侵犯 CRM 者）即使进行术前短期放射治疗，其局部复发率仍较高[14]，为降低局部复发率，推荐更积极的新辅助疗法。1991 年 Krook 等[15]研究发现放射治疗联合化学治疗可以降低进展期肿瘤患者的局部复发率，提高整体生存率，另外两项研究也建议新辅助治疗应联合化学治疗和放射治疗，可以降低局部复发率[16-17]，且与术后化学治疗相比，其疗效更显著[16]。2004 年 Sauer 等[18]证实与术后化学治疗相比，术前化学治疗联合放射治疗有利于局部复发率控制及降低药物毒性。因此，对局部进展期直肠癌最好应进行长期新辅助放射治疗，联合化学治疗作为放射治疗增敏剂。

长期以来，进展期肿瘤（高 CRMs 侵犯风险）的筛选是根据直肠指检（肿瘤固定）或内镜超声，但两者评估肿瘤侵犯 CRMs 的精确性均不高。荷兰的 TME 研究试图在术前排除进展期肿瘤，术后病理仍发现有 16% 侵犯 CRMs，可能与术前对大肿瘤的评级偏低有关。2000 年初开始应用 MRI 评估直肠癌，可精确显示直肠系膜腔及肿瘤与 CRM 的关系，能很好地分辨肿瘤是否侵犯或接近直肠系膜筋膜[2, 19-24]，此项技术有助于 CRM 的确定，是医学的重大进步[11]。

除 CRM 之外，淋巴结转移是局部复发的重要危险因素，但影像学无法进行淋巴结受累的精确诊断，因淋巴结受累的主要诊断标准是淋巴结大小，直肠癌中许多直径小于 5mm 的淋巴结可发生微小转移[25]。MRI 中引入淋巴结特异性对比剂有利于受累淋巴结的检测[26]，MRI 技术的发展、精确判断 CRM 及根据淋巴结转移的肿瘤分级有助于制订更加个体化的治疗方案，根据局部复发风险选择最适于个体患者的治疗方案，理论上个体化治疗可更好地控制局部复发率，同时降低直肠癌整体的治疗相关性风险发生率。

荷兰一项根据 MRI 结果进行直肠癌个体化治疗及手术效果评估的多中心前瞻性研究正在进行，3 年局部复发率的最终结果不久将问世。在这项研究中，所有直肠癌患者术前均进行 MRI 检查，评估肿瘤复发可能性（如 CRM、淋巴结转移和肿瘤厚度等），根据 MRI 结果进行分层次治疗：低风险组单纯手术治疗，中风险组术前 5×5Gy 放射治疗联合手术治疗，高风险组术前行长期联合放化疗（CRT）。这项研究的目的是为了证实对直肠癌患者进行分层次治疗，可获得更佳的治疗效果及减少治疗相关并发症，初步研究结果显示 2 年的局部复发率为 2.8%，提示分层次治疗是安全有效的[27]。

目前，许多研究结果用于指导治疗方案的制订，如对新辅助 CRT 的反应程度，据报道有高达 25% 的完全缓解率，且有更高比例的患者肿瘤变小或分级降低[28]。目前治疗的趋势是对术前 CRT 反应良好者采取侵犯小、器官骚扰小的手术方式，对完全缓解的患者可采取"等等看"的策略[29-31]。在这种治疗策略中，MRI 的精确使用在 CRT 治疗后对肿瘤的重新分期至关重要。

应用 MRI 对直肠癌进行分期

肿瘤分期

直肠癌的肿瘤分期可分为 4 类：T1 期是指肿瘤侵犯黏膜下层；T2 期是指肿瘤侵犯固有肌层；T3 期是指肿瘤侵犯直肠系膜脂肪组织；T4 期是指肿瘤侵犯临近器官。应用 MRI 对肿瘤进行分期的精确性，不同的研究差异性较大，从 67%～83% 不等[32]，这种差异性的原因部分是由于 MRI 不能显示黏膜下层，因此不能很好地区分 T1 和 T2 期肿瘤，在这方面直肠内超声可靠性更高[32]；另外 MRI 辨别 T2～T3 期肿瘤也有困难。MRI 上显示完整的低信号肌层时，多提示肿瘤未侵犯直肠系膜脂肪（阳性率为 86%～91%）[33]，然而对处于 T2～T3 期之间且伴有结缔组织增生的病例，MRI 不能精确区分结缔组织增生伴有肿瘤细胞转移（pT3）和结缔组织增生不伴肿瘤细胞转移（pT2）（图 4.9a，b）。MRI 可精确区分 T3 和 T4 期肿瘤，敏感性为 74%～82%，特异性为 76%～96%。

环周切缘（CRM）

直肠系膜筋膜在 MRI 的 T2 加权横断面上表现为低信号线性结构，是外科医师进行直肠癌根治术需切除的结构，术前可精确评估 CRM，一项对 7 个独立中心研究结果的 meta 分析显示其敏感性为 60%～88%，而特异性为 73%～100%[1]，且被 Mercury Study Group 的一项大宗的多中心前瞻性研究所证实，总体精确性为 88%，表明应用 MRI 来判断 CRM 是可靠的（图 4.10）[35]。

淋巴结转移

直肠癌的系膜和系膜外淋巴结转移对治疗策略至关重要。以往直肠癌是根据淋巴结大小来区分有无淋巴结转移，这种方法有其自身的限制性，因为小淋巴结（<5mm）也可出现转移，且在直肠癌中这类转移的淋巴结占多数[25]；其他方法如淋巴结边界和异质性也曾被用于判断淋巴结转移，良性淋巴结多边界清晰、内部信号均匀，而恶性淋巴结边界多不规则、内部信号不均匀，随着这些准则的提高，其敏感性在 36%～85%，特异性在 95%～100%[36-37]。然而必须认识到，上述各项准则在判断小淋巴结上是有困难的，因此各种精确判断淋巴结状态的 MRI 对比剂及弥散加权 MRI 正在研究中，超小顺磁氧化铁是一种淋巴结特异性 MR 对比剂，研究证实其具有可靠性及较高的阴性检出率[38]；虽然结果是令人振奋的，但超小顺磁氧化铁尚不能广泛应用于临床。

新辅助放化疗后再分期

对新辅助疗法反应良好的局部进展期肿瘤，如侵犯直肠系膜筋膜者经治疗后肿瘤缩小，外科医师会考虑选择损伤范围小的手术方式，因此目的是为保留器官、神经而行局部切除或对完全缓解、接近完全缓解患者进行"等等看"的策略时，肿瘤重新分期非常必要。

yT 和 yN 分期

对新辅助治疗后完全缓解的患者进行 MRI 分期，只能进行 T 和 N 分期[39-41]，治疗后进行 MRI 分期评估的难点在于低信号瘢痕组织的形成，无法将瘢痕组织与残留肿瘤细胞的瘢痕组织区分开，因

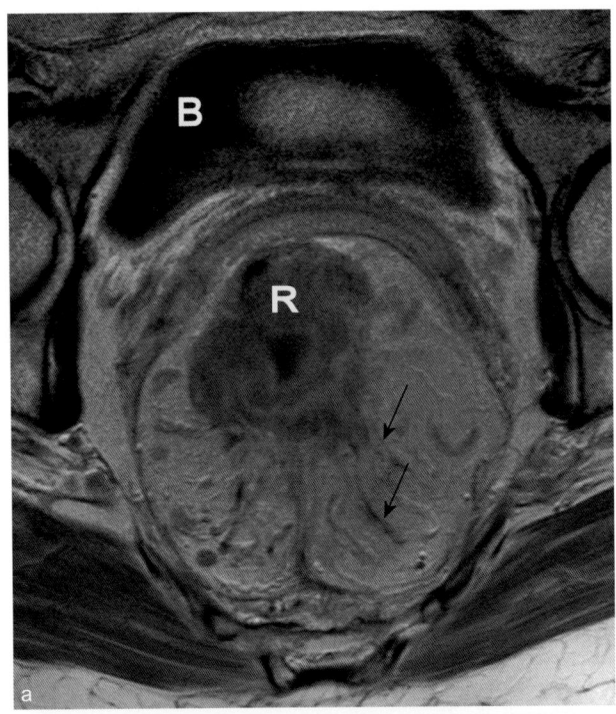

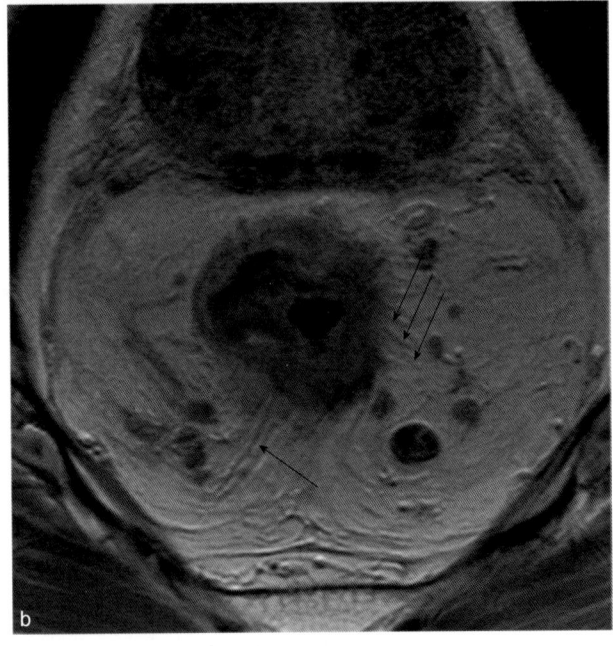

图 4.9 （a，b）为 MRI 的 T1 加权像，快速自旋回波（TR/TE 为 612/15ms），轴向对比增强。均显示对直肠癌的结缔组织增生反应（黑色箭头），但不能区分结缔组织增生伴（b）肿瘤细胞（T3 期肿瘤）和结缔组织增生不伴（a）肿瘤细胞（T2 期肿瘤）。两图均显示直肠系膜淋巴结。R：直肠肿瘤；B：膀胱（Reprinted with permission from Beets-Tan et al.[21]）

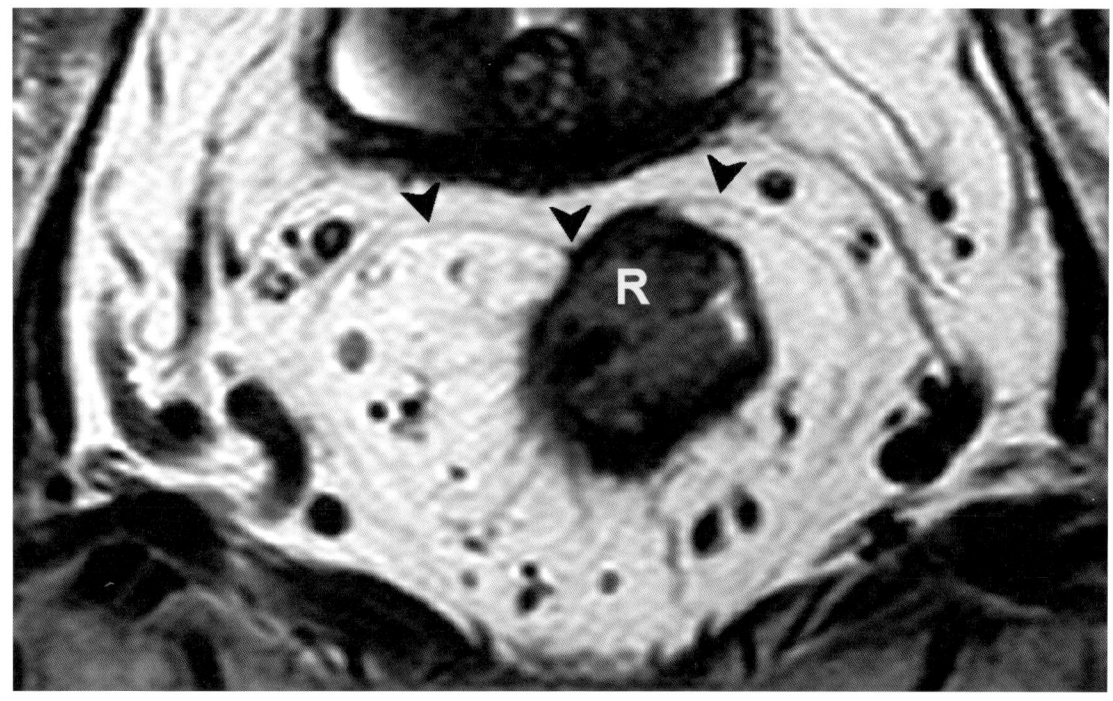

图 4.10　轴向 MRI 图像，T2 加权，快速自旋回波（TR/TE 为 3427/150ms），显示直肠癌（R）及直肠前方的直肠系膜筋膜（黑色箭头）

此有相当多的完全缓解肿瘤患者再次行 MRI 检查时，影像学医师为了安全起见作出过度分期的诊断。但是外科手术主要想了解肿瘤是否局限于肠壁而无淋巴结转移，精确的 T 和 N 分期反而是次要的。一项近期研究显示，对治疗完全缓解的患者进行 MRI 检查，结合治疗前后形态学和体积特征进行分析，专家和新手对 ypT0～2 期肿瘤（局限于肠壁适合局部切除）的诊断准确率相似[33]，阳性率高达 94%。另外一项多中心前瞻性研究显示，通过 MRI 对比剂来筛选 ypT0～2 期肿瘤患者，可显著降低分期不足的风险，这意味着选择适宜病例进行局部切除是可行的[42]。Lahaye 也证实了 ypN0 分期的安全性[43]。

肿瘤治疗后与直肠系膜筋膜关系

Mercury Study Group 的一项多中心研究显示，经放化疗完全缓解者，对其进行再分期的准确率为 77%，尤其是其阴性诊断率高达 98%[44]，后者是该研究中心对另两个独立中心研究的肯定[45]。Vliegen 等致力于研究放化疗后完全缓解后的转归，可分为 4 个类型：类型 1，形成厚达 2mm 的脂肪垫；类型 2，在肿瘤与直肠系膜筋膜间形成锯齿状结构；类型 3，形成弥散的低密度纤维组织；类型 4，形成弥散的等信号或高信号组织。类型 1、2 高度提示肿瘤已经远离直肠系膜筋膜，而类型 3 则有 50% 侵犯直肠系膜筋膜，类型 4 明确侵犯直肠系膜筋膜，提示需扩大切除范围。

MRI 检查直肠癌的策略

新一代的体内相控阵线圈有较高的信噪比，可以提供较高的空间和对比分辨率，可对直肠癌进行标准的成像。检查前不需要进行肠道或其他准备，因对比剂对原发灶和放化疗完全缓解后分期没有帮助[47]；不建议使用直肠内对比剂，因为这样会扩张直肠壁，从而压缩直肠系膜脂肪，使肿瘤原发灶、淋巴结分期及放化疗后分期变得困难。MRI 的 T2 加权快速自旋回波二维图像可以用于 3 个平面，首先对肿瘤进行矢状面成像，而后冠状面和横断面垂直成像，可精确计算肿瘤体积，使原发灶分期准确，还可以计算肿瘤至直肠系膜筋膜的距离。同时可采用薄层扫描（4mm 或更薄），也可调整视角从头到尾观察骶岬至肛管，从前到后观察耻骨至骶骨。

肛门直肠瘘

肛门直肠瘘

肛门直肠瘘是指直肠或肛管与会阴部皮肤的异常解剖通路，这些异常通路多是由肛管皮下的肛门腺感染后播散形成肛周脓肿，可进一步形成肛瘘。肛瘘可分为简单肛瘘和复杂肛瘘，前者只有一个简单的或原发的瘘管，后者还包含脓肿破溃形成的继发瘘管，多见于克罗恩病和复发性肛瘘（见第22章）。

1976年，Parks等将肛瘘分为4个亚型[48]：第1个亚型是括约肌间型肛瘘，瘘管只穿过肛门内括约肌，开口于会阴部皮肤，距离肛门较近；第2个亚型是经括约肌肛瘘，瘘管经肛门内外括约肌到达坐骨直肠窝；第3个亚型是括约肌上肛瘘，瘘管向上穿过肛提肌，然后向下经坐骨直肠周围脂肪，穿透皮肤；第4个亚型是括约肌外肛瘘，瘘管在较高的水平穿过肛门内外括约肌，穿过坐骨直肠周围脂肪，向下穿透会阴部皮肤，同时向上于坐骨直肠窝穿透直肠。

肛瘘术后有复发的倾向，最常见的原因是术中未能准确找到内口或瘘管分支。术前进行影像学检查，尤其是MRI有助于明确复杂肛瘘的瘘管数量、是否伴发肛周脓肿，避免术中遗漏，对反复多次手术的病例尤为适用。术前MRI检查可能影响手术方式选择，显著降低复发率，从而提高手术成功率[49-50]。

传统的肛瘘影像学检查方法是瘘管造影，但该方法并不可靠，其最大的缺点是不能显示瘘管与括约肌复合体的关系，因为后者在瘘管造影片上不能辨别，而只能推测；且如果瘘管被粪渣堵住，则不能在X线片上显影，可能造成复杂肛瘘的漏诊。

2004年，Buchanan等[50]通过肛管内超声（EAUS）、直肠指检、MRI等方法检查肛瘘，研究发现MRI的准确率为90%，EAUS和直肠指检分别为81%和61%，虽然EAUS在诊断肛瘘内口的准确率高于MRI（分别为97%和91%），但MRI诊断肛瘘整体优于EAUS，2008年Sahni等[52]通过一项系统的回顾性研究证实了这一点。

文献对于诊断肛瘘应该用体内或体外相控阵MRI是存在争议的，肛管内线圈在确诊原发的简单瘘管方面更准确，但复杂性瘘管和继发行脓肿往往因超过其检测范围而不能被检测到[54-55]，手术过程中也容易将其忽视，因此体外MRI对肛瘘的诊断治疗有显著益处。

MRI检查肛瘘的策略

与直肠MRI成像相似，肛瘘的高分辨率MRI成像也需要体外的相控阵线圈产生的高信噪比。MRI的T2加权快速自旋回波二维图像可以用于3个平面，首先进行矢状面成像，而后进行冠状面和横断面垂直成像。和人体纵轴相比，肛管略微向前倾斜，对肛管进行冠状面和横断面垂直成像至关重要，因为肛管的倾斜使得分辨其解剖结构和瘘管位置变得困难。脂肪抑制成像和快速自旋回波（FSE）T2加权像结合有利于瘘管的检测，同时视野应该从骶前间隙至会阴。有时瘘管会向上或向下延伸（有的会到达大腿的皮下组织），因此有时需增大视野。有时瘘管向上达到肛提肌水平，需对直肠进行冠状面和横断面垂直成像，从而来评估肛瘘内口与直肠的关系，如图4.11a，b中显示，经T2加权快速自旋回波MRI证实的经括约肌肛瘘和括约肌外肛瘘。

结论和展望

MRI对直肠癌和直肠肛门瘘进行初次或再次手术治疗的作用非常突出。对局部进展期的直肠癌患者，贯彻新辅助疗法前后进行MRI检查，有利于个体化治疗方案的建立，取得良好的治疗效果，减少治疗并发症。目前，人们正致力于保留器官功能的治疗策略研究，MRI能够筛选适宜治疗的及治疗反应良好的病例。随着成像技术的进步和诊断精确性的提高，局部切除小肿瘤（原发或经新辅助放化疗降阶的肿瘤），甚至对新辅助放化疗完全缓解的患者采取"等等看"策略都是安全的。

对直肠肛门瘘来说，外科治疗的目的是消灭复杂性瘘管、降低复发率，同时保留功能，专科MRI检查可以指导手术治疗。如果经检查证实为肛提肌水平以上病变，则需要选择的手术方案为修补内口和括约肌复合体，此时如选择经坐骨直肠窝引流往往是不恰当的，可能会引发医源性的括约肌外或括约肌上肛瘘，将很难治愈。

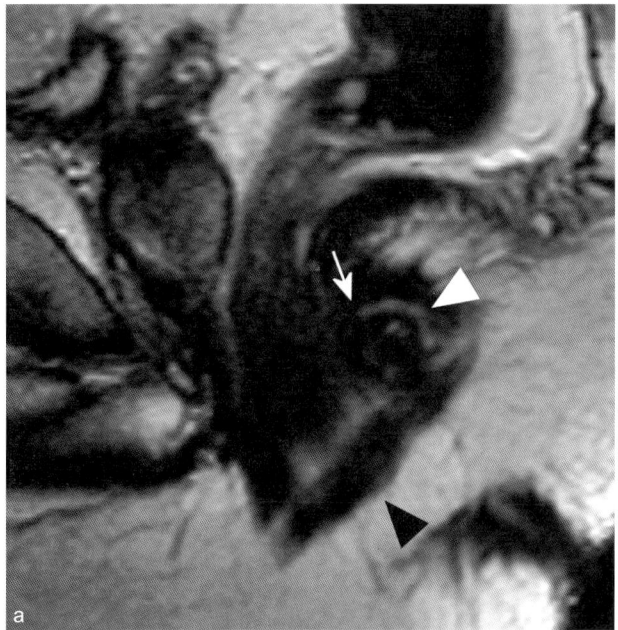
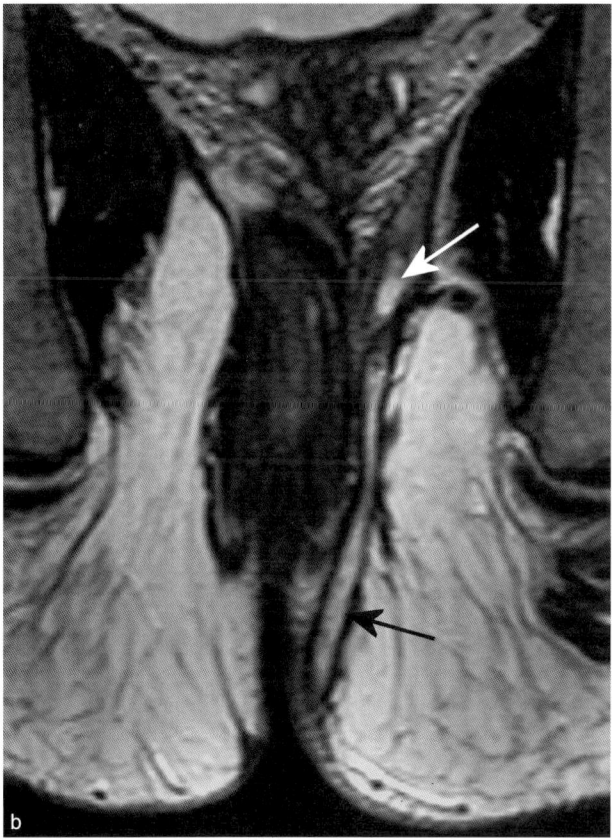

图 4.11 （a）T2 加权矢状位，快速自旋回波（TR/TE 为 3427/150ms）MRI 显示肛管（黑色箭头）后方高信号的经括约肌瘘管（白色箭头），肛门括约肌用白色箭头标记。（b）T2 加权冠状位，快速自旋回波（TR/TE 为 3427/150ms）MRI 显示高信号的括约肌外肛瘘瘘管（黑色箭头）。瘘管终止于左侧盆腔的一个脓腔（白色箭头）（Reprinted with permission from Beets-Tan et al.[56]）

参考文献

1. Lahaye MJ, Engelen SM, Nelemans PJ, Beets GL, van de Velde CJ, van Engelshoven JM, et al. Imaging for predicting the risk factors – the circumferential resection margin and nodal disease – of local recurrence in rectal cancer: a meta-analysis. Semin Ultrasound CT MR. 2005;26(4):259–68.
2. Bissett IP, Fernando CC, Hough DM, Cowan BR, Chau KY, Young AA, et al. Identification of the fascia propria by magnetic resonance imaging and its relevance to preoperative assessment of rectal cancer. Dis Colon Rectum. 2001;44:259–65.
3. Dworak O. Morphology of lymph nodes in the resected rectum of patients with rectal carcinoma. Pathol Res Pract. 1991;187:1020–4.
4. Moriya Y, Sugihara K, Akasu T, Fujita S. Importance of extended lymphadenectomy with lateral node dissection for advanced lower rectal cancer. World J Surg. 1997;21:728–32.
5. Engelen SM, Beets-Tan RG, Lahaye MJ, Kessels AG, Beets GL. Location of involved mesorectal and extramesorectal lymph nodes in patients with primary rectal cancer: preoperative assessment with MR imaging. Eur J Surg Oncol. 2008;34:776–81.
6. Church JM, Raudkivi PJ, Hill GL. The surgical anatomy of the rectum – a review with particular relevance to the hazards of rectal mobilisation. Int J Colorectal Dis. 1987;2:158–66.
7. Havenga K, DeRuiter MC, Enker WE, Welvaart K. Anatomical basis of autonomic nerve-preserving total mesorectal excision for rectal cancer. Br J Surg. 1996;83:384–8.
8. Boyle P, Ferlay J. Mortality and survival in breast and colorectal cancer. Nat Clin Pract Oncol. 2005;2:424–5.
9. Ferlay J, Autier P, Boniol M, Heanue M, Colombet M, Boyle P. Estimates of the cancer incidence and mortality in Europe in 2006. Ann Oncol. 2007;18:581–92.
10. Heald RJ, Ryall RD. Recurrence and survival after total mesorectal excision for rectal cancer. Lancet. 1986;1(8496):1479–82.
11. Nagtegaal ID, Quirke P. What is the role for the circumferential margin in the modern treatment of rectal cancer? J Clin Oncol. 2008;26:303–12.
12. Kapiteijn E, Marijnen CA, Nagtegaal ID, Putter H, Steup WH, Wiggers T, et al. Preoperative radiotherapy combined with total mesorectal excision for resectable rectal cancer. N Engl J Med. 2001;345:638–46.
13. Sebag-Montefiore D, Steele RJ, Quirke P, Grieve R, Khanna S, Monson JR. Routine short course pre-op radiotherapy or selective post-op chemoradiotherapy for resectable rectal cancer? Preliminary results of the MRC CR 07 randomized trial. J Clin Oncol. 2006;24(18S):3511.
14. Marijnen CA, Nagtegaal ID, Kapiteijn E, Kranenbarg EK, Noordijk EM, van Krieken JH, et al. Radiotherapy does not compensate for positive resection margins in rectal cancer patients: report of a multicenter randomized trial. Int J Radiat Oncol Biol Phys. 2003;55:1311–20.
15. Krook JE, Moertel CG, Gunderson LL, Wieand HS, Collins RT, Beart RW, et al. Effective surgical adjuvant therapy for high-risk rectal carcinoma. N Engl J Med. 1991;324:709–15.
16. Bosset JF, Collette L, Calais G, Mineur L, Maingon P, Radosevic-Jelic L, et al. Chemotherapy with preoperative radiotherapy in rectal cancer. N Engl J Med. 2006;355:1114–23.
17. Gerard JP, Conroy T, Bonnetain F, Bouche O, Chapet O, Closon-Dejardin MT, et al. Preoperative radiotherapy with or without concurrent fluorouracil and leucovorin in T3-4 rectal cancers: results of FFCD 9203. J Clin Oncol. 2006;24:4620–5.
18. Sauer R, Becker H, Hohenberger W, Rodel C, Wittekind C, Fietkau R, et al. Preoperative versus postoperative chemoradiotherapy for rectal cancer. N Engl J Med. 2004;351:1731–40.
19. Brown G, Richards CJ, Newcombe RG, Dallimore NS, Radcliffe AG, Carey DP, et al. Rectal carcinoma: thin-section MR imaging for staging in 28 patients. Radiology. 1999;211:215–22.

20. Blomqvist L, Machado M, Rubio C, Gabrielsson N, Granqvist S, Goldman S, et al. Rectal tumour staging: MR imaging using pelvic phased-array and endorectal coils vs endoscopic ultrasonography. Eur Radiol. 2000;10:653–60.
21. Beets-Tan RG, Beets GL, Vliegen RF, Kessels AG, Van Boven H, De Bruine A, et al. Accuracy of magnetic resonance imaging in prediction of tumour-free resection margin in rectal cancer surgery. Lancet. 2001;357(9255):497–504.
22. Beets-Tan RG, Beets GL. Rectal cancer: how accurate can imaging predict the T stage and the circumferential resection margin? Int J Colorectal Dis. 2003;18:385–91.
23. Peschaud F, Cuenod CA, Benoist S, Julie C, Beauchet A, Siauve N, et al. Accuracy of magnetic resonance imaging in rectal cancer depends on location of the tumor. Dis Colon Rectum. 2005;48:1603–9.
24. Salerno G, Daniels IR, Moran BJ, Wotherspoon A, Brown G. Clarifying margins in the multidisciplinary management of rectal cancer: the MERCURY experience. Clin Radiol. 2006;61:916–23.
25. Wang C, Zhou Z, Wang Z, Zheng Y, Zhao G, Yu Y, et al. Patterns of neoplastic foci and lymph node micrometastasis within the mesorectum. Langenbecks Arch Chir. 2005;39:312–8.
26. Will O, Purkayastha S, Chan C, Athanasiou T, Darzi AW, Gedroyc W, et al. Diagnostic precision of nanoparticle-enhanced MRI for lymph-node metastases: a meta-analysis. Lancet Oncol. 2006;7:52–60.
27. Engelen SM, Lahaye MJ, Beets-Tan RG, Jansen RL, Lammering G, De Bruine AP, et al. Tailored treatment of primary rectal cancer based on MRI: does it reduce the number of incomplete resections? Ann Oncol. 2008;19 Suppl 1:i17–8.
28. O'Neill BD, Brown G, Heald RJ, Cunningham D, Tait DM. Non-operative treatment after neoadjuvant chemoradiotherapy for rectal cancer. Lancet Oncol. 2007;8:625–33.
29. Habr-Gama A, Perez RO, Proscurshim I, Campos FG, Nadalin W, Kiss D, et al. Patterns of failure and survival for nonoperative treatment of stage c0 distal rectal cancer following neoadjuvant chemoradiation therapy. J Gastrointest Surg. 2006;10:1319–29.
30. Lezoche G, Baldarelli M, Guerrieri M, Paganini AM, De Sanctis A, Bartolacci S, et al. A prospective randomized study with a 5-year minimum follow-up evaluation of transanal endoscopic microsurgery versus laparoscopic total mesorectal excision after neoadjuvant therapy. Surg Endosc. 2008;22:352–8.
31. Maas M, Nelemans PJ, Valentini V, Das P, Rodel C, Kuo LJ, et al. Long-term outcome in patients with a pathological complete response after chemoradiation for rectal cancer: a pooled analysis of individual patient data. Lancet Oncol. 2010;11:835–44.
32. Beets-Tan RG, Beets GL. Rectal cancer: review with emphasis on MR imaging. Radiology. 2004;232:335–46.
33. Dresen RC, Beets GL, Rutten HJ, Engelen SM, Lahaye MJ, Vliegen RF. Locally advanced rectal cancer: MR imaging for restaging after neoadjuvant radiation therapy with concomitant chemotherapy. Part I. Are we able to predict tumor confined to the rectal wall? Radiology. 2009;252:71–80.
34. Bipat S, Glas AS, Slors FJ, Zwinderman AH, Bossuyt PM, Stoker J. Rectal cancer: local staging and assessment of lymph node involvement with endoluminal US, CT, and MR imaging – a meta-analysis. Radiology. 2004;232:773–83.
35. MERCURY Study Group. Extramural depth of tumor invasion at thin-section MR in patients with rectal cancer: results of the MERCURY study. Radiology. 2007;243:132–9.
36. Brown G, Richards CJ, Bourne MW, Newcombe RG, Radcliffe AG, Dallimore NS, et al. Morphologic predictors of lymph node status in rectal cancer with use of high-spatial-resolution MR imaging with histopathologic comparison. Radiology. 2003;227:371–7.
37. Kim JH, Beets GL, Kim MJ, Kessels AG, Beets-Tan RG. High-resolution MR imaging for nodal staging in rectal cancer: are there any criteria in addition to the size? Eur J Radiol. 2004;52:78–83.
38. Lahaye MJ, Engelen SM, Kessels AG, de Bruine AP, von Meyenfeldt MF, van Engelshoven JM, et al. USPIO-enhanced MR imaging for nodal staging in patients with primary rectal cancer: predictive criteria. Radiology. 2008;246:804–11.
39. Chen CC, Lee RC, Lin JK, Wang LW, Yang SH. How accurate is magnetic resonance imaging in restaging rectal cancer in patients receiving preoperative combined chemoradiotherapy? Dis Colon Rectum. 2005;48:722–8.
40. Kuo LJ, Chern MC, Tsou MH, Liu MC, Jian JJ, Chen CM, et al. Interpretation of magnetic resonance imaging for locally advanced rectal carcinoma after preoperative chemoradiation therapy. Dis Colon Rectum. 2005;48:23–8.
41. Allen SD, Padhani AR, Dzik-Jurasz AS, Glynne-Jones R. Rectal carcinoma: MRI with histologic correlation before and after chemoradiation therapy. AJR Am J Roentgenol. 2007;188:442–51.
42. Engelen SM, Beets-Tan RG, Lahaye MJ, Lammering G, Jansen RL, van Dam RM, et al. MRI after chemoradiotherapy of rectal cancer: a useful tool to select patients for local excision. Dis Colon Rectum. 2010;53:979–86.
43. Lahaye MJ, Beets GL, Engelen SM, Kessels AG, de Bruine AP, Kwee HW. Locally advanced rectal cancer: MR imaging for restaging after neoadjuvant radiation therapy with concomitant chemotherapy. Part II. What are the criteria to predict involved lymph nodes? Radiology. 2009;252:81–91.
44. Mercury Study Group. Diagnostic accuracy of preoperative magnetic resonance imaging in predicting curative resection of rectal cancer: prospective observational study. BMJ. 2006;333(7572):779.
45. Vliegen RF, Beets GL, Lammering G, Dresen RC, Rutten HJ, Kessels AG, et al. Mesorectal fascia invasion after neoadjuvant chemotherapy and radiation therapy for locally advanced rectal cancer: accuracy of MR imaging for prediction. Radiology. 2008;246:454–62.
46. Kulkarni T, Gollins S, Maw A, Hobson P, Byrne R, Widdowson D. Magnetic resonance imaging in rectal cancer downstaged using neoadjuvant chemoradiation: accuracy of prediction of tumour stage and circumferential resection margin status. Colorectal Dis. 2008;10:479–89.
47. Vliegen RF, Beets GL, von Meyenfeldt MF, Kessels AG, Lemaire EE, van Engelshoven JM, et al. Rectal cancer: MR imaging in local staging – is gadolinium-based contrast material helpful? Radiology. 2005;234:179–88.
48. Parks AG, Gordon PH, Hardcastle JD. A classification of fistula-in-ano. Br J Surg. 1976;63:1–12.
49. Beets-Tan RG, Beets GL, van der Hoop AG, Kessels AG, Vliegen RF, Baeten CG, et al. Preoperative MR imaging of anal fistulas: does it really help the surgeon? Radiology. 2001;218:75–84.
50. Buchanan GN, Halligan S, Bartram CI, Williams AB, Tarroni D, Cohen CR. Clinical examination, endosonography, and MR imaging in preoperative assessment of fistula in ano: comparison with outcome-based reference standard. Radiology. 2004;233:674–81.
51. Kuijpers HC, Schulpen T. Fistulography for fistula-in-ano. Is it useful? Dis Colon Rectum. 1985;28:103–4.
52. Sahni VA, Ahmad R, Burling D. Which method is best for imaging of perianal fistula? Abdom Imaging. 2008;33:26–30.
53. de Souza NM, Gilderdale DJ, Coutts GA, Puni R, Steiner RE. MRI of fistula-in-ano: a comparison of endoanal coil with external phased array coil techniques. J Comput Assist Tomogr. 1998;22:357–63.
54. Stoker J, Hussain SM, van Kempen D, Elevelt AJ, Lameris JS. Endoanal coil in MR imaging of anal fistulas. AJR Am J Roentgenol. 1996;166:360–2.
55. Halligan S, Bartram CI. MR imaging of fistula in ano: are endoanal coils the gold standard? AJR Am J Roentgenol. 1998;171:407–12.
56. Beets-Tan RG, Beets GL, van der Hoop AG, Kessels AG, Vliegen RF, Baeten CG, van Engelshoven JM. Preoperative magnetic resonance imaging of anal fistulas: does it really help the surgeon? Radiology. 2001;218(1):75–84.

第 5 章　结肠直肠再手术前内镜评估

Kok Sun Ho · Francis Seow-Choen
汪志明 译　李 宁 审校

摘 要

本章界定了内镜检查在再次手术患者术前评估中的作用与其他影像检查互补，为再次手术的患者提供了新的评估方法，特别是评估癌肿复发和明确肠道吻合后出现的问题，并将其创新性应用于炎症性肠病的诊治。内镜检查可以直接观察肠腔黏膜，并行活组织检查，可助于肿瘤复发的诊断，并对不典型增生性病变作出评估、说明及外科决策。本章概述了内镜在这些复杂患者中的应用，为需要再次手术或结直肠重建的患者提供决策的依据，并为再手术的高风险的患者放置结肠支架提供帮助。

关键词

内镜评价；结肠镜；结直肠再手术；吻合口漏；肿瘤；贮袋炎；吻合口狭窄

引 言

外部影像技术可帮助外科医生比较准确地了解腹部情况，评估患者再手术的风险。尽管目前的 CT、MRI 及结肠成像等技术已比较完善，但结肠镜检查可以直观地显示肠腔黏膜表面，仍然是患者再手术前评估的重要内容。内镜能直接观察病变及正常结肠和小肠的腔内结构，并且可以行组织学检查。在某些情况下还能做一些治疗，能减少患者行困难且危险的再手术的机会。

内镜在术后早期的作用

出 血

吻合口出血及吻合口瘘是结直肠术后的两个潜在并发症。吻合口出血的发生率为 0.5%～4%[1-4]。有研究在术后常规行肠镜检查，发现术后吻合口出血的发生率为 5%～10%[5-6]。这些报道的差异可能是因为这些内镜检查出的出血大部分能自发停止，并不引起临床症状（图 5.1）。

在直肠术后发现严重出血，外科医生可以选择内镜治疗或者再次手术。有医生担心术后立即行内镜检查有吻合口裂开的风险，但迄今为止并尚无此类报道[2,4]。有研究者常规或者选择性在术中通过内镜检查吻合口，并不增加并发症发生率[5-6]。在采用内镜治疗吻合口出血的研究中，也无发生吻合口瘘的报道[1,2,4,7]。

内镜下止血方法包括黏膜下注射肾上腺素、电凝止血和钛夹止血等[2,4,7]。止血的成功率可达 80%[1-2]；内镜止血不成功可再行手术治疗。若出血位置不在吻合口，内镜检查还能对病灶进行定位，为手术做好准备。

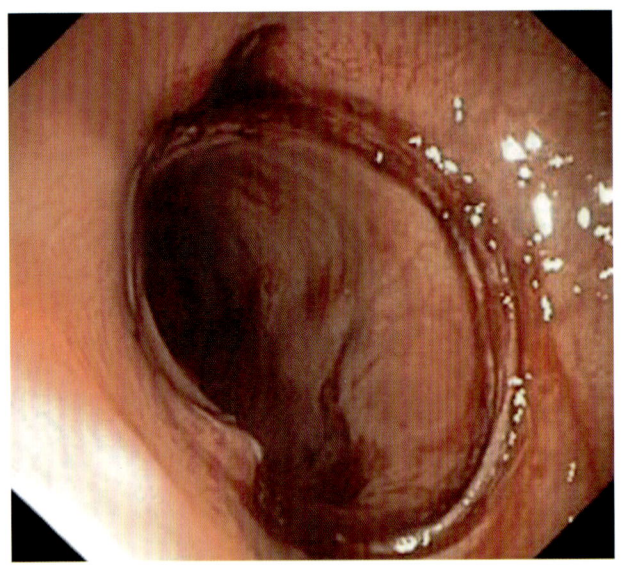

图 5.1　手术中的吻合口视图

吻合口瘘

临床上显著的结直肠或结肠肛管吻合口瘘的发生率为 0.1%~9%，临床或放射学检查发现瘘的发生率为 0.4%~19.2%[8-13]，主要治疗方法包括保守治疗、经皮穿刺引流及结肠改道（保留或者拆除吻合口）等。行手术切除吻合口的患者，常常不考虑肠吻合恢复肠道连续性[12]。当吻合口瘘的患者出现脓毒症时，因担心吻合口开裂或者感染扩散，外科医生很少会考虑内镜治疗。

许多内镜治疗方法已被用于治疗吻合口瘘。在内镜下经肛门行负压辅助直肠引流（endosponge，内吸海绵），是治疗腹膜外的直肠吻合口瘘的一种新方法。对于低位直肠切除术后瘘的患者，这种方法可以避免手术，达到骶骨前的引流的效果，成功率达到 88%[14-17]。这种方法吻合口愈合相当慢，但可能有效，泄漏之后保留了部分功能，需要多次更换海绵（有或者没有内镜辅助）。该技术也被应用于放射治疗相关性瘘道的治疗[18]。内吸海棉的问题将在第 49 章中详述。经肛显微外科手术甚至钛夹修补吻合口的方法也有报道[19]。使用覆膜支架封堵缺损、促进愈合可能是将来的发展方向[20]。

在术前或术中都可行内镜检查，既可以评估黏膜的活力，也可以确定病变的位置及范围。但在术中检查时往往并不很直观，尤其是吻合口位于在盆腔深部时。吻合口表面可能被炎性物质或者感染组织覆盖，较难辨认。内镜检查可以帮助决定是拆除吻合口还是加强缝合。内镜还可以评价近端肠管的粪便量，决定是否需要术中行肠道清理。

结直肠术后晚期并发症的内镜干预

需要再次手术的常见问题包括肿瘤复发、贮袋炎、吻合口狭窄和结肠瘘等。

肿瘤复发

单纯使用内镜检查肿瘤复发有其局限性，因为大部分肿瘤复发在腔外。即使没有肿瘤复发迹象，内镜对于异时性病变的检测仍很重要。PET/CT 可以检查肿瘤是否广泛复发。肿瘤切除术后常有局部复发，通常复发从腔外开始，表现为转移小结节、区域淋巴结或盆腔壁受累，肿瘤最后才侵犯到肠腔内部。如果内镜发现吻合口未受侵犯，说明复发只是广泛转移的一个局部表现（图 5.2）。先前的吻合口瘘是吻合口复发的一个危险因素[11, 21, 22]。内镜检查和活检要同时进行，并综合其他影像资料来判断肿瘤是否侵及到腔内。

有时肿瘤复发从吻合口开始，这可能是经肛手术或者经肛内镜显微手术操作过程中的种植转移，这种转移常见于 T2 期黏膜层肿瘤或低分化肿瘤[23]。这些事件促使许多结直肠专家在吻合前用直肠灌洗来杀死肿瘤细胞[23]。孤立的腔内吻合口转移预后好于腔外转移。腔内转移不伴腔外病灶的病例是再次

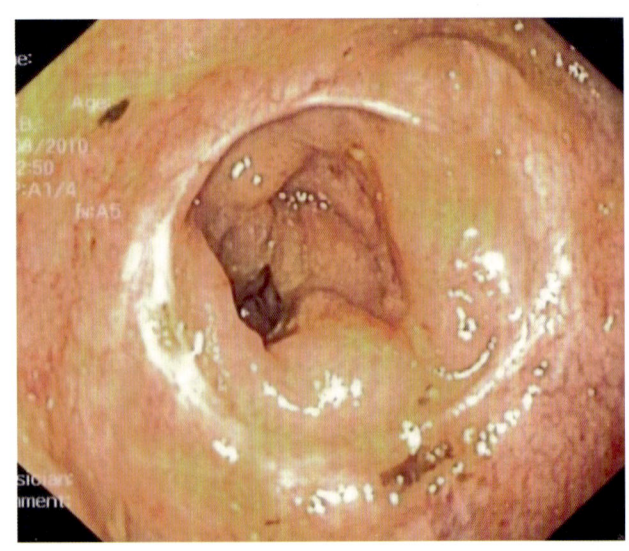

图 5.2　肠腔外的复发导致先前结肠吻合口上方肠腔狭窄

行根治性手术的指征。有时复发肿瘤邻近吻合口，但不在吻合口。这些病例结合其他影像检查，未见其他转移，提示为异时癌。这时肠镜检查意义重大，有助于确定最适当的手术方式和手术范围。

回肠贮袋炎

内镜是目前可用于评估贮袋结构异常的工具之一，可以发现贮袋入口或出口狭窄、贮袋瘘、窦道和瘘口。结合 CT 小肠造影、胃加芬液®（显影剂产品—Gastrografin®）灌肠、MRI 等影像学检查，可提高内镜检查的准确性[25]。如果 J 形贮袋盲端渗漏，则需要超声或 CT 引导下置管引流。一些患者需要反复的影像学检查，这些患者选择 MRI 可以减少辐射的次数。CT 小肠造影对于小肠狭窄或贮袋入口狭窄诊断的准确性低，而 MRI 对于贮袋窦道诊断的准确性差，结合内镜的检查，可以增加这些诊断的准确性。内镜检查的优越性还体现在可以行组织学检查，一例之前诊断为溃疡性结肠炎的患者通过组织学检查可能会被确诊为克罗恩病，家族性息肉病患者术后通过肠镜活检可能会发现黏膜组织发育不良。内镜可以监测贮袋黏膜的变化，为贮袋炎分级并指导治疗；在此过程中还能帮助决策是否需要切除贮袋。

吻合口狭窄

结直肠术后的吻合口狭窄发生率为 30%[26-28]，内镜可以直视观察狭窄的位置、性质、长度及狭窄程度，并取活检。放射或内镜检查偶尔可以发现无症状的狭窄，这些狭窄并不需要干预。术后早期的狭窄有可能随着时间的推移而扩张。有症状的狭窄，根据患者症状及病因需要进一步的评估及处理，必要时可行经内镜球囊扩张术，成功率可达 90%~100%（图 5.3、图 5.4、图 5.5）[27, 29, 30]。上述治疗无效的患者还可以使用伞状自膨式金属支架。最近，Forshaw[31] 等报道了一组重度吻合口狭窄的患者经内镜行狭窄切除术，该组患者住院时间短，少数患者因出血、微穿孔等并发症需要再手术，如果吻合口处的肠管角度大则操作困难。也有一些报道介绍内镜电切技术，使用乳头切开刀、钩刀并联合使用荧光内镜来辨认近端肠管，特别是初始采用端侧吻合者[32-35]，但有些技术发生再狭窄的概率较高[32]。

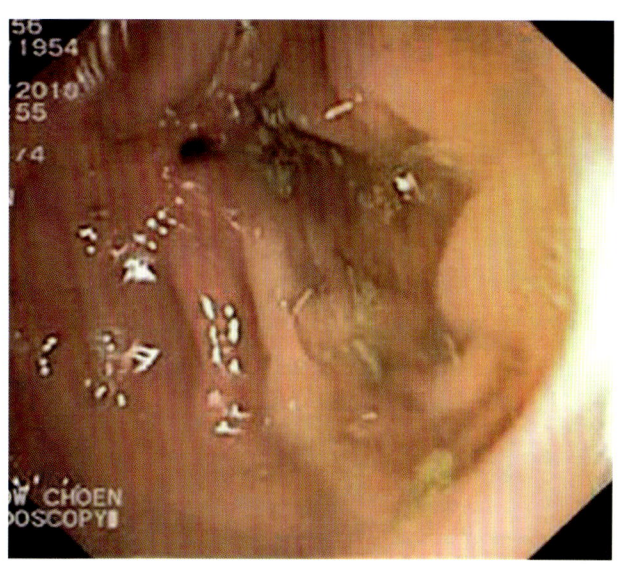

图 5.3　结肠镜检查的狭窄图像

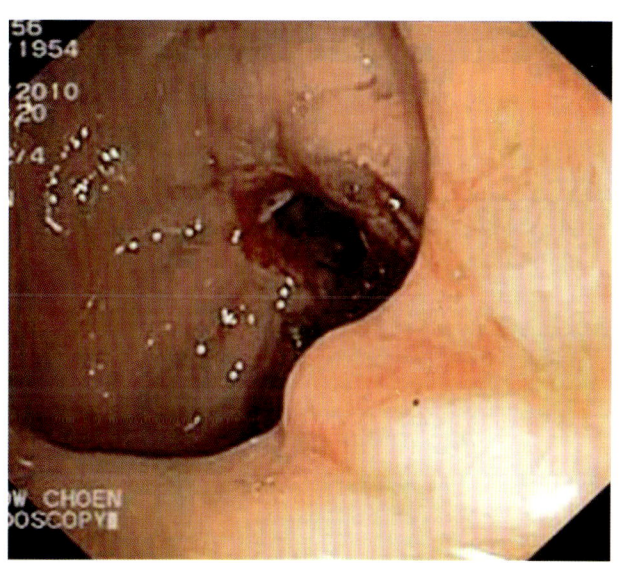

图 5.4　内镜尝试通过后的狭窄图像

其他治疗方法包括内镜下注射激素治疗克罗恩病的狭窄，单次注射并不减少扩张的次数，大多数病例至少需要注射 2 次以上[36]。最近已有可降解生物支架临床应用的报道，但是支架使用前扩张的次数与狭窄症状复发之间的关系并不明确[29, 37, 38]。扩张后的患者常有一些症状，如肠蠕动加快、腹胀、腹痛、便秘或腹泻，同时伴有与健康相关的生活质量的下降，这种生活质量的下降在一定程度上与狭窄扩张后内镜评估时间的推迟无关[39]。这可能与放射和内镜方法定义的狭窄严重程度和长度，以及与患者的临床症状并不一致有关。

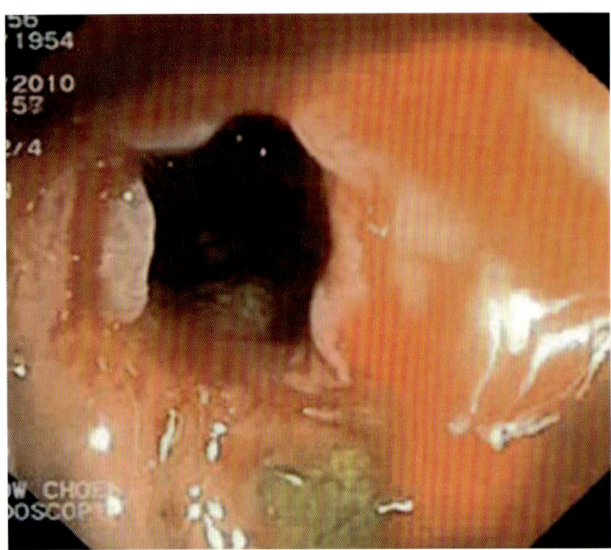

图 5.5　内镜扩张后的狭窄图像

重复扩张与支架置入术受首次扩张的时间（尤其是术后 4 个月内）因素的影响，男性患者发生狭窄的概率更高，尽管这些研究并没有区分患者是否接受放射治疗及疾病的良恶性。另外，扩张后临床症状的改善率要高于手术成功率，一些早期的狭窄患者并没有症状[40-41]。

结　论

内镜的引入对低位直肠吻合口瘘的治疗有重要影响，部分患者可能通过保守治疗治愈，而不需要手术干预。对吻合口狭窄的内镜治疗包括电切术、病灶内注射激素（适用于克罗恩病患者）、支架（可同时进行扩张），手术成功率较高，但是许多患者需要多次扩张，生活质量会有所下降。

参考文献

1. Cirocco WC, Golub RW. Endoscopic treatment of postoperative hemorrhage from a stapled colorectal anastomosis. Am Surg. 1995;61:460–3.
2. Malik AH, East JE, Buchanan GN, Kennedy RH. Endoscopic haemostasis of staple-line haemorrhage following colorectal resection. Colorectal Dis. 2008;10:616–8.
3. Linn TY, Moran BJ, Cecil TD. Staple line haemorrhage following laparoscopic left-sided colorectal resections may be more common when the inferior mesenteric artery is preserved. Tech Coloproctol. 2008;12:289–93.
4. Martínez-Serrano MA, Parés D, Pera M, Pascual M, Courtier R, Egea MJ, et al. Management of lower gastrointestinal bleeding after colorectal resection and stapled anastomosis. Tech Coloproctol. 2009;13:49–53.
5. Ishihara S, Watanabe T, Nagawa H. Intraoperative colonoscopy for stapled anastomosis in colorectal surgery. Surg Today. 2008;38:1063–5.
6. Li VK, Wexner SD, Pulido N, Wang H, Jin HY, Weiss EG, et al. Use of routine intraoperative endoscopy in elective laparoscopic colorectal surgery: can it further avoid anastomotic failure? Surg Endosc. 2009;23:2459–65.
7. Perez RO, Sousa Jr A, Bresciani C, Proscurshim I, Coser R, Kiss D, et al. Endoscopic management of postoperative stapled colorectal anastomosis hemorrhage. Tech Coloproctol. 2007;1:64–6.
8. Eriksen MT, Wibe A, Norstein J, Haffner J, Wiig JN, Norwegian Rectal Cancer Group. Anastomotic leakage following routine mesorectal excision for rectal cancer in a national cohort of patients. Colorectal Dis. 2005;7:51–7.
9. Lim M, Akhtar S, Sasapu K, Harris K, Burke D, Sagar P, et al. Clinical and subclinical leaks after low colorectal anastomosis: a clinical and radiologic study. Dis Colon Rectum. 2006;49:1611–9.
10. Matthiessen P, Hallböök O, Rutegård J, Simert G, Sjödahl R. Defunctioning stoma reduces symptomatic anastomotic leakage after low anterior resection of the rectum for cancer: a randomized multicenter trial. Ann Surg. 2007;246:207–14.
11. Law WL, Choi HK, Lee YM, Ho JW, Seto CL. Anastomotic leakage is associated with poor long-term outcome in patients after curative colorectal resection for malignancy. J Gastrointest Surg. 2007;11:8–15.
12. Khan AA, Wheeler JM, Cunningham C, George B, Kettlewell M, Mortensen NJ. The management and outcome of anastomotic leaks in colorectal surgery. Colorectal Dis. 2008;10:587–92.
13. Fernández-Cebrián JM, Gil P, Hernández-Granados P, Fiuza C, Ochando F, Loinaz C, et al. Initial surgical experience in laparoscopic total mesorectal excision for middle and lower third rectal cancer: short-term results. Clin Transl Oncol. 2009;11:460–4.
14. Weidenhagen R, Gruetzner KU, Wiecken T, Spelsberg F, Jauch KW. Endoscopic vacuum-assisted closure of anastomotic leakage following anterior resection of the rectum: a new method. Surg Endosc. 2008;22:1818–25.
15. Glitsch A, von Bernstorff W, Seltrecht U, Partecke I, Paul H, Heidecke CD. Endoscopic transanal vacuum-assisted rectal drainage (ETVARD): an optimized therapy for major leaks from extraperitoneal rectal anastomoses. Endoscopy. 2008;40(3):192–9. Epub 2008 Jan.
16. Bemelman WA. Vacuum assisted closure in coloproctology. Tech Coloproctol. 2009;13:261–3.
17. Arezzo A, Miegge A, Garbarini A, Morino M. Endoluminal vacuum therapy for anastomotic leaks after rectal surgery. Tech Coloproctol. 2010;14:279–81.
18. von Bernstorff W, Glitsch A, Schreiber A, Partecke LI, Heidecke CD. ETVARD (endoscopic transanal vacuum-assisted rectal drainage) leads to complete but delayed closure of extraperitoneal rectal anastomotic leakage cavities following neoadjuvant radiochemotherapy. Int J Colorectal Dis. 2009;24:819–25.
19. Beunis A, Pauli S, Van Cleemput M. Anastomotic leakage of a colorectal anastomosis treated by transanal endoscopic microsurgery. Acta Chir Belg. 2008;108:474–6.
20. Tsereteli Z, Sporn E, Geiger TM, Cleveland D, Frazier S, Rawlings A, et al. Placement of a covered polyester stent prevents complications from a colorectal anastomotic leak and supports healing: randomized controlled trial in a large animal model. Surgery. 2008;144:786–92.
21. Chang SC, Lin JK, Yang SH, Jiang JK, Chen WC, Lin TC. Long-term outcome of anastomosis leakage after curative resection for mid and low rectal cancer. Hepatogastroenterology. 2003;50:1898–902.
22. Ptok H, Marusch F, Meyer F, Schubert D, Gastinger I, Lippert H, Study Group Colon/Rectum Carcinoma (Primary Tumour). Impact of anastomotic leakage on oncological outcome after rectal cancer resection. Br J Surg. 2007;94:1548–54.
23. Ganai S, Kanumuri P, Rao RS, Alexander AI. Local recurrence after transanal endoscopic microsurgery for rectal polyps and early

cancers. Ann Surg Oncol. 2006;13:547–56.
24. Kodeda K, Holmberg E, Jörgren F, Nordgren S, Lindmark G. Rectal washout and local recurrence of cancer after anterior resection. Br J Surg. 2010;97:1589–97.
25. Tang L, Cai H, Moore L, Shen B. Evaluation of endoscopic and imaging modalities in the diagnosis of structural disorders of the ileal pouch. Inflamm Bowel Dis. 2010;16(9):1526–31.
26. De Lusong MA, Shah JN, Soetikno R, Binmoeller KF. Treatment of a completely obstructed colonic anastomotic stricture by using a prototype forward-array echoendoscope and facilitated by SpyGlass (with videos). Gastrointest Endosc. 2008;68:988–92.
27. Ambrosetti P, Francis K, De Peyer R, Frossard JL. Colorectal anastomotic stenosis after elective laparoscopic sigmoidectomy for diverticular disease: a prospective evaluation of 68 patients. Dis Colon Rectum. 2008;51:1345–9.
28. McKee R, Pricolo VE. Stapled revision of complete colorectal anastomotic obstruction. Am J Surg. 2008;195:526–7.
29. Araujo SE, Costa AF. Efficacy and safety of endoscopic balloon dilation of benign anastomotic strictures after oncologic anterior rectal resection: report on 24 cases. Surg Laparosc Endosc Percutan Tech. 2008;18:565–8.
30. Geiger TM, Miedema BW, Tsereteli Z, Sporn E, Thaler K. Stent placement for benign colonic stenosis: case report, review of the literature, and animal pilot data. Int J Colorectal Dis. 2008;23:1007–12.
31. Forshaw MJ, Maphosa G, Sankararajah D, Parker MC, Stewart M. Endoscopic alternatives in managing anastomotic strictures of the colon and rectum. Tech Coloproctol. 2006;10:21–7.
32. Shimada S, Yagi Y, Yamamoto K, Matsuda M, Baba H. Novel treatment of intractable rectal strictures associated with anastomotic leakage using a stenosis-cutting device. Int Surg. 2007;92:82–8.
33. Mukai M, Kishima K, Iizuka S, Fukumitsu H, Fukaswa M, Yazawa N, et al. Endoscopic hook knife cutting before balloon dilatation of a severe anastomotic stricture after rectal cancer resection. Endoscopy. 2009;41 Suppl 2:E193–4.
34. Morris ML, Tucker RD, Baron TH, Song LM. Electrosurgery in gastrointestinal endoscopy: principles to practice. Am J Gastroenterol. 2009;104:1563–74.
35. Curcio G, Spada M, di Francesco F, Tarantino I, Berrsi L, Burgio G, et al. Completely obstructed colorectal anastomosis: a new non-electrosurgical endoscopic approach before balloon dilatation. World J Gastroenterol. 2010;16:4751–4.
36. East JE, Brooker JC, Rutter MD, Saunders BP. A pilot study of intrastricture steroid versus placebo injection after balloon dilatation of Crohn's strictures. Clin Gastroenterol Hepatol. 2007;5:1065–9.
37. Lykke J, Meisner S. Treatment of benign postoperative anastomotic strictures of the colon and rectum with self-expanding coated plastic stents. Ugeskr Laeger. 2008;170:1255.
38. Janík V, Horák L, Hnaní ek J, Málek J, Laasch HU. Biodegradable polydioxanone stents: a new option for therapy-resistant anastomotic strictures of the colon. Eur Radiol. 2011;21(9):1956–61.
39. Nguyen-Tang T, Huber O, Gervaz P, Dumonceau JM. Long-term quality of life after endoscopic dilation of strictured colorectal or colocolonic anastomoses. Surg Endosc. 2008;22:1660–6.
40. Dai Y, Chopra SS, Wysocki WM, Hünerbein M. Treatment of benign colorectal strictures by temporary stenting with self-expanding stents. Int J Colorectal Dis. 2010;25(12):1475–9.
41. Keränen I, Lepistö A, Udd M, Halttunen J, Kylänpää L. Outcome of patients after endoluminal stent placement for benign colorectal obstruction. Scand J Gastroenterol. 2010;45:725–31.

第 6 章 直肠肛门疾病再次手术的压力测定、直肠肛管抑制反射和顺应性评估

Luigi Brusciano · C. Di Stazio · F. Lucido · A.Del Genio

刘建磊 译 姜 军 审校

本章主要介绍传统的直肠肛管功能评估方法：直肠肛管测压、直肠感觉和顺应性、矢量容积测压和神经电生理学方法，尤其是在再次手术或重建病例中的应用。同时 Andrew P.Zbar 还对各种检测方法在直肠肛门疾病中应用的优缺点进行详细解读。

摘 要

近年来，对再手术患者进行直肠肛管生理功能的评估逐渐减少，这是因为术前的测压结果与术后功能并无直接关联。本章主要介绍直肠肛管测压、矢量容积测压和直肠肛管抑制反射的检测、意义及其应用的局限性。直肠重建后新直肠顺应性评估的方法包括阻抗容积描记法、听觉反射法和恒压评估法。对这些检测方法应充分了解、合理应用，尤其是进行肠管贮袋 – 肛管重建的患者，部分患者术后功能恢复差，且可能伴发吻合口瘘、腹腔感染。大便失禁患者已经不用传统的肌电图检测，术中神经生理评估逐渐恢复活力，随着骶神经调节技术的引入，通过短期的神经刺激治疗后，筛选出适宜进行永久性神经刺激器植入的病例。本章和下一章主要介绍测压法和神经生理学对于适宜进行重建手术的病例的临床应用，以及其内在的生理局限性。

关键词

直肠肛管测压法；直肠肛管抑制反射；直肠感觉；顺应性；矢量容积测压法；神经生理学检测；再手术；重建

引 言

直肠肛管测压是一种客观的检测方法，可以评估直肠肛管肌肉的控便能力和感觉功能，是直肠肛管病理生理学功能评估的手段之一，是检查肛管括约肌完整性的辅助方法。但测压结果和临床症状的关联性较差，因此对初次手术的直肠肛管疾病患者进行生理学（直肠肛管测压）评估是有争议的，鉴于其影响治疗方案制订的讨论，用其对再次手术者进行评估可能引发更多争议。

部分患者存在显著的盆底形态学异常，但功能性检测结果变化不显著，此时外科手术纠正形态学异常往往不能达到预期效果。伴有直肠前突的便秘患者，测压结果往往表现为直肠感觉异常、耻骨直肠肌痉挛或直肠肛管抑制反射（RAIR）的改变，对于此类患者，外科手术虽然能够改善直肠排便，如未能改善伴随的功能学异常，往往认为手术方案是不合理的。同样，对括约肌损伤的大便失禁患者，可以进行括约肌完整性修复的手术，如果术后患者仍存在显著的功能学异常，如无法自主收缩肛门外

括约肌，那么认为该手术方式存在缺陷。可以通过传统的测压法对排便协同异常进行评估，如用力收缩肛门时伴随臀肌或腹肌异常收缩，对这类患者行括约肌成形术后需进行生物反馈辅助治疗。

因此，Rao 等[1]对排便异常患者进行直肠肛管功能的系统性检测，评估其对治疗效果的影响，研究显示直肠肛管功能评估在 88% 的患者中显示异常信息，经治疗后 76% 有改善。直肠肛管测压检查不但可以提供客观的诊断，还可很好地了解潜在的病理生理异常，为功能性缺陷患者进行外科重建手术提供依据；此外，压力测定结果可能影响排便异常患者的治疗方案及效果。我们认为对直肠肛管功能的评估不能代替详细的体格检查（包括临床的直肠肛管生理检测），肛管测压可在术前为部分病例提供重要信息，决定治疗方案，甚至预测术后效果。

技术细节

虽然目前有许多测压的检测方法[2]，除了检测体位，没有形成统一的检测方法。由于没有任何一种方法能被广泛接受，比较不同研究中心的测压数据存在困难，因此我们建议每个医疗中心建立自己的正常参考值。

测压有几种方法，但基本原则是应用压力传感器来记录远端直肠和肛管的压力，目前有水囊或气囊、袖状导管、压力传感器和水灌注导管等几种方法。

微气囊装置的导管上绑有一个乳胶气囊，形成两个独立的腔室，每个气囊腔室通过塑料导管与压力感受器相连，同时直肠内置入另外一个气囊。测压装置置于直肠内，使内部气囊被肛门内括约肌（IAS）环绕，外部气囊被肛门外括约肌（EAS）的皮下部环绕[3]。理论上这种装置可以分别感受 IAS 和 EAS 的压力，但由于 IAS 和 EAS 两者有较多的重叠部分而无法完全区别开。微气囊装置不能反映辐射状压力变化，只能反映平均压，并且球囊本身会影响平均压力的准确性。

水灌注系统是目前应用最广泛的装置，由多根塑料导管组成，通过微量灌注系统注入蒸馏水，我们也是应用此系统[4]。该系统的原理是通过导管内持续注入的水流感受该处括约肌的压力，注水速率必须恒定 [通常为 0.3ml/（通道·分钟）]，高速率注水会导致直肠内液体积聚，影响试验的可重复性，低速率注水往往不能迅速反映腔内压力的变化。随着注水量的增加，达到最大容积，液体会进入直肠壶腹或经肛门漏出，当直肠内间隙充满液体后，为克服最初的抵抗而需要的压力称为极限压[5]。随着肛管内压力增高，黏膜层与导管的测孔接触，阻止水流，极限压也就成为克服黏膜阻力的压力，可通过压力传感器转变为电信号。

水灌注导管的最大优点是同一测压导管上有多个注水通道（通常 4~8 个），根据研究目的的不同，导管上的通道可以呈辐射状排列（静息时测量）或阶梯式螺旋状排列（肛管平均压力）。不同肛肠中心的检测方法也不同，测压导管可固定在一个位置（静息技术）、间断退出导管（静息 - 拖出技术）或连续退出导管（连续手动 / 自动拖出技术）。手动拖出技术在每个位置测压之前先稳定一段时间，可以获得更精确的数据，牵拉技术可以提供肛管的纵行压力分布，因肛管的不同位置压力变化较大，所以牵拉技术很重要。

导管持续牵拉会刺激括约肌，引起假性张力变化，如果通过自动牵拉装置牵拉充分润滑的导管，假性张力变化会降至最小。间断牵拉技术可以提供可靠的肛管静息压，而持续牵拉技术可恰当地评估肛管压力分布及功能性括约肌长度。

评论：传统的直肠肛管测压与移动式直肠肛管测压
Andrew P. Zbar

大多数结直肠医院的肛肠研究所都有直肠肛管测压（ARM）这一项目，可为研究括约肌提供客观的方法，但由于患者的症状与测压结果之间关系不密切，因此其在临床应用是有争议的[1-2]。通过直肠指检来评估肛管静息压和最大收缩压的敏感性、特异性和预测价值不足[3]，而压力测定具有可重复性及客观性，可进行括约肌损伤风险评估，并可前瞻性预测某些治疗措施的治疗效果，如括约肌修补、骶神经刺激等，然而测压法尚未用于指导超低位结直肠吻合中新贮袋的建立。此外如直肠全层脱垂患者伴有显著地肛管静息压降低和RAIR消失（作为IAS活力的检测指标，详见下文），其治疗效果往往较差。同时进行经肛括约肌牵引术或者直肠前切除术，应避免对此类疾病经会阴行手术治疗[4]。在考虑行IAS切断术治疗慢性肛裂前应进行直肠肛管压力检测，因为有证据显示术前肛门张力正常或者偏低者，往往出现术后功能不良[5-6]。

如本章中Brusciano等报道，虽然直肠肛管测压应用广泛，目前尚缺乏标准的操作技术[7]，每个实验室需要建立自己的正常参考值。近来随着固态微传感器技术的发展，将其直接安装在测压导管上，不需要注水、牵拉，且与传统的水灌注测压相关性较好，为移动测压提供了可能；但固态测压设备价格高，易损坏[8]。传统的测压导管是聚乙烯材质，导管细而灵活，其上辐射状或纵行排列多个通道侧孔（通常为4~8个），辐射状排列的导管是用于静态压力评估，或者移动它来观察肛管的上下缘；阶梯式螺旋状排列的导管适用于记录肛管的纵行压力分布，这种导管可以通过手动或者机器牵拉，从而记录肛管全长的压力分布，并可降低静态测压产生的不对称性，如痔切除术后肛管变形、括约肌切开术后部分括约肌消融。

在传统的直肠肛管测压基础上衍生出其他设备，如动态直肠肛管测压法（AARM），可以更好地观察各种状态下直肠肛管功能，如体位改变、咳嗽、排尿、睡眠等，有助于了解贮袋 – 肛管吻合术后夜间急迫排便状态下的压力变化。下消化道动力的检测最初是应用无线遥测胶囊，但是仪器产生的射频会使观测信号衰减[9]，新式胶囊安装了压力敏感性微传感器，并可产生固定频率的信号[10-11]。AARM设备是由Miller等[12]和Kumar等[13]单独发明，Kumar发明了一种特殊的方法，可以进行睡眠时ARM检测，这种设备包括测压电极仓、压力传感器、信号放大器和便携式记录仪，压力数据是通过不同的脉冲间隔记录在磁带上，脉冲间隔组成了脉冲序列，磁带上的信息可解码成信号标记，与被检者的日常活动（粪便自制、疼痛等）相对应，通过检查发现原发性大便失禁患者的IAS一过性松弛频率高[14]。这种数字化技术可以将峰值过滤，就像动态心电图一样（Holter）使得波形流畅，清除高频和低频的伪波。最近发明一种新型的便携式可手持的AARM，是一种带微传感器的可充气微球囊装置，可进行中短期的肛管静息压、收缩压和咳嗽压力的跟踪分析[15-18]。

正常状态下，直肠每分钟收缩5~10次，餐后出现收缩频率降低，约3次/min，间隔20~30min出现，同时每90min出现直肠复合运动，后者是缓慢的推进式收缩，与小肠移行性复合运动的第Ⅲ期相似[19]。肛管压力在觉醒状态和睡眠状态差异较大，睡眠时肛管活动基本静止，清醒及排便前会叠加每分钟1~2次的慢波或超慢波[20]，有时会出现强有力的孤立收缩，这种收缩是随意的，并且与直肠活动无关。这些记录的数据与粪便性状和情绪状态有关[21]。与同龄对照组相比，便秘患者的直肠及肛管的活动均变慢，尤其是在餐后，这种检测方法对有便秘病史而传统的传输试验检查结果不能确诊的患者有帮助[22]。因家族性息肉病或溃疡性结肠炎行全结直肠切除的患者，夜间出现污粪现象与AARM中贮袋活动增多有关[23]；部分结肠J形贮袋患者也有同样表现[24]。AARM可以提供贮袋的重要生理信息，为新直肠贮袋的建立及个性化贮袋的设计提供参考[25]，同时有助于痔切除术后效果不佳原因的阐明，虽然测压结果与失禁患者的排便记录相关性差，但术后污粪患者常出现AARM压力降低伴有慢波活动减少[26]。目前，AARM仍作为实验设备，可为那些压力正常或降低、括约肌完整、结肠运输时间正常的便秘或失禁患者提供帮助[27]。AARM尚不能为新直肠或贮袋提供足够多的生理信息，但术前可以提供重要信息，以排除效果不好的结肠肛管吻合方式。

动态数据采集设备如图6.1所示。

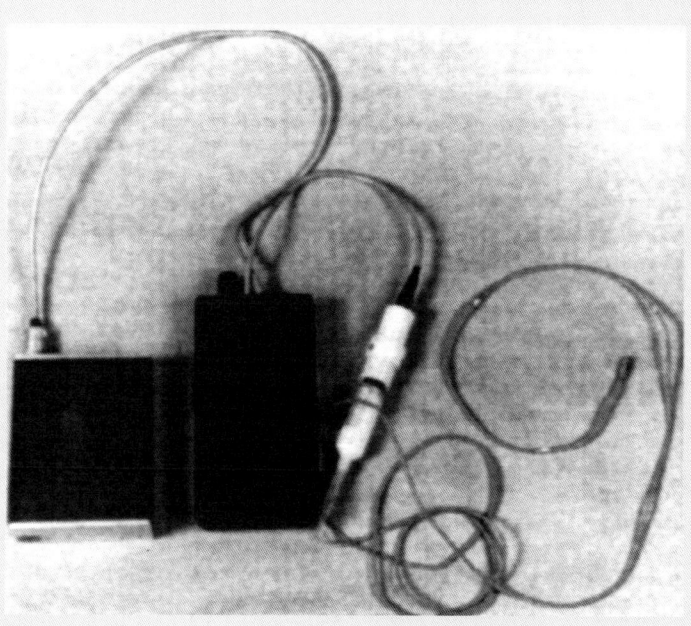

图6.1 动态数据采集设备（Reprinted with permission from Kumar et al.[75]）

参考文献

1. Carty NJ, Moran B, Johnson CD. Anorectal physiology measurements are of no value in clinical practice. True or false? Ann R Coll Surg Engl. 1994;76:276–80.
2. Vaizey CJ, Kamm MA. Prospective assessment of the clinical value of anorectal investigations. Digestion. 2000;61:207–14.
3. Eckardt VF, Elmer T. Reliability of anal pressure measurements. Dis Colon Rectum. 1991;34:772–7.
4. Glasgow SC, Birnbaum EH, Kodner IJ, Fleshman JW, Dietz DW. Preoperative anal manometry predicts continence after perineal proctectomy for rectal prolapse. Dis Colon Rectum. 2006;49:1052–8.
5. Pescatori M, Maria G, Anastasio G. "Spasm related" internal sphincterotomy in treatment of anal fissure. A randomized prospective study. Coloproctology. 1991;1:20–2.
6. Renzi A, Izzo D, DiSarno G, Talento P, Torelli F, Izzo G, et al. Clinical, manometric and ultrasonographic results of pneumatic balloon dilatation vs. Lateral internal sphincterotomy for chronic anal fissure: a prospective, randomized, controlled trial. Dis Colon Rectum. 2008;51:121–7.
7. Swash M. Henry MM. Coloproctology and the pelvic floor. Oxford: Butterworth Heinemann Ltd; 1992.
8. Miller R, Bartolo DC, Roe AM, Mortensen NJ. Assessment of microtransducers in anorectal manometry. Br J Surg. 1988;75:40–3.
9. Connell AM, McCall J, Misiewicz J, Rowlands E. Observation of the clinical use of radiopills. Br Med J. 1963;ii:771–4.
10. Browning C, Valori R, Wingate DL, Maclachlan D. A new pressure sensitive ingestible radiotelemetric capsule. Lancet. 1981;ii:509–15.
11. Womack NR, Williams NS, Holmfield JHM, Morrison JFB, Simpkins KC. New method for the dynamic assessment of anorectal function in constipation. Br J Surg. 1985;72:994–8.
12. Miller R, Lewis GT, Bartolo DCC, Cervero F, Mortensen NJ. Sensory discrimination and dynamic activity in the anorectum: evidence using a new ambulatory technique. Br J Surg. 1988;75:1003–7.
13. Kumar D, Waldron D, Williams NS, Browning C, Hutton MRE, Wingate DL. Prolonged anorectal monitoring and external anal sphincter electromyography in ambulant human subjects. Dig Dis Sci. 1990;35:641–8.
14. Sun WN, Read NW, Miner PB, Kurgan DD, Donnelly TC. The role of transient internal anal sphincter relaxation in faecal incontinence. Int J Colorectal Dis. 1997;12:296–7.
15. Dent JA. A new technique for continuous sphincter pressure measurement. Gastroenterology. 1976;71:263–7.
16. Orrom WJ, Williams JG, Rothenberger DA, Wong WD. Portable anorectal manometry. Br J Surg. 1990;77:876–7.
17. Bollard RC, Gardiner A, Duthie GS. Outpatient hand held manometry: comparison of techniques. Colorectal Dis. 2001;3:13–6.
18. Duthie GS. Ambulatory monitoring in anorectal disease [Thesis]. University of Aberdeen, Aberdeen, UK; 1992.
19. Szurszewski JH. A migrating electric complex of the canine small intestine. Am J Physiol. 1969;217:1757–63.
20. Kumar D, Williams NS, Waldron D, Wingate DL. Prolonged manometric recording of anorectal motor activity in ambulant human subjects: evidence of periodic activity. Gut. 1989;30:1007–11.
21. Wilgan P, Mishkinpour H, Becker M. Effect of anger on colon motor and myoelectric activity in irritable bowel syndrome. Gastroenterology. 1988;94:1105–6.
22. Ferrara A, Pemberton JH, Grotz RL, Hanson RB. Prolonged ambulatory recording of anorectal motility in patients with slow-transit constipation. Am J Surg. 1994;167:73–9.

23. Miller R, Orrom WJ, Duthie GS, Bartolo DCC, Mortensen NJM. Ambulatory anorectal physiology in patients following restorative proctocolectomy for ulcerative colitis and familial polyposis: a comparison of three reservoir designs. Br J Surg. 1985;72:470–4.
24. Romanos J, Stebbing JF, Smilgin Humphreys MM, Takeuchi N, Mortensen NJ. Ambulatory manometric examination in patients with colonic J pouch and in normal controls. Br J Surg. 1996;83:1744–6.
25. Ho Y-H, Tan M, Leong AFPK, Sedow-Choen F. Ambulatory manometry in patients with colonic J-pouch and straight coloanal anastomosis. Randomized controlled trial. Dis Colon Rectum. 2000;43:793–9.
26. Ho YH, Tan M. Ambulatory anorectal manometric findings in patients before and after haemorrhoidectomy. Int J Colorectal Dis. 1997;12:296–7.
27. Ronholt C, Rasmussen OO, Christiansen J. Ambulatory manometric recording of anorectal activity. Dis Colon Rectum. 1999;42:1551–9.

压力参数

直肠肛管压力参数包括肛门肌肉张力、直肠顺应性、直肠肛管感觉和直肠肛管抑制反射（RAIR），测压报告要包括直肠肛管测压流程，并且应包含所有可给医师提供参考的信息（如肛门外括约肌对肌肉激动剂或拮抗剂无反应）。另外一项评估测压过程的指标是会阴防御反射。这个生理反射是由于腹内压力增高引发盆底和腹部肌肉收缩活动[6]，被检者做咳嗽动作，检查者观察会阴部肌肉收缩，如压力生理性增加提示反射阳性，压力病理性降低提示反射阴性，压力降低明显者可能伴随排尿、排气。咳嗽时肛门内压力增高，但正常值随性别、年龄而变化，与检测模式及被检者的耐受性有关。因此，一份测压报告需包含测压全过程及所有直肠肛管功能[7]，表6.1是本中心门诊测压报告。

肛门肌肉张力

利用拖出法测量的肛管内最高压力定义为肛管最大静息压，也称之为平均基础压力（MBP），因检测方法多种多样、报道的正常人数据少且变化范围大，因此很难建立其正常参考值。肛管高压带在解剖上是与肛门内括约肌纤维聚集区对应，女性（2.0～3.0cm）较男性（2.5～3.5cm）偏短[8]。我们认为正常男性MBP在60～70mmHg，正常女性MBP在50～60mmHg，距肛缘1.5cm处压力最大。肛管静息压是由以下几部分组成：肛门内括约肌占50%～85%，外括约肌占20%～30%，余下的15%是由肛垫膨胀产生。平滑肌能够连续最大收缩，是由于其内在的肌源性和外在的自主神经源性特征，

表6.1 本中心直肠肛管测压报告

评估参数	结果	正常参考值（n.v.）
肛管长度（高压带）	4cm	
静息压（ARP）	72mmHg	60～70mmHg
最大主动收缩压（MCV）：增幅	增加60mmHg	n.v.>117mmHg
最大主动收缩压（MCV）：持续期	20s	n.v.（15～25s）
直肠肛管抑制反射（RAIR）吹气法	存在	
阈值	30cc	
松弛时间（RT）	14s	
复原时间	12s	
反应总时间	26s	
直肠容积		
感觉阈值	30cc	（n.v.25～30cc）
便意阈值	60cc	（n.v.40～60cc）
最大耐受量	120cc	（n.v.80～160cc）

结论：测得肛管长度为4cm，静息压正常，最大主动收缩压的增幅及持续期不足，肛门外括约肌复原能力差，拮抗肌活动增强（臀肌及外展肌），轻度直肠高敏感性；模拟排便反射时松弛不完全；RAIR存在，且其振幅、松弛及恢复时间正常；年龄松弛率为70%（残余压力18mmHg）

因此肛门内括约肌可自发地控制无意识的粪便排出。内括约肌因直肠扩张而松弛，且随直肠适应扩张刺激后而恢复张力。肛管静息压在白天和夜间呈规律性波动，且受直肠内粪便及躯体姿势影响，呈纵向或横向变化。静息压及收缩压均呈现功能性不对称，这是由于肛管周围肌肉不对称分布所致；肛管近端背侧压力高于腹侧，这是因耻骨直肠肌导致；肛管中段压力分布均匀；肛管远端腹侧压力高于背侧，这些不同平面的压力梯度有助于粪便自制。

主动收缩

肛门外括约肌的主动收缩可使肛管内压力升高，通常为静息压的 2～3 倍（100～180mmHg），且在肛管远端外括约肌主体所在处压力最高。由于肌肉的疲劳性，最大收缩压只能维持 40～60s。肛管最大收缩压（MSP）男性高于女性，且随年龄增大而降低，女性在年龄相关的压力降低表现更为明显。收缩压主要由肛门外括约肌收缩产生，部分来自肛提肌收缩。疲劳指数作为一个测压参数，可用于评估肛管括约肌的功能[9]，即括约肌由静息状态至完全疲劳，再恢复至静息压水平的时间。我们研究发现，健康志愿者的平均疲劳指数为 3.3min，便秘患者为 2.8min，污粪患者为 2.3min，大便失禁患者为 1.5min。事实上，部分大便失禁患者的收缩压开始是正常的，随之迅速显著下降，部分外括约肌萎缩、阴部神经病变导致的大便失禁内镜超声检查无异常，疲劳指数有助于这部分患者的鉴别。Brusciano 等[10]在对排便障碍患者进行盆底康复治疗研究时，将疲劳指数作为一个有用的评估因子。

肛门外括约肌和盆底肌有 3 种类型的活动，即静息张力、反射性收缩和主动收缩[11]。通常骨骼肌在静息状态下是不活动的，但肛门外括约肌与之不同，在静息状态保持连续的无意识的电活动，这可能是马尾神经反射的一部分。当腹内压力增高或直肠扩张时，EAS 和耻骨直肠肌反射性、甚至进一步主动收缩，从而避免粪便渗漏[12]。

评论：肛垫对肛门密闭性的重要性
Andrew P. Zbar

肛垫是由位于齿状线上的黏膜及黏膜下的组织形成的复合体，包括结缔组织和弹性组织[1]。通过对患者进行清醒及全麻下测压，排除 IAS 的干扰，同时记录 EAS 的肌电图活动，从而阐明外括约肌的功能[2]，肛垫功能的评估是利用逐渐增粗的灌注式导管来进行压力测定，从而描述括约肌张力与肛管直径的线性关系，并把这种关系外推至坐标轴，横坐标表示张力[1,3-5]。这个假设很重要，因为肛垫区是粪便自制的重要机制。近期研究出一种人造肛垫，即生物强化装置，包含胶原、戊二醛、硅胶、碳微粒和自体脂肪，通过局部射频对其支持，应用于主要因 IAS 损伤导致大便失禁的患者，取得中短期的成功。这种 IAS 生物增强装置在第 33 章有详细阐述。

肛管静息压产生机制很复杂，不能单纯应用肛垫来解释。测压检查发现从肛管近端向远端压力逐渐升高，最大静息压是在距肛缘 1～2cm 处，这一高压带在解剖上与聚集的平滑肌纤维束相对应，但这一纤维束并非真正意义的组织学可辨别的括约肌[6]。通过三维软件发现肛管近端背侧的扇形高压区是由耻骨直肠肌和 IAS 产生，远端腹侧的高压区可能是由 EAS 的浅部和皮下部产生[7]。最初认为肛管压力纵行及环形分布不对称，反映了肛管括约肌的解剖分布，从而可以解释粪便自制的机制的观点太过简单[8]，并且组织学[9]及括约肌分布的解剖学[10]也不支持这一观点。括约肌的解剖分布可通过更加高级的专用成像技术来检测：可利用三维重建的超声技术或表面相控阵磁共振成像技术检测[11]。

绝大多数观点认为最大主动收缩压由 EAS 产生，做收缩动作时，须仔细观察记录的压力（尤其是大便失禁患者行括约肌修补术后），因为检测结果的可重复性与检查者相关。鉴于外括约肌收缩的本质，在持续收缩或重复收缩时需作出特殊说明，而且收缩的幅度依赖于检查者的判断，明确有无臀部或大腿肌肉的参与。疲劳指数表示主动收缩的能力，是开始收缩至收缩压恢复至静息压的时间，在那些大便失禁患者可作为一项评估失禁严重度的指标[12-13]。括约肌及耻骨直肠肌的解剖分布形成粪便自制的"三环"学说，Shafik 认为 EAS 的深部因附着于耻骨支下缘将肛管向前牵拉，EAS 的中部因附着于尾骨将肛管向后牵拉，EAS 皮下部因附着于会阴部皮肤将肛管向前牵拉[14]。这一观点逐渐得到生理学[15]的认可，并且成为教科书上粪便自制的机制，IAS 的重要性被忽视了。通过研究刺激排便时肌电图变化，Shafik 等[16]进一步提出，肛提肌收缩时缩短，从正侧面提升肛管，但是这一理论已被驳斥，动态 CT 和 MRI 检查发现，肛提肌收缩时产生与上述相反的变化[17-21]。

IAS 作为粪便自制的机制被忽视，大多数人认为可以部分切断 EAS（如肛瘘切除术）而不发生排便相关并发症[22-26]，这些理论被证明是错误的，微小的控便机制损伤均可影响生活质量[27]，慢性肛裂行 IAS 切开术，术后因 IAS 切断导致主动收缩功能障碍[28-29]。同时有些慢性肛裂患者行 IAS 切开术前，行肛门内三维 MRI 检查发现 EAS 皮下部有缺陷，在行 IAS 切开术后肛管远端功能受损，如术前有 EAS 缺陷，往往预示术后功能障碍[30]。静息状态单纯的括约肌收缩尚不能完成控便功能，肛柱、黏膜及黏膜下痔组织等辅助闭合肛门的机制如也参与其中，肛垫作为维持粪便自制的机制尤为重要。Gibbons 等[1]发现括约肌张力和肛管直径间存在线性关系，与拉普拉斯定律（Law of Laplace）一致。而实际重要的原理是帕斯卡定律（Pascal's law），即在密闭的容器内，施加于静止液体上的压强将以等值同时传到各点；然而在体内系统，肛管不同部位的张力是不同的。根据拉普拉斯定律在肛管的形状一定的情况下，其张力、压力和半径有明确的关系[31]，也就是说，肛管也可以像心、肺一样，应用数学模型来评估，即通过肛管的几何学特征可以评估其张力-压力关系，如果肛管为球形，则两个参数的预测与实际最接近。直线斜率可因 EAS 收缩而增加，因 IAS 松弛而降低，当肛管张力为 0 时，括约肌的弹性指数或肛管内直径也会发生变化。认为肛垫有助于肛门闭合不仅仅是理论上的，部分病例因括约肌切开术或痔切除术而出现排便障碍，就是因为手术方式改变了肛门闭合机制。

拉普拉斯定律仅适用于圆柱形装置，肛管的形状决定了其环行及纵行张力，肛管完全塌陷需要一个负压（像肺一样），黏膜皱襞使得肛管的几何形状变得复杂，从而影响环行张力，皱襞间的液体使得肛管顺应性增加，也改变了静息状态下肛管的圆周。肛管直径越小的地方，液体覆盖的黏膜及管腔的表面张力越重要，此处的弹性系数会增加，在管腔闭合处管壁的厚度和张力增加，在该处形成阀门的作用。近来 Thekkinkattil 等通过研究特发性大便失禁患者的肛垫面积发现内在差异[32]，但痔切除术后大便失禁的原因复杂，所以对其研究应持审慎的态度，他们认为肛门闭合机制存在个体差异性，部分患者术后出现括约肌间脓肿（也许是术前漏诊）、直肠肛管抑制反射改变、直肠肛管压力梯度紊乱、内括约肌损伤（尤其是微创操作未将 IAS 与黏膜下层分离）、痔脱垂者术前排便习惯及黏膜敏感性改变[33-36]。

参考文献

1. Gibbons C, Trowbridge EA, Bannister JJ, Read NW. Role of anal canal cushions in maintaining continence. Lancet. 1986;1:886–8.
2. Schweiger M. Method for determining individual contributions of voluntary and involuntary anal sphincters to resting tone. Dis Colon Rectum. 1979;22:415–6.
3. Allen ML, Zamani S, Dimarino AJ, Sodhi S, Miranda LA, Nusbaum M. Manometric measurement of anal canal resting tone: comparison of a rectosphincteric balloon probe with a water-perfused catheter assembly. Dig Dis Sci. 1998;43:1411–5.
4. Sangwan YP, Solla JA. Internal anal sphincter: advances and insights. Dis Colon Rectum. 1998;41:1297–311.
5. Zbar AP, Jayne DG, Mathur D, Ambrose NS, Guillou PJ. The importance of the internal anal sphincter (IAS) in maintaining continence: anatomical, physiological and pharmacological considerations. Colorectal Dis. 2000;2:193–202.
6. Fritsch H, Brenner E, Lienemann A, Ludwikowski B. Anal sphincter complex: reinterpreted morphology and its clinical relevance. Dis Colon Rectum. 2002;45:188–94.
7. Williams AB, Kamm MA, Bartram CI, Kmiot WA. Gender differences in the longitudinal pressure profile of the anal canal related to anatomical structure as demonstrated on three-dimensional anal sonography. Br J Surg. 2001;87:1675–9.
8. Taylor BM, Beart RW, Phillips SF. Longitudinal and radial variations of pressure in the human anal sphincter. Gastroenterology. 1984;86:693–7.
9. Zbar AP, Aslam M, Hider A, Toomey P, Kmiot WA. Comparison of vector volume manometry and conventional manometry in anorectal dysfunction. Tech Coloproctol. 1998;2:84–90.
10. Goes RN, Simons AJ, Masri L, Beart RW Jr. Gradient of pressure and time between proximal anal canal and high-pressure zone during internal anal sphincter relaxation: its role in the fecal continence mechanism. Dis Colon Rectum. 1995;38:989–96.
11. Morren GL, Beets-Tan RG, Van Engelshoven JM. Anatomy of the anal canal and perianal structures as defined by phased-array magnetic resonance imaging. Br J Surg. 2001;88:1506–12.
12. Telford KJ, Ali AS, Lymer K, Hospker GL, Kiff ES, Hill J. Fatigability of the external anal sphincter in anal incontinence. Dis Colon Rectum. 2004;47:746–52.
13. Bilali S, Pfeifer J. Anorectal manometry: are fatigue rate and fatigue rate index of any clinical importance? Tech Coloproctol.

2005;9:225–8.
14. Shafik AA. A new concept of the anal sphincter mechanism and physiology of defecation. IX. Single loop continence: a new theory of the mechanism of anal continence. Dis Colon Rectum. 1980;23:37–46.
15. Dalley II AF. The riddle of the sphincters. The morphophysiology of the anorectal mechanism reviewed. Am Surg. 1987;53:298–306.
16. Shafik A, Gamal el-Din MA, el-Sibaei O, Abdel Hamid Z, el-Said B. Involuntary action of the external anal sphincter. Manometric and electromyographic studies. Eur Surg Res. 1992;24:188–96.
17. Li D, Guo M. Morphology of the levator ani muscle. Dis Colon Rectum. 2007;50:1–9.
18. Guo M, Li D. Pelvic floor images: anatomy of the levator ani muscle. Dis Colon Rectum. 2007;50:1647–55.
19. Zbar AP, Guo M, Pescatori M. Anorectal morphology and function: analysis of the Shafik legacy. Tech Coloproctol. 2008;12:191–200.
20. Zbar AP, Guo M, Pescatori M. Anorektale morphologie und function: analyse der arbeiten von Shafik. Coloproctology. 2009;31:269–81.
21. Guo M, Gao C, Li D, Guo W, Shafik AA, Zbar A, et al. MRI anatomy of the anal region. Dis Colon Rectum. 2010;53:1542–8.
22. Milligan ETC, Morgan CN. Surgical anatomy of the anal canal with special reference to ano-rectal fistulae. Lancet. 1934;2:1213–7.
23. Gorsch RV. Anorectal fistula: anatomical considerations and treatment. Am J Surg. 1936;32:302–7.
24. Morgan CN, Thompson HR. Surgical anatomy of the anal canal with special reference to the surgical importance of the internal sphincter and conjoint longitudinal muscle. Ann R Coll Surg Engl. 1956;19:88–114.
25. Oh C, Kark AE. Anatomy of the external anal sphincter. Br J Surg. 1972;59:717–23.
26. Thompson JP, Ross AH. Can the external anal sphincter be preserved in the treatment of trans-sphincteric fistula-in-ano? Int J Colorectal Dis. 1989;4:247–50.
27. Casillas S, Hull TL, Zutshi M, Trzcinski R, Bast JF, Xu M. Incontinence after a lateral internal sphincterotomy: are we underestimating it? Dis Colon Rectum. 2005;48:1193–9.
28. Zbar AP, Aslam M, Allgar V. Faecal incontinence after internal sphincterotomy for anal fissure. Tech Coloproctol. 2000;4:25–8.
29. Shafik A, el-Sibai O, Shafik AA. Is myoelectric activity transmittable from one muscle to another: an experimental study. Int J Surg Investig. 2000;2:165–70.
30. Zbar AP, Kmiot WA, Aslam M, Williams A, Hider A, Audisio RA, et al. Use of vector volume manometry and endoanal magnetic resonance imaging in the adult female for assessment of anal sphincter dysfunction. Dis Colon Rectum. 1999;42:928–33.
31. Richeson AW. Laplace's contribution to pure mathematics. Natl Math Mag. 1942;17:73–8.
32. Thekkinkattil DK, Dunham RJ, O'Herlihy S, Finan PJ, Sagar PM, Burke DA. Measurement of anal cushions in idiopathic faecal incontinence. Br J Surg. 2009;96:680–4.
33. Ho YH, Seow-Choen F, Goh HS. Haemorrhoidectomy and disordered rectal and anal physiology in patients with prolapsed haemorrhoids. Br J Surg. 1995;82:596–8.
34. Zbar AP, Beer-Gabel M, Chiappa AC, Aslam M. Fecal incontinence after minor anorectal surgery. Dis Colon Rectum. 2001;44:1610–2.
35. Zbar AP. Measurement of anal cushions in idiopathic faecal incontinence. Br J Surg. 2009;96:1373–4.
36. Zbar A, Murison R. Transperineal ultrasound in the assessment of haemorrhoids and haemorrhoidectomy: a pilot study. Tech Coloproctol. 2010;14:175–9.

直肠肛管抑制反射（RAIR）

RAIR 是指直肠扩张会引起 IAS 一过性松弛，肛管内压力短暂降低，随后恢复至基线的反射活动[13]，RAIR 的引出表示神经反射弧是完整的，反射弧的感受器位于直肠壁内，传出神经位于骶丛内，人们认为 RAIR 为取样反射，可以辨别气体、液体、固体粪便[14]。图 6.2 是一典型的 RAIR。

RAIR 可产生直肠肛管压力梯度，为排便动作准备。先天性巨结肠（Hirchsprung's disease）患者该反射消失，低位直肠切除及回肠贮袋肛管吻合术后早期该反射也可能为阴性，结肠肛管手工吻合及低位吻合器吻合术后神经可能再生[15-16]。虽然有许多方法可以评估 RAIR，但尚缺乏标准方法，我们应用的方法是向传感器末端的球囊（置于直肠）内注入 60ml 水或者空气，观察肛管的反应。如果 RAIR 存在，直肠扩张后会引起 EAS 反射性收缩，随之 IAS 松弛。这种检测技术受检查者及检查方法影响，近、中、远处括约肌的松弛程度也不同，近端 IAS 松弛度最大。

RAIR 和直肠肛管兴奋反射的潜伏期就是从球囊膨胀开始，到引出反射所需的时间，以 s 为单位，许多学者都研究过 RAIR 及其各项参数的重要性，包括潜伏期、反射持续时间、反射发生时括约肌近远端的振幅等[17-18]。

大便失禁患者扩张直肠时会出现明显的括约肌松弛[19-20]，鉴于此，Zbar 等[21]比较大便失禁及便秘患者的兴奋和抑制反射的潜伏期、最大兴奋和抑制压力、振幅和抑制斜率、斜率和压力恢复时间、抑制曲线下面积，他们发现不同患者在不同检测平面抑制曲线恢复时间均不同，大便失禁患者恢复时

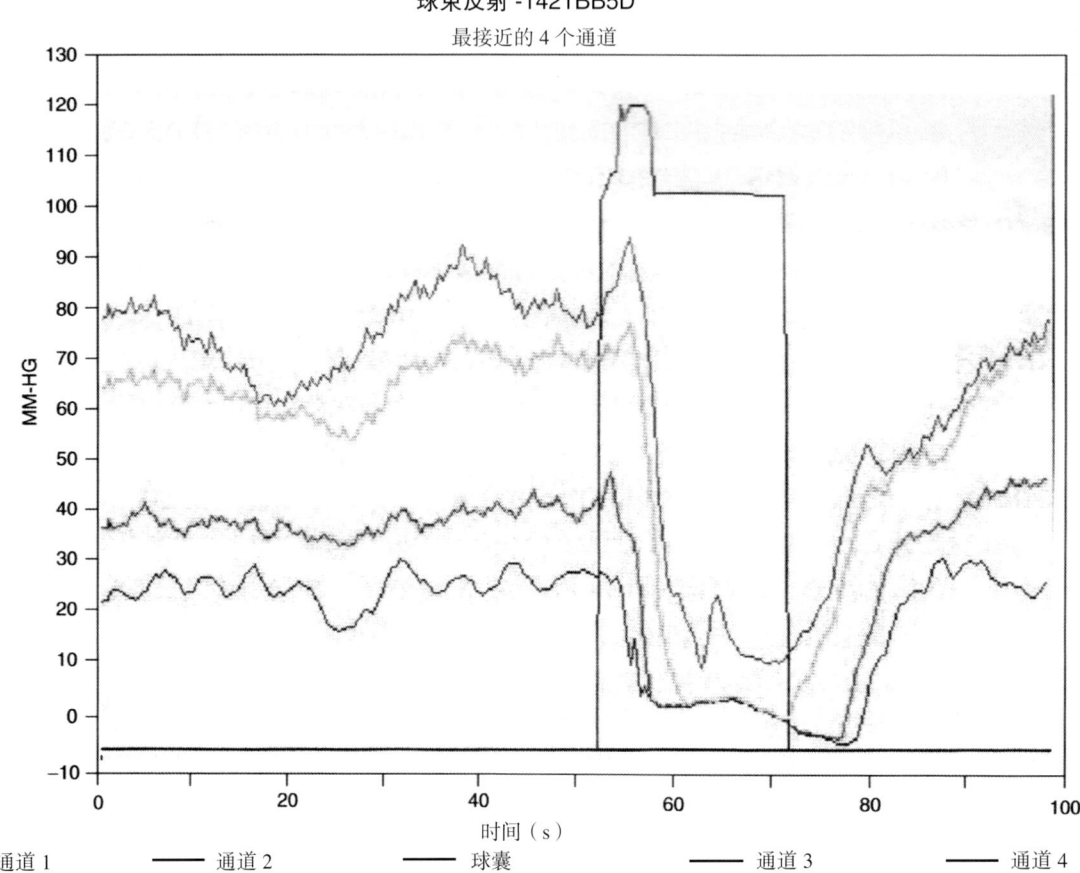

图 6.2　正常的 RAIR（Reprinted with permission from Roberts.[76]）

间最短，因此他们推断粪便自制可能部分依靠直肠肛管抑制反射，RAIR 的某些参数也许可以预测直肠低位吻合术后的功能变化。

低位直肠前切除、结肠肛管吻合、回肠贮袋肛管吻合术后，RAIR 通常会消失，不论是手工或吻合器吻合，随着时间推移、功能改善、夜间排便次数减少，该反射可逐渐恢复[15-16]。据报道，低位直肠吻合术后 6~12 个月，只有 21% 的患者存在 RAIR，术后 2 年有 85% 的 RAIR 为阳性[22]。因为 RAIR 的神经反射通路位于肠壁内，直肠切除将其损伤，所以术后早期 RAIR 消失，有学者认为术后 6 个月吻合口处的神经再生[23]，另有学者认为 RAIR 的恢复是盆底张力感受器再生的结果。

评论：RAIR
Andrew P. Zbar

RAIR 是指直肠膨胀时肛管内压力降低，主要与 IAS 松弛有关，1877 年 Gowers[1] 首次提出，随后于 1935 年由 Denny-Brown 和 Robertson 进一步证实。定义为当直肠内球囊快速膨胀时，肛管静息压一过性降低，且超过静息压的 25%，随后压力恢复至静息状态。这一反射的神经生理学尚不清楚，但脊髓损伤、马尾综合征、全直肠切除或骶前神经阻滞后该反射仍然存在，因此推断 RAIR 受壁内神经丛调控[3-4]。RAIR缺失对先天性巨结肠具有诊断意义[5-6]，但在新生儿应用尚有局限性[7-8]。在低位直肠前切除吻合术后2年左右RAIR恢复，且大致与排便功能恢复、急迫排便次数减少相一致[9-10]。RAIR的引出与检查者高度相关，且与直肠和球囊的顺应性、直肠的几何形状及物理膨胀作用有关。如果静息压偏低或者直肠敏感性降低，则可能出现假阴性结果，并且该反射存在易疲劳性，两次重复操作间需有休息间隔。

有些文献报道RAIR引出之前有一过性压力升高，称为直肠肛管兴奋反射，在肛管远端比较明显，有些人认为该反射与潜在的阴部神经病变及其严重度有关[10-11]。RAIR可以重复引出，由于直肠肛管兴奋反射的存在，引出RAIR可能需要高于常规容积的气体，可能会刺激括约肌收缩，从而增加反应初始的压力。研究认为，NO是RAIR的主要神经递质，由壁内的非胆碱能、非肾上腺素能神经元产生[12]，且RAIR的机器感受器位于黏膜，因为利用局麻药凝胶涂于黏膜[13]或神经节阻滞剂[14]可以抑制该反射的引出。

RAIR的引出有许多方法，包括一系列的导管和球囊、以水或气作为媒介。通常是应用螺旋式导管及充气法，以直肠初始感觉阈值作为基础的充气量，当肛管内压力较静息压升高或降低两个标准差时，认为直肠肛管兴奋或抑制反射存在。在肛管的近中远部，RAIR的引出有明显差异，通常在肛管近端引出RAIR时肛管松弛率最大。大多数实验室对RAIR的描述都是存在或缺失，但RAIR曲线是有个体差异性的，包括反射引出的潜伏期、反射斜率、压力恢复斜率、恢复时间及抑制曲线下面积等，目前的测压分析软件已经具备了计算上述各项指标功能，也许可以找出某些疾病的特异性RAIR变化[15]。有些实验室发现大便失禁患者有其特异性RAIR变化曲线，如肛门外括约肌损伤的患者肛管远端无兴奋反射，而近端抑制反射正常；特发性大便失禁患者远端兴奋反射抑制，而近端抑制反射正常。RAIR和一些其他功能性指标（如IAS变薄或损伤）结合可以对术后功能进行预测，筛选出适宜进行直肠超低位切除、吻合的病例，同时对行IAS保留手术的儿童也有益处[16]，对顽固性肛裂患者行括约肌消融治疗前也应该进行这些功能评估，因部分患者术后功能差。

参考文献

1. Gowers WR. The automatic action of the sphincter ani. Proc R Soc Lond B Biol Sci. 1877;26:77–84.
2. Denny-Brown D, Robertson EG. An investigation of the nervous control of defaecation. Brain. 1935;58:256–310.
3. Roberts PL. Rectoanal inhibition. In: Wexner SD, Zbar AP, Pescatori M, editors. Complex anorectal disorders: investigation and management. London: Springer; 2005. p. 39–47.
4. Lubowski DZ, Nicholls RJ, Swash M, Jordan MJ. Neural control of internal anal sphincter function. Br J Surg. 1987;74:688–90.
5. Lanfranchi GA, Bazzocchi G, Federici S, Brignola C, Campieri M, Rossi F, et al. Anorectal manometry in the diagnsos of Hirschprung's disease – comparison with clinical and radiological criteria. Am J Gastroenterol. 1984;79:270–5.
6. De Lorijn F, Kremer LC, Reitsma JB, Benninga MA. Diagnostic tests in Hirschprung;s disease: a systematic review. J Pediatr Gastroenterol Nutr. 2006;42:496–505.
7. Kawahara H, Kubota A, Hasegawa T, Okuyama H, Ueno T, Watanabe T, et al. Anorectal sleeve micromanometry for the diagnosis of Hirschprung's disease in newborns. J Pediatr Surg. 2007;42:2075–9.
8. Huang Y, Zheng S, Xiao X. Preliminary evaluation of anorectal manometry in diagnosing Hirschsprung's disease in neonates. Pediatr Surg Int. 2009;25:41–5.
9. Suzuki H, Matsumoto K, Amano S, Fujioka M, Honzumi M. Anorectal pressure and rectal compliance after low anterior resection. Br J Surg. 1980;676:655–7.
10. O'Riordain MG, Molloy RG, Gillen P, Sangwan Y, Coller JA, Barrett RC, et al. Distal rectoanal excitatory reflex: a reliable index of pudendal neuropathy. Dis Colon Rectum. 1995;38:916–20.
11. Sangwan YP, Coller JA, Barrett RC, Murray JJ, Roberts PL, Schoetz DJ Jr. Prospective comparative study of abnormal distal rectoanal excitatory reflex, pudendal nerve terminal motor latency and single fiber density as markers of pudendal neuropathy. Dis Colon Rectum. 1996;39:894–8.
12. O'Kelly TJ, Brading AF, Mortensen NJM. Nerve mediated relaxation of the human internal anal sphincter: the role of nitric oxide. Gut. 1993;34:689–93.
13. Meunier P, Mollard P. Control of the internal anal sphincter (manometric study of human subjects). Pflugers Arch. 1977;370:233–9.
14. Kumar D, Phillips SF. Human myenteric plexus: confirmation of unfamiliar structures in adults and neonates. Gastroenterology. 1989;9:1021–8.

15. Zbar A, Ramesh J. Parameters of the rectoanal inhibitory reflex in different anorectal disorders. Dis Colon Rectum. 2003;46:557–8.
16. Lin CL, Chen CC. The rectoanal relaxation reflex and continence in repaired anorectal malformations with and without an internal sphincter saving procedure. J Pediatr Surg. 1996;31:630–3.

模拟排便

测压检查有助于发现模拟排便时的异常表现[24]，做排便动作时直肠内压力增高，同时肛管内压力降低（很大程度上靠 EAS 松弛），该动作受意识支配，并且需后天学习获得。如果不能协调完成排便动作提示排便功能障碍，原因可能为直肠收缩障碍、肛管矛盾收缩、肛管松弛障碍或以上三者都有。

鉴于此，Rao 等[25]将排便功能障碍分为 3 类：①排便动力充足型，即排便时腹内压及直肠内压力增高，同时肛管压力矛盾性收缩；②排便动力不足型，排便时推动力不足，即直肠内压力不增加，且有肛管矛盾性收缩；③排便时推动力正常（直肠内压力升高），但肛管不松弛（肛管内压力未降低）或松弛不全（松弛率 <20%）。

以上均可能导致排便时直肠肛管推动力不足，但有些被检者是因为检查环境影响，肛管不能正常松弛。Rao 等[25]发现行移动式家庭测压检查时，80% 的患者括约肌松弛良好，22% 的健康人在左侧卧位检查时有出口梗阻表现，而坐于马桶检查时，其中 95% 表现正常。因此，如果被检者在卧位检查时有出口梗阻表现，最好让其采取坐位重复检查；如有必要，可将球囊置入直肠，向内充气产生膨胀感觉，模拟直肠内有粪便到达。

上述分类不能作为排便运动异常的诊断标准，排便动作存在男女差异，男性的排便指数高于女性，但两者比较无统计学差异；同时，男性较女性发生排便功能障碍的概率低。老年人排便指数降低且球囊排出时间延长，提示年龄与盆底功能减退有关。当咳嗽、打喷嚏或吹气球时，腹内压力增高，反射性引起肛门内压力增高，该反射受骶神经调控，有助于判断大便失禁患者神经损伤的解剖平面。因为通过咳嗽引发该反射存在个体差异性，并且可控制性及可重复性均较差，现在通常应用吹气球的方法来诱导。

肛门松弛压是指被检者做排便动作时，基础压力与肛管内最小压力的差值，出口梗阻型排便障碍患者的肛管残余压高于静息压，肛管松弛率的计算公式为：肛管松弛率（%）= 肛管松弛压 / 肛管静息压 ×100。为全面评估诱导排便时直肠肛管内压力变化，应用排便指数，计算公式为：排便指数 = 直肠内最大压力（力排）/ 肛管内最小压力（力排）。

直肠感觉

直肠感觉是指间断膨胀直肠可以引起初始感觉、排便感觉、急迫感及不适感的最小气体量，通常是将球囊置入直肠，逐渐向内增加注气或注水量，记录患者最初感觉到球囊、排便感觉和达到最大耐受程度的容积。直肠低敏感性是指直肠初始感觉阈值及最大耐受量增高，常见于便秘患者；直肠高敏感性常见于急迫性大便失禁[7]。

评论：直肠肛管黏膜的敏感性
Andrew P. Zbar

除了基础的球囊实验，文献还报道了其他直肠肛管黏膜敏感性实验。据推测，直肠肛管敏感性对排便及控便有重要意义，但是目前对其神经传导通路知之甚少，且检测方法有限，只是知道它在一系列肛门疼痛综合征中起重要作用，如肠易激综合征、痉挛性肛门痛、特发性肛门痛等。Duthie 和 Gairns[1] 从解剖学上阐述直肠肛管内神经末梢的重要意义；早在 20 世纪 50 年代，Sotolo[2] 和 Fan[3] 就分别提出这一观点。它们最初集中在肛管移行区，该处感觉神经末梢称为麦氏（Meissner）触觉小体、克氏（Krause）终末小体、摩擦小体、戈－马（Golgi-Mazzoni）压力小体、帕氏（Paccinian）膨胀小体，与皮肤内的神经末梢相似。表浅的压力感受器位于黏膜层，信号传至骶前神经节，深层（包括浆膜和系膜）的压力感受器通过盆腔内脏神经传入，神经突触位于腰髓内，伤害性刺激信号经交感和副交感神经神经传入，经下腹上和下腹下神经丛传至 L_1/L_2，腰麻或阴部神经阻滞后不良刺激无法传入。有些感受器对扩张刺激敏感，其他感受器可能对化学、机械和热刺激敏感[4]。

黏膜敏感性的评估是顺应性和压力评估的部分内容，直肠内球囊膨胀时被检者要求对初始感觉、排便感觉、最大耐受量作出判断，这样评估比较粗略，不能提供直肠容积、顺应性或肠壁硬度的精确信息[5]。直肠对内容物的感知和直肠充盈的感觉不同，他们共同反应直肠弹性，但不能明确反应黏膜敏感性，这些差异有助于说明正常值的范围，初始感觉阈值是 40～90ml，急迫排便阈值是 140～160ml，最大耐受量是 200～300ml[6]。通常肠易激综合征直肠敏感性增高[7]，在腹泻为主或便秘为主的肠易激综合征中均很明显[8]；但在炎性结直肠病中增高不明显[9]；而顽固性特发性便秘，尤其是慢传输型便秘[10-11]直肠敏感性降低；排便失禁者直肠敏感性的变化是混合型的。

然而，在直肠低顺应性时直肠敏感性经常出现异常，反映了直肠容积降低，在直肠脱垂修补术后则反映了直肠黏膜复位[12]。肛管敏感性的明确评估是有困难的，Duthie 和 Gairns[1] 曾应用毛发、针刺及不同温度的金属盆来评估肛门敏感性，Rogers[13] 和 Miller 等[14-15] 分别改进了检测技术，通过灌注不同温度的液体来评估；Siegel[17] 最初设计产生不同强度方波电流的电极；Roe 等[16] 首次应用这种电极来评估肛门敏感性，被称为黏膜电敏感性技术（MES），可以检测许多不同的传入神经通路[18]。该系统是使用一种特殊设计的 10-Fr 导管，其上间隔 1cm 装有 2 个铂丝电极，采用 100ms 直流电，5 次/s 连续刺激，电流从 1mA 逐渐增加至 20mA，直到被检者感受到刺激（通常为麻刺感），正常值为 2～7mA，且与年龄有关，年龄增大敏感性降低[19]。排便失禁者 MES 增高，有 EAS 缺陷者表现尤为突出；顺产后 MES 是增加的，这种增加是可逆的[20]；排便梗阻者 MES 增加[21]；慢性肛裂的 MES 降低；痔疮患者 MES 增高，行痔切除术后会更高；直肠脱垂行直肠固定术后，MES 变化不明显；结肠肛管吻合术后因切除肛管移行区，MES 降低，因此在行吻合器下低位贮袋肛管吻合时，保留直肠黏膜有助于术后功能和感觉的保留[22-24]；回肠贮袋肛管吻合术后因切除直肠黏膜 MES 降低，术后污粪发生率较显著[24]，虽然污粪发生与年龄相关[25]。

参考文献

1. Duthie HL, Gairns FW. Sensory nerve endings and sensation in the anal region of man. Br J Surg. 1960;67:585–9.
2. Sotolo JR. Nerve endings of the walls of the descendent colon and rectum. Z Zellforsch. 1954;41:S101–11.
3. Fan WW. Histological studies of sensory nerves in the sigmoid and rectum. Arch Fur Jap Chir. 1955;24:567–74.
4. Rogers J, Hayward M, Henry M, Misiewicz JJ. Temperature gradient between the rectum and anal canal: evidence against the role of temperature sensation as a sensory modality in the anal canal of normal subjects. Br J Surg. 1988;75:1083–5.
5. Broens PMA, Penninckx FM, Lestar B, Kerremans R. The trigger for rectal filling sensation. Int J Colorect Dis. 1994;9:1–4.
6. Felt-Bersma RJF. Anorectal sensitivity. In: Wexner SD, Zbar AP, Pescatori M, editors. Complex anorectal disorders: investigation and management. London: Springer; 2005. p. 137–52.
7. Ritchie J. Pain from distension of the pelvic colon by inflating a balloon in the irritable bowel syndrome. Gut. 1973;14:125–32.
8. Prior A, Maxton DG, Whorwell PJ. Anorectal manometry in irritable bowel syndrome: differences between diarrhoea and constipation predominant subjects. Gut. 1990;31:458–62.
9. Chang L, Munakata J, Mayer EA, Schmulson MJ, Johnsons TD, Bernstein CN, et al. Perceptual responses in patients with inflammatory and functional bowel disease. Gut. 2002;47:497–505.
10. Mertz H, Naliboff B, Mayer EA. Physiology of refractory constipation. Am J Gastroenterol. 1999;94:609–15.
11. Penning C, Steens J, van der Schaar PJ, Kuyvenhoven J, Delamarre JB, Lamers CB, et al. Motor and sensory function of the rectum in different subtypes of constipation. Scand J Gastroenterol. 2001;36:32–8.
12. Siproudhis L, Bellissami E, Juguet F, Mendier M-H, Allain H, Bretagne J-F, et al. Rectal adaptation to distension in patients with overt rectal prolapse. Br J Surg. 1998;85:1527–32.
13. Rogers J. Rectal and anal sensation. In: Swash M, Henry MM, editors. Coloproctology and the pelvic floor. Oxford, UK: Butterworth Heinemann; 1992. p. 54–60.
14. Miller R, Bartolo DCC, Cervero F, Mortensen NJM. Anorectal temperature sensation: a comparison of normal and incontinent patients. Br J Surg. 1987;74:511–5.

15. Miller R. The measurement of anorectal sensation. In: Kumar D, Waldron D, Williams NS, editors. Clinical measurement in coloproctology. London: Springer-Verlag; 1991. p. 60–6.
16. Roe AM, Bartolo DCC, Mortensen NJM. New method for the assessment of anal sensation in various anorectal disorders. Br J Surg. 1986;73:310–2.
17. Siegel H. Cutaneous sensory threshold stimulation with high frequency square wave current. J Invest Dermatol. 1951;18:441–5.
18. Vierck CJ, Greenspan JD, Ritz LA, Yeomans DC. The spinal pathways contributing to the ascending conduction and descending modulations of pain sensation and reactions. In: Yaksh TL, editor. Spinal Afferent Processing. New York: Plenum Press; 1986. p. 275–329.
19. Felt-Bersma RJF, Poen AC, Cuesta MA, Meuwissen SGM. Anal sensitivity test: what does it measure and do we need it? Dis Colon Rectum. 1997;40:811–6.
20. Cornes H, Bartolo DC, Stirrat GM. Changes in anal canal sensation after childbirth. Br J Surg. 1991;78:74–7.
21. Solana A. Roig JV, Villoslada C, Hinojosa J, Lledo S. Anorectal sensitivity in patients with obstructed defecation. Int J Colorect Dis. 1996;11:65–70.
22. Holdsworth PJ, Johnston D. Anal sensation after restorative proctocolectomy for ulcerative colitis. Br J Surg. 1988;75:993–6.
23. Komatsu J, Oya M, Ishikawa H. Quantitative assessment of anal canal sensation in patients undergoing low anterior resection for rectal cancer. Surg Today. 1995;25:867–73.
24. Miller R, Bartolo DCC, Cervero D, Mortensen NJM. Does preservation of the anal transitional zone influence sensation after ileal-anal anastomosis for ulcerative colitis? Clin Controversies Inflamm Bowel Dis Bologna: Tipografia Negri SRL; 1987: 205A.
25. Tonita R, Igarashi S. Assessments of anal canal sensitivity in patients with soiling 5 years or more after colectomy, mucosal proctectomy and ileal J pouch-anal anastomosis for ulcerative colitis. World J Surg. 2007;31:210–6.

直肠顺应性

顺应性是用来评估直肠的扩张能力，也就是直肠在一定压力下能容纳的粪便量，以及推迟排便的能力，是通过人工向直肠内乳胶气囊注气、注水，或通过恒压器向直肠内高顺应性聚乙烯球囊注气、注水，观察直肠内压力与容积的关系来评估的。直肠测压时应用乳胶球囊有一定局限性，乳胶球囊自身的顺应性会影响结果，所以建议使用恒压模式向直肠内球囊注气来扩张直肠，可引起腔内压力升高，随后压力缓慢降低，当直肠适应了增加的容积后，压力维持稳定状态，每次注气后直肠内压力要进行校正，需减去球囊膨胀升高的压力，描绘球囊容积（dV）与直肠内压力（dP）变化的曲线，直肠顺应性可以通过计算该曲线斜率得出，计算公式：顺应性 =dV/dP cc mmHg。直肠顺应性有助于评估放射性直肠损伤、新直肠功能失调、回肠贮袋及回肠贮袋肛管吻合术后不明原因排便次数增多；然而文献上对直肠顺应性正常值的报道差异较大，并且有许多缺陷。

评论：直肠顺应性评估法的缺陷—阻抗容积描记法、恒压法、肛管反射计法
Andrew P. Zbar

目前对直肠的功能和形态学进行了许多研究，但对直肠容积的研究尚处于起步阶段，如何来测量正常人及病患的直肠膨胀性存在相当大的争议，Brusciano 等认为最简单的评估方法就是直肠顺应性，是用物理学方法来定义的，即单位容积的压力变化（$\Delta P/\Delta V$），但这种单纯的物理学表达不能充分反映直肠的生物力学特征。顺应性是应用可扩张的有高度顺应性的球囊，绘制压力 - 容积曲线，曲线的斜率即为直肠顺应性[1]，这一简单的检测方法被广泛用于评估肠易激综合征[2]和放射性直肠损伤[3]的直肠功能，并有一系列年龄、性别差异的报道[4]，但目前尚缺乏标准的检测方法，国际上对其正常值的报道相差 4 倍[5-7]。

许多物理因素会影响顺应性的测量[8-11]，如球囊的材质和大小、膨胀技术（连续或阶梯式）、膨胀速度和注入的媒介物（气或水），通过对受试者进行分析，Madoff 等[8]指出在非线性的压力 - 容积曲线图上无法计算出单一的数字，必须在曲线上确定一点（上升支、下降支或平台期），才能计算出其斜率[12]，同时对中空脏器膨胀还要考虑一系列复杂的数学因素，因此在不同状态下作出的顺应性报告

是有问题的。

Madoff 等[8]指出在进行顺应性检测时,是把直肠假想为一个密闭的容器,而实际上它是未封闭的圆柱状结构,标准的顺应性检测应是假设球囊无线性或者挤压效果,且直乙交界封闭,这样检测的直肠顺应性没有考虑直肠内的几何形状及球囊材质自身的顺应性。Madoff 还指出直肠内腔的大小可能影响顺应性:巨结肠患者的直肠壁僵硬且没有弹性,但因内腔较大,单位压力的改变需要较大容积,因此顺应性高;直肠内腔较小者虽然是正常的,但检测结果可能显示低顺应性和肠壁弹性差,这些可能是错误的结果,这也说明了顺应性和容积的区别,直肠容积是粪便自制的重要机制,在压力-容积评估中并没有反映直肠容积。另外,直肠外组织的弹性也被忽略,可影响顺应性的检测,因此将直肠切除后进行检测与体内结果比较是不同的[13]。

神经生理学家 Hans Gregersen[14-15]还强调与中空器官(如直肠、肛管、输尿管、主动脉或十二指肠)扩张相关的许多生物学因素可能影响顺应性,直肠作为可扩张的器官,也具有生物工程学的复杂性,因此需要发展和应用更加先进的方法来检测其特性。对中空脏器的体内或体外研究,膨胀性可通过恒压法来测定,容积通过直肠成像来测定,这是 Gregersen 采用的最新方法,可在直肠扩张、几何形状发生改变时检测其容积,直肠成像可通过 B 型超声或者磁共振来完成[16-17],成像后体积信息是通过计算脏器腔内的横截面积(CSA)来获得,在体内无法有效的测量脏器壁,通常忽略其厚度,为了进一步检测该脏器扩张后的各项指标变化,必须采用等压或等容的方法,膨胀刺激为阶梯式或渐进式增加。通过比较视觉模拟量表(初始感觉、排便感觉、最大耐受量)发现,在等压条件下男性可耐受更大容积,而女性在膨胀/压缩循环中容积变化较大,即所谓的滞后现象,老年女性表现更为突出。可重复性是对反复、均衡膨胀过程的适应性和稳定性,即所谓的"组织预处理"现象[18-19]。直肠扩张的本质在于其稳定的黏弹性,即软组织突然受压的能力,扩张初期直肠内容积在低压力状态下快速增加,这是直肠自身顺应性的标志,随后进入压力-容积曲线的平台期,此时容积更大,扩张的阻力来自直肠内结缔组织,代表直肠的容积或渐进顺应性。这两种顺应性彼此不相关,最后的报告取决于计算的那个顺应性。

这样的检测是基于器官均质性的基础上,即所有的组分(黏膜层、黏膜下层、黏膜肌层、固有肌层和浆膜层)具有相似的机械特性,而与压力来自的方向无关。在胃肠道上述假设不成立,因为组织是非均质性的[20]。可膨胀球囊的表面必须与要膨胀的器官完全接触,因此球囊必须足够大,它本身的弹性才不会影响检测结果,同时球囊的滞后现象也被忽略不计。球囊的大小和力学特征很重要,短球囊提供局限的膨胀刺激,可模拟直肠内的粪团;大球囊(或小且顺应性好的球囊)可以延伸,从而提供足够大的容积变化,虽有形状改变,但不对压力产生影响,提示容积测定作为一项参数,其评估意义可能不如 CSA 测定。

然而生物工程学方法非常复杂,并且包括许多肠道相关的物理学术语,如张力(描述形变)、压力(描述标准的力)和刚度(弹性系数),从理论上讲,将这些参数和特异的直肠疾病联系起来很有价值,如直肠炎影响肠壁刚度。Gregersen[14-15]指出直肠膨胀时主要的压力计算公式为:$\tau = \Delta P r / h$,其中 τ 为压力,ΔP 为透壁压力,r 为腔内半径,h 为肠壁厚度,可以是直肠壁的原始厚度或变形之后的肠壁厚度。这个方程式就是所谓的拉普拉斯定律[21],可对形状规则、均匀材质进行压力检测。拉普拉斯定律很复杂,假定肠壁上所有点的张力相同,直肠内压力变化与肠壁外压力平衡,且直肠的长宽比值较高,因此在体内环境下是不切实际的。该定律也没有考虑直肠在体内的形状,并假定直肠壁很薄,在膨胀过程中没有僵硬的弯曲,但直肠与刻板的圆柱体、椭圆形和球形[22]不同。在不同情况下,尤其是疾病状态,直肠壁的刚度、直肠容积、肠壁厚度不同,因此应用同样的顺应性评估方法不准确。

张力和压力是向各个方向的,肠管扩张时暴露在压力负荷中,直肠圆周上的压力增加、肠壁变薄、肠壁延展,后者是与肠壁性质相关,因此变形后会出现力的三维构成,即正、负张力及切应力,在压力（σ）和张力（ε）间产生一个比例常数，这就是弹性系数，即 Young 系数，为生物工程学参数，反应 σ 随 ε 变化的速度，是从胡克定律（Hooke's law）衍生而来，该定律适用于可变形的弹性材料，σ/ε 呈线性关系。弹性力学的 Young 系数依赖于直肠所受的力、直肠初始的 CSA、变形后变化的长度及变形前初始长度，但有些参数在体内是无法测量的，由于人体组织的各向异性，该系数在体内为非线性关系，不容易定义其压缩性（横向收缩、轴向压缩）。非线性实际上容易伸展性，体内正常生理条件下粪团运输时，肠腔内压力升高，防止直肠不可逆性变形。为了确定人类直肠的这种非线性关系，需根据任何压力下两测量点间增加的张力来计算增加的弹性系数，确定中空器官的有效刚度，建立能对直肠机械特性进行更准确描述的方程式[23]。每一个系数都是在生物材料经过预处理和滞后现象进行检验，施加于生物组织如直肠的张力和压力是时间依赖性的，不可能瞬间施加或消除，后者会引发压力松弛（突然膨胀后压力随时间降低）和蠕变（快速施加压力后持续变形）。上述任一在生物组织上发生的现象（压力松弛、蠕变、滞后现象）都是组织自身黏滞性特征，在正常人和患者的直肠均可发现。

鉴于直肠顺应性检测的局限性和较差的可重复性，人们试图寻找其他可以客观评估直肠刚度和容积的指标。阻抗面积描计法（IP）是一项用于检测中空脏器腔内 CSA 的技术，通过逐渐向有顺应性的球囊内注入导电液体，记录两个电极间的电阻[24]，这个方法是基于欧姆定律，即磁场衰变原理，最初是 Harris 等[25] 将其应用于评估输尿管尿流，将针形电极刺入输尿管，在电极之间通电，电压与腔内 CSA 呈相反的变化趋势。后来 Mortensen 等[26] 采用了一个球囊，将电流限制在球囊装置内的液体里。Gregersen 等[27] 对这一装置进一步改造，用以测量猪直肠的电阻，后逐步应用于人类直肠[28]。后来这种装置商品化（GMC，APS Hornslet，丹麦），但其主要用于科研，采用特殊设计的多电极导管，可测量阻抗，长约 20cm，外附有球囊，同时给予连续的交流电，测量阻抗的电极位于中间，在兴奋电极之间。IP 应用的导管是中空的聚乙烯氯化物或聚氨酯管，内附有压力传感器。大多数装置的导管外都有 4 个不锈钢环形电极，通过向球囊内注入恒温、低浓度、低传导性的盐水（将生理盐水用蒸馏水稀释 1000 倍）来记录 CSA。环形电极和压力感受器与记录装置、电脑相连，可实时记录数据，CSA 是通过计算球囊内液体阻抗来计算获得[29]，并应用于胃肠道的各个部分[30]。

在 IP 测量中应用欧姆定律，测量导管上排列多个电极，并在一定容积的导体内接入交流电，计算公式为 $V=I \cdot Z$，V 为电压，I 为电流，Z 为液体阻抗。在检测电极周围产生均匀的电场，电场强度与电极间距离及液体导电性相关，因所有的参数均可保持恒定，可得出 $V=\kappa CSA^{-1}$，在 IP 系统中测得的电压与 CSA 呈反比。这种装置对低阻抗的膨胀液体、电流强度的稳定性和导管的位置提出了几个重要的假设；探针应采取中轴线的位置；对球囊性质也有几个基本假设：球囊应该足够大、囊壁薄、不可延伸、不导电、低弯曲硬度及膨胀时较小的线性挤压度。考虑到这些局限性，IP 检测时直肠内复杂的几何形状较顺应性对检测结果影响小，后者主要检测直肠硬度和容积。

IP 中提供的数据可通过最小二乘法来标绘，从而建立指数关系，曲线的斜率即弹性（E），表示直肠膨胀时的关系，提供一个描述直肠膨胀及其黏弹性的数学模型[31-33]。IP 仍处于实验阶段，临床中在直肠顺应性检测中获得的直肠压力要低于 IP 检测的数据，这可能反映了两种检测技术不同的膨胀方法，最大 CSA 的变异及其与直肠感觉、最大耐受量之间的关系[34-35]。Dall 等[28] 最初研究正常的直肠，并建立了研究方法，后这些方法逐渐用于临床，对大便失禁[36]、排便功能障碍[37] 以及脊髓损伤患者[38-39] 进行研究。有证据显示脊髓或马尾损伤后直肠张力增高，提示中枢神经的脊髓抑制作用，也提示了骶神经调节治疗的一个中枢神经机制。

此外，还有一项商业化的临床应用技术，即恒压装置，最初是由 Whitehead 和 Delveaux[40] 设计的，用于评估直肠均匀膨胀时压力 - 容积特性及直肠感觉间的联系，从而试图确定直肠壁刚度与容积。该技术应用一个薄壁的聚乙烯直肠球囊，利用电子扩张技术将其扩张至一定容积，通过计算机控制的膨胀反馈系统，调节压力在 $0 \sim 40$mmHg 之间变化时扩张的球囊产生最小的变化，扩张刺激可以通过控制容积或者压力来完成。球囊被认为有无限的顺应性，可通过持续或阶梯式扩张方式，恒压装置在反馈机制下维持一恒定压力，从而来检查膨胀循环中压力 – 容积特性[41]。该设备作为一个等压的容积装置，在扩张容积的每一步维持压力平衡，可获得一"S"形曲线，曲线和直肠初始感觉、初始排便感觉、最大耐受量相关[42]。曲线的起始部表示直肠肌肉对被动膨胀时反应性收缩，随膨胀增加收缩活动减弱，反应肠道结缔组织的被动张力。恒压球囊内体积受直肠容积的限制，任何压力下球囊内体积是用标准化直肠体积（直肠容积 – 测量的直肠体积/直肠容积）来表示。这个参数和IP检查中的张力（σ）有些类似，是一个比直肠顺应性更有用的参数。

在正常环境中恒压装置下的压力 – 容积曲线与性别、体重指数或年龄无关，在40mmHg压力下直肠容积和顺应性与容积变更的校正直接相关，可使测得直肠顺应性的标准差降低，提示该参数更加可靠、可重复性好。在正常患者中，恒压方法测得的直肠容积不受恒压膨胀的连续性、速率或类型影响。研究发现餐后直肠内球囊体积呈标准化降低[43]，并可预测药物作用后张力变化的幅度，如新斯的明可增加局部收缩、胰高血糖素可产生相反的作用，阿托品对肛管近远端产生不同的抑制作用。

恒压装置对直肠疾病的诊断尚缺乏特异性。大便失禁患者直肠膨胀时的收缩反应不具有速率依赖性，在较低的感觉阈值下增加膨胀的持续时间，且与对照组相比直肠容积和顺应性均显著降低[44]。骶神经调节治疗后，恒压法测得的初始感觉阈值、初始排便感觉阈值和最大耐受量均有所降低，同时所有灌注感觉的压力阈值和张力均降低，但对顺应性没有显著作用，提示恒压装置在确定骶神经调节治疗后感觉功能改善方面起到重要作用[45]。通过恒压装置，我们发现顽固性便秘直肠感觉功能受损及顺应性改变，但这一发现并非普遍现象[46]，可能有助于便秘患者的分类，特发性慢传输型便秘有直肠感觉和顺应性改变，但耻骨直肠肌矛盾收缩有直肠敏感性增加、缺乏顺应性改变[9]。应用恒压装置对全直肠系膜切除直肠重建术后直肠容积评估，发现术后1年顺应性逐渐改善，与术后早期阵发性排便急迫和大便失禁没有显著联系[47]；而术后晚期发展的大便失禁与新直肠容积下降及RAIR缺失有关，通常发生在肛门括约肌功能减弱之前。利用恒压装置随访经肛门内镜微创手术（TEMS）术后患者时，会发现直肠顺应性改变，即使在RAIR、直肠敏感性和肛管静息压恢复后顺应性仍未恢复[48]，也许这可以解释在TEMS后只有3/4的患者能完全恢复粪便自制。可能提示TEMS后发生大便失禁的因素包括术前IAS缺陷、术前静息压低、全层TEMS切除、超过50%的环形切除等，但目前这些术前检查结果能否预测TEMS术后大便失禁的发生尚不明确[49]。

这些新设备的原理虽然相似，但需利用不同的假设，如恒压装置利用无限顺应性的大球囊，在一定范围压力内检测囊内体积，从而反映直肠受阶梯式膨胀后其生物力学特性。膨胀早期直肠内体积在低压力状态下快速增加，可以感受到直肠松弛；达到直肠容积后直肠顺应性即为压力 – 容积曲线的最大斜率，这一模型建立在直肠的几何形状不影响结果的假设之上。目前在大便失禁者中发现恒压结果差异包括低容积下直肠僵硬、扩张直肠时的收缩反应（与速率无关）、感知时间的增加、不同扩张速率效应不同、直肠容积和顺应性降低、直肠可扩张性降低、感觉阈值降低及感觉期延长。近期恒压结果显示肠易激综合征[50]患者的静息顺应性差异显著，痔切除术后直肠的膨胀性和感觉会显著降低[51-52]，克罗恩病患者直肠感觉阈值显著改变，即使是在睡眠时[53]。最近，应用类似的检测方法来评估肛管的膨胀性及刚性，称为反射测量仪，证实了肛管的黏弹性，原理是通过高度顺应性的聚氨酯球囊，将其绑在数字信号传感器上，向球囊内发送带状声波，反射回来的声波通过扩音器接受，再通过Waki公式来计算CSA[54]。该装置检测显示肛管有一个滞后的环，对突然扩张的刺激具有抵抗作用，在随访放射性直肠炎及结肠肛管吻合术后均发现其重要性[55]。

图6.3a显示IP人用系统，图6.3b显示临床IP测量中CSA和压力曲线。

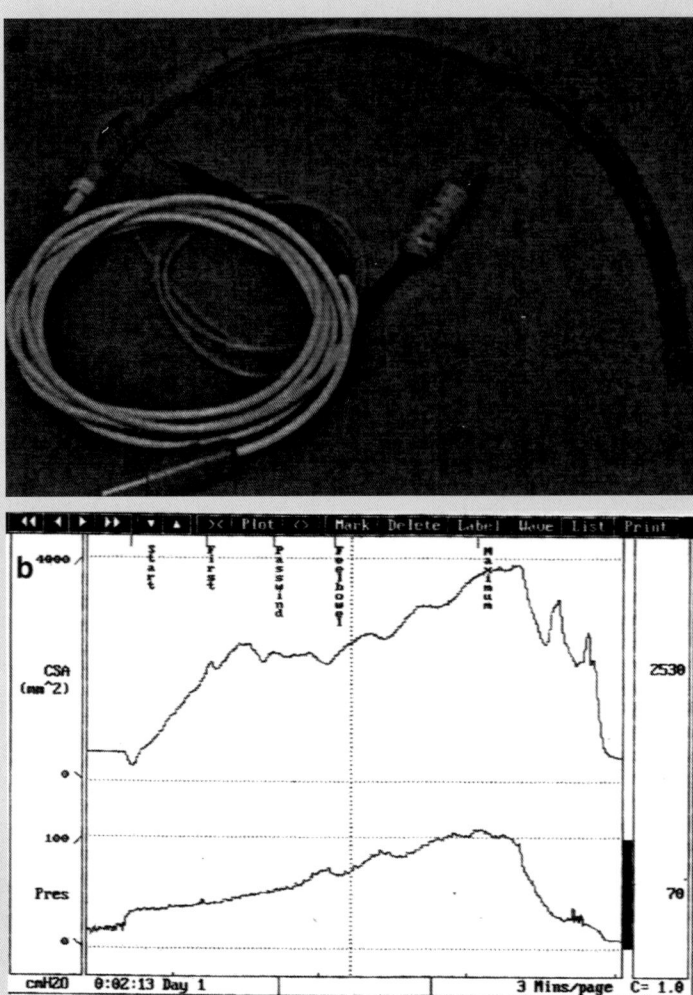

图 6.3 （a）示人用 IP 系统；（b）示临床应用 IP 系统、CSA 及压力变化曲线（Reprinted with permission from Duthie and Gardiner.[77]）

参考文献

1. Varma JS, Smith AN. Reproducibility of the proctometrogram. Gut. 1986; 27:288–92.
2. Kendall GP, Thompson DG, Day SJ, Lennard-Jones JE. Inter- and intra-individual variation in pressure-volume relations of the rectum in normal subjects and patients with irritable bowel syndrome. Gut. 1990;31:1062–8.
3. Varma JS, Smith AN, Busuttil A. Correlation of clinical and manometric abnormalities of rectal function following chronic radiation injury. Br J Surg. 1985;72:875–8.
4. Sorensen M, Rasmussen OO, Tetzschner T, Christiansen J. Physiological variation in rectal compliance. Br J Surg. 1992;79:1106–8.
5. Suzuki H, Fujioka M. Rectal pressure and rectal compliance in ulcerative colitis. Jpn J Surg. 1982;12:79–81.
6. Rasmussen O, Christensen B, Sorensen M, Tetzschner T, Chritiansen J. Rectal compliance in the assessment of patients with fecal incontinence. Dis Colon Rectum. 1990;33:650–3.
7. Felt-Bersma RJ, Sloots CE, Poen AC, Cuesta MA, Meuwissen SG. Rectal compliance as a routine measurement: extreme volumes have direct clinical impact and normal values exclude rectum as a problem. Dis Colon Rectum. 2000;43:1732–8.
8. Madoff RD, Orrom WJ, Rothenberger DA, Goldberg SM. Rectal compliance: a critical appraisal. Int J Colorectal Dis. 1990;5:37–40.
9. Toma TP, Zighelboim J, Phillips SF, Talley NJ. Methods for studying intestinal sensitivity and compliance: in vitro studies of balloons and a barostat. Neurogastroenterol Motil. 1996;8:19–28.
10. Krogh K, Ryhammer AM, Lundby L, Gregersen H, Lauerberg TS. Comparison of methods used for measurement of rectal compliance. Dis Colon Rectum. 2001;44:199–206.
11. Madoff RD, Shelton AA. Clinical rectal compliance measurement. In: Wexner SD, Zbar AP, Pescatori M, editors. Complex anorectal disorders: investigation and management. London: Springer; 2005. p. 63–71.
12. Rao GN. Evaluation of rectal dynamics and viscoelasticity in health and disease [MD Thesis]. University of Hull, Cottingham, United Kingdom; 1998.

13. Thayer ML, Madoff RD, Jacobs DM, Bubrick MP. Comparative intrinsic and extrinsic compliance: characteristics of S, J and W ileoanal pouches. Dis Colon Rectum. 1991;34:404–8.
14. Gregersen H, Kassab G. Biomechanics of the gastrointestinal tract. Neurogastroenterol Motil. 1996;8(4):277–97.
15. Gregersen H, Barlow J, Thompson DG. Development of a computer-controlled tensiometer for real-time measurements of tension in tubular organs. Neurogastroenterol Motil. 1999;11:109–18.
16. Dal Lago A, Minetti AE, Biondetti P, Corsetti M, Basilisco G. Magnetic resonance imaging of the rectum during distension. Dis Colon Rectum. 2005; 48:1220–7.
17. Frokjaer JB, Liao D, Bergmann A, McMahon BP, Steffensen E, Drewes AM, et al. Three-dimensional biomechanical properties of the human rectum evaluated with magnetic resonance imaging. Neurogastroenterol Motil. 2005;17:531–40.
18. Bouchoucha M, Jais JP, Arhan P, Landais P, Faverdin CL, Pellerin D. Variation of rheological properties of the human rectal wall with distending volume. Clin Invest Med. 1994;17:107–14.
19. Arhan P, Faverdin C, Persoz B, Devroede G, Dubois F, Dornic C, et al. Relationship between viscoelastic properties of the rectum and anal pressure in man. J Appl Physiol. 1976;41(5 Pt 1):677–82.
20. Sacks MS, Sun W. Multiaxial mechanical behavior of biological materials. Annu Rev Biomed Eng. 2003;5:251–84.
21. Richeson AW. Laplace's contribution to pure mathematics. Natl Math Mag. 1942;17:73–8.
22. Regen DM. Tensions and stresses of ellipsoidal chambers. Ann Biomed Eng. 1996;24:400–17.
23. Rao GN, Drew PJ, Monson JRT, Duthie GS. Incremental elastic modulus – a challenge to compliance. Int J Colorectal Dis. 1997;12:33–6.
24. Gregersen H, Andersen MB. Impedance measuring system for quantification of cross-sectional area in the gastrointestinal tract. Med Biol Eng Comput. 1991;29:108–10.
25. Harris JH, Thirkelsen EE, Zinner NR. Electrical measurement of ureteral flow. In: Boyarsky S, Tanagho EA, Gottschalk CW, Zimskind PD, editors. Urodynamics. London: Academic Press; 1971. p. 465–72.
26. Colstrup H, Mortensen SO, Kristensen JK. A probe for measurements of related cross-sectional area and pressure in the resting female urethra. Urol Res. 1983;11:139–43.
27. Dall FH, Jørgensen CS, Djurhuus JC, Gregeresen H. Biomechanical wall properties of the porcine rectum: a study using impedance planimetry. Dig Dis Sci. 1991;9:346–52.
28. Dall FH, Jørgensen CS, Houe D, Gregeresen H, Djurhuus JC. Biomechanical wall properties of the human rectum. A study with impedance planimetry. Gut. 1993;34:1581–6.
29. Gregersen H, Djurhuus JC. Impedance planimetry. A new approach to biomechanical wall properties in the intestine. Dig Dis. 1991;9:332–40.
30. Gregersen H, Stodkilde-Jorgensen H, Djurhuus JC, Mortensen SO. The four electrode impedance technique: a method for investigation of compliance in luminal organs. Clin Phys Physiol Meas 1988;9(Suppl A):61–4.
31. Andersen MB, Stodkilde-Jorgensen H, Gregersen H. Versatile software system for analysis of gastrointestinal pressure recordings. Dig Dis Sci. 1991;9:382–8.
32. Rao GN, Drew PJ, Monson JRT, Duthie GS. Physiology of rectal sensations: a mathematic approach. Dis Colon Rectum. 1997;40:298–306.
33. Gregersen H. Impedance planimetry: application for studies of rectal function. In: Wexner SD, Zbar AP, Pescatori M, editors. Complex anorectal disorders: investigation and management. London: Springer-Verlag; 2005. p. 72–104.
34. Zbar A. Compliance and capacity of the normal human rectum – physical considerations and measurement pitfalls. Acta Chir Iugosl. 2007;54:49–57.
35. Duthie GS, Gardiner AB. Clinical impedance planimetry. In: Wexner SD, Zbar AP, Pescatori M, editors. Complex anorectal disorders: investigation and management. London: Springer-Verlag; 2005. p. 105–13.
36. Salveoli B, Bharucha AE, Rath-Harvey D, Pemberton JH, Phillips SF. Rectal compliance, capacity and rectoanal sensation in fecal incontinence. Am J Gastroenterol. 2001;96:58–68.
37. Gosselink MJ, Hop WCJ, Schouten WR. Rectal compliance in females with obstructed defecation. Dis Colon Rectum. 2001;44:991–7.
38. Krogh K. Colorectal function in patients with spinal cord lesions [Thesis]. Aarhus University, Aarhus, Denmark; 2000.
39. Zbar AP. The role of impedance planimetry in anorectal assessment. Dis Colon Rectum 2008;51:1584–5; author reply 1586. Epub 2008 Aug 1.
40. Whitehead WE, Delveaux M. Standardization of barostat procedures for testing smooth muscle and sensory thresholds in the gastrointestinal tract. The Working Team of Glaxo-Wellcome Research, UK. Dig Dis Sci. 1997;42: 223–41.
41. Bell AM, Pemberton JH, Zinsmeister AR. Variations in muscle tone of the human rectum: recordings with an electromechanical barostat. Am J Physiol. 1991;260:G17–25.
42. Fox M, Thumshirn M, Fried M, Schwizer W. Barostat measurement of rectal compliance and capacity. Dis Colon Rectum. 2006;49:360–70.
43. Bharucha AE, Dhamija S, Japp A, Seide B, Walters B, Stroetz R, et al. Contractile response to colonic distension is influenced by oscillation frequency. Neurogastroenterol Motil. 2005;17:64–75.
44. Bharucha AE, Fletcher JG, Seide B, Riederer SJ, Zinsmeister AR. Phenotypic variation in functional disorders of defecation. Gastroenterology. 2005;128:1199–210.
45. Bharucha AE, Fletcher JG, Harper CM, Hough D, Daube JR, Stevens C, et al. Relationship between symptoms and disordered continence mechanisms in women with idiopathic faecal incontinence. Gut. 2005;54:546–55.
46. Iludag O, Morren GL, Dejong CH, Baeten CG. Effect of sacral neuromodulation on the rectum. Br J Surg. 2005;92:1017–23.
47. Mochiki E, Nakabayashi T, Suzuki H, Haga N, Fujita K, Asao T, et al. Barostat examination of proximal site of the anastomosis in patients with rectal cancer after low anterior resection. World J Surg. 2001;25:1377–82.
48. Herman RM, Richter P, Walega P, Popiela T. Anorectal sphincter function and rectal barostat study in patients following transanal endoscopic microsurgery. Int J Colorectal Dis. 2001;16:370–6.

49. Kennedy ML, Lubowski DZ, King DW. Transanal endoscopic microsurgery excision: is anorectal function compromised? Dis Colon Rectum. 2002;45:601–4.
50. Gregersen H, Liao D. New perspectives of studying gastrointestinal muscle function. World J Gastroenterol. 2006;12:2864–9.
51. Park JH, Baek YH, Park DI, Kim HJ, Cho YK, Sohn CI, et al. Analysis of rectal dynamic and static compliances in patients with irritable bowel syndrome. Int J Colorectal Dis. 2008;23:659–64.
52. Filho FL, Macedo GM, Dos Santos AA, Rodrigues LV, Oliveira RB, Nobre E Souza MA. Stapled haemorrhoidopexy transiently decreases rectal compliance and sensitivity. Colorectal Dis. 2011;13:219–24.
53. Faure C, Giguère L. Functional gastrointestinal disorders and visceral hypersensitivity in children and adolescents suffering from Crohn's disease. Inflamm Bowel Dis. 2008;14:1569–74.
54. Mitchell PJ, Klarskov N, Hosker G, Lose G, Kiff ES. Anal acoustic reflectometry: a new technique for assessing anal sphincter function. Colorectal Dis. 2010;12:692–7.
55. Mitchell PJ, Klarskov N, Telford KJ, Hosker GL, Lose G, Kiff ES. Anal acoustic reflectometry: a new reproducible technique providing physiological assessment of anal sphincter function. Dis Colon Rectum. 2011;54:1122–8.

排便刺激实验

被检测者要求努力排出模拟粪便，同时记录排便时间。通常采取盐水控便及球囊排出的形式，分别用以评估粪便自制机制及有无排便梗阻。

盐水控便试验及球囊排出试验

盐水控便试验试图将 800ml 生理盐水注入直肠内，记录肛门开始漏水时（漏水超过 10ml）注水的容积，计算注水量与漏水量的差值，计算公式为：保留百分比 = 保留的盐水体积 / 注入的盐水体积 × 100。

盐水注入试验在临床上未能广泛应用，在大便失禁[27]或间歇性漏粪[28]的直肠炎患者中存在显著的肛管重叠反应，但盐水注入实验对 RAIR 和松弛的 EAS 收缩有作用，可刺激主要控便机制的恢复[26]。球囊排出试验结果在排便功能障碍患者中有差异，但尚不足以辨别排便梗阻综合征（ODS）和盆底失迟缓。对那些没有临床异常检查结果或盆底异常的排便困难患者也许有意义[29]；同时，每个肛肠中心需要建立各自的正常参考值[30-31]。

单元推荐

测压在直肠重建及直肠脱垂治疗中的应用

大多数子宫脱垂患者会伴有不同程度的大便失禁，当其咨询直肠切除术后疗效时，术前测压检查非常必要，尤其是对年轻或生活方式多样的患者，文献报道直肠脱垂患者术前最大收缩压 >60mmHg 者，将近 90% 术后可取得预期效果，而术前最大收缩压 <60mmHg 者最好只进行脱垂的局部纠正治疗，这样不损伤直肠的贮便功能，不会出现术中（如直肠固定术）进一步损伤括约肌的风险。并非所有测压结果低于正常者在经会阴直肠切除术后排便功能均不能改善，但压力极低者或经 RAIR 证实 IAS 功能缺失者不宜行经会阴直肠切除术（阿尔特迈耶术）[32]。

评估直肠脱垂的参数包括 MBP、MSP、RAIR 和直肠感觉，Poen 等[33]研究发现，腹腔镜直肠固定术后 MBP 明显增高，但 MSP 术后没有显著改变，括约肌长度稍增加，但变化不显著。Delemarre 等[34]曾证实经腹直肠固定术后 MSP 增加，但该结果的改善与术后远期复发率无关。术后 MBP 增幅虽小，但较术前变化显著，提示 IAS 功能的恢复，控便功能显著改善。MAP 显著增加，提示 IAS 功能显著改善，也许是术后控便改善的因素之一。MBP（代表 IAS 功能）和 MSP（代表 EAS 功能）与大便失禁息息相关[35,36]。人们认为术后 MBP 的增加是由于直肠脱垂术后，成功切除脱垂的肠管，RAIR 的恢复所致[37]。脱垂患者肛管静息压降低，而直肠固定术后显著增加[36]，RAIR 术后由阴性恢复至阳性，且小容积即可诱导其产生。经腹腔镜直肠固定术后直肠敏感性没有显著变化，且排便正常及失禁患者间无显著差异。神经反射、EAS 和耻骨直肠肌的主动收缩与手术无显著联系[38]，详见第 51 章复发性直肠脱垂。

测压在混合痔及直肠出口梗阻中的应用

直肠前突和排便梗阻综合征（ODS）的主要测压表现为直肠低敏感性，具有重要的临床意义，在排便频次减少、排便障碍或两者均有的患者中 23% 表现为直肠低敏感，而没有便秘症状的患者中只有 5% 有类似表现。排便梗阻患者因直肠前突或直肠黏膜内套叠所致的机械性梗阻，使得直肠低敏感性表现更为突出，Reboa 等[39]研究发现纠正直肠前突可以使超过 90% 的患者直肠敏感性增加及恢复直肠感觉。

痔切除术后发现直肠敏感性也会改善、初始感觉阈值降低、收缩压增高。Reboa[39]还发现切除直肠壁的厚度与术后 RAIR 的诱发阈值呈反比；同时 Behboo 等[40]发现切除直肠壁的表面积与 RAIR 诱发阈值显著相关，提示直肠充盈感受器分布于直肠黏膜，切除直肠壁越多，RAIR 诱发阈值越高，部分吻合器黏膜切除术后排便急迫可能与之相关。

90% 的直肠前突患者手术纠正前突后直肠敏感性增加、直肠感觉阈值降低，前突未纠正的患者只有 44% 的表现敏感性增加，Boccasanta 等发现前突患者行吻合器下直肠切除术（STAAR）后也会出现直肠顺应性恢复及感觉阈值降低的现象[41]。这些现象说明直肠前突和（或）直肠黏膜内套叠纠正后，临床便秘评分也会出现极大的改善。相反，Renzi 等[42]对 68 例直肠前突患者行手术治疗，其中 61 例（89.7%）临床效果满意，但手术前后直肠敏感性没有显著差异。Frascio 等[43]也发现类似现象，术前直肠感觉阈值正常，而最大耐受量降低，提示直肠敏感性增加，似乎与 ODS 患者的表现相反；并且术后直肠感觉反射研究显示排便感觉阈值没有变化，但诱发腹痛的阈值明显增高，从压力测定的角度均提示直肠敏感性降低、ODS 症状加重。最近 Wong[44] 和 Suttor[45] 等发现，部分 ODS 患者伴有肠易激综合征的症状，这部分患者行 STARR 术后功能恢复要差。我们研究认为 STARR 手术前后肛门静息压和收缩压变化不显著，而直肠敏感性显著增加、球囊排出功能改善，提示成功排便能力的改善。

排便梗阻综合征（ODS）的测压表现和肛门痉挛

肛门痉挛可以引起或加重 ODS 症状，近来 Faried 等[46]通过对比生物反馈训练、注射肉毒毒素 A 及耻骨直肠肌部分切断术治疗肛门痉挛的疗效，发现在注射肉毒毒素 A 组中肛管松弛即静息压降低者占 75%，而生物反馈训练治疗组中仅占 55%，耻骨直肠肌部分切断术组中占 95%[31]。此项研究显示生物反馈训练效果有限，肉毒毒素 A 注射短期治疗效果好，耻骨直肠肌部分切断术有效率最高且并发症发生率低。

排便失禁的测压表现

粪便自制是在耻骨直肠肌、肛门括约肌、结肠运动和直肠肛管敏感性的综合作用下完成的。直肠肛管测压和肛门内超声是最有效的体外检测大便失禁的手段，Keating 等[47]对仅凭病史和体格检查诊断为大便失禁患者进行测压检查发现，19% 的诊断及 50% 的治疗需要更改，同样，Rao 等发现直肠肛管测压有助于了解大便失禁潜在的病例生理机制、指导个性化治疗[25]。测压检查还可以筛选能从生物反馈训练治疗中获益的患者，虽然许多研究均发现治疗前的测压结果与治疗效果间没有统计学意义[1]，这可能也反映了大便失禁复杂的病因学，括约肌功能仅仅是一个方面，直肠功能和敏感性、粪便性状、神经系统完整性及认知状态均对排便有影响。而且没有证据显示针对改善直肠敏感性（感觉训练）的恢复训练效果优于力量训练。测压检查能筛选出预测大便失禁预后的参数，评估生物反馈联合/不联合肛门电刺激治疗效果。通过直肠肛管测压结果和直肠敏感性阈值的变化来评估治疗效果，有研究显示生物反馈训练治疗较盆底训练更能增加肛管收缩压，且减少提肛时的腹部张力。

应用器械辅助是生物反馈治疗成功的必要手段。Solomon 等[48]研究发现直肠指检的同时进行语言反馈治疗仅适用于轻中度大便失禁患者，对重度失禁患者的疗效有待观察。良好的括约肌功能和轻中度失禁症状是提示生物反馈联合肛门电刺激治疗有效的预后指标，直肠敏感性改善也提示症状改善。虽然生物反馈及肛门电刺激治疗有助于直肠肛管功能恢复、改善括约肌收缩功能，部分研究显示经治疗失禁症状改善，但未发现静息压及 MSP 变化，人们对这些治疗的真正机制产生疑问。生物反馈治疗的临床效果与括约肌收缩功能的改变无关，提示保守治疗方法的非特异性效果，同时生物反馈恢复治疗不必像药物和健康－饮食－行为治疗那样一定要产生良好的功能结果[49]。

测压与骶神经刺激

骶神经刺激（SNS）（详见第 35 章）可以通过刺激盆底收缩而影响直肠感觉，从而改善大便失禁者的控便功能，Kenefick 和 Christiansen[50]通过前瞻性研究发现，SNS 可以提高静息压及收缩压，是盆底张力增加的表现，通过影响自主神经及体神经改变 IAS（自主神经支配）、EAS 及盆底（体神经支配）功能，但 SNS 确切的作用机制目前尚不清楚[51]。除了传出神经直接作用于运动神经元外，还与刺激位于盆底的张力感受器引发传入神经信号增强，传至脊髓及大脑有关，从而导致所有传至控便器官的传出刺激增强，Otto 等[52]研究认为 SNS 可影响直肠感觉，即感觉阈值、排便感觉和最大耐受量，在电刺激的过程中增加直肠内容积，但并不影响直肠内压力和顺应性；这提示 SNS 可引发直肠松弛，不影响直肠的弹力学特性，从而增加直肠容积，改善控便功能。

众所周知，进食通过胃结肠反射影响结直肠的动力，SNS 可以降低大便失禁者餐后直肠内张力，继而减弱胃结肠反射，但不影响直肠的位相性运动，Michelsen 等[53]发现 SNS 可以改变排便时结直肠传输时间，通过骶髓的副交感神经纤维影响左半结肠和直肠、迷走神经的副交感神经纤维影响右半结肠；SNS 还可以影响慢性特发性便秘患者的结肠运输功能，这些结果表明 SNS 不但通过骶神经根，而且通过中枢神经系统的脊上水平施加影响[53]。

测压在大便失禁外科治疗中的应用

对怀疑肛门括约肌损伤的患者，需进行影像学及神经肌肉功能学检测，了解其是否适宜行标准的手术修复治疗。在这种情况下肛门超声和直肠肛管测压检查互相补充，有助于确定大便失禁是解剖性或功能性，超声可以明确诊断括约肌损伤，而测压结果中静息压降低提示 IAS 缺陷，收缩压降低提示 EAS 缺陷，EAS 缺陷的程度和 MSP 呈负相关。Leeuw 等[54]对顺产或初次手术导致肛门括约肌损伤的患者研究发现，肛门测压和腔内超声的关系，以及其与患者特异的直肠肛管主诉间的相互关系提示，在行腔内超声检查后，测压几乎不能提供有助于治疗的额外信息。然而，对因分娩导致括肛门约肌损伤的患者进行随访发现，测压和腔内超声检测结果存在争议[55]，有些研究显示括约肌损伤后静息压和收缩压降低，而其他研究显示只有一项指标有差异或者均无差异[56]。肛门括约肌损伤伴或不伴不适主诉的患者之间肛门测压无差异，鉴于以上结果，对肛门括约肌损伤的患者进行直肠敏感性检测的临床意义有限[57]；肛门括约肌复合体的异常超声结果多提示分娩时肛门括约肌损伤，但研究结果之间也有一些矛盾，有些研究提示肛门内超声结果与肛门直肠不适主诉密切相关，而其他研究发现并没有这种联系。虽然大便失禁患者术前进行肛门测压及肛门内超声检查有助于治疗方案的制订，但术后测压结果的预后指示意义较差。括约肌修补术后可以发现测压的反常表现，如静息压、收缩压和肛管长度等，这些表现支持对括约肌严重缺陷及肛门张力差的患者进行括约肌重叠成形术。Gearhart 等[55]发现没有单一的测压参数可以预测括约肌成形术后的效果，但术前平均静息压、收缩压以及肛管长度与术后参数呈负相关。Zutshi 等[56]对手术治疗大便失禁患者术后行肛门测压检查发现，测压结果与大便失禁严重度评分、大便失禁生活质量评分无关，但括约肌修补术后大便失禁严重度评分降低、大便失禁生活质量评分升高[56]。Nordenstam 等[57]对因产伤行手术修补的绝经前的初产妇进行直肠肛门测压检查发现，直肠敏感性是大便失禁的主要因素。

括约肌重叠修补术后平均 MSP 和括约肌长度均增加，但只有收缩压的差异与功能性结果相关[58-59]。大便失禁的临床症状改善，与直肠肛管测压参数的显著变化不相关，Elton 和 Stoodley[59] 发现术后测压结果间没有显著差异，且许多研究中[60-61]术后测压结果间是矛盾的。虽然 Fleshman 等[62] 认为只要括约肌长度、平均静息压和 MSP 可以恢复正常，就可以维持良好的控便功能；Van Tets 和 Kuijpers 报道肛门括约肌修补术后 30%～40% 的患者排便功能改善，但与术后测压结果间的一致性较差，提示临床症状的改善最有可能是建立了局部的狭窄，或部分由于心理安慰作用[63]；Ooi 等[64] 发现术后排便"显著"改善的患者平均静息压、MSP 及平均括约肌长度也显著改善，而术后排便"轻度"改善的患者测压结果没有显著变化。临床症状显著改善与测压结果间没有任何联系，这种现象难以解释，提示在建立会阴体时仔细排列耻骨直肠肌和尾骨肌形成"会阴夹"而起到一定的作用，此外在括约肌重叠成形术中进行盆底筋膜成形术没有任何压力或临床症状改善[65]。

测压和肛瘘

肛瘘术后控便功能会受到较大影响，这是因为手术损伤括约肌，影响肛管的压力，肛门超声可以检测到。因此术前评估是否存在括约肌的缺陷非常重要，有助于适当手术方式的选择：肛瘘挂线或者肛瘘切开／切除术。Roig 等[66] 发现肛瘘术前伴有大便失禁者较不伴有者术后静息压降低更显著，而两组在 MSP 上没有区别。肛瘘术后失禁评分与平均静息压、MSP 降低密切相关，肛管长度在手术前后变化不显著。同时手术方式的选择会影响测压结果：肛瘘切开术可致静息压及收缩压均显著降低，肛瘘切除后立即进行括约肌修补可致 MSP 显著降低但不影响平均静息压，肛瘘挂线术、肛瘘切开术致平均静息压显著下降，不影响 MSP。肛瘘不伴有 IAS 损伤者较伴有者术后平均静息压降低更多，且平均静息压较后者更低；同样，肛瘘伴有 EAS 损伤者较不伴有或萎缩较轻者术后 MSP 低。

测压在回肠贮袋肛管吻合中的应用

术前评估静息压有助于外科医师向病患说明盆底贮袋术后预期结果，年龄和测压不是建立贮袋的禁忌。术前大便失禁可能与直肠活动性疾病有关，而回肠贮袋肛管吻合术（IPAA）后失禁没有急迫症状，多是由于括约肌功能不良。术前括约肌静息张力低与术后失禁有关，但围术期进行了许多研究，如肛门括约肌张力、贮袋顺应性、感觉以及阴部神经运动功能等，上述各项因素与术后失禁的关系尚不明确[67-69]，术前静息压低可能提示括约肌内在缺陷，但这种缺陷往往没有临床表现或因原发病的其他症状而被忽视。

Church 等[70] 发现术前肛管括约肌静息压越高，IPAA 术后压力降低幅度越大，较大的压力降低幅度与术后较差的功能性结果相关，术前和术后静息压有助于预测手术效果。围术期静息压远远大于 40mmHg 与 IPAA 术后良好功能及生活质量相关，但静息压低并不意味 IPAA 术后效果差。

测压在直肠切除治疗直肠癌的应用

直肠癌行括约肌保留的术式，术中需对盆底彻底游离，有可能损伤到括约肌或肛提肌，许多行低位前切除术的患者出现排便习惯改变[71]，同时术后肛管静息压降低，MSP 变化不大，大部分患者 RAIR 消失，但可逐渐恢复，所有患者直肠容积和顺应性降低[72]。Kakodkar 等[72] 认为 RAIR 的缺失、最大容积和高压带低于 5% 的正常值，均是术后功能差的独立危险因素。Koda[73] 等认为肛管长度与术后功能有关。三维测压检测的环形高压带可以作为保留括约肌的直肠癌根治术后括约肌损伤的指标，静息状态下环形高压带（≥20mmHg）的长度可作为术后严重排便功能不良（Wexner 评分超过 10）的指标[74]，直肠肛管测压与保留括约肌的直肠癌根治术后大便失禁的康复治疗有关。直肠低位前切除联合结肠肛管吻合术前后肛管压力变化不大，但临床评估提示 Wexner 失禁评分改善或恶化。

评论：再手术病例的直肠肛管测压检测

Andrew P. Zbar

直肠肛管测压在初次手术病例中的应用尚存争议，更不可能作为再手术或重建手术效果预判工具。从法医学的角度来说希望测压可提供客观的依据，尤其是在肛瘘外科治疗中括约肌有损伤风险者的测压记录，及 SNS 或生物反馈治疗成功的监测。然而没有数据来支持这种想法，许多中心放弃对 SNS 治疗者进行测压评估，因为该治疗主要依赖感觉反馈，目前尚不清楚个别测压参数能否预测治疗效果。现在还没有客观证据证明测压可以指导手术方式的选择，但直肠脱垂患者行经会阴直肠乙状结肠切除术及 ODS 患者行经肛门吻合器手术术后出现静息压降低及 RAIR 的缺失。目前，对伴有顽固性肛裂且已行局部手术治疗的直肠癌患者，是否保留括约肌还是依靠直觉，是否应在测压及超声指导下选择手术方式，还没有充足的证据[1]。

参考文献

1. Zbar AP. The role of functional evaluation before anorectal surgery. Società Italiana di Chirurgia ColoRettale. 2005;9:74–83. Position paper www.siccr.org.

参考文献

1. Sangwan YP, Coller JA, Schoetz Jr DJ, Murray JJ, Roberts PL, Rao SS, et al. How useful are manometric tests of anorectal function in the management of defecation disorders? Am J Gastroenterol. 1997;92:469–75.
2. Zbar AP, Kmiot WA. Anorectal investigation. In: Phillips RKS, editor. A companion to specialist surgical practice; colorectal surgery. 1st ed. London: WB Saunders; 1997. p. 1–33.
3. Schuster MM. Colon motility and anosphincteric manometric recordings by air-filled balloon technique. In: Smith LE, editor. Practical guide to anorectal testing. 2nd ed. New York: Igaku-Shoin; 1995. p. 37–50.
4. Smith LE. Practical guide to anorectal testing. 2nd ed. New York: Igaku-Shoin; 1995.
5. Harris LD, Winans CS, Pope CE. Determination of yield pressure: a method for measuring anal sphincter competence. Gastroenterology. 1996;50:754–60.
6. Brusciano L, Limongelli P, del Genio G, Rossetti G, Sansone S, Healey A, et al. Clinical and instrumental parameters in patients with constipation and incontinence: their potential implications in the functional aspects of these disorders. Int J Colorectal Dis. 2009;24:961–7.
7. Gruppo Lombardo per lo Studio della Motilita Intestinale. Anorectal manometry with water-perfused catheter in healthy adults with no functional bowel disorders. Colorectal Dis. 2009;12:220–5.
8. Jorge JMN, Wexner SD. Anorectal manometry: techniques and clinical applications. South Med J. 1993;86:924–31.
9. Marcello PW, Barrett RC, Coller JA, Schoetz Jr DJ, Roberts PL, Murray JJ, et al. Fatigue rate as a new measurement of external sphincter function. Dis Colon Rectum. 1998;41:336–43.
10. Brusciano L, Limongelli P, del Genio G, Sansone S, Rossetti G, Maffettone V, et al. Useful parameters helping proctologists to identify patients with defaecatory disorders that may be treated with pelvic floor rehabilitation. Tech Coloproctol. 2007;11:45–50.
11. Garavoglia M, Borghi F, Levi AC. Arrangement of the anal striated musculature. Dis Colon Rectum. 1993;36:10–5.
12. Farouk R, Duthie GS, Bartolo DCG. Functional anorectal disorders and physiological evaluation. In: Beck DE, Wexner SD, editors. Fundamentals of anorectal surgery. New York: McGraw-Hill; 1992. p. 173–83.
13. Lowry AC, Simmang CL, Boulos P, Farmer KC, Finan PJ, Hyman N, American Society of Colon and Rectal Surgeons; Association of Coloproctology of Great Britain and Ireland; Coloproctology Surgical Society of Australia, et al. Consensus statement of definitions for anorectal physiology and rectal cancer. Colorectal Dis. 2001;3:272–5.
14. Miller R, Bartolo DCC, Cervero F. Anorectal sampling: a comparison of normal and incontinent patients. Br J Surg. 1998;75:44–7.
15. Lane RH, Parks AG. Function of the anal sphincters following colo-anal anastomosis. Br J Surg. 1977;64:596–9.
16. O'Riordain MG, Molloy RG, Gillen P, Horgan A, Kirwan WO. Rectoanal inhibitory reflex following low stapled anterior resection of the rectum. Dis Colon Rectum. 1992;35:874–8.
17. Sangwan YP, Coller JA, Barrett RC, Murray JJ, Roberts PL, Schoetz Jr DJ. Distal rectoanal excitatory reflex: a reliable index of pudendal neuropathy. Dis Colon Rectum. 1995;38:916–22.
18. Sangwan YP, Coller JA, Schoetz Jr DJ, Murray JJ, Roberts PL. Latency measurement of rectoanal reflexes. Dis Colon Rectum. 1995;38:1281–5.
19. Kaur G, Gardiner A, Lee PW et al.; Increased sensitivity to the rectoanal reflex is seen in incontinent patients. Colorectal Dis. 1999; Suppl 1:39A–40A
20. Kaur G, Gardiner A, Duthie GS. Rectoanal reflex parameters in incontinence and constipation. Dis Colon Rectum. 2002;45:928–33.
21. Zbar AP, Aslam M, Gold DM, Gatzen C, Gosling A, et al. Parametrs of the rectoanal inhibitory reflex in patients with idiopathic fecal incontinence and chronic constipation. Dis Colon Rectum. 1998;41:200–8.
22. Sagar PM, Holdsworth PJ, Johnston D. Correlation between laboratory findings and clinical outcome after restorative proctocolectomy: serial studies in 20 patients with end-to-end pouch anal anastomosis. Br J Surg. 1991;78:67–70.
23. Horgan AF, Molloy RG, Coulter J, Sheehan M, Kirwan WO. Nerve regeneration across colorectal anastomosis after low anterior resec-

tion in a canine model. Int J Colorectal Dis. 1993;8:167–9.
24. Satish SC, Rao SS. Constipation: evaluation and treatment of colonic and anorectal motility disorders. Gastrointest Endosc Clin N Am. 2009;19:117–39.
25. Rao SS, Hatfield R, Soffer E, Rao S, Beaty J, Conklin JL. Manometric tests of anorectal function in healthy adults. Am J Gastroenterol. 1999;94:773–83.
26. Haynes WG, Read NW. Ano-rectal activity in man during rectal infusion of saline: a dynamic assessment of the anal continence mechanism. J Physiol. 1982;330:45–56.
27. Read NW, Haynes WG, Bartolo DC, Hall J, Read MG, Donnelly TC, et al. Use of anorectal manometry during rectal infusion of saline to investigate sphincter function in incontinent patients. Gastroenterology. 1983;85:105–13.
28. Rao SS, Read NW, Stobart JA, Haynes WG, Benjamin S, Holdsworth CD. Anorectal contractility under basal conditions and during rectal infusion of saline in ulcerative colitis. Gut. 1988;29:769–77.
29. Bordeianou L, Savitt L, Dursun A. Measurements of pelvic floor dyssynergia: which test result matters? Dis Colon Rectum. 2011; 54:60–5.
30. Fleshman JW, Dreznik Z, Cohen E, Fry RD, Kodner IJ. Balloon expulsion test facilitates diagnosis of pelvic floor outlet obstruction due to nonrelaxing puborectalis muscle. Dis Colon Rectum. 1992;35:1019–25.
31. Dedeli O, Turan I, Öztürk R, Bor S. Normative values of the balloon expulsion test in healthy adults. Turk J Gastroenterol. 2007; 18:177–81.
32. Glasgow SC, Birnbaum EH, Kodner IJ, Fleshman JW, Dietz DW. Preoperative anal manometry predicts continence after perineal proctectomy for rectal prolapse. Dis Colon Rectum. 2006;49:1052–8.
33. Poen AC, De Brauw M, Felt-Bersma RJF, de Jong D, Cuesta MA. Laparoscopic rectopexy for complete rectal prolapse. Clinical outcome and anorectal function tests. Surg Endosc. 1996;10:904–8.
34. Delemarre JB, Gooszen HG, Kruyt RH, Soebhag R, Geesteranus AM. The effect of posterior rectopexy on fecal continence. A prospective study. Dis Colon Rectum. 1991;34:311–6.
35. Brodon G, Dolk A, Holmström B. Recovery of the internal anal sphincter following rectopexy: a possible explanation for continence improvement. Int J Colorectal Dis. 1988;3:23–8.
36. Felt-Bersma RJF, Klinkenberg-Knol EC, Meuwissen SGM, Felt-Bersma RJF, Klinkenberg-Knol EC, Meuwissen SGM, Felt-Bersma RJF, Klinkenberg-Knol EC, Meuwissen SGM. Anorectal function investigations in incontinent and continent patients. Differences and discriminatory value. Dis Colon Rectum. 1990; 33:479–86.
37. Zbar AP, Takashima S, Hasegawa T, Kitabayashi K. Perineal rectosigmoidectomy (Altemeier's procedure): a review of physiology, technique and outcome. Tech Coloproctol. 2002;6:109–16.
38. Madden MV, Kamm MA, Nicholls RJ, Santhanam AN, Cabot R, Speakman CT. Abdominal rectopexy for complete prolapse: prospective study evaluating changes in symptoms and anorectal function. Dis Colon Rectum. 1992;35:48–55.
39. Reboa G, Gipponi M, Ligorio M, Marino P, Lantieri F. The impact of stapled transanal rectal resection on anorectal function in patients with obstructed defecation syndrome. Dis Colon Rectum. 2009; 52:1598–604.
40. Behboo R, Zanella S, Ruffolo C, Vafai M, Marino F, Scarpa M. Stapled haemorrhoidopexy: extent of tissue excision and clinical implications in the early postoperative period. Colorectal Dis. 2011;13(6):697–702. doi:10.1111/j.1463-1318.2010.02247.x. Epub 2010 Feb 24.
41. Boccasanta P, Venturi M, Salamina G, Cesana BM, Bernasconi F, Roviaro G. New trends in the surgical treatment of outlet obstruction: clinical and functional results of two novel transanal stapled techniques from a randomised controlled trial. Int J Colorectal Dis 2004;19:359–369.
42. Renzi A, Talento P, Giardiello C, Angelone G, Izzo D, Di Sarno G. Stapled trans-anal rectal resection (STARR) by a new dedicated device for the surgical treatment of obstructed defaecation syndrome caused by rectal intussusception and rectocele: early results of a multicenter prospective study. Int J Colorectal Dis. 2008;23:999–1005.
43. Frascio M, Stabilini C, Ricci B, Marino P, Fornaro R, De Salvo L, et al. Stapled transanal rectal resection for outlet obstruction syndrome: results and follow-up. World J Surg. 2008;32:1110–5.
44. Wong RK, Palsson OS, Turner MJ, Levy RL, Feld AD, von Korff M, et al. Inability of the Rome III criteria to distinguish functional constipation from constipation-subtype irritable bowel syndrome. Am J Gastroenterol. 2010;105:2228–34.
45. Suttor VP, Prott GM, Hansen RD, Kellow JE, Malcolm A. Evidence for pelvic floor dyssynergia in patients with irritable bowel syndrome. Dis Colon Rectum. 2010;53:156–60.
46. Faried M, El Nakeeb A, Youssef M, Omar W, El Monem HA. Comparative study between surgical and non-surgical treatment of anismus in patients with symptoms of obstructed defecation: a prospective randomized study. J Gastrointest Surg. 2010;14:1235–43.
47. Keating JP, Stewart PJ, Eyers AA, Warner D, Bokey EL. Are special investigations of value in the management of patients with fecal incontinence? Dis Colon Rectum. 1997;40:896–901.
48. Solomon MJ, Pager CK, Rex J, Roberts R, Manning J. Randomized, controlled trial of biofeedback with anal manometry, transanal ultrasound, or pelvic floor retraining with digital guidance alone in the treatment of mild to moderate fecal incontinence. Dis Colon Rectum. 2003;46:703–10.
49. Boselli AS, Pinta F, Cecchini S, Costi R, Marchesi F, Violi V, et al. Biofeedback therapy plus anal electrostimulation for fecal incontinence: prognostic factors and effects on anorectal physiology. World J Surg. 2010;34:815–21.
50. Kenefick NJ, Christiansen J. A review of sacral nerve stimulation for the treatment of faecal incontinence. Colorectal Dis. 2004;6:75–80.
51. Amend B, Matzel KE, Abrams P, de Groat WC, Sievert KD. How does neuromodulation work. Neurourol Urodyn. 2011;30:762–5. doi:10.1002/nau.21096.
52. Otto SD, Burmeister S, Buhr HJ, Kroesen A. Sacral nerve stimulation induces changes in the pelvic floor and rectum that improve continence and quality of life. J Gastrointest Surg. 2010;14:636–44.
53. Michelsen H-B, Worsoe J, Krogh K, Lundby L, Christensen P, Buntzen S, et al. Rectal motility after sacral nerve stimulation for faecal incontinence. Neurogastroenterol Motil. 2009;22:36–46.
54. de Leeuw JW, Vierhout ME, Struijk PC, Auwerda HJ, Bac DJ, Wallenburg HC. Anal sphincter damage after vaginal delivery relationship of anal endosonography and manometry to anorectal complaints. Dis Colon Rectum. 2002;8:1004–10.
55. Gearhart S, Hull T, Floruta C, Schroeder T, Hammel J. Anal manometric parameters: predictors of outcome following anal sphincter repair? J Gastrointest Surg. 2005;9:115–20.
56. Zutshi M, Salcedo L, Hammel J, Hull T. Anal physiology testing in fecal incontinence: is it of any value? Int J Colorectal Dis. 2010; 25:277–82.
57. Nordenstam JF, Altman DH, Mellgren AF, Rothenberger DA, Zetterström JP. Impaired rectal sensation at anal manometry is associated with anal incontinence one year after primary sphincter repair in primiparous women. Dis Colon Rectum. 2010;53:1409–14.
58. Ha HT, Fleshman JW, Smith M, Read TE, Kodner IJ, Birnbaum EH. Manometric squeeze pressure difference parallels functional outcome after overlapping sphincter reconstruction. Dis Colon Rectum. 2001;44:655–60.
59. Elton C, Stoodley BJ. Anterior anal sphincter repair: results in a district general hospital. Ann R Coll Surg Engl. 2002;84:321–4.
60. Sitzler PJ, Thompson JP. Overlap repair of damaged anal sphincter. A single surgeon's series. Dis Colon Rectum. 1996;39:1356–60.
61. Oliveira L, Pfeifer J, Wexner SD. Physiological and clinical outcome of anterior sphincteroplasty. Br J Surg. 1996;83:502–5.
62. Fleshman JW, Peters WR, Shemesh EL, Fry RD, Kodner IJ. Anal sphincter reconstruction: anterior overlapping muscle repair. Dis Colon Rectum. 1991;34:739–43.
63. Van Tets WF, Kuijpers JHC. Pelvic floor procedures produce no consistent changes in anatomy or physiology. Dis Colon Rectum. 1998;41:365–9.

64. Ooi BS, Tjandra JJ, Tang CL, et al. Anorectal physiology testing before and after a successful sphincter repair: a prospective study. Colorectal Dis. 2000;2:220–8.
65. Evans C, Davis K, Kumar D. Overlapping anal sphincter repair and anterior levatorplasty: effect of patient's age and duration of follow-up. Int J Colorectal Dis. 2006;21:795–801.
66. Roig JV, Jorda J, García-Armengol J, Esclapez P, Solana A. Changes in anorectal morphologic and functional parameters after fistula-in-ano surgery. Dis Colon Rectum. 2009;52:1462–9.
67. Nicholls RJ, Belliveau P, Neill M, Wilks M, Tabaqchali S. Restorative proctocolectomy with ileal reservoir: a pathophysiological assessment. Gut. 1981;22:462–8.
68. Nasmyth DG, Johnston D, Godwin PG, Dixon MF, Smith A, Williams NS. Factors influencing bowel function after ileal pouch–anal anastomosis. Br J Surg. 1986;73:469–73.
69. Scott NA, Pemberton JH, Barkel DC, Wolff BG. Anal and ileal pouch manometric measurements before ileostomy closure are related to functional outcome after ileal pouch–anal anastomosis. Br J Surg. 1989;76:613–6.
70. Church JM, Saad R, Schroeder T, Fazio VW, Lavery IC, Oakley JR, et al. Predicting the functional result of anastomoses to the anus: the paradox of preoperative anal resting pressure. Dis Colon Rectum. 1993;36:895–900.
71. Efthimiadis C, Basdanis G, Zatagias A, Tzeveleki I, Kosmidis C, Karamanlis E, et al. Manometric and clinical evaluation of patients after low anterior resection for rectal cancer. Tech Coloproctol. 2004;8 Suppl 1:205–7.
72. Kakodkar R, Gupta S, Nundy S. Low anterior resection with total mesorectal excision for rectal cancer: functional assessment and factors affecting outcome. Colorectal Dis. 2006;8:650–6.
73. Koda K, Yasuda H, Hirano A, Kosugi C, Suzuki M, Yamazaki M, et al. Evaluation of postoperative damage to anal sphincter/levator ani muscles with three-dimensional vector manometry after sphincter-preserving operation for rectal cancer. J Am Coll Surg. 2009;208:362–7.
74. Pucciani F, Ringressi MN, Redditi S, Masi A, Giani I. Rehabilitation of fecal incontinence after sphincter-saving surgery for rectal cancer: encouraging results. Dis Colon Rectum. 2008;51:1552–8.
75. Kumar D, Hallan RI, Womack NR, O'Connell PR, Miller R. Measurement of anorectal function, ch 3. In: Kumar D, Waldron DJ, Williams NS, editors. Clinical measurement in coloproctology. London: Springer; 1991. p 40.
76. Roberts PL. Rectoanal inhibition, ch 2.2. In: Wexner SD, Zbar AP, Pescatori M, editors. Complex anorectal disorders: investigation and management. London: Springer; 2005.
77. Duthie GS, Gardiner AB. Impedance planimetry: clinical impedance planimetry, Ch 2.5 (ii). In: Wexner SD, Zbar AP, Pescatori M, editors. Complex anorectal disorders: investigation and management. London: Springer; 2005.

第 7 章 再手术病例中向量测压和神经生理评估时的建议

Andrew P. Zbar

倪 玲译 姜 军审校

摘 要

历年来对于再手术患者进行肛门直肠的生理评估已减少；很明显的是功能预后与术前测压没有直接的相关性。本章介绍了向量测压和神经生理检测的解读技术和测定，以及评估时的局限性，尤其是对于再手术的病例。

关键词

向量测压；神经生理检测（NPT）；再手术；重建的；皮质体感诱发电位（CSSEPs）

向量测压

纵向压力的表面光度测定是标准尿动力学检查[1]的一部分，也是抗反流手术前后[2]评估下段食道括约肌的生理基础。然而，它在肛门直肠疾病[3]中应用很局限。Taylor等[4]为了规范男性和女性的肛门压力，最初记录了在肛管长度不同的患者中，肛管横截面上的纵向压力不对称。他们利用一种可滑动的双腔导管来同时测定纵向和径向的压力。在静息相和持续用力相，高压区（HPZ）的传统评估：高压区的长度代表了该部分括约肌承受压力超过了最大压力的50%，它最多只是大致反映了生理括约肌程度的中间水平，不能反映不同性别间的不对称，也不能反映患者已有的或产后肛门外括约肌（EAS）的缺陷。

最近介绍了一种引导传统肛门直肠测压（ARM）的自动化快速"拖出"方法用来减少功能性肛门括约肌长度的预计差异，后者通常会影响测量值[5-6]。这种叫作向量测压（VVM）的新式纵向压力表面光度测定技术，使用了一种直径为4.8mm的特制聚乙烯导管，并且有平均至少8个径向排列的扇形孔（前、右、后、左）；当使用的光流越大时，在导管撤退中得到的数据点越多，因此计算机软件得到用来创建肛门括约肌区的三维构象的数学插值就越少（Polygram Lower GI edition software 5.05, C4 version, Synectics Medical, Inc., Irving, TX），后者也叫作向量图。该计算机软件使用指定的向量计算将数据转换成一种三维的三联坐标，后者主要取决于探针的轴向位置。在这里，X和Y坐标记录在远离肛管中心点的角点，而Z轴是垂直的，因此对于任何给定的三维压力点有一个扇形压力多边形对应于向量体积，公式如下：

$$\text{向量体积} = \sum_{i=1}^{8/t=1} d \cdot \sin(45)\{P_1P_2 + P_2P_3 + P_2P_4 + \ldots\ldots P_8P_1\}$$

其中，1是肛缘以上水平的可记录压力，d是测量点之间的距离，P是各个扇形区的压力向量。sin（正弦）45用了8个不同的方向，而当有更多的方向时会有相应改变。因此，在指定的导管撤退速度上，没有一个体积参数代表向量多边形的总积分。计算机与一个高分辨率的监视屏相连，它有梯度调色板来建立一个颜色编码的可旋转向量图，用来评估图形缺口，后者代表了增加的总的扇形压力[7-8]。对于平均括约肌长度，当撤退速度为 1cm/s 时，样条曲线插值提供的平滑三维图上有平均 15 000 个独立数据点用来建立向量图。因此，当方向点增加时，数据插值减少，图像边缘更平滑。向量图也可以从开放的网状或固态设计中得到。图 7.1 展示了向量体积组成的物理原理。

对于健康人群[9]和患者[10]，几乎没有传统的肛门直肠测压和向量体积测压之间的对比。已有人

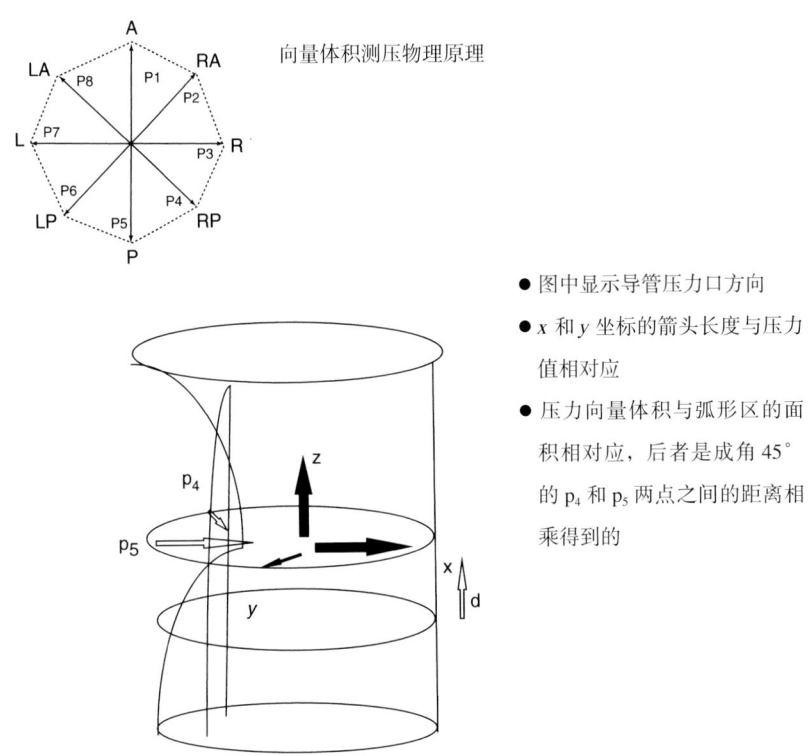

图 7.1 向量体积组成 / 测压的物理原理。使用 8 个不同方向径向排列的聚乙烯导管，在撤退速度恒定时，它提供一个 45°的扇形多边形的总压力，用来测定向量体积和建立向量图。L：左侧；LA：左前；LP：左后；A：前侧；RA：右前；R：右侧；RP：右后；P：后侧（Reproduced with permission from Zbar et al.[9]）

对比研究一般患者的传统肛门直肠测压和向量体积测压，如被动大便失禁、全层直肠脱垂、慢性肛裂，测量了平均静息向量体积（MRVV）、平均收缩向量体积（MSVV）、HPZ 长度（在静息和收缩时）、静息时的最大平均压（MR）、持续收缩时的最大平均压（MPS）和不对称百分比，后者是从完整圆圈中整合的截面百分偏差。扇形压力用来分析和建立右、左、前、后的平均压力。如预期所示，与传统的肛门直肠测压相比，在静息时和收缩时的 MRVV、MSVV、MPR、MPS 差异明显；然而，总体来讲，MPR 超过肛门静息压，MPS 低于平均收缩压。有可能在传统的肛门直肠测压中，当导管自动撤退时，肛门括约肌的自发收缩引起记录到的 MMPR 高于平均肛门静息压；也有可能是灌注泄漏引起。传统的肛门直肠测压中，MPS 值低于平均收缩压，可能反映了在向量体积技术中，持续充分地收缩有较大的难度（见下表）[11]。

尽管在大小便失禁并且有高张力的肛裂患者中有既定的扇形顺序，并且在肛裂患者前侧的扇形压力有增高的趋势，但是在不同的肛门直肠状况下并没有证据显示先天的扇形差异。有人研究了这些扇形的差异[12-14]，在图 7.2a, b 中显示。传统和向量体积的静息和收缩相关性差异证实，HPZ 长度的测量的两种方法间强烈相关（表 7.1）。然而，扇形不对称之间无相关性，并且有显著的肛门外括约肌(EAS)缺陷[15]，或在慢性肛裂患者肛门内括约肌（IAS）分离后[16]，尽管近期的研究数据显示 VVM 可以用来确定上述疾病患者直到肛管最后 1cm 的肛门外括

向量体积测压和传统测压之间在静息和最大收缩时的相关性和 P 值

	MRAP	MRVV	HPZ	MPR
MRVV	0.51 (<0.001)			
HPZ(length)	0.17 (0.07)	0.43 (<0.001)		
MPR	0.79 (<0.001)	0.70 (<0.001)	0.19 (0.05)	
Asymmetry (%)	−0.21 (0.027)	−0.24 (0.009)	−0.07 (0.45)	−0.29 (0.003)
	MSP	MSVV	HPZ	% asymmetry
MSVV	0.59 (<0.001)			
Asymmetry (%)	−0.13 (0.18)	−0.24 (0.01)		
HPZ(length)	−0.14 (0.14)	0.26 (0.006)		−0.04 (0.72)
MPS	0.86 (<0.001)	0.78 (<0.001)	−0.11 (0.26)	−0.19 (0.05)

MRVV：最大静息向量体积；HPZ：高压区（静息或最大收缩时）；MPR：静息时的平均向量体积压力；MSVV：平均收缩向量体积；MPS：收缩时的平均向量体积压力；MRAP：传统的平均肛门静息压；MSP：传统的平均收缩压

约肌缺陷[17-18]。似乎早期的超声不能确诊和修复的括约肌损伤，而 VVM 的超声图像使用有可能偏失了其最初目的[19-20]。进一步的近期研究数据显示，在总的向量静息参数，如静息时的 HPZ 长度和静息时的不对称百分比中有显著的差异；在局部抵抗慢性肛裂的肛门内括约肌分离的大多数收缩变量中也有差异[16]，或者是术后可控制和不可控制的排便患者，尤其是静息时的 HPZ 长度有显著的不同。后者显示肛门内括约肌切开术被大量施行，这在之前行超声内镜时可以观察到[21]，并且发现肛门内括约肌分离程度远远超过术前预计。在排便可控制的术后患者，静息不对称百分比趋势上升了 6.7%，而大便失禁的术后患者趋势下降了 3.1%。这些收缩参数的变化原因尚不清楚，但可以推测术后存在过多的括约肌自发疲劳（甚至在排便可控制的患者也是如此），此时因为直肠动力被忽视，内容物进入直肠后可发生泄漏。后面这种现象在"肛门直肠抽样调查"中被发现，在排气和排便中区别，这在第 6 章直肠肛门抑制反射中有讨论；并被认为是肛门内括约肌的功能之一[22]。也有人认为某些患者的皮下构成有缺陷，并且与肛门外括约肌的部分有重叠（这在某些肛裂患者术前行肛门内核磁共振显像时可以观察到[23]），因此，肛门内括约肌远端分离使得肛管远端无以支撑导致大便失禁，并且有可能伴随术后收缩功能缺陷[24]。此时，VVM 仍必须被看做是一种试验性检测，尽管它提供了一种有趣的方式来学习扇形括约肌的不对称性。这种仪器和软件很昂贵，并且没有广泛应用，但是作为一种测压工具，VVM 是很有效的[25]。可以想象，在未来使用这种仪器评估肛裂患者，可以确定哪些在肛门内括约肌被分离后功能较差，并且有助于确定保留括约肌术式的选择[26-27]。未来特定的参数评估可以描绘出功能不良的细微差别，它对应于在某些肛门直肠术后大便失禁的直接生物反馈治疗，可以更好地确定哪些患者更适合于直肠贮袋的重建，哪些不适合于因直肠脱垂行经会阴直肠乙状结肠切除术[28-30]。

神经生理检测

传统的肛管神经生理检测（NPT）由下面几部分组成：痛苦的同心针状肌电图（CNEMG）和单纤维肌电图（SFEMG）；肛门外括约肌修复手术中使用的一些技术。这其中也需要使用接触肌电图（EMG）来评估肛门内会阴部神经末端的载体潜伏期（PNTML），通常认为广泛的（尤其是两侧的）会阴部神经病变是大便失禁患者括约肌成形术后远期成功率的一个反向指标。在第 1 个案例中，肛门内超声的出现已经替代 CNEMG 和 SFEMG[31-32]，而 PNTML 并没有完全取代括约肌修复术的成功应用[33]。随着对大便失禁中动力肌成形术机制的进一步认识（本书中其他章节有叙述），NPT 重新开始流行，这其中需要将肌肉生理学与预估手术成功率关联起来。骶神经调节和外周神经刺激技术被越来越多地应用，多数用于治疗大便失禁，也有部分是慢传输或正常传输的严重便秘，其中体感诱发体位的中枢机制评估对于预测远期成功率有价值。这些结论主要来自于对尿动力学的神经生理和神经解剖的认知。使用 NPT 技术的标准检测曾经是常规肛门直肠检查的一部分，如今仅应用于大便失禁时的治疗和评估术后患者[34]。

神经传导和肌电图研究测量传出神经分布；传入神经的损伤比较难以定量。1930 年，Beck[35] 最

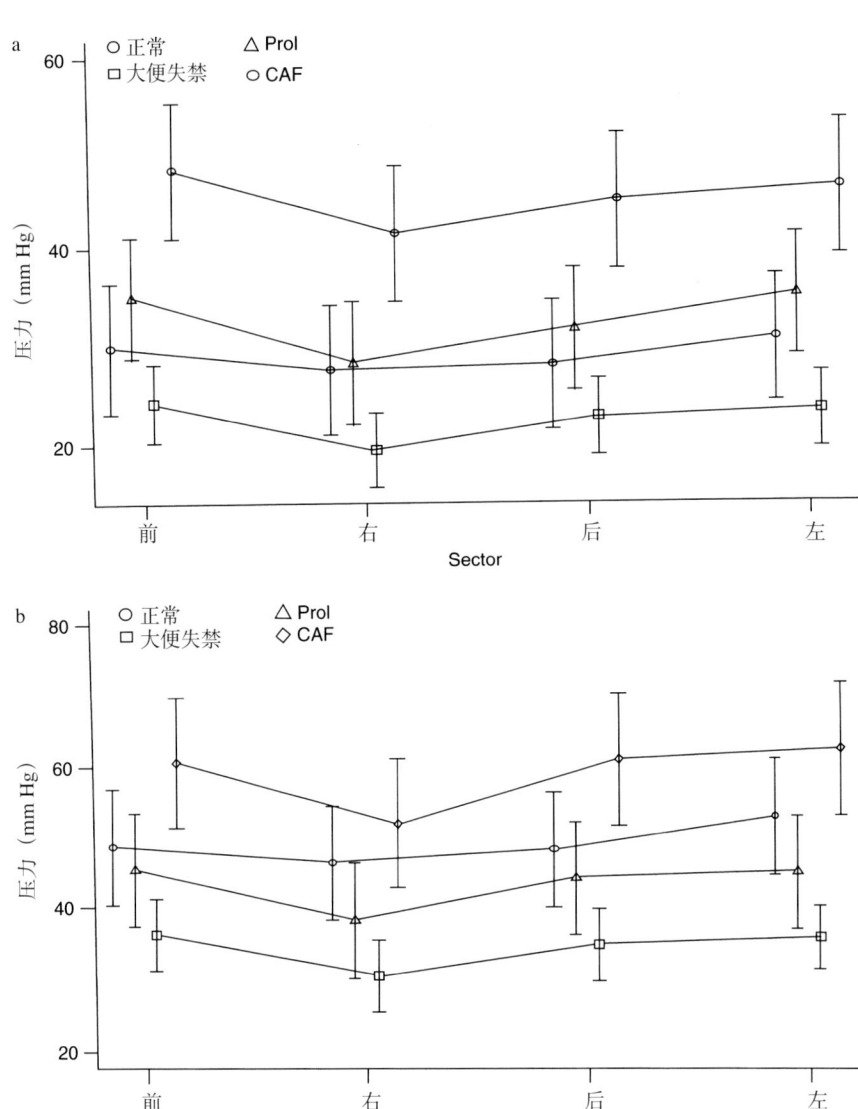

图 7.2 (a) 不同肛门直肠情况下使用向量体积测压得到的静息时扇形压力（平均值和 95% 可信区间）；(b) 不同肛门直肠情况下使用向量体积测压得到的持续收缩时扇形压力（平均值和 95% 可信区间）。Prol：脱垂；CAF：慢性肛裂（Reprinted with permission from Zbar et al.[9]）

早描述了传统肌电图，Adrian[35] 使用了同心针设计，Bronck[36] 在 1929 年对其改装；这些早期记录中仪器基础技术无太多差别。在此认知基础上，运动肌单位由以下部分组成：单个前角细胞、所有的外周神经纤维、运动神经终板以及其支配的肌纤维。一条肌纤维（MF）由一个运动神经元（MN）支配，但是一个运动神经元可以支配很多条肌纤维。肌纤维的功能不同，其组成也不同。典型的横纹肌纤维被分为两大类，Ⅰ型和Ⅱ型。Ⅰ型肌纤维是慢增强纤维，而Ⅱ型纤维是快时相性纤维[37]。本文中，肛提肌肌纤维主要是Ⅰ型纤维来持续增强肌力，而Ⅱ型肌纤维更广泛分布于肛周和尿道周围[38]。动力薄肌成形术是刺激肛门括约肌的一种技术，用于不同情况下，使Ⅱ型优势肌纤维转变为Ⅰ型，在某些成功案例中使用免疫组织病理检查已经证实此种转变。

为了便于记录，在独立肌单位的自发收缩中，这些肌单位组成一个运动单位电位（MUP），其获得的单个信号幅度包含各个单根纤维电位，而信号的性状取决于同时放电的纤维数。信号的持续时间主要是指记录到的首次偏离到其回到基线的时间。对于肛门而言，肌电图可以在体表进行，包括同心针（CN）、单根纤维（SF）和金属电极。用来标记肛门括约肌的肌电图被更多地认为是一种不必要的侵入性操作，而耻骨直肠肌的肌电图可能更准确，尤其是在刺激性操作时，因此大部分被动态核磁共振检查取代。如果说肌电图的价值，那就是在曾经减少的实验室数量中扮演特殊角色，而如今这些应用已被限制。它可以解释肌纤维的去神经和神经支配恢复，在括约肌完整性中也有一定作用，但对比应用超声和核磁共振仍有疑问。在一些失败的括约肌成形术中，后者可显示的结果很少，因为很多患者被判断为骶神经刺激，而不去考虑括约肌的完整性。该区域的中间值仍然没有可用性，通常包括一些折衷组的患者不能严格地用于对比[39]。这有可能是在某些肛门直肠畸形修复后功能性恢复不好，为了得到较好的临床结果做出的肌电图记录[40]。

肛门外括约肌的 CNEMG（图 7.3）最早被应用，用于评估自发性、复原模式和 MUP 波形。同心针由一个直径为 0.7mm 的铂金金属外套一金属插管组成，外管直径为 65mm，所以内层的金属被完全绝缘。理想记录的频率范围为 10Hz～10kHz，敏感度为 100～500mV，每个记录段如静息、收缩、紧绷和咳嗽时的清除速度为 20ms。CN 电极的引入用于括约肌左右两侧伴随着反应性 MUP 的释放，这与最初的插入放电不同，当患者在过程中放松时这种变化迅速消失。在去神经时，正常的 MUP 活性被纤维颤动去神经电位取代，伴随独立的肛门外括约肌和耻骨直肠肌记录。随着针的进和退，这些活性在刺激性操作中是独立的。去神经时，当肌纤维数量减少，异常波形变得明显。保护轴发生神经恢复变化时，运动单位幅度变大，持续时间边长，更具多相性。肌病状态下，运动单位总体幅度减小，持续波形变短。这也可以用来更好地解释矛盾耻骨直肠肌综合征在紧绷状态时活性增大[41]。产后或创伤性肛门外括约肌损伤时，幅度和活性总体下降。在一些深层神经疾病时会出现自发性纤维颤动和肌痉挛[42]。

SFEMG 最早由 Stålberg 和 Trontelj 报道[43]，它记录单个肌纤维活动电位，是 CNEMG[43] 的补充部分。这种电极有一个较小的针，表面仅有 25μm，能够探测仅 0.0003mm² 记录表面的电信号。与 CNEMG 相比，单个纤维电位（SFPs）持续时间较短，振幅更大，快速上升时间更长，为纤维密度提供更特殊信息（同一肌肉在不同位置测得肌纤维电位分析的平均值）。记录到的单个纤维电位（>100μV）的上升表示神经支配开始恢复，这是神经再生的结果，表示局部的轴突在刺激新的肌纤维，相比于 CNEMG 的变化，纤维密度的上升更多。这些数据与年龄相关，超过 60 岁的人群，纤维密度上升的趋势高于正常值的（1.5±0.16）[44-46]。最近，肛门括约肌肌电图再次被用于诊断非典型帕金森病，此时外周没有发现明显的神经病变，而肛门外括约肌的运动诱发电位有轻微变化[47]。在脊髓手术[48]和自主神经疾病[49]的术中也被使用。高密度表面的肌电图用于诊断确定肛门外括约肌支配的特定区域，而其在临床中的应用尚未发现[50]。利用普通肌电图改良的新模型，其探针更新，更有选择性，能够提供更快的不同发布长度的蜕变和探测到更微小的信号[52]，Bayesian 分析法比起一般的"正常"与"异常"视觉上的区别[51]，前者似乎更好地描述了肌电图 MUP。

会阴神经刺激（即会阴神经末端运动潜伏期试验 PNTML）最早由 Kiff 等提出[53]，用于评估盆底肌肉末梢运动神经支配，主要测量神经刺激到肌肉反应的时间间隔（图 7.4）。基于此种目的，研究发明了一种可置换、自带黏性的电极，并获得专利（Dantec Electronic Tonsbakken 16-18 DK-2740, Skovlunde Denmark and St. Mark's Hospital）。这种电极被预先连接到手套的示指掌侧，并在标准距离的手指根部放置记录电极，从而组成一个双极刺激电极。示指沿着坐骨棘移动，同时以 1s 的间隔提供一个 0.1～0.2ms 且不高于 15mA 的方形刺激，直到获得信号，从而形成记录的方向。将检查的手指 180°旋转用于左侧会阴神经的测量，得到一个颠倒的波形图。正常的 PNTML 值为两侧各是（2.0±0.2）ms；经阴道分娩后或者直肠脱垂，以及随着年龄的增长，该数值增大[54]。在会阴神经病变时，尤其是双侧的神经病变影响了括约肌的成功修复，但近来认为这种病变只是相对禁忌，仅仅作为大便失禁患者进行长期治疗的失利因素中咨询的一部分[33, 45, 55]。然而，双侧耻骨直肠肌和肛门外括约肌，在大便失禁评分、MUP 恢复以及 PNTML 测量值之间有明显的相关性[56]。这种相关比较复杂：延长的会阴神经末端运动潜伏期和异常的单纤维肌电图并不总是对应于大便失禁评分。在便秘患者，评估 MUP 的恢复可以让患者放松其括约肌，同心针状肌电图有助于诊断矛盾耻骨直肠肌收缩和不完全松弛。肌电图在这种特异性诊断中发挥作用。如肛裂时肛门内括约肌的价值在肛门直肠实验时不再重视[56]。如今，用于肛门内插入和记录不同深度信号的多通道表面肌电图侵入性操作较少，通过使用创新圆周信号技术可提供各种准确的信息，如神经支配区域、纤维长度、振幅、单个 MUP 的重复放电频率和传导速度。这在诊断肛门内超声不能确诊的括约肌完整性和排便困难的

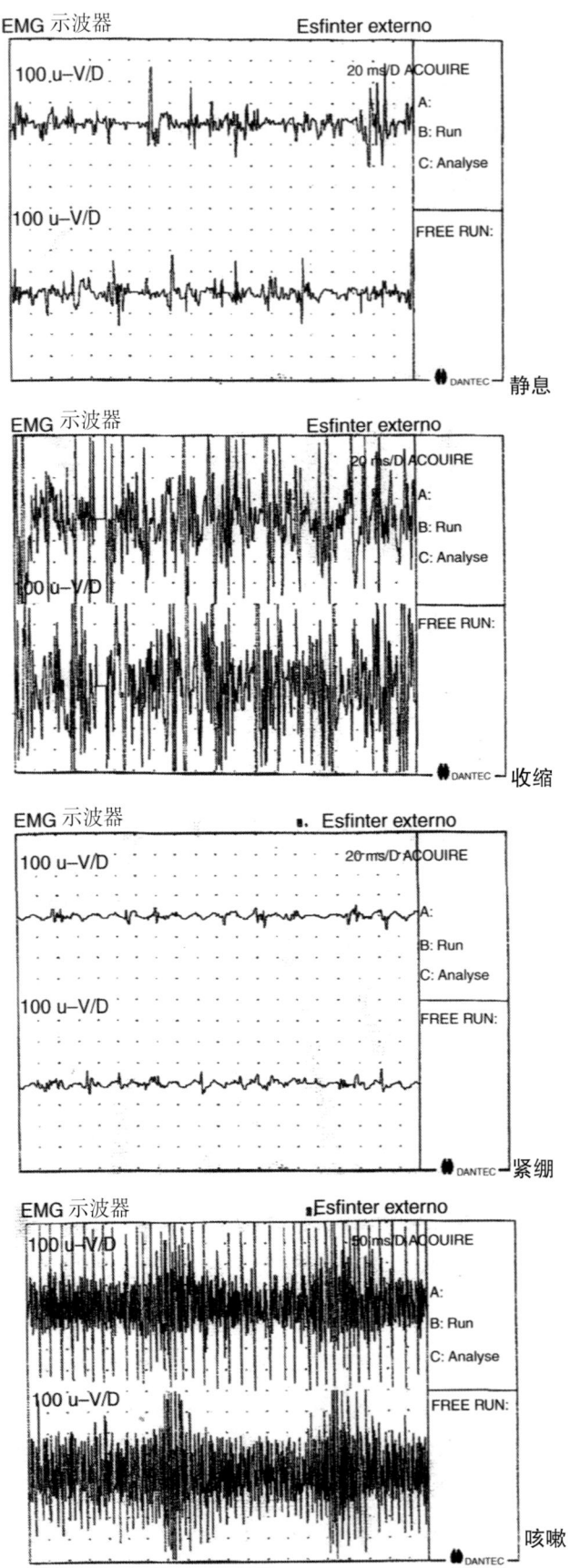

图 7.3 肛门外括约肌的同心针肌电图记录（Reprinted with permission from Rosato and Lumi.[46]）

第 7 章 再手术病例中向量测压和神经生理评估时的建议

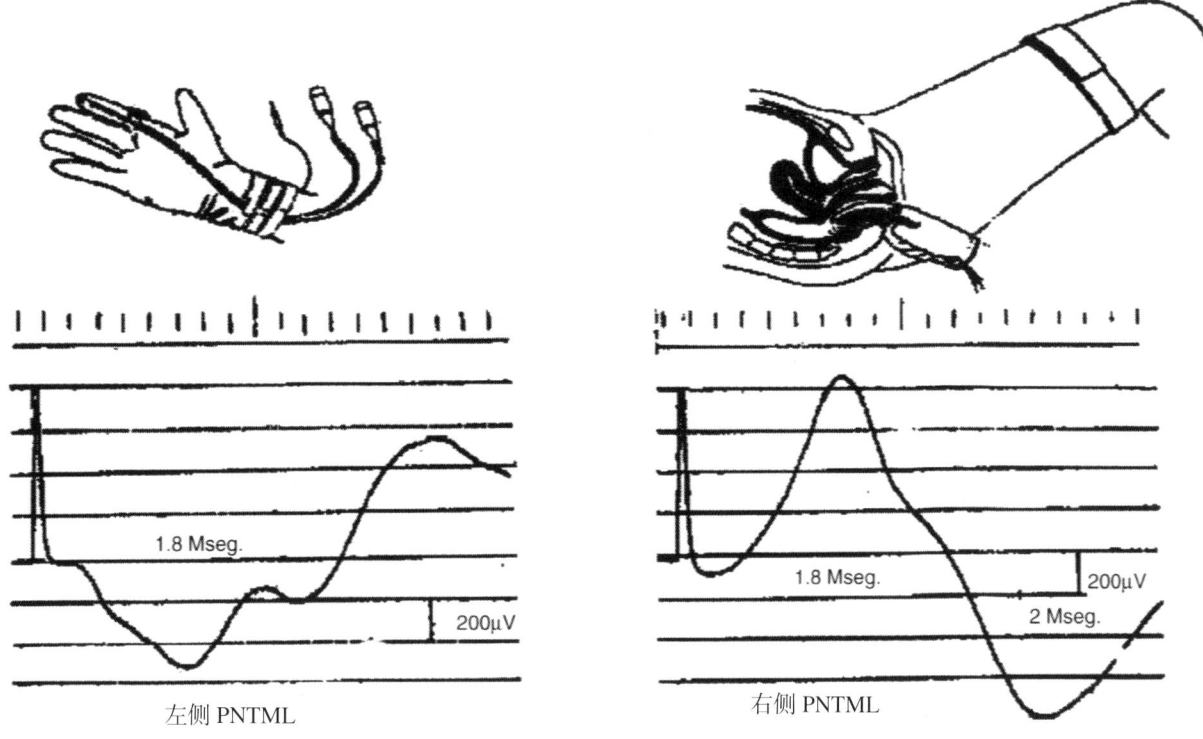

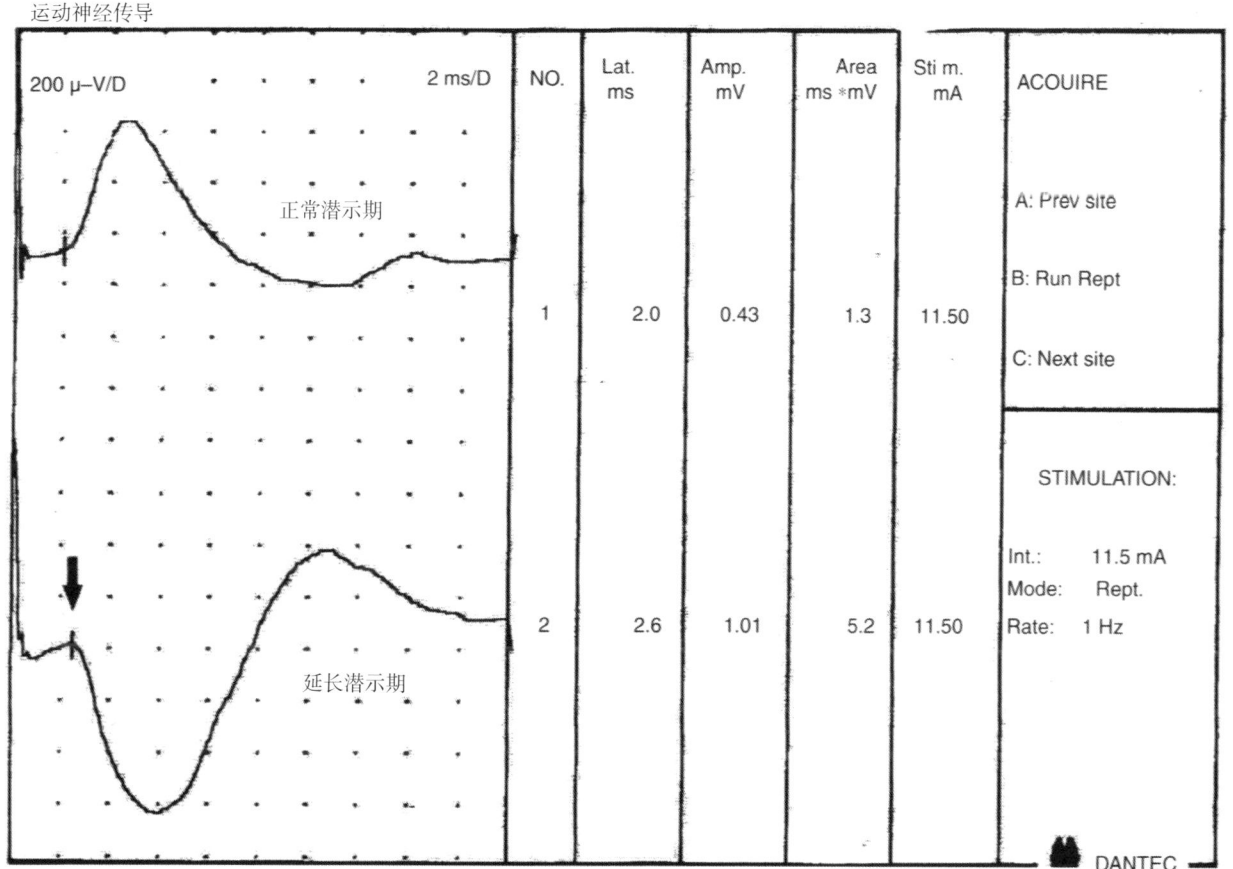

图 7.4 会阴神经末端运动潜伏期测量技术图（Reprinted with permission from Rosato and Lumi.[46]）

肛门痉挛时有帮助；同时对功能性疾病的康复治疗也可提供一些客观数据[57-58]。

皮质体感诱发电位

在一些实验室，人们使用皮质体感诱发电位（CSSEPs）来测定患者体内的骶神经调节，尤其是针对顽固性大便失禁患者。在本书的第35章有更详尽的叙述，但是关于骶神经刺激（SNS）的机制目前了解得不多[59]。CSSEPs被广泛用于排出障碍疾病，包括大便失禁的频率、迫切程度和欲望的症状，尿潴留以及膀胱疼痛综合征[60]，正电子发射断层扫描参数图分析应答者与无应答者之间的感兴趣区，检查刺激关闭、神经刺激的预期值和初始刺激来显示应答者内杏仁核和额叶皮质的二次刺激，以及右侧前运动皮质的强烈失活下沉默运动前区、体感循环和辅助运动皮质[61]。同样，骶神经和周围神经刺激的核心作用很明显，但是对其理解得不透彻，骶神经刺激使得会阴体感诱发电位潜伏期在同侧和对侧的首次偏离明显缩短。因此，骶神经刺激在传入皮质感觉区水平调节皮质活性，也被认为是成功的骶神经刺激传出的预测因子[62]。类似的结果在表面骶神经电刺激中也得到证实[60]。

对于脊髓横断小鼠的实验研究显示与脊髓横断相关的泌尿反射亢进被经皮骶神经刺激阻断，并且与不同的神经肽如P物质、神经肽A、降钙素基因（与神经节背根肽释放相关）的上升减缓相关，提示传入神经纤维C活性的阻断是骶神经刺激作用的机制之一[63]。尽管如此，这种作用的化学机制还不是很清楚，比较复杂；对右侧前扣带回和右侧额下回的额叶区进行单个光子发射计算机断层扫描分析显示存在灌注损伤，这也与SNS作用相关，后者参与老年男性的自主排尿过程。因此，存在外周和中枢的神经肽——脑轴来对刺激起应答作用[64-65]。

对植入神经刺激器表现为急迫性尿失禁的女性进行评估也得到上述结论，它作用于外周感受器，相应的脊髓和皮质区尚不清楚。由于最初没有得到理想结果，结论弹性较大。在骶神经刺激评估时使用正电子发射断层扫描，扣带回中间、腹内侧前额叶皮质、中脑和相邻丘脑中线的脑血流量显著下降，背外侧的前额叶皮质中血流量上升。骶神经刺激的早期存在差异，当初始刺激时，小脑中间的脑血流量下降；右侧中央后回、岛状区和腹内侧前额叶皮

质血流量上升。在慢性植入时，正因为有这种转变使得感觉皮质、运动前皮质和小脑之间存在差异，这三种区域均参与学习行为。这种作用很有可能是通过脊髓对大脑中参与学习行为的区域再教育，因此急性骶神经刺激调节参与感觉学习的区域，而在慢性骶神经刺激过程中这种作用减弱[66]。此时，尽管近来对于前颞叶变性和尿失禁患者的运动前区/前扣带回和壳核/屏状核/岛状区进行正电子发射断层扫描存在差异，但是对于肛门括约肌的中枢性功能的认识远没有其在尿失禁中的作用深刻[67]。在最近的一个研究大便失禁的直肠下神经损伤的动物模型中，Pierce等[68]证实皮质体感诱发电位下降，但没有神经形态学上的变化结果，这提示作为过程修改的一种形式，皮质意识的变化在中枢而不是外周。这改变了二级神经元的刺激和中枢传入。有确凿的证据（利用脑电波）显示在健康人体内，使用表面电极的骶神经刺激后产生CSSEP；Sheldon等[69]证实传入感受器活性的外周神经损伤有改变，在没有外周神经髓鞘形成时也可能发生[69]。

运动通路的电生理活性也可像电刺激一样被磁力激发[70]，这种作用在皮质被前腰骶神经刺激或会阴神经刺激加强，甚至两者叠加[71]。这种作用具有会阴刺激主导的不对称性，可以发挥更大效果，从而中枢路径受到既有的会阴神经状态的影响[72]。解释上述结论需谨慎，因为它依赖于骶部磁性刺激的部位和使用的有限磁性区强度[73]。这种类型的刺激生理学减少了直肠的体积/容积，当重复刺激下评估运动阈值、内皮质化、皮质沉默期时，与外周肌肉相比，肛门直肠肌肉的中枢作用不同[74]。这些问题不仅复杂，且取决于刺激发生的频率和长期性；在骶神经的成功刺激中，皮质图像显示表达和整体的兴奋性在骶神经刺激开始后立即下降，但是在骶神经刺激去除后这种下降就消失了。肛门肌电图使用头皮网状覆盖双边内侧皮质来代表这种多点的皮质刺激[75]，但这与任何已有的改良肛门直肠测压无明确相关性。

结　论

皮质体感诱发电位（CSSEPs）具有实验性和特殊性，但是未来研究可能会发现骶神经刺激和外周神经刺激之间的协调和分化，主要用于结直肠学

中，尤其是用于传统的研究方法无效的顽固性大便失禁的患者。

参考文献

1. Klopper PJ, de Haas F, Dijkhuis T. Computerized experimental multichannel urethral pressure profilometry. World J Urol. 1990;8:159–62.
2. Bombeck CT, Vaz O, DeSalvo J, Donahue PE, Nyhus LM. Computerized axial manometry of the esophagus: a new method for the assessment of antireflux operations. Ann Surg. 1987;206:465–72.
3. Perry RE, Blatchford GJ, Christensen MA, Thorson AG, Attwood SEA. Manometric diagnosis of anal sphincter injuries. Am J Surg. 1990;159:112–7.
4. Taylor BM, Beart RW, Phillips SF. Longitudinal and radial variations of pressure in \the human anal sphincter. Gastroenterology. 1984;86:693–7.
5. Coller JA. Clinical application of anorectal manometry. Surg Clin N Am. 1987;16:17–33.
6. Coller JA, Sangwan Y. Computerized anal sphincter manometry performance and analysis. In: Smith LE, editor. Practical guide to anorectal testing. 2nd ed. New York: Igaku-Shoin; 1995. p. 51–100.
7. Dijkhuis T, Bendiman WA, van der Hulst VPM, Klopper PJ. Graphical representation of eight-channel pressure profiles on a personal computer. Med Biol Eng Comput. 1990;28:502–4.
8. Waegermaekers CTBJ. Profilemeting van de distal oesophagus sphincter [thesis]. University of Amsterdam, Amsterdam, 1980
9. Zbar AP, Aslam M, Hider A, Toomey P, Kmiot WA. Comparison of vector volume manometry and conventional manometry in anorectal dysfunction. Tech Coloproctol. 1998;2:84–90.
10. Zbar A. Vectorvolume manometry. In: Wexner SD, Zbar AP, Pescatori M, editors. Complex anorectal disorders: investigation and management. New York: Springer; 2005. p. 48–62.
11. Braun JC, Trentner KH, Drew B, Klimaszewski M, Schumpelick V. Vector manometry for differential diagnosis of fecal incontinence. Dis Colon Rectum. 1994;37:989–96.
12. Keck JO, Staniunas RJ, Coller JA, Barrett RC, Oster ME. Computer-generated profiles of the anal canal in patients with anal fissure. Dis Colon Rectum. 1995;38:72–9.
13. Williams N, Barlow J, Hobson A, Scott N, Irving M. Manometric asymmetry in the anal canal in controls and patients with faecal incontinence. Dis Colon Rectum. 1995;38:1275–80.
14. Williams N, Scott A, Irving M. Effect of lateral sphincterotomy on internal anal sphincter function: a computerized vector manometric study. Dis Colon Rectum. 1995;38:700–4.
15. Sultan AH, Kamm MA, Nicholls RJ, Bartram CI. Prospective study of the extent of internal anal sphincter division during lateral sphincterotomy. Dis Colon Rectum. 1994;37:1031–3.
16. Zbar AP, Aslam M, Allgar V. Faecal incontinence after internal sphincterotomy for anal fissure. Tech Coloproctol. 2000;4:25–8.
17. Grande M, Caddedu F, Sileri P, Ciano P, Attina GM, Selvaggio I, et al. Anal vector volume analysis: an effective tool in the management of pelvic floor disorders. Tech Coloproctol. 2011;15:31–7. Epub 2010 Dec 14.
18. Schizas AMP, Emmanuel AV, Williams AB. Anal canal vector volume manometry. Dis Colon Rectum. 2011;54:759–68.
19. Zbar AP. Reading too much into anal vectorvolumetric parameters: correspondence for "anal vector volume analysis: an effective tool in the management of pelvic floor disorders". Tech Coloproctol. 2011;15(4):473–4. Epub 2011 Nov 9.
20. Zbar AP. Anal vectorvolumetry: a bridge too far. Dis Colon Rectum. 2011;54(10):e258. author reply e258.
21. Sultan AH, Kamm MA, Nicholls RJ, Bartram CI. Prospective study of the extent of internal anal sphincter division during lateral sphincterotomy. Dis Colon Rectum. 1994 Oct;37(10):1031–3.
22. Miller R, Bartolo DCC, Cervero F, Mortensen NJ. Anorectal sampling: a comparison of normal and incontinent patients. Br J Surg. 1988;75:44.
23. Zbar AP, Kmiot WA, Aslam M, Williams A, Hider A, Audisio RA, et al. Use of vector volume manometry and endoanal magnetic resonance imaging in the adult female for assessment of anal sphincter dysfunction. Dis Colon Rectum. 1999;42:928–33.
24. Zbar AP, Khaikin M. For debate: should we care about the internal anal sphincter? Dis Colon Rectum. 2012;55(1):105–8.
25. Yang Y-K, Wexner SD. Anal pressure vectography is of no apparent benefit for sphincter evaluation. Int J Colorectal Dis. 1994;9:92–5.
26. Hussein AM, Shehata MAS, Zaki Y, El Seweify MEA. Computerized anal vector manometric analysis in patients with tailored lateral sphincterotomy for anal fissure. Tech Coloproctol. 2000;4:143–9.
27. Giordano P, Gravante G, Grondona P, Ruggiero B, Porrett T, Lunniss PJ. Simple cutaneous advancement flap anoplasty for resistant chronic anal fissure: a prospective study. World J Surg. 2009;33:1058–63.
28. Pucciani F, Rottoli ML, Bologna A, Cianchi F, Forconi S, Cutelle M, et al. Pelvic floor dyssynergia and bimodal rehabilitation: results of combined pelviperineal kinesitherapy and biofeedback training. Int J Colorectal Dis. 1998;13:124–30.
29. Glasgow SC, Birnbaum EH, Kodner IJ, et al. Preoperative anal manometry predicts continence after perineal proctectomy for rectal prolapse. Dis Colon Rectum. 2006;49:1052–8.
30. Zbar AP, Nguyen H. Management guidelines in the treatment of full-thickness prolapse. In: Altomare D, Pucciani F, editors. Rectal Prolapse: Diagnosis and Clinical Management. Rome: Springer; 2008. p. 201–6.
31. Tjandra JJ, Milsom JW, Schroeder T, Fazio VW. Endoluminal ultrasound is preferable to electromyography in mapping anal sphincteric defects. Dis Colon Rectum. 1993;36:689–92.
32. Sultan AH, Kamm MA, Talbot IC, Nicholls RJ, Bartram CI. Anal endosonography for identifying external anal sphincter defects confirmed histologically. Br J Surg. 1994;81:463–5.
33. Chen AS, Luchtefeld MA, Senagore AJ, MacKeigan JM, Hoyt C. Pudendal nerve latency: does it predict outcome after of anal sphincter repair? Dis Colon Rectum. 1998;41:1005–9.
34. Rosato GO, Lumi CM, Miguel AA. Anal sphincter electromyography and pudendal nerve terminal motor latency assessment. Semin Colon Rectal Surg. 1992;3:68–74.
35. Beck A. Electromyographische untersuchungen am sphincter ani. Arch Physiol. 1930;224:278–92.
36. Adrian ED, Bronk DW. The discharge of impulsesd in motor nerve fibers. II. The frequency of discharge in reflex and voluntary contractions. J Physiol. 1929;67:119–51.
37. Buchtal F. The general concept of the motor unit: neuromuscular disorders. Res Publ Assoc Res Nerv Ment Dis. 1961;38:3–30.
38. Pette D. Fiber transformation and fiber replacement in chronically stimulated muscle. J Heart Lung Transplant. 1992;11:S299–305.
39. Chan MK, Tjandra JJ. Sacral nerve stimulation for fecal incontinence: external anal sphincter defect vs. intact anal sphincter. Dis Colon Rectum. 2008;51:1015–25.
40. Iwai N, Kanida H, Taniguchi H, Tsuto T, Yanigahara J, Takahashi T. Postoperative continence assessed by electromyography of the external sphincterin anorectal malformations. Z Kinderchir. 1985;40:87–90.
41. Wexner SD, Cheape JD, Jorge JMN, Heymen S, Jagelman DG. A prospective assessment of biofeedback for the treatment of paradoxical puborectalis contraction. Dis Colon Rectum. 1992;35:145–50.
42. Fowler CJ. Pelvic floor neurophysiology. Meth Clin Neurophysiol. 1991;2:1–20.
43. Stålberg E, Trontelj J. Single fiber electromyography. Surrey: Mirvalle; 1979.
44. Snooks SJ, Swash M. Nerve stimulation techniques. In: Henry MM, Swash M, editors. Coloproctology and the pelvic floor: pathophysi-

ology and management. London: Butterworths; 1985. p. 184–206.
45. Lauerberg S, Swash M. Effects of ageing on anorectal sphincters and their innervations. Dis Colon Rectum. 1989;32:737–42.
46. Rosato O, Lumi CM. Neurophysiology in pelvic floor disorders. In: Wexner SD, Zbar AP, Pescatori M, editors. Complex anorectal disorders: investigation and management. London: Springer; 2005. p. 153–69.
47. Winge K, Jennum P, Lokkegaard A, Werdelin L. Anal sphincter EMG in the diagnosis of Parkinsonian syndromes. Acta Neurol Scand. 2010;121:198–203. Epub 2009 Sept 24.
48. Khealanai B, Husain AM. Neuwophysiologic intraoperative monitoring during surgery for tethered cord syndrome. J Clin Neurophysiol. 2009;26:76–81.
49. Sakakibara R, Uchiyama T, Yamanishi T, Kishi M. Sphincter EMG as a diagnostic tool in autonomic disorders. Clin Auton Res. 2009;19:20–31.
50. Mesin L, Gazzoni M, Merletti R. Automatic localisation of innervations zones: a simulation study of the external anal sphincter. J Electromyogr Kinesiol. 2009;19:e413–21.
51. Pino LJ, Stashuk DW, Podnar S. Bayesian characterization of external anal sphincter muscles using quantitative electromyography. Clin Neurophysiol. 2008;119:2266–73.
52. Mesin L, Gervasio R. Detection volume of simulated electrode systems for recording sphincter muscle electromyogram. Med Eng Phys. 2008;30:896–904.
53. Kiff ES, Swash M. Normal proximal and delayed distal conduction in the pudendal nerves of patients with idiopathic (neurogenic) faecal incontinence. J Neurol Neurosurg Psychiatry. 1984;47:820–3.
54. Ryhammer AM, Lauerberg S, Hermann P. Long-term effect of vaginal deliveries on anorectal function in normal perimenopausal women. Dis Colon Rectum. 1996;39:852–9.
55. Sangwan YP, Coller JA, Barrett RC, Roberts PL, Murray JJ, Rusin L. Unilateral pudendal neuropathy. Impact on outcome of anal sphincter repair. Dis Colon Rectum. 1996;39:686–9.
56. Sorensen M, Nielsen MB, Pedersen JF, Christiansen J. Electromyography of the internal anal sphincter performed under endosonographic guidance. Description of a new method. Dis Colon Rectum. 1994;37:138–43.
57. Merletti R, Bottin A, Cescon C, Farina D, Gazzoni M, Martina S, et al. Multichannel surface EMG for the non-invasive assessment of the anal sphincter muscle. Digestion. 2004;69:112–22.
58. Enck P, Hinninghofen H, Merletti R, Azpiroz F. The external anal sphincter and the role of surface electromyography. Neurogastroenterol Motil. 2005;17 Suppl 1:60–7.
59. Matzel K, Matzel KE. Sacral nerve stimulation for fecal disorders: evolution, current status, and future directions. Acta Neurochir. 2007;97(Pt 1):351–7. Review.
60. Matsushita M, Nakasato N, Nakagawa H, Kanno A, Kaiho Y, Arai Y. Primary somatosensory evoked magnetic fields elicited by sacral surface electrical stimulation. Neurosci Lett. 2008;431:77–80.
61. Malaguti S, Spinelli M, Giardello G, Lazzeri M, Van Den Hombergh U. Neurophysiological evidence may predict the outcome e of sacral neuromodulation. J Urol. 2003;170(6 Pt 1):2323–6.
62. Govaert B, Melenhorst J, Nieman FH, Bols EM, van Gemert WG, Baeten CG. Factors associated with percutaneous nerve evaluation and permanent sacral nerve modulation outcome in patients with fecal incontinence. Dis Colon Rectum. 2009;52:1688–94.
63. Shaker H, Wang Y, Loung D, Balbaa L, Fehlings MG, Hassouna MM. Role of C-afferent fibres in the mechanism of action of sacral root neuromodulation in chronic spinal cord injury. BJU Int. 2000;85:905–10.
64. Griffiths D. Clinical studies of cerebral and urinary tract function in elderly people with urinary incontinence. Behav Brain Res. 1998;92:151–5.
65. Blok BF, Stums LM, Holstege G. Brain activation during micturition in women. Brain. 1998;121(Pt 11):2033–42.
66. Blok BF, Groen J, Bosch JL, Veltman DJ, Lammertsmaa AA. Different brain effects during chronic and acute sacral neuromodulation in urge incontinent patients with implanted neurostimulators. BJU Int. 2006;98:1238–43.
67. Perneczky R, Diehl-Schmid J, Forstl H, Drzezga A, May F, Kurz A. Urinary incontinence and its functional anatomy in frontotemporal lobar degenerations. Eur J Nucl Med Mol Imaging. 2008;35:605–10.
68. Pierce C, Healy CF, O'Herlihy C, O'Connell PR, Jones JFX. Reduced somatosensory cortical activation in experimental models of neuropathic fecal incontinence. Dis Colon Rectum. 2009;52:1417–22.
69. Sheldon R, Kiff ES, Clarke A, Harris ML, Hamdy S. Sacral nerve stimulation reduces corticoanal excitability in patients with faecal incontinence. Br J Surg. 2005;92:1423–31.
70. Pellicione G, Scarpinoi O, Piloni V. Motor evoked potentials recorded from external anal sphincter by cortical and lumbo-sacral magnetic stimulation: normative data. J Neurol Sci. 1997;149:69–72.
71. Hamdy S, Enck P, Aziz Q, Rothwell JC, Uengdergil S, Hobson A, et al. Spinal and pudendal nerve modulation of human corticoanal motor pathways. Am J Physiol. 1998;274(2 Pt 1):G419–23.
72. Hamdy S, Enck P, Aziz Q, Unergoergil S, Hobson A, Thompson DG. Laterality effects of human pudendal nerve stimulation on corticoanal pathways: evidence for functional asymmetry. Gut. 1999;45:58–63.
73. Morren GL, Walter S, Lindehammar H, Halböök O, Sjödahl R. Evaluation of the sacroanal motor pathway by magnetic and electrical stimulation in patients with fecal incontinence. Dis Colon Rectum. 2001;44:167–72.
74. Morren GL, Walter S, Halböök O, Sjödahl R. Effects of magnetic sacral root stimulation on anorectal pressure and volume. Dis Colon Rectum. 2001;44:1827–33.
75. Lefaucheur JP. Excitability of the motor cortical representation of the external anal sphincter. Exp Brain Res. 2005;160:268–72.
76. Harris ML, Singh S, Rothwell J, Thompson DG, Hamdy S. Rapid rate magnetic stimulation of human sacral nerve roots alters excitability within the cortico-anal pathway. Neurogastroenterol Motil. 2008;20:1132–9.

第二篇
肛门直肠重建手术的决策制定

引 言

Robert D. Madoff

不管是良性还是恶性疾病，保留患者的肛门直肠功能对其预后或患者满意度都是一个关键因素。本篇接下来的部分介绍了在有挑战性的情况下决定行肛门直肠重建手术相关的关键问题。

对于复杂肛门直肠疾病患者的综合治疗来说，手术只是其中一个单独的因素，尤其是对于癌症和炎性肠病的患者。在手术前，外科医生在决定某些关键问题时扮演了关键的角色，如决定手术的替代方案，何时进行干预治疗（尤其是对于"还凑合"或是药物治疗失败的炎性肠病患者），以及在手术前还能采取哪些其他的干预措施，特别是对于直肠癌患者采取新辅助放化疗。

外科医生第一个与手术有关的决定就是手术方式的选择。第1例报道的腹腔镜结肠切除术至今仅仅只有20年。在那时，腹腔镜结肠切除术得到了很多试验的支持（其中包括重要的随机试验，如COST和CLASICC试验），并被广泛接受。机器人结直肠手术的发展很大程度上代表了腹腔镜手术的发展，这种主要用于盆腔手术的方法，一开始是由几个独立的团队首先使用，但现在在国际上得到越来越多人的接受。虽然我们还需要等待几项大型随机试验的结果，但在患者的选择和手术技术上已经达成了公认的标准。本部分还讨论了3个特别的挑战：腹腔镜手术疑难病例的解决方法、腹腔镜再次手术及机器人手术的注意事项。

随着环形吻合器的使用和能达到解剖学切除的全系膜切除术被广泛接受，直肠癌的手术发生了巨大的改变。在因癌症进行直肠切除的过程中，保留括约肌一直是我们的一个主要目标，超低位吻合的技术也得到了巨大的发展。但是，进行低位吻合，尤其是在进行新辅助治疗或是辅助治疗的患者中，经常会导致肠道功能不良——"低位前切除术综合征"，很多学者建议用重建技术来改善缓解这种问题，包括端-侧吻合、结肠J形贮袋以及结肠成形术，在本部分中都进行了介绍。此外，虽然现在还没有进行大范围的实践，但完全直肠肛门重建为保留合理的肛门功能而不行结肠造口术提供了希望，即使接受了腹会阴联合切除术。最后，尽管解剖学直肠手术和能减少局部复发的放射治疗得到了巨大发展，但肿瘤的局部复发仍是一个重要问题，成功治愈需要根治性切除，而这经常需要多器官切除。来自美国和澳大利亚的权威专家编写了两个单独的章节来介绍这个有挑战性的问题。

自从首次报道Nigro放化疗方案到今天的40多年间，肛管癌作为一种不同的疾病，其治疗方法发生了翻天覆地的变化。在那时，手术治疗作为一种二级治疗用于放化疗无效或是放化疗后肿瘤复发的患者。然而肛管癌的手术同复发性直肠癌的手术一样，会引起特别的挑战，因为手术需要对之前进行过放射治疗的盆腔进行广泛的切除，还时常需要切除周围受侵犯的器官。最近，尤其是自从AIDS开始流行以来，肛管癌的流行病学特点发生了变化，男性和年轻人的发病率增加。随着人们更加了解人乳头瘤病毒，肛管癌的生物学基础变得更清楚，人乳头瘤病毒是大多数病例的病原体。人们还发现了高风险的群体，包括男同性性接触者及免疫抑制的患者，如艾滋病和移植术后的患者。肛管上皮内瘤变现在被视为肛管癌的前期病变，本部分还对肛门上皮内瘤变的筛查和治疗方法进行了讨论。

第 8 章 外科直肠重建：超低位吻合术的术式选择

Mary R. Kwaan · Robert D. Madoff
陈启仪 译　李 宁 审校

摘 要

虽然中长期的数据显示直肠功能获益方面存在诸多争议，但是不同外科术式的选择仍被新直肠重建常规使用。预后较差的结果和低位直肠前切除综合征的发生率较报道更为常见。这些问题的原因比较复杂，包括吻合口破裂，吻合口周围的感染，贮袋容积小，重建期间括约肌的损伤以及放射治疗对括约肌的影响等。括约肌保留观点的盛行使得在临床工作中对复杂患者的评估和重建更为重要，并更注重术后生活质量的客观评估。本章主要阐述低位直肠切除重建后的功能，并比较不同直肠重建的方法，以及疑难病例的管理等。

关键词

直肠重建；超低位吻合；端 – 端直肠肛管吻合；结肠 – 直肠吻合；结肠 J 形贮袋；端 – 侧或 "Baker" 吻合；横结肠成形术；Heineke-Mikulicz

引 言

大部分直肠局部肿瘤的患者可以通过外科手术治愈。对于非常低位的直肠癌患者，仍需要进行腹会阴联合切除，导致永久性的结肠造口。最近 10 年间，我们取得了一系列的进步，努力保留肛门括约肌，恢复患者肠道的连续性，包括进行直肠癌手术的外科医生专业化程度增加，增加高分辨率的术前影像学的使用，外科缝合器械设计的进步，可接受手术切缘更靠近肿瘤远端边缘，新辅助放化疗能够使较大和固定的肿瘤萎缩，使得更适合标准化的手术治疗。缝合技术的进步使一些直肠癌患者的局部复发率明显降低，并改善这些患者与癌症相关的存活率[1-3]。

有括约肌功能不全的患者，直肠切除术面临着排便功能急剧的改变，包括肠道运动频率增加，里急后重感和排便不尽感等。对于一些患者，这些改变作为直肠前切除综合征的一部分，影响其生活质量和性功能，最终影响其生理和社会功能[4-6]。目前也无有效的干预措施改变直肠前切除综合征，许多患者只能经过滴定式的调整饮食方式，服用止泻剂或泻剂，间断使用肛垫和规律地进行排便功能锻炼等。理解直肠癌治疗后生活质量的一个主要方面是需了解术后肠道功能的改变。

本章回顾和比较直肠切除重建后外科医师使用的改善肠道功能的技术，侧重于低结直肠或结肠 – 肛管吻合术。验证这些技术吻合的并发症和详细阐述功能性结果，包括放射治疗对于总体功能的结果。

直肠重建技术

肿瘤切除后，保留的直肠能通过几种方式重建结构，包括端－端结肠肛管或直肠－肛管吻合（人工缝合或吻合器吻合）术（图 8.1）。其他的技术是通过模拟增加直肠直径的宽度以提供近端肛管的储便功能。这些技术包括结肠 J 形贮袋（与全结肠直肠切除术后回肠 J 形贮袋类似），它通过折叠近端结肠并闭合结肠的系膜形成。贮袋折叠的顶点可吻合于肛管或远端直肠（图 8.2）。贮袋长度为 6~9cm，增加贮袋的长度容易导致排便时间的延长[7]。端－侧吻合或"Baker"吻合[8]近端结肠留一盲端以储存大便，从结肠切除系膜的远端 3~4cm 用于吻合至直肠或肛管（图 8.3）。横结肠成形术是通过纵向的结肠切开并通过 Heineke-Mikulicz 的方式横向修补结肠，形成近端结肠更大的肠腔，直肠和肛管残端的端－端吻合形成远端的结肠成形术（图 8.4）。最终术式的选择除了受患者剩余结肠和盆腔的解剖及体型影响外，外科医师必须考虑这些重建技术对术后并发症及功能的影响。肿瘤的结果并不受重建类型的影响。

吻合口并发症

一项 meta 分析统计了 8 项随机试验的 866 例患者，比较了结肠 J 形贮袋与直接的吻合术，结果显示两者吻合口瘘的发生率并无显著差异。另一项由 Heriot 等进行的随机和非随机的系统分析（大部分是前瞻性的），纳入了 3 项研究的 154 例患者，结果发现结肠 J 形贮袋与直接的吻合术之间吻合口瘘发生率并无显著差异，但更倾向于行结肠 J 形贮袋术。同时他还系统性分析了 2 项研究的 66 例患者，结果显示两种吻合方式对吻合口狭窄并发症的发生率

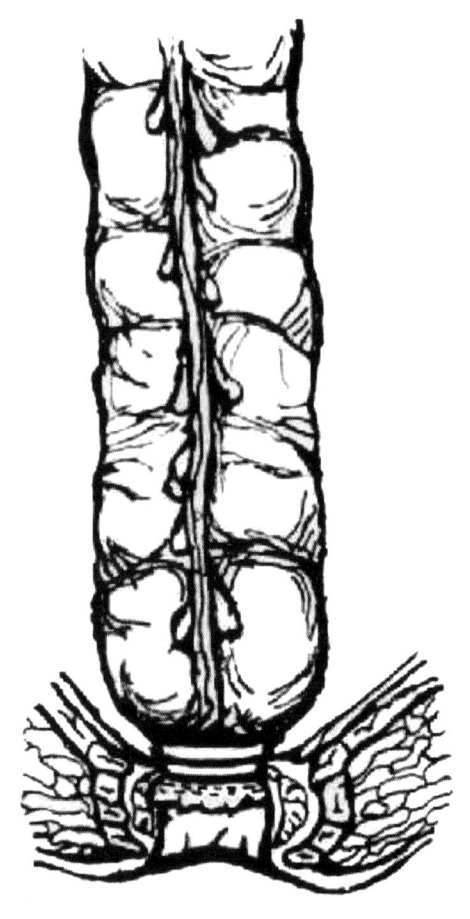

图 8.1　直接端－端吻合

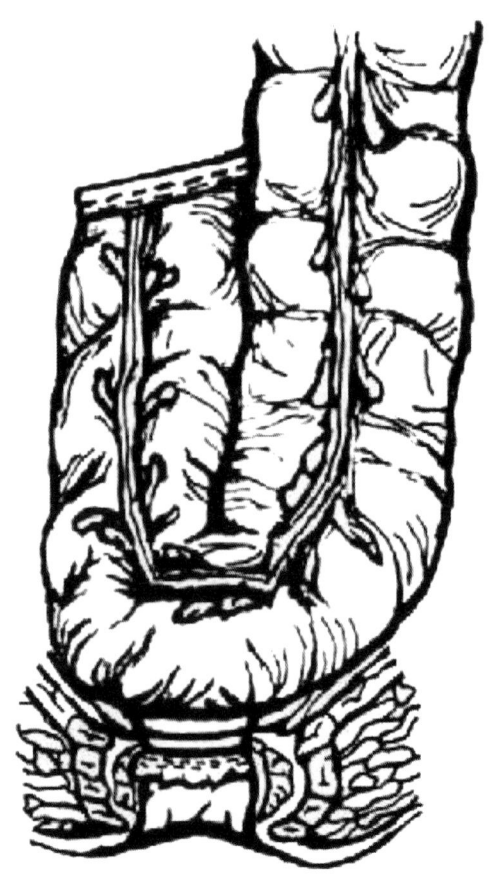

图 8.2　结肠 J 形贮袋吻合

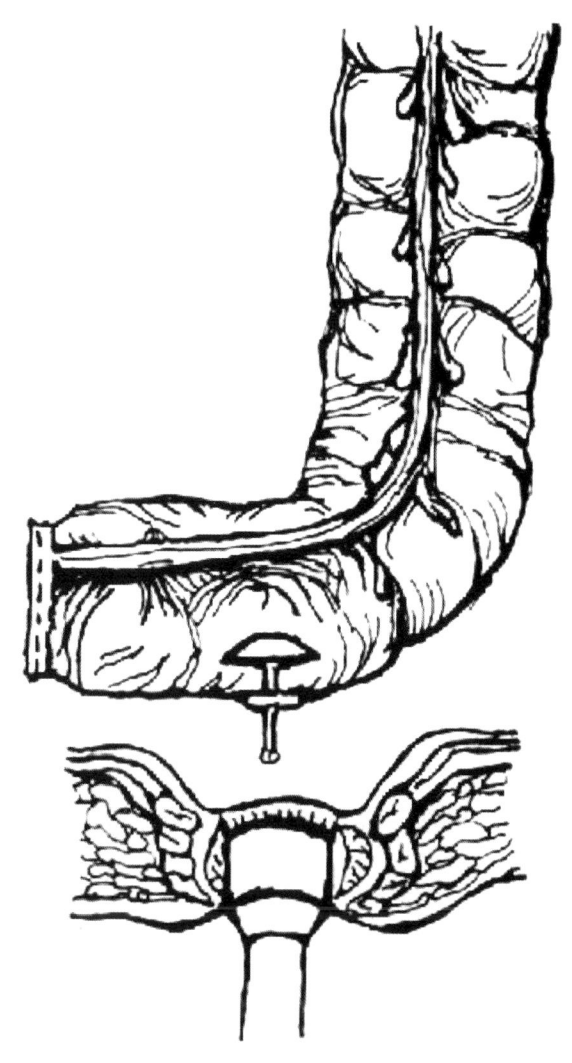 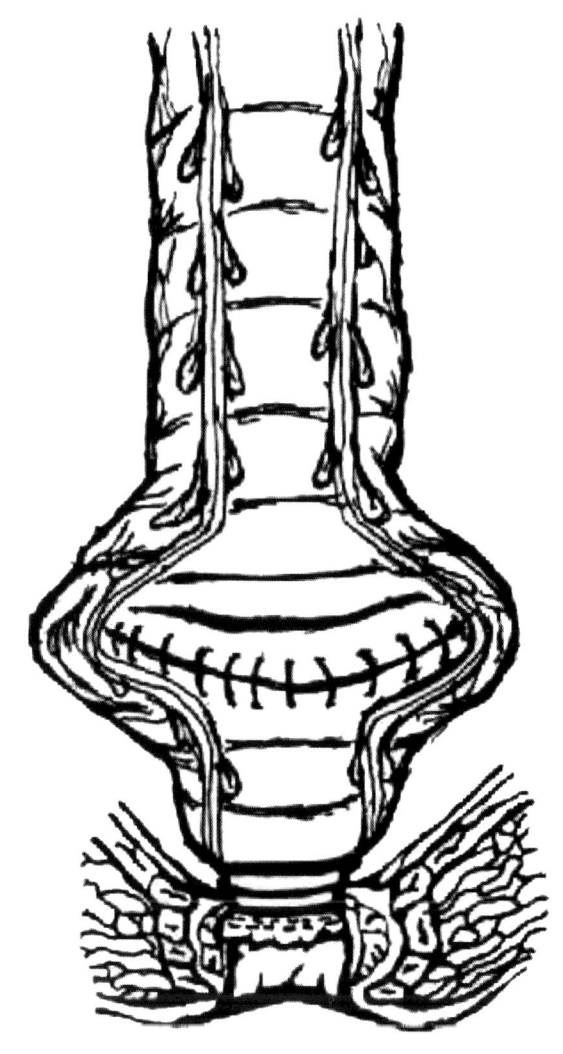

图 8.3　侧 – 端吻合　　　　　　　　　图 8.4　端 – 端横结肠成形术

也无显著差异。一些学者认为，由于当一侧结肠切开行结肠 J 形贮袋术或侧 – 端吻合时系膜断裂或损伤较少，因此近端的吻合具有更好的血供。Koh 等[11]的一项 meta 分析，纳入了 7 项随机研究发现，直接吻合将增加吻合口瘘的发生风险（风险比为 0.36，95%CI：0.12～1.08）；但该结果主要受 Hallböök 等进行的一项包括 100 例患者的单中心随机试验的影响[12]。在这项研究中，直接吻合与结肠 J 形贮袋吻合的瘘发生率分别为 15% 和 2%（P=0.03）。其他的研究结果表明，直接结肠 – 肛管吻合和结肠 J 形贮袋吻合术吻合口瘘的发生率分别为 8%～16% 和 8%～9%[13-15]。

另一项 meta 分析纳入了 3 项随机试验的 215 例患者，比较了结肠 J 形贮袋与侧 – 端吻合术，并未发现吻合口瘘发生率的差异[9]。端 – 侧吻合吻合口瘘的发生率为 7%～10%[16-17]。在 Jiang 的一项研究中发现，一例端 – 侧吻合的患者出现侧支坏死[18]，2003 年 Machado 等进行的一项随机试验研究发现端 – 侧吻合术的患者吻合口狭窄发生率为 4%[17]。另一项随机试验纳入 40 例患者，比较侧端长度为 3cm 和 6cm 的端 – 侧吻合术吻合口瘘的发生情况，结果显示侧端为 6cm 的患者吻合口瘘发生率为 10%，而 3cm 长患者未见吻合口瘘[19]。

一项随机试验发现横结肠成形术具有更高吻合口瘘发生率[20]，该研究吻合口距离肛门 3.4cm，常规使用预防性回肠造口术，44 例横结肠成形术吻合口瘘发生率为 16%，而结肠 J 形贮袋无 1 例发生（P=0.01），所有横结肠成形术瘘口均在结肠肛管吻合口远端的前方。Ho等推测，增加结肠切口与远端的距离可能保留端－端吻合口的血供，从而降低吻合口瘘的风险；他们认为，切开的纵轴与横断端的距离至少需4cm。克利夫兰医院同意该观点并建议横结肠成形术结肠造口与重建远端边缘的距离为4~6cm[21]。克利夫兰医院的另一项回顾性研究表明，结肠成形术吻合器吻合的吻合口瘘和吻合口狭窄的发生率均为4.8%，而人工缝合具有更高的吻合口瘘发生率（28.5%）[22]。但作者认为，导致吻合口并发症的原因可能为低位的手工缝合而非吻合重建技术本身。本研究也报道了结肠J形贮袋的手工缝合出现44%和22%的吻合口瘘和吻合口狭窄的并发症。来自克利夫兰医院主持的多中心随机试验结果发现，无法行结肠J形贮袋而行结肠成形术患者吻合口裂开和吻合口狭窄发生率分别为8.5%和12.8%，而行结肠J形贮袋患者的吻合口裂开和吻合口狭窄发生率分别为4.6%和3.8%[23]。

在一项meta分析研究了3项随机试验的158例患者，结果表明结肠J形贮袋与结肠成形术之间吻合口瘘的发生率无显著差异[10]，Liao等分析了4项随机对照研究的316例患者证实了这一结论。该meta分析结果表明，结肠J形贮袋与横结肠成形术之间的总吻合口瘘发生率分别为5%和10%，两者之间并无显著统计学差异[24]。随后的meta分析结果显示，结肠J形贮袋与结肠成形术两种技术间吻合口狭窄的发生率分别为5.5%和4%，且无显著统计学差异。

总之，多项研究表明，尽管统计学上无显著差异，但与其他技术相比，结肠J形贮袋具有更低的吻合口瘘发生率；相反，由于吻合口狭窄的相关数据较少，至于哪种技术可降低吻合口狭窄并发症，目前尚不明确。尽管横结肠成形术有更多的并发症，但当结肠J形贮袋难以实施如系膜较短或盆腔狭窄等因素时，可选择横结肠成形术作为替代的术式。该两种术式对于重建的直肠容量以及敏感性，尚未见显著差异[25]。与结肠－直肠的直接吻合与结肠－肛管的吻合术相比，贮袋重建术式已经越来越受欢迎，尽管结肠J形贮袋可能降低吻合口瘘的发生率，但最合适的结肠的选择、贮袋的大小、最佳的吻合部位及如何避免排便困难、长期愈后（>2年）与老年患者的手术指征等多方面仍然存在诸多矛盾[26]。

直肠重建后肠功能的评估

对于直肠良恶性肿瘤患者，对排便功能进行量化和测量相对困难。大多数功能需要进行评估，但是单一的测量、评分或问卷调查均很难充分评估直肠肛门的功能。目前已有两种工具经过科学的设计和严格的验证，但还未得到研究者的广泛采纳。Bakx等[27]设计和验证的结直肠功能结果问卷表及Temple等[28]设计的纪念Sloan Kettering癌症中心的肠道功能仪，主要用于直肠癌患者。目前文献报道的肠道功能评估的组成详见表8.1。报道中，肠道蠕动频率或每天蠕动的次数是最主要的参数。

排便不尽感是术后常见的并发症，包括肛周粪便污染、排气不尽感、松软大便或成形大便。研究中使用排便不尽的严重程度和频率进行评分。其中Kirwan-Fazio是最简单的评分系统[29]，它包括无不尽感（Ⅰ）、排气不尽感（Ⅱ）、水样便（Ⅲ）及频繁的大便污染（Ⅳ）4个分级。Hallböök评分系统[12]和排便不尽严重指数（FISI）包括不尽感不同程度的频率，分数越高程度越重[30]。FISI评分系统详见表8.2。

排便不尽是指无法在特定时间内（如>15min）将肠道粪便排空。成簇排便是指感觉排便完全，随后很快又需再次排便一次到几次。排便紧迫感是感觉需立即进行排便，且伴有害怕排便失禁的心理。排便紧迫可通过询问患者可延迟多长时间排便进行评估。肛门感觉损害是指患者无法辨别是排气还是排便，并可通过询问患者排气是否存在安全感心理进行评估。排便功能的其他评估措施包括询问患者

表8.1 直肠肛门功能相关综合征

肠道蠕动频率	
大便失禁	
排便不尽	
成簇排便	
排便紧迫感	
肛门感觉异常	判断排气和排便的能力
调节饮食控制排便	
使用护垫	
使用止泻药	
使用泻剂	

表 8.2 大便失禁的严重程度指数（FISI）

	≥2次/天	1次/天	≥2次/周	1次/周	1~3次/月
气体	12	11	8	6	4
黏液便	12	10	7	5	3
液体便	19	17	13	10	8
固体便	18	16	13	10	8

对排便功能失常所采取的一些措施，如调节或限制饮食、使用护垫、止泻药、泻剂或灌肠。一些研究报道了排便功能对生活方式影响的问卷调查，包括是否影响离开家庭参与社会活动、对肠道功能是否满意以及对术后性生活的满意度等。

放射治疗

术前或术后放射治疗已经被证实可改善癌症相关的愈后，特别是对于直肠癌外科切除术后局部复发率具有明显的效果。但放射治疗并未改善总体和与疾病无关的生存率。另外，放射治疗对于改善短期和长期的预后（如较差的愈后及肠梗阻）存在疑问。对于括约肌保留手术，术前和术后放射治疗对肠功能有很长且持久的不良反应。这些影响的作用机制与盆腔软组织的纤维化、直肠周围神经及肛门括约肌有关。

在长期随访研究中发现，无论是短期疗程（25Gy，超过5天）还是长期疗程（50Gy，超过4~6周）的术前放射治疗与排便功能有关。来自斯德哥尔摩的一项1级和2级试验[31]分析了64例患者，其中21例患者接受术前放射治疗（25Gy），平均随访时间为14年，离肛门的距离平均为10cm，这一结果表明，放射治疗可增加肠道蠕动频率和大便失禁（放射治疗与非放射治疗组，57% vs 26%，$P=0.01$）。作为荷兰全直肠系膜切除研究[32]的一部分，362例低位直肠前切除的患者随访5年，结果显示，术前放射治疗（25Gy）导致更差的排便频率（3.69 vs 3.03/天，$P=0.011$），增加排便失禁（62% vs 38%，$P<0.001$），已经使用护垫频率更高，这些症状在低位肿瘤患者（距肛缘5~10cm）表现更为明显。更大比例的放射治疗患者研究报道了放射治疗对于肠功能的影响（放射治疗组与非放射治疗组，34% vs 22%，$P=0.01$）。目前尚缺乏术前长期疗程的放化疗对于直肠肛门的功能影响的详细数据。波兰的一项直肠癌研究，将患者随机分为术前长期疗程的放化疗和短期疗程的放射治疗，并随访12个月，结果显示肠功能在两组间均较差，大便失禁发生率在短期疗程患者组是42%，而在长期疗程患者组是50%[33]。该研究排便紧迫感的发生率接近60%，而成簇排便发生率高达90%。

一项术后放射治疗的长期随访研究表明，与未接受放射治疗的患者相比，这些患者常伴有慢性腹泻、排便紧迫感、成簇排便以及大便失禁等症状。Kollmorgen[34]等报道了直肠切除术行放化疗，40个月的随访结果显示41例患者出现了上述症状。19世纪80年代丹麦的研究学者Lundby[35]等也有类似发现，经过17年随访发现15例患者出现上述症状，该结果于2005年被报道。

另一项由Fazio[23]指导、Parc[36]等执行的随机试验，比较了低位直肠癌的患者行结肠成形术与J形贮袋或直接吻合术，并评估了新辅助化学治疗对肠功能的影响。共计364例患者纳入了该研究，58%接受术前放射治疗，88%接受化学治疗。新辅助化学治疗的患者未进行随机化。在术后4个月，术前行放射治疗的患者24h排便频率更高；在4和12个月的夜间排便频率也增加；术后4和24个月，术前放射治疗的患者排便紧迫感更明显。

直接吻合重建与结肠J形贮袋重建间的直肠功能比较

我们常把结肠J形贮袋与直接的端-端吻合术作比较（在第9章也进行了描述）。总而言之，大部分的研究更倾向于使用结肠J形贮袋[26]。少部分的研究进行了长期随访（2年或超过2年），结果表明这两种技术之间排便功能的差异较小。

排便频率

短期的随访（<12个月）结果显示，行结肠J

形贮袋术的患者排便频率明显改善。一项 meta 分析结果显示，7 项研究中的 5 项随机试验表明结肠 J 形贮袋吻合的患者肠蠕动频率更低，这项结果与一项中长期的随访（8~18 个月）结果相似[9]。除了 1 项研究，其余研究中吻合口与肛缘的距离均小于 5cm。一项系统分析[10]评估了随机和非随机的研究，且大部分是前瞻性研究，同样发现每天的 J 形贮袋吻合肠道蠕动频率更低，在随访的 6 个月为 1.88/天（$P=0.011$）和随访 12 个月为 1.35/天（$P=0.001$）。另一项仅纳入 2 项试验的 meta 分析，24 个月的随访，其中一项表明 J 形贮袋具有更好的结果。这项试验中 19%J 形贮袋患者排便次数超过 4 次 / 天，而 37% 的直接吻合患者出现排便次数超过 4 次 / 天[37]。Heriot 系统阐述了 5 项研究的 331 例患者，结果发现，24 个月随访显示两者间排便的差异为 0.74 次 / 天（$P=0.01$）。

大便失禁

在一项 meta 分析中[9]，仅一项研究报道了术前放射治疗[12]，大多数的研究中只有一小部分患者进行了术后放射治疗。因此，该荟萃分析的患者放射治疗后对排便的不良反应不可能与现在典型放射治疗后的不良反应相同。在 7 项研究中（除了 2 项）进行 8~18 个月的随访研究显示，在 J 形贮袋吻合患者中更少发生大便失禁以外，其余研究均认为直接吻合与结肠 J 形贮袋吻合术大便失禁的发生率相同[9]。Hallböök 等进行的 2 个月 ~1 年的随访研究显示，与直接吻合相比，结肠 J 形贮袋吻合更少发生大便失禁[12]。一项对直肠切除患者的回顾性分析研究发现，在术后 6 个月时直接结肠肛管吻合的 Wexner 排便失禁评分较结肠 J 形贮袋更差（平均 5.3 vs 2.0；$P<0.05$）。但在 1 年和 2 年后，两者无显著统计学差异[38]。长期随访显示，这种大便失禁并不严重，大部分患者很少或偶尔发生。

排便紧迫感

诸多研究发现，如果患者经过结肠 J 形贮袋重建术，则很少发生排便紧迫感。Brown 等[9]的荟萃分析显示，6 项随机试验中的 3 项研究结果显示，短期随访发现结肠 J 形贮袋重建具有更少的排便紧迫感，在中长期随访中仅有一项研究认为结肠 J 形贮袋重建有更少的排便紧迫感，而在长期随访中则发现显著差异[9]。Heriot 等[10]系统分析 8 项为期 6 个月和 12 个月的研究的随访结果显示，结肠 J 形贮袋重建的排便紧迫感相对较低，但在 3 项为期 2 年的随访中则未见显著差异[10]。

排便功能的其他监测手段

排便不尽在荟萃分析中很难进行比较和统一监测[9]，尽管 Heriot 等进行的荟萃分析中没有指标的讨论，但在 4 项研究中并未发现排便功能差异显著[10]。

其 他

低位吻合的患者是容易引起排便功能变差。Hida 等进行的 5 年随访发现[39]，尽管放射治疗的使用并未阐述，但结肠 J 形贮袋重建比端 - 端重建具有更好的排便功能。通过 17 类特异性非随机研究的评分系统对排便功能进行评估，结果显示，距肛缘 5~8cm 的结肠 J 形贮袋重建和直接重建之间的排便功能无显著差异。该研究强调了低位肿瘤或吻合的患者行结肠 J 形贮袋重建可能具有持久的改善排便功能。

端 - 侧重建与结肠 J 形贮袋重建

结肠 J 形贮袋重建的一个局限是损伤排便功能。当结肠 J 形贮袋大于 10~12cm 时就出现该问题。一项随机试验探讨了端侧重建排便不尽是否要少于结肠 J 形贮袋。

基于 5 项已发表的研究中的 4 项研究的 meta 分析发现，根据短期、中长期及长期临床随访结果显示，端侧重建与结肠 J 形贮袋重建间未见显著差异[9]。在 Machado 等的一项研究中，吻合口与肛缘的平均距离为 4cm[17]，但是在其他研究中均大于 4cm[16, 18]。来自瑞典的 Machado 等的一项纳入 100 例患者的随机对照研究显示，大部分患者接受了术前放化疗，但是在其他研究中并未使用。Huber 等[16]的研究中显示，行 J 形贮袋重建的患者术后 6 个月排便频率明显改善（2.3 vs 3.1 次 / 天；$P<0.05$）。在一些相同的研究中，只有小部分行端侧重建的患者在术后 3 个月有排便不尽感（1/30 vs 7/29）。但随着结肠 J 形贮袋组症状的改善，术后 6 个月随访结果显示两组间未见统计学差异。

大部分研究发现，排便不尽感可随着时间推移而减轻。Machado 等[17]对结肠 J 形贮袋进行术后随访 6 个月，结果显示排便不尽感由 33% 下降至 21%。端侧重建随访 2 年后发现排便不尽感由 50% 下降至 31%。台湾的一项研究[18]观察了 48 例行结肠 J 形贮袋和端侧重建的患者，结果显示两组间排便不尽感发生率均为 50%。

总之，现有证据表明，在排便功能上，端侧重建与结肠 J 形贮袋重建两者相同；但是目前研究并未包括超低位吻合的患者[40]。

结肠 J 形贮袋与横结肠成形术

自 Z'graggen 提出创新术式横结肠成形术以来[41]，已经有大量的研究报道了相关的结果。横结肠成形术并不如结肠 J 形贮袋或端侧重建术那么复杂，因为它不需要使用结肠外或肠系膜组织进行重建。另外，同直接端侧重建一样，它对于系膜缘较短的患者是有益的。由于患者选择的偏差，结肠 J 形贮袋与横结肠成形术之间很难进行比较，因为重建困难的患者如盆腔狭窄、系膜肥胖或其他解剖因素等将不考虑行结肠 J 形贮袋重建术[42]。由于倾向性问题，仍有 7% 行结肠 J 形贮袋重建术。一项多中心随机试验中，26% 的患者由于距肛缘 <3cm 的低位直肠肿瘤而无法行结肠 J 形贮袋重建术[23]。

在一项荟萃分析中，3 项随机试验比较了结肠 J 形贮袋与结肠成形术，研究结果表明在短期和中长期的随访中，排便频率无明显差异，但是结肠 J 形贮袋重建患者排便紧迫感更差[20]。

在一项对结肠成形的试验中，排除行结肠 J 形贮袋的患者，比较结肠成形和直接端-端重建，当患者解剖上允许行结肠 J 形贮袋，则可进行结肠 J 形贮袋和结肠成形术的比较研究。58% 的患者进行了术前放射治疗，大部分患者接受了新辅助化学治疗。这是目前最大的一项对横结肠成形术的研究，纳入了 268 例患者。结果表明，结肠 J 形贮袋重建比结肠成形术具有更好的功能，如在术后 4、12 和 24 个月随访显示，其具有更低的排便次数，在术后 24 个月更少的成簇排便（40% vs 63%；$P<0.03$）。术后第 4 个月随访结果显示，J 形贮袋重建也有更少的排便不连续以及更低的 FISI 评分（39.5 vs 51；$P=0.001$），第 24 个月随访结果相同（31.1 vs 36.8；$P=0.04$）。

横结肠成型与直接端-端吻合重建

目前，仅有一项比较横结肠重建与直接吻合的随机对照研究[23]，选择低位直肠癌无法行结肠 J 形贮袋吻合的患者。这些患者较可行结肠 J 形贮袋的患者具有更高的 BMI（30.5% vs 64%）。在术后第 4、12 和 24 个月的随访中，并未发现直肠肛门功能的差异。但术后 4 个月随访显示，结肠成形术组中排便的连续性较差。

直肠肛门生理学评估

大部分研究认为，如结肠 J 形贮袋、横结肠成形术及端-侧吻合等重建技术，直肠肛门的功能可干预肠壁上的神经信号，这些信号的异常可导致结肠收缩变迟钝或被废除。重建的直肠具有储存大便的功能，但是重建的直肠容积影响肠道的功能。与直接端-侧吻合重建相比，结肠 J 形贮袋储便容量更大。关于这一点，Mantyh 等[21]发现结肠 J 形贮袋的平均容量为 150ml，结肠成形为 117ml，而直

表 8.3 最大耐受容量（ml）

	直接端-端	结肠 J 形贮袋	端-侧	P	术前或术后放射治疗（%）	术后至监测的时间间隔（月）
Hida 等[39]	76.3	101.7		0.004	ND	60
Jiang 等[10]		157.5	171.5	NS	ND	12
Huber 等[8]		296	243	<0.05	ND	6
Machado 等[30]		178	126	<0.001	78	24
Furst 等[5]	120	107		0.76	65	6
Hallböök 等[12]	128	258		<0.001	6	12
Ho 等[20]	123[a]	108		NS	9	12
Joo 等[28]	138	156		NS	20	12

ND，NS：无显著统计学差异；a：结肠成形术患者

接吻合重建为83ml。其他的储便容量比较详见表8.3。在一些研究中，比较了结肠 J 形贮袋与直接吻合重建之间的储便容积，表明结肠 J 形贮袋具有更大的储便容积[16-18]，Machado 等进行的 2 年随访结果显示，结肠 J 形贮袋储便容积较端 - 侧吻合重建更大（178 vs 126ml）[17]。但在另一些报道中，这些重建术的储便容量并无明显差异[15, 20, 38]。Jiang 等[18]的研究发现，与术前相比，重建术后储便容积明显降低，但是结肠 J 形贮袋患者的储便容积迅速恢复。

大部分研究发现，与重建技术无关的是，直肠重建术后肛门静息压明显降低，并能随时间而恢复。一项随机试验比较了 J 形贮袋与直接吻合重建[43]（17% 患者进行了放疗）。Heah[44]等进行的一项随机研究，比较了乙状结肠和横结肠 J 形贮袋重建，Ho[20]等比较了 J 形贮袋与结肠成形术之间的肛门静息压，结果均表明重建后静息压降低。Jiang 等的一项研究比较了端 - 侧吻合与结肠 J 形贮袋重建，结果显示在重建术 1 年后，静息压和排粪压均明显增加，且端 - 侧吻合增加更为明显[18]。但是两年后这两种压力明显下降。另一项研究比较了端 - 侧吻合重建 6cm 和 3cm 的侧支，表明重建术 1 年后静息压和排粪压均升高[19]。

对于评估直肠重建后肛门生理的变化是热点话题，但是这些研究结果并无一致性，这可能与无法评估的解剖因素的差异导致肠道功能不同有关。这一问题较重建的直肠储便容量更为复杂，虽然直肠敏感性的阈值与排便不连续评分有一定相关性，但这些数据与功能缺陷无相关性[45]。贮袋的扩张能力和它的协调性以及传输对贮袋的储便能力有重要影响，尤其是对于手工吻合或吻合器吻合后远端括约肌损伤的患者[46-47]。

结 论

目前的证据表明，如有条件，则结肠 J 形贮袋对于外科医生是一种更好的选择，因该重建具有更好的肠道功能，可允许更低的吻合。端 - 侧吻合重建术可作为一种备选术式，但是目前大多数研究主要用于直肠低位吻合。应当放弃应用横结肠成形术，因为它较结肠 J 形贮袋效果差，且在有困难的盆腔时并不优于直接吻合重建。尽管大多数的研究关注直肠癌术后肠道功能的话题，但是我们对于术前放射治疗和术后肠道功能的理解还存在诸多问题。多数放射治疗主要关注短期效果，大部分的这些研究中，还不清楚除了直接端 - 端吻合以外还有其他重建方式。虽然本章致力于关注对括约肌保留的问题，但患者重建术后肠道功能不良的生活质量不应当被忽视，应权衡生活质量和永久性造口之间的利弊。目前针对这一问题进行的生活质量调查研究，在某种程度上是对患者阐明及应用上的一种挑战[48]。

参考文献

1. Anwar S, Fraser S, Hill J. Surgical specialization and training – its relation to clinical outcome for colorectal cancer surgery. J Eval Clin Pract. 2012;18:5–11. Epub 2010 Aug 4.
2. Rojo A, Sancho P, Alonso O, Encinas S, Toledo G, García JF. Update on the surgical pathology standards on rectal cancer diagnosis, staging and quality assessment of surgery. Clin Transl Oncol. 2010;12:431–6.
3. Weiss J, Moghanaki D, Plastaras JP, Haller DG. Improved patient and regimen selection in locally advanced rectal cancer: who, how, and what next? Clin Colorectal Cancer. 2009;8:194–9.
4. Kakodkar R, Gupta S, Nundy S. Low anterior resection with total mesorectal excision for rectal cancer: functional assessment and factors affecting outcome. Colorectal Dis. 2006;8:650–6.
5. Hoerske C, Weber K, Goehl J, Hohenberger W, Merkel S. Long-term outcomes and quality of life after rectal carcinoma surgery. Br J Surg. 2010;97:1295–303.
6. Ho VP, Lee Y, Stein SL, Temple LK. Sexual function after treatment for rectal cancer: a review. Dis Colon Rectum. 2011;54:113–25.
7. Köninger JS, Butters M, Redecke JD, Z'graggen K. Evacuation of neorectal reservoirs after TME. Recent Results Cancer Res. 2005;165:180–90.
8. Nakada I, Kawasaki S, Sonoda Y, Watanabe Y, Tabuchi T. Abdominal stapled side-to-end anastomosis (Baker type) in low and high anterior resection: experiences and results in 69 consecutive patients at a regional general hospital in Japan. Colorectal Dis. 2004;6:165–70.
9. Brown CJ, Fenech DS, McLeod RS. Reconstructive techniques after rectal resection for rectal cancer. Cochrane Database Syst Rev. 2008:CD006040.
10. Heriot AG, Tekkis PP, Constantinides V, Paraskevas P, Nicholls RJ, Darzi A, Fazio VW. Meta-analysis of colonic reservoirs versus straight coloanal anastomosis after anterior resection. Br J Surg. 2006;93:19–32.
11. Koh P-K, Tang C-L, Eu K-W, Samuel M, Chan E. A systematic review of the function and complications of colonic pouches. Int J Colorectal Dis. 2007;22:543–8.
12. Hallböök O, Påhlman L, Krog M, Wexner SD, Sjödahl R. Randomized comparison of straight and colonic J pouch anastomosis after low anterior resection. Ann Surg. 1996;224:58–65.
13. Benoist S, Panis Y, Boleslawski E, Hautefeuille P, Valleur P. Functional outcome after coloanal versus low colorectal anastomosis for rectal carcinoma. J Am Coll Surg. 1997;185:114–9.
14. Barrier A, Martel P, Gallot D, Dugue L, Sezeur A, Malafosse M. Long-term functional results of colonic J pouch versus straight coloanal anastomosis. Br J Surg. 1999;86:1176–9.
15. Furst A, Burghofer K, Hutzel L, Jauch KW. Neorectal reservoir is not the functional principle of the colonic J-pouch: the volume of a

short colonic J-pouch does not differ from a straight coloanal anastomosis. Dis Colon Rectum. 2002;45:660–7.
16. Huber FT, Herter B, Siewert JR. Colonic pouch vs. side-to-end anastomosis in low anterior resection. Dis Colon Rectum. 1999;42:896–902.
17. Machado M, Nygren J, Goldman S, Ljungqvist O. Similar outcome after colonic pouch and side-to-end anastomosis in low anterior resection for rectal cancer: a prospective randomized trial. Ann Surg. 2003;238:214–20.
18. Jiang JK, Yang SH, Lin JK. Transabdominal anastomosis after low anterior resection: a prospective, randomized, controlled trial comparing long-term results between side-to-end anastomosis and colonic J-pouch. Dis Colon Rectum. 2005;48:2100–10.
19. Tsunoda A, Kamiyama G, Narita K, Watanabe M, Nakao K, Kusano M. Prospective randomized trial for determination of optimum size of side limb in low anterior resection with side-to-end anastomosis for rectal carcinoma. Dis Colon Rectum. 2009;52:1572–7.
20. Ho YH, Brown S, Heah SM, Tsang C, Seow-Choen F, Eu KW, Tang CL. Comparison of J-pouch and coloplasty pouch for low rectal cancers: a randomized, controlled trial investigating functional results and comparative anastomotic leak rates. Ann Surg. 2002;236:49–55.
21. Mantyh CR, Hull TL, Fazio VW. Coloplasty in low colorectal anastomosis: manometric and functional comparison with straight and colonic J-pouch anastomosis. Dis Colon Rectum. 2001;44:37–42.
22. Remzi FH, Fazio VW, Gorgun E, Zutshi M, Church JM, Lavery IC, Hull TL. Quality of life, functional outcome, and complications of coloplasty pouch after low anterior resection. Dis Colon Rectum. 2005;48:735–43.
23. Fazio VW, Zutshi M, Remzi FH, Parc Y, Ruppert R, Fürst A, Celebrezze Jr J, Galanduik S, Orangio G, Hyman N, Bokey L, Tiret E, Kirchdorfer B, Medich D, Tietze M, Hull T, Hammel J. A randomized multicenter trial to compare long-term functional outcome, quality of life, and complications of surgical procedures for low rectal cancers. Ann Surg. 2007;246:481–8.
24. Liao C, Gao F, Cao Y, Tan A, Li X, Wu D. Meta-analysis of the colon J-pouch vs transverse coloplasty pouch after anterior resection for rectal cancer. Colorectal Dis. 2010;12:624–31.
25. Matsuoka H, Masaki T, Kobayashi T, Sato K, Sugiyama M, Atomi Y. Comparison of functional and clinical outcomes: colonic J-pouch vs. coloplasty in patients with low rectal cancer. Hepatogastroenterology. 2010;57:70–2.
26. Hida J, Okuno K. Pouch operation for rectal cancer. Surg Today. 2010;40:307–14.
27. Bakx R, Sprangers MA, Oort FJ, van Tets WF, Bemelman WA, Slors JF, van Lanschot JJ. Development and validation of a colorectal functional outcome questionnaire. Int J Colorectal Dis. 2005;20:126–36.
28. Temple L, Bacik J, Savatta SG, Gottesman L, Paty PB, Weiser MR, Guillem JG, Minsky BD, Kalman M, Thaler HT, Schrag D, Wong WD. The development of a validated instrument to evaluate bowel function after sphincter-preserving surgery for rectal cancer. Dis Colon Rectum. 2005;48:1353–65.
29. Kirwan WO, Turnbull RB, Fazio VW, Weakley FL. Pull-through operation with delayed anastomosis for rectal cancer. Br J Surg. 1978;65:695–8.
30. Rockwood TH, Church JM, Fleshman JW, Kane RL, Mavrantonis C, Thorson AG, et al. Patient and surgeon ranking of the severity of symptoms associated with fecal incontinence. Dis Colon Rectum. 1999;42:1525–32.
31. Pollack J, Holm T, Cedermark B, Holmström B, Mellgren A. Long-term effect of preoperative radiation therapy on anorectal function. Dis Colon Rectum. 2006;49:345–52.
32. Peeters KC, van de Velde CJ, Leer JW, Martijn H, Junggeburt JM, Kranenbarg EK, Steup WH, Wiggers T, Rutten HJ, Marijnen CA. Late side effects of short-course preoperative radiotherapy combined with total mesorectal excision for rectal cancer: increased bowel dysfunction in irradiated patients–a Dutch colorectal cancer group study. J Clin Oncol. 2005;23:6199–206.
33. Pietrzak L, Bujko K, Nowacki MP, Kepka L, Oledzki J, Rutkowski A, Szmeja J, Kladny J, Dymecki D, Wieczorek A, Pawlak M, Lesniak T, Kowalska T, Richter P, Polish Colorectal Study Group. Quality of life, anorectal and sexual functions after preoperative radiotherapy for rectal cancer: report of a randomised trial. Radiother Oncol. 2007;84:217–25.
34. Kollmorgen CF, Meagher AP, Wolff BG, Pemberton JH, Martenson JA, Illstrup DM. The long-term effect of adjuvant postoperative chemoradiotherapy for rectal carcinoma on bowel function. Ann Surg. 1994;220:676–82.
35. Lundby L, Krogh K, Jensen VJ, Gandrup P, Qvist N, Overgaard J, Laurberg S. Long-term anorectal dysfunction after postoperative radiotherapy for rectal cancer. Dis Colon Rectum. 2005;48:1343–9.
36. Parc Y, Zutshi M, Zalinski S, Ruppert R, Furst A, Fazio VW. Preoperative radiotherapy is associated with worse functional results after coloanal anastomosis for rectal cancer. Dis Colon Rectum. 2009;52:2004–15.
37. Ho Y, Seow-Choen F, Tan M. Colonic J-pouch function at six months versus straight coloanal anastomosis at two years: randomized controlled trial. World J Surg. 2001;25:876–81.
38. Joo JS, Latulippe JF, Alabaz O, Weiss EG, Nogueras JJ, Wexner SD. Long-term functional evaluation of straight coloanal anastomosis and colonic J-pouch: is the functional superiority of colonic J-pouch sustained? Dis Colon Rectum. 1998;41:740–6.
39. Hida J, Yoshifuji T, Tokoro T, Inoue K, Matsuzaki T, Okuno K, Shiozaki H, Yasutomi M. Comparison of long-term functional results of colonic J-pouch and straight anastomosis after low anterior resection for rectal cancer: a five-year follow-up. Dis Colon Rectum. 2004;47:1578–85.
40. Siddiqui MR, Sajid MS, Woods WG, Cheek E, Baig MK. A meta-analysis comparing side to end with colonic J-pouch formation after anterior resection for rectal cancer. Tech Coloproctol. 2010;14:113–23.
41. Z'graggen K, Maurer K, Mettler D, et al. A novel colonic reservoir for rectal reconstruction: description of the technique. Gastroenterology. 1997;112:A1487.
42. Ulrich AB, Seiler CM, Z'Graggen K, Löffler T, Weitz J, Büchler MW. Early results from a randomized clinical trial of colon J pouch versus transverse coloplasty pouch after low anterior resection for rectal cancer. Br J Surg. 2008;95:1257–63.
43. Sailer M, Fuchs K-H, Fein M, Thiede A. Randomized clinical trial comparing quality of life after straight and pouch coloanal reconstruction. Br J Surg. 2002;89:1108–17.
44. Heah SM, Seow-Choen F, Eu KW, Ho YH, Tang CL. Prospective, randomized trial comparing sigmoid vs. descending colonic J-pouch after total rectal excision. Dis Colon Rectum. 2002;45:322–8.
45. Schuld J, Kreissler-Haag D, Remke M, Steigemann N, Schilling M, Scheingraber S. Reduced neorectal capacitance is a more important factor for impaired defecatory function after rectal resection than the anal sphincter pressure. Colorectal Dis. 2010;12:193–8.
46. Willis S, Hölzl F, Wein B, Tittel A, Schumpelick V. Defecation mechanisms after anterior resection with the J-pouch-anal and side-to-end anastomosis in dogs. Int J Colorectal Dis. 2007;22:161–5.
47. Kobayashi Y, Yagi M, Iiai T, Tani T, Maruyama S, Hatakeyama K. Comparison of colonic J-pouch and transverse coloplasty pouch in patients with rectal cancer after an ultralow anterior resection using fecoflowmetric profiles. Int J Colorectal Dis. 2009;24:1321–6.
48. Hallböök O, Nystrom P-O, Sjodahl R. Physiologic characteristics of straight and colonic J pouch anastomosis after rectal excision for cancer. Dis Colon Rectum. 1997;40:332–8.

第 9 章 新直肠贮袋及其修正手术

Olof Hallböök

陈启仪 译 李 宁 审校

摘 要

本章讨论直肠癌不同的直肠重建的发展和功能结果。这些数据主要用于讨论低位肿瘤患者保留括约肌，以及增加暂时性近端转流造口和新辅助化学治疗的使用等。

关键词

新直肠贮袋；直肠切除；远端肠管功能；结肠贮袋；横结肠成形术；端–侧结肠肛管吻合术

引 言

1886 年，Kraske[1] 首次尝试将乙状结肠与直肠残端吻合的保肛术。该手术使用后路切口，但经常发生包括粪瘘在内的严重并发症，并伴有一定的围术期死亡率的发生。为了减少吻合的风险，1892 年，Muansell[2] 报道一种腹前位拖出式结直肠吻合术，该术式是将肛管外翻进行结肠 – 肛管吻合，可减少进入盆腔的操作。由于该术式拖出的操作（包括 Cutait-Turnbull 术，是一种延迟的结肠 – 直肠吻合术，在左半结肠优先通过肛门后进行结肠肛管吻合），其功能恢复差，所以应用并不广泛[3]。这些术式目的只是去除肠管的病变，而对肿瘤播散的机制未做考虑，故其肿瘤学预后很差。而后，在 1908 年 Miles[4] 基于他所作的病理学研究对这些术式作了进一步的修正，即放弃原有保留括约肌的切除术，改做腹腔腹膜切除术，这是多数低位直肠肿瘤的黄金标准术式。

目前，直肠癌的外科治疗目的是在完整切除肿瘤的同时，对于合适的患者避免进行永久性造口。前切除吻合的观念是在 20 世纪 40 年代由 Dixon[5] 提出，这使得结肠造口率有缓慢下降的趋势。由此，Parks[6] 描述了一种结 – 直肠吻合术，这使外科医生可以通过肛门行吻合术。20 世纪 70 年代，由于环状钉合吻合器及其改良技术（包括双钉[7] 及三钉[8] 技术）的应用和推广，各种水平上的吻合术变得容易实施。保肛的实施必须以其肿瘤学改变为出发点，本章我们主要讨论这方面的问题。

远端肠道的功能

中枢神经系统的调控、肠管运动的协调（结直肠为主）、良好的直肠储存功能以及完善的肛门括约肌，组成了一个复杂的功能体系，以维持远端肠管功能正常。在这个复杂的运作体系中，各种功能都十分重要，而其中任何一种或几种功能的紊乱，都会导致大便失禁或急迫感。另外，当存在明显括约肌损伤时，如果其他因素依然完好，大便连续性仍可能保持正常。直肠内压与肛门内压之间的协调十分重要，在肛门管与远端肠管间持续存在的正压力梯度可以防止大便外漏。远端肠管的腔内压取决于由自主神经控制的结肠运动动力以及直肠壁的张力。直肠壁的弹性和适应性的松弛可以由压力与容量来反映，即直肠的顺应性，而在活体中，压力/容量不足以描述直肠或者重建的直肠贮袋的弹力属性[9-10]。贮袋连续性在1948年首次由Gaston[11]提出，通过测量直肠填充时容受性舒张反应来定义贮袋功能。该反应由内生性非肾上腺素能、非胆碱能硝基能以及其他神经递质共同介导[12]。结肠的适应性松弛的能力比直肠差很多，所以在直肠切除术后保留结肠的远端（乙状结肠或降结肠）是一种不完美的直肠替代物。

直肠切除术后远端肠管功能

外科医生很久以前即认识到保留远端贮袋至少6～8cm长度的重要性[13]。在此方面，Matzel等[14]发现大便次数与吻合口水平直接相关。因此，在满足肿瘤学原则的基础上，应当尽可能多保留直肠残端。然而，由于技术原因，在进行全结肠系膜切除术时，在肛管顶部横向切除也比较常见，这将切除大部分直肠贮袋，尽管肿瘤位于直肠的中段1/3处。

很多接受过渡性结肠直肠直接吻合的患者已经脱离了一种致死性疾病，并避免了永久性造口，据报道排便控制功能可接受。然而，为了避免结肠造口需付出一定代价。继发的"前切除综合征"可以表现为大便紧迫感、大便失禁、大便断裂以及大便次数增多，许多研究证实绝大多数患者（超过90%）可能会受到影响[15-17]。术后功能恢复难以预期，尽管经过多年的适应，这些症状可能仍然存在[17]。除此之外，建立低位吻合，直肠贮袋缺失，这也会伴随术后功能不良的报道[15]。

这些手术术后常常出现直肠括约肌损伤（常表现为静息肛门压的降低）；然而，直肠切除术后肠功能损伤主要来源于重建直肠容量的降低，而肛门括约肌损伤的影响则相对较小[14, 28]。与降低的静息压力相关的临床文献报道并不统一，这可能在某种程度上与粪便的黏度有一定关系[19]。接受回肠贮袋肛管吻合术的患者，为排除更多的松软粪便，需要肛门括约肌有更大的张力。吻合口瘘和盆腔脓肿均有可能导致肠功能障碍。Hallböök和Sjödahl[20]的病例对照研究比较了多年前曾有吻合口瘘的患者与无并发症的患者。尽管在肛门括约肌功能上无显著差异，曾有吻合口瘘的患者出现了贮袋容量及顺应性的下降，同时伴随有长期及短期的肠功能障碍。

结肠贮袋

前切除综合征的改善会增加重建直肠的顺应性[15, 21]。在前述各种因素中，直肠贮袋的缺失是目前唯一可以通过外科重建恢复的。吸取回肠贮袋的经验后，这些重建方式中最接近生理的可能为尝试进行低位结直肠或者结肠肛管的吻合。Lazorthes[22]与Parc[23]在1986年各自独立报道使用结肠J形贮袋。早期的结果似乎符合其假设，即大便的次数、不尽感以及紧迫感均有显著的下降。该贮袋是将建立一短的末端结肠反折，经贮袋顶端送入吻合器行结肠壁的侧-侧吻合（图9.1）。环形吻合器常用来与肛管吻合。与直接吻合不同，结肠贮袋可使贮存容量恢复、改善顺应性以及重建直肠的感觉[24]（图9.2）。与正常直肠相比，结肠贮袋尽管有足够的容量，但仍存在感觉障碍以及顺应性的下降[25]。可能被解释为清空障碍，这是结肠贮袋的一个缺点，1986年的一个法国患者的系列研究中曾报道过[23]。在这项研究中，25%患者存在自发的排空障碍，需要经常使用灌肠液辅助排空。

在过去的20年中，有很多报道评价结肠贮袋的优点。2006年发表的一篇全面的综述对比了接受结肠贮袋或直接吻合的1050例患者的资料[26]。尽管该系统分析由于包含了随机和观察性研究导致公众偏见的缺陷，但它得出的结论与随后的（2008年）一项循证医学分析结果类似[27]。这项系统仅纳入了9项（共473例患者）随机对照试验。总之，两项系统分析表明贮袋优于直接吻合，主要表现在排便频率、排便不连续、排便紧迫感及重建术18个月后是否需要止泻剂等方面。但是，由于超过两年随访的病例数太少，很难得出何种重建更有优势的结论。关于术后并发症未见明显差异的内容将在随后的章节中进行详细讨论。

应当记住的是这些手术是针对平均年龄约70岁、与癌症相关的恶性疾病在第一个2年的死亡率为20%～40%的人群。但这存在一定的争议，如果这些患者的寿命超过预期后存在肠功能的问题，甚至在第一个2年能短暂获益也是值得的。在结肠贮袋的患者中，10%～25%的患者存在排气排便的问题[23, 28]。开始，贮袋一般大于12cm，但最近研究中多使用75mm的吻合钉将结肠贮袋重建为5～6cm长（图9.1）。目前有两项随机试验证实，随

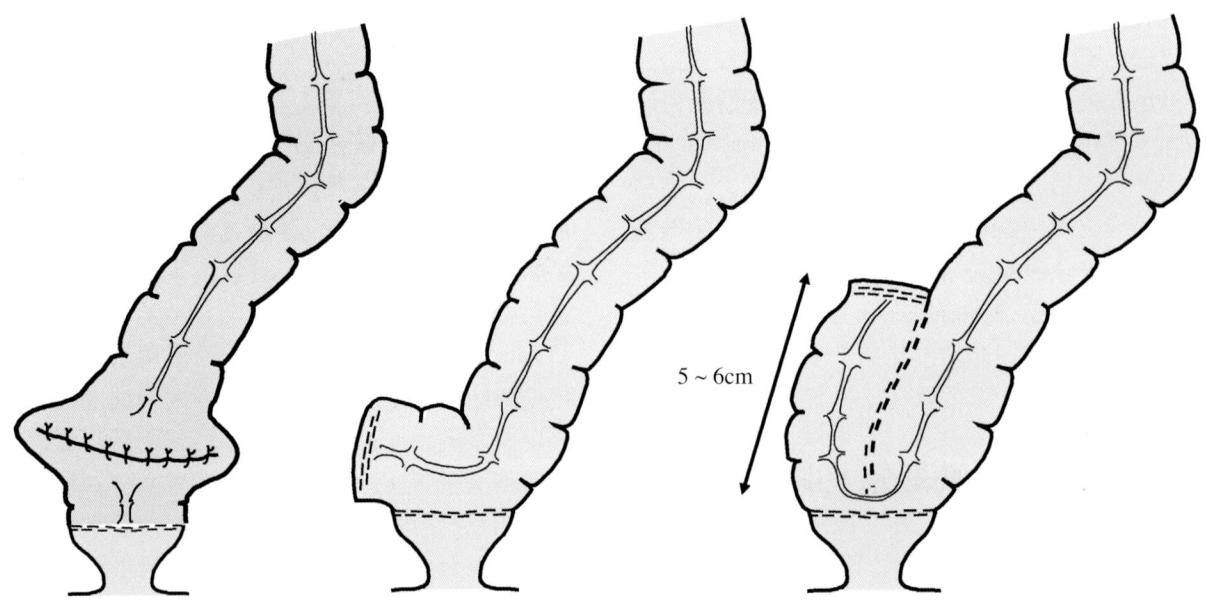

图9.1 3种结肠-肛管吻合术,从左至右:横结肠成形术,Baker/端-侧吻合术,结肠J形贮袋术

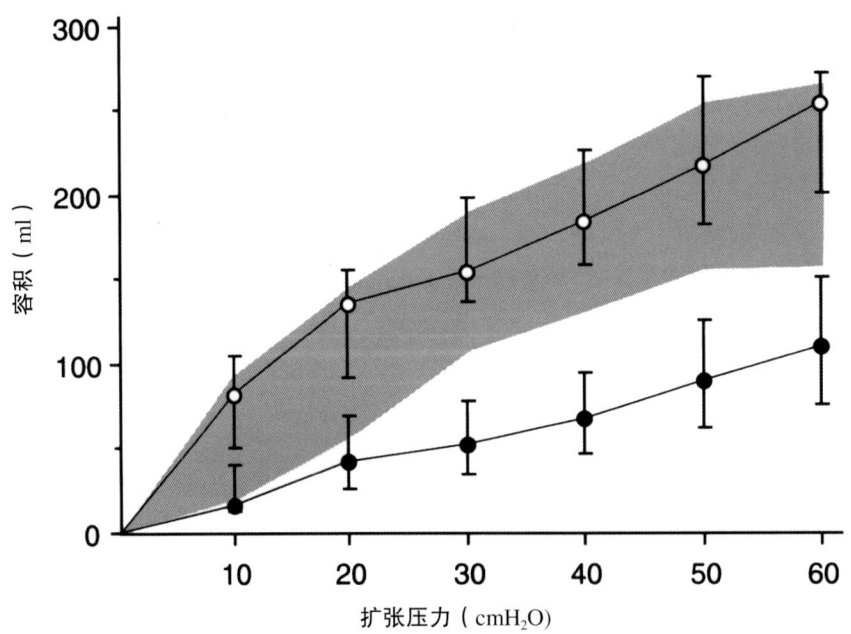

图9.2 新的直肠容积用机械性恒压获得的扩张压力表示。患者行直肠前切除术1年后。空白环表示使用90mm吻合钉行结肠贮袋术患者($n=21$),实心环表示端-端吻合患者($n=21$)。数值以均数表示,四分位间距表示误差线。阴影区域是健康者直肠的四分位间距($n=39$)(From Hallböök.[51])

着贮袋长度的增加,排气排便相关并发症将增加[29]。Hida等研究将患者随机分为贮袋为5cm和10cm两组患者,结果发现虽然两组患者间排便频率和排便紧迫感无明显差异,但结肠贮袋短的患者排气排便相关并发症比10cm组少[30]。Lazorthes等比较了结肠贮袋为6cm和10cm的患者并得出了相同的结论[31]。Hallböök和Sjödahl等进行的一项研究结果表明,使用75mm的吻合钉较90mm的吻合钉排气排便的相关并发症少[25]。吻合钉型号的降低对排便频率、排便紧迫感及排便不连续等无明显的影响。

选择乙状结肠和将结肠行贮袋术对结肠动力和憩室疾病的影响也不尽相同。此外，高位的次级肠系膜动脉结扎可能导致乙状结肠缺血及无法行吻合的结果。除了手术中关于长度和血管的问题（它需在术中判断）以外，目前很少有证据表明选择哪一段肠管更优。一项证据尚不足的试验，患者的结肠贮袋随机选择乙状结肠和降结肠，在这项研究中并未发现选择乙状结肠和降结肠进行贮袋对肠功能及重建的直肠功能有明显的差异[32]。

根据1986年的一项研究，结肠贮袋仅用于直肠肛管重建术的患者。图9.3示一例患者结肠贮袋与直肠远端壶腹部吻合代替肛管吻合，患者的结肠贮袋由于排便困难而拆除。

结肠贮袋术式选择

横结肠成形术

有时不适合、甚至不可能进行结肠贮袋，重建肠道的连续性。这可能与剩余结肠长度较短、肠道的活动度、脂肪组织导致肠道折叠困难或狭窄的盆腔无足够的空间进行贮袋重建有关。自1999年提出的横结肠成形术为这一类患者提供了新的术式选择[33]。现有3项随机试验比较了结肠J形贮袋和结肠成形术，根据短期和中长期的随访结果表明，两种术式对肠道功能的影响无显著差异。其中一项研究认为，结肠成形术增加了吻合口瘘的风险[34]，但是这项研究结果尚未得到其他研究的证实[27]。在随后的一项纳入4项随机试验的系统分析中，比较了结肠J形贮袋与结肠成形术之间的差异[35]。在这项研究中，27%的患者由于在术中判断不可行结肠J形贮袋而行结肠成形术和直接吻合术，经过2年的随访，结果显示，虽然在所有组中外科并发症发生率相同，但结肠J形贮袋有更少的排便频率、更少的成簇排便及更少的排便不连续发生，因此该研究者认为结肠J形贮袋较结肠成形术和直接吻合术更优。结肠J形贮袋的优势在2年以后的随访中表现更为明显。

在技术上，结肠成形重建是据结肠横断的末端4～6cm处纵向切8～10cm的切口（图9.1）。结肠切开处通过Mikulicz的方式横向缝合，结肠与远端直肠残端行端-端吻合。结肠成形重建的倡议者指出，这是一更为简单的重建术。尽管其优势并未在相关的研究中证实，但排便排气相关并发症较结肠J形贮袋重建少。

端-侧吻合

端-侧吻合的概念在胃肠外科很容易理解。这一术式是在1950年由Baker在直肠前切除术背景下首次提出的[36]，其合理性是能代偿不同肠腔的直径。

在技术上，端-侧直肠肛管吻合较结肠J形贮袋更为简单，端-侧吻合同横结肠成形术一样，在患者存在结肠长度较短、肥胖以及盆腔狭窄等因素时有一定的优势。在1999年Machado等的一项研究比较端-侧吻合与结肠J形贮袋吻合的随机试验中[27]，吻合口侧端位于结肠末端3～4cm处，吻合口通过肛门双排吻合钉进行吻合[37]。Jiang等的吻合在腹腔中进行，并不在肛门进行，以避免操作损伤肛门括约肌[38]。相反，Huber等经腹以吻合钉吻合和手工经肛门吻合，且后者吻合居多[39]。

尽管有不同的吻合技术，但在研究中，主要与结肠J形贮袋的6个月随访结果进行比较。Huber等发现结肠J形贮袋排便频率降低，但其他的肠道功能如排便排气功能与端-侧吻合无明显差异[39]；另外的两项随机试验中进行了2年的随访[37-38]。

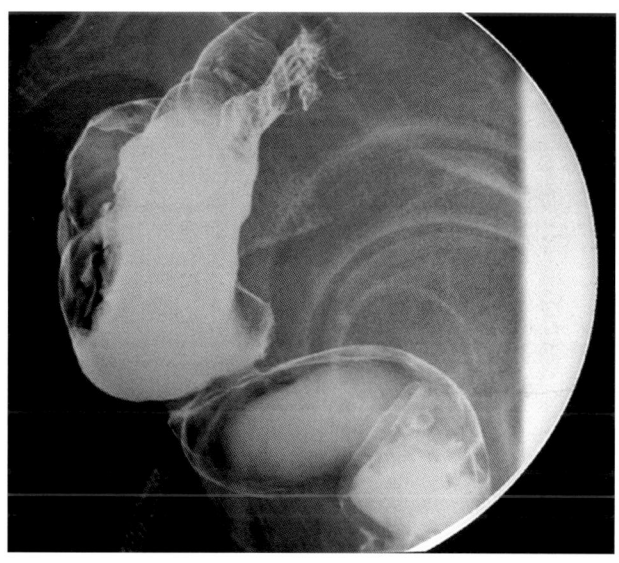

图9.3 钡灌肠造影检查显示不恰当的结肠J形贮袋术；贮袋连接位置太高，即代替肛管的直肠过低。图中贮袋因为严重的并发症被迫去除

新直肠储便袋的生理功能

总之，可能除了直接吻合以外，所有的其他 3 项吻合直肠重建技术包括结肠 J 形贮袋、横结肠成形术及端－侧吻合技术均有相同的临床结果。起初，术式的探讨主要是基于重建的直肠容量或并发症为主要关注点。在这一背景下，肛门直肠的生理研究表明，回肠贮袋有更好的结果；但是回肠不同于结肠，且末端回肠排出粪便也有很大不同。其他直肠重建后的功能分析是观察不同吻合对推动力的影响，即评估远端直肠的压力而不是容积。

在吻合口上建立压力袋的问题的提出是基于使用移动测压法研究结肠肛管吻合[40-41]。近期，通过恒压器监测 10min 的方法研究端－侧或结肠 J 形贮袋重建的直肠动力，较传统研究方法相比，需更长的时间。Bakx 等的研究结果表明，新直肠的功能可能与延迟推进运动更为密切，而非新直肠容积的增加[42]。这可能表示良好的新直肠功能的关键是更多地中断蠕动活性，而非产生更大的贮袋。这一效果可以通过以下几种方式实现：①折叠或横断结肠；②横结肠造口术；③在结肠末端重建几公分的侧吻合口。

吻合口瘘

理论上讲，在结肠侧边形成的吻合如结肠 J 形贮袋和端－侧吻合重建对于重建的直肠容量有一定优势。①结肠侧边较末端肠管具有更好的微循环[43]；②结肠 J 形贮袋或端－侧吻合重建术中，肠系膜可更好地填充盆腔吻合口后方的死腔，可降低因液体聚集而导致的感染的风险。有趣的是，起初的研究发现，端－侧吻合口重建的瘘发生率较端－端吻合重建低。尽管如此，最近 20 年中大量的研究尚无法证实这些重建技术间并发症包括吻合口瘘的发生率有显著差异[26-27]。

暂时性粪便转流

现有研究无法证实上述重建技术对吻合口瘘的发生率有显著差异，医生对于暂时性造口的态度也不一样。目前一项最大的随机研究的数据清晰表明，预防性造口降低了低位切除术患者吻合口瘘发生率[44]。一项随访研究表明，使用临时性造口对肠功能无明显影响[53]。

吻合口瘘和开放性直肠重建的处理

吻合口瘘的处理主要依赖于病情的严重程度，如临床症状、发生的速度、是否存在生命威胁，残端肠管裂开，逐渐发展为脓腔（肠道或吻合口污染物所致）。转移性造口可发挥重要作用，它不仅能改善总体预后，还能降低吻合口瘘的发生率。

虽然吻合口瘘是保留括约肌的直肠切除术中非常严重的并发症，但是目前还较少涉及吻合口瘘的处理和需行永久性造口的风险。下表总结了 3 类不同患者行 J 形贮袋后吻合口瘘的不同处理方式[45-47]。近期，一项新的技术——经肛真空负压引流——用于治疗回肠肛管吻合后的骶前脓肿[48]。在其他的行直肠前切除出现吻合口瘘的患者中，该技术可使 29 例患者中 22 例患者的吻合口瘘最终关闭。这可能是一项被看好的技术，有助于消除脓腔以及避免形

结肠 J 形贮袋吻合口瘘患者的处理

	Machado 等[45]	Maggiori 等[45]	Kruschewski 等[47]
患者总数	161	200	128
吻合口瘘 n%	17(11)a	41(20)b	15(12)a
临时性造口比例	–	95%	100%
仅给予抗生素或无任何其他治疗	1	20	–
经皮或经肛引流	5	10	3
腹腔镜或开腹引流	8	8	12
吻合口紧急切除	3	3	–

a：仅吻合口瘘症状

b：吻合口瘘症状和放射性吻合口瘘

成盆腔慢性窦道。

一项来自 Hallböök O 的尚未发表的研究，纳入 104 例结肠 J 形贮袋吻合口的患者，有 83 例患者贮袋超过 2 年或直至死亡，7 例患者回肠造口无法关闭，14 例患者贮袋被去除。贮袋去除的原因是早期的吻合口瘘（$n=5$）、晚期的管状瘘（$n=1$）、贮袋功能差（$n=4$）、局部肿瘤的再发（$n=2$）以及新的结肠肿瘤（$n=2$）。由于高龄和恶性疾病的出现，在有吻合口瘘的严重并发症时，放弃经肛排便的可能性远高于年轻的回肠袋患者。低位直肠前切除术行永久性造口风险的研究主要引证于预防性造口的随机试验[48]。234 例患者中，有 45 例患者平均在术后 22 个月由临时性造口改为永久性造口。出现吻合口瘘导致永久性造口患者的发生率为 53%，而无吻合口瘘的患者行永久性造口的风险为 11%。另一项来自法国的研究结果表明，出现吻合口瘘后行永久性造口的概率为 22%，而未出现吻合口瘘行永久性造口的概率为 3%[46]。来自德国的一项研究结果类似表明，22% 的患者因为吻合口瘘或盆腔脓肿行永久性造口，这项研究结果也表明原位造口较因并发症而被迫造口有更好的耐受性[49]。

除了外科因素，文化差异是可能影响保肛手术决定的一重要因素。最近一项来自 11 个国家的 13 个研究所的研究结果显示，文化、地域和种族的差异影响永久性造口患者的生活质量，且比年龄、性别和教育影响更大[50]。

结 论

目前有几种术式可供保留括约肌的直肠切除的直肠重建。基于目前的研究，结肠 J 形贮袋或端 – 侧吻合较直接的端 – 端吻合或结肠成形更有优势[51-52]。尽管当发生并发症时，25%～50% 的临时性造口患者将被迫行永久性造口，但行暂时性的造口可降低吻合口瘘发生的风险。

参考文献

1. Kraske P. Zur Extirpation hochsitzender Mastdarmskrebse. Arch F Klin Chir (Berl). 1886;33:563–73.
2. Maunsell HW. A new method of excising the two upper portions of the rectum and the lower segment of the sigmoid flexure of the colon. Lancet. 1892;2:473–6.
3. Cutait DE, Cutait R, Ioshimoto M, da Hyppólito Silva J, Manzione A. Abdominoperineal endoanal pull-through resection. A comparative study between immediate and delayed colorectal anastomosis. Dis Colon Rectum. 1985;28:294–9.
4. Miles EW. A method of performing abdomino-perineal excision for carcinoma of the rectum and of the terminal portion of the pelvic colon. Lancet. 1908;ii:1812–3.
5. Dixon CF. Anterior resection for malignant lesions of the upper part of the rectum and of the sigmoid. Ann Surg. 1948;128:425–42.
6. Parks AG. Transanal technique in low rectal anastomosis. Proc R Soc Med. 1972;65:475–9.
7. Knight CD, Griffen FD. An improved technique for low anterior resection of the rectum using the EEA stapler. Surgery. 1980;88:710–4.
8. Moran BJ, Docherty A, Finnis D. Novel stapling technique to facilitate low anterior resection for rectal cancer. Br J Surg. 1994;81:1230.
9. Madoff RD, Orrom WJ, Rothenberger DA, Goldberg SM. Rectal compliance: a critical appraisal. Int J Colorectal Dis. 1990;5:37–40.
10. Zbar AP. Compliance and capacity of the normal human rectum – physical considerations and measurement pitfalls. Acta Chir Iugosl. 2007;54:49–57.
11. Gaston EA. The physiology of faecal continence. Surg Gynecol Obstet. 1948;87:280–9.
12. Stebbing JF, Brading AF, Mortensen NJM. Nitrergic innervation and relaxant response of rectal circular smooth muscle. Dis Colon Rectum. 1996;39:294–9.
13. Goligher JC, Hughes ESR. Sensibility of the rectum and colon: its role in the mechanism of anal continence. Lancet. 1951;i:543–8.
14. Matzel KE, Stadelkmaier U, Muehldorfer S, Hohenberger W. Continence after colorectal reconstruction following resection: impact of level of anastomosis. Int J Colorectal Dis. 1997;12:82–7.
15. Williams NS, Price R, Johnston D. The long term effect of sphincter preserving operations for rectal carcinoma on function of the anal sphincter in man. Br J Surg. 1980;67:203–8.
16. McDonald PJ, Heald RJ. A survey of postoperative function after rectal anastomosis with circular stapling devices. Br J Surg. 1983;70:727–9.
17. Lewis WG, Holdsworth PJ, Stephenson B, Finan PJ, Johnston D. Role of the rectum in the physiological and clinical results of colo-anal and colo-rectal anastomosis after anterior resection for rectal carcinoma. Br J Surg. 1992;79:1082–6.
18. Lustosa SA, Matos D, Atallah AN, Castro AA. Stapled versus handsewn methods for colorectal anastomosis surgery. Cochrane Database Syst Rev. 2001:CD003144.
19. Williamson MER, Lewis WG, Miller AS, Holdsworth PJ, Johnston D. Recovery of physiologic and clinical function after low anterior resection of the rectum for carcinoma: myth or reality? Dis Colon Rectum. 1995;38:411–8.
20. Hallböök O, Sjödahl R. Anastomotic leakage and functional outcome after anterior resection of the rectum. Br J Surg. 1996;83:60–2.
21. Pedersen IK, Hint K, Olsen J, Christiansen J, Jensen P, Mortensen PE. Anorectal function after low anterior resection for carcinoma. Ann Surg. 1986;204:133–5.
22. Lazorthes F, Fages P, Chiotasso P, Lemozy J, Bloom E. Resection of the rectum with construction of a colonic reservoir and colo-anal anastomosis for carcinoma of the rectum. Br J Surg. 1986;73:136–8.
23. Parc R, Tiret E, Frilaux P, Moszkowski E, Loygue J. Resection and colo-anal anastomosis with colonic reservoir for rectal carcinoma. Br J Surg. 1986;73:139–41.
24. Hallböök O, Nyström PO, Sjödahl R. Physiological characteristics of straight and colonic J-pouch anastomoses after rectal excision for cancer. Dis Colon Rectum. 1997;40:332–8.
25. Hallböök O, Sjödahl R. Comparison between the colonic J-pouch-anal anastomosis and healthy rectum: clinical and physiological

function. Br J Surg. 1997;84:1437–41.
26. Heriot AG, Tekkis PP, Constantinides V, Paraskevas P, Nicholls RJ, Darzi A, et al. Meta-analysis of colonic reservoirs versus straight coloanal anastomosis after anterior resection. Br J Surg. 2006;93:19–32.
27. Brown CJ, Fenech D, McLeod RS. Reconstructive techniques after rectal resection for rectal cancer. Cochrane Database Syst Rev. 2008;(2):CD006040.
28. Hallböök O, Påhlman L, Krog M, Wexner SD, Sjödahl R. Randomized comparison of straight and colonic J pouch anastomosis after low anterior resection. Ann Surg. 1996;224:58–65.
29. Hida J, Yasutomi M, Maruyama T, Tokoro T, Wakano T, Uchida T. Enlargement of colonic pouch after proctectomy and coloanal anastomosis: potential cause for evacuation difficulty. Dis Colon Rectum. 1999;42:1181–8.
30. Hida J, Yasutomi M, Fujimoto K, Okuno K, Ieda S, Machidera N, et al. Functional outcome after low anterior resection with low anastomosis for rectal cancer using the colonic J-pouch. Dis Colon Rectum. 1996;39:989–91.
31. Lazorthes F, Gamagami R, Chiotasso P, Istvan G, Muhammad S. Prospective, randomized study comparing clinical results between small and large colonic J-pouch following coloanal anastomosis. Dis Colon Rectum. 1997;40:1409–13.
32. Heah SM, Seow-Choen F, Eu KW, Ho YH, Tang CL. Prospective, randomized trial comparing sigmoid vs. descending colonic J-pouch after total rectal excision. Dis Colon Rectum. 2002;45:322–8.
33. Z'graggen K, Maurer CA, Buchler MW. Transverse coloplasty pouch. Dig Surg. 1999;16:363–6.
34. Ho YH, Brown S, Heah SM, Tsang C, Seow-Choen F, Eu KW, Tang CL. Comparison of J-pouch and coloplasty pouch for low rectal cancers: a randomized, controlled trial investigating functional results and comparative anastomotic leak rates. Ann Surg. 2002;236:49–55.
35. Fazio VW, Zutshi M, Remzi FH, Parc Y, Ruppert R, Fürst A, Celebrezze Jr J, Galanduik S, Orangio G, Hyman N, Bokey L, Tiret E, Kirchdorfer B, Medich D, Tietze M, Hull T, Hammel J. A randomized multicenter trial to compare long-term functional outcome, quality of life, and complications of surgical procedures for low rectal cancers. Ann Surg. 2007;246:481–90.
36. Baker JW. Low end to side recto-sigmoidal anastomosis: description of the technique. Arch Surg. 1950;61:143–57.
37. Machado M, Nygren J, Goldman S, Ljungqvist O. Similar outcome after colonic pouch and side-to-end anastomosis in low anterior resection for rectal cancer. Ann Surg. 2003;238:214–20.
38. Jiang J-K, Yang S-H, Lin J-K. Transabdominal anastomosis after low anterior resection: a prospective, randomized, controlled trial comparing long-term results between side-to-end anastomosis and colonic J-pouch. Dis Colon Rectum. 2005;48:2100–10.
39. Huber FT, Herter B, Sievert JR. Colonic pouch vs. side-to-end anastomosis in low anterior resection. Dis Colon Rectum. 1999;42:896–902.
40. Williamson MER, Lewis WG, Holdsworth PJ, Finan PJ, Johnston D. Decrease in the anorectal pressure gradient after low anterior resection of the rectum: a study using continuous ambulatory manometry. Dis Colon Rectum. 1994;37:1228–31.
41. Romanos J, Stebbing JF, Smiligin Humphreys MM, Takeuchi N, Mortensen NJ. Ambulatory manometric examination in patients with colonic J pouch and in normal controls. Br J Surg. 1996;83:1744–6.
42. Bakx R, Doeksen A, Slors JF, Bemelman WA, van Lanschot JJ, Boeckxstaens GE. Neorectal irritability after short-term preoperative radiotherapy and surgical resection for rectal cancer. Am J Gastroenterol. 2009;104:133–41.
43. Hallböök O, Johansson K, Sjödahl R. Laser-Doppler blood flow measurement in rectal resection for carcinoma – comparison between the colonic pouch and straight reconstruction. Br J Surg. 1996;83:389–92.
44. Matthiessen P, Hallböök O, Rutegård J, Simert G, Sjödahl R. Defunctioning stoma reduces symptomatic anastomotic leakage after low anterior resection of the rectum for cancer. Ann Surg. 2007;246:207–14.
45. Machado M, Hallböök O, Goldman S, Nystrom PO, Järhult J, Sjodahl R. Defunctioning stoma in low anterior resection with colonic pouch for rectal cancer: a comparison between two hospitals with different policy. Dis Colon Rectum. 2002;45:940–5.
46. Maggiori L, Bretagnol F, Lefevre JH, Ferron M, Vicaut E, Panis Y. Conservative management is associated with a decreased risk of definitive stoma after anastomotic leakage complicating sphincter-saving resection for rectal cancer. Colorectal Dis. 2010. doi:10.1111/j.1463-1318.2010.02252.x.
47. Kruschewski M, Gröne J, Vogel N, Zimmermann M, Buhr HJ. Management and results of complications after anterior resection with colonic pouch reconstruction for rectal cancer. Colorectal Dis. 2010. doi:10.1111/j.1463-1318.2009.01935.x.
48. Van Koperen PJ, Van Berge Henegouwen MI, Slors JF, Nemelman WA. Endo-sponge treatment of anastomotic leakage after ileo-anal pouch anastomosis: report of two cases. Colorectal Dis. 2008;10:943–4.
49. Fischer A, Tarantino I, Warschkow R, Lange J, Zerz A, Hetzer FH. Is sphincter preservation reasonable in all patients with rectal cancer? Int J Colorectal Dis. 2010;25:425–32.
50. Holzer B, Matzel KE, Schiedeck T, Christiansen J, Christensen P, Rius J, Richter P, Lehur PA, Masin A, Kuzu MA, Hussein A, Oresland T, Roche B, Rosen HR, Study Group for Quality of Life in Rectal Cancer. Do geographic and educational factors influence the quality of life in rectal cancer patients with a permanent colostomy? Dis Colon Rectum. 2005;48:2209–16.
51. Hallböök O. Colonic pouch anastomosis after rectal excision for cancer. Medical dissertation. Linköping: Linköping University; 1996.
52. Steffen T, Tarantino I, Hetzer FH, Warschkow R, Lange J, Zünd M. Safety and morbidity after ultra-low coloanal anastomoses: J-pouch vs end-to-end reconstruction. Int J Colorectal Dis. 2008;23:277–81.
53. Lindgren R, Hallböök O, Rutegård J, Sjödahl R, Matthiessen P. Does a defunctioning stoma affect anorectal function after low rectal resection? Results of a randomized multicenter trial. Dis Colon Rectum. 2011 Jun;54(6):747–52. PubMed PMID: 21552061.
54. Lindgren R, Hallböök O, Rutegård J, Sjödahl R, Matthiessen P. What is the risk for a permanent stoma after low anterior resection of the rectum for cancer? A six-year follow-up of a multicenter trial. Dis Colon Rectum. 2011 Jan;54(1):41–7. PubMed PMID: 21160312.

第 10 章 放射性损伤直肠的重建

Vikram Reddy · Walter E.Longo

韦 瑶 译 李 宁 审校

摘 要

直肠癌术前影像学应用的增多导致更多新辅助放化疗的应用；另外，其他临近器官（如前列腺、子宫）恶性肿瘤的辅助放射治疗也导致结直肠损伤。本章概述结直肠专家对这一特殊问题的解决方案，并着重介绍不同的结直肠重建术式。

关键词

放射性直肠损伤；重建；放射治疗；手术切除；直肠恶性肿瘤；瘘；出血；狭窄

引 言

1895 年威廉·伦琴发现了 X 线。两周后，他妻子安娜·贝莎手部的 X 片问世，她直呼看到了自己的尸骨。这一发现后的两年，放射线对肠道的损伤被人们发现，并进行了描述[1]。从那时起，射线对不同器官、系统的作用被广泛学习和探究。人们注意到，放射线对胃肠道的损伤最为明显，尤其是对小肠、结肠和直肠。

尽管存在损伤，放射线无论在疾病的诊断还是治疗中均发挥了重要作用，放射治疗（radiation therapy, XRT）更是成为如宫颈癌、前列腺癌、睾丸癌、膀胱癌、直肠癌、肛管癌等恶性肿瘤综合治疗的重要手段之一。治疗性的骨盆照射指经过 5~8 周的放射治疗，最大程度地破坏瘤细胞，同时能让正常组织从放射损伤中恢复过来[2]。根据瘤体大小（镜下癌及肉眼癌）的不同，放射剂量从 45~80Gy 不等[3]。

尽管人们认识到放射治疗对正常组织的损伤性，并在技术上做了大量改进，以减少或避免这类损伤，但那些意外的放射性损伤仍是潜在的问题。

直肠放射治疗的理论基础

直肠受到照射主要是在治疗肛管直肠恶性肿瘤或者在治疗其他盆腔恶性肿瘤时受累。放射治疗是恶性肿瘤多学科综合治疗的重要组成手段之一，术前、术后均可实施。放射治疗可以降低局部肿瘤复发率，提高直肠病灶切除率；对于低位直肠肿瘤患者，放射治疗使保肛手术成为可能。一系列临床实验都证实了放射治疗在直肠恶性肿瘤治疗中的地位。

20 世纪七八十年代，一系列的试验证明术后放射治疗联合化学治疗比单一化学治疗降低局部复发率，并提高总体生存率[4-9]。术后放射治疗的优势在于治疗主要考虑病理分期分级而非术前不完全可靠的临床分期。基于胃肠道肿瘤研究组织和北部中心癌症治疗协作组的研究结果，美国国立卫生研究院推荐术后联合放化疗应用于直肠癌 II、III 期的患者[5, 7, 10]。欧洲对围术期放射治疗的效果进行了广泛研究，表明经放射治疗后局部复发率降低了 50%~60%[11-18]。在这些研究中，一项荷兰直肠癌临床试验发现行全系膜切除术的患者，经术后辅助放射治疗，局部复发率仅 5.6%。这一研究中，35% 的患者为淋巴结转移阳性的Ⅲ期患者，经过放射治疗后局部复发率比对照组显著下降（10.6% vs 20.6%），其他期别的患者局部复发率仅小幅下降，无显著统计学差异。另外两个亚组的局部复发率也显著下降：一组是低位直肠前切除的（相比 Haetmann 术式及腹会阴联合直肠癌根治术）；另一组是肿瘤边缘距离肛周 5～10cm 范围内的患者（相比肿瘤边缘距肛周更近或者更远者）。尽管上述研究表明局部复发率降低，但总体生存率并没有显著差异。瑞典[11,13,17]、斯德哥尔摩Ⅱ[11,13,17]及曼彻斯特[11,13,17]的研究表明总体生存率提高。这些在局部复发率和总体生存率上显现的不同结果恰好说明了一些在放射治疗过程中非直肠癌致死因素（尤其是心血管系统致死因素）的存在，如在斯德哥尔摩Ⅱ试验中看到的结果，或者由于肿瘤远处转移到一定程度，手术和放射治疗的确降低局部复发率，但对于总体生存率却几乎没有帮助。

术前放射治疗的疗程影响肿瘤降期。波兰的一项研究表明，相比长程放射治疗，短程放射治疗仅部分降低肿瘤分期，尤其对于那些有淋巴结转移的患者[14]。不同的放射治疗时程对于总体生存率无明显影响，但短程放射治疗后局部复发率低，长程放射治疗后肠道狭窄的发生率高。

一些研究表明，联合放化疗无论在局部复发率还是肛门括约肌功能保护上，都较单一治疗有更好的疗效。欧洲癌症研究诊疗组织的一项研究表明：化学治疗（术前或术后）联合长程放射治疗相比单独放射治疗显著降低局部复发率[12]。FFCD 9203 试验表明新辅助放化疗在降低局部复发率上具有显著疗效[15]。

另一些研究点集中在放射治疗和手术时间的问题上。Frykholm 等[19]的研究表明，在Ⅱ、Ⅲ期直肠癌患者，术前短程放射治疗在控制局部复发方面较术后长程放射治疗为好。一项德国的试验显示，术前放射治疗在控制局部复发方面显著优于术后放射治疗，且毒性更低[20]。

直肠放射性损伤的临床表现

直肠放射性损伤的真正发生率很难准确估算。在接受盆腔照射的患者中，50%～70% 出现急性症状如腹痛、腹泻、里急后重和直肠出血等。多数大型研究认为慢性放射性直肠损伤发生率波动于 5%～20%[5,21-24]。

放射性直肠损伤的外科治疗

手术切除和重建直肠的指征主要包括直肠恶性肿瘤和放射性肠损伤所致的并发症如瘘、出血和狭窄。

直肠恶性肿瘤

全系膜切除术是根治性切除直肠恶性肿瘤原发灶的标准术式，但本章内不做详细论述[25-26]。根据肿瘤与肛周括约肌的位置关系不同，直肠癌的手术方式主要分为低位直肠前切除术（LAR）及腹会阴联合直肠癌根治术（APR）。在过去的 20 年里，大多数中低位直肠癌的患者接受了保留括约肌功能的手术（结肠-肛管、低位或者超低位结直肠吻合术）。经腹会阴直肠癌根治术的唯一绝对手术适应证是肿瘤侵犯肛门外括约肌。肿瘤侵犯肛门内括约肌的患者仍可实施括约肌间切除术，并取得良好的效果。肿瘤边缘侵犯肛管或者距离括约肌小于 1cm 的患者需行腹会阴联合直肠癌根治术。肿瘤距离齿状线 2cm 以上的患者，可以实施保留括约肌的切除术；肿瘤边缘距离齿状线 1～2cm 者可以实施括约肌间切除术，以达到清除病灶的目的；距肛门少于 5cm 的肿瘤，即使实施 Heald 等[25,28,29]提出的全系膜切除术，仍需保留 2cm 的阴性切缘[27]。即使肿瘤的位置允许实施保留括约肌的术式，但由于病史过长及检查等导致的括约肌永久性失功等情况，则必须实施腹会阴联合直肠癌根治术[30]。肥胖或骨盆深、窄的患者实施经腹低位或超低位结直肠吻合在技术上相对困难，可能需要经会阴行结-直肠吻合术。

接下来讨论保留括约肌的肠道重建术式的选择问题。吻合口可以手工缝线缝合，也可以应用吻合器吻合。重建方式包括直接结-直肠吻合、结肠-肛管吻合或者结肠贮袋（结肠贮袋-肛管吻合、结肠成形术和端-侧吻合）。这些问题将在探讨直肠重建的不同术式中分别论述。

吻合技术

一旦切除直肠，则需要通过各种不同术式重建肠道连续性。术式取决于肿瘤边缘的位置、括约肌的功能、患者的体型及术者的经验等。

结-直肠和结肠-肛管吻合器吻合

结肠-肛管吻合的位置仍在争论之中，主要是由于难以明确外科肛管（指从肛门口至肛提肌）与解剖肛管（指从肛门口至齿状线）之间的不同。有些学者认为游离至肛提肌，将结肠与外科肛管做吻合应定义为结肠-肛管吻合，但也有学者认为应该与齿状线即解剖肛管做吻合才是结肠-肛管吻合（他们认为外科肛管吻合应该是低位或者超低位的结-直肠吻合）。

随着吻合器的出现，低位直肠前切除+结肠-肛管吻合实施起来容易了许多[33]。主要技术要点包括自盆底游离直肠并以线型切割闭合器切断直肠，直肠残端与结肠或贮袋以圆形吻合器自肛门途径吻合。以管状吻合器切除直肠残端的技术使得吻合口没有张力地移动到齿状线附近。由于有了贮袋，低位吻合口的功能进一步提高，这将在后面详细论述。

结肠-肛管手工吻合

在圆形吻合器出现之前，手工缝合行结肠-肛管吻合是标准术式。这种吻合可以采多种缝合方式，但无一例外都需要经腹松解、游离直肠，然后再经会阴或骶骨吻合。这样的手术方式可以联合是由Parks和Percy[35-36]于20世纪80年代早期提出的黏膜切除术，使得一些低位直肠肿瘤患者避免行腹会阴联合直肠癌根治术。腹部直肠松解、游离完成后，会阴部分直肠的解剖分离就需要借助Lone Star拉钩或者Parks拉钩的帮助。直肠黏膜需要浸润在肾上腺素溶液中，以达到无出血切除。在齿状线上几厘米切断直肠，其残端与通过盆地肌肉的远端结肠或结肠贮袋以丝线在齿状线上间断缝合行结肠-肛管吻合。

手工吻合也可以外翻直肠残端而不做黏膜切除[37]。在这种情况下，关闭的直肠残端需要经腹在分界线以上进行充分游离，然后再经肛门将其外翻，并游离齿状线以上部分。随后经肛管下拉结肠或贮袋，再进行手工吻合。这种体外吻合的方式肠道通畅性好，且并发症少[38]。

对于非常低位的肿瘤（肛提肌上1~2cm），需要实施经腹会阴联合直肠癌根治术，Schiessel[39]等报道切除内括约肌，手工行结肠-肛管吻合术后并发症极少。这样的术式需要腹腔内广泛游离松解，直至括约肌水平，然后行经肛门的括约肌间切除术，远端结肠手工缝闭。研究表明，对于直肠肛管交界处的肿瘤，这一术式术后肛门功能及肠道通畅性完好，是经腹会阴直肠癌根治术的替代方案之一[40-41]。

其他的吻合方式包括Localio、Baron[43]及Mason[44]描述的经括约肌间吻合术[42]。括约肌间吻合术需要患者取右侧卧位，抬高左腿以暴露会阴部；经左下腹斜行切口充分松解游离腹部后，从骶尾关节至肛门做正中切口，切除尾骨，切断肛提肌，切断时标记括约肌；充分游离远端直肠，然后行结肠-肛管吻合，再重建括约肌。

完全或部分切除内括约肌行结肠-肛管吻合术后肛门功能是否完好保留尚存在争议。一些结果显示肛门功能良好[45-47]，但也有研究显示相比保留内括约肌的结肠-肛管吻合术，切除内括约肌后患者控便能力差，生活质量下降。

低位直肠前切除术后结肠贮袋

低位前切除后直接吻合可以引起严重的肛门功能障碍，即"低位切除综合征"，由于失去了直肠功能，表现为急便、便频和气、大便失禁[49-50]，这与吻合的位置有关[49]。大部分症状于术后一年有所缓解[51]，但也有研究表明术后持续存在排便问题[52]。结肠贮袋可以视为新直肠，从而提高LAR患者肠管功能。接下来将按照使用的频率依次介绍不同的贮袋方式。

结肠J形贮袋

1986年，Parc等[53-54]和Lazorthes等[53-54]分别报道了结肠J形贮袋成功替代直肠的功能。结肠J形贮袋的制作过程主要包括下列步骤：游离结肠系膜，结肠浆肌层相对，纵行切开并置肠壁，分别吻合肠管前后壁（可采用器械吻合或手工缝合），最后将贮袋固定于肛管。为了使吻合口没有张力，游离脾区的结肠系膜是必要的。贮袋的理想长度约5cm，大于5cm的贮袋容易排空不畅而需要灌肠或予以缓泻剂[55]。几项前瞻性随机对照研究显示，结肠J形贮袋吻合术后肛门功能要优于直接行结肠-肛管吻合[56-58]。结肠J形贮袋形成的新直肠顺应性好，容量大，提高了LAR术后患者直肠功能[59]。结肠J形贮袋已经成为世界很多中心采用的标准术式。

无法实施结肠J形贮袋的技术因素主要有窄骨盆（在男性患者）、大容量J形贮袋、结肠系膜缩短、左半结肠憩室、结肠过短、妊娠或者括约肌肥厚的长肛管。结肠成形术在理论上可以解决上述问题。

结肠成形术

1999年Z'graggen等[61]首次描述了结肠成形术，以替代存在技术困难无法实施的J形贮袋[62-63]。操作主要步骤包括：在结肠对系膜缘距离结肠切断残端4~6cm处始纵行切开结肠约8~10cm，然后以3-0可吸收缝线缝合切口，然后做端-端吻合。

结肠成形术的优势在于操作简单（结肠游离范围小），相比J形贮袋所需骨盆空间小，容易延伸。功能上与J形贮袋相当[64-65]，甚至最近有研究表明结肠成形术具有较低的吻合口裂开的发生率[65]。但结肠成形术具有较高的瘘发生率，所以至今没有被广泛认可。

端-侧吻合

端-侧吻合术的提出是为了解决结、直肠不同的肠管直径的问题。采用双重闭合的方式：直肠残端以线型闭合器闭合，管状吻合器针底座自远端结肠的对系膜缘穿出与之吻合[66-67]。

回肠间位贮袋

Jean Quenu 在1933年最先描述由一段介于结肠和直肠残端之间的回盲肠重建切断的直肠。在之前以及后来20世纪30年代的经验基础之上，回肠或回盲肠间位贮袋在实验及临床上均重新被描述[68-69]。制作这样的贮袋，需要一段血供良好的回肠代替切断的直肠，且回肠需逆时针旋转180度置于结肠与直肠之间。

这一术式的倡导者认为，相比配对的自愿者，这种新直肠的重建方式保留了内外的神经支配，并具有比较好的排空功能[68-72]。缺点是没有上述重建方式优越性，并且需要额外的肠吻合，使得这一需要更多技术和外科操作的术式接受度很低。

结肠 H 形贮袋

J形贮袋的排空困难随贮袋长度的缩短而减少，外科医师认为逆蠕动的吻合臂是导致贮袋排空功能不佳的原因，顺行的吻合壁对维持正常贮袋功能更加有利。因此，顺行的H形贮袋应运而生[73]。距结肠末端8cm处切断结肠，并行侧-侧吻合做成一个长约6cm的贮袋。然后将H形贮袋与直肠残端行端-端吻合。制作该贮袋技术上有难度，但在功能上较J形贮袋没有提高，因此H形贮袋已经几乎被弃用了。

放射导致的直肠并发症

直肠放射性损伤可以是急性损伤，亦可以是慢性损伤。与急性损伤不同，慢性放射性肠损伤表现为一个放射治疗后3月~30年的、无痛的、渐进的过程[74]。慢性损伤与进程相关，表现为在急性损伤性改变基础上出现的闭塞性血管炎及黏膜下纤维化。这些可以导致肠腔不同程度的狭窄及闭塞。放射治疗导致的并发症与总的放射治疗剂量及照射野范围大小有关[75]。一些研究表明，表现急性放射毒性的患者易发生慢性放射性损伤[76]。但没有出现急性放射性毒性不代表不会发生慢性损伤。在糖尿病、高血压及既往盆腔手术等情况下，直肠发生慢性放射性肠损伤的风险增加，推测可能与粘连及肠管位置固定等有关[74,77]。

经历过盆腔放射治疗的患者，75%在治疗期间就会出现直肠症状，20%将有慢性表现，大约5%出现一些严重的并发症，如直肠周围瘘、狭窄或控便力下降等[78]。直肠出血是最常见的慢性放射性肠损伤的表现，而超过50%的患者在盆腔放射治疗初始或放射治疗前即出现出血症状，往往合并有其他疾病（12%为肿瘤）[79]，因此需要内镜检查明确诊断。内镜检查可以明确肠黏膜的脆性、颗粒度和黏膜下毛细血管扩张的程度[80]。组织学表现为严重的血管改变（特征性表现为内膜下纤维化导致的微动脉狭窄、毛细血管扩张、内皮退化和血小板性微血栓的形成）伴黏膜固有层纤维化及隐窝变形[81]。

尽管药物治疗取得了很大的进步，但外科手术仍然是一些难治病例或并发症（瘘、狭窄、梗阻）的首选治疗方式。手术主要指征最常见的是直肠狭窄、直肠阴道或直肠尿道瘘。大部分患者实施转流手术也是因为上述并发症的发生，手术治疗的有效率达72%[82]。还有一些患者经历重建肠道连续性的手术，常常需要在近端先做一个保护性造口。总之，手术干预率非常高，波动于30%~65%，术后病死率达6.7%~25%[82-83]。直肠重建的各种术式将在下面一章叙述。

直肠梗阻和狭窄

直肠狭窄或梗阻可以通过直肠扩张、近端肠造口、Hartmann 术式、腹会阴联合切除、低位直肠前切除、结肠肛管吻合或 Bricker 术式等解决。选择何种术式要遵从个体化原则，根据患者不同特点而决定。手术之前，需要常规内镜检查并活检排除肿瘤。低位直肠狭窄可采用肛指扩张，而高位狭窄需采用 Hegar 扩张器、Savary 探条或者内镜下球囊扩张。这些方式均具有较高的复发率，常需要每 3～4 个月重复扩张一次。转流性造口常用在重症患者或急性梗阻患者。转流性造口的目的常常是为了消除受累直肠的炎症水肿，以期进一步行确定性重建手术。永久性结肠造口适用于高龄、身体状况较差的患者，相比重建肠道通畅性手术更加安全。低位直肠前切除并吻合的术式在一些病例可以应用，但吻合口可能再狭窄，且吻合口瘘的发生率也较高。一些重建性的手术仍需要在近端做保护性造口，以减少吻合口瘘的发生。重建方式将在下面具体描述。

Parks 结肠-肛管套袖式吻合术

1978 年，Parks[84] 等将结肠-肛管套袖式吻合术进行改进。这一术式最初是由 Ravitch 和 Sabiston[85] 等为修补直肠阴道瘘提出的。这一术式的成功使得外科医师将其应用于治疗放射治疗导致的其他并发症[86-89]。保留括约肌正常功能是保证重建成功的重要基础。这一术式的技术要点主要包括：切除狭窄肠段；充分游离近端结肠，使结肠-肛管吻合口无张力；切除直肠-肛管残端黏膜，将近端健康结肠套入直肠残端，并在齿状线或齿状线以上进行吻合[84]。近端结肠做保护性造口，以避免吻合口瘘发生。

Bricker 修补

1979 年，Bricker 和 Johnston[90] 提出一项新技术来解决直肠阴道瘘及直肠狭窄。对直肠狭窄的患者，与狭窄垂直对折近端健康结肠，直至肠管对系膜缘形成一个类似带蒂的移植物，以增加狭窄肠腔的腔内直径。所有患者都需要做暂时性造口。Bricker[90] 等报道该术式并发症发生率约 50%，而 73% 患者控便能力满意。近年线性闭合器的应用，使得这种手术方式获得不错的疗效[92]。

改良 Duhamel 术式

Martin 改良的 Duhamel 术式也应用于放射治疗导致的直肠狭窄[93]。这一术式在狭窄以上分段处理直肠。直肠充分游离直至狭窄处，游离好的近端结肠下拉至直肠第 3 段，在肛缘上 3～4cm 处经肛门切开直肠后壁约 0.5cm 大小，然后下拉的结肠通过这个开口与直肠吻合。经肛管置入一把长 Kocher 钳并通过直肠后壁及结肠前壁之间吻合口，使得结直肠间开口扩大。在这项报道中，直肠和膀胱均保留了正常的感觉及功能。新的内切割器具有相似的效果，且肠瘘及吻合口再狭窄的发生率较低，在既往没有肠瘘的患者约 6.4%。

直肠瘘

一旦排除肿瘤复发是导致肠瘘的原因，常常需要手术治疗来解决这一令人头痛的问题。直肠瘘可以表现为直肠阴道瘘、直肠尿道瘘和直肠膀胱瘘（直肠尿道瘘及其治疗方式在第 39 章探讨）。直肠阴道瘘是其中最常见的，但这个问题无法通过直肠或阴道皮瓣推移解决，因为这些推移的组织也接受过照射。修补只能采用没有被照射的组织，不同的重建方式将在下面讨论。

Parks 结肠-肛管套袖式吻合术

较大的直肠阴道瘘需要行 Parks 结肠-肛管套袖式吻合术。这一术式是最常用的经腹治疗直肠阴道瘘的方法。将结肠脾区及降结肠充分游离，目的是尽量切除累及的直肠。如果直肠与阴道紧密粘连而无法分开，则尽量游离至直肠远端，经肛管切除直肠黏膜或经腹刮除、电灼黏膜。近端结肠套入直肠并在齿状线或其上进行吻合。75% 的患者术后控便较好，并持续至术后 5 年[84-95]。术前深入学习并理解括约肌功能对实施这一术式非常重要。

Bricker 修补

Bricker 修补适用于大的直肠阴道瘘或者瘘合并狭窄的患者。随着 Bricker 修补技术的进步，逐渐发展了 3 类手术方式：

第 I 类或"补片"：近端结肠游离好后，健康结肠成环状至于瘘的位置，结肠-直肠行端侧吻合，然后在结肠环顶端行结肠-结肠吻合，恢复肠道通畅性。

第Ⅱ类或"圆角或折叠"：这一术式对于有很长狭窄伴或不伴有瘘的患者非常有用。自近端健康结肠开始到远端越过狭窄直肠，于肠对系膜缘切开，结肠对折后以可吸收材料连续缝合形成一个长的缝合线路，近端结肠与形成的缝合线路做吻合，重建肠道通畅性。

第Ⅲ类：在瘘或狭窄的起始处切断直肠和远端结肠，近端结肠与直肠在直肠瘘起始处作吻合，以形成一个广口径的结直肠吻合口。

对所有病例均应做暂时性造口。正如前面提到的，这一术式的效果也很好[90-92, 96]。

Martius 皮瓣

Martius 皮瓣是修补膀胱阴道瘘的一种方法，最早在20世纪20年代末被提出[97]。这一术式在治疗放射导致的直肠阴道瘘上取得了巨大成功[98]。从提出至今，已经发展了几种改良的术式。最著名的是改良 Martius 皮瓣，这一术式以大阴唇代替球海绵体肌[99]。手术时患者取截石位，从阴道开始分离。直肠阴道瘘找到后，将阴道黏膜自瘘上分离下来，直肠阴道瘘的中隔分离后以可吸收缝线横向缝闭直肠缺损。垂直切割大阴唇并将皮瓣提起。游离球海绵体肌脂肪垫，注意保护外侧及内侧的阴部前、后动脉。游离的皮瓣经皮下打隧道补于阴道缺损，以3-0可吸收缝线间断缝合。然后将阴道黏膜覆于其上。对于放射损伤的患者，需要做保护性造口以利于充分愈合。Boronow[100]报道了良好的治疗效果，84%的患者成功闭合瘘口。但其他学者报道的长期随访结果并不令人满意，主要问题包括脓毒症、阴道狭窄、性交困难及肠蠕动过快等[101]。为了解决阴道狭窄及性较困难的问题，一些医生提出应用大腿中部的全层皮瓣进行瘘口修补[102]。

直肠尿道瘘

随着治疗前列腺癌的放射治疗技术的发展（近距放射疗法及体外光束放射治疗），直肠尿道瘘已经非常少见，但仍是一种严重的并发症[103-104]。自发性闭合很少，放射损伤导致的直肠尿道瘘自愈更未见相关报道。虽然经肛管或经括约肌间的术式已成功用于修补直肠尿道瘘[104-106]（经直肠肛管前、后、矢状面或经直肠括约肌），但没有一种术式成功用于放射治疗导致的直肠尿道瘘。在修补的尿道与直肠之间间隔一些没有被照射的组织，如网膜[104]、股薄肌瓣[107]（最常用的是颊黏膜[108-109]）有助于直肠尿道瘘的愈合。也可以经腹（结肠-直肠吻合或 Turnbull-Cutait 技术[110-111]）或经会阴[108-109]进行直肠修补。均必须行保护性造口及尿道改道，以保证愈合良好。股薄肌置入可以使80%以上的放射治疗导致的直肠阴道瘘闭合[109]。

结 论

随着直肠癌治疗的发展，盆腔手术的开展实施越来越多。环状吻合器的出现使得结肠-直肠吻合更加容易方便。结肠贮袋技术解决了直肠切除后肛门失功的问题。尽管盆腔放射治疗技术一直在进步，但放射治疗导致的直肠损伤仍是持续存在的问题。很多新技术涌现出来，以解决放射治疗导致的各种直肠并发症。治疗主要包括减轻受照射直肠炎症水肿的转流性造口和后期直肠-肛管吻合，重建肠道通畅。

参考文献

1. Walsh D. Deep tissue traumatism from Roentgen Ray exposure. Br Med J. 1897;2(1909):272–3.
2. Hall E. Radiobiology for the radiologist. Philadelphia: Lippincott William and Wilkins; 2000.
3. Halperin EC, Perez C, Brady L, Schmidt-Ullrich R. Principles and Practice of Radiation Oncology. The discipline of radiation oncology. In: Perez C, Brady L, Schmidt-Ullrich R, Halperin EC, editors. Philadelphia: Lippincott Williams and Wilkins; 2004.
4. Gastrointestinal Tumor Study Group. Prolongation of the disease-free interval in surgically treated rectal carcinoma. N Engl J Med. 1985;312:1465–72.
5. Russell AH, Harris J, Rosenberg PJ, Sause WT, Fisher BJ, Hoffman JP, Kraybill WG, Byhardt RW. Anal sphincter conservation for patients with adenocarcinoma of the distal rectum: long-term results of radiation therapy oncology group protocol 89–02. Int J Radiat Oncol Biol Phys. 2000;46:313–22.
6. Fisher B, Wolmark N, Rockette H, Redmond C, Deutsch M, Wickerham DL. Postoperative adjuvant chemotherapy or radiation therapy for rectal cancer: results from NSABP protocol R-01. J Natl Cancer Inst. 1988;80:21–9.
7. Krook JE, Moertel CG, Gunderson LL, Wieand HS, Collins RT, Beart RW. Effective surgical adjuvant therapy for high-risk rectal carcinoma. N Engl J Med. 1991;324:709–15.
8. Tveit KM, Guldvog I, Hagen S, Trondsen E, Harbitz T, Nygaard K, Nilsen JB, Wist E, Hannisdal E, Norwegian Adjuvant Rectal Cancer Project Group. Randomized controlled trial of postoperative radiotherapy and short-term time-scheduled 5-fluorouracil against surgery alone in the treatment of Dukes B and C rectal cancer. Br J Surg. 1997;84:1130–5.
9. Wolmark N, Wieand HS, Hyams DM, Colangelo L, Dimitrov NV,

Romond EH, Wexler M, Prager D, Cruz Jr AB, Gordon PH, Petrelli NJ, Deutsch M, Mamounas E, Wickerham DL, Fisher ER, Rockette H, Fisher B. Randomized trial of postoperative adjuvant chemotherapy with or without radiotherapy for carcinoma of the rectum: National Surgical Adjuvant Breast and Bowel Project Protocol R-02. J Natl Cancer Inst. 2000;92:388–96.
10. NIH consensus conference. Adjuvant therapy for patients with colon and rectal cancer. JAMA. 1990;264:1444–50.
11. Marsh PJ, James RD, Schofield PF. Adjuvant preoperative radiotherapy for locally advanced rectal carcinoma. Results of a prospective, randomized trial. Dis Colon Rectum. 1994;37:1205–14.
12. Medical Research Council Rectal Cancer Working Party. Randomised trial of surgery alone versus radiotherapy followed by surgery for potentially operable locally advanced rectal cancer. Lancet. 1996;348(9042):1605–10.
13. Swedish Rectal Cancer Trial. Improved survival with preoperative radiotherapy in resectable rectal cancer. N Engl J Med. 1997;336:980–7.
14. Martling A, Holm T, Johansson H, Rutqvist LE, Cedermark B. The Stockholm II trial on preoperative radiotherapy in rectal carcinoma: long-term follow-up of a population-based study. Cancer. 2001;92:896–902.
15. Bosset JF, Collette L, Calais G, Mineur L, Maingon P, Radosevic-Jelic L, Daban A, Bardet E, Beny A, Ollier JC, EORTC Radiotherapy Group Trial 22921. Chemotherapy with preoperative radiotherapy in rectal cancer. N Engl J Med. 2006;355:1114–23.
16. Bujko K, Nowacki MP, Nasierowska-Guttmejer A, Michalski W, Bebenek M, Kryj M. Long-term results of a randomized trial comparing preoperative short-course radiotherapy with preoperative conventionally fractionated chemoradiation for rectal cancer. Br J Surg. 2006;93:1215–23.
17. Gerard JP, Conroy T, Bonnetain F, Bouche O, Chapet O, Closon-Dejardin MT, et Untereiner M, Leduc B, Francois E, Maurel J, Seitz JF, Buecher B, Mackiewicz R, Ducreux M. Preoperative radiotherapy with or without concurrent fluorouracil and leucovorin in T3-4 rectal cancers: results of FFCD 9203. J Clin Oncol. 2006;24:4620–5.
18. Peeters KC, Marijnen CA, Nagtegaal ID, Kranenbarg EK, Putter H, Wiggers T, Rutten H, Pahlman L, Glimelius B, Leer JW, van de Velde CJ, Dutch Colorectal Cancer Group. The TME trial after a median follow-up of 6 years: increased local control but no survival benefit in irradiated patients with resectable rectal carcinoma. Ann Surg. 2007;246:693–701.
19. Frykholm GJ, Glimelius B, Pahlman L. Preoperative or postoperative irradiation in adenocarcinoma of the rectum: final treatment results of a randomized trial and an evaluation of late secondary effects. Dis Colon Rectum. 1993;36:564–72.
20. Sauer R, Becker H, Hohenberger W, Rodel C, Wittekind C, Fietkau R, Martus P, Tschmelitsch J, Hager E, Hess CF, Karstens JH, Liersch T, Schmidberger H, Raab R, German Rectal Cancer Study Group. Preoperative versus postoperative chemoradiotherapy for rectal cancer. N Engl J Med. 2004;351:1731–40.
21. Buchi K. Radiation proctitis: therapy and prognosis. JAMA. 1991;265:1180.
22. Otchy DP, Nelson H. Radiation injuries of the colon and rectum. Surg Clin North Am. 1993;73:1017–35.
23. Cho KH, Lee CK, Levitt SH. Proctitis after conventional external radiation therapy for prostate cancer: importance of minimizing posterior rectal dose. Radiology. 1995;195:699–703.
24. Schultheiss TE, Lee WR, Hunt MA, Hanlon AL, Peter RS, Hanks GE. Late GI and GU complications in the treatment of prostate cancer. Int J Radiat Oncol Biol Phys. 1997;37:3–11.
25. Heald RJ, Ryall RD. Recurrence and survival after total mesorectal excision for rectal cancer. Lancet. 1986;1(8496):1479–82.
26. MacFarlane JK, Ryall RD, Heald RJ. Mesorectal excision for rectal cancer. Lancet. 1993;341(8843):457–60.
27. Pollett WG, Nicholls RJ. The relationship between the extent of distal clearance and survival and local recurrence rates after curative anterior resection for carcinoma of the rectum. Ann Surg. 1983;198:159–63.
28. Heald RJ, Husband EM, Ryall RD. The mesorectum in rectal cancer surgery – the clue to pelvic recurrence? Br J Surg. 1982;69:613–6.
29. Heald RJ. Total mesorectal excision is optimal surgery for rectal cancer: a Scandinavian consensus. Br J Surg. 1995;82:1297–9.
30. Church JM, Saad R, Schroeder T, Fazio VW, Lavery IC, Oakley JR, Milsom JW, Tuckson W. Predicting the functional result of anastomoses to the anus: the paradox of preoperative anal resting pressure. Dis Colon Rectum. 1993;36:895–900.
31. The American Society of Colon and Rectal Surgeons. Practice parameters for the treatment of rectal carcinoma. Dis Colon Rectum. 1993;36:989–1006.
32. Porter GA, Soskolne CL, Yakimets WW, Newman SC. Surgeon-related factors and outcome in rectal cancer. Ann Surg. 1998;22:157–67.
33. Knight CD, Griffen FD. An improved technique for low anterior resection of the rectum using the EEA stapler. Surgery. 1980;88 710–4.
34. Benoist S, Panis Y, Boleslawski E, Hautefeuille P, Valleur P. Functional outcome after coloanal versus low colorectal anastomosis for rectal cancer. J Am Coll Surg. 1997;185:114–9.
35. Parks AG, Percy JP. Resection and sutured colo-anal anastomosis for rectal carcinoma. Br J Surg. 1982;69:301–4.
36. Parks AG, Percy JP. Rectal carcinoma; restorative resection using a sutured colo-anal anastomosis. Int Surg. 1983;68:7–11.
37. Hautefeuille P, Valleur P, Perniceni T, Martin B, Galian A, Cherqui D, Hoang C. Functional and oncologic results after coloanal anastomosis for low rectal carcinoma. Ann Surg. 1988;207:61–4.
38. Velez JP, Villavicencio RT, Schraut W, Lee K. Outcome analysis of external coloanal anastomosis. Am J Surg. 1999;177:467–71.
39. Schiessel R, Karner-Hanusch J, Herbst F, Teleky B, Wunderlich M. Intersphincteric resection for low rectal tumours. Br J Surg. 1994;81:1376–8.
40. Rullier E, Zerbib F, Laurent C, Bonnel C, Caudry M, Saric J, Parneix M. Intersphincteric resection with excision of internal anal sphincter for conservative treatment of very low rectal cancer. Dis Colon Rectum. 1999;42:1168–75.
41. Saito N, Ono M, Sugito M, Ito M, Morihiro M, Kosugi C, Sato K, Kotaka M, Nomura S, Arai M, Kobatake T. Early results of intersphincteric resection for patients with very low rectal cancer: an active approach to avoid a permanent colostomy. Dis Colon Rectum. 2004;47:459–66.
42. Lazorthes F, Fages P, Chiotasso P, Bugat R. Synchronous abdominotrans-sphincteric resection of low rectal cancer: new technique for direct colo-anal anastomosis. Br J Surg. 1986;73:573–5.
43. Localio SA, Baron B. Abdomino-transsacral resection and anastomosis for mid-rectal cancer. Ann Surg. 1973;178:540–6.
44. Mason AY. Transsphincteric approach to rectal lesions. Surg Annu. 1977;9:171–94.
45. Schiessel R, Novi G, Holzer B, Rosen HR, Renner K, Hölbling N, Feil W, Urban M. Technique and long-term results of intersphincteric resection for low rectal cancer. Dis Colon Rectum. 2005;48:1857–8.
46. Chamlou R, Parc Y, Simon T, Bennis M, Dehni N, Parc R, Tiret E. Long-term results of intersphincteric resection for low rectal cancer. Ann Surg. 2007;246:912–6.
47. Yamada K, Ogata S, Saiki Y, Fukunaga M, Tsuji Y, Takano M. Long-term results of intersphincteric resection for low rectal cancer. Dis Colon Rectum. 2009;52:1065–71.
48. Bretagnol F, Rullier E, Laurent C, Zerbib F, Gontier R, Saric J. Comparison of functional results and quality of life between intersphincteric resection and conventional coloanal anastomosis for low rectal cancer. Dis Colon Rectum. 2004;47:832–8.
49. Karanjia ND, Schache DJ, Heald RJ. Function of the distal rectum after low anterior resection for carcinoma. Br J Surg. 1992;79:114–6.
50. Miller AS, Lewis WG, Williamson ME, Holdsworth PJ, Johnston D, Finan PJ. Factors that influence functional outcome after coloanal anastomosis for carcinoma of the rectum. Br J Surg.

1995;82:1327–30.
51. Keighley MR, Matheson D. Functional results of rectal excision and endo-anal anastomosis. Br J Surg. 1980;67:757–61.
52. Paty PB, Enker WE, Cohen AM, Minsky BD, Friedlander-Klar H. Long-term functional results of coloanal anastomosis for rectal cancer. Am J Surg. 1994;167:90–5.
53. Parc R, Tiret E, Frileux P, Moszkowski E, Loygue J. Resection and colo-anal anastomosis with colonic reservoir for rectal carcinoma. Br J Surg. 1986;73:139–41.
54. Lazorthes F, Fages P, Chiotasso P, Lemozy J, Bloom E. Resection of the rectum with construction of a colonic reservoir and colo-anal anastomosis for carcinoma of the rectum. Br J Surg. 1986;73:136–8.
55. Ho YH, Yu S, Ang ES, Seow-Choen F, Sundram F. Small colonic J-pouch improves colonic retention of liquids – randomized, controlled trial with scintigraphy. Dis Colon Rectum. 2002;45:76–82.
56. Hallbook O, Pahlman L, Krog M, Wexner SD, Sjodahl R. Randomized comparison of straight and colonic J pouch anastomosis after low anterior resection. Ann Surg. 1996;224:58–65.
57. Ho YH, Tan M, Seow-Choen F. Prospective randomized controlled study of clinical function and anorectal physiology after low anterior resection: comparison of straight and colonic J pouch anastomoses. Br J Surg. 1996;83:978–80.
58. Lazorthes F, Chiotasso P, Gamagami RA, Istvan G, Chevreau P. Late clinical outcome in a randomized prospective comparison of colonic J pouch and straight coloanal anastomosis. Br J Surg. 1997;84:1449–51.
59. Ortiz H, Armendariz P. Anterior resection: do the patients perceive any clinical benefit? Int J Colorectal Dis. 1996;11:191–5.
60. Harris GJ, Lavery IJ, Fazio VW. Reasons for failure to construct the colonic J-pouch. What can be done to improve the size of the neo-rectal reservoir should it occur? Dis Colon Rectum. 2002;45:1304–8.
61. Z'graggen K, Maurer CA, Buchler MW. Transverse coloplasty pouch. A novel neorectal reservoir. Dig Surg. 1999;16:363–6.
62. Fazio VW, Mantyh CR, Hull TL. Colonic "coloplasty": novel technique to enhance low colorectal or coloanal anastomosis. Dis Colon Rectum. 2000;43:1448–50.
63. Mantyh CR, Hull TL, Fazio VW. Coloplasty in low colorectal anastomosis: manometric and functional comparison with straight and colonic J-pouch anastomosis. Dis Colon Rectum. 2001;44:37–42.
64. Furst A, Suttner S, Agha A, Beham A, Jauch KW. Colonic J-pouch versus coloplasty following resection of distal rectal cancer: early results of a prospective, randomized, pilot study. Dis Colon Rectum. 2003;46:1161–6.
65. Remzi FH, Fazio VW, Gorgun E, Zutshi M, Church JM, Lavery IC, Hull TL. Quality of life, functional outcome, and complications of coloplasty pouch after low anterior resection. Dis Colon Rectum. 2005;48:735–43.
66. Machado M, Nygren J, Goldman S, Ljungqvist O. Similar outcome after colonic pouch and side-to-end anastomosis in low anterior resection for rectal cancer: a prospective randomized trial. Ann Surg. 2003;238:214–20.
67. Machado M, Nygren J, Goldman S, Ljungqvist O. Functional and physiologic assessment of the colonic reservoir or side-to-end anastomosis after low anterior resection for rectal cancer: a two-year follow-up. Dis Colon Rectum. 2005;48:29–36.
68. Garavoglia M, Fioramonti J, Gentilli S, Borghi F, Bueno L. Myoelectric activity of an ileal isoperistaltic or antiperistaltic loop interposed between colon and rectum: an experimental study in pigs. Eur Surg Res. 1993;25:46–51.
69. von Flue M, Harder F. New technique for pouch-anal reconstruction after total mesorectal excision. Dis Colon Rectum. 1994;37:1160–2.
70. von Flue MO, Degen LP, Beglinger C, Hellwig AC, Rothenbuhler JM, Harder FH. Ileocecal reservoir reconstruction with physiologic function after total mesorectal cancer excision. Ann Surg. 1996;224:204–12.
71. Degen LP, von Flue MO, Collet A, Hamel C, Beglinger C, Harder F. Ileocecal segment transposition does not alter whole gut transit in humans. Ann Surg. 1997;226:742–6.
72. Hamel CT, Metzger J, Curti G, Degen L, Harder F, von Flüe MO. Ileocecal reservoir reconstruction after total mesorectal excision: functional results of the long-term follow-up. Int J Colorectal Dis. 2004;19:574–9.
73. Goere D, Benoist S, Penna C, Nordlinger B. H-pouch: new isoperistaltic colonic pouch for coloanal anastomosis after rectal resection for cancer: a pilot study. Dis Colon Rectum. 2004;47:1740–4.
74. Kennedy GD, Heise CP. Radiation colitis and proctitis. Clin Colon Rectal Surg. 2007;20:64–72.
75. Nussbaum ML, Campana TJ, Weese JL. Radiation-induced intestinal injury. Clin Plast Surg. 1993;20:573–80.
76. Eifel PJ, Levenback C, Wharton JT, Oswald MJ. Time course and incidence of late complications in patients treated with radiation therapy for FIGO stage IB carcinoma of the uterine cervix. Int J Radiat Oncol Biol Phys. 1995;32:1289–300.
77. Dorr W, Hendry JH. Consequential late effects in normal tissues. Radiother Oncol. 2001;61:223–31.
78. Hayne D, Vaizey CJ, Boulos PB. Anorectal injury following pelvic radiotherapy. Br J Surg. 2001;88:1037–48.
79. Andreyev HJ, Vlavianos P, Blake P, Dearnaley D, Norman AR, Tait D. Gastrointestinal symptoms after pelvic radiotherapy: role for the gastroenterologist? Int J Radiat Oncol Biol Phys. 2005;62:1464–71.
80. Reichelderfer M, Morrissey JF. Colonoscopy in radiation colitis. Gastrointest Endosc. 1980;26:41–3.
81. Haboubi NY, Schofield PF, Rowland PL. The light and electron microscopic features of early and late phase radiation-induced proctitis. Am J Gastroenterol. 1988;83:1140–4.
82. Anseline PF, Lavery IC, Fazio VW, Jagelman DG, Weakley FL. Radiation injury of the rectum: evaluation of surgical treatment. Ann Surg. 1981;194:716–24.
83. Pricolo VE, Shellito PC. Surgery for radiation injury to the large intestine. Variables influencing outcome. Dis Colon Rectum. 1994;37:675–84.
84. Parks AG, Allen CL, Frank JD, McPartlin JF. A method of treating post-irradiation rectovaginal fistulas. Br J Surg. 1978;65:417–21.
85. Ravitch MM, Sabiston Jr DC. Anal ileostomy with preservation of the sphincter; a proposed operation in patients requiring total colectomy for benign lesions. Surg Gynecol Obstet. 1947;84:1095–9.
86. Cooke SA, de Moor NG. The surgical treatment of the radiation-damaged rectum. Br J Surg. 1981;68:488–92.
87. Borkowski A, Nowacki M. Simultaneous repair of post-irradiation vesicovaginal and rectovaginal fistulas. J Urol. 1982;128:926–8.
88. Gazet JC. Parks' coloanal pull-through anastomosis for severe, complicated radiation proctitis. Dis Colon Rectum. 1985;28:110–4.
89. Nowacki MP, Szawlowski AW, Borkowski A. Parks' coloanal sleeve anastomosis for treatment of postirradiation rectovaginal fistula. Dis Colon Rectum. 1986;29:817–20.
90. Bricker EM, Johnston WD. Repair of postirradiation rectovaginal fistula and stricture. Surg Gynecol Obstet. 1979;148:499–506.
91. Bricker EM, Kraybill WG, Lopez MJ. Functional results after postirradiation rectal reconstruction. World J Surg. 1986;10:249–58.
92. Steichen FM, Barber HK, Loubeau JM, Iraci JC. Bricker-Johnston sigmoid colon graft for repair of postradiation rectovaginal fistula and stricture performed with mechanical sutures. Dis Colon Rectum. 1992;35:599–603.
93. Starr DS, Lawrie GM, Morris GC. Treatment of postradiation stricuture of the rectum by the modified Duhamel procedure. Am J Surg. 1979;137:795–7.
94. Shimada S, Yagi Y, Yamamoto K, Matsuda M, Baba H. Novel treatment of intractable rectal strictures associated with anastomotic leakage using a stenosis-cutting device. Int Surg. 2007;92:82–8.
95. Cooke SA, Wellsted MD. The radiation-damaged rectum: resection with coloanal anastomosis using the endoanal technique. World J Surg. 1986;10:220–7.

96. Bricker EM, Johnston WD, Kraybill WG, Lopez MJ. Reconstructive surgery for the complications of pelvic irradiation. Am J Clin Oncol. 1984;7:81–9.
97. Martius H. Die operative Widerherstellung der volkommen fehlenden Harnorare und des Schliessmuskls derslben. Zentralbl Gynakol. 1928;52:480–6.
98. White AJ, Buchsbaum HJ, Blythe JG, Lifshitz S. Use of the bulbocavernosus muscle (Martius procedure) for repair of radiation-induced rectovaginal fistulas. Obstet Gynecol. 1982;60:114–8.
99. Elkins TE, DeLancey JO, McGuire EJ. The use of modified Martius graft as an adjunctive technique in vesicovaginal and rectovaginal fistula repair. Obstet Gynecol. 1990;75:727–33.
100. Boronow RC. Repair of the radiation-induced vaginal fistula utilizing the Martius technique. World J Surg. 1986;10:237–48.
101. Aartsen EJ, Sindram IS. Repair of the radiation induced rectovaginal fistulas without or with interposition of the bulbocavernosus muscle (Martius procedure). Eur J Surg Oncol. 1988;14:171–7.
102. Margolis T, Elkins TE, Seffah J, Oparo-Addo HS, Fort D. Full-thickness Martius grafts to preserve vaginal depth as an adjunct in the repair of large obstetric fistulas. Obstet Gynecol. 1994;84:148–52.
103. Nyam DC, Pemberton JH. Management of iatrogenic rectourethral fistula. Dis Colon Rectum. 1999;42:994–9.
104. Chrouser KL, Leibovich BC, Sweat SD, Larson DW, Davis BJ, Tran NV, Zincke H, Blute ML. Urinary fistulas following external radiation or permanent brachytherapy for the treatment of prostate cancer. J Urol. 2005;173:1953–7.
105. Vidal Sans J, Palou Redorta J, Pradell Teigell J, Banús Gassol JM. Management and treatment of eighteen rectourethral fistulas. Eur Urol. 1985;11:300–5.
106. Garofalo TE, Delaney CP, Jones SM, Remzi FH, Fazio VW. Rectal advancement flap repair of rectourethral fistula: a 20-year experience. Dis Colon Rectum. 2003;46:762–9.
107. Ryan JA, Beebe HG, Gibbons RP. Gracilis muscle flap for closure of rectourethral fistula. J Urol. 1979;122:124–5.
108. Zinman L. The management of the complex recto-urethral fistula. BJU Int. 2004;94:1212–3.
109. Vanni AJ, Buckley JC, Zinman LN. Management of surgical and radiation induced rectourethral fistulas with an interposition muscle flap and selective buccal mucosal onlay graft. J Urol. 2010;184:2400–4.
110. Lane B, Stein D, Remzi F, Strong S, Fazio V, Angermeier K. Management of radiotherapy induced rectourethral fistula. J Urol. 2006;175:1382–8.
111. Remzi FH, El Gazzaz G, Kiran RP, Kirat HT, Fazio VW. Outcomes following Turnbull-Cutait abdominoperineal pull-through compared with coloanal anastomosis. Br J Surg. 2009;96:424–9.

第 11 章　复发性直肠癌的手术切除

Michael John Solomon · Peter Jun Myung Lee · Kirk Austin

范朝刚 译　李　宁 审校

摘　要

本章概述了可切除性复发性直肠癌患者的治疗方法，着重介绍有关盆腔脏器切除术的患者诊治路径。复发性直肠癌的治疗需要多学科参与，包括肿瘤内科、造口治疗、骨科、泌尿外科、血管外科和结直肠外科。此类复杂的手术具有一组广泛的适应证，目前正被日益频繁地施行，相关的技术难点将在本章讨论。建议阅读本章的读者同时参考反映美国同行观点的第 12 章。

关键词

手术切除；复发性直肠癌；盆腔脏器切除术；局限性盆腔疾病；无不可治愈的转移性疾病；ASA 评分；患者的偏好；姑息性盆腔脏器切除术

引　言

有关复发性直肠癌的根治性切除和盆腔脏器切除术的文献自 1948 年起就有报道，但是一般都认为这些手术具有极高的手术技术难度，患者术后生活质量差，伴有相当大的手术并发症与死亡的风险。近 20 年来，因为在先进的影像技术的辅助下对盆腔解剖的理解有了进一步的提高，关于如何治疗复发性直肠癌的观念已经发生了转变，治疗策略从选择非手术治疗转为手术治疗。由于这些转变，目前已积累了相当多的病案系列报道，证明此类手术具有可接受的并发症发病率、死亡率和生活质量指数。更重要的是这些临床研究显示，相比于相关的可供替代的非手术治疗，如化学治疗、放射治疗和其他姑息治疗，手术切除具有更优越的生存结果。正因为有了这些研究证据，人们对盆腔脏器切除术这个唯一有可能治愈复发性直肠癌，且生活质量可接受甚至更好的治疗方法重新燃起了兴趣。这个趋势可以从目前专业癌症中心的全世界施行盆腔脏器切除术的数目得到佐证。本章所阐述的观点属于我们机构治疗策略的一部分，需要与第 12 章的内容对比阅读。

当前大部分复发性直肠癌患者可选择的治疗方法包括姑息性化学治疗、放射治疗和支持治疗。这些治疗方法的疗效最好也不会超过 4% 的 4 年生存率，中位生存期 10～17 个月[1-2]。而且，复发性直肠癌患者因肿瘤浸润导致严重的局部症状而死得特别痛苦。这些恶性肿瘤可能会向前方扩展浸润膀胱、阴道、子宫、精囊和前列腺，向后方浸润骶前筋膜、骶骨和骶神经，或者向侧方浸润盆侧壁软组织、输尿管、大血管和神经。盆腔脏器和组织的受侵会导致盆腔疼痛、坐骨神经痛、肠梗阻、下肢血管阻塞，以及膀胱、阴道或肠道的癌性瘘管形成。

这些恶性肿瘤引起的症状和并发症只能通过化学治疗和放射治疗得到暂时的缓解[3]。此外，由于大多数患者在初始治疗中已经接受过大剂量的放射治疗，所以可能无法将姑息性放射治疗作为一种治疗方案。虽然放化学治疗能在一定程度上缓解患者的症状，但根治性手术切除能最大程度地缓解由肿瘤浸润盆骨引起的疼痛和神经痛，尽管我们联合根治性和姑息性治疗也很难达到这种根治性切除。在这一点上，尸检分析已经证实了25%~50%的患者死亡时病变局限于盆腔，这有可能进一步支持了盆腔脏器切除术较非手术治疗所具有的优势[4]。

复发性直肠癌手术治疗的科学理由

衡量一个手术疗效的最好办法是观察相关的并发症发生率、死亡率、术后生活质量和生存数据，在某些经挑选的病例，应考虑选择观测无进展生存期而不是无病生存期。但是，对于复发性直肠癌治疗方法的大部分知识最多只能算观察性的知识，相关的随机临床试验很难设计与操作，并且不大可能实施，因为此类患者群体的内部差异性很大，执行完整的随访工作的后勤保障也相当困难。不仅如此，患者的数量也比较少，因此很难解释不同治疗方法的疗效差异。如果不同的治疗方法及其疗效之间存在显著差异，采用严格的随机临床试验来评价不同的治疗方法已经被证明很困难[5]。

过去10年间，盆腔脏器切除术的逐渐发展已经证明该手术可以安全施行，伴有可接受的死亡率与并发症发病率，但是手术需要严谨周密的计划和多学科合作。手术的目标是完成镜下切缘阴性的完整切除（R0），但是实现该目标的任务相当艰巨，原因在于手术解剖受骨盆空间的限制，并且既往手术或放射治疗消除了正常解剖平面。来自Sloan Kettering癌症中心的研究数据显示，与R0切除相比，切缘阳性（镜下阳性/R1或巨检阳性/R2）患者术后远期生存结果明显更差，R0切除患者术后5年生存率可达35%~65%，而R1与R2切除患者分别仅22%与14%[6]。来自日本的包括83例局部复发性直肠癌的研究结论也支持上述研究结果，即不能取得阴性切缘会导致较差的术后生存率[7]。

目前的研究数据显示，复发性直肠癌接受根治性手术治疗可取得34%~40%的5年生存率，与此相比，目前以姑息性化学治疗与放射治疗为手段的标准治疗方案，其5年死亡率为100%。在这点上，Heriot等[8]对1569例接受盆腔脏器切除术的直肠癌复发病例作了全面的荟萃分析，结果显示平均5年总体生存率达30.7%，切缘阴性（R0）的病例可获得更高的5年生存率（38.2%）。这个研究结果与其他盆腔脏器切除术病例研究的结果一致。一项包括160例直肠癌局部复发病例的研究发现，行盆腔脏器切除治疗后5年生存率可达36%~46%，取得切缘阴性（R0切除）可以作为预后较好的预测因子[2]。该研究还显示盆腔脏器切除术可以安全施行，手术死亡率约0.6%，并发症发病率约27%，尚属可接受范围；同时该研究还发现，采用盆腔脏器切除术治疗令人生畏的盆腔侧壁复发也具有可行性，R0切除率可达到53%。Heriot等[2]发现术后46%的患者无复发，平均无病生存期达到30个月；不仅如此，在平均随访19个月后，65%的患者存活，围术期和术后30天死亡率为0[2,8-11]。

与良好的肿瘤学疗效同样重要的研究结果是，盆腔脏器切除治疗后的存活者可取得与初次手术治疗后患者相近的远期生活质量（FACT-C问卷，106 vs 107）。根治性盆腔脏器切除术后患者的普适生活质量评分（基于第2版36项简表问卷测算）与澳大利亚的普通民众的评分相似；不过该研究发现，盆腔脏器切除术患者的36项简表问卷中体能测评部分评分较普通民众更低（44.7），但是精神部分的测量得分较高，与普通民众相当（53.5）[12]。该研究结果与Miller等[13]对接受不同治疗的局部复发性直肠癌患者的生活质量及成本效益的研究结果更是相互补充，Miller等的研究结论是盆腔脏器切除术作为确定性治疗方案，与非手术和姑息性治疗方案相比，具有成本效益优势。

显然，对于局部复发直肠癌患者而言，接受盆腔脏器切除治疗后唯一的、最重要的生存预测因素就是获得R0切除或切缘阴性。世界范围的文献报道盆腔脏器切除术R0切除率为20%~70%，对来自专业诊疗中心的局部复发性直肠癌手术治疗的数据进行广泛的分析研究，可以发现围术期死亡率约0~18%，术后30天内死亡率为10%~30%，并发症发生率在可接受范围[14-15]。

盆腔脏器切除术的手术指征

直肠癌复发患者需要同时接受外科与内科治疗团队的评估，以确定是否适合接受盆腔脏器切除术这样彻底的切除手术。目前复发性直肠癌行盆腔脏器切除术的手术指征包括[16-17]：

1. 局限于盆腔的复发性疾病：癌症复发范围必须局限于盆腔。过去10年中盆腔脏器切除术的解剖学手术禁忌证发生了巨大的改变。传统的观念认为癌性病灶浸润骨骼与重要的神经或大血管是行盆腔脏器切除术的相对禁忌证，但是，目前的研究资料显示，许多这样的病例通过术前MRI影像资料辅助准确设计手术计划及多学科术前综合治疗，R0切除在技术上是可实现的。

2. 不存在不可治愈的转移性病灶：对于伴有可治愈的转移病灶的局部复发性患者也可选择性地考虑盆腔脏器切除术。MRI和PET/CT全身扫描可以更准确地评估病情，并确定因转移灶已经不可治愈而不应考虑盆腔脏器切除术的患者。相关的转移病灶的处理包括对肝、肺、卵巢、大脑等不同部位病灶的选择性治疗[18-22]。

3. ASA评分1~3级：ASA评分可以用来挑选身体状况能够耐受如此高级别大手术的患者，伴有严重威胁生命的不适合盆腔脏器切除术的系统性疾病的患者。

4. 患者本人在完全知情的情况下同意选择盆腔脏器切除术：患者需要经历相当深入的医患沟通后才能做出最终的选择。知情同意书需要详尽而系统地讨论手术治疗和非手术治疗可能预期的生活质量、与手术伴随的死亡风险和并发症风险，以及手术治疗相关的会阴与生殖系统的重建的性质[23]。应该为患者提供专门的心理支持治疗来帮助他们应对疾病和接下来的大手术。如果有可能邀请一位经历过盆腔脏器切除术的病友来作患者对患者的咨询服务，将会对患者起到很大的心理帮助作用。

针对肿瘤相关性局部的、难以控制症状的姑息性治疗将来也可能成为盆腔脏器切除术的一个适应证。这些症状包括肿瘤浸润所致的重度持续性坐骨神经痛或骨性疼痛、癌性瘘管所致的盆腔感染及因肿瘤占位所致的梗阻。一些医疗小组已经证明这种姑息性盆腔脏器切除术可以改善患者生活质量和控制疼痛，并且可能只需要将肿瘤肉眼大体切除就能实现症状缓解[24-26]。盆腔脏器切除术与目前的"标准治疗"——姑息性化学治疗与放射治疗相比，关键的区别在于手术治疗可获得30%~50%的5年生存率，而姑息治疗的结果是5年100%死亡。

对拟行盆腔脏器切除治疗的转诊患者的诊疗路径

如果需要行盆腔脏器切除治疗，患者需要转给多学科专家治疗小组接受评估，该多学科小组应包括以下专业的专家：结直肠外科、泌尿外科、整形外科、骨外科、血管外科、内科、放射治疗科及造口治疗科。首次评估应包括同患者会谈、复习病史和最近可用于疾病分期的影像资料，PET/CT资料可用于重新分期并排除不可治愈的转移性疾病，盆腔MRI资料可用于确定病灶是否可以切除以及明确骶骨浸润范围。专科会诊在某些情况下是必要的，例如患者需要切除膀胱并重建泌尿道连续性，或者需要切除供应与回流下肢血液的大血管，或者需要切除骶骨或其他骨盆的骨性结构。整形外科医师通常也是治疗组的重要成员，会阴区的皮瓣重建以及肿瘤切除后遗留下来的巨大组织缺损修补需由他们来完成。

成功的治疗需要采取多学科团队协作的策略，治疗的决策基础是对患者病情的准确评估与严谨周密的手术方案设计。在初始评估后，还需要将病情提交到多学科讨论会议上进一步讨论，与会专家应包括：

- 结直肠外科医师
- 泌尿外科医师
- 骨外科医师
- 整形外科医师
- 血管外科医师
- 影像专业医师
- 肿瘤内科医师
- 放射治疗科医师
- 各专科的培训医师（fellows）与住院医师（registars）
- 专科护士
- 造口治疗师
- 麻醉师
- 营养师和膳食专家
- 病房与手术室护士
- 理疗师
- 心理咨询师

这样的专题讨论会议汇集了各个相关专业的专家，系统复习患者的病史、血液检查结果及最新的影像资料，有助于就患者的治疗做出快速的决策。必须复习 PET/CT 资料以确定是否有转移性疾病存在，复习 MRI 资料确定病灶是否可以切除。如果患者因为已经发生不可治愈的转移性疾病或因技术上不具有切除可行性而判定为不能切除，则接下来由肿瘤内科与放射治疗科医师共同来评估是否适合姑息性化学治疗和放射治疗。值得注意的是，有些患者在原发灶的治疗中已经接受了最大剂量的放射治疗而不适合接受更多的放射治疗。图 11.1 显示了复发性直肠癌典型的团队治疗路径[27]。

那些被确定为适合行盆腔脏器切除术的患者接下来需要被告知多学科会议的决策结果。这一步骤有利于从容有序地获得知情同意协议。当患者和家属不得不考虑一个大规模的切除手术并将之与其他治疗方法权衡比较时问题变得比较复杂。这些患者需要相当多的医疗咨询与心理支持。同意手术的患者然后被介绍去接受术前评估。术前评估包括以下步骤：

- 麻醉前病情复习与常规检查（胸片与心电图、伴或不伴肺功能检查、血气分析、心脏超声检查及呼吸/心脏功能评估）
- 造口治疗评估
- 营养与膳食评估
- 社会心理评估、支持和咨询，在这个过程中患者会获得与其他经历过盆腔脏器切除的患者联系交流的机会

下表例举了可供将要行盆腔脏器切除术的患者参考的有关手术与住院的具体信息。

患者术后应转送至重症监护病房（ICU）接受术后早期治疗，盆腔脏器切除术后患者在 ICU 平均

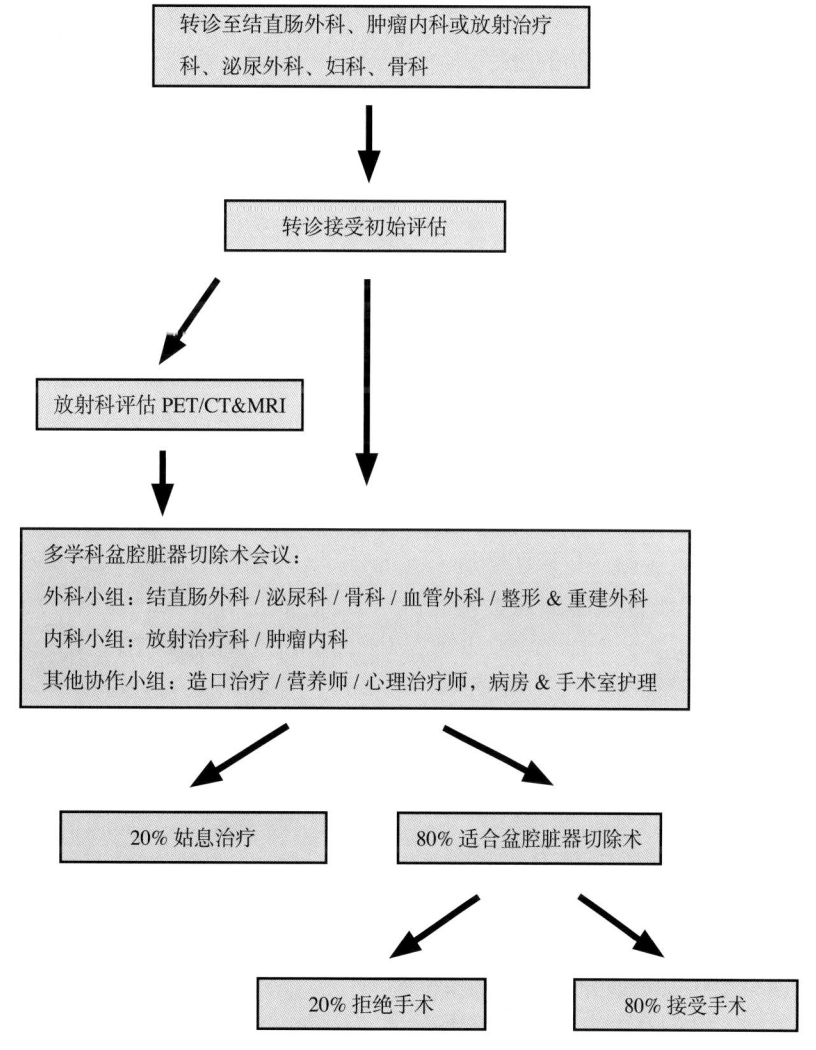

图 11.1　**典型的评估路径图例**

盆腔脏器切除术的手术与住院具体情况[9]	
中位手术时间	9h（3～16h）
中位输血量	6.6u（0～17u）
参与手术的专科平均数	3（1～5）
重症监护病房中位住院天数	3天（0～11天）
中位住院天数	25天（5～126天）

接受2～3天的治疗。在ICU住院期间的日常治疗应包括：

- 重症监护治疗
- 结直肠外科医师负责的基本术后处理
- 其他专科的术后处理（负责的医师可能包括泌尿外科医师/整形外科医师/骨外科医师/血管外科医师，专科培训医师，专科住院医师，住院医师）
- 造口治疗
- 护理与其他相关协作医疗人员（膳食师、理疗师、全肠外营养支持专科护士）的治疗

值得重视的是，接受了骶骨切除或腹直肌纵向皮瓣会阴重建或骶骨缺损修补手术治疗的患者必须采取30度角侧倾体位以避免对相关手术部位的压迫。当病情稳定后患者可以转送至配备拥有护理与治疗此类患者丰富经验的护士与相关医护人员的专科病房继续治疗。盆腔脏器切除术后患者平均需要住院22天，然后转送至康复治疗机构治疗。在专科病房住院期间，患者的日常治疗包括：

- 结直肠外科治疗组的诊疗
- 其他相关专科治疗组的诊疗（泌尿外科医师/整形外科医师/骨外科医师/血管外科医师，专科培训医师，专科住院医师，住院医师）
- 专科护理（这些患者需要特殊的加强护理，通常需要2名护士同时看护）
- 造口治疗
- 其他相关协作医疗人员的诊疗（膳食师、理疗师、全肠外营养支持专科护士、社会工作者、牧师）

出院后前3个月患者视病情需要每月门诊复诊1次或多次，复诊时所有相关的参与患者治疗的专家都需要在场为患者诊疗。3个月后，患者一般已充分康复，可以转回给最初的转诊专家继续接受每6个月1次的门诊复诊。这些患者此后的随访至少应该包括CEA血清水平的监测。再手术后CT扫描结果往往难以解释，原因在于解剖结构异常与放射治疗并发症会导致瘢痕组织与肿瘤复发灶鉴别困难。PET/CT和MRI检查可能是更有用的术后影像学随访工具，因为同时进行PET扫描有助于鉴别瘢痕组织、解剖变异和肿瘤复发。

盆腔脏器切除术的分类

局部复发性直肠癌的治疗是一项艰难而复杂的任务，手术的目标是完成R0切除，将恶性组织连同周围部分正常组织从盆腔完整切除。盆腔脏器切除术中需要和恶性肿瘤整块切除的器官或组织可能包括膀胱、前列腺、子宫与输卵管、阴道、直肠、盆腔血管与神经或骨盆的骨性结构（如骶骨）。如此彻底的手术留下的巨大组织缺损需要转移大块肌皮瓣行重建和修复。

从盆腔结构受侵范围的角度看，局部复发性直肠癌患者是一个异质性的群体，因此手术切除范围是不恒定的，需要个体化处理，故而此类手术没有标准而固定的手术流程，而是根据肿瘤的部位、大小和受累器官的数目而有变动。为便于理解手术方法，骨盆可以分成4个主要区域，用来指示盆腔复发病灶的部位（图11.2）[28-29]。

1. 骨盆前腔内组分包括膀胱、前列腺、精囊、输精管、尿道、尿生殖膈、背静脉丛、闭孔内外肌、盆底肌群前部（耻骨尾骨肌和耻骨直肠肌的部分）、

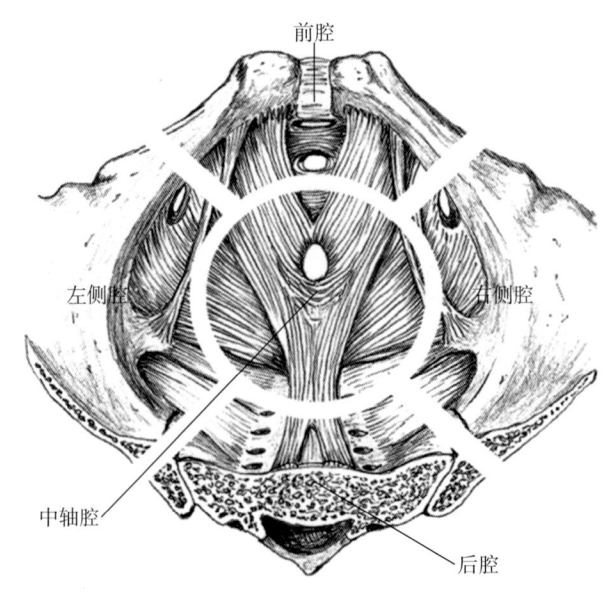

图11.2 图解骨盆前腔、中轴腔、后腔和侧腔

部分盆腔骨骼（耻骨联合、耻骨上下支）和闭孔神经与血管。

2. 骨盆中轴腔内组分包括阴道、子宫、卵巢、输卵管、阔韧带、子宫圆韧带、直肠和盆底肌（髂骨尾骨肌）。

3. 骨盆后腔内组分包括直肠、盆底肌（尾骨肌）、髂内血管的分支、梨状肌、骶神经 $S_1 \sim S_4$、骨盆骨骼（骶骨和尾骨）、坐骨尾骨韧带的前部和骶结节韧带与骶棘韧带的内侧部。

4. 骨盆侧腔内组分包括骨盆侧壁结构、输尿管、髂内血管、髂外血管、坐骨棘附近的梨状肌与闭孔内肌、尾骨肌、坐骨附近的骶结节韧带与骶棘韧带、坐骨（包括坐骨结节和坐骨棘）、腰骶干和远离坐骨棘的坐骨神经。

广义而言，理解这些腔室最好的途径是掌握它们的解剖中心位点，因为各腔室的周边部分有相互重叠。骨盆前腔的解剖中轴是尿道，骨盆中轴腔的中心点是尾骨尖，骨盆后腔的中心点是第 3 骶椎，骨盆侧腔的中心点是坐骨棘。盆腔脏器切除术的关键在于将受累腔室内的器官与组织完整切除，包括骨性边缘。

鉴于手术切除范围具有较大的差异性，此类手术可以被定义为部分或全盆腔脏器切除术（PE）。全 PE 的定义是将原发或复发性肿瘤（连或不连相依附的骨骼）和所有的残留盆腔脏器整块切除，即切除骨盆所有 4 个腔室的内容物。部分 PE 的定义是将原发或复发性肿瘤（连或不连相依附的骨骼）和最多 3 个骨盆腔室内的内容物整块切除。

PE 通常需要采取经腹途径施行，手术的结尾阶段往往经会阴操作，此阶段的操作采用膀胱截石体位或俯卧位。骨盆前腔、中轴腔和侧腔的切除最好采取经腹和经会阴截石体位操作。切除后方 S_4 以下的骶骨以及骶棘韧带可以彻底切除盆底组织，该部的切除操作采用经腹途径视野比俯卧体位更好。

因为骶髂关节连接的特性，第 3 骶椎（S_3）及其上方的骶骨如果受累，手术切除需要采取俯卧位，除非仅仅需要切除第 5 腰椎（L_5）椎体前方和骶椎上部的骨皮质（此操作可以通过经腹途径完成）。侧方高位骶骨切除和 S_2、S_3 椎体的完整切除需要采取俯卧体位经后方入路完成。

根据受肿瘤侵犯的盆腔脏器的数目与种类，手术的实施需要组织一个由多专业的技术熟练的外科医师组成的团队，包括结直肠外科、血管外科、泌尿外科、骨外科和整形修复外科专业。结直肠外科医师主导实施手术，其他专业的医师适时参与手术。手术还需要专业的麻醉师和手术护士，手术可能需要持续 8~20h，平均约 9h。如果需要切除一侧的骨盆侧室或双侧的血管神经组织，手术平均时间会延长到约 12h。

复发直肠癌的手术方法

盆腔前部复发

盆腔前部局部复发灶可能浸润骨盆前腔内的任何组织结构。在评估肿瘤对盆腔前部结构的浸润程度以及与骨性结构的固定程度之前，应首先沿后方平面［全直肠系膜（TME）或骶前平面］与侧方平面（坐骨棘至闭孔内肌平面）游离。

如果子宫、阴道或两者都受到肿瘤浸润，则需要将双侧输卵管、卵巢、子宫、部分阴道后壁或阴道全部与肿瘤及直肠整块切除。依据阴道或会阴切除范围的大小，可能行一期缝合伴阴道重建，或者行肌皮瓣转移会阴重建。医生一般会更倾向于采用肌皮瓣重建会阴，因为此类手术的会阴伤口通常很大，也因为经常患者既往接受过放射治疗。另外，复发灶与肛门的距离决定需要行超低位前切除结肠 J 形贮重建还是根治性腹会阴联合切除术。

如果膀胱顶部或更高部位受肿瘤浸润，可以将部分膀胱、肿瘤复发灶及直肠整块切除，行一期膀胱修补。如果膀胱下部或三角区以下、前列腺或两者同时受肿瘤浸润，必须行根治性全膀胱切除术或全膀胱前列腺切除术伴回肠或结肠代膀胱术。如果肿瘤紧临或已经侵入耻骨，手术切除盆腔前部组织结构时需要更彻底的切缘。需要广泛暴露而不是广泛切开肛提肌前部，暴露范围外侧需达耻骨下支，后方需达坐骨结节，手术入路需选择经会阴入路。将股收肌与股薄肌从耻骨下支侧缘的附着处分离，进一步分离闭孔筋膜进入盆腔。耻骨下支用震荡骨锯或季氏线锯自前方从耻骨前部锯开（图 11.3，切线 A），后方从坐骨锯开（图 11.3，切线 B）。

如有必要，可将部分或全部耻骨联合与肿瘤整块切除。如果行部分切除，暴露并横截双侧耻骨下支（图 11.3，切线 C），将之与后方的坐骨分离；在前方沿耻骨上支下缘将耻骨的下半部分横断。

耻骨联合的上半部分与耻骨联合上支共同维持

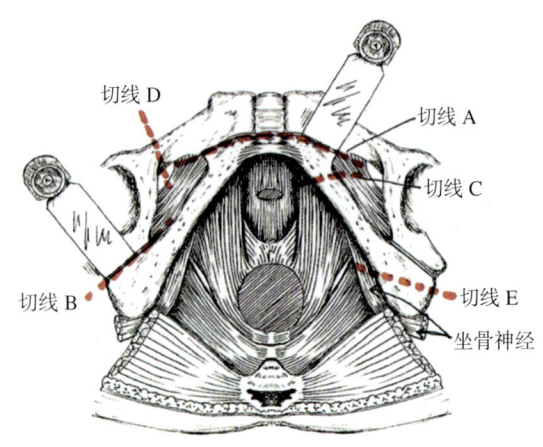

图 11.3 横截耻骨的不同切线

骨盆的稳定性。施行耻骨联合全切除需要横断双侧耻骨下支（图 11.3，切线 C）并尽量靠外侧横断耻骨上支（图 11.3，切线 D）。重建骨盆结构采用聚丙烯补片将耻骨支的四个断端连接并用肌皮瓣或旋转皮瓣覆盖。坐骨结节可沿切线 E（图 11.3）切除，但必须仔细保护从坐骨结节后外侧经过的坐骨神经，此处手术操作需要腹部医生与会阴部医生协作以辨认与保护坐骨神经。

盆腔中央复发

盆腔中央复发又叫中轴区复发，通常包括吻合口复发和新直肠系膜区的复发。为确保环周切缘阴性往往需要广泛切除周围的组织，因此通常必须施行包括广泛盆底与会阴连同 S_4 椎体切除的根治性腹会阴联合切除术。S_4 椎体的切除可以经腹于骶棘韧带水平用骨刀完成，或者偶尔采用俯卧体位操作。更近侧的复发灶也可以采用超低位前切除结肠 J 形贮重建手术治疗。但是，由于复发性直肠癌具有较大的异质性，这些中央复发灶的切除治疗经常需要同时切除邻近的器官，包括子宫、输卵管和卵巢、阴道、膀胱、精囊和前列腺。当遇到这些情况时操作如前所述。

盆腔侧壁复发

盆腔侧壁复发以前被认为是施行盆腔脏器切除术的禁忌证。盆腔侧壁复发的手术解剖入路需要循髂内血管外侧的平面，并需要将髂内血管周围组织部分或全部与肿瘤整块切除。这个解剖平面提供了整块分离与切除盆腔侧壁结构的入路，包括闭孔内肌和梨状肌、骶结节和骶棘韧带及骶神经根；同时也提供了切除盆壁骨性结构的入路，包括骶骨、髂骨、坐骨，这些结构可以通过前入路切除，也可以通过俯卧侧刀体位切除。

彻底探查腹腔排除转移灶与分离腹腔粘连后，从主动脉和下腔静脉水平开始解剖分离，分别解剖并用血管阻断带标记输尿管、髂总和髂外血管。从腹主动脉分叉开始清扫淋巴结，范围包括腹主动脉分叉、髂总血管、髂外血管旁淋巴组织直至髂内血管根部。髂内血管旁淋巴组织此刻不清扫，留待与血管和肿瘤整块切除。

输尿管松解术

接下来该通过观察与触摸来确定远端输尿管在盆腔内的走行以及与肿瘤的关系。如果一侧或双侧输尿管都已受到肿瘤侵犯，需要此时决定选择施行输尿管膀胱再植术还是根治性膀胱切除回肠或结肠代膀胱术。如果决定行根治性膀胱切除术，输尿管应在更晚些时候离断。如果没有发现输尿管受侵的证据，将单侧或双侧输尿管自骨盆上口松解直至膀胱壁。盆腔段输尿管完全游离后，用血管阻断带套住松解后的输尿管，这样在整个漫长的手术过程中，当盆腔结构被离断或切除时都可以很容易地辨认出输尿管。如果输尿管需要在手术早期横断，则在双侧输尿管断端留置 8-Fr 婴儿喂养管，将喂养管连接到导管测量包以便每小时测量尿量。

血管游离和髂内动脉结扎

游离并用血管阻断带标识髂总动脉（CIA）和髂总静脉（CIV）后，将髂外动脉（EIA）和髂外静脉（EIV）游离至腹股沟韧带，评估大血管与肿瘤的相对关系或受侵犯程度。如果大血管受肿瘤浸润，需要决定将受累血管部分切除还是全部切除，以及用补片修补还是血管间置移植修补血管缺损。图 11.4 显示血管间置移植修复 EIA。

通过在受累血管段以外最近端与远端分别留置血管阻断带来实现髂外血管的远端控制，这样在此后的血管解剖或断流的操作中如有需要就可控制血流。接着需要辨认出髂内动脉（ⅡA）的根部，并留置血管阻断带以实现近心端血流控制。为了获得安全操作髂内静脉（ⅡV）和 CIV 的手术入路，在游离髂外血管之前，必须先在根部或第一分支远端结扎并离断ⅡA，否则几乎不可能对远端血管进行手术操作。依次结扎和离断ⅡA和ⅡV是盆腔侧壁手术中最重要的步骤之一，可以让术者由此进入到一个新的更外侧的组织平面，并可将髂总和髂外血管向外侧牵引而移出盆腔或手术解剖平面。图 11.5 显示髂总和髂外血管被移出盆腔。

盆腔血管断流

盆腔血管断流通过离断和缝扎病灶侧ⅡA和ⅡV实现，如果需要行骶骨切除术，则需要离断双侧ⅡA和ⅡV。ⅡA和ⅡV需要在处理远端分支前先予离断。所有通往深部的血管需要缝扎，一般使用 5-0 的 Prolene 缝线。解剖平面内其他通外后外侧的分支也需要离断和缝扎处理。重要的一点是，对手术技巧要求最高的操作是将通往后方与侧方的小静脉在它们进入后方的肌肉与骨骼前从ⅡV后壁离断。这步操作完成后，如有需要，可以将髂外血管依据受侵程度离断或部分切除。在离断血管前于血管的近端与远端分别放置血管夹。在结扎和离断髂外血管前，需要向 EIA 的远端注入肝素以降低下肢动脉与静脉血管内血栓的风险。偶尔，髂血管并不需要全部切除，而是仅仅需要将静脉的后内侧壁与肿瘤整块切除。腿部的血运重建可以采用一段 Goretex（聚四氟乙烯）人造血管/补片或取一段大隐静脉或股浅静脉移植物修补髂外血管来实现。如果无法实现上述操作，可施行股－股动脉 Goretex（聚四氟乙烯）人工血管交叉搭桥术或腋－股动脉 Goretex（聚四氟乙烯）人工血管搭桥术。我们更倾向于血管断流后在继续切除操作前立即恢复下肢血液循环以降低血栓、骨筋膜室综合征和再灌注损伤的风险。值得注意的是，搭桥术或修补术有时候会因为肿瘤巨大而受限或受阻，从而使下肢的血运重建在某些病例不能早期实现。

骶神经根解剖

手术进行至此，已经可以在ⅡA和ⅡV外侧进行解剖，盆筋膜已直接暴露于视野中，该筋膜覆盖着腰骶丛神经、S_1 和 S_2 的坐骨神经上干和位于神经根后方的梨状肌，同时暴露的还有盆底骨骼肌的骨骼附着处（图 11.6 和图 11.7 a, b）。

然后解剖坐骨神经干并将之向侧方牵引，以便必要时切除肌肉和骨盆骨骼。如果肿瘤已经浸润至坐骨神经水平，将受累段神经与肿瘤整块切除。在直视下解剖平面从神经根越过进入至梨状肌。可以采用超声刀（Ethicon Endosurgery Inc., Johnson & Johnson）将梨状肌、肛提肌和闭孔内肌从盆侧壁切除。超声刀有助于取得更好的止血效果，并可以将骨骼肌直接从骨骼剥离。该解剖平面可以使盆侧壁的解剖取得清晰的巨视下阴性切缘，当盆侧壁复发源于髂内淋巴结系统时尤其有用。如果肿瘤向前外侧沿坐骨大孔、坐骨棘或坐骨小孔浸润骨性结构或韧带结构，用骨刀或电刀将受侵骨骼、骶棘韧带和骶结节韧带切除。

通常将膀胱向内侧游离以使之与盆侧壁和耻骨分离。该盆腔前部的解剖为闭孔内肌及血管的解剖

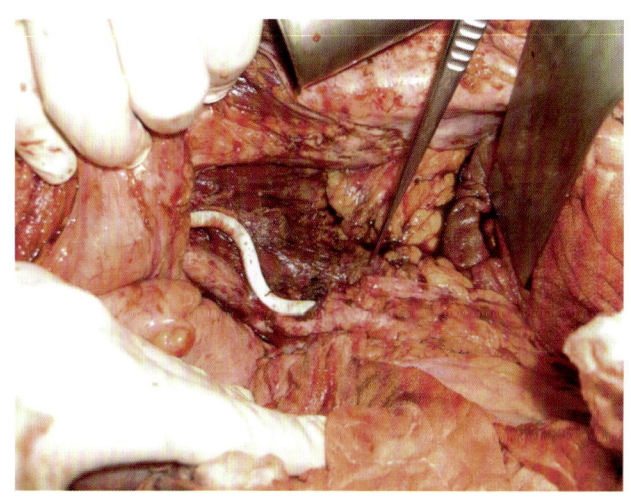

图 11.4　聚四氟乙烯人造血管间置修复右侧髂外动脉

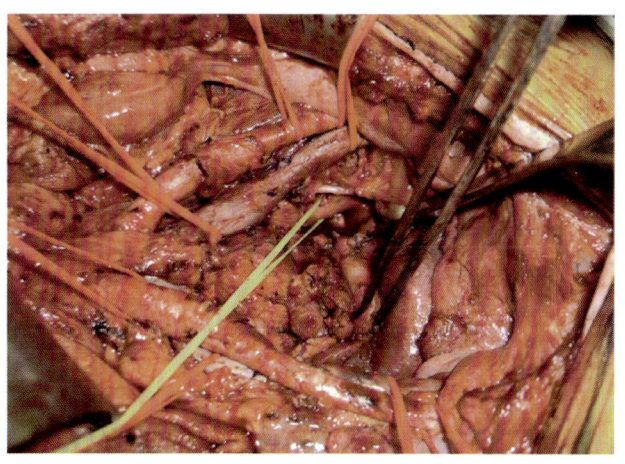

图 11.5　解剖双侧髂血管，抬举髂外血管，暴露腰骶神经干（黄色血管阻断带标记）。注意神经干表面的闭孔神经

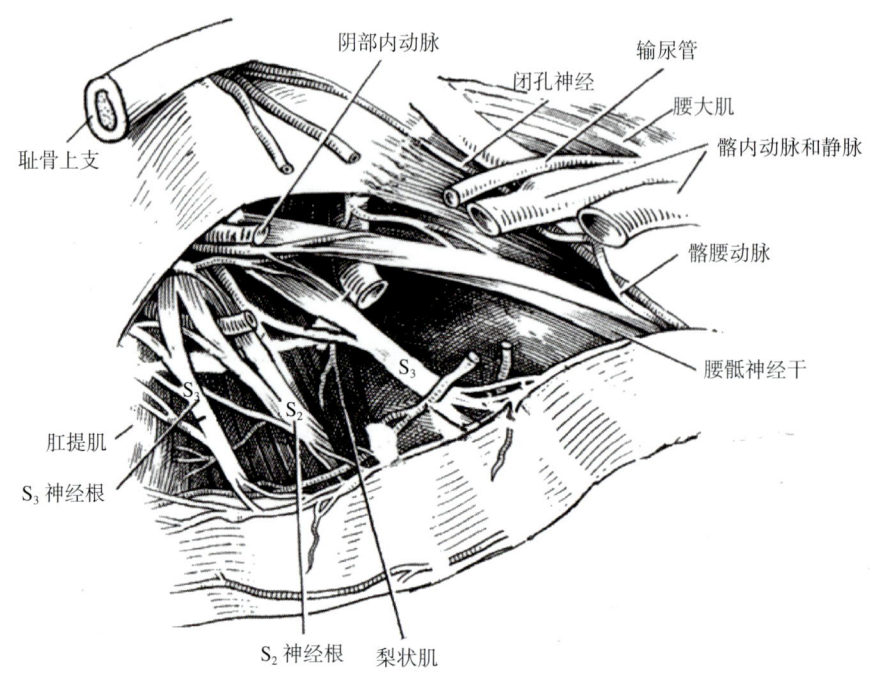

图 11.6　髂外血管外侧的骨盆侧壁解剖结构与相互关系

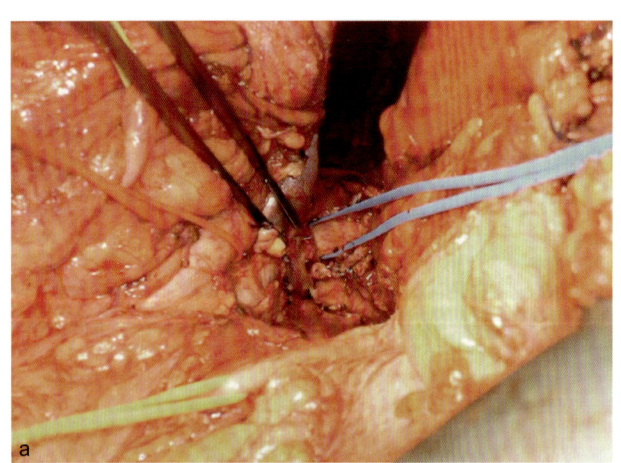
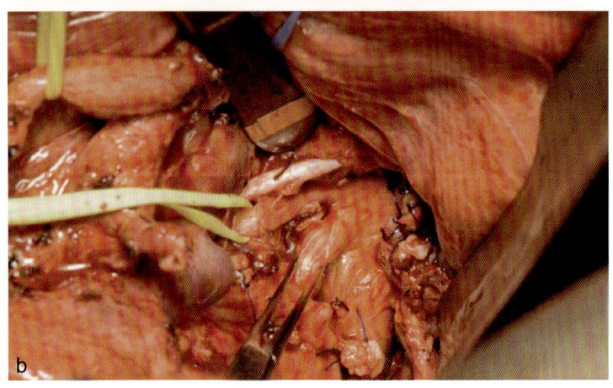

图 11.7　髂内血管外侧解剖平面（a），髂内血管结扎后解剖出 S_1、S_2、S_3 神经（b）

或切除操作提供了通畅的解剖入路。梨状肌和闭孔内肌一旦游离，就取得了进一步解剖骶棘韧带、骶结节韧带、盆底肌（肛提肌和尾骨肌）和骶骨的手术入路。接下来根据侧壁复发灶向内侧的浸润程度进行经盆腔或会阴的盆底和骶骨的不同组合的广泛切除。

盆腔后部复发

盆腔后部的复发通常需要腹会阴联合切除加骶骨切除，但是，如果复发灶仅累及骶骨筋膜，可以通过骨膜剥离，将之与肿瘤及盆腔后部的其他结构整块切除。如果骶骨受侵，需要行骶骨切除，切除的范围根据骶骨受侵的范围而定。因为骶髂关节连接的特性，第 3 骶椎（S_3）及以上椎体如果受侵，一般需要采取俯卧体位行手术切除，除非仅仅第 5 腰椎（L_5）和骶骨上部椎体前面的骨皮质需要切除（这种情况需要经腹切除）。骶骨侧上部和 S_2 和 S_3 椎体全部切除需要采用俯卧位后方入路操作。

盆腔后部复发灶切除手术中前方的解剖平面与腹会阴联合切除术相同，除非肿瘤已经侵犯阴道或膀胱。在这些情况下，需要施行阴道后壁或全部切除、膀胱部分或全部切除。一般而言，初次手术如果是腹会阴联合切除，盆腔脏器切除术就需要切除膀胱和骨盆前腔的结构。与侧壁复发相似，往往需要行双侧输尿管松解、侧壁血管游离和血管断流以清除盆腔病灶或减少骶骨切除时的出血。

S_3 及以上水平的骶骨切除手术中，经腹只需要对髂内血管施行近端结扎，远端分支血管的结扎可以在骶骨切除阶段施行。但是，S_3 及以下水平的骶骨切除术中，需要在骶骨切除水平将髂内血管的远端分支结扎。需要注意，S_3 以下水平的骶骨切除术后很少发生排尿功能障碍。但是单侧 S_1 和 S_2 切除会导致轻度膀胱功能障碍，而双侧 S_1 和 S_2 切除会导致膀胱完全丧失功能。因此，由于功能原因必须行膀胱全部切除加回肠或结肠代膀胱术。

低位盆腔后部复发需要广泛切除整个盆底后部结构，切除范围侧方起自坐骨棘，内侧达 $S_3 \sim S_4$ 交界处（以骶棘韧带深部为界）。如果有肿瘤浸润，梨状肌和骶神经的外侧段也需要部分切除。梨状肌和骶神经从盆侧壁离断后，暴露 S_3 和 S_4 结合处，离断纵向韧带和中线区的肌肉。横断骶骨前，会阴区的手术者自后方解剖尾骨、骶骨至 S_3 水平。接着用 20mm 的加长型骨刀和骨锤经腹腔横断骶骨，操作方法是从中线向两侧推进，并沿着骶棘韧带直至坐骨棘（图 11.8 和图 11.9）。

如果位于梨状肌表面的腰骶神经干和高位骶神经干与肿瘤没有邻接或受侵犯，可予以保留。通过腹会阴区的联合解剖、会阴前部的解剖平面与后外侧平面汇合，将切除标本从会阴伤口移走。

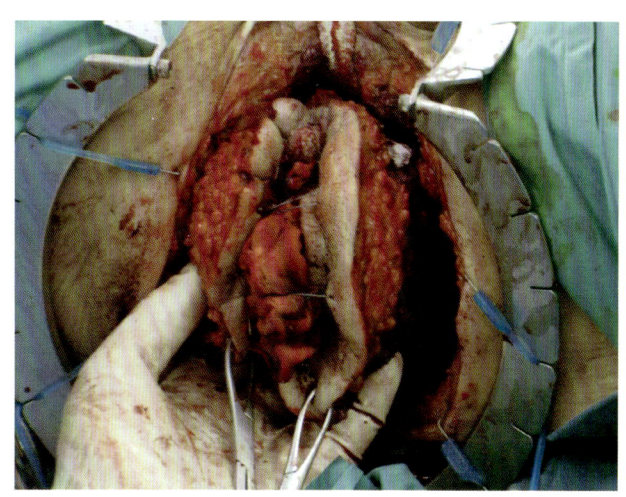

图 11.9 经会阴移走切除标本

$S_2 \sim S_3$ 水平的骶骨切除需要在经腹腔手术操作部分完成后，将患者摆放于俯卧铡刀位操作。在关闭腹腔前，按图 11.10 所示方法，用一个骶骨钉标记骶骨横断的位置。

有了该标记，在患者被摆放于俯卧位后可以用经侧面摄片的方法确认骶骨横断位置。在转成俯卧体位前，还需要在膀胱截石体位经会阴完成前方的游离，并将会阴切口采用连续缝合的方法临时关闭。必须注意，S_1 全部切除会中断骨盆的支撑，不管尝试何种固定装置，目前还不能成功地切除和修复。S_1 椎体的前半部可以经腹用骨刀予以切除，然后改俯卧体位经 $S_1 \sim S_2$ 融合线横截骶骨，保留 S_1 椎体的后半部分，从而保留骨盆的稳定性（图 11.11a, b）。

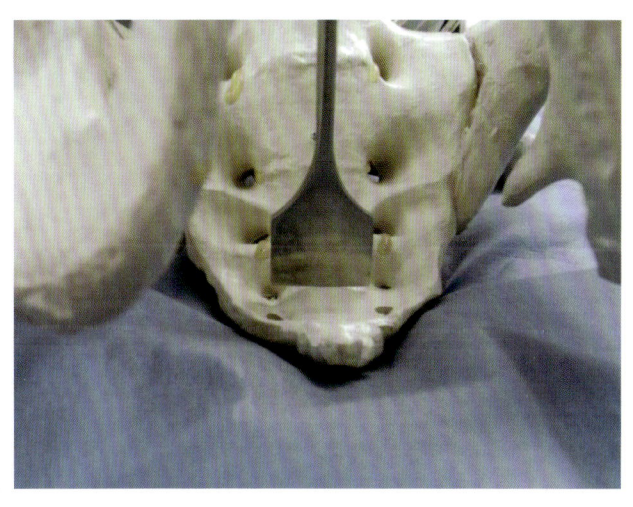

图 11.8 经腹腔用骨刀自 S_3 以下横截骶骨

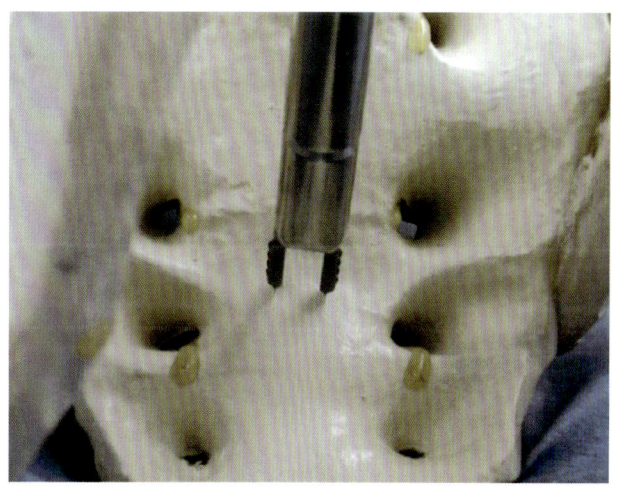

图 11.10 嵌置骶钉

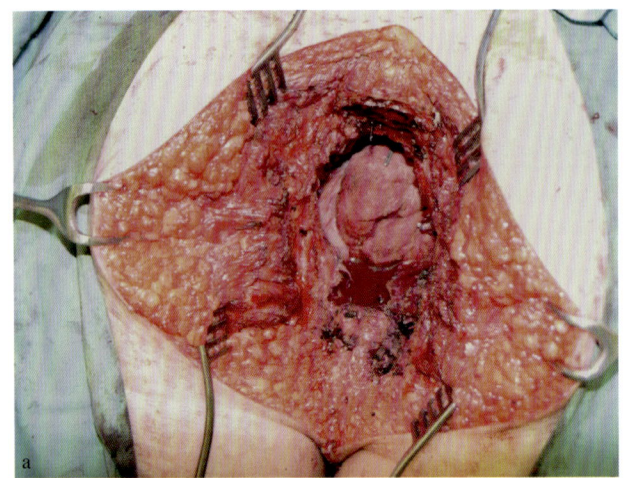

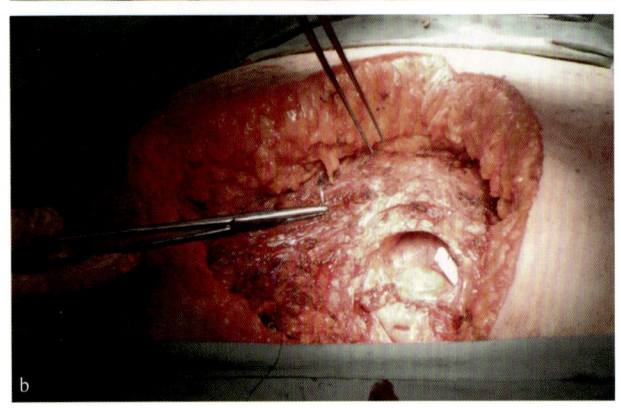

图 11.11 俯卧位自 S_3 以上骶骨切除（a），完成后入路骶骨切除（b）

会阴重建

肌皮瓣能够保护小肠，预防会阴疝，最重要的是提高了会阴切口一期愈合的成功率。VRAM 肌皮瓣是最好、最常用的重建皮瓣，原因在于与其他皮瓣相比，该皮瓣具有充足的组织体积来填补会阴和骶骨缺损区，并且可以很方便地翻转入会阴和骶骨区。采用 VRAM 肌皮瓣的另一个好处是它为一个易于发生切口愈合障碍的区域提供了新的、未受放射损伤、血供充足的组织促进愈合。

有一些病理因素会妨碍 VRAM 肌皮瓣的应用，这些因素包括既往或现在有腹壁造口、既往腹壁手术切口（尤其是耻骨上横切口、阑尾手术横切口和开放性腹股沟疝修补术切口）。病理性肥胖和血管疾病也可能影响到制作 VRAM 所必需的腹壁血管的通畅程度。在这些情况下，需要行腹壁 CT 血管造影来了解腹壁血管的通畅程度。

需要注意，可供选择的股薄肌肌皮瓣通常不够结实，且体积一般不足以覆盖盆腔脏器切除术后的会阴伤口。可以在俯卧体位的情况下采用臀大肌肌皮瓣，但是，如果术中施行了盆侧壁髂内血管切除或结扎，臀大肌主要血管会被断流而依赖于侧支循环，所以这种情况下应避免采用臀大肌肌皮瓣。腹直肌皮瓣在骨盆前腔器官被切除时使用更方便，但是即使保留了膀胱，该皮瓣仍然可以使用，不过需要将一侧膀胱游离后向内侧推开，以便肌皮瓣可以经耻骨膀胱前间隙通过。

术前标记好肌皮瓣的位置很重要，如果患者需要两处腹壁造口，肌皮瓣供应区同侧的造口位置需要设置在传统位置的更外侧，方法是自中线切口向传统的造口位置画线，将造口位置从传统位置外移 5cm。如果患者需要两处腹壁造口，VRAM 供皮区对侧的造口位置也需要在开腹前标记好。在经腹手术操作阶段，需要很仔细地确保轻柔地牵拉腹直肌，这样腹壁下血管仅仅受到最小程度的压迫。在将 VRAM 肌皮瓣绕轴旋转穿过盆腔置入会阴或骶骨区伤口时，必须高度谨慎以避免扭曲腹壁下血管蒂。将肌皮瓣置入预定位置后必须检查它的位置、张力和活力。可以对皮瓣进行必要的修剪，然后将之缝合固定（图 11.12、图 11.13 和图 11.14）。

如果患者因为腹壁下血管狭窄或腹壁造口的原因不适合采用 VRAM 肌皮瓣修复，则臀大肌肌皮瓣修复是一个不错的选择。如果需要采用臀大肌肌皮瓣，在游离和切除髂内血管时必须保留臀上血管以保存臀大肌充足的血供（图 11.15 a,b）。

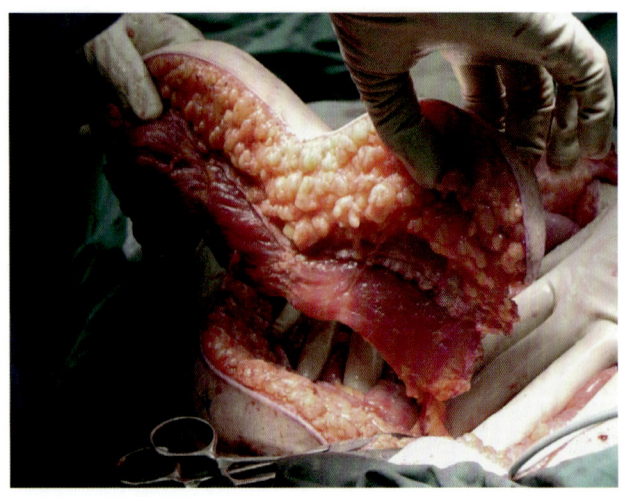

图 11.12 基于腹壁下血管蒂的纵向腹直肌肌皮瓣游离完成

第 11 章 复发性直肠癌的手术切除

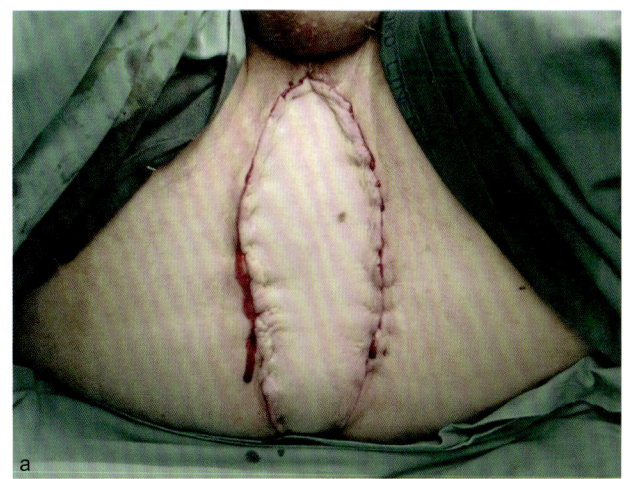

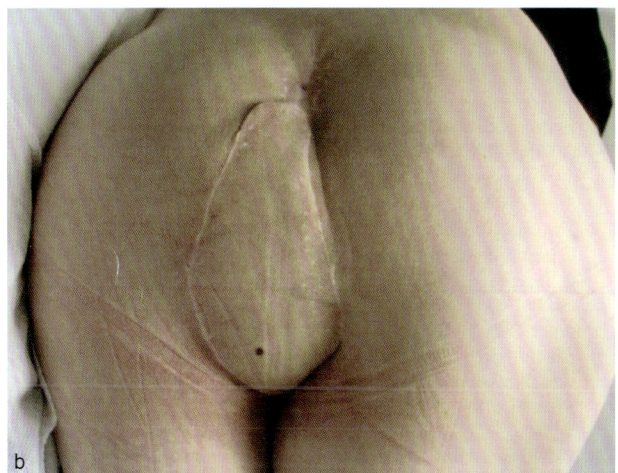

图 11.13 （a,b）纵向腹直肌肌皮瓣修补会阴和骶骨区伤口

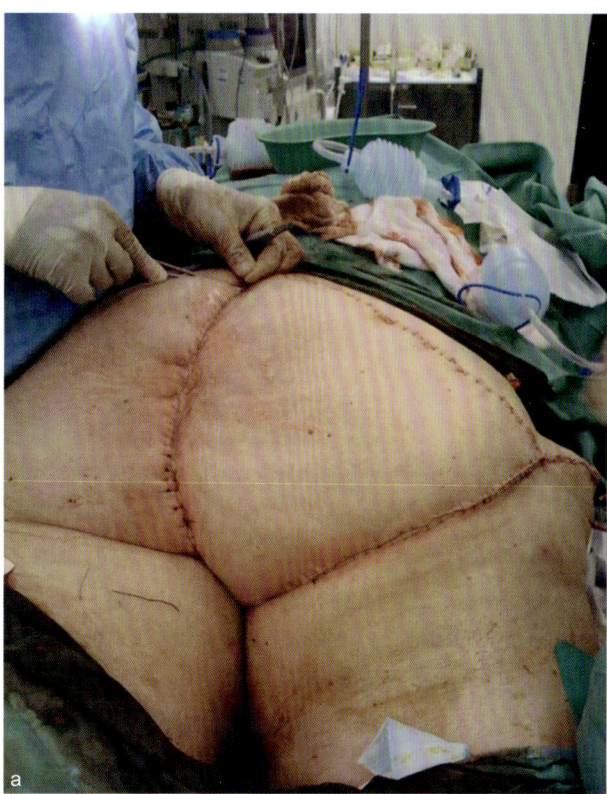

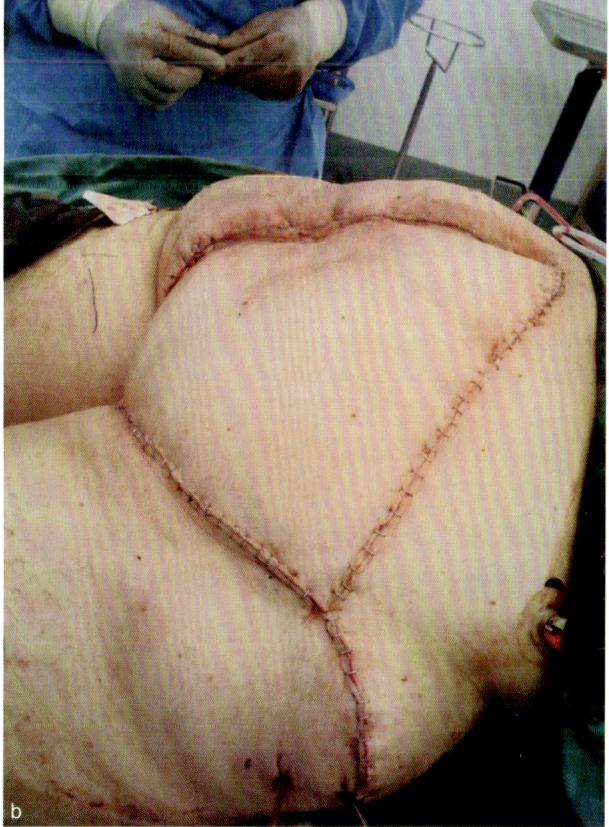

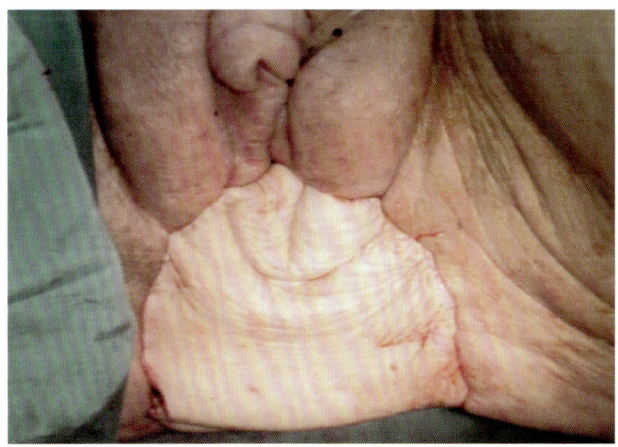

图 11.14 纵向腹直肌肌皮瓣重建阴道后壁

图 11.15 （a,b）臀大肌肌皮瓣修补伤口

结 论

直肠复发代表一个重要的外科难题。以治愈为目的的手术切除涉及多学科协作，并且经常需要复杂的修复和重建手术治疗。在某些病例，局部复发灶切除联合单发转移灶切除可能具有一定的治疗价值，患者有可能获得长期生存[30]。骨盆的解剖构造为直肠癌复发灶设定了一个狭小的空间，虽然直肠癌手术的 TME 标准化已经在一定程度上消除了复发的风险。从这个意义上说，局部复发经常预示全身复发[31]，它可能起因于淋巴管的隐匿性转移灶、初次手术时从原发灶脱落的癌细胞、不合格的 TME 标本阳性环周切缘或术中对肿瘤的不合适的触碰。低位直肠癌、穿孔性直肠癌和初次手术需要多器官切除的直肠癌局部复发风险增高。术后随访和复发灶的可切除性的评估通常需要采用 PET 和 MRI 进行影像学分期[22]。在某些病例，术前充分的评估可能会提示需要计划行输尿管支架置入，支架本身可能并不能预防术中输尿管损伤，但会有利于术中及时发现并修补输尿管损伤[32]。

应该将局部复发病灶归类于不同的骨盆腔室，骨盆腔室分类可以决定手术的方式。盆腔骨盆中央型复发病灶累及新直肠、吻合口或会阴，浸润范围局限于盆腔脏器而无关于骨骼或盆腔侧壁结构；盆腔前部复发病灶累及子宫、宫颈、阴道、膀胱、精囊、前列腺或尿道；盆腔后部复发病灶累及骶骨；盆腔侧壁复发通常累及手术操作难度最大的盆侧壁的神经和血管结构，并经常穿透坐骨大孔、梨状肌或两者同时。

通过采取更积极的切除方法，并对切缘不充分的病例采取术中放射治疗或大剂量组织间近距离放射治疗，一些传统的直肠癌局部复发手术切除的禁忌证，包括盆腔侧壁结构受累、髂血管受压或受浸润、下肢水肿、坐骨神经或骶骨受侵和局限性腹膜种植转移，已经被消除[34-35]。一些以前的绝对手术禁忌证现在已经成为相对禁忌证，包括环髂血管浸润＞180°、肿瘤穿透坐骨切迹及下肢淋巴静脉大管道受阻。盆腔脏器切除术的手术并发症相当普遍，导致一些患者需要长时间住院治疗、大量的造口支持治疗及就术后较高的局部与全身复发风险作大量的咨询服务，尤其是在手术没有达到 R0 切除的情况下。综合抗肿瘤治疗也伴随有相当大的并发症风险，主要有外周神经损伤、输尿管狭窄、小肠梗阻、放射性骨坏死及切口并发症[14]。

参考文献

1. Cass AE, Million RR, Pfaff WW. Patterns of recurrence following surgery alone for adenocarcinoma of the colon and rectum. Cancer. 1976;37:2861–5.
2. Heriot AG, Byrne CM, Lee P, Dobbs B, Tilney H, Solomon MJ, Mackay J, Frizelle F. Extended radical resection: the choice for locally recurrent rectal cancer. Dis Colon Rectum. 2008;51:284–91.
3. Temple WJ, Saettler EB. Locally recurrent rectal cancer: role of composite resection of extensive pelvic tumours with strategies for minimizing risk of recurrence. J Surg Oncol. 2000;73:47–58.
4. Cohen A, Minsky B. Aggressive Surgical Management of Locally advanced primary and recurrent rectal cancer. Current Status and Future Directions. Dis Colon Rectum. 1990;33:432–8.
5. Solomon MJ, McLeod RS. Should we be performing randomized controlled trials evaluating surgical operations? Surgery. 1995;118:459–67.
6. Hahnloser D, Nelson H, Gunderson LL, Hassan I, Haddock MG, O'Connell MJ, Cha S, Sargent DJ, Horgen A. Curative potential of mulitimodality therapy for locally recurrent rectal cancer. Ann Surg. 2003;237:502–8.
7. Yamada K, Ishizawa T, Niwa K, Chuman Y, Akiba S, Aikou T. Patterns of pelvic invasion are prognostic in the treatment of locally recurrent rectal cancer. Br J Surg. 2001;88:988–93.
8. Heriot AG, Tekkis PP, Darzi A, Mackay J. Surgery for local recurrence of rectal cancer. Colorectal Dis. 2006;8:733–47.
9. Austin KKS, Solomon MJ. Pelvic exenteration with En-bloc iliac vessel resection for lateral pelvic wall involvement. Dis Colon Rectum. 2009;52:1223–33.
10. Wanebo HJ, Antoniuk P, Koness J, Levy A, Vezeridis M, Cohen SI. Pelvic resection for recurrent rectal cancer. Dis Colon Rectum. 1999;42:1438–48.
11. Moriya Y, Akasu T, Fujita S, Yamamoto S. Total pelvic exenteration with distal sacrectomy for fixed recurrent rectal cancer in the pelvis. Dis Colon Rectum. 2004;47:2047–54.
12. Austin KKS, Young JM, Solomon MJ. Quality of life of survivors after pelvic exentration for rectal cancer. Dis Colon Rectum. 2010;53:1121–6.
13. Miller AR, Cantor SB, Peoples GE, Pearlstone DB, Skibber JM. Quality of life and cost effectiveness analysis of therapy for locally recurrent rectal cancer. Dis Colon Rectum. 1998;43:1695–701.
14. Hellinger MD, Santiago CA. Reoperation for recurrent colorectal cancer. Clin Colon Rectal Surg. 2006;19:228–38.
15. Mimezami AH, Sagar PM, Kavanagh D, Witherspoon P, Lee P, Winter D. Clinical algorithms for the surgical management of locally recurrent rectal cancer. Dis Colon Rectum. 2010;53:1248–57.
16. Hansen MH, Balteskard L, Dorum LM, Eriksen MT, Vonen B. Norwegian Colorectal Cancer Group. Locally recurrent rectal cancer in Norway. Br J Surg. 2009;96:1176–82.
17. Rodriguez-Bigas MA, Chang GJ, Skibber JM. Multidisciplinary approach to recurrent/unresectable rectal cancer: how to prepare for the extent of resection. Surg Clin N Am. 2010;19:847–59.
18. Tascieri AM, Elli M, Vignatti GA, et al. Repeated liver resection for recurrent metastases from colorectal cancer. Hepatogastroenterology. 2003;50:472–4.
19. Ike H, Shimada H, Ohki S, Togo S, Yamaguchi S, Ichikawa Y. Results of aggressive resection of lung metastases from colorectal carcinoma detected by intensive follow-up. Dis Colon Rectum. 2002;45:468–75.
20. Young-Fadok TM, Wolff BG, Nivatvongs S, Metzger PP, Ilstrup DM. Prophylactic oophorectomy in colorectal carcinoma: preliminary results of a randomized, prospective trial. Dis Colon Rectum.

1998;41:277–85.
21. Messiou C, Chalmers A, Boyle K, Sagar P. Surgery for recurrent rectal carcinoma: the role of preoperative magnetic resonance imaging. Clin Radiol. 2006;61:250–8.
22. Desai D, Zervos E, Arnold M, Burak W, Mantil J, Martin E. Positron emission tomography affects surgical management in recurrent colorectal cancer patients. Ann Surg Oncol. 2003;10:59–64.
23. Gleeson N, Baile W, Roberts WS, Hoffman M, Fiorica JV, Barton D, Cavanagh D. Surgical and psychosexual outcome following vaginal reconstruction with pelvic exenteration. Eur J Gynaecol Oncol. 1994;15:89–95.
24. Deckers P, Olsson C, Williams L, Mozden P. Pelvic exenteration as palliation of malignant disease. Am J Surg. 1976;131:509–15.
25. Yeung R, Moffat F, Falk R. Pelvic exenteration of recurrent and extensive primary colorectal adenocarcinoma. Cancer. 1993;72:1853–8.
26. Brophy P, Hoffman J, Eisenberg B. The role of palliative pelvic exenturation. Am J Surg. 1994;167:386–90.
27. Obias VJ, Reynolds Jr HL. Multidisciplinary teams in the management of rectal cancer. Clin Colon Rectal Surg. 2007;20:143–7.
28. de Witt JHW, Vermaas M, Ferenschild FTJ, Verhoef C. Management of locally advanced primary and recurrent rectal cancer. Clin Colon Rectal Surg. 2007;20:255–63.
29. Mirnezami AH, Sagar PM. Surgery for recurrent rectal cancer: technical notes and management of complications. Tech Coloproctol. 2010;14:209–16.
30. Pramateftakis MG, Hatzigianni P, Kanellos D, Vrakas G, Kanellos I, Sgelopoulos S, Ouzounidis N, Lazaridis C. Brain metastases in colorectal cancer. Tech Coloproctol. 2010;14(Suppl):S67–8.
31. Rodriguez-Bigas M, Stulc J, Davidson B, Petrelli N. Prognostic significance of anastomotic recurrence from colorectal adenocarcinoma. Dis Colon Rectum. 1992;35:838–42.
32. Sheikh F, Khubchandani I. Prophylactic ureteric catheters in colon surgery – how safe are they? Report of three cases. Dis Colon Rectum. 1990;33:508–10.
33. Suzuki K, Dozois RR, Devine RM, et al. Curative reoperation for locally recurrent rectal cancer. Dis Colon Rectum. 1996;39:730–6.
34. Shoup M, Guillem J, Alektiar K, Liau K, Paty PB, Cohen AM, Wong WD, Minsky BD. Predictors of survival in recurrent rectal cancer after resection and intraoperative radiotherapy. Dis Colon Rectum. 2002;45:585–92.
35. Kuehne J, Kleisi T, Biernacki P, Girvigian M, Streeter O, Corman ML, Ortega AE, Vukasin P, Essani R, Beart RW. Use of high dose rate brachytherapy in the management of locally recurrent rectal cancer. Dis Colon Rectum. 2003;46:695–9.
36. Nuyttens JJ, Kolkman-Deurloo IK, Vermaas M, Ferenschild FT, Graveland WJ, De Wilt JH, Hanssens PE, Levendag PC. High-dose-rate intraoperative radiotherapy for close or positive margins in patients with locally advanced or recurrent rectal cancer. Int J Radiat Oncol Biol Phys. 2004;58:106–12.

第 12 章 廓清术及重建

Patrick S. Sullivan · Eric J. Dozois

王绪林 译　李　宁 审校

摘　要

目前的盆腔廓清术较以前已进行多次改进，以改善肿瘤治疗效果、减少并发症及改善生活质量。本章讨论盆腔廓清术的适应证、禁忌证及手术方案，并列出各种重建技术，同时还包括多学科综合治疗方案，其中着重介绍盆腔廓清和重建所涉及的问题，包括软组织修复、恢复胃肠道及尿路的通畅性，以及生殖系统重建。本章应参照第 11 章阅读。

关键词

盆腔廓清；重建手术；复发性直肠癌；复发性肛管癌；直肠；新直肠；前路廓清；后路廓清；前后路联合廓清

引　言

盆腔廓清术是指针对盆腔局部进展期肿瘤进行两个及两个以上的盆腔器官的整块切除。文献中盆腔廓清术有多种不同的定义，所以比较彼此之间的治疗效果比较困难。盆腔廓清术特指将全部或部分盆腔内的生殖器官、泌尿器官、下消化道器官切除。若骶骨受侵犯，也同时需进行骨骼肌肉系统的切除。

过去，盆腔廓清术是多种盆腔肿瘤的初始治疗方法，因为那时患者大多到了肿瘤晚期，肿瘤已经侵犯盆腔多个器官才就诊。现今盆腔廓清术主要针对复发性的肿瘤。盆腔廓清术分为两个阶段：廓清阶段，即整块切除盆腔脏器；重建阶段，包括软组织修复、恢复胃肠道及尿道通畅性，有时还包括生殖系统重建。

目前的盆腔廓清术较以前已进行多次改进，以改善肿瘤治疗效果、减少并发症及改善生活质量。尽管围术期死亡率显著下降，可并发症发生率仍然较高。近来对软组织重建的重视降低了伤口相关并发症发生率。尽管盆腔廓清术可能会有风险，但却能给患者带来缓解甚至治愈的机会。

廓清术前患者和医生应充分交流，使患者对术后情况有清晰的认识。手术会显著影响患者的性功能、膀胱功能、肠道功能，所以术前可以让患者进行心理咨询。由于手术的复杂性，将患者转诊到有经验的多学科治疗中心可以保证肿瘤治疗效果及手术安全。盆腔廓清术可用于多种盆腔疾病，本章我们主要讨论其在晚期或复发性的直肠癌和肛管癌的应用。

历史回顾

1948 年，妇科医生 Alexander Brunschwig[1] 首次报道了为缓解晚期肿瘤进行的盆腔脏器切除术。他描述了一种 3 步手术方式：第 1 步为粪便转流，第 2 步为经皮肾造瘘行尿路转流，第 3 步为切除盆腔受累器官。由于3个独立的步骤增加了并发症发生率，他又将其改为1步完成，并报道了在22例患者的应用结果[1]。同一时期，Appleby报道了8例患者进行直肠膀胱切除、结肠代膀胱术[2]。Brintnall和Flocks则首次报道9例晚期直肠癌的盆腔脏器切除[3]。后来Bricker又发明了回肠代膀胱术[4]。现代的盆腔廓清术就是基于这些早期的手术基础，而手术技术有了提高，降低了并发症的发生。

解剖学考虑

了解盆腔的解剖结构，包括软组织、血管、神经、骨骼结构，对评价和处理复杂盆腔肿瘤非常重要。既往手术史、盆腔放射治疗史以及巨大肿瘤都会改变盆腔的正常解剖结构，增加盆腔分离操作风险。盆腔内一些重要血管和神经，损伤或切除它们将严重影响神经肌肉功能及生理机能。

出血是盆腔廓清术中严重手术并发症之一。术者应熟悉直肠、泌尿系、女性生殖系统的动静脉解剖，以便安全地游离结扎相应的血管。分离盆腔侧壁时将遇到髂内血管的分支，稍不注意则会导致大出血。若为盆腔再次手术或曾有放射治疗史，血管通常为纤维组织包裹，当肿瘤切除或骶骨切除需分离血管时，最好由有经验的血管外科医生协助。

若需行骶骨切除，则需了解硬膜囊、骶神经根、坐骨神经、梨状肌、骶结节韧带及骶棘韧带的解剖关系。若需进行扩大的骶骨骨盆切除，骨科或脊柱肿瘤外科医生的帮助能更好地保护神经根，并保证肿瘤切除的肌肉骨骼边界。

适应证和禁忌证

决定行廓清术前必须考虑手术目标。若为姑息性手术，则手术能够缓解症状的可能性应较大，同时不应导致显著的并发症。若为治愈性手术，则手术应切缘阴性的可能性应比较大。查看患者情况时应考虑以下几点：

1. 患者的身体是否有足够的生理储备应对大手术、大量失血以及长时间麻醉？
2. 达到切缘阴性的可能性有多大？
3. 手术是否能延长生存时间或改善生活质量？

如何选择患者，对降低手术的死亡率和并发症发生率至关重要。年龄也是重要的风险因素，但年龄本身并不是绝对禁忌证。相对于年龄，患者的生理状态更为重要。一些研究表明65岁以上的患者盆腔廓清术后恢复可与年轻患者类似[5-6]。伴有严重并发疾病的患者，如未控制的糖尿病、严重冠脉疾病、营养不良、终末期器官功能不全等，手术风险较高。

需要行盆腔廓清术的直肠癌或肛管癌是由复发导致。30%～50%的直肠癌复发局限于盆腔内，故切除后可能达到治愈的效果[7]。若患者的身体条件允许手术，则要进一步权衡手术对肿瘤的益处与手术风险。很多研究表明，肿瘤学治疗益处主要决定于是否能达到切缘阴性（R0）切除。术前首先要评价这一点。肿瘤多处固定则难以达到切缘阴性，而术前评价时有这种情况的患者治疗效果较差[8]。复发肿瘤由中心向前浸润（侵犯泌尿生殖系器官）的患者达到切缘阴性切除的可能性最大，手术效果好[8]。若肿瘤向后方或侧后方浸润，侵犯骨盆侧壁，达到切缘阴性的可能性则会减小。这种情况下，切缘阳性的可能性最大，除非进一步扩大手术范围，如行半骨盆切除术[9]。与复发性直肠癌切除术后效果不佳相关的预后因素列于表12.1。

关于直肠肛管癌行盆腔廓清术的禁忌证，不同医院及不同手术之间都不尽相同。表12.2中列出了我们认为的相对及绝对禁忌证。若无法完全切除肿瘤导致肉眼肿瘤残余，则手术对患者的生存益处有限，因此无法完全切除肿瘤是主要的手术禁忌证。术中放射治疗可改善显微镜下切缘阳性患者的局部治疗效果[10]。在某些情况下，若想达到切缘阴性，只有扩大手术范围，如行高位骶骨切除或半骨盆切除。这种情况下，若医生认为手术相对安全，患者则需要权衡为了获得治愈机会是否值得承受手术带

表12.1 盆腔廓清术治疗复发性直肠癌疗效差的相关预后因素

无法达到R0切除[33]
初次手术方式（腹会阴联合切除差于低位前切除）[8,47]
癌胚抗原升高[48]
原发肿瘤分期晚，如T4、淋巴结转移[40]
无复发间期<12月[40]
高位骶骨侵犯（S_2以上）[44]
肿瘤与骨盆多处固定[8]
大量输血，神经浸润[33]
骶骨皮质及骨髓受累[33]
术前存在疼痛（坐骨神经）[40]

表 12.2　廓清术的绝对及相对禁忌证

绝对禁忌证	相对禁忌证
远处转移无法切除	单侧骨盆壁侵犯严重
侵犯双侧骨盆壁	无法达到 R0 切除
身体状态差	高于 S_3 的骶骨受累
	包裹髂血管

来的残疾（如下肢截肢、神经肌肉功能严重受损等）。目前扩大范围的手术对肿瘤治疗效果的数据还很少，不足以给予指导意见。我们选择性地进行这种手术，疗效令人鼓舞[9]。

术前评价和手术方案制定

考虑给患者进行盆腔廓清术之前需详细询问病史及体检，还要了解之前的治疗情况（包括手术及辅助放化疗）。疼痛及神经功能受损提示肿瘤处于较晚期，可能无法切除[8]。双下肢水肿提示静脉或淋巴管受阻。应行结肠镜排除结肠其他部位病变。若直肠完整，应行直肠指检以评价肿瘤与前列腺或阴道后壁的关系。女性患者需行妇科检查以评价局部浸润的范围。还要膀胱镜检查评价膀胱侵犯的位置及范围。

需行实验室检查，查看贫血情况及营养状态。白蛋白、前白蛋白、转铁蛋白能反映患者的蛋白储备情况，可影响患者术后并发症及死亡率。根据病情需要，行营养支持治疗可改善患者术后的康复情况，尤其是切口愈合情况。对于结直肠癌患者还应查癌胚抗原（CEA）水平。CEA 升高与盆腔廓清术后生存时间缩短相关（如前述），因此遇到这种情况时，应连同其他指标一起考虑是否行手术治疗[11]。

近 50% 直肠癌局部复发的患者伴有远处转移，这种情况手术将无法达到治愈效果[8]。术前行影像学检查评价局部和远处转移情况是术前检查的重要部分。我们检查肿瘤转移项目包括 PET/CT 检查。近来研究表明 18-FDG PET 检查能提高发现结直肠局部复发及转移的敏感性[12-14]。Ogunbiyi 等[15]对 58 例晚期或复发性结直肠癌的研究发现，PET 检查的敏感性和特异性分别为 91% 和 100%。Selzner 等[16]发现联合 PET 及 CT 检查对发现直肠癌复发的敏感性达 89%，而单用 CT 的敏感性为 64%。这项研究中 PET/CT 联合检查导致 21% 患者的治疗方案改变。

盆腔磁共振（MRI）是评价神经肌肉骨骼侵犯、制定手术计划的首选检查。特别是对向后方及侧方进展的肿瘤，MRI 能评价骶骨侵犯的高度、腰骶神经的受累情况以及在骨盆侧壁是否存在边界（图 12.1）。而且还需行脊髓 MRI，以显示肿瘤对神经根及椎间孔的侵犯情况、硬膜囊的压迫情况。磁共振血管成形还可以显示血管的受累情况，以决定是否需要血管外科医生介入。

术前制定手术计划存在的一个重要问题是，直肠癌和肛管癌复发灶可能位置分散，且影像学难以界定。复发灶可能浸润至正常组织或呈薄片状，有时复发灶中还间隔存在岛状的正常组织。因此，术前很难明确界定肿瘤边界。术中情况可能与术前影像学检查情况大不一致，故应做好术中改变手术方案的准备。因此，对于复发性直肠癌的手术应行术

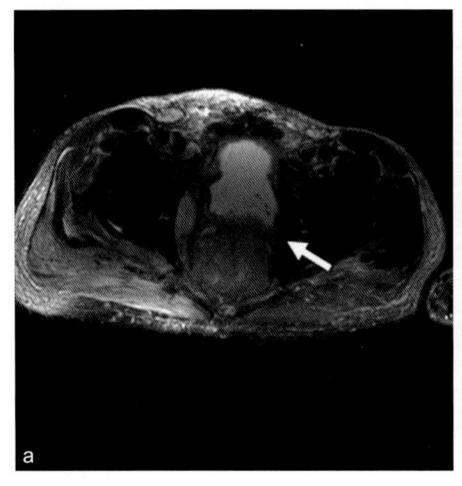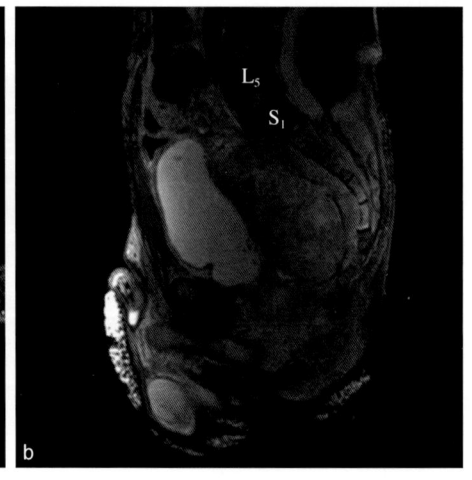

图 12.1　复发性直肠癌患者盆腔磁共振 T2 加权的轴位片和矢状位片。轴位片显示了距离很近但未侵犯的左侧盆壁边界（a，箭头）。矢状位片显示肿块骶骨侵犯的近端位于第 1 骶椎（S_1）椎体平面

中冰冻病理切片检查，必要时进一步扩大手术保证切缘阴性。相对于前方浸润来说，向后方及侧方浸润更易出现这种情况。对于前方浸润的肿瘤，单用 CT 检查通常就足以制定术前手术方案（图 12.2）。

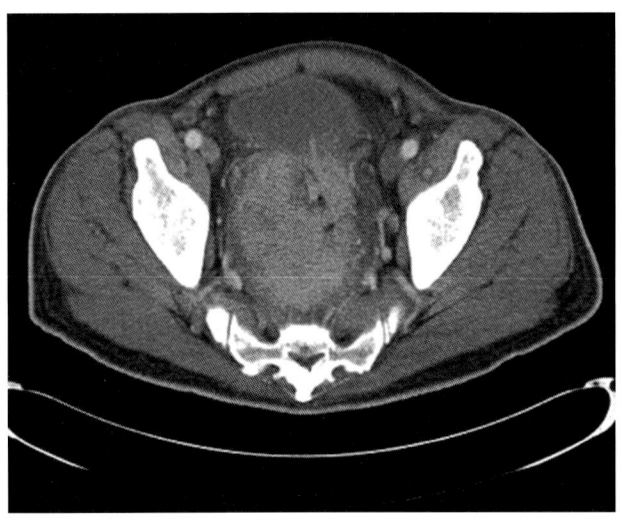

图 12.2　轴位 CT 片显示原发性局部进展期直肠癌向前方浸润膀胱

还有一个困难是如何在影像学检查图像中区分复发性直肠癌与术后纤维粘连以及放射治疗导致的纤维粘连。T2 加权的 MRI 上纤维与肿瘤的信号密度不同，因此有助于进行鉴别[17]。据报道钆剂增强的 MRI 对盆腔复发的敏感性和特异性分别为 87% 和 100%，而标准 MRI 的敏感性和特异性分别为 80% 和 86%[12]。

还有一些方法也能用来区分肿瘤与术后的炎症性改变。我们动态观察患者影像学改变，尤其关注病变大小随时间的变化，连同 CEA 水平的变化一起观察。CT 引导下经皮穿刺活检可以确诊复发，但阴性结果并不能排除复发。若无组织学诊断，CEA 水平升高，加上影像学上病变大小随时间明显改变，应考虑为肿瘤复发。

廓清术分类

廓清术这个词的概念有些模糊，因为通常所说的廓清术并不包括盆腔脏器全切除。而且，通常廓清术的分类中也不包括骶骨及骨盆的切除。根据切除器官的不同，廓清术也有一些变化。Rodriguez-Bigas 和 Petrelli[18] 描述了 4 种廓清术：全盆腔、前部、后部、肛提肌上。

根据本章的主题，我们将直肠或重建的直肠作为肿瘤发展的基点对廓清术进行分类。前部廓清术的切除范围包括直肠或重建的直肠（若既往手术为低位前切除或结肠－肛管吻合）以及所有直肠前方受累的脏器，如生殖器官、膀胱（图 12.3）。后部廓清的切除范围包括直肠或重建的直肠及其后方及侧方受累的组织，如肌肉骨骼组织和神经血管结构（图 12.4）。前后部廓清术包括前部和后部的组织结构，还包括骶骨骨盆的骨性结构（图 12.5）。

多学科团队

需要有经验的多学科团队进行盆腔廓清术的术前评价、制定手术计划、执行手术，这点非常重要。我们团队包括以下学科的外科专家：普外科和结直肠外科、骨肿瘤科、脊柱骨科、泌尿肿瘤科、整形和重建外科、血管外科。团队其他重要成员还包括骨骼肌肉放射性专家、肿瘤内科专家、进行术中放射治疗的肿瘤放射治疗专家，以及有经验的麻醉医师。具有多学科专家的外科团队能保证手术安全，提高手术效率，还能扩大手术范围。团队在每次手术前都应开会讨论手术的适应证、辅助治疗的作用、手术切除的界限。还应在复杂手术术后进行讨论，以利于明确以后可改善的方面。

综合治疗的作用

综合治疗包括全身放射治疗、体外放射治疗、术中电子放射治疗（IOERT）等，对改善局部晚期直肠癌及复发性直肠癌的治疗效果有重要作用，研究表明 5 年生存率可达到 25% ~ 36%[8, 19, 20]。术前化学治疗及放射治疗能增加切缘阴性切除的可能性[20]。对于复发性直肠癌，若患者之前未曾接受过放射治疗，给予 50.4Gy 的体外放射治疗，同时给予同步化学治疗。对于曾接受放射治疗的化学治疗，术前还要给予 20 ~ 30Gy 的体外放射治疗[21-22]。术前还给予 5-氟尿嘧啶为基础的化学治疗，化学治疗方案根据患者之前曾接受的方案进行调整。

研究表明 IOERT 可控制肿瘤局部进展，提高生存率[10]。根据术中切缘的情况决定 IOERT 的剂量。

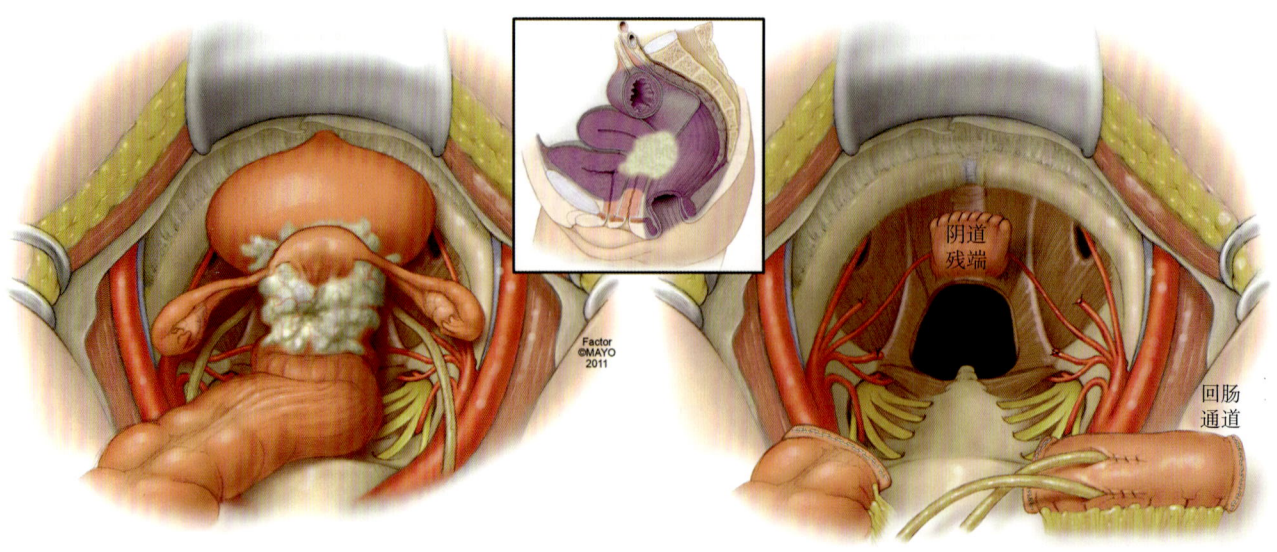

图 12.3　前部廓清术。整块切除直肠或重建的直肠、泌尿生殖器官，和（或）女性生殖器官；切除后组织缺损需要重建。© 2011，copyright Mayo Clinic, used with permission

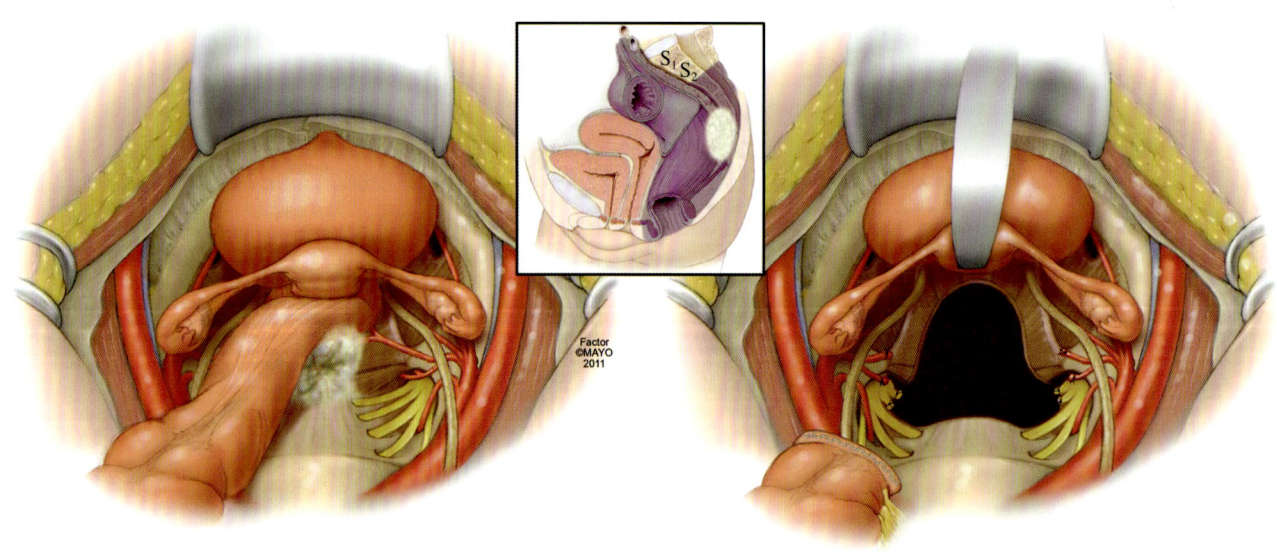

图 12.4　后部廓清术。整块切除直肠或重建的直肠、骶骨；切除后组织缺损需要重建。© 2011，copyright Mayo Clinic, used with permission

通常 R0 切除给予 12.5Gy，R1 切除给予 15Gy，R2 切除给予 20Gy（表 12.3）。术中当肿瘤标本切除后，外科医师、病理科医师及放射治疗科医师联合评价标本情况，并判断哪些区域肿瘤复发的风险较高。根据我们的经验，若术后出现肿瘤局部复发，复发的位置通常在 IOERT 照射区之外[10]。

手术技术

前部廓清

对于再次手术患者及盆腔广泛放射治疗的患者，我们使用输尿管支架。使用 Lloyd-Davies 体位

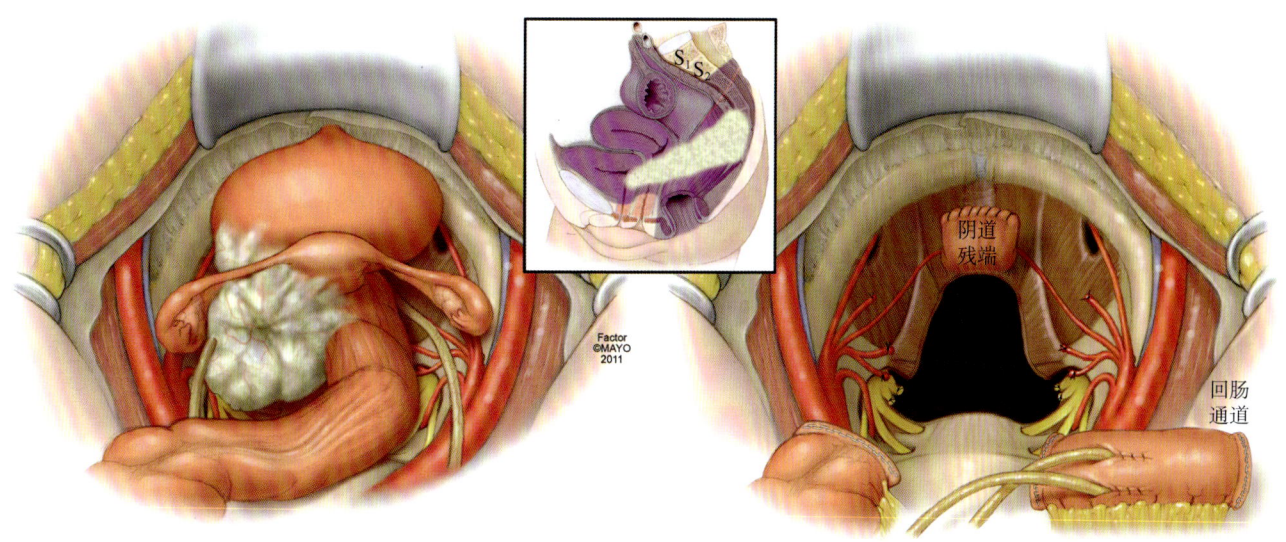

图 12.5 前后部廓清术。整块切除前部和后部的结构；切除后组织缺损需要重建。© 2011，copyright Mayo Clinic, used with permission

表 12.3 术中电子放射治疗剂量（IOERT）与切缘的关系

切缘	IOERT 剂量（Gy）
R0（<5mm）	750～1250
R1	1000～1500
局限性的 R2	1500～2000

以进行会阴部操作。对上下肢进行充分护垫保护，防止神经损伤。采用腹部正中切口入腹探查，确认盆腔外无病变，并判定盆腔肿瘤的可切除性。对任何可疑的盆腔外病变进行活检并行冰冻切片检查。若活检标本提示盆腔外有转移，将无法进行治愈性切除。任何粘连在盆腔肿瘤上的组织（多为小肠）都应整块切除。

游离左半结肠，在恰当的位置切断肠管，以备手术后期的结肠造口。分离盆腔深部至骶前间隙，并向后沿着主动脉下段、髂血管、输尿管进行分离（图 12.6）。悬吊牵引输尿管及血管。再次手术的盆腔瘢痕严重、解剖结构已改变，应仔细分离，避免副损伤及大出血。分离左髂总血管最易导致大出血，应小心分离。腰动脉后方分支的撕裂若未发现，也可导致大量出血。

进一步确定前方及侧方切除的范围（根据术前影像学检查而定），充分游离此范围内的器官及结构，以进行整块切除。进一步在骶骨前方分离骶前

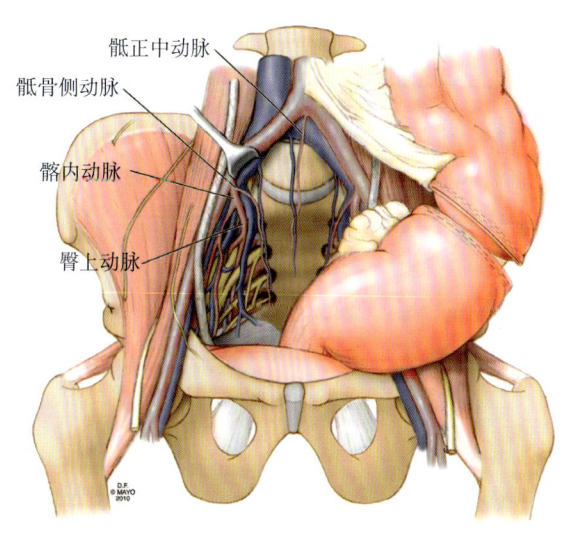

图 12.6 直肠游离后骶前间隙的解剖结构。为显示神经血管结构，未画出 Waldeyer 筋膜。© 2011，copyright Mayo Clinic, used with permission

间隙，分离操作要在 Waldeyer 筋膜前方。然后进行盆壁的侧方分离，注意保护腰骶丛和髂内血管。

在肿瘤前部浸润的女性患者，有时需切除阴道后壁，这种操作需要经阴道和经腹腔同时进行。而男性患者的前部浸润常累及膀胱三角区级前列腺，因此常需行膀胱前列腺切除术。少数患者行膀胱部分切除术就已足够。切除膀胱时，尽量靠近膀胱游

离输尿管,以保证输尿管重建时有足够的长度。进入 Retzius 间隙,充分游离膀胱前方。沿着骨盆侧壁依次结扎髂内血管走向膀胱的动静脉分支,切断膀胱的血供。切开膀胱两侧的腹膜,找到双侧管道并钳夹。然后分离两侧输尿管,一直分到膀胱,然后钳夹切断,提出盆腔。远端切缘要送病理检查确认阴性。输尿管分离并提出盆腔后,输尿管蒂放到膀胱和前列腺上。然后进行前部分离。打开双侧盆腔内筋膜,然后结扎背侧静脉复合体,到达尿道,拔出导尿管,离断尿道。

后部廓清(骶骨切除术)

第一阶段:前入路

输尿管支架置入后,从正中切口入腹探查,确认盆腔外无病变以及盆腔内肿瘤的可切除性。游离左半结肠,在恰当的位置切断,留待后期行结肠造口。显露骶前间隙。沿主动脉下段、髂血管及输尿管进行盆腔后部的分离。明确前方及侧方切除的范围(根据术前影像学结果),充分游离此范围内的器官和结构,以便于进一步整块切除。根据需要,进行骶骨切缘上段水平的冰冻切片检查以确认切缘阴性。

血管的显露除了需要游离髂血管外,通常还要游离主动脉和腔静脉下段。需对髂总及髂外动脉环周游离以利于显露静脉。首先逐步分离结扎髂内动脉分支,一直向下到臀上动脉后支起始部,臀上动脉后支需要保留以保证臀肌瓣血供(图12.7)。控制髂内静脉主干后,结扎髂内静脉分支。应先结扎分支,后结扎主干,以防静脉充盈导致大出血。分离结扎骶骨侧静脉及骶骨中静脉的分支,这些静脉回流至左髂总静脉或下腔静脉分叉处后方。粗短的髂内分支最好予以缝扎。沿骶骨两侧进行血管分离,直到盆底。

在前部操作过程中,根据需要进行结肠造口及结肠代膀胱术。然后准备腹直肌的肌皮瓣,以便后续的会阴重建。术中 X 线透视确定骶骨切除平面,并在此水平把骶骨前部切开。骶骨切开处放置螺钉,以利于后部操作时 X 线透视定位(图 12.8)。在关腹及改变患者体位之前,将一厚硅胶片置入骶骨和血管之间,避免在后部进行骶骨切除时导致损伤(图12.9)。然后关腹,进行造口(肠道、尿路),然后

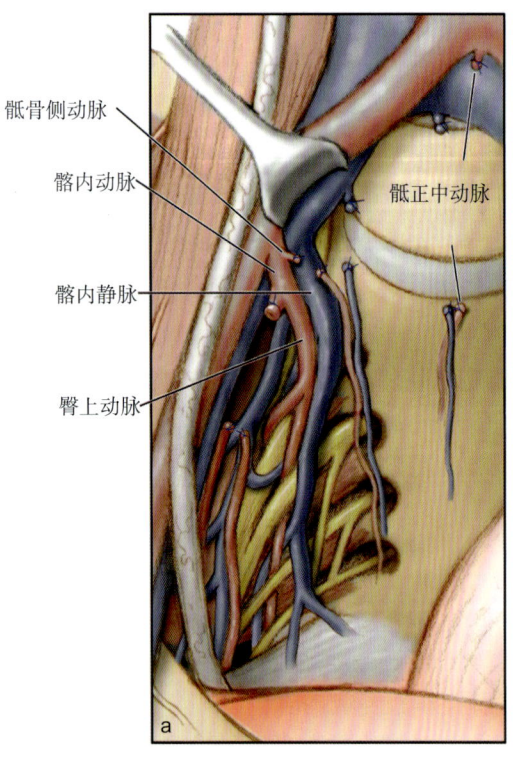
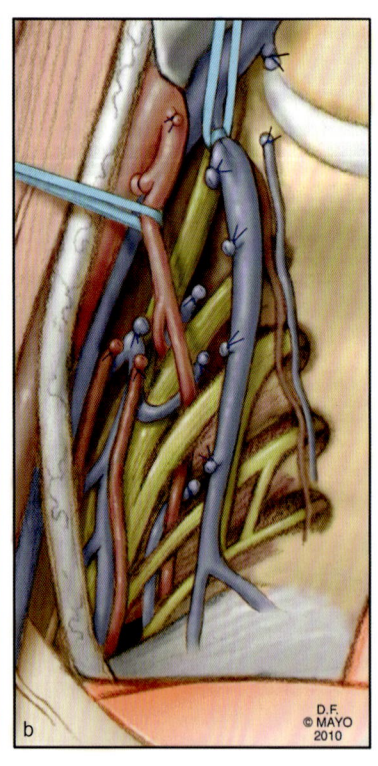
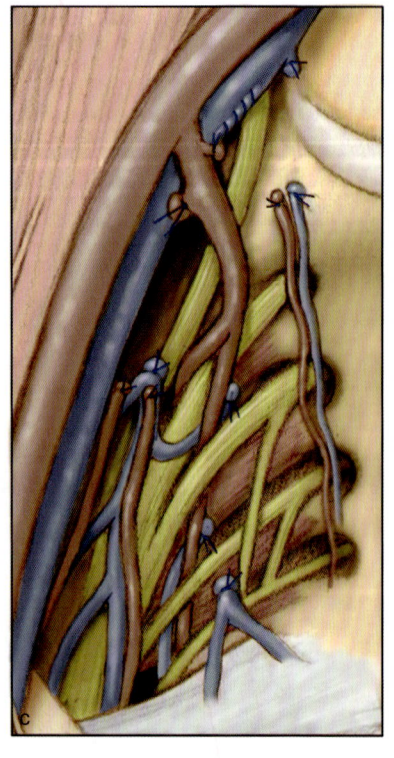

图 12.7 血管显露和分离。(a) 髂内动脉已结扎,保留臀肌血供;(b) 结扎髂内静脉的骶骨侧分支,直到骶骨下段;(c) 高位结扎髂内静脉。© 2010,copyright Mayo Clinic, used with permission

第 12 章　廓清术及重建　　131

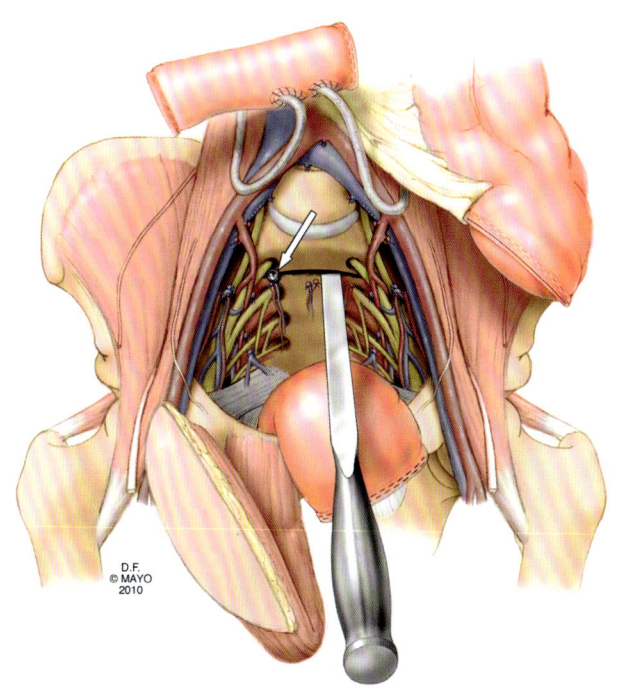

图 12.8　单皮质横向截骨，以螺钉（箭头）做标记，以利于后部分离操作时透视定位。© 2010，copyright Mayo Clinic, used with permission

将患者改成俯卧位。

第二阶段：后入路

第二阶段患者要采用俯卧位。在骶骨中段做正中切口，离断臀大肌在骶骨的附着。然后离断骶棘韧带和骶结节韧带，从后部进入盆腔（图 12.10）。

离断梨状肌，注意保护坐骨神经和阴部神经。然后椎板切除、结扎硬膜囊、切除骶骨（图 12.11）。骶骨切除要根据影像学检查，保证切缘无肿瘤。标本切除后病理医师及整个手术团队都要评价切除的彻底性。后部的伤口已带蒂腹直肌皮瓣重建（图 12.12）。根据手术范围及手术每阶段耗时，整个手术可在 1 天完成，也可分成几天完成。

前后部联合廓清

前后部联合廓清时，按照前述的步骤进行。具体步骤的先后顺序受多因素影响，但一般来说，先进行前部廓清再进行后部廓清。若进行高位骶骨切除或扩大的骶骨骨盆切除，手术需分多步在多个手术日完成。通常，第 1 天进行前部分离，48h 后进行后部廓清并切除肿瘤，如果需要，脊柱骨盆重建在 14 天后进行。

廓清后重建

盆腔廓清后重建包括尿路重建、胃肠道重建及会阴重建。在女性患者，若阴道后壁一起切除，还需行阴道重建。扩大盆腔切除术后，会阴部伤口并发症是术后常见的并发症。扩大盆腔切除术后，会阴部伤口不愈合发生率在 7% ~ 66%[23]。放射治疗导致 41% 的直肠癌患者行会阴部切除后出现切口并发症[24]。廓清术，包括骶骨骨盆切除术，其伤口的充

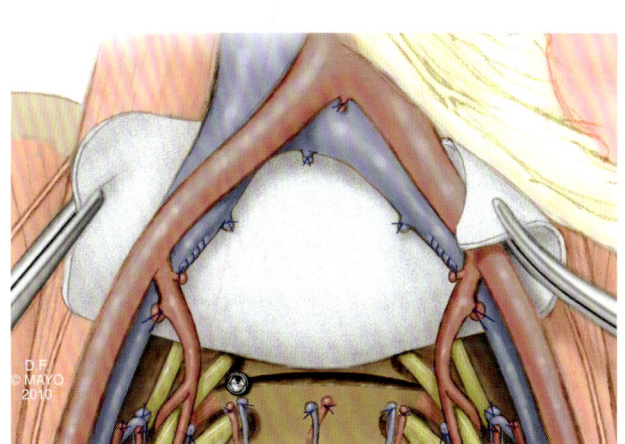

图 12.9　放置硅胶片保护前方血管，防止后部骨切开时误伤。© 2010，copyright Mayo Clinic, used with permission

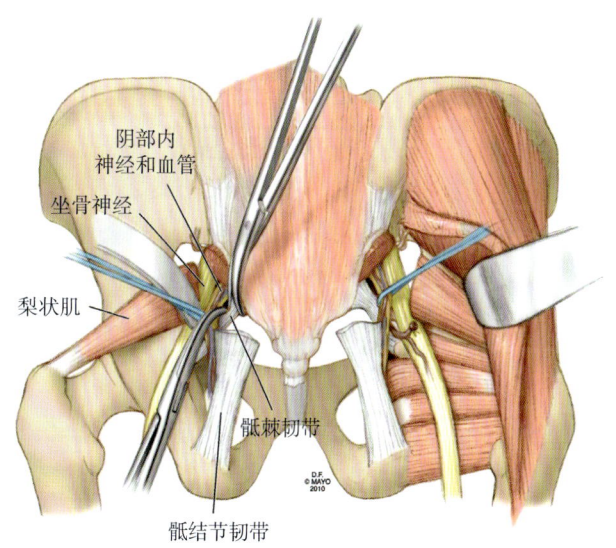

图 12.10　分离骶棘韧带、骶结节韧带和梨状肌。© 2010，copyright Mayo Clinic, used with permission

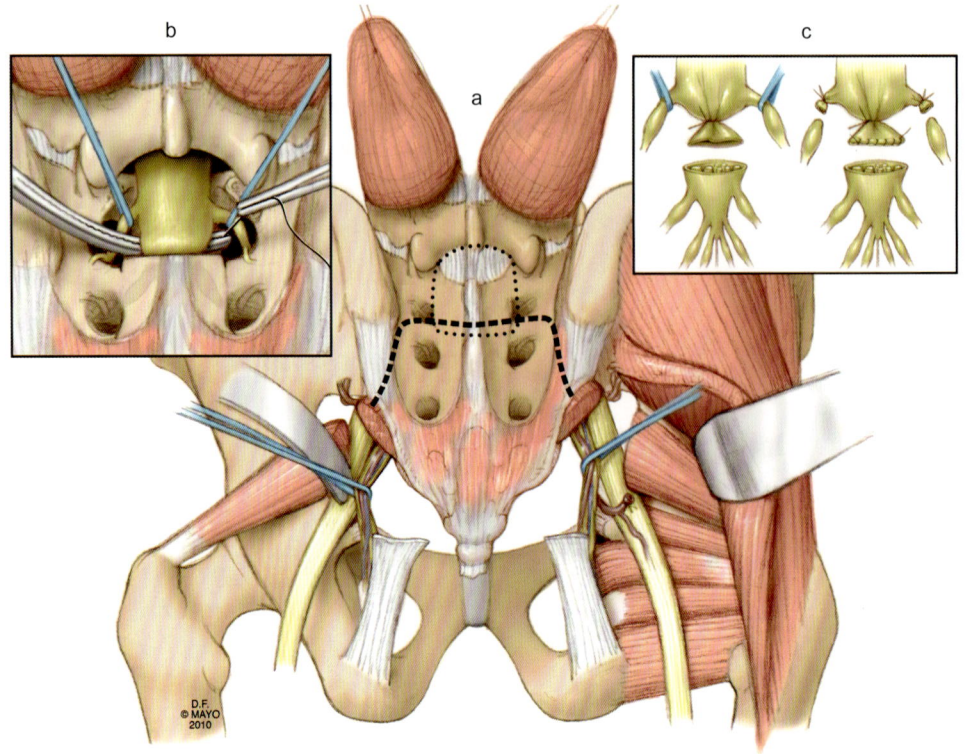

图 12.11 后部骶骨切开（a），椎板切除（b）及硬膜囊结扎（c）。© 2010，copyright Mayo Clinic, used with permission

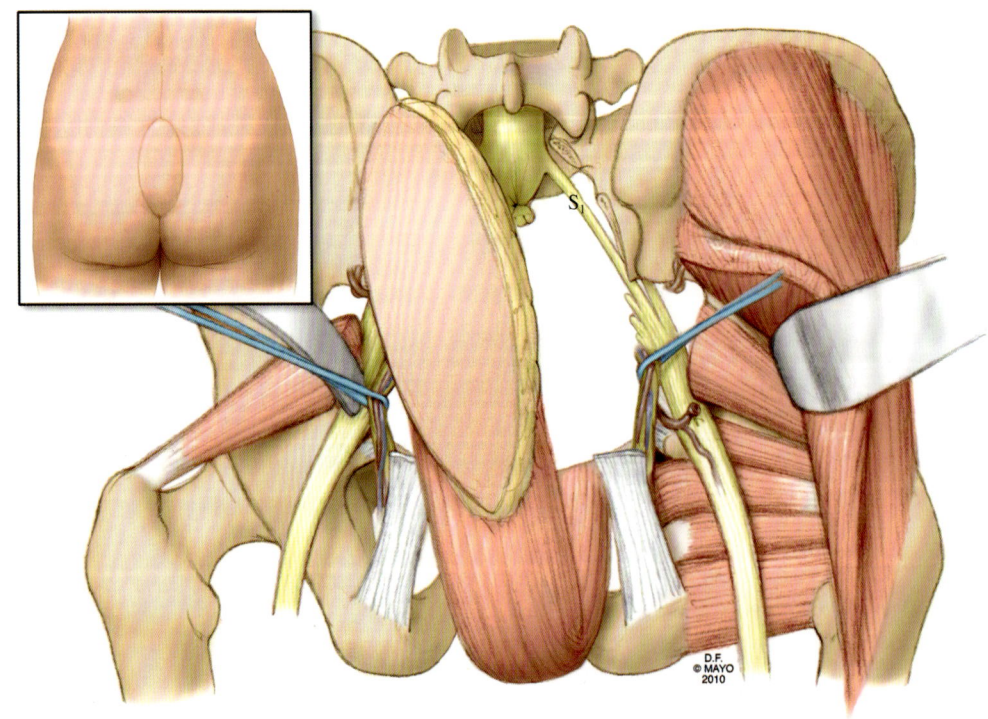

图 12.12 经会阴部转移带蒂腹直肌肌皮瓣，以便会阴部重建。© 2010，copyright Mayo Clinic, used with permission

填和覆盖极为困难，富有挑战。

网膜瓣

带蒂网膜瓣的主要优点在于能够充填廓清术后的盆腔死腔[25]。这种用有血供的组织充填盆腔，能减少盆腔脓肿的风险，并能防止小肠粘连于局部及由此导致的粘连性肠梗阻。游离网膜，根据蒂的长度和大小选择保留网膜左侧或右侧为血管蒂。可在胃侧游离胃网膜血管弓直至胃网膜右血管或胃网膜左血管根部，以延长网膜瓣，对侧的胃网膜血管予以切断结扎。因胃网膜右血管更为粗大且分支较多，有些选择保留右侧。可于横结肠系膜开窗，以使网膜瓣更接近盆腔。

腹直肌肌皮瓣

腹直肌肌皮瓣（vertical rectus abdominus myocutaneous，VRAM）血管良好、体积较大，可以用来充填盆腔内死腔、重建会阴部，是我们用来进行盆腔廓清术后会阴部软组织重建的首选。Chessin 等[23]对直肠肛管癌术前放射治疗后腹会阴联合切除的59 例患者以 VRAM 瓣重建或直接缝合，并对结果进行了对比研究。以 VRAM 瓣重建的患者会阴部伤口并发症发生率明显降低（15.8%vs44.1%），进行肌皮瓣取除的部位也没有腹壁疝及感染。Radice 等[26]对比了直接缝合、带蒂网膜充填及 VRAM 瓣重建，发现 VRAM 瓣等患者伤口感染率及住院时间都明显减少。

游离 VRAM 瓣要切取脐上的一块皮肤，连同其下的脂肪组织及腹直肌。腹直肌前鞘要连同肌皮瓣一同切取，保留后鞘进行关腹。要仔细分离，保留通过前鞘的穿支血管，最大程度地减少筋膜去除范围。VRAM 瓣的血供来自腹壁下血管，因此要游离腹壁下血管作为血管蒂。VRAM 瓣大小要适合重建会阴伤口，旋转 VRAM 瓣以通过腹腔进入盆腔，并使皮肤部分朝向会阴。将 VRAM 瓣与会阴部缝合时要注意不能过分扭转，也不能张力太大（图12.13）。

臀大肌肌皮瓣

臀大肌肌皮瓣基于臀下动脉蒂。可通过游离并

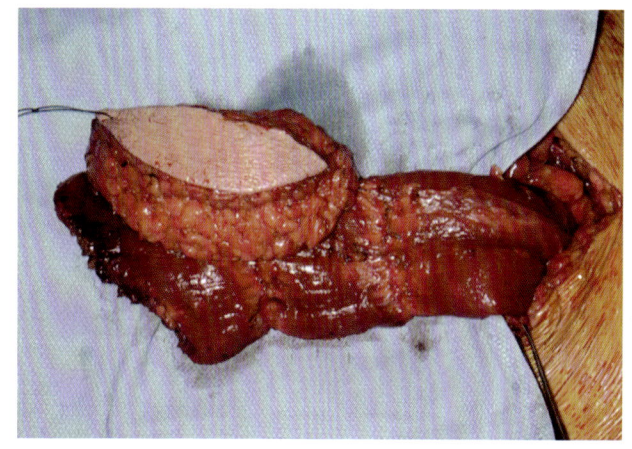

图 12.13　切取的腹直肌肌皮瓣，蒂长足以能够进行盆腔重建

局部推进技术或 V-Y 推进肌皮瓣制作臀大肌肌皮瓣。操作方法包括上提和推进臀大肌浅部及其皮肤。要制作两个臀大肌肌皮瓣，并保留臀大肌深部的50%。将切取的两个肌皮瓣提出，将其中一个肌皮瓣内侧部分去上皮化，然后将其填入盆部缺损，这样，即使骶骨部分切除后的较大腔隙也可以完全充填。将另一个肌皮瓣推进到中线部，并和第一个肌皮瓣进行缝合，完成中线部分重建。肌皮瓣切取后的缺损以 V-Y 方法进行缝合。对于骶骨切除后巨大的会阴部缺损，可以在下方以 VRAM 瓣，并联合两侧筋膜 V-Y 推进瓣进行修复。

股薄肌瓣

若无法应用 VRAM 瓣，股薄肌也可用来充填部分骨盆缺损。股薄肌血供不稳定，选择程度也有限，而且体积较小，不易完全充填盆腔内死腔。它通过股中部纵行切口来获取。它的血供来源于股深动脉近端的血管蒂，其远端来源隐动脉的血管蒂要予以结扎。若使用股薄肌肌皮瓣，在切取肌肉和相应的皮肤后，要把它旋转到会阴部切口（图 12.14）。

全股部肌皮瓣

半骨盆切除术后可利于截肢后废肢的软组织制作股部肌皮瓣（图 12.15）。后部半骨盆切除后肌皮瓣的设计基于臀上和臀下血管。在保留臀部血管的前提下，可以把包含臀肌的巨大后部肌皮瓣旋转覆

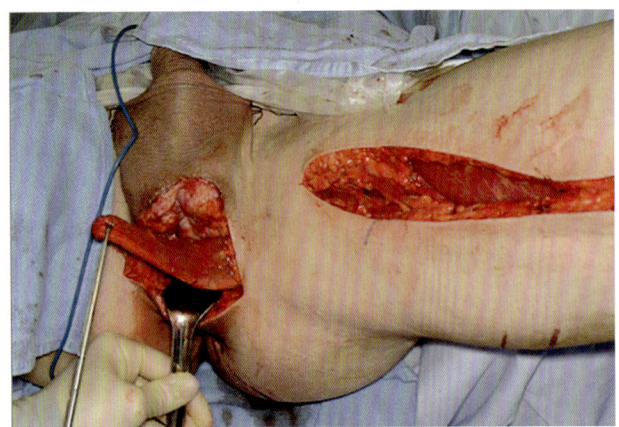

图 12.14　股薄肌瓣

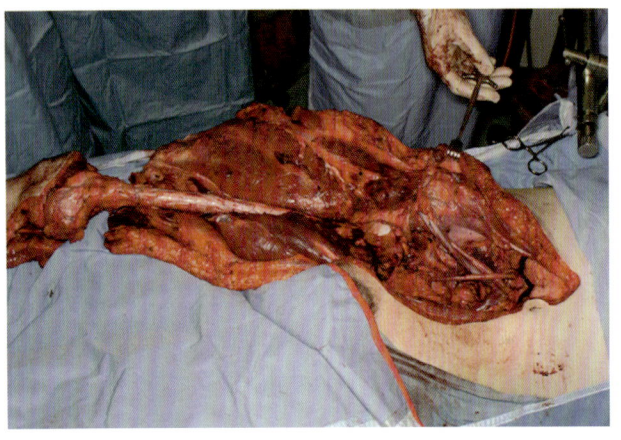

图 12.15　切除股骨后的全股部肌皮瓣

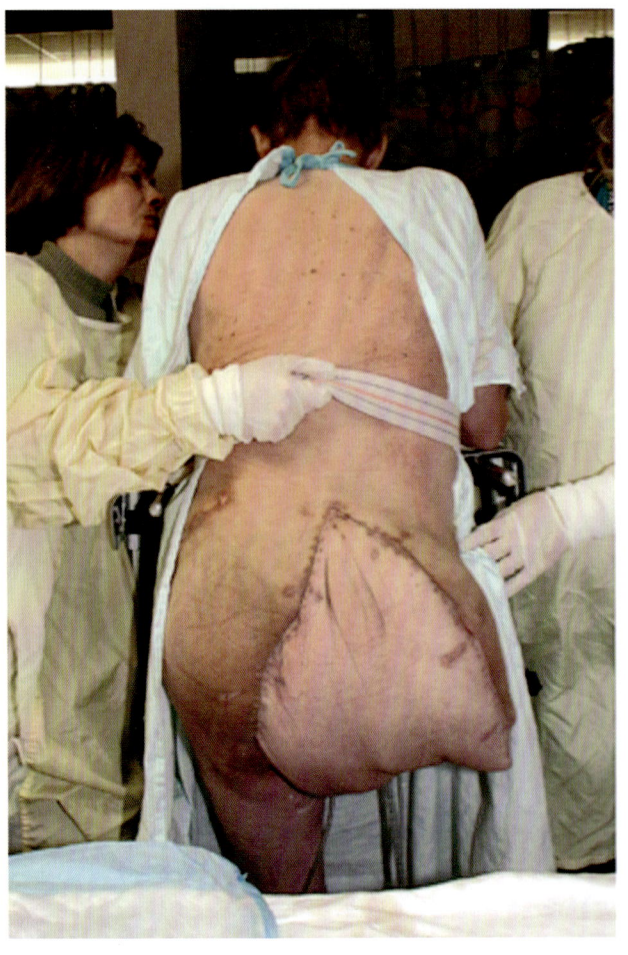

图 12.16　全股部肌皮瓣充填缺损愈合后

盖骨性骨盆切除后的骨盆缺损。如果肿瘤学方面合适，保留髂内血管可增加后部肌皮瓣的血供，减少瓣的坏死。局限性的骨性骨盆切除可保留骶骨穿支血管。

前部半骨盆切除的肌皮瓣为前部肌肉组织肌皮瓣。这些瓣的血管来自股浅动脉的肌内分支。这种轴向的肌皮瓣血供来源于股血管的分支，包括来自股深动脉的旋股内侧动脉和旋股外侧动脉。这种长肌皮瓣包含股四头肌，体积较大，能较好地填充盆腔缺损。

全半盆切除后肌皮瓣要用到大部分股部肌肉，其血供来源于股浅和股深血管，保护这两个血管可以使大量的肌肉组织得以保留。股深动脉的旋动脉分支穿过大收肌走向后部及侧部的肌肉间室，也能为全股部肌皮瓣提供血供。全股部肌皮瓣可提供最大体积的有血供组织，以对巨大缺损进行软组织重建（图 12.16）。

尿路重建

若需性膀胱切除，则需重建尿路通道，以收集并排除尿液。重建方式包括可控制排尿的手术（Koch 贮袋、Indiana 贮袋），或不可控制排尿的尿路造口术。大部分针对结直肠恶性肿瘤的廓清术后不能行可控制排尿的手术方式，因此尿路重建的方式主要包括回肠代膀胱、结肠代膀胱或输尿管结肠吻合/输尿管乙状结肠吻合。若直肠上动脉完整，我们通常用乙状结肠，因为它较易游离，上腹部两侧都可以做造口，而且这种术式也避免了做小肠吻合。若肠系膜下动脉已切除，则用回肠代膀胱。

阴道重建

部分女性患者行扩大前部廓清术时需要切除部分阴道壁，以保证切缘阴性。前部盆腔廓清术后阴道重建的术式有多种。我们优先选用腹直肌肌皮（RAM）瓣进行阴道重建，因其血供稳定，而且能充分充填盆腔死腔（图 12.17）。Soper 等[27] 回顾分析了 32 例廓清术后以 RAM 瓣行阴道重建的患者（85% 曾接受放射治疗），发现肌皮瓣相关的并发症发生率为 32%，仅 1 例患者出现阴道硬化。以 RAM 瓣行阴道重建减少了会阴部并发症，也能维持患者的自我性心理印象。

骶骨骨盆重建

若肿瘤向后侵犯骶骨、骨盆侧壁及坐骨结节，为达切缘阴性，可能需行骶骨骨盆切除或半骨盆切除。半骨盆切除的类型决定于肿瘤的范围。我们通常做的半骨盆切除包括 4 型，即全骶骨切除（第 1 型）、半骶骨切除（第 2 型）、半骶骨切除 + 外侧半骨盆切除（第 3 型）、全骶骨切除 + 半骨盆切除（第 4 型），第 1 型和第 3 型最常用（图 12.18）。对于某些患者，手术需要破坏脊柱骨盆的连续性，破坏腰骶干、切除髋关节，则行外半骨盆切除术（髂腹间切断术）。有些患者肿瘤范围稍局限，则可仅切除部分骶骨和髂骨内侧部分，保留下肢。切除骨性部分后，有多种重建术式可用来维持脊柱稳定性。某些情况下可以用有血供的腓骨加钛棒重建脊柱骨盆的稳定性[28]（图 12.19）。

廓清术后并发症

对有选择的患者行盆腔廓清术后，总体死亡率在 0～9%[8, 29-34]。死亡原因包括术中无法控制的大出血、盆腔感染、肾衰竭、心血管功能障碍[35-36]。24%～68% 的患者会出现并发症，大部分为会阴部切口愈合问题[9, 19, 29, 32, 35, 36]。并发症发生率随着切除范围增大而增加[9, 35]。行骶骨切除、半骨盆切除或行术中放射治疗的患者并发症发生率更高，大部分与后部切口相关[8]。IOERT 的重要不良反应包括与剂量相关的周围神经病（16%～34%）和输尿管硬化（6%）。

报道较多的并发症包括盆腔脓肿、小肠梗阻、瘘、会阴部切口问题和输尿管梗阻。Henry 等[38] 报道 53% 盆腔复发性肿瘤的患者切除术后出现并发症，其中近 1/3 为感染相关的并发症，盆腔感染发生率为 9.2%，腹部切口感染为 5.7%，会阴部切口感染为 3.4%。

大部分浅表感染可通过局部引流和伤口护理治愈。盆腔脓肿通常在前部或后部行经皮穿刺置管引

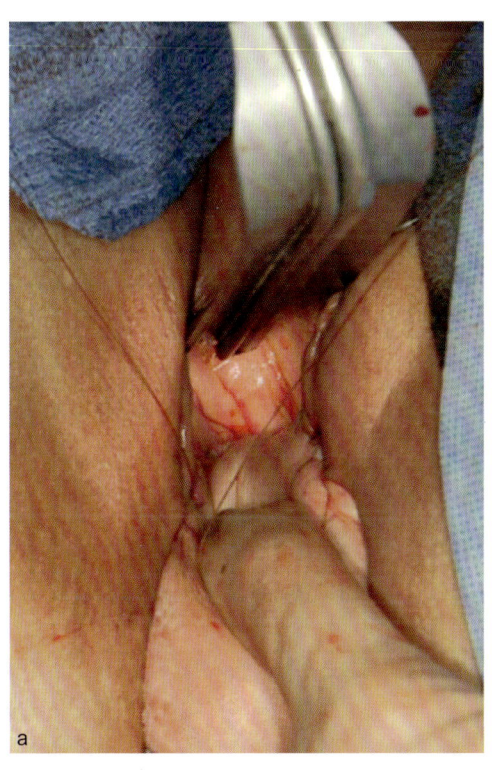
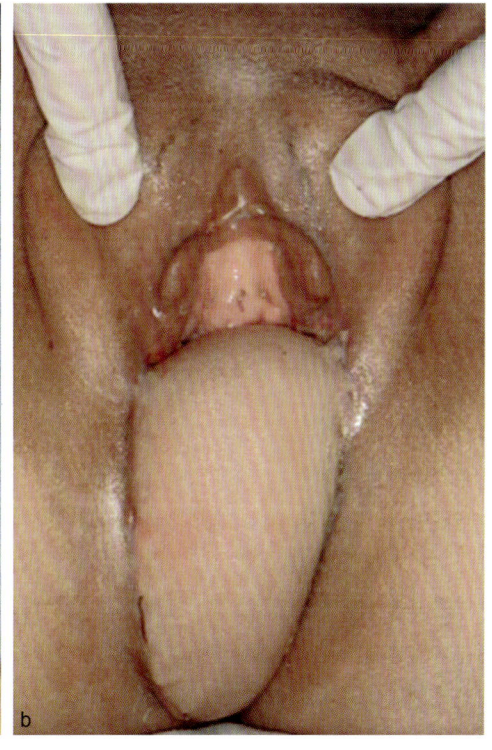

图 12.17 （a）扩大前部廓清术后以腹直肌肌皮瓣（VRAM）填充阴道后壁缺损；（b）愈合后的 VRAM 瓣重建的阴道后壁

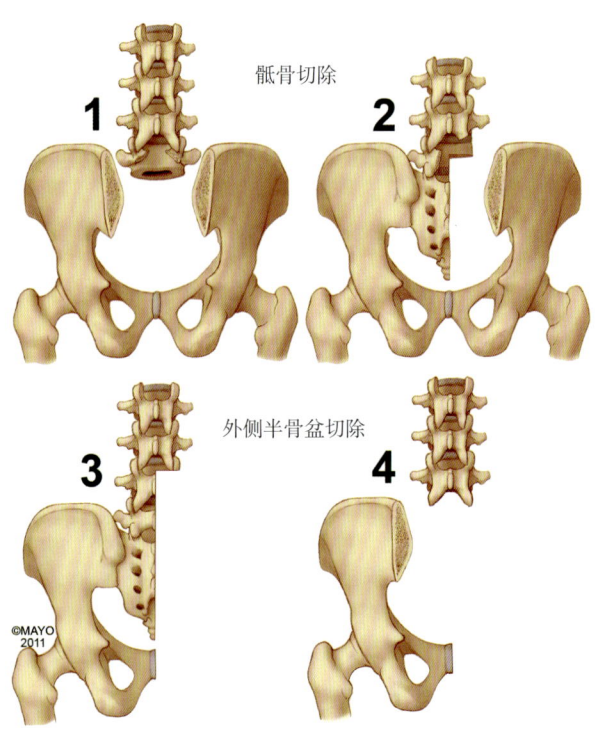

图 12.18 骶骨骨盆切除的分型（1～4 型）。© 2011, copyright Mayo Clinic, used with permission

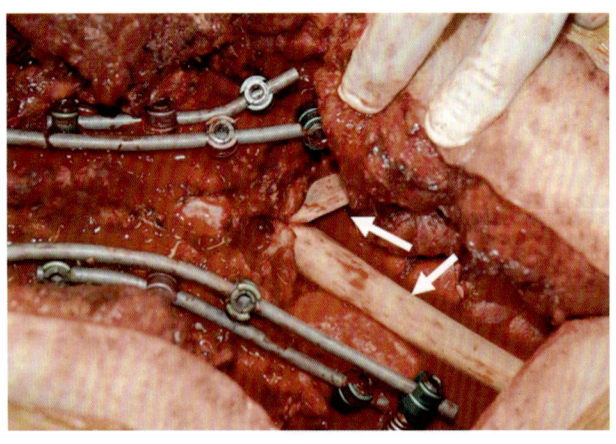

图 12.19 第 1 型切除（全骶骨切除）后重建术中照片。术中双侧用血管化的腓骨（白箭头）联合钛棒进行重建

流。低位的盆腔脓肿不能行 CT 引导下经皮穿刺引流,可通过手术经会阴部或经肛管引流。Chessin 等[23]发现用 RAM 瓣行会阴部重建后,会阴部伤口并发症发生率降低,从 44% 降至 16%。随着有血供的组织瓣应用的增加,感染相关的并发症会继续降低。

尿路并发症也是常见的并发症。若行尿路重建,可能发生输尿管梗阻和输尿管瘘[36]。后部廓清术后可能发生永久性膀胱功能不全,需要间断性地导尿或膀胱造口。游离输尿管或盆腔放射治疗导致输尿管硬化,继而导致肾功能不全,这种情况也有报道[39]。CT 尿路成像可以用来诊断大部分尿路并发症。放置双 J 管是解决输尿管梗阻导致的肾积水的最佳选择。若无法经膀胱镜放置双 J 管,但仍需性尿液转流治疗尿瘘,也可以放置肾输尿管支架或经皮肾造口。

廓清术后肿瘤学治疗效果

因各种廓清术的分类标准不甚一致,其肿瘤学治疗效果不易对比。目前发表的文献中,患者的病情也不相同。若肿瘤复发位于前部（生殖器官、膀胱）,通常可以达到 R0 切除,术后生存时间也较长。Moore 等[40]发现 72% 前部复发的患者可达到 R0 切除,相比之下,侧部和后部复发的患者的 R0 切除率分别为 50% 和 36%。Stocchi 等[41]报道连同尿路整块切除的患者 3 年生存率为 45%。前部复发的肿瘤固定于骨性骨盆的情况较少,更易于完全切除,因此术后生存时间更长。

侧部和后部复发与骨盆固定更多, R0 切除的可能性更小[8,40]。新近研究报道侧部和后部复发的患者, R0 切除率能达到 51%～100%[9,33,35,42,43],这些患者的 5 年生存率为 20%～39%。R0 切除是 5 年最重要的生存率预测指标[8,35]（表 12.4）。

低位骶骨切除可使部分患者达到长期生存, 5 年生存率可达 37%[8]。因低位骶骨侵犯可达到这种治疗效果,有些人研究在高位骶骨侵犯的患者是否能达到类似效果。Wanebo 等[44-45]报道了两组复发性直肠癌高位骶骨切除的病例, 5 年生存率分别为 33% 和 31%。我们研究组为 9 例复发性直肠癌患者进行了高位骶骨切除, 5 年生存率为 30%, 2 例患者 5 年后仍存活;而且无手术导致的死亡,并发症也可接受,手术对肿瘤的局部控制较好,仅有 1 例患者术后再次出现盆腔复发[9]。

与未接受 IOERT 的复发性直肠癌患者相比,术中行 IORT 的患者生存情况更好[46]。研究显示,综合治疗方案中加用 IOERT 可使生存率提高 15%[39]。目前尚无手术联合 IORT 与仅用手术治疗的随机对照研究,但资料显示加用 IORT 不仅对切缘阴性的患者有益,对显微镜下切缘阳性和肉眼切缘阳性的患者也有益。Haddock 等[10]新近报道了梅奥诊所复发性结直肠癌综合治疗的结果，综合治疗方案包括 IOERT。R0、R1、R2 切除的预期 5 年生存率分别为 46%、27% 和 16%。对于仔细选择过的复发性盆腔肿瘤，廓清术后 5 年生存率可高达 39%，与肺、肝、脑的孤立性转移切除术后的结果类似 [35]。

结　论

对于部分晚期原发性或及局部复发性结直肠癌、肛管癌的患者，盆腔廓清术仍是治疗选择之一。术前影像学检查有助于制定手术方案。仔细选择患者，并由一个多学科外科治疗团队来治疗患者，能减少死亡率及并发症发生率，达到最佳的肿瘤切除效果。现代辅助治疗方案，包括 IOERT 能进一步改善肿瘤治疗效果。目前的数据支持对有选择的患者施行盆腔廓清术，使患者获得长期生存。

参考文献

1. Brunschwig A. Complete excision of pelvic viscera for abdominal carcinoma. Cancer. 1948;1:177–88.
2. Appleby LH. Proctocystectomy; the management of colostomy with ureteral transplants. Am J Surg. 1950;79:57–60.
3. Brintnall ES, Flocks RH. En masse "pelvic viscerectomy" with ureterointestinal anastomosis. Arch Surg. 1950;61:851–68.
4. Bricker EM. Bladder substitution after pelvic evisceration. Surg Clin North Am. 1950;30:1511–21.
5. Lichtinger M, Averette H, Penalver M, Sevin BU. Major surgical procedures for gynecologic malignancy in elderly women. South Med J. 1986;79:1506–10.
6. Matthews CM, Morris M, Burke TW, Gershenson DM, Wharton JT, Rutledge FN. Pelvic exenteration in the elderly patient. Obstet Gynecol. 1992;79:773–7.
7. Gunderson LL, Sosin H. Areas of failure found at reoperation (second or symptomatic look) following "curative surgery" for adenocarcinoma of the rectum. Clinicopathologic correlation and implications for adjuvant therapy. Cancer. 1974;34:1278–92.
8. Hahnloser D, Nelson H, Gunderson LL, Hassan I, Haddock MG, O'Connell MJ, et al. Curative potential of multimodality therapy for locally recurrent rectal cancer. Ann Surg. 2003;237:502–8.
9. Dozois EJ, Privitera A, Holubar SD, Aldrete JF, Sim FH, Rose PS, Walsh MF, Bower TC, Leibovich BC, Nelson H, Larson DW. High sacrectomy for locally recurrent rectal cancer: can long-term survival be achieved? J Surg Oncol. 2011;103(2):105–9.
10. Haddock MG, Miller RC, Nelson H, Pemberton JH, Dozois EJ, Alberts SR, et al. Combined modality therapy including intraoperative electron irradiation for locally recurrent colorectal cancer. Int J Radiat Oncol Biol Phys. 2011;79:143–50.
11. Wang JY, Tang R, Chiang JM. Value of carcinoembryonic antigen in the management of colorectal cancer. Dis Colon Rectum. 1994;37:272–7.
12. Whiteford MH, Whiteford HM, Yee LF, Ogunbiyi OA, Dehdashti F, Siegel BA, et al. Usefulness of FDG-PET scan in the assessment of suspected metastatic or recurrent adenocarcinoma of the colon and rectum. Dis Colon Rectum. 2000;43:759–70.
13. Arulampalam T, Costa D, Visvikis D, Boulos P, Taylor I, Ell P. The impact of FDG-PET on the management algorithm for recurrent colorectal cancer. Eur J Nucl Med. 2001;28:1758–65.
14. Moore HG, Akhurst T, Larson SM, Minsky BD, Mazumdar M, Guillem JG. A case-controlled study of 18-fluorodeoxyglucose positron emission tomography in the detection of pelvic recurrence in previously irradiated rectal cancer patients. J Am Coll Surg. 2003;197:22–8.
15. Ogunbiyi OA, Flanagan FL, Dehdashti F, Siegel BA, Trask DD, Birnbaum EH, et al. Detection of recurrent and metastatic colorectal cancer: comparison of positron emission tomography and computed tomography. Ann Surg Oncol. 1997;4:613–20.
16. Selzner M, Hany TF, Wildbrett P, McCormack L, Kadry Z, Clavien P-A. Does the novel PET/CT imaging modality impact on the treatment of patients with metastatic colorectal cancer of the liver? Ann Surg. 2004;240:1027–36.
17. Torricelli P, Pecchi A, Luppi G, Romagnoli R. Gadolinium-enhanced MRI with dynamic evaluation in diagnosing the local recurrence of rectal cancer. Abdom Imaging. 2003;28:19–27.
18. Rodriguez-Bigas MA, Petrelli NJ. Pelvic exenteration and its modifications. Am J Surg. 1996;171:293–8.
19. Heriot AG, Byrne CM, Lee P, Dobbs B, Tilney H, Solomon MJ, et al. Extended radical resection: the choice for locally recurrent rectal cancer. Dis Colon Rectum. 2008;51:284–91.
20. Dresen RC, Gosens MJ, Martijn H, Nieuwenhuijzen GA, Creemers G-J, Daniels-Gooszen AW, et al. Radical resection after IORT-containing multimodality treatment is the most important determinant for outcome in patients treated for locally recurrent rectal cancer. Ann Surg Oncol. 2008;15:1937–47.
21. Mohiuddin M, Marks G, Marks J. Long-term results of reirradiation for patients with recurrent rectal carcinoma. Cancer. 2002;95:1144–50.
22. Valentini V, Morganti AG, Gambacorta MA, Mohiuddin M, Doglietto GB, Coco C, et al. Preoperative hyperfractionated chemoradiation for locally recurrent rectal cancer in patients previously irradiated to the pelvis: a multicentric phase II study. Int J Radiat Oncol Biol Phys. 2006;15(64):1129–39.
23. Chessin DB, Hartley J, Cohen AM, Mazumdar M, Cordeiro P, Disa J, et al. Rectus flap reconstruction decreases perineal wound complications after pelvic chemoradiation and surgery: a cohort study. Ann Surg Oncol. 2005;12:104–10.
24. Bullard KM, Trudel JL, Baxter NN, Rothenberger DA. Primary perineal wound closure after preoperative radiotherapy and abdominoperineal resection has a high incidence of wound failure. Dis Colon Rectum. 2005;48:438–43.
25. Liebermann-Meffert D. The greater omentum. Anatomy, embryology, and surgical applications. Surg Clin North Am. 2000;80:275–93.
26. Radice E, Nelson H, Mercill S, Farouk R, Petty P, Gunderson L. Primary myocutaneous flap closure following resection of locally advanced pelvic malignancies. Br J Surg. 1999;86:349–54.
27. Soper JT, Secord AA, Havrilesky LJ, Berchuck A, Clarke-Pearson DL. Rectus abdominis myocutaneous and myoperitoneal flaps for neovaginal reconstruction after radical pelvic surgery: comparison of flap-related morbidity. Gynecol Oncol. 2005;97:596–601.
28. Rose PYM, Dekutoski M, Sim F. Classification of spinopelvic resections: oncologic and reconstructive implications. Combined Musculoskeletal Tumor Society/International Society for Limb Salvage meeting 2008. Boston, MA. 2008.
29. Kakuda JT, Lamont JP, Chu DZJ, Paz IB. The role of pelvic exenteration in the management of recurrent rectal cancer. Am J Surg. 2003;186:660–4.
30. Estes NC, Thomas JH, Jewell WR, Beggs D, Hardin CA. Pelvic exenteration: a treatment for failed rectal cancer surgery. Am Surg. 1993;59:420–2.
31. Magrini S, Nelson H, Gunderson LL, Sim FH. Sacropelvic resection and intraoperative electron irradiation in the management of recurrent anorectal cancer. Dis Colon Rectum. 1996;39:1–9.

32. Law WL, Chu KW, Choi HK. Total pelvic exenteration for locally advanced rectal cancer. J Am Coll Surg. 2000;190:78–83.
33. Ike H, Shimada H, Ohki S, Yamaguchi S, Ichikawa Y, Fujii S. Outcome of total pelvic exenteration for locally recurrent rectal cancer. Hepatogastroenterology. 2003;50:700–3.
34. Melton GB, Paty PB, Boland PJ, Healey JH, Savatta SG, Casas-Ganem JE, et al. Sacral resection for recurrent rectal cancer: analysis of morbidity and treatment results. Dis Colon Rectum. 2006;49:1099–107.
35. Weber KL, Nelson H, Gunderson LL, Sim FH. Sacropelvic resection for recurrent anorectal cancer. A multidisciplinary approach. Clin Orthop Relat Res. 2000;372:231–40.
36. Moriya Y, Akasu T, Fujita S, Yamamoto S. Total pelvic exenteration with distal sacrectomy for fixed recurrent rectal cancer in the pelvis. Dis Colon Rectum. 2004;47:2047–54.
37. Gunderson LL, Nelson H, Martenson JA, Cha S, Haddock M, Devine R, et al. Locally advanced primary colorectal cancer: intraoperative electron and external beam irradiation +/− 5-FU. Int J Radiat Oncol Biol Phys. 1997;37:601–14.
38. Henry LR, Sigurdson E, Ross EA, Lee JS, Watson JC, Cheng JD, et al. Resection of isolated pelvic recurrences after colorectal surgery: long-term results and predictors of improved clinical outcome. Ann Surg Oncol. 2007;14:2000–9.
39. Bouchard P, Efron J. Management of recurrent rectal cancer. Ann Surg Oncol. 2010;17(5):1343–56.
40. Moore HG, Shoup M, Riedel E, Minsky BD, Alektiar KM, Ercolani M, et al. Colorectal cancer pelvic recurrences: determinants of resectability. Dis Colon Rectum. 2004;47:1599–606.
41. Stocchi L, Nelson H, Sargent DJ, Engen DE, Haddock MG. Is en-bloc resection of locally recurrent rectal carcinoma involving the urinary tract indicated? Ann Surg Oncol. 2006;13:740–4.
42. Saito N, Koda K, Takiguchi N, Oda K, Ono M, Sugito M, et al. Curative surgery for local pelvic recurrence of rectal cancer. Dig Surg. 2003;20:192–200.
43. Schurr P, Lentz E, Block S, Kaifi J, Kleinhans H, Cataldegirmen G, et al. Radical redo surgery for local rectal cancer recurrence improves overall survival: a single center experience. J Gastrointest Surg. 2008;12:1232–8.
44. Wanebo HJ, Antoniuk P, Koness RJ, Levy A, Vezeridis M, Cohen SI, et al. Pelvic resection of recurrent rectal cancer: technical considerations and outcomes. Dis Colon Rectum. 1999;42:1438–48.
45. Wanebo HJ, Koness RJ, Vezeridis MP, Cohen SI, Wrobleski DE. Pelvic resection of recurrent rectal cancer. Ann Surg. 1994;220:586–97.
46. Dresen RC, Gosens MJ, Martijn H, Nieuwenhuijzen GA. Radical resection after IORT-containing multimodality treatment is the most important determinant for outcome in patients treated for locally recurrent rectal cancer. Ann Surg Oncol. 2008;15:1937–47.
47. Tilney HS, Tekkis PP, Sains PS, Constantinides VA, Heriot AG, Association of Coloproctology of Great Britain and I. Factors affecting circumferential resection margin involvement after rectal cancer excision. Dis Colon Rectum. 2007;50:29–36.
48. Schneebaum S, Arnold MW, Young D, LaValle GJ, Petty L, Berens MA, et al. Role of carcinoembryonic antigen in predicting resectability of recurrent colorectal cancer. Dis Colon Rectum. 1993;36:810–5.

第 13 章　首次腹腔镜手术后再手术

Mariano Laporte · Nicolás A. Rotholtz
王　刚译　李　宁审校

摘　要

在择期结直肠癌切除手术中，已经证明腹腔镜手术具有较好的疗效。目前，有许多前瞻性随机试验表明，腹腔镜手术应用于结直肠癌患者是安全的。很多研究都对腹腔镜手术和传统的开腹手术进行了比较，这些研究已经证实，腹腔镜技术应用于结肠切除术从肿瘤学角度考虑是安全的，而且将腹腔镜应用于复杂结直肠疾病、结直肠的急诊手术和术后并发症同样有效。

关键词

再次手术；再次腹腔镜手术；首次腹腔镜手术；腹膜炎；吻合口瘘；肠漏；腹腔镜检查；剖腹手术

引　言

首例腹腔镜结肠切除术报道于 1991 年[1]。随后，有多项研究验证了腹腔镜操作微创的优势；然而，1994 年，Berends 等[2] 报道了将腹腔镜应用于 14 例早期结肠癌的患者中，有 3 例出现伤口复发。随着对腹腔镜手术操作熟练程度的提高以及吻合技术的优化，这种并发症的发生率已明显减少[3-6]。

目前有许多前瞻性随机试验表明，腹腔镜手术可以安全地用于大肠癌，很多研究都对腹腔镜术和常规的开腹手术进行了比较[7-10]。这些研究已经证实，腹腔镜辅助结肠切除术与并发症发生率的增加无关，并且它是一种安全可行的手术方法[10]；UK CLASSIC 研究的一项长期随访报道，两组中肿瘤复发率相似[11]。腹腔镜技术应用结肠手术使肺部感染及伤口感染的发生率明显减少，但是任何一项技术都有可能带来其他潜在的并发症，如吻合口瘘（AL）、肠梗阻和术后出血等[5-7, 12]。在复杂的结直肠手术以及治疗腹腔镜结直肠切除术后并发症中，腹腔镜已经广泛应用[13]。

腹膜炎的腹腔镜管理

多年以来，腹膜炎被认为是腹腔镜手术的禁忌证；但是，随着时间的推移，这种观点已经改变；现在外科医生已经认识到，采用腹腔镜可以很容易达到并灌洗腹部的所有区域。伤口感染是腹膜炎患者常见的并发症之一，在多项研究中，已证实腹腔镜手术可以减少这种事件的发生率[7-9, 14]。理论上讲，二氧化碳造成的气腹可能诱发菌血症[14]；但大多数临床和实验研究却得出相反的结论，与开腹手术比较，腹腔镜的全身性炎症反应少、创伤小、细胞因子反应少、组织损伤少[14-20]。目前的证据表明，腹腔镜手术在不同紧急情况都有很多优势，并在消化性溃疡穿孔、急性胆囊炎、急性复杂憩室炎、急性阑尾炎和盆腔炎病例中频繁使用[13, 21]。

普通外科术腹腔镜后并发症的管理

腹腔镜手术后,并发症的发生率为 0.05%~8%[14, 22, 23]。术中最好能及时发现损伤,但有些热损伤一般会延迟出现。而且,腹部影像证明约有 50% 的病例出现术后腹腔感染[24];再次腹腔镜手术展现了腹腔镜的优越性,并报道感染来源的诊断准确度为 93%~100%[25]。但是,由传统的开腹手术进行腹部探查时,腹腔内感染和术后长期疼痛的风险将增加,术后肠梗阻的发生率较高,伤口并发症更多,住院时间延长[24]。

有腹部手术史的患者再次行急诊手术的机率是 1%~4.4%,而这些病例往往会在胃肠手术后出现[26-27]。在 Unalp 等发表的研究中[28],4410 例患者中有 81 例进行了再次剖腹手术,紧急行再次剖腹探查术最常见的适应证为吻合口瘘或肠瘘。研究表明,早期诊断这些术后并发症并快速决策行再次手术,可降低腹腔感染和多器官衰竭的发病率[29]。

使用再次腹腔镜手术,可能会帮助并加快手术的决定,并使得微创优势达到最佳。在现有的文献中,当通过剖腹手术进行再手术,原手术和再手术之间的间隔时间相当长,这可能意味着患者在腹腔镜手术结束后不久不愿进行剖腹手术[30]。众所周知,再次腹腔镜术在许多病例中是一种有效的方法,术中没有发现阳性症状,也不会增加并发症发生率。当在术后早期决定做再次腹腔镜手术时,以前的戳孔没有完全愈合,可以利用戳孔再次建立气腹[24];但是,目前已经发表了许多手术相关的并发症的研究,包括气腹针、套管和其他医源性损伤扩张的肠管[25]。

自 20 世纪 90 年代以来,就有关于腹腔镜胆囊切除术后再次行腹腔镜术的描述[30-31],类似的方法也可以用于治疗上消化道手术后的并发症。Iqbal 等[32] 描述了腹腔镜抗逆流手术后进行再手术,可以安全地进行重复腹腔镜术,手术结果令人满意。Calmes 等[33] 在初始腹腔镜减肥手术后使用了这种方法;研究者描述了 49 例患者在腹腔镜下 Roux-en-Y 胃旁路手术后接受了再次微创手术,普遍获得了成功。

Kirshtein 等[25] 在一般性综述中报道了 64 例患者接受腹腔镜再手术后发生多种并发症。最初的手术包括 49 例腹腔镜手术,14 例剖腹手术和 1 例内窥镜手术。在这些手术中,51(80%)例在初次手术后 76h 内进行了再手术。需要进行再次手术的患者中,多数经历了腹腔镜胆囊切除术,其中包括 7 例胆漏、5 例血肿感染、2 例肝下脓肿和 1 例小肠穿孔。18 例(28.1%)患者,再次腹腔镜术中没有发现腹腔内有病理改变;其中,86% 的手术通过腹腔镜完成。有 9 例患者中转开腹,需行小肠切除、造口,以及胃、结肠和小肠的穿孔修补等。Kirshtein 等得出结论,腹腔镜手术是处理开腹和腹腔镜术后并发症的一种有效工具,并且避免了延误诊断和不必要的剖腹手术。

腹腔镜结直肠手术的并发症

吻合口瘘(AL)是结直肠手术中最严重的并发症,通常需要再次进行手术。所有大肠癌手术中,有 3.4%~6% 发生吻合口瘘,大多数(2.9%~15.3%)发生在低位直肠的保肛手术。发生吻合口瘘后的死亡率为 6%~39.3%[34-36]。虽然术中建议进行吻合口充气实验,但是值得注意的是,即使进行了检测和修复,并不能完全阻止 AL 的识别或发生[37]。此外,虽然大家都同意利用吻合器可以更快速地进行操作,但是吻合器和手工缝制吻合的并发症发生率、死亡率和吻合口瘘的发生率相似[38]。末端回肠分流造口术虽然并不能防止 AL,却会降低需要再次进行手术的风险。多项研究表明发生 AL 的危险因素包括男性、营养状况不良、肥胖、大量输血及吻合位置等[12, 39-41]。

人们普遍认识到,将常规手术和腹腔镜手术进行比较,其并发症发生率和死亡率之间并没有显著差异。美国的一项前瞻性随机对照研究[42] 对 621 例接受常规手术和 627 例腹腔镜手术的患者进行了比较。两组的并发症发生率相似,总并发症发生率分别为 21% 和 20%,并且该研究结果与其他研究的结果也相似[43-46]。然而,最近的一项荟萃分析[47] 对开腹手术和腹腔镜结直肠手术进行了比较,并对所有随机对照研究进行了评估,腹腔镜组表现出较高的术中并发症发生率(odds ratio, 1.37;P=0.01)和较高的肠管损伤率(odds ratio, 1.88;P=0.2)(2159 例患者接受腹腔镜手术,1896 例患者接受开腹手术)。此外,腹腔镜技术应用于结直肠手术可以明显降低粘连的风险[48],因此降低了粘连相关性小肠梗阻[49] 和腹疝[50] 的发生。

有多项研究对比了腹腔镜技术和开腹手术应用于直肠癌切除手术，结果显示，并发症发生率或死亡率没有显著差异[8, 11, 35, 44, 45, 51]。Laurent等[45]报道了471例进展期直肠癌的患者；其中，238例经腹腔镜手术治疗，233例经开腹手术治疗，术后并发症发生率和死亡率无显著差异。腹腔镜组盆腔感染（包括吻合口瘘、脓肿、缺血）的发生率为11.8%，常规组为12.9%（P值没有显著差异）。Kirchhoff等[37]分析了1316例择期腹腔镜结直肠手术术中和术后并发症的可能相关的危险因素，他们发现，术后并发症的发生率明显受到男性、年龄>75岁、ASA评分>3、肿瘤疾病和外科医生经验等因素影响。经研究发现，腹腔镜手术对于肥胖患者[53]及晚期的结直肠癌患者是选择性有效的[52]，对于复杂的非恶性疾病也是如此，包括子宫内膜异位症[54]和Crohn病[55]。在后一种情况下，最近的Cochrane系统评价表明，本组腹腔镜手术的伤口相关并发症发生率降低，非疾病相关再手术的总体发生率降低。

结直肠术后并发症的腹腔镜管理

再手术最常见的原因为粘连性小肠梗阻，在传统开腹手术后很常见。由于减少了对小肠的操作和气腹的原因，腹腔镜手术可以减少粘连的发生[56]。有研究显示，通过腹腔镜手术处理开腹手术后急性肠梗阻的成功率达到66%，早期通过再次腹腔镜手术将这些患者转变为单带或局限黏连性病变十分重要[57]。梗阻的常见原因是肠管在戳孔位置发生嵌顿，通过腹腔镜手术可以很容易地修补腹壁缺损来解除梗阻。还有一类特殊的患者，他们在进行腹腔镜下辅助性回肠造口术后，发生了小肠梗阻，在这些患者中，早期术后梗阻可能是由一些可预防原因导致，包括回肠造口扭曲、造口近端的粘连性肠扭转、造口通过的筋膜开口过于紧密[58]。粘连松解时，小肠可能会发生损伤，虽然腹腔镜修补肠管损伤是可行的，但是小切口取出肠道进行修补似乎更为安全[56]。因此，在缝合戳孔时将腹膜关闭是预防各种特殊并发症的关键因素。

出血是腹腔镜结直肠术后可能威胁生命的一种并发症。虽然需要考虑到血流动力学稳定，但众所周知，应当避免在血流动力学不稳定的患者中进行腹腔镜术，对于这类患者来说，传统的开腹手术更为合理[28, 59, 60]。另外，可以使用EndoCatch袋（美国手术，康涅狄格州诺沃克；泰科医疗集团，马萨诸塞州曼斯菲尔德）收集血块，通过腹腔镜来控制有限的出血，使其能够通过套管针部位进行传递[56]。经证明，这种方法已经用于治疗胆囊切除后和防逆流过程中的出血并发症[61-63]。

吻合口瘘无疑是结直肠手术后最具威胁性的一种并发症，并具有很高的发生率和死亡率。在某些特定的患者中，再次腹腔镜方法可以解决这个问题。Wind等[64]报道了10例在首次腹腔镜结直肠手术后出现AL的患者，用再次腹腔镜手术的方法成功地进行治疗。其中有2例患者没有中转开腹，与其他病例相比，他们在重症监护病房中的时间更短，较早恢复正常饮食，并较早的首次造口排便。其他人也报道了这种再次腹腔镜的方法，包括我们的研究小组[65-68]，但需要随机对照试验进一步验证其优势。Wind等的研究中，低位直肠吻合后行预防性回肠造口术，而当这些患者发生吻合口瘘时，回肠造口可作为最终造口。与15例开腹手术后进行再次剖腹手术的患者相比，腹腔镜组在术后30天表现出更低的死亡率和更短的住院时间。

Pera等[69]进行了一项研究，低位直肠吻合口瘘的及时治疗在绝大多数病例中是可行的。在10例患者中，有3例可以成功地通过经皮穿刺引流治疗，而其他7例患者则进行腹腔灌洗和分流造口术。4例患者经腹腔镜微创治疗，术后早期使用腹腔镜未造成并发症。同样，2009年，Joh等[67]的研究报道了17例患者（占研究人数的58%）接受了腹腔镜直肠切除，并有手术后AL，其中大部分可以通过腹腔镜成功治疗；对轻微或中度腹腔内污染的患者行腹腔灌洗和回肠造口分流术。1例患者因为吻合口坏死进行了再次吻合术，而在另一病例中，由于发生了严重的腹腔感染进行了剖腹探查和Hartmann手术。手术30天内无死亡病例发生，79.3%的患者分流回肠造口再次还纳。

2009年，我们发表了经验性研究[66]，报道了17例患者接受腹腔镜再手术的结果，并将其与10例接受再次常规开腹手术的患者相比。这两组最初进行了腹腔镜吻合术。微创组进行再次手术的最常见原因为AL（13例）；需要进行多次腹腔灌洗、引流和回肠造口术。该试验组中，只有1例患者需要进行中转开腹。其他需要再次腹腔镜手术的患者包括小肠穿孔、内疝伴肠梗阻、1例结肠皮肤瘘、1例切口疝。关于住院时间的长短或术后并发症的发生率，各组间无显著差异。

基于最初的这一小部分证据，如果患者没有达到预期恢复，在首次腹腔镜手术后进行腹腔镜再次探查似乎较为合理，这是判断 AL 或其他可能出现的并发症的一种早期诊断工具。这种早期的再次介入可能会阻止严重的全身性腹膜炎及全身败血症。腹腔镜再次探查的一个显著和重要的优势是伤口并发症的发生率降低，包括早期伤口裂开和晚期切口疝。对于再次手术，应通过以前的戳孔位置建立气腹。当怀疑戳孔位置存在小肠粘连阻塞时，使用开放技术进入腹腔再建立气腹似乎更为安全，常常在左上腹进行。也有报道描述了成功在远离戳卡的位置采用气腹针建立气腹[56]。进腹后，必须仔细检查腹部。手术台应能允许采取多种体位来减少对肠管的操作，能因此减少医源性肠损伤的风险。如果发生肠损伤，可通过腔镜下缝合技术修复，但这通常比较耗时，也可以通过小切口取出肠管，并在体外进行缝合。

研究者经验

在我们的研究（结果尚未发表）中，从 2000 年 6 月至 2010 年 7 月共有 860 例患者进行结直肠手术，其中 458 例（53.3%）为男性。平均年龄为 58.7 岁（16～92 岁），其中有 447 例患者（52%）为恶性肿瘤，413 例患者（48%）为良性疾病。平均手术时间为 181min（60～510min），平均住院天数为 4.3 天。218 例患者中，有 244 例发生并发症（28.3%），其中，208 例（85.2%）患者为早期，36 例（14.8%）为晚期。39 例患者（3.6%）需要进行再次手术：29 例（74.3%）患者通过腹腔镜进行再手术，10 例（25.7%）进行剖腹手术。如表 13.1 所示，74%（29/39）的再次手术患者进行了肠切除术，其中大部分进行左半结肠切除术。

通过打开第一种方法中所使用的端口位点，进行气腹再手术。应仔细处理肠管，以避免内脏损伤。腹腔镜再手术组的中转开腹率为 13.8%（4/29）。1 例患者由于降结肠缺血需要进行剖腹手术，另有 2 例患者由于继发于全身性腹膜炎的显著性肠道扩张不能建立气腹，需要进行中转开腹。在腹腔镜再手术中，有 20 例患者（69%）发现有 AL（表 13.2 和表 13.3）。这些病例大部分（n=18）能够进行严格的腹腔灌洗，腹腔引流的位置靠近吻合口裂开处。

表 13.1　腹腔镜和开腹手术的主要操作[66]

	腹腔镜术 (n)	剖腹术 (n)
肠节段切除	23	6
左半结肠	18	4
右半结肠	5	1
横结肠	–	1
直肠前切除术	4	1
结肠次全切除术	–	2
全结肠切除术	2	–
回盲部切除术	–	1

表 13.2　行再次探查手术的原因[66]

并发症	腹腔镜术 (n=29)	剖腹术 (n=10)
吻合口瘘	20 (69)	2 (20)
切口疝	3 (10.3)	–
小肠穿孔	2 (6.9)	4 (40)
腹腔内出血	1 (3.4)	1 (10)
结肠皮肤瘘	1 (3.4)	–
内疝	1 (3.4)	–
病理阴性	1 (3.4)	–
狭窄裂开	–	1 (10)
Ogilvie 综合征	–	1 (10)
粘连	–	1 (10)

数值显示为 n (%)

表 13.3　手术探查结果及治疗[66]

调查结果	n	治疗	n
吻合口瘘	18	腹腔灌洗，引流＋回肠造口术	18
切口疝	3	修补	3
吻合口瘘＋结肠缺血	2	节段性结肠切除术＋回肠造口术	2
小肠损伤	2	小肠段切除，回肠造口术	2
内疝	1	修补	1
结肠皮肤瘘	1	节段性结肠切除术	1
出血	1	腹腔冲洗	1
无	1		

这证实了左半结肠和直肠前切除后发生的 AL，可以很容易地通过腹腔镜再手术治疗。3 例患者的瘘口很容易被发现，进行了吻合口瘘的腹腔镜下缝合。所有的患者均在右下腹戳卡位置行预防性回肠造口术（图 13.1）。1 例患者由于肠内容物引起的腹膜炎需要进行第二次探查手术，并进行了 Hartmann 手术。

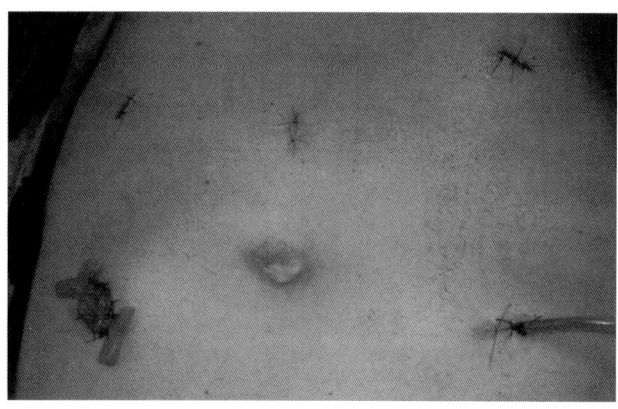

图 13.1 再次腹腔镜手术后患者。将戳卡放置在原手术中使用的相同位点。在右下腹进行保护性回肠造口术

术后第 2~3 个月之间，行灌肠检查证实了吻合口的完整性，并进行造口还纳手术。

3 例患者戳卡切口处（脐周、上腹或耻骨上）持续存在严重的术后疼痛并伴有明显的腹胀，他们再次行腹腔镜探查手术。这 3 例患者都是一种急性疝，采用腹腔镜方法进行腹膜缺损封堵，可以很容易减少其发生。2 例患者由于肠道损伤需要进行再手术，这可能是由对以往多次手术的粘连进行松解所导致的。虽然腹部手术史不是腹腔镜探查的绝对禁忌证，但必须认真松解粘连，以避免肠管损伤。根据我们的经验，一般都能够找到肠穿孔，并通过腹腔镜对其进行缝合。

结 论

虽然与常规手术相比，腹腔镜结直肠手术可能会减少一些不良事件，但术后并发症仍然存在。在许多情况下，在首次腹腔镜手术后，使用腹腔镜进行再手术似乎是可行的，并值得进行进一步的前瞻性随机对照研究，特别是当发生 AL 时。对于经验丰富的术者，早期粘连性小肠梗阻通常很容易通过腹腔镜手术进行治疗[70-74]。

参考文献

1. Jacobs M, Verdeja JC, Goldstein HS. Minimally invasive colon resection (laparoscopic colectomy). Surg Laparosc Endosc. 1991;1:144–50.
2. Berends FJ, Kazemier G, Bonjer HJ, Lange JF. Subcutaneous metastases after laparoscopic colectomy. Lancet. 1994;344:58.
3. Senagore AJ, Luchtefeld MA, Mackeigan JM. What is the learning curve for laparoscopic colectomy? Am Surg. 1995;61:681–5.
4. Schlachta CM, Mamazza J, Seshadri PA, Cadeddu M, Gregoire R, Poulin EC. Defining a learning curve for laparoscopic colorectal resections. Dis Colon Rectum. 2001;44:217–22.
5. Li JC, Hon SS, Ng SS, Lee JF, Yiu RY, Leung KL. The learning curve for laparoscopic colectomy: experience of a surgical fellow in an university colorectal unit. Surg Endosc. 2009;23:1603–8.
6. Tekkis PP, Senagore AJ, Delaney CP, Fazio VW. Evaluation of the learning curve in laparoscopic colorectal surgery: comparison of right-sided and left-sided resections. Ann Surg. 2005;242:83–91.
7. The Clinical Outcomes of Surgical Therapy Study Group (COST). A comparison of laparoscopically assisted and open colectomy for colon cancer. N Engl J Med. 2004;350:2050–9.
8. Guillou PJ, Quirke P, Thorpe H, Walker J, Jayne DG, Smith AM, Heath RM, Brown JM, MRC CLASICC trial group. Short-term endpoints of conventional versus laparoscopic-assisted surgery in patients with colorectal cancer: multicentre, randomised controlled trial. Lancet. 2005;365(9472):1718–26.
9. Bonjer HJ, Hop WC, Nelson H, Sargent DJ, Lacy AM, Castells A, Guillou PJ, Thorpe H, Brown J, Delgado S, Kuhrij E, Haglind E, Påhlman L, Transatlantic Laparoscopically Assisted vs Open Colectomy Trials Study Group. Laparoscopically assisted vs. open colectomy for colon cancer: a meta-analysis. Arch Surg. 2007;142:298–303.
10. Gervaz P, Inan I, Perneger T, Schiffer E, Morel P. A prospective, randomized, single-blind comparison of laparoscopic versus open sigmoid colectomy for diverticulitis. Ann Surg. 2010;252:3–8.
11. Jayne DG, Thorpe HC, Copeland J, Quirke P, Brown JM, Guillou PJ. Five-year follow-up of the Medical Research Council CLASICC trial of laparoscopically assisted versus open surgery for colorectal cancer. Br J Surg. 2010;97:1638–45.
12. Kirchhoff P, Clavien PA, Hahnloser D. Complications in colorectal surgery: risk factors and preventive strategies. Patient Saf Surg. 2010;4:5.
13. Champagne B, Stulberg JJ, Fan Z, Delaney CP. The feasibility of laparoscopic colectomy in urgent and emergent settings. Surg Endosc. 2009;23:1791–6.
14. Agresta F, Ciardo LF, Mazzarolo G, Michelet I, Orsi G, Trentin G, Bedin N. Peritonitis: laparoscopic approach. World J Surg. 2006;1:9.
15. Evasovich M, Clark T, Horattas M, Holda S, Treen L. Does pneumoperitoneum during laparosocopy increase bacterial translocation? Surg Endosc. 1996;10:1176–9.
16. Are C, Talamini MA, Murata K, De Maio A. Carbon dioxide pneumoperioneum alters acute-phase response induced by lipopolysaccharide. Surg Endosc. 2002;16:1464–7.
17. Horattas MC, Haller N, Ricchiutti D. Increased transperitoneal bacterial translocation in laparoscopic surgery. Surg Endosc. 2003;17:1464–7.
18. Hanly EJ, Mendoza-Sagaon M, Murata K, Hardacre JM, De Maio A, Talamini MA. CO_2 pneumoperitoneum modifies the inflammatory response to sepsis. Ann Surg. 2003;237:343–50.
19. Hanly EJ, Bachman SL, Marohn MR, Boden JH, Herring AE, De Maio A, Talamini MA. CO_2 pnueomoperitoneum-mediated attenuation of the inflammatory response is independent of systemic acidosis. Surgery. 2005;137:559–66.
20. Hanly EJ, Fuentes JM, Aurora AR, Bachman SL, De Maio A, Marohn MR, Talamini MA. Carbon dioxide pneumoperitoneum prevents mortality from sepsis. Surg Endosc. 2006;20:1482–7.
21. Sauerland S, Agresta F, Bergamaschi R, Borzellino G, Budzynski A, Champault G, Fingerhut A, Isla A, Johansson M, Lundorff P, Navez B, Saad S, Neugebauer EAM. Laparoscopy for abdominal emergencies. Surg Endosc. 2006;20:14–29.
22. Schrenk P, Woisetschlager R, Rieger R, Wayand W. Mechanism, management, and prevention of laparoscopic bowel injuries. Gastrointest Endosc. 1996;43:572–4.
23. Schafer M, Lauper M, Krahenbuhl L. Trocar and Veress needle injuries during laparoscopy. Surg Endosc. 2001;15:275–80.

24. Kirshtein B, Roy-Shapira A, Domchik S, Mizrahi S, Lantsberg L. Early relaparoscopy for management of suspected postoperative complications. J Gastrointest Surg. 2008;12:1257–62.
25. Kirshtein B, Domchik S, Mizrahi S, Lantsberg L. Laparoscopic diagnosis and treatment of postoperative complications. Am J Surg. 2009;197:19–23.
26. Ching SS, Murlikrishnan VP, Whiteley GS. Relaparotomy: a five year review of indications and outcome. Int J Clin Pract. 2003;57:333–7.
27. Hutchins RR, Gunning MP, Lucas DN, Allen-Mersh TG, Soni NC. Relaparotomy for suspected intraperitoneal sepsis after abdominal surgery. World J Surg. 2004;28:137–41.
28. Unalp HR, Kamer E, Kar H, Bal A, Peskersoy M, Onal MA. Urgent abdominal reexplorations. World J Surg. 2006;1:10.
29. Dexter SPL, Miller GV, Davides D, Martin IG, Ling HMS, Sagar PM, Larvin M, McMahon MJ. Relaparoscopy for the detection and treatment of complications of laparoscopic cholecystectomy. Am J Surg. 2000;178:316–9.
30. Deziel DJ, Millikan KW, Economou SG. Complications of laparosopic cholecystectomy: a national survey of 4292 hospitals and an analysis of 77604 cases. Am J Surg. 1993;163:9–14.
31. Dexter SP, Miller GV, Davides D, Martin IG, Sue Ling HM, Sagar PM, Larvin M, McMahon MJ. Relaparoscopy for the detection and treatment of complications of laparoscopic cholecystectomy. Am J Surg. 2000;179:316–9.
32. Iqbal A, Awad Z, Simkins J, Shah R, Haider M, Salinas V, Turaga K, Karu A, Mittal SK, Filipi CJ. Repair of 104 failed anti-reflux operations. Ann Surg. 2006;244:42–51.
33. Calmes JM, Giusti V, Suter M. Reoperative laparoscopic Roux-en-Y gastric bypass: an experience with 49 cases. Obes Surg. 2005;15:316–22.
34. Chambers WM, Mortensen NJ. Postoperative leakage and abscess formation after colorectal surgery. Best Pract Res Clin Gastroenterol. 2004;18:865–80.
35. Aziz O, Constantinides V, Tekkis PP, Athanasiou T, Purkayastha S, Paraskeva P, Darzi AW, Heriot AG. Laparoscopic versus open surgery for rectal cancer: a meta-analysis. Ann Surg Oncol. 2006;13:413–24.
36. Joh YG, Kim SH, Hahn KY, Stulberg J, Chung CS, Lee DK. Anastomotic leakage after laparoscopic proctectomy can be managed by minimally invasive approach. Dis Colon Rectum. 2009;52:91–6.
37. Kirchhoff P, Dincler S, Buchmann P. A multivariate analysis of potential risk factors for intra and postoperative complications in 1316 elective colorectal procedures. Ann Surg. 2008;248:259–65.
38. Zorcolo L, Covotta L, Carlomagno N, Bartolo DCC. Safety of primary anastomosis in emergency colorectal surgery. Colorectal Dis. 2002;5:262–9.
39. Walker KG, Bell SW, Rickard MJ, Mehanna D, Dent OF, Chapuis PH, Bokey EL. Anastomotic leakage is predictive of diminished survival after potentially curative resection for colorectal cancer. Ann Surg. 2004;240:255–9.
40. Murrell ZA, Stamos MJ. Reoperation for anastomotic failure. Clin Colon Rectal Surg. 2006;19:213–6.
41. Konishi T, Watanabe T, Kishimoto J, Nagawa H. Risk factors for anastomotic leakage after surgery for colorectal cancer: results of prospective surveillance. J Am Coll Surg. 2006;202:439–44.
42. Veldkamp R, Kuhry E, Hop WC, Colon cancer Laparoscopic or Open Resection Study Group (COLOR). Laparoscopic surgery versus open surgery for colon cancer: short-term outcomes of a randomized trial. Lancet Oncol. 2005;6(7):477–84.
43. Larach SW, Patankar SK, Ferrara A, Williamson PR, Perozo SE, Lord AS. Complications of laparoscopic colorectal surgery. Analysis and comparison of early vs. latter experience. Dis Colon Rectum. 1997;40:592–6.
44. Milsom JW, Böhm B, Hammerhofer KA, Fazio V, Steiger E, Elson P. A prospective, randomized trial comparing laparoscopic versus conventional techniques in colorectal cancer surgery: a preliminary report. J Am Coll Surg. 1998;187:46–55.
45. Laurent C, Leblanc F, Wütrich P, Scheffler M, Rullier E. Laparoscopic versus open surgery for rectal cancer: long-term oncologic results. Ann Surg. 2009;250:54–61.
46. Robinson CN, Chen GJ, Balentine CJ, Sansgiry S, Marshall CL, Anaya DA, Artinyan A, Albo D, Berger DH. Minimally invasive surgery is underutilized for colon cancer. Ann Surg Oncol. 2011;18(5):1412–8.
47. Sammour T, Kahokehr A, Srinivasa S, Bissett IP, Hill AG. Laparoscopic colorectal surgery is associated with a higher intraoperative complication rate than open surgery. Ann Surg. 2011;253:35–43.
48. Dowson HM, Bong JJ, Lovell DP, Worthington TR, Karanija ND, Rockall TA. Reduced adhesion formation following laparoscopic versus open colorectal surgery. Br J Surg. 2008;95:909–14.
49. Rosin D, Zmora O, Hoffman A, Khaikin M, Bar Zakai B, Munz Y, Shabtai M, Ayalaon A. Low incidence of adhesion-related bowel obstruction after laparoscopic colorectal surgery. J Laparoendosc Adv Surg Tech A. 2007;17:604–7.
50. Duepree HJ, Senagore AJ, Delaney C, Fazio VW. Does means of access affect the incidence of small bowel obstruction and ventral hernia after bowel resection? Laparoscopy versus laparotomy. J Am Coll Surg. 2003;197:177–81.
51. Delaney CP, Change E, Senagore AJ, Broder M. Clinical outcomes and resource utilization associated with laparoscopic and open colectomy using a large national database. Ann Surg. 2008;247:819–24.
52. Verheien PM, Stevenson AR, Lumley JW, Clark AJ, Stitz RW, Clark DA. Laparoscopic resection of advanced colorectal cancer. Br J Surg. 2011;98:427–30.
53. Kamoun S, Alves A, Bretagnol F, Lefevre JH, Valleur P, Panis Y. Outcomes of laparoscopic colorectal surgery in obese and nonobese patients: a case-matched study of 180 patients. Am J Surg. 2009;198:450–5.
54. Serrachioli R, Poggioli G, Pierangeli F, Manuzzi L, Gualerzi B, Savelli L, Remorgida V, Mabrouk M, Venturoli S. Surgical outcome and long-term follow-up after laparoscopic rectosigmoid resection in women with deep infiltrating endometriosis. BJOG. 2007;114:889–96.
55. Dasari BV, McKay D, Gardiner K. Laparoscopic versus open surgery for small bowel Crohn's disease. Cochrane Database Syst Rev. 2011:CD006956.
56. McCormick JT, Simmang CL. Reoperation following minimally invasive surgery: are the rules different? Clin Colon Rectal Surg. 2006;19:217–22.
57. Wang Q, Hu ZQ, Wang WJ, Zhang J, Wang Y, Ruan C. Laparoscopic management of recurrent adhesive small-bowel obstruction: long-term follow-up. Surg Today. 2009;39:493–9.
58. Ng KH, Ng DC, Cheung HY, Wong JC, Yau KK, Chung CC, Li MC. Obstructive complications of laparoscopically created defunctioning ileostomy. Dis Colon Rectum. 2008;51:1664–8.
59. Agresta F, De Simone P, Bedin N. The Laparoscopic approach in abdominal emergencies. A single-center 10-year experience. JSLS. 2004;8:25–30.
60. Warren O, Kirnoss J, Paraskeva P, Darzi A. Emergency laparoscopy – current best practice. World J Surg. 2006;1:24.
61. Yau P, Watson D, Devitt P, Game P, Jamieson G. Early reoperation following laparoscopic antireflux surgery. World J Emerg Surg. 2000;179:172–6.
62. Tsalis K, Zacharakis E, Vasiliadis K. Bile duct injuries during laparoscopic cholecystectomy: management and outcome. Am Surg. 2005;71:1060–5.
63. Ying F, Shuodong W, Hong Y, Yang S, Jing K, Yu T, Amos SE. Lessons learnt after 12 years experience in laparoscopic cholecystectomy at a single center. Hepatogastroenterology. 2010;57:202–6.
64. Wind J, Koopman AG, van Berge Henegouwen MI, Slors JFM, Gouma DJ, Bemelman WA. Laparoscopic reintervention for anastomotic leakage after primary laparoscopic colorectal surgery. Br J Surg. 2007;94:1562–6.
65. Ten Broek RP, Van Goor H. Laparoscopic reintervention in colorectal surgery. Minerva Chir. 2008;63:161–8.
66. Rotholtz NA, Laporte M, Lencinas SM, Bun ME, Aued ML,

Mezzadri NA. Is a laparoscopic approach useful for treating complications after primary laparoscopic colorectal surgery? Dis Colon Rectum. 2009;52:275–9.
67. Joh YG, Kim SH, Hahn KY, Stulberg J, Chung CS, Lee DK. Anastomotic leakage after laparoscopic proctectomy can be managed by a minimally invasive approach. Dis Colon Rectum. 2009;52:91–8.
68. Kwak JM, Kim SH, Son DH, Kim J, Lee SI, Min BW, Um JW, Moon HY. The role of laparoscopic approach for anastomotic leakage after minimally invasive surgery for colorectal cancer. J Laparoendosc Adv Surg Tech A. 2011;21(1):29–33.
69. Pera M, Delgado S, Garcia-Valdecasas JC, Castells A, Pique JM, Bombuy E, Lacy AM. The management of leaking rectal anastomosis by minimally invasive techniques. Surg Endosc. 2002;16:603–6.
70. Schlachta CM, Mamazza J, Gregoire R, Burpee SE, Poulin EC. Could laparoscopic colon and rectal surgery become the standard of care? A review and experience with 750 procedures. J Can Chir. 2003;46:432–40.
71. Rotholtz NA, Laporte M, Zanoni G, Bun ME, Aued L, Lencinas S, Mezzadri NA, Pereyra L. Predictive factors for conversion in laparoscopic colorectal surgery. Tech Coloproctol. 2008;12:27–31.
72. Rotholtz NA, Bun ME, Tessio M, Lencinas SM, Laporte M, Aued ML, Peczan CE, Mezzadri NA. Laparoscopic colectomy: medial versus lateral approach. Surg Laparosc Endosc Percutan Tech. 2009;19:43–7.
73. Rotholtz NA, Montero M, Laporte M, Bun M, Lencinas S, Mezzadri N. Patients with less than three episodes of diverticulitis may benefit from elective laparoscopic sigmoidectomy. World J Surg. 2009;33:2444–7.
74. Poon JT, Law WL. Laparoscopic resection for rectal cancer: a review. Ann Surg Oncol. 2009;16:3038–47.

第 14 章 探讨困难性腹腔镜手术的解决途径

Joshua R. Karas · Roberto Bergamaschi

赵 坤 译　江志伟 审校

摘 要

本章概述了如何解决因腹腔内病变或粘连导致的腹腔镜下结直肠手术中面临的难题。在腹腔镜技术更为发达的今天，其并发症及禁忌证将被进一步讨论。本章就如何解决困难性腹腔镜手术，尽量减少手术并发症和如何处理术中并发症方面介绍目前的理念。

关键词

困难性腹腔镜手术；多次开腹手术；致密的粘连；疏忽的器官损伤；解剖改变；出血；抗凝治疗；再次手术

引 言

困难性腹腔镜手术往往被定义成：在手术中，那些能被预见到的不良事件往往会在下列情况下发生，包括多次开腹手术造成的腔镜入路困难、致密的粘连、变化的解剖位置有可能导致无意间器官损伤的风险及必须接受抗凝治疗的患者有出血的风险。

随着腹腔镜手术经验的增加及相关器械的改进，可以通过腹腔镜技术安全实施很多干预措施。以往一直被视为腹腔镜手术禁忌的复杂病例，如今也被许多掌握丰富先进腔镜技术的外科医生成功治疗。

本章主要介绍当前关于如何完成困难性腹腔镜手术及尽量减少手术并发症（包括位于腹部皮肤与结、直肠之间的器官）的观点。但对于那些并非结、直肠疾病专业的专科医生而言，本文的观点或许不易被理解和接受。我们试图让读者简要了解英语文献中可获得的证据。本章并不是一个提供此主题的综述，而是突出一些相关问题，并概述腹腔镜外科在这具有挑战性的形势下所扮演的角色。

基本原理

腹腔镜手术展现出诸多优点，包括减轻术后疼痛、缩短术后肠梗阻时间、加速恢复进食固体食物、较低的切口感染率、降低切口疝发生率以及更好的美容效果。鉴于这些优点，腹腔镜手术正逐步被认可，用来取代开腹手术来处理复杂的再手术病例。外科医生对于中转开腹应放低门槛，中转不应当被视为失败，而是表明拥有良好的临床判断。

通路（第一个入路）

对于再手术病例，建立安全通路进入腹腔是关键的一步。尽管外科医生会根据自己的偏好选择开放进入或者盲穿（气腹针）技术，但很多与通路相关的并发症也随着第一个穿刺套管的进入接踵而来，这些并发症可以被分为以下几类。

有手术史的腹部

Hasson 技术最初被描述为一种可以进入有手术史的患者腹腔的方法[1]。通过一种称之为下切的技术，手术者可以将一种钝尖穿刺套管在直视下置入腹腔，而不是用气腹针盲目进入。大多数外科医生在做这类手术时都比较喜欢这种切开技术[2]。当遇见一个有手术史的病例时，避开原切口瘢痕是一种明智的选择，因为这会降低意外损伤腹腔脏器的风险。设想一例患者曾经接受过正中剖腹手术（这是最常见的情况），第一个穿刺套管应位于腹直肌外侧，胸腔下缘腋前线水平与髂前上棘连线的中点。手术者必须注意不能将穿刺器放置得过于靠外侧，因为这容易损伤降结肠而且视野暴露不足。详细了解患者的既往手术情况有助于确定第一个穿刺套管最佳的穿刺点。如患者曾经接受过左半结肠切除术，那第一个穿刺点应选在腹部的右侧。这种理念同样适用于曾经接受过右侧腹部手术的患者。

为了帮助手术者有效确定穿刺点，光纤接入穿刺套管系统已于最近研发出来。它能让手术者随着穿刺套管进入腹腔的同时看清楚腹壁层的情况。研发这种系统的目的就是在获得腹腔镜通路的同时尽量减少脏器损伤的风险。目前有两种光学穿刺套管：一种使用刀片，另一种使用的是旋转、锋利、塑料制的透明尖端；两种型号都是在腹腔镜直视下置入穿刺套管。不管手术者选择何种型号的穿刺套管，这种穿刺技术都只需很小的力量，而且整个进腹过程都是直视的。这些新型的穿刺套管也能和 EndoAssist 机械设备匹配，这样就能代替人工辅助，同时能让手术者在穿刺套管进腹及主要操作过程中获得更大的手术操作空间[3]。

有烧伤史的腹壁

曾经遭受过腹壁大范围烧伤（Ⅲ~Ⅳ度）的患者也对腹腔镜入路构成了重大挑战（图 14.1）。手术者必须要意识到网膜可能会紧密粘连于前腹壁的腹膜壁层。建议使用 Hasson 技术，谨慎引导第一个穿刺套管于下腹部最低位（右侧或左侧）进入腹腔，因为此处最不可能存在大网膜的粘连。然后手术者必须仔细地将网膜从壁层腹膜上分离下来，以便其

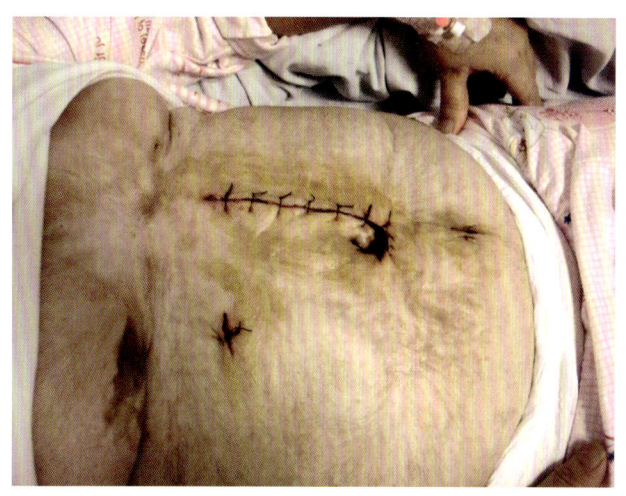

图 14.1 烧伤的腹壁

进一步置入其他穿刺套管。

视野类型

对于这类复杂的手术而言，0°镜通常没有任何作用，因为手术者通常需要环视粘连处的周边，而不是直接看前方。最低要求的镜头角度是 30°，但有时 45°镜会更有用处。尖端可以偏转的镜头或许是一种不错的选择，但操作镜头的医师必须熟悉这种设备。我们喜欢使用一种视野与摄像头之间没有界面的视频腹腔镜设备，而不是一个光学系统；因为后者可能形成烟雾，而当电缆软管被固定以后很难保证无菌。此外，手术者需注意摄像芯片是固定在视频腹腔镜的尖端；而在以往的系统，摄像芯片则是置于患者腹部之外。

血管损伤

尽管 Hasson 技术不能完全消除损伤主要血管的风险，但有证据显示这种风险因 Hasson 技术更加常规的使用而降低[4]。尽管血管损伤很少见，但需要开腹手术立即发现并修补损伤的血管[5]。在中转开腹之前，术者也许可以尝试用 Satinsky 夹控制出血的血管（图 14.2）。大量的与穿刺套管插入相关的血管损伤证据都来自个案报道。在一份回顾分析 629 例穿刺套管不良事件的报告中，有 408 例伴有主要血管损伤，致死 26 例，其中最常受损的是主动脉（23%）和腔静脉（15%）[6]。在这份分析报告中，有些外科医生使用了光学视图端口，暗示这类

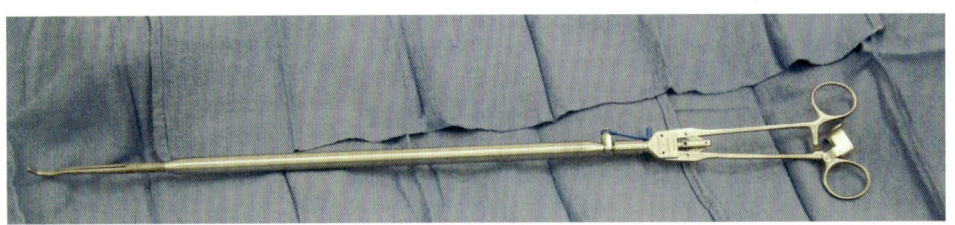

图 14.2　内镜使用的 Satinsky 夹

入路也不能完全避免穿刺套管插入导致的损伤。

肠道损伤

不过，不管是肠道损伤的发生率还是与之相关的死亡率，都没有因 Hasson 技术的使用而下降。值得强调的是 Hasson 技术应在远离原先疤痕的位点实施[7]。据报道，将近 40% 的肠管贯通伤是由穿刺套管置入之后导致[8]。因此，必须在直视下置入穿刺套管，同时要有充分的腹腔内视野，这就要求麻醉医生提供充分的腹壁肌肉松弛度。

气 腹

毫无疑问，为避免损伤，需要一个充分的气腹环境。一个外科医生需要进行思考，一步一步评估气腹不充分的所有可能原因。一旦所有常见的原因被排除后，手术者需与麻醉医生沟通，以确保前腹壁得到了充分的麻痹。尽可能降低腹腔内压力对于准备手术的患者而言是有益的，尽管在暴露状态下，提供腹腔内 10mmHg 压力与 15mmHg 压力几乎没有区别[9]。如果有手术史的患者接受的是骨盆内手术，那气腹压不超过 10mmHg 也许就足够了，因为骨盆相对不可延展。

当诱导和维持气腹时，外科医生必须要考虑患者的体型。如果腹壁厚度达到 10cm 或者更厚些，需要 15cm 而不是普通的 10cm 长的入路。如果穿刺套管太短而不能穿过腹壁，置入的气体很可能会导致明显的皮下气肿以及随后的潮气量增加。特殊的身体状况，包括阻塞性肺疾病及其他的呼吸系统疾病、充血性心脏疾病等，也许可被视为长时间气腹的禁忌证。在这些情况下，随着气腹压的增加，内脏器官的血流、心输出量、肾皮质血流会随之减少，从而导致局部或广泛的腹腔室隔综合征[10]。对于这些患有特定疾病的患者，或许可以选择一氧化二氮或者氦气建立气腹，当然要考虑到这些气体分别是可燃和不可溶解的。

操作步骤

暴 露

我们喜欢将患者置于截石位，将其手臂包裹于一边的衬垫上。截石位不仅为术中乙状结肠镜检查或者结肠镜检查创造了条件，而且也方便子宫操作。为了避免手术者的肘受到任何干扰，且术中可以使用较长的腹腔镜器械，患者的双膝高度不得高于腹部。对于肥胖的患者，手术者应当考虑将其胸部束缚于手术台上，因为在消毒之前，手术者必须要确定已经将患者安全地固定在手术台上。若是想将患者置于头低脚高位，可以通过遥控手术台完成。

要想安全地完成再次手术，手术者必须会正确地处理粘连、大网膜、肠管及其他器官。一般来说，轻柔的外科操作会降低意外损伤器官的风险。在这方面，不给肠钳上齿的做法应该应用于所有的肠管。适当的暴露可以通过使用闭合的器械推开粘连完成，而不是通过夹持肠管；膨胀明显的肠管会加大暴露的难度，延长手术时间。在这种情况下，应避免以氮为基础的麻醉，因为这样会扩张小肠。其他可以帮助暴露和压缩肠管的方法包括倾斜手术台和间断手动压迫腹壁。最终，手术者应当果断增加额外的入路以达到适当的暴露。

额外增加的入路

额外增加的入路不需要开放置入，但必须在直视下插入。入路之间的几何关系应尽可能呈三角形。当第一个入路置入以后，因为致密粘连的存在，腹腔内空间将会受到限制。我们之所以不推荐无刀片穿刺套管，是因为这类穿刺套管进腹时需要较大的力量，这会导致腹壁向腹腔内隆起；我们比较倾向于刀片穿刺套管或超声引导端口[11-12]。在结、直肠手术中多重穿刺套管的置入已被单孔技术取代[13-14]。

分 离

前腹壁与腹腔内脏器的粘连应当由冷剪刀在腹腔镜花生撑开器创造的一个平面里进行分离。外科医生有时会遇见小肠袢与前腹壁之间形成极端致密粘连的情形，不可能创造一个安全的分离平面。因此，有必要考虑切除一部分腹膜壁层及筋膜来松解肠袢，正如在开腹手术中处理这类情况一样。此外，基于能量（基于单极高频、电凝、超声）设备导致的损伤比较隐匿，导致其使用受到限制[15]。这些能量设备无意间导致中空器官的损伤往往看不见，因此也就不能被意识到。

粘连小肠的扩张

粘连的形成是导致肠梗阻和肠扩张的主要原因。最初，肠梗阻是腹腔镜手术的禁忌证。扩张的肠管会限制视野，也会增加肠管意外损伤的风险。但自从1991年，第1例腹腔镜下粘连松解报道以来[16]，腹腔镜手术已逐渐成为外科医生治疗这类普通疾病的选择。关于腹腔镜下处理粘连性小肠梗阻的数据很有限，而且差异也很显著。一份由Levard等组织实施、针对308例患者、耗时8年以上、涵盖35个中心的大范围、多中心的、回顾性的分析报告表明，成功实施腹腔镜手术的占54.6%，中转开腹的占45.4%[17]。研究表明，有过1~2次手术史的患者相对于有过3次及以上手术史的接受腹腔镜手术的成功率要明显增高（56% vs 37%；$P<0.05$）。某些作者为成功实施腹腔镜下粘连性小肠梗阻松解制作了一个相对临床参数列表，包括：①置放鼻胃管后反复发作的小肠梗阻；②一定的腹胀；③近端梗阻；④既往手术局限于腹部某一区域；⑤既往手术未发现致密粘连的存在；⑥能够安全地安置入路；⑦梗阻部分并未固定于腹膜后[18]。

止 血

对于有过手术史的腹腔镜手术，止血无疑是一大难题。大出血在再次手术过程中并不少见，往往由之前并存的疾病或术中探查时引起。粘连会改变解剖结构，这会导致分离的复杂化。一些药物，如泼尼松、血小板聚集抑制剂及抗凝剂，会降低组织的稳定性，从而增加渗血的风险，会影响视野。术中探查导致出血，往往是由于不能妥善处理好组织或由于设备故障导致的暴露不够充分。预防出血需要从正确理解解剖及选择合适的器械开始。下面介绍的止血材料应该是手术室为再次手术提前预备：

- 血管夹
- 网状胶原蛋白
- 电凝治疗仪（双极和单极）
- 镜下圈扎环、纤维蛋白黏合剂
- 缝合线
- 血管夹闭设备

在配合再次手术之前，手术室所有成员应当接受相应的培训以懂得使用上述设备。手术团队，包括器械护士和巡回护士，应当在术前讨论处理急性出血事件程序，并且要熟悉这些设备的名称。如出现了喷射性出血情况，控制镜头的医生应当立即将镜头撤回到穿刺套管内，以避免视野受干扰。手术者应该用不做重要操作的那只手给予压迫以临时控制出血。对于静脉出血，可以通过10mm的穿刺套管置入海绵进行压迫即可有效止血。对于最大直径小于7mm的动脉出血，可以通过镜下圈扎环、血管夹、使用腹腔内打结器完成的贯穿缝合，或者通过血管夹闭设备达到有效止血。在最终确定止血之前，手术者一定要证实出血的血管是否可以废用。若此血管不允许废用，可以使用腔镜下Satinsky血管夹临时控制出血，同时着手进行腹腔镜下血管重建术。

来自肝、胰腺、脾、肠系膜或腹膜后的渗血可以通过压迫和使用网状胶原蛋白及纤维蛋白黏合剂得到有效控制。在使用止血药之前，应进行充分的压迫止血。对于复杂的再次手术，引流管的使用值得好好考虑。一根具有主动吸引作用的引流管是有效果的，但不能直接被置于先前出血点的附近。每位开展腹腔镜下再次手术的外科医生应该熟练掌握镜下缝合和打结的技术。

肠破裂

肠损伤是腹腔镜再手术最严重的并发症之一。本章不介绍大肠或直肠穿孔伤。未发现的肠破裂是一种危及生命的并发症，它可能导致灾难性的后果。虽然这些不良事件也可以发生于传统手术，但在腹腔镜手术中发生肠破裂而未发觉的风险更大。如前所述，一个无法识别的小肠损伤的常见原因是利用能量设备进行腹腔镜下的粘连松解术。在一项回顾性配对分析比较的结果中接受腹腔镜手术和传统手术的小肠梗阻患者，肠穿孔率分别为27%和13.5%[19]。其他的研究没有显示出总体发病率和死亡率在这两种方法上的差异[20]。肠破裂发生后应能被识别，我们推荐应进行思考，区分不同原因导致的穿孔，包括各种能量器械（单极、超声刀或双极）所造成的穿孔，以及剪刀或由于钳子的张力所导致的机械性穿孔。对于后者，外科医生可以安全地进行手工缝合修复。修复过程是通过腹腔镜还是开腹手术，应取决于外科医生的专业知识和腹腔镜下的打结和缝合技术是否熟练。体外打结不推荐，因为有撕裂肠壁的危险。如果肠破裂是由热损伤导致的，不应考虑缝合修复，手术切除是标准的方式。在小肠内容物明显溢出的地方确定肠破裂的位置，我们建议考虑应用腹腔镜夹夹住肠破裂的近端（图14.3）。

尿道损伤

虽然腹腔镜手术中输尿管损伤率仍然是未知的，但在再次盆腔手术中经常发生[21]。我们建议腹腔镜再次手术中常规使用输尿管支架系统，更倾向使用软支架，腹腔镜手术结束必须取出，因为他们是无空隙的。输尿管支架不一定保护输尿管免受伤害，而是帮助外科医生确定输尿管损伤，尤其是当患者经历过放射治疗或多次腹部手术。当外科医生担心输尿管损伤而又不愿使用支架，可以通过静脉注射靛蓝染料来识别位置[21]。腹腔内出现蓝色染料就可以确诊。重要的是要立即发现并修复输尿管损伤，同时外科医生必须区分输尿管的部分断裂和完全断裂。虽然完全断裂的输尿管可以用腹腔镜完成修复，但由于必须涉及泌尿科专家，所以并不建议[22]。而输尿管的部分横断可以在腹腔镜下用5-0可吸收缝线进行修复。放置支架预防狭窄是必要的，腹腔内引流是为了避免术后尿漏（图14.4）。术中可能发生膀胱损伤，可以用3-0可吸收编织缝线再修复两层。Foley导管必须放置至膀胱尿道排泄造影完成（图14.5）。

术中内镜检查

术中内镜检查是可以为再次手术带来帮助的工具，最好是在手术开始前就开始进行肠镜。再次手术期间的术中胃镜和肠镜检查不太容易发现结直肠疾病。应该使用术中胃镜检查对小肠扩张进行评估。减少小肠扩张的方法包括用腹腔镜在屈氏韧带以下近端空肠放置动脉夹，或内镜检查时使用二氧化碳充气。根据病情，术中肠镜检查最好采用推进式小肠镜技术，其使用相对简单，并有较低的资金投资和维护。一方面，双气囊小肠镜需要专门的培训，需大量的资金投入和时间消耗。螺旋管式小肠镜，它采用对小肠深插管的一种特殊套管，目前正在评估[23-24]。

将患者摆成截石位的一个优势是使术中结肠镜容易可行。术中结肠镜检查对评估缺血、穿孔、术前形成的肿瘤[25]和吻合是必需的。在这种情况下，防止大肠的长期扩张，二氧化碳气腹是首选。硬式直肠镜检查对于急诊结直肠病是必需的，因为它是评估直肠理想的手段。

戳口的关闭

成功的腹腔镜再次手术操作后，不应轻视戳口的关闭，因为它可能导致严重的并发症。切口疝的程度可以从无症状的筋膜缺损至嵌顿/绞窄性疝。外科医生应该尝试关闭所有戳口。筋膜缺损10mm或更大应该缝合，即使在斜套管针插入的病例。筋膜关闭是使用开放技术并用一个粗大的针（UR6）

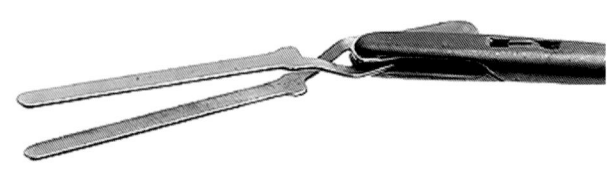

图14.3 内镜用的bulldog

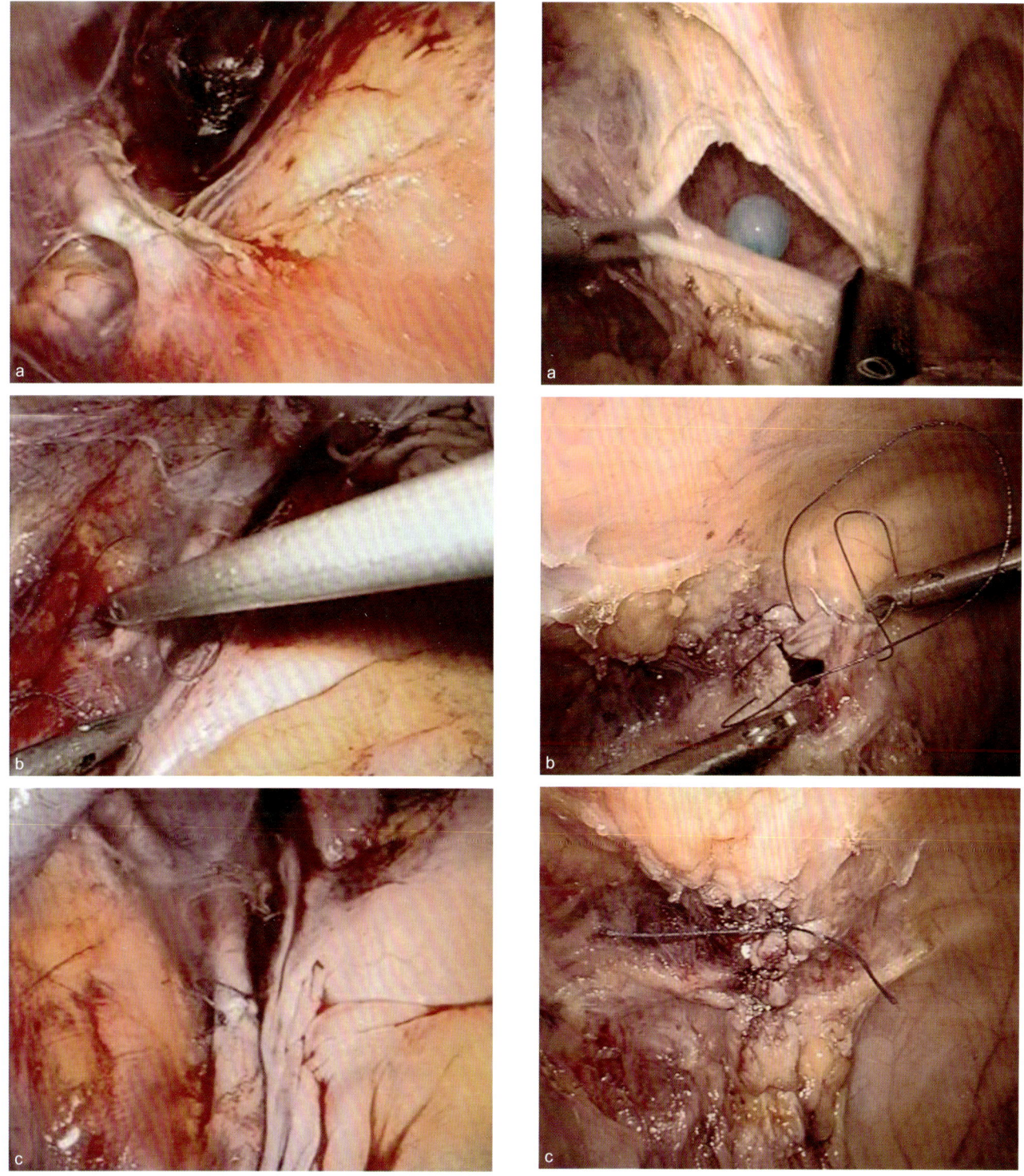

图14.4 （a）伴有尿漏的输尿管损伤；（b）内镜下缝合输尿管；（c）输尿管损伤的最终修复

图14.5 膀胱损伤和修复。（a）可以看到Foley导尿管球囊的膀胱穿孔；（b）腹腔内下缝合修复；（c）膀胱的最后修复

来减少针断裂在腹壁内的机会。开放缝合5mm的戳口常常是不可能的，除非患者体质指数低。因此，在大多数情况下，首选腹腔镜使用缝线Passer关闭5mm的缺陷。如果患者有一个大的、早已存在的切口疝并需放置补片修补，修补将推迟。若再手术中发生肠破裂和进行了肠切除，也应推迟修复。

结 论

在决定给患者采用腹腔镜手术方法时，应从临床疗效的角度进行谨慎评估，而不是替代结果的措施。对一个困难性或再次手术的病例选择使用腹腔镜手术，需要优先考虑患者的利益。即使在腹腔镜手术有明显优势的情况下，是否决定进行腹腔镜手术也应该依赖于外科医生的经验、设备是否齐全、辅助人员对于腹腔镜是否熟悉。必须明确告知患者，为了保护他们，中转开腹的门槛可能会降低。

参考文献

1. Hasson HM. A modified instrument and method for laparoscopy. Am J Obstet Gynecol. 1971;110:886–7.
2. Vignali A, Di Palo S, De Nardi P, Radaelli G, Orsenigo E, Staudacher C. Impact of previous abdominal surgery on the outcome of laparoscopic colectomy: a case-matched control study. Tech Coloproctol. 2007;11:241–6.
3. Gilbert JM. The EndoAssist robotic camera holder as an aid to the introduction of laparoscopic colorectal surgery. Ann R Coll Surg Engl. 2009;91:389–93.
4. Kazemier G, Hazebroek EJ, Lange JF, Bonjer HJ. Vascular injuries during laparoscopy. J Am Coll Surg. 1998;186:604–5.
5. Nordestgaard AG, Bodily KC, Osborne RW, Buttorff JD. Major vascular injuries during laparoscopic procedures. Am J Surg. 1995;169:543–5.
6. Bhoyrul S, Vierra MA, Nezhat CR, Krummel TM, Way LW. Trocar injuries in laparoscopic surgery. J Am Coll Surg. 2001;192:677–83.
7. Bergamaschi R. Minimizing complication rates in laparoscopic surgery for benign colorectal diseases. Tech Coloproctol. 2000;4:103–7.
8. Hashizume M, Sugimachi K. Needle and trocar injury during laparoscopic surgery in Japan. Surg Endosc. 1997;11:1198–201.
9. Neudecker J, Sauerland S, Neugebauer E, Bergamaschi R, Bonjer HJ, Cuschieri A, Fuchs KH, Jacobi C, Jansen FW, Koivusalo AM, Lacy A, McMahon MJ, Millat B, Schwenk W. The European Association for Endoscopic Surgery clinical practice guidelines on the pneumoperitoneum for laparoscopic surgery. Surg Endosc. 2002;16:1121–43.
10. Hunter JG. Laparoscopic pneumoperitoneum: the abdominal compartment syndrome revisited. J Am Coll Surg. 1995;181:469–70.
11. String A, Berber E, Foroutani A, Macho JR, Pearl JM, Siperstein AE. Use of the optical access trocar for safe and rapid entry in various laparoscopic procedures. Surg Endosc. 2001;15:570–3.
12. Stitz RW. Optimal port site placement. Tech Coloproctol. 2010;14:273–6.
13. Keshava A, MacKenzie S, Al-Kubati W. Single-port laparoscopic right colonic resection. ANZ J Surg. 2010;80:30–2.
14. Leblanc F, Champagne BJ, Augestad KM, Stein SL, Maderstein E, Reynolds HL, Delaney C. Single incision laparoscopic colectomy: technical aspects, feasibility and expected benefits. Diagn Ther Endosc. 2010;2010:913216.
15. Essani R, Bergamaschi R. Laparoscopic management of adhesive small bowel obstruction. Tech Coloproctol. 2008;12:283–7.
16. Bastug DF, Trammell SW, Boland JP, Mantz EP, Tiley 3rd EH. Laparoscopic adhesiolysis for small bowel obstruction. Surg Laparosc Endosc. 1991;1:259–62.
17. Levard H, Boudet MJ, Msika S, Molkhou JM, Hay JM, Laborde Y, Gillet M, Fingerhut A, French Association for Surgical Research. Laparoscopic treatment of acute small bowel obstruction: a multicentre retrospective study. ANZ J Surg. 2001;71:641–6.
18. Wang Q, Hu ZQ, Wang WJ, Zhang J, Wang Y, Ruan CP. Laparoscopic management of recurrent adhesive small-bowel obstruction: long-term follow-up. Surg Today. 2009;39:493–9.
19. Wullstein C, Gross E. Laparoscopic compared with conventional treatment of acute adhesive small bowel obstruction. Br J Surg. 2003;90:1147–51.
20. Duron JJ, du Montcel ST, Berger A, Muscari F, Hennet H, Veyrieres M, Hay JM, French Federation for Surgical Research. Prevalence and risk factors of mortality and morbidity after operation for adhesive small bowel obstruction. Am J Surg. 2008;195:726–34.
21. Corman ML. Carcinoma of the rectum. In: Corman ML, editor. Colon and rectal surgery. 5th ed. Philadelphia: Lippincott Williams & Wilkins; 2004. p. 948.
22. Gözen AS, Cresswell J, Canada AE, Ganta S, Rassweiler J, Teber D. Laparoscopic ureteral reimplantation: prospective evaluation of medium-term results and current developments. World J Urol. 2010;28:221–6.
23. Morgan D, Upchurch B, Draganov P, Binmoeller KF, Haluszka O, Jonnalagadda S, Okolo P, Grimm I, Judah J, Tokar J, Chiorean M. Spiral enteroscopy: prospective U.S. multicenter study in patients with small-bowel disorders. Gastrointest Endosc. 2010;72:992–8.
24. Soria F, Lopez-Albors O, Morcillo E, Sarria R, Carballo F, Perez-Cuadrado E, Sanchez F, Latorre R. Experimental laparoscopic evaluation of double balloon versus spiral enteroscopy in an animal model. Dig Endosc. 2011;23:98.
25. Conaghan P, Maxwell-Armstrong C, Garrioch M, Hong L, Acheson A. Leaving a mark: the frequency and accuracy of tattooing prior to laparoscopic colorectal surgery. Colorectal Dis. 2011;13:1184–7.
26. Del Rio P, Dell'Abate P, Gomes B, Fumagalli M, Papadia C, Coruzzi A, Leonardi F, Pucci F, Sianesi M. Analysis of risk factors for complications in 262 cases of laparoscopic colectomy. Ann Ital Chir. 2010;81:21–30.
27. Rotholtz NA, Laporte M, Zanoni G, Bun ME, Aued L, Lencinas S, Mezzadri NA, Peyreyra L. Predictive factors for conversion in laparoscopic colorectal surgery. Tech Coloproctol. 2008;12:27–31.
28. Pinto RA, Shawki S, Narita K, Weiss EG, Wexner SD. Laparoscopy for recurrent Crohn's disease: how do the results compare with the results for primary Crohn's disease? Colorectal Dis. 2011;13(3):302–7.
29. Li JC, Lee JF, Ng SS, Yu RY, Hon SS, Leung WW, Leung KL. Conversions in laparoscopic-assisted colectomy for right colon cancer: risk factors and clinical outcomes. Int J Colorectal Dis. 2010;25:963–8.

第 15 章 机器人手术的思考

Hester Y. S. Cheung · Cliff C. C. Chung · Michael K. W. Li
赵　坤 译　江志伟 审校

摘　要

本章概述机器人在结直肠手术中的应用，描述其优点及操作装置。机器人辅助下结直肠手术已经成为高端腹腔镜技术的自然延伸，因为它能提供更为广阔的手术视野及增加操作器械的灵活性。这些优点特别适用于视野局限的盆腔手术，能够提供更为精确的操作以及良好的组织分离，其在前列腺癌手术方面的经验也逐步运用到盆腔肛肠领域。

关键词

机器人辅助腹腔镜手术；全直肠系膜切除术（TME）；直肠癌；保留肛门括约肌的 TME

引　言

在治疗直肠癌方面，手术相关的因素非常重要，不仅要实现局部切除，也要做到功能保护。膀胱和性功能障碍是直肠手术后重要的常见并发症。在全直肠系膜切除术（TME）的技术引进前，这些并发症发生率高，文献报道 10%～30% 膀胱功能障碍和 40%～60% 性功能障碍[1-4]。这些功能障碍的主要原因可能是骨盆和沿主动脉远端的神经损伤。

随着 TME 技术引入（直肠癌切除的"金标准"）并认识到自主神经需要保护，膀胱和性功能障碍的发生率似乎有所减少。然而，由于患者的运行模式和神经纤维的大小存在个体差异，神经识别很困难，尤其肥胖或狭窄骨盆的患者。最近的研究表明，即使应用 TME "神经配对"技术，泌尿和性功能障碍的发生率分别为 12% 和 10%～35% 之间[5-10]。

在过去的 20 年中，各种腹腔镜腹部手术已成为公认的技术，短期获益包括减少术后疼痛、住院时间短，并改善外观效果[11]。然而，由于腹腔镜学习起来比较困难，同时存在一些固有的困难，包括图像是二维的、有限的灵活性和缺少触觉，意味着在某些复杂的手术如直肠癌手术中，腹腔镜技术仍然是一个挑战。

近年来，机器人辅助腹腔镜手术一直倡导提高外科医生的视野、灵巧度和舒适度。这种技术特别适合在狭小的空间进行解剖，如骨盆，需要精确的活动和精细的组织解剖[12]。毫不奇怪，机器人手术已在前列腺手术产生巨大的影响，在过去的几年里，全世界有超过 30 000 例的机器人辅助前列腺根治性切除术的报道[13]。

从理论上讲，机器人技术可能在涉及重建和功能保存的盆腔手术中更有优势。2001 年报道第 1 例机器人结肠切除术[14]，2006 年报道第 1 例机器人 TME[15]。机器人结直肠手术是一个迅速崛起的领域，与常规腹腔镜手术相比，可以解决一些固有的困难[14]。到目前为止，已经有 22 项临床研究（13 项病例系列研究、

8项对照研究和1项随机对照试验[16])的文献报道，证明机器人结直肠手术是安全和可行的。实施的操作包括右半结肠切除术、左半结肠切除术、直肠癌切除术，以及次全和全结肠切除术。

在直肠癌手术中，机器人技术提供了一个稳定的三维成像摄像平台；机器人手柄将外科医生的手部运动转换为连接仪器的运动，克服手眼协调的不自然和腹腔镜器械的刚性限制。它也可以给外科医生提供一个舒适的、符合人体工程学的理想手术操作位置。机器人辅助腹腔镜保留肛门括约肌的全直肠系膜切除术将在下面进一步讨论。

机器人辅助腹腔镜下全直肠系膜切除术的适应证和患者的选择

机器人辅助腹腔镜下保留肛门括约肌全直肠系膜切除可以用于大部分中低直肠病变的根治性治疗，这些病变进行保留括约肌的切除术是可行的。对位于中位直肠的可疑病变，是否采取普通切除或TME，应在游离全部直肠后决定。如果在游离全直肠后肿瘤和盆底之间的距离小于5cm，则只能施行TME手术。在实践中，如果低位前切除术（即切除时必须完全切开盆腔腹膜反折并分离外侧韧带）是以治愈为目的，这就意味着几乎所有的病例都应行TME。如果是姑息性手术，如转移性疾病的患者，全直肠系膜切除术是不必要的，在这些情况下，腹腔镜低位前切除术并保留2cm的远端壁边缘通常就足够了。

像腹腔镜前切除术一样，伴有邻近器官受累的局部进展期疾病是机器人辅助腹腔镜保留括约肌TME的禁忌证。需要广泛的整块切除——超过TME的切除范围。放射学提示T3或T4晚期的患者，应考虑术前放化疗，之后还应评估腹腔镜保留括约肌的切除术是否仍然可能。对于有多次下腹部手术史或心肺储备差，不能耐受长时间的气腹的患者，机器人辅助腹腔镜直肠癌切除术也不可取。对于已患泌尿生殖功能障碍的患者，并不需要使用机器人辅助技术，因为精确的保护骨盆和骶前神经是次要的。

术前评估与准备

术前评估与准备同常规开放手术基本相同。常规CT扫描有助于排除局部进展期肿瘤和提供选择更好的患者，特别是对于初学者。慢性肺疾病应评估肺功能。如果预期进行低位切除或需要行回肠造口术，术前应进行穿刺孔位置的选择。患者应接受标准的机械性肠道准备，围术期应用抗生素，并常规预防深静脉血栓的形成。然而，亚急性梗阻或内镜下梗阻性肿瘤的患者，良好的肠道准备可诱发急性梗阻，阻碍腹腔镜下解剖。在这种情况下，不推荐使用标准口服制剂的肠道准备；而重点应放在饮食限制（如手术前2~3天低渣饮食）。

操作团队和设备安装

机器人辅助腹腔镜直肠癌手术从来不是单一外科医生完成的手术。在一个专业小组中，两名机器人外科医生是必不可少的；有经验的麻醉师、护士、熟悉手术过程的技术人员、各种腹腔镜和机器人处理文书，以及配套的多功能性技术团队都是其中的组成部分。

同其他先进的腹腔镜手术一样，机器人辅助腹腔镜直肠癌手术在一个集成的机器人腹腔内镜治疗手术室中进行，配有一个通用并且即插即用的各种内镜和腹腔镜的系统（包括机器人腹腔镜），其中还应包括三维显示器。推荐的工具包括：

1. 一个12mm的戳卡（Ethicon Endo-Surgery公司，辛辛那提，OH）的机器人摄像机的透镜系统

2. 一个5mm的超声解剖装置如谐波ACE（Ethicon Endo-Surgery公司）或5mm Ligasure™装置（泰科医疗集团，博尔德，CO）

3. 腹腔镜双极电凝镊（佳乐医药有限公司，加的夫，英国），5mm的尺寸

4. 内镜钛夹钳和钛夹

5. 肠道切割闭合器

6. 机器人耗材：prograsp™钳，马里兰双极镊子，永久电钩

7. 亚历克西斯创口牵开器（应用医学，圣塔玛格丽塔，CA）悬垂在标本作为腹壁保护

8. 肠吻合器

操作技术

"完全"机器人的方法最初是由受过训练的外科医生使用。早期的经验表明，与传统的腹腔镜手术相比，这种方法的手术时间明显延长，很快就发

现操作时间延长的主要原因是该过程中涉及机器人的对接[17-19]，在盆腔解剖的实际"操作时间消耗"只有60min左右。为此，其他研究人员已经改为"混合"的方式，试图减少机器人重设期间的对接时间。

使用三臂技术混合的方法步骤描述如下（视频见 springerlinks.com）：

1. 减少拥挤和防止机器人手臂和腹腔镜随后的碰撞。戳孔的位置应该在一把尺子和标记的帮助下精心划定。下腹部机器人手臂预定戳孔（R_1、R_2、R_3）之间要有足够的间距（图15.1）。腹腔镜的初始阶段，5mm的戳孔是通过下腹部这些预标记位点进行穿刺的，通过这些戳孔游离乙状结肠。在准备好机器人对接阶段后，将这些5mm的戳孔改为8mm戳孔。

2. 腹腔镜阶段：30°腹腔镜经脐下12mm戳孔进入。腹腔镜游离乙状结肠是通过右髂窝两个5mm的戳孔，辅助医生通过左髂窝5mm的戳孔提供对抗牵引力。游离乙状结肠后，使用标准技术控制和分离肠系膜下血管蒂[20]。为乙状结肠吻合提供预期的水平可以在无张力下达到真骨盆，完整地游离脾曲并不总是必需的。取下全部脾曲只是表明长度不足（结肠或乙状结肠肠系膜）、乙状结肠不健康（如术前放疗）或疾病（如慢性憩室炎）。即使需要游离脾曲，也最好推迟到游离全直肠后，因为充分游离的左半结肠往往掉入骨盆，阻碍了机器人后续解剖盆腔。

3. 对接：在左半结肠被充分分离出来，将下腹部的3个5mm的戳孔替换为8mm戳孔。30°腹腔镜移除，对接进行。随着经验的积累，对接时间可短至5min。机器人相机镜头系统最后通过脐下12mm戳孔插入（图15.1）。机器人的位置、监测和操作团队，如图15.2所示。

4. 机器人阶段：通过腹腔镜的视野，组织钳通过3号臂进入（R_3），永久烙钩和马里兰双极钳臂分别通过1号臂（R_1）和2号臂（R_2）进入（图15.1）。外科医生在操纵台用抓钳抓起直肠，用1号臂和2号进行分离。由助手通过上腹部的两个戳孔进行另外的回缩和吸/灌（图15.1）。首先进行后部的解剖，联合使用锐性和钝性分离，剥离直肠系膜筋膜缘，随后是直肠系膜和骶前筋膜之间的平面。完善止血应在术中任何时间进行。应识别和保护骶前筋膜腹下神经。随着解剖的不断深入，解剖平面向前转弯，可以将30°腹腔镜向上旋转180°。在两边外侧解剖后进行后部的解剖，在直肠和直肠系膜缘仔细解剖勃起神经。向前将直肠与迪氏筋膜分离，迪氏筋膜包覆着男性精囊或女性的阴道。盆腔解剖的终点是盆底（后方）和男性的前列腺和精囊或女性的阴道（前方）。应能清楚地看到直肠远端穿过盆底的肌肉。随着经验的积累，操作时间可以限制到1h内。

图15.1 戳孔位置的混合技术。最初的腹腔镜阶段期间，5mm的戳卡通过臂1（R_1）、臂2（R_2）和臂3（R_3），用于腹腔镜下解剖。后来改为8mm的戳卡与机器人相对接。C 摄影透镜系统

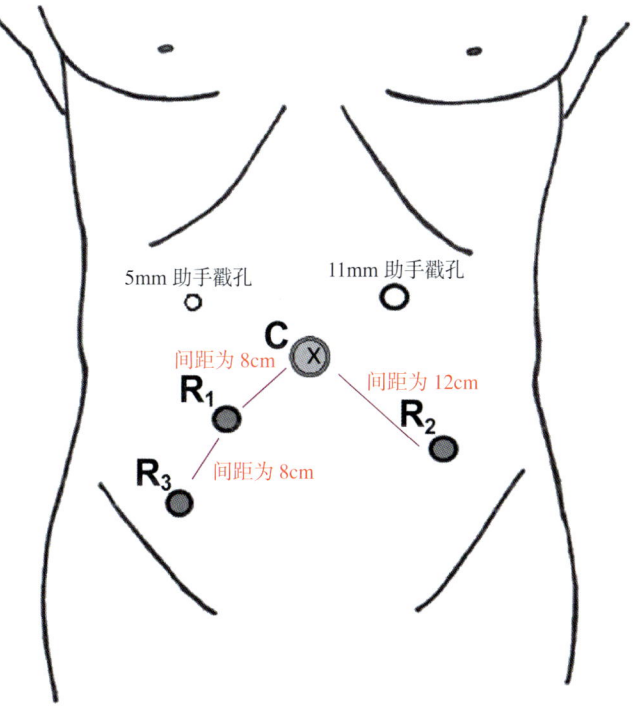

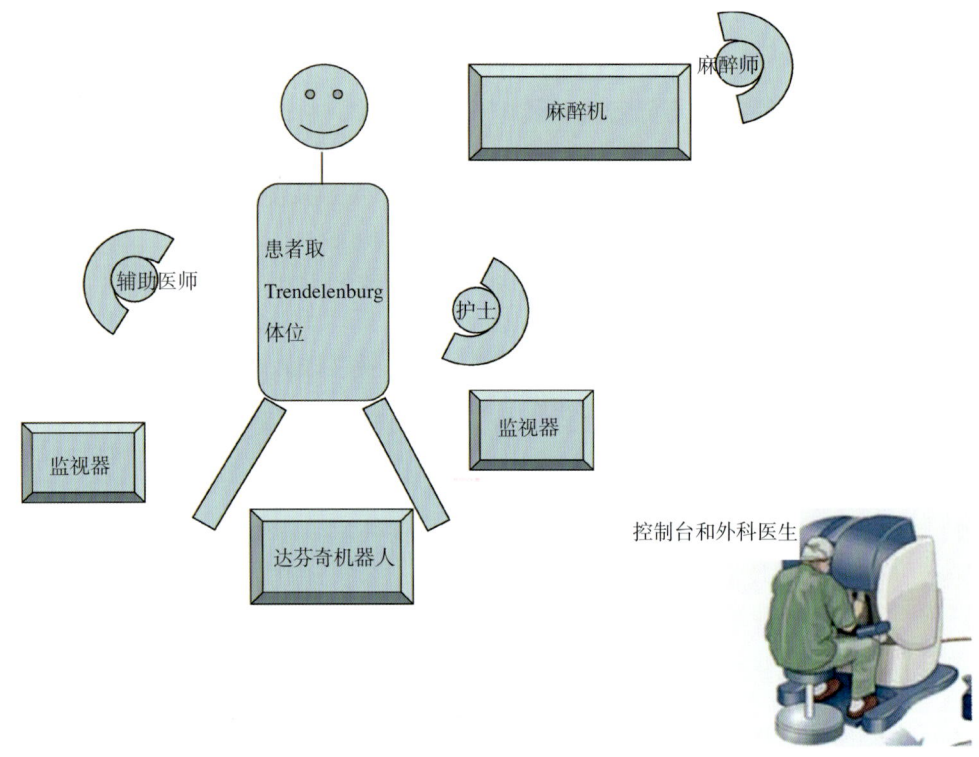

图 15.2　操作团队的位置。整个手术过程中，患者采用 Trendelenburg 体位，右低倾斜位

5. 移除：充分清扫盆腔后，移除系统。

6. 在移除机器人工具后，将右髂窝的 8mm 戳孔（R_3）改为 5～12mm 戳孔，腔镜下闭合器经此进入并离断直肠（直肠肿瘤远侧）。

7. 标本切除和取出：4～6cm pfannestiel 切口取标本。如果肿瘤很小，也可以通过右髂窝下预定的回肠造口处取出。标本取回期间使用切口保护器进行腹壁保护。

8. 腔内吻合：气腹重建，使用标准的腹腔镜环形吻合器完成腔内吻合。

9. 在预标记吻合处进行覆盖回肠造口。

10. 骶前间隙放置引流并固定。

11. 应关闭所有腹膜缺损大于 5mm 的戳孔，以防止切口疝的发生。

术后处理

机器人辅助腹腔镜的直肠癌根治术后处理与传统的手术本质上类似。通常不要求放置鼻胃管；如果术中放置了鼻胃管，术后应拔除。导尿管放置1～2天。去除气动加压袜以弹力袜代替。术后患者可以补充液体，大部分术后第 2 或第 3 天发展到正常饮食。鼓励他们术后第 2 天下床活动，一旦患者活动，应去除弹力袜。如果引流量不多，通常术后第 2 天去除引流管。对于覆盖回肠造口的患者，应教授其造口护理技术。机器人辅助直肠手术后，患者通常只有轻至中度疼痛，尽量减少麻醉药的使用。大多数人术后第 5～7 天都能够排便。覆盖造口的患者，应进行造影来确定吻合的完整性。在初次手术后 2 周，可以关闭回肠造口。

结　论

毫无疑问，机器人直肠癌手术非常可行。外科手术机器人的许多优点，如改进的灵活性和视野，人体力学上更加舒适，代表未来微创手术的重大飞跃。缺少大量腹腔镜经验、却又想掌握复杂的腹腔全直肠系膜切除术的结直肠外科医生，可以从这种新技术中受益。目前，最主要关注的仍然是肿瘤学的预后。CLASSIC 试验的数据显示，腹腔镜全直肠系膜切除术与开放手术相比，患者的径向切缘阳性的比率少量增加（12% 和 6%，虽然并没有统计学意义）[21]。目前,由于缺乏长期数据，机器人辅助直肠癌切除术的肿瘤学预后是否与常规腹腔镜手术具有可比性（或优于）还不确定[22-23]。除此之外，机器的体积庞大且笨重，所以应优先选用空间宽敞的手术室。一个精心设计的、人性化的内镜机器人系统和充分的团队训练至关重要。此外，当前的达芬奇机器人系统不提供触觉反馈的操作，虽然到目前为止还没有证明其并发症发生率比标准腹腔镜手术高，但仍有无意中损伤组织的风险，因为外科医生必须依靠视觉来估计施加在组织上的张力。人们希望技术的进一步发展将给我们带来更小、更便宜、更快、更安全且改进触觉反馈的机器人系统。目前，机器人辅助的右半结肠切除术已被证明可行[24-25]，虽然与标准腹腔镜切除术相比，手术时间和成本的优势尚未证实；内括约肌直肠切除术[26]、腹会阴联合切除术[27]、直肠结肠切除修复术[28]、憩室切除术[29]，甚至存在转移的患者同样适用[30]。还有可能进行机器人辅助的单孔操作[31]；EndoAssist设备可改进手术辅助并稳定手术视野[32]，如果有的医师对这种新技术缺乏经验，其他医师可以通过机器人中心进行远程的遥控。目前，仍迫切需要有关的功能预后、肿瘤学预后和长期生存的数据，来证明手术机器人可以广泛应用。

参考文献

1. Fazio VW, Fletcher J, Montague D. Prospective study of the effect of resection of the rectum on male sexual function. World J Surg. 1980;4:149–52.
2. Chang PL, Fan HA. Urodynamic studies before and/or after abdominoperineal resection of the rectum for carcinoma. J Urol. 1983;130:948–51.
3. Kinn AC, Ohman U. Bladder and sexual function after surgery for rectal cancer. Dis Colon Rectum. 1986;29:43–8.
4. Santangelo ML, Romano G, Sassaroli C. Sexual function after resection for rectal cancer. Am J Surg. 1987;154:502–4.
5. Masui H, Ike H, Yamaguchi S, Oki S, Shimada H. Male sexual function after autonomic nerve-preserving operation for rectal cancer. Dis Colon Rectum. 1996;39:1140–5.
6. Havenga K, Enker WE, McDermott K, Cohen AM, Minsky BD, Guillem J. Male and female sexual and urinary function after total mesorectal excision with autonomic nerve preservation for carcinoma of the rectum. J Am Coll Surg. 1996;182:495–502.
7. Enker WE, Havenga K, Polyak T, Thaler H, Cranor M. Abdominoperineal resection via total mesorectal excision and autonomic nerve preservation for low rectal cancer. World J Surg. 1997;21:715–20.
8. Maas CP, Moriya Y, Steup WH, Kiebert GM, Kranenbarg WM, Van de Velde CJ. Radical and nerve-preserving surgery for rectal cancer in The Netherlands: a prospective study on morbidity and functional outcome. Br J Surg. 1998;85:92–7.
9. Nesbakken A, Nygaard K, Bull-Njaa T, Carlsen E, Eri LM. Bladder and sexual dysfunction after mesorectal excision for rectal cancer. Br J Surg. 2000;87:206–10.
10. Kim NK, Aahn TW, Park JK, Lee KY, Lee WH, Sohn SK, Min JS. Assessment of sexual and voiding function after total mesorectal excision with pelvic autonomic nerve preservation in males with rectal cancer. Dis Colon Rectum. 2002;45:1178–85.
11. Martel G, Boushey RP. Laparoscopic colon surgery: past, present and future. Surg Clin North Am. 2006;86:867–97.
12. Lanfranco AR, Castellanos AE, Desai JP, Meyers WC. Robotic surgery: a current perspective. Ann Surg. 2004;239:14–21.
13. Patel VR, Chammas Jr MF, Shah S. Robotic assisted laparoscopic radical prostatectomy: a review of the current state of affairs. Int J Clin Pract. 2007;61:309–14.
14. Ballanttbe GH, Merola P, Weber A, et al. A robotic solutions to the pitfalls of laparoscopic colectomy. Osp Ital Chir. 2001;7:405–12.
15. Pigazzi A, Ellenhorn JD, Ballantyne GH, Paz IB. Robotic-assisted laparoscopic low anterior resection with total mesorectal excision for rectal cancer. Surg Endosc. 2006;20:1521–5.
16. Baik SH, Ko YT, Kang CM, Lee WJ, Kim NK, Sohn SK, Chi HS, Cho CH. Robotic tumor-specific mesorectal excision of rectal cancer: short-term outcome of a pilot randomized trial. Surg Endosc. 2008;22:1061–8.
17. Delaney CP, Lynch AC, Senagore AJ, Fazio VW. Comparison of robotically performed and traditional colorectal surgery. Dis Colon Rectum. 2003;46:1633–9.
18. Anvari M, Virch DW, Bamehriz F, Gryfe R, Chapman T. Robotic-assisted laparoscopic colorectal surgery. Surg Laparosc Endosc Percutan Tech. 2004;14:311–5.
19. Spinoglio G, Summa M, Priora F, Quarati R, Testa S. Robotic colorectal surgery: first 50 cases experience. Dis Colon Rectum. 2008;51:1627–32.
20. Chung CC, Ha JPY, Tsang WWC, Li MKW. Laparoscopic-assisted total mesorectal excision and colonic J pouch reconstruction. Surg Endosc. 2001;15:1098–101.
21. Guillou PJ, Quirke P, Thorpe H, Walker J, Jayne DG, Smith AM, Heath RM, Brown JM, MRC CLASICC trial group. MRC CLASICC trial group. Short-term endpoints of conventional versus laparoscopic-assisted surgery in patients with colorectal cancer (MRC CLASICC trial): multicenter randomised controlled trial. Lancet. 2005;365:1718–26.
22. Baek JH, McKenzie S, Garcia-Aguilar J, Pigazzi A. Oncologic outcomes of robotic-assisted total mesorectal excision for the treatment of rectal cancer. Ann Surg. 2010;251:882–6.
23. Ng KH, Lim YK, Ho KS, Ooi BS, Eu KW. Robotic-assisted surgery for low rectal dissection: from better views to better outcome. Singapore Med J. 2009;50:763–7.
24. D'Annibale A, Pernazza G, Morpurgo E, Monsellato I, Pende V, Lucandri G, Termini B, Orsini C, Sovernigo G. Robotic right colon resection: evaluation of first 50 consecutive cases for malignant disease. Ann Surg Oncol. 2010;17:2856–62.
25. de Souza AL, Prasad LM, Park JJ, Marecik SJ, Blumetti J, Abcarian H. Robotic assistance in right hemicolectomy: is there a role? Dis Colon Rectum. 2010;53:1000–6.
26. Leong QM, Son DN, Cho JS, Baek SJ, Kwak JM, Amar AH, Kim SH. Robot-assisted intersphincteric resection for low rectal cancer: technique and short-term outcome for 29 consecutive patients. Surg Endosc. 2011;25(9):2987–92.
27. Patel CB, Ramos-Valadez DI, Haas EM. Robotic-assisted laparoscopic abdominoperineal resection for anal cancer: feasibility and technical considerations. Int J Med Robot. 2010;6:399–404.
28. Pedraza R, Patel CB, Ramos-Valadez DI, Haas EM. Robotic-assisted laparoscopic surgery for restorative proctocolectomy with ileal J pouch-anal anastomosis. Minim Invasive Ther Allied Technol. 2011;20(4):234–9.
29. Ragupathi M, Ramos-Valadez DI, Patel CB, Haas EM. Robotic-assisted laparoscopic surgery for recurrent diverticulitis: experience in consecutive cases and a review of the literature. Surg Endosc. 2011;25:199–206.
30. Patriti A, Ceccarelli G, Bartoli A, Spaziani A, Lapalorcia LM, Casciola L. Laparoscopic and robot-assisted one-stage resection of

colorectal cancer with synchronous liver metastases: a pilot study. J Hepatobiliary Pancreat Surg. 2009;16:450–7.
31. Gilbert JM. The EndoAssist robotic camera holder as an aid to the introduction of laparoscopic colorectal surgery. Ann R Coll Surg Engl. 2009;91:389–93.
32. Sebajang H, Trudeau P, Dougall A, Hegge S, McKinley C, Anvari M. The role of telementoring and telerobotic assistance in the provision of laparoscopic colorectal surgery in rural areas. Surg Endosc. 2006;20:1389–93.

第 16 章 完全肛门重建

J. Manuel Devesa・Javier Die・Rosana Vicente
邹长林 译　王西墨 审校

摘 要

完全肛门直肠重建的目的是在肛门直肠根治切除后最大限度地恢复其生理功能和外观。本章针对那些接受过腹会阴联合切除患者的完全肛门直肠重建方法作一概述，并讨论了括约肌替代和增强方法的技术问题和结局。

关键词

完全肛门重建（TAR）；腹会阴联合切除术（APR）；自控排便；新建直肠；内括约肌；外括约肌；顺行节制性灌肠（ACE）

引 言

自 Krase 做了第一例保留肛门和括约肌的直肠切除手术以来，已有超过 125 年的时间，尽管直肠癌患者的保肛手术已经取得了巨大进步，但如今仍会有很大一部分患者将不可避免地接受全肛门直肠切除而行永久性腹部结肠造口术。作为肿瘤治愈的小代价，虽然很多患者乐于接受这一术式，但其严重影响了他们的生活质量，并且造瘘口相关并发症会伴其一生：大约有 10% 的患者需要接受额外的手术。此外，腹会阴联合切除术（APR）具有较高的术后会阴伤口并发症，报道发生率在 40%～60% 之间，尤其是术前会阴部实施过放射治疗者[1]。

APR 术后完全肛门重建（TAR）的目的是恢复因永久性造瘘带来的身体外观和生理机能的改变。1930 年，Chittenden[2] 首次发表了其尝试利用臀大肌皮瓣作为新建肛门括约肌施行可控性会阴造瘘作为 TAR 的手术。20 年后，Margottini[3] 报道了一组 90 例行会阴造瘘的患者，然而由于疗效不尽如人意，这些手术并没有获得广泛接受。直至 20 世纪 80 年代中期，随着新的手术技巧的发展和技术的进步，给这一领域带来了新的可能性。

排便自控力的机制较为复杂，仍不完全清楚，而良好的自控力有赖于恢复解剖完整性和以下结构的正常功能：

1. 直肠是具有比结肠更低扩张阈值的适应性储器，能贮存内容物直至找到恰当的排泄时机；

2. 肛门直肠括约肌，包括内括约肌发挥静息状态的动态关闭机制和外括约肌在直肠内压超过静息压时作为主动动态控制系统，可防止直肠内容物的溢出；

3. 直肠黏膜，当直肠/盆腔感受器完整时，能传递直肠对其内容物的感觉，可识别出直肠内容物的性状，区分气体、液体或固态粪便。

任何这些结构的解剖学或功能上的缺陷均可导致不同程度的大便失禁，后者通常与伴随的缺陷程度成正比。于是，尽可能地恢复这些功能并符合生理的 TAR 方法应引起重视。

肛门直肠重建

APR 术后已不可能恢复肛门的感觉，但是利用降结肠再造新的直肠贮袋、自体肌肉再造的新括约肌或者人工括约肌等方法能够使那些接受过全肛门直肠切除的患者的 TAR 变得可行。此外，利用阑尾造瘘或放置回 / 结肠导管施行顺行结肠灌洗（单独或者同时伴随其他任何重建手术）会使相当多数量的患者达到一种假可控性的状态[4]。下面我们将对新直肠和新括约肌再造的 TAR 的不同选择，以及顺行节制性灌肠技术做回顾和分析。

直肠再造

直肠的主要功能是充当储器，并传导直肠扩张的感觉，其容量在健康成人大约有 300ml。临床证据显示，当直肠被切除并被一段具有生理性推进波和有限存储能力的降结肠所取代，会出现令人不安的里急后重感，增加排便次数，从而导致便急、遗粪和大便失禁的发生。虽然很多接受结肠 - 肛管吻合的患者仍具有直肠肛门抑制反射，能感知新建直肠内的固体粪便，甚至能区分气体、液体和固体，但是，仍然有一些患者的感觉功能丧失。这是继发于直肠内特殊感受器的切除和盆腔神经不可避免的损毁[5]。当患者肛门直肠感觉完全丧失，被动性失禁几乎不可避免，可是那些尚存直肠感觉的病例中，新建直肠的益处更多体现在减少了新建直肠的运动而不单单是其潜在的储器作用。

从这一点来说，对那些接受直肠切除，并行超低位结直肠或结肠 - 肛管吻合患者，已证实建立短的结肠 J 形贮袋对减少术后里急后重和排便次数有效。2000 年，Fazio 等[6] 报道其成功实施了针对低位结直肠或结肠 - 肛管吻合口进行加强的结肠成形术，从此，结肠贮袋或结肠成形术成为直肠切除术后的常规术式。尽管已经在本书第 8 章和第 9 章做了详尽探讨，这两种术式的功能性结果还是大致相似的。业已证实，至少在随访评估的 2 年以内，结直肠贮袋或结肠成形术的患者的排便次数有改善，直肠扩张的耐受容量提高，相比那些直接结直肠吻合或结肠 - 肛管吻合的患者具有更好的功能和更低的大便失禁发生率。

TAR 过程中一旦建立贮袋，新建直肠的外形必须适应重建的解剖结构，结肠远端的 3～4cm 被新建括约肌包裹。尽管犬的 J 形贮袋联合股薄肌新建肛门括约肌已有报道[7]，但这一情况中，从技术角度讲，贮袋应位于新建括约肌之上。另一组报道的两例患者中[8]，6cm 的 C 形贮袋或侧方贮袋[9-10] 就建立于新建肛门括约肌水平之上。Geerdes 等[11] 报道了另一类型储器，他们在紧贴股薄肌包绕的近端打开结肠对系膜缘 15cm，并利用一段孤立的末段回肠肠段像补丁一样进行覆盖，以此来建立贮袋。然而，这是一个更加复杂却没有体现出任何功能性益处的操作。Williams 等[12] 报道了一例之前做过结直肠切除术的患者，行三联回肠贮袋（臂长 15cm）联合激活股薄肌成形术的 TAR，利用一个 Silastic® 塞置入贮袋的输出口。Devesa 等[13] 推荐一些相对简单的 TAR 选择包括在结肠 - 肛管吻合口上 6～7cm 实施的横向 Fazio 结肠成形术，或实施旨在减少降结肠蠕动力的新建括约肌近端的纵向肌层切开术[14]。

评论和建议

令人惊讶的是，大部分 TAR 的报道均围绕于新建括约肌，而很少关注建立储器或远端低张力肠段这些替代直肠生理功能的尝试。虽然尚未有与 TAR 手术中新建直肠的益处和哪种贮袋功能性更好的有力证据[8,9,11]，但简单结肠成形术或新建括约肌近端肌层切开术似乎并没有明显增加并发症，且能促进功能状态，效果类似于超低位结直肠或结肠 - 肛管吻合术后的状态。TAR 的其他类型的贮袋报道，在技术上更复杂，更有挑战性，并且在没有功能获益的情况下严重并发症更多，进一步的研究仍然是有必要的[15-16]。

括约肌替代物

括约肌替代物的内容在本书第 5 章也有描述。

内括约肌

内括约肌维持正常排便控制的作用有限，并具有争议性；但是却有临床证据表明，那些接受直肠手术的患者，术中有意或无意的内括约肌损害会引发令人烦恼的遗粪或不同程度的大便失禁[17-18]。进一步的证据表明内瘘手术中对内括约肌的保留与提高术后功能相关[19-20]。Torres 等[21] 报道了 TAR 后重建新内括约肌的初步尝试，他在一例患者身上应用了平滑肌新括约肌转置的技术；此项技术又被 Schmidt[22] 和 Fedorov 等[23] 进一步发展，在他们的方法中，平滑肌新建内括约肌包裹在拖出结肠的螺旋装置里。此项技术里，远端 3~4cm 的结肠周围脂肪被剔除，浆肌层从黏膜层剥离，制成一个平滑肌套，螺旋状切开制成宽 1.5cm、长 5~7cm 带蒂的肌肉瓣。这个瓣套在肠管外并靠 3-0 可吸收线间断缝合固定，制成一个位于结肠终端的长 3~4cm 的锥状的平滑肌翻边。初步数据显示 20 例患者获得满意的功能性效果。

此后，Pescatori 等[24]、Elias 等[25]、Lasser 等[26]、Gamagmi 等[27] 和 Portier 等[28] 也发表了直肠切除术后利用结肠平滑肌替代肛门内括约肌的修复性手术。最近的一项研究中，Lorenzi 等[29] 描述了此项手术的功能性效果，并报道了括约肌替代技术的研究结果，操作方法为先剥除结肠末端黏膜，然后将其外翻 1.5cm 与会阴皮肤的新建肛门做吻合。在一组 27 例患者的报道中，Fedorov 等[23] 描述了平滑肌新建括约肌，Vorobiev 等[10] 证明翻转包裹水平的肠腔内压增加了 38%，这与 Portier 等报道的结果接近，后者显示在翻转包裹水平存在 40cm 水柱的压力梯度。

评论和建议

尽管学者们报道的研究结果令人鼓舞，但是在临床实践中仍然难以判断 TAR 技术中再造一个新的内括约肌的真正功能性获益到底有多少。而且，如果利用游离移植制作平滑肌翻边，既无内在也无外在神经支配，那么其作用机制可能导致其仅仅类似于生物学 Thiersch 移植，仅提供了一定程度的排便屏障。为了澄清这一点，进行做与不做平滑肌新建括约肌的 TAR 的前瞻性对比研究是很必要的。同时，无论对结果有什么影响，利用结肠平滑肌再造新内括约肌都值得尝试，因为此方法很容易实施，而且不像 TAR 相关的其他技术操作一样，它并不显著增加外科相关并发症。

外括约肌

臀大肌

自从 1902 年 Chetwood 首次描述臀大肌成形术治疗肛门失禁以来，各种利用单侧或双侧臀大肌转置的技术已经用于治疗大量肛门失禁的患者，并取得了不同程度的成功[31-32]。Chittenden[2] 率先行直肠癌肛门直肠切除后利用臀大肌进行肛门括约肌重建，此后 Knapp[33] 也做了报道，但两项研究结果不尽如人意。Farid 等[34] 描述了对一小组先天性或神经系统疾病的年轻患者行利用阔筋膜增强的单边臀大肌成形术。最近，Cong 等[35] 报道了对生物反馈治疗和长期的功能锻炼后的低位直肠癌患者，成功应用臀大肌行肛门括约肌重建。根据 Devesa[32] 和 Guelinkx[31] 等发表的数据显示，虽然利用电刺激臀大肌成形术进行肛门括约肌重建能获取更满意的结果，但这一手术还没有专门应用于 TAR。

长收肌

Fedorov 和 Shelygin[36] 报道了一组 48 例 TAR 后利用股长收肌再造括约肌的患者，82% 的患者取得了满意的远期功能性结果。然而，尚缺乏足够的文献支持，且无此肌肉有关的进一步报道。

股薄肌

1952 年，Pickrell 等[37] 描述了用股薄肌行括约肌重建手术治疗肛门失禁。然而最初报道的成功并没有被其他学者所证实，因为简单的股薄肌包裹被认为难以维持长时间的肌肉张力。Jacob 等[38] 在 1976 年首次报道了一例先天性肛门直肠异常行 TAR 中静态股薄肌成形术的病例。Simonsen 等[39] 在同年也报道了一例因肿瘤行腹会阴联合切除术后行此手术的病例。然而，直至 1990 年电刺激技术的发展之前，上述手术很难奏效，当时 Baeten 等[40] 和 Williams 等[41] 通过植入神经激发装置来使肌肉处于持续收缩状态。从那以后，电刺激股薄肌成形术成为肌肉括约肌替代的手术选择。

目前已经报道了各种各样的单侧或双侧股薄肌成形术技术。Wong 和 Wee[42]、Ho 和 Seow-Choen[43] 分别设计了将肌腱固定在同侧耻骨或筋膜上的类似 α 环的缝合方法。另一项研究中，Mander 等[8] 则应用了不同的设计，在一组患者中，肌肉被从后方拉至并绕过肛管，肌腱与同侧坐骨结节固定，形成类似于 α 形状的环；另一组患者，则将肌肉从新建肛管前方穿过，肌腱固定在对侧坐骨结节，形成 γ 状装置。有一例患者的肌肉从肛管后方穿过并与对侧坐骨结节固定，形成 ε 状装置。Cavina 等[45] 在 α

环额外增加了第二条股薄肌装置,一条肌肉与坐骨结节固定,而另一条肌肉与耻骨固定。Geerdes 等[11]将双侧股薄肌成形术进行改造,没有利用肌腱,将肌肉拉至并绕过新建直肠,同时进行盆底和肛门括约肌再造。这一装置中,双侧肌肉从后方拉至肛管,从残端近侧 3~4cm 处肠系膜开孔穿过,并互相固定。

接受 TAR 的患者可以同步进行电刺激治疗,或者等到患者康复且会阴部伤口彻底愈合再进行。Violi 等[46]在确定性的肌肉移植手术之前进行生物反馈训练,目的是将并发症降到最低,并节约医疗资源。

评论和建议

肌肉转置是复杂的手术。TAR 是利用臀大肌再造新括约肌,效果仍然不确切,并缺乏真实数据。臀大肌成形术的技术实施困难,且常伴有来自于肌张力方面的并发症,可出现肌肉环的断裂、神经支配障碍、肌肉萎缩等,尽管 Farid 等[34]声称已经解决了这些问题。总之,电刺激股薄肌成形术获得了比臀大肌成形术更好的功能性结果,成为针对新括约肌成形术、肛门失禁和 TAR 等情况较受推崇的选择方案,尤其在 APR 术后大便失禁的治疗具有较高的成功率[11,41,45]。至于股薄肌成形术的类型,每一位研究者都有其各自推崇的方案是完全可以理解的,但尚无科学依据可以声称某一种特殊装置优于另一种。虽然 α 环是最常用的装置,但最佳的新建括约肌仍然有待研究来验证。另一个尚无定论的问题为双侧转置是否优于单侧转置,而一些数据提示双侧股薄肌成形术对肛管直肠重建并非理想的方式[48]。关于 TAR 所报道的最大的病例数的电刺激股薄肌成形术由 Cavina 等[45]发表,其报道在最长 55 个月的随访期中,98 例患者的成功率为 87%,但是本组患者的并发症发生率(37%)较高。很多研究证实了针对肛门失禁的电刺激性股薄肌成形术的有效性,但是无论采用什么技术,都伴有较高的并发症,频繁需要再手术。最严重的并发症为肛管或新建肛管的坏死,其较之治疗单纯大便失禁,更多的发生于 APR 后实施该手术时[49]。由于所报道的高并发症发生率和不令人满意的成本效益关系,电刺激的股薄肌成形术在美国已经不再是治疗选择了。

括约肌加强

人工肛门括约肌

肛周成功植入人工肛门括约肌用于治疗大便失禁是在 1987 年由 Christiansen 和 Lorentzen 发表的。不过专门设计的肠括约肌产品(Action®,American Medical Systems,Minneapolis,MN)直至 1996 年才上市。单个研究和多中心试验证实了临床效果优于电刺激股薄肌成形术[51]。在此技术良好的效果的鼓舞下,Romano 等[52]将之应用于一组以往接受过 APR 的 8 例患者的 TAR 中,他们客观评价了此项技术,除 1 例之外,其他患者获得了很好的排便控制力,并在 6~28 个月的随访中未发现任何并发症。随后进一步的研究中,Devesa 等[13]和 Ocares 等[53]也分别发表了 1 例和 4 例初步成功的结果。然而,与人工肛门括约肌装置相关的并发症发生率较高,导致 47% 的患者需要取出装置[54],而且晚期并发症随着时间延长仍继续增多[55]。

肛门环缩术(Thiersch 手术)

1891 年,Thiersch[56]描述了一种利用银线环扎肛管治疗直肠脱垂的简单方法。此后,出现了很多关于肛门环扎主要材料的形状和种类(筋膜、肌腱、丝线、Feflon® 网、硅树脂)技术改良方面的报道。Horn 等[57]和 Larach 等[58]发表了此项技术在一组大便失禁和直肠脱垂患者中令人满意的结果。然而,尽管此简单且低成本的技术拥有令人鼓舞的结果,但并没有获得广泛接受,最可能的原因是环扎物的频繁断裂和术后大便嵌塞的严重问题。

最近,笔者的研究小组发表了利用弹性硅胶带肛门环扎治疗一组 33 例大便失禁患者的研究结果[59]。整组患者的功能性结果与一组 53 例病情相似接受 Action® 植入的患者进行比较。手术应用于两例治愈性 APR 患者作为后续手术的 TAR 中,其中一例纳入到此研究中,而另一例随后施行该手术。此技术与 Fazio 结肠成形术和旨在结肠顺行灌洗的阑尾造瘘术同时进行,两例均取得非常好的结果:一例患者获得很好的排便控制力且完全不再需要灌肠,而另一例术后已经有一年终止灌肠了(结果尚未发表)。

评价和建议

除了中、重度肛门失禁患者在大多数报道中所取得的极佳的功能预后以外，Romano 等[52]在接受 TAR 的患者中也报道了同样效果，但是与植入物高度相关的高并发症发病率使得此项技术已被摒弃，且该材料已经不再生产。据我们所掌握的知识，除 Devesa 等[59]提出该手术之外，还没有其他关于改良 Thiersch 手术的报道，于是也就尚无定论。如果吊索装置能够改进，那么在两例患者均能在无需顺行灌肠的情况下，自主排便的研究才能得以授权，进一步开展临床试验。

顺行节制性灌肠

1990 年，针对先天性肛门直肠发育不良儿童令人烦恼的排便困难，Malone 等[61]介绍了利用阑尾造瘘来进行顺行节制性灌肠（ACE）技术的概念。Malone 手术在本书第 24 章有确切讨论，Malone 使 75% 的这些儿童达到了"假排便困难"。最近，Ardelean 等[62]也发表了一组类似患者实施这一操作的结果，认为 ACE 对于保持大便失禁患者的清洁是一项可靠的治疗选择。操作的实施较为简单且由患者自己实施，仅有轻微或完全没有不舒服的感觉。靠重力压力注入结肠的温水量为 750~1000ml，且在 30min 内完成全结肠排空。最初，两次灌肠间隔 24h，而一段时间以后，很多患者发现间隔 48h 也能获得相同效果。

对于无再造括约肌的会阴结肠造瘘患者获得满意的结肠灌洗效果的是由 Chiotasso 等[63]在 1992 年报道的，他们提示患者只经历了很少的体像紊乱。2007 年，Farroni 等[64]比较了一组类似患者接受会阴结肠造瘘术联合阑尾造瘘术与腹壁结肠造瘘术后的症状、功能状态、生活质量和自感健康情况，结果表明会阴结肠造瘘加阑尾造瘘行 ACE 对于选择性的病例来说，相对于永久性腹壁造瘘是一项有效的、可以接受的选择。他们进一步证实，腹壁结肠造瘘患者存在大量造瘘口相关问题（中位数，38.1 个问题），而阑尾造瘘或盲肠导管患者的问题则很有限（中位数，8.7 个问题）。当无法实施阑尾造瘘术的时候，回肠的再造阑尾造瘘[65]、盲肠皮瓣[66]或结肠导管[67]都可供选择。这些改造是根据针对尿失禁的可控性尿流改道术（Mitrofanoff 手术）[68]的泌尿科文献演化而来，已经有人报道了联合 Mitrofanoff 手术和 ACE 操作提供完全排便控制的尝试[69]。

评价和建议

已经证实 ACE 是一项有用的、安全的操作，能使晚期大便失禁或会阴部结肠造瘘的患者达到满意的假可控状态，并且可以避免便秘，且症状较轻，可是比在行 TAR 外括约肌重建或替代手术后的持久性大便失禁来说要更常见。此外，在排便可控和生活质量方面，ACE 相对于逆行灌肠能提供更好的功能性预后。无论是作为独立操作，还是作为复杂重建的补充，TAR 时行阑尾造瘘或回肠/盲肠/结肠导管做顺行结肠灌洗的益处是显而易见的。Malone 手术虽然对于 TAR 较其他选择介绍得较晚，但很有可能在不久的将来在会阴部结肠造瘘术后的治疗中扮演重要角色。

TAR 相关技术：发病率和预后

所有 TAR 的报道都是对实施手术结果的回顾性分析，且报道患者的数量很少，所做的随访时间也相应比较短。就这一点来说，数据收集和评价的方法（例如评分系统、生活质量评估）也不一致或不足(甚至没有)。很多此类报道没有关注便秘的影响，后者经常发生且可能影响患者的生活质量。此外，很多手术包括种类繁多的重建手术，病因情况使得必须要做 APR，这也使得不同的研究难以评价解释。因此，TAR 的不同术式预后的科学对比不可能解决这些问题。此种情况下唯一能做的分析是明确每一种技术的并发症发生率和功能性评价，而有些研究没有给出客观的评分。另一个对所实施手术表示满意的方法是对比那些存在腹部造口或恢复成会阴部造口的患者的生活质量评分，但是这种分析研究少得可怜[70]。在这一点上，Violi 等[71]检查了 TAR 后患者的月度记录，显示患者相关症状是在保持整体患者评分的情况下由术者进行客观纠正的，评分往往高丁传统 Wexner 排便控制评分，所报道的排便控制事件和排便困难之间不存在真实的相关性。这将意味着调整评分体系可能要求提供更多经过验证的评价工具。

在下面的章节中，我们回顾和细致分析报道的针对 TAR 的单独或是联合使用不同方法的发病率和功能性结局。附表罗列了现有的最重要的研究，并根据研究者报道的数据总结的结果。

括约肌重建

电刺激和非电刺激股薄肌成形术

表 16.1 显示了电刺激和非电刺激股薄肌成形术的并发症和功能结果。APR 后应用电刺激股薄肌成形术进行肛门直肠重建术的累积发病率报道为 20%~90%。特殊并发症包括肛门直肠糜烂、肠穿孔、会阴脓毒症、结肠残端绞窄，肌肉坏死合并肛门或人造肛门的狭窄或坏死。另外，相当数量的并发症与植入物相关，尤其是植入物的糜烂和感染。这些并发症在电刺激股薄肌成形术中尤其明显，在某报道中植入物的移除率可达 32%[72]。

尽管评估排便控制的方法在不同的方法中没有严格的可比性。据报道，动力性股薄肌成形术的好的结果占全部病例的 0[8]~87%[45] 之间，但是正常的排便控制据 Rosen 等[44] 报道仅有 20%。Violi 等[46] 指出一个重要的特征是结果会随着时间推移而逐渐改善，而据 Ho 等[43] 报道在患者能够完全控制固体或水样便之前平均要花 20 个月的时间。

有些意外的是，应用非电刺激股薄肌成形术

表 16.1 通过单独括约肌重建进行完全肛门重建：电刺激股薄肌成形术 (D)/ 非电刺激股薄肌成形术 (A)

研究者（年）	患者（n）（总数/被评估数）	D/A	并发症	功能状态
Williams 等 (1991)[41]	12	8/0		62% 控制固体和液体粪便 1 例患者使用肛门栓
Santoro 等 (1994)[73]	14/11	0/14	1 无改善	73% 显示出足够的排便控制
Mander 等 (1996)[8]	10/9	10/0	80% 并发症发生率 1 外植体	所有患者经历了排便失禁发作期并且用垫以坚持排便
Geerdes 等 (1997)[11]	16/12	16/0	4 无改善	31% 灌肠控制满意；75% 患者每日行灌肠可控
Cavina 等 (1998)[45]	31/26	98/0	37% 并发症发生率 1 无改善 4 外植体	87% 患者达到控制固体和液体粪便
Rullier 等 (2000)[48]	15/12	0/15	73% 并发症发生率 3 无改善	78% 控制固体，偶尔液体失禁
Rosen 等 (2002)[44]	35	35/0	60% 并发症发生率 6 外植体 5 无改善	20% 控制固体、液体和气体； 66% 仅控制固体
Lirici 等 (2004)[76]	3/3	3/0		基于 36 项内容的满意控制
Koch 等 (2004)[72]	28/28	28/0	53% 并发症发生率 32% 外植体	35% 满意控制 (7% 肠道灌洗)
Ho 等 (2005)[43]	17/11	17/0	40% 并发症发生率 2 用电量解释	55% 盆底功能问题 9 例患者没有刺激而控制良好
Simonsen 等 (2005)[39]	24/22	0/24	22% 较大并发症发生率 65% 较小并发症发生率 1 无改善 2 拒绝腹部造瘘关闭	77% 固体或软便潴留
Violi 等 (2005)[46]	23/16	15/8	37% 并发症发生率	75% Jorge-Wexner 评分 ≤ 8 (5 年生存率达 100%) 87% 动力性 37.5% 非动力性

取得的结果在3种参考方法中相当一致，固体粪便的充分控制占总病例的73%~78%[39, 48, 73]。在Ho等[43]报道中这些结果与受刺激的对照组具有可比性，82%进行电刺激股薄肌成形术的患者可以达到无刺激而控制排便。

这些结果几乎与Violi等报道一致[46]，而Williams等[41]发现当刺激物被去除时，所有患者会完全大便失禁。这些矛盾的结果很难解释，可能源于所选患者的多种不同因素的影响，包括执行方案的类型，所用评估技术手段的不同，随访过程中的可变性。从某种程度上来看电刺激和与非电刺激股薄肌成形术相比，电刺激股薄肌成形术可能不会带来明确的益处。

如果事实情况就是这样的话，股薄肌成形术的功能性结局应归咎于股薄肌的生物环扎而不是刺激本身；否则，大多数的经刺激物移植治疗的会阴造口将会面临重新移植或者重新改做经腹造口术。因为失败或其他原因，25%的患者[11]重新改做新的经腹造口，在另一组[46]中的23例患者中的2例则拒绝造口关闭。

除了大便失禁，便秘也是TAR之后一个需要考虑的重要问题，几项研究发现股薄肌成形术后明显的盆底功能问题需要结肠灌洗，以促进改善并避免经腹部结肠造口术。这个功能缺陷几乎只发生在刺激组，可影响高达55%的患者[44]。

平滑肌肛门括约肌假体与结肠灌洗

表16.2显示了应用结肠平滑肌外套的会阴部结肠造瘘术并行结肠灌洗的并发症和功能结果。早期特殊并发症主要是会阴局部伤口裂开、造瘘口周围感染、会阴吻合口坏死、结肠缺血和结肠阴道瘘。在一些患者中，这些并发症可能导致最终不得不改成经腹结肠造口。黏膜脱垂和人造肛门狭窄是后期最主要的并发症。

Gamagami等[27]通过测压技术证实新建肛门袖口部存在一个持续高压的区域，通常压力均值为39cm·H_2O，另外Lasser等[26]发现60%的患者出现新建括约肌强直性痉挛；然而，两项研究中的所有患者都进行了结肠灌洗，因此，假可控状态很大程度上可能是由于从会阴结肠造口进行每日或隔日灌洗达到的，而不是由于新建内括约肌本身达到的。Lasser等还指出不出现痉挛并不总是意味着较差的功能性结果，而平滑肌性的新括约肌对自控排便的贡献与为了避免出现大量漏出的环扎术的效应更加相关。Portier等[28]对18例腹会阴直肠癌切除术后的患者实施了会阴结肠造瘘加Malone手术，在6个月的随访过程中，平均自控排便评分为6.4（满分为20），平均大便失禁生活质量总分为12.5（满分为16）。没有患者因为较差的功能性成果而要求

表16.2 平滑肌肛门括约肌假体与结肠灌洗

研究者（年）	患者数（n）（总数/评估数）	并发症	功能状态
Lasser等(1997)[26]	40/38	55%并发症发生率 2例无改善	11%一般控制 87%高度满意 5%完全失禁(恢复经腹部结肠造口术)
Gamagami等(1999)[27]	63/46	65%并发症发生率 3例无改善	59%满意控制 4%失禁
Portier等(2005)[28]	18/17	33%并发症发生率	平均Jorge-Wexner评分6.5/20 平均大便失禁/生活质量总分12.5/16 无改善
Pocard等(2007)[74]	12/12	没有报道	中位Vaizey大便失禁评分11/24 92%污染护具 生活质量评分(QLQ C-30)相当于结肠-肛门吻合术(n=38)和经会阴结肠造口术(n=12)
Hirche等(2010)[75]	44/27	围术期并发症： 40%较小并发症发生率， 7%较大并发症发生率 长期并发症： 23%较小并发症发生率， 7%较大并发症发生率 3例无改善	所有患者的静息压与收缩压相比具有显著统计学差异 修正Holschneider评分：22例患者控制良好，5例患者部分控制 生存质量分析显示高于全球健康和疾病状态平均分

进行腹部结肠造口术。在这项研究中，比较令人惊讶的是没有会阴并发症，这可能用由拖出的结肠带入盆腔的组织是没受过放射损伤的这一事实来解释。Pocard 等[74]比较了结肠-肛管吻合术和利用结肠平滑肌游离瓣会阴部造口周围自体移植的会阴结肠造口术患者的功能性结果和生活质量，后一手术是由 Lasser 等[26]描述的，他发现两种技术在功能性结果和生活质量方面的结果具有可比性。这些研究都没有显示患者进行灌肠治疗与否的功能状态比较结果。在最近的一篇文章中，Hirche 等[75]报道了一项长期研究的结果，27 例患者进行了联合会阴和新括约肌训练的新括约肌重建[23]，进行至少 6 个月的会阴造口的外部电刺激、生物反馈治疗（大多数病例）和结肠灌洗。客观评估后认定实现正常自控排便的患者达到了 80%，所有患者的静息压和缩窄压具有统计学显著差异。

人造括约肌

表 16.3 显示了为建立一个可控的经会阴结肠造口而植入的人造括约肌的并发症和功能结果。Romano 等报道的病例数最多，包含 8 例患者，括约肌植入后均没有并发症发生（随访时间，6～28 个月）。其余报道的结果呈多样化，许多患者最后不得不因为皮肤或结肠糜烂而拆除植入物。

括约肌重建和贮袋

在 TAR 手术中贮袋的重建只在几篇文献中报道了少量病例，仅仅作为括约肌再造术的一个附加手术，相关的并发症发生率没有被提及。不幸的是，仍然缺乏客观对比患者做或不做贮袋的研究。在这些研究中贮袋的类型不同而使分析十分困难。

Geerdes 等[11]对比了 4 例进行贮袋联合双电刺激性股薄肌成形术的患者与 11 例没有贮袋的患者，发现排便控制没有得到改善。在另外一项包含 26 例患者的研究中，Vorobiev 等[10]描述了一项肛门内括约肌联合结肠 C 形贮袋的平滑肌成形术，据报道在回肠造口关闭术后 12 个月其完美控制排便率达 85%。平均肛门静息压 3 个月时是 39 mmHg，1 年后可达到 54 mmHg。Vorobiev 等也观察到了人造肛门直肠耐受容量的初始值和最大值具有类似的变化规律。结肠成形术联合内括约肌再造和人造括约肌的植入中的作用，我们的研究[13]尚无法客观阐明。

在一项实验研究当中，Hughes 等对 7 只狗进行经腹会阴直肠切除术，术后研究了结肠 J 形贮袋肌肉电刺激联合电刺激股薄肌的效果，研究表明电刺激贮袋产生收缩和足够的肌肉压力使贮袋排空。这项技术目前还没有在人体内应用。

顺行节制性灌肠：Malone 技术及其他

表 16.4 显示了 ACE 单独或与其他技术联合应用的并发症和功能效果，除了平滑肌括约肌假体重建，其余已经在表 16.2 中说明。最常见的与 Malone 技术有关的早期并发症包括脓肿和阑尾坏死，两种情况均需要重新干预并行盲肠造口术。回肠\盲肠\结肠管道方法从技术上说更复杂并且具有很高的发病率，尤其是当有腹腔内吻合口存在的时候。远期并发症通常与造口狭窄有关，其很容易通过临时性导管或通过外科 V-Y 成形术解决。其他远期并发症包括造口漏和反流。为预防造口狭窄和黏膜脱垂，Ardelean 等[77]进行了 VQZ 成形术，为预防漏和反流，Levitt 等[78]使盲肠围绕阑尾或阑尾假体，类似 Nissen 胃底折叠术。Williams 等[79]描述了一个结肠内带有 Kock 类型瓣膜的管状结构来

表 16.3 人造括约肌

研究者（年）	患者数量（n）（全部/被评估的）	并发症	功能结果
Romano 等（2003）[52]	8/8	没有严重并发症	87% 良好控制（Jorge-Wexner 评分范围：3～9） 生活质量明显改善
Lirici 等（2004）[76]	3/3	1 例皮肤糜烂 2 例结肠糜烂植入物移除	固体粪便控制良好，移除前有胃肠胀气
Devesa 等（2005）[13]	1/1	1 例皮肤糜烂，植入物移除	Jorge-Wexner 评分：6
Ocares 等（2009）[53]	1/1	1 例感染糜烂，植入物移除	没有评价

表 16.4

研究者（年）	程序	患者数（n）（总数/评估数）	并发症	功能状态
Saunders 等（2004）[67]	CCC+ESGN	14/14	ESGN 的并发症发生率为 71% CCC 发生率为 36%	50% 患者对固态和液态粪便可节制 6 例无改善
Farroni 等（2007）[64]	技术（n=10） 盲肠管道（n=3）	13/13	没有报道	85% 无排泄物渗漏 无改善
Ardelean 等（2009）[62]	ACE（n=6） ACE+PSARP（n=1） ACE+PSARVP（n=2）	9/9	没有报道	所有患者都很干净

CCC：可控的结肠导管；ESGN：电刺激腹薄肌合成；ACE：顺行结制性灌肠；PSARP：臀部矢状肛门直肠成形术；PSARVP：臀部矢状肛门直肠阴道成形术

预防废物的反流。总而言之，对于小直径的造口而言，其排便控制的并发症发生率较高，但大多数并发症相对容易处理[80]。

Saunders 等[67]提议将电刺激股薄肌和可控的结肠导管相结合以应对 TAR。14 例患者中的 7 例在接受治疗并进行足够的随访后发现能够很好地控制固体及液体粪便。在经会阴结肠造口术和韦尔氏手术中，Farroni 等[64]报道了在对 13 例患者中的 11 例进行顺行结肠灌洗后发现超过 1h 没有排便；其他患者报道仅仅少量排便。随访过程中没有患者要求转成经腹部造瘘。在另一组因肛门直肠畸形而行二次手术的患者当中，Alderlean 等[62]报道了应用 Malone 技术的 9 例患者都能保持干便至少 24h。当外部括约肌被重建或代替的时候，ACE 技术有利于避免 TAR 后便秘的发生。在 ACE 中，好的功能效果看起来是由于结肠灌洗而不是此项技术的其他方面，而研究者们并没有报道给予和不给予结肠灌洗患者的相关状况。

谁是进行 TAR 的合适人选，并且何时实施更为适合？

所有这些回顾性资料分析表明，进行经腹会阴联合直肠切除然后行全肛门直肠重建术的患者，宁愿选择经会阴结肠造口也不愿意采用经腹部结肠造口，即使其功能达不到最理想的效果。可是需要考虑的问题是所有的患者均来自研究组而没有随机对照的研究来比较这两种情况的差异。众所周知在结肠肛门吻合术后，大量患者都会面临不同程度的功能失调，尤其是在进行放化疗治疗的时候[81]。关于这点，格鲁曼等[82]报道了行经腹会阴直肠切除术的患者具有更好的生存质量，与那些行直肠癌低位前切除和结肠肛门吻合术患者对比。尽管这项研究存在方法学缺陷，它强调括约肌尽量保留操作后的生活质量的重要性，直肠癌的研究应更注重有关这些参数的标准，而不是广泛的保肛率[83-85]。

撇开这些从前的注意事项，毫无疑问的是多数进行 APR 的患者宁愿选择经会阴结肠造口术，即使其不能保证良好的排便控制。选择到最理想的患者是关乎手术成败的关键。有二组行全直肠肛门重建术的候选病例：分别是具有先天严重直肠肛门畸形的儿童和那些直肠和肛门被完全切除的患者。第一组所有的患者均是做重建手术的潜在候选人，但是经腹会阴联合直肠切除术后行全直肠肛门重建术的适应证是具有争议的。首先，没有证据表明 TAR 会对癌症患者的生存造成不利影响；其次，所有患者必须知道术后很少能做到完美的排便控制，或者说永远也达不到，而通过一个造口作为替代来实现定期结肠灌洗还是比较容易实现的；再者，必须要患者知道的是此手术方法的并发症发生率，并且需要接受一个准确的评估，以不给围术期增添额外的风险。在此，细致的咨询和工作以便确信真正的了解 TAR 过程的风险收益比。高龄、肥胖、伴随疾病、会阴放疗，以及导致复发风险的所有因素均应在考虑之中。

TAR 可以同步或者在 APR 数年后施行。将简单的会阴部结肠造瘘联合 Malone 技术作为直肠 APR 手术的一个环节，要比延迟手术更简单易行。最近的一项研究证实[86]，与会阴部结肠造瘘术相关的盆腔会阴并发症和伤口裂开的发生率较一期会阴缝合更少。然而，只有那些没有接受过放疗的T1-2N0期的动机性良好的肿瘤患者适合做同步重建。对于延迟手术，TAR应至少在APR两年后才能实施，因为此时盆腔复发的风险已经很小。同步重建仍存在争议，认为其仅仅是利用超声内镜进行盆腔复发检查的早期诊断，从而提供了更好监控的可能，而并非其本身。同步重建和延迟重建之间的生活质量评分差异目前尚无报道。

结 论

避免永久性结肠造口是患者的梦想，也是外科医生的目标。腹会阴联合直肠切除术后的TAR在技术上是可行的，但它是困难、具有挑战性的手术，具有较高的并发症发生率，且功能性预后不尽如人意。此类手术应由那些具有专门技术的医生承担，术前必须挑选动机性良好的患者，并充分告知可能的益处和风险。

对不同术式的回顾性分析得出如下认识。同时性重建手术仅限应用于T1-2N0的直肠癌，二期重建必须要等到盆腔复发的风险降到最低时再进行。为了达到完美的排便控制力，虽然对丧失结构和相应功能的恢复是必需的，但再造一个有效的、永久的新括约肌似乎是TAR最重要的环节。目前，难以想象还有比臀大肌或股薄肌更适合的其他肌肉，但是这两种选择都有较高的并发症发生率，且臀大肌的功能性结果不理想。虽然还没有对比研究，非电刺激股薄肌成形术的效果可能优于非电刺激性臀大肌成形术，和电刺激股薄肌成形术相似；而后一种选择在很多国家已经很少应用了。由于其高并发症发生率和高昂的成本，人工括约肌植入几乎已经被摒弃。针对避免和减少被动性粪漏的新内括约肌重建术应仅仅视为其他手术的补充。直肠的替代必须旨在获得一个低张的远端段，而不是一个大容量储器。

总之，联合Malone手术的会阴结肠造瘘是最简单、最安全，也是最便宜的手术，是现行的术式当中能提供最好功能性的选择。对此特殊类型患者群的功能性结果来说，无论是以恰当装置对新建肛门简单环绕的内括约肌重建术，还是贮袋、结肠成形术或降结肠远端的肌切开术，都尚未得到证实。

参考文献

1. Bullard KM, Trudel JL, Baxter NN, et al. Primary perineal wound closure after preoperative radiotherapy and abdominoperineal resection has a high incidence of wound failure. Dis Colon Rectum. 2005;48:438–43.
2. Chittenden AS. Reconstruction of anal sphincter by muscle slips from glutei. Ann Surg. 1930;92:152–4.
3. Margottini M. L'amputazione abdomino-perineale del retto con abbassamento del colon al perineo. LII Congr SIC. 1950;181–6.
4. Penninckx F, D'Hoore A, Vanden Bosch A. Perineal colostomy with antegrade continence enemas as an alternative after abdominoperineal resection for low rectal cancer. Ann Chir. 2005;130:327–30.
5. Abercrombie JF, Rogers J, Williams NS. Total anorectal reconstruction results in complete anorectal sensory loss. Br J Surg. 1996;83:57–9.
6. Fazio VW, Mantyh CR, Hull TL. Colonic. "coloplasty": novel technique to enhance low colorectal or coloanal anastomosis. Dis Colon Rectum. 2000;43:1448–50.
7. Hughes SF, Scott SM, Pilot MA, Williams NS. Electrically stimulated colonic reservoir for total anorectal reconstruction. Br J Surg. 1995;82:1321–6.
8. Mander BJ, Abercrombie JF, George BD, Williams NS. The electrically stimulated gracilis neosphincter incorporated as part of total anorectal reconstruction after abdominoperineal excision of the rectum. Ann Surg. 1996;224:702–11.
9. Rouanet P, Senesse P, Bouamrirene D, Toureille E, Veyrac M, Astre C, Bacou F. Anal sphincter reconstruction by dynamic gracilloplasty after abdominoperineal resection for cancer. Dis Colon Rectum. 1999;42:451–6.
10. Vorobiev GI, Odaryuk TS, Tsarkov PV, Talalakin AI, Rybakov EG. Resection of the rectum and total excision of the internal anal sphincter with smooth muscle plasty and colonic pouch for treatment of ultralow rectal carcinoma. Br J Surg. 2004;91:1506–12.
11. Geerdes BP, Zoetmulder FA, Heineman E, Vos EJ, Rongen MJ, Baeten CG. Total anorectal reconstruction with a double dynamic gracilloplasty after abdominoperineal reconstruction for low rectal cancer. Dis Colon Rectum. 1997;40:698–705.
12. Williams NS, Hallan RI, Koeze TH, Watkins ES. Construction of a neorectum and neoanal sphincter following previous proctocolectomy. Br J Surg. 1989;76:1191–4.
13. Devesa JM, López-Hervás P, Vicente R, Rey A, Die J, Fralle A. Total anorectal reconstruction: a novel technique. Tech Coloproctol. 2005;9:149–52.
14. Devesa JM, Botella JI, López-Hervás P, Rey A, Die J, Calero A. Ultrashort bowel syndrome: surgical management and long-term results of an exceptional case. J Pediatr Surg. 2008;43:5–9.
15. Baeten CG, Rongen MJ. Total anorectal reconstruction – fact or fiction. Swiss Surg. 1997;3:262–5.
16. Violi V, Boselli AS, De Bernardinis M, Costi R, Sarli L, Iusco D, Roncoroni L. Functional outcome of total anorectal reconstruction: incontinence or constipation? Acta Biomed. 2003;74 Suppl 2: 103–7.
17. Casillas S, Hull TL, Zutshi M, Trzcinski R, Bast JF, Xu M. Incontinence after a lateral internal sphincterotomy: are we underestimating it? Dis Colon Rectum. 2005;48:1193–9.
18. Ortiz H, Marzo J, Armendáriz P, DeMiguel M, Blasi ML. Fissure-in-ano. Alterations in continence and quality of life during disease and at six months after lateral subcutaneous internal sphincterotomy. Cir Esp. 2005;77:91–5.
19. Zbar AP, Ramesh J, Beer-Gabel M, Salazar R, Pescatori M. Conventional cutting vs. internal anal sphincter-preserving seton for high trans-sphincteric fistula: a prospective randomized manometric and clinical trial. Tech Coloproctol. 2003;7:89–94.
20. Athanasiadis S, Helmes C, Yazigi R, Köhler A. The direct closure of the internal fistula opening without advancement flap for trans-sphincteric fistulas-in-ano. Dis Colon Rectum. 2004;47:1174–80.

21. Torres RA, Gonzalez MA. Perineal continent colostomy. Report of a case. Dis Colon Rectum. 1988;31:957–60.
22. Schmidt E. The continent colostomy. World J Surg. 1982;6:805–9.
23. Fedorov VD, Odaryuk TS, Shelygin YA, Tsarkov PV, Frolov SA. Method of creation of a smooth-muscle cuff at the site of perineal colostomy after extirpation of the rectum. Dis Colon Rectum. 1989;32:562–6.
24. Pescatori M, Caracciolo F, Anastasio G. Restoration of intestinal continuity after rectal excision by electrostimulated smooth and striated muscles. BAM. 1991;1:259–62.
25. Elias D, Lasser P, Leroux A, Rougier P, Comandella MG, Deraco M. Colostomies perineales pseudo-continente apres amputacion rectal pour cancer. Gastroenterol Clin Biol. 1993;17:181–6.
26. Lasser PH, Dubé P, Grillot JM, et al. Colostomie perineale pseudo-continente. J Chir. 1997;134:174–9.
27. Gamagami RA, Chiotasso P, Lazorthes F. Continent perineal colostoy after abdominoperineal resection: outcome after 63 cases. Dis Colon Rectum. 1999;42:626–31.
28. Portier G, Bonhomme N, Platonoff I, Lazorthes F. Use of Malone antegrade continence enema with perineal colostomy after rectal resection. Dis Colon Rectum. 2005;48:499–503.
29. Lorenzi M, Vernillo R, Garzi A, Vindigni C, D'Onofrio P, Angeloni GM, Stefanoni M, Picchianti D, Genovese A, Lorenzi B, Iroatulam AJ. Experimental internal anal sphincter replacement with demucosated colonic plication. Tech Coloproctol. 2003;7:9–16.
30. Chetwood CH. Plastic operation for restoring of the sphincter ani with report of a case. Med Rec. 1902;61:529.
31. Guelinckx PJ, Sinsel NK, Gruwez JA. Anal sphincter reconstruction with the gluteus maximus muscle: anatomic and physiologic considerations concerning conventional and dynamic gluteoplasty. Plast Reconstr Surg. 1996;98:293–302.
32. Devesa JM, Fernandez JM. Bilateral gluteoplasty for anal incontinence. Semin Colon Rectal Surg. 1997;8:103–9.
33. Knapp LS. Plastic repair for postoperative anal incontinence. Ann Surg. 1939;109:146–50.
34. Farid M, Moneim HA, Mahdy T, Omar W. Augmented unilateral gluteoplasty with fascia lata graftin fecal incontinence. Tech Coloproctol. 2003;7:23–8.
35. Cong J, Chen CH, Zhang H, et al. Using the gluteus muscle to reconstruct the anal sphincter for very low rectal cancer. Chin J Clin Oncol. 2007;4:98–102.
36. Fedorov VD, Shelygin YA. Treatment of patients with rectal cancer. Dis Colon Rectum. 1989;32:138–45.
37. Pickrell KL, Broadbent TR, Masters FW, Metzger JT. Construction of a rectal sphincter and restoration of anal continence by transplanting the gracilis muscle: report of four cases in children. Ann Surg. 1952;135:853–6.
38. Jacob ET, Shapira Z, Bar-Natan N, Berant M. Total anorectal reconstruction following congenital anorectal anomaly. Dis Colon Rectum. 1976;19:172–7.
39. Simonsen OS, Stolf NA, Aun F, Raia A, Habr-Gama A. Rectal sphincter reconstruction in perineal colostomies after abdominoperineal resection for cancer. Br J Surg. 2005;63:389–91.
40. Baeten C, Spaans F, Fluks A. An implanted neuromuscular stimulator for fecal continence following previously implanted gracilis muscle. Report of a case. Dis Colon Rectum. 1988;31:134–47.
41. Williams NS, Patel J, George BD, Hallan RI, Watkins ES. Development of an electrically stimulated neoanal sphincter. Lancet. 1991;338:1166–9.
42. Wong SK, Wee JT. Reconstruction of an orthotopic functional anus after abdominoperineal resection. Aust N Z J Surg. 1984;54:575–8.
43. Ho KS, Seow-Choen F. Dynamic graciloplasty for total anorectal reconstruction after abdominoperineal resection for rectal tumour. Int J Colorectal Dis. 2005;20:38–41.
44. Rosen HR, Urbarz C, Novi G, Zöch G, Schiessel R. Long-term results of modified graciloplasty for sphincter replacement after rectal excision. Colorectal Dis. 2002;4:266–9.
45. Cavina E, Seccia M, Chiarugi M. Total anorectal reconstruction supported by electrostimulated gracilis neosphincter. Recent results. Cancer Res. 1998;146:104–13.
46. Violi V, Boselli A, De Bernardinis M, Costi R, Pietra N, Sarli L, Roncoroni L. Anorectal reconstruction by electrostimulated gracilplasty as part of abdominoperineal resection. Eur J Surg Oncol. 2005;31:250–8.
47. Madoff RD, Rosen HR, Baeten CG, LaFontaine LJ, Cavina E, Devesa M, Rouanet P, Christiansen J, Faucheron JL, Isbister W, Köhler L, Guelinckx PJ, Påhlman L. Safety and efficacy of dynamic muscle plasty for anal incontinence: lessons from a prospective, multicenter trial. Gastroenterology. 1999;116:549–56.
48. Rullier E, Zerbib F, Laurent C, Caudry M, Saric J. Morbidity and functional outcome after double dynamic graciloplasty for anorectal reconstruction. Br J Surg. 2000;87:909–13.
49. Cera SM, Wexner SD. Muscle transposition: does it still have a role? Clin Colon Rectal Surg. 2005;18:46–54.
50. Christiansen J, Lorentzen M. Implantation of artificial sphincter for anal incontinence. Lancet. 1987;2:244–5.
51. Wong WD, Congliosi SM, Spencer MP, Corman ML, Tan P, Opelka FG, Burnstein M, Nogueras JJ, Bailey HR, Devesa JM, Fry RD, Cagir B, Birnbaum E, Fleshman JW, Lawrence MA, Buie WD, Heine J, Edelstein PS, Gregorcyk S, Lehur PA, Michot F, Phang PT, Schoetz DJ, Potenti F, Tsai JY. Safety and efficacy of the artificial bowel sphincter for fecal incontinence: results of a multicenter cohort study. Dis Colon Rectum. 2002;45:1139–53.
52. Romano G, La Torre F, Cutini G, Bianco F, Esposito P, Montori A. Total anorectal reconstruction with the artificial bowel sphincter: report of eight cases. A quality of life assessment. Dis Colon Rectum. 2003;46:730–4.
53. Ocares M, Caselli G, Caselli B. Artificial bowel sphincter for anorectal reconstruction. Preliminary report and review of surgical technique. Rev Chil Cir. 2009;61:350–5.
54. Ruiz MD, Alos R, Roig JV. Long-term results of artificial bowel sphincter for the treatment of severe faecal incontinence. Are they what we hoped for? Colorectal Dis. 2009;11:831–7.
55. Wexner SD, Hin HY, Weiss E, Nogueras JJ, Li VK. Factors associated with failure of the artificial bowel sphincter: a study over 50 cases from Cleveland Clinic Florida. Dis Colon Rectum. 2009;52:1550–7.
56. Thiersch (1891) quoted in Carrasco AB. Contribution a l'etude du Prolapsus du Rectum Masson. Paris; 1943.
57. Horn HR, Schoetz Jr DJ, Coller JA, Veidenheimer MC. Sphincter repair with a Silastic® sling for anal incontinence and rectal procidentia. Dis Colon Rectum. 1985;28:868–72.
58. Larach S, Vazquez B. Modified Thiersch procedure with silastic mesh implant: a simple solution for fecal incontinence and severe prolapsed. South Med J. 1986;79:307–9.
59. Devesa JM, López-Hervás P, Vicente R, Rey A, Die J, Moreno I, Teruel D. Anal encirclement with a simple rectal sling for faecal incontinence. Tech Coloproctol. 2011;15:17–22.
60. Devesa JM, Rey A, Lopez-Hervas P, Halawa KS, Larrañaga I, Svidler L, Abraira V, Muriel A. Artificial anal sphincter: complications and functional results of a large personal series. Dis Colon Rectum. 2002;45:1154–63.
61. Malone PS, Ransley PG, Kiely EM. Preliminary report: the antegrade continence enema. Lancet. 1990;336:1217–8.
62. Ardelean M-A, Bauer J, Schimke C, Ludwikowski B, Schimpl G. Improvement of continence with reoperation in selected patients after surgery for anorectal malformation. Dis Colon Rectum. 2009;52:112–8.
63. Chiotasso P, Schmitt L, Juricic M. Acceptation des stomies perineales. Gastroenterol Clin Biol. 1992;16:200.
64. Farroni N, Van den Bosch A, Haustermans K, Van Cutsem E, Moons P, D'hoore A, Penninckx F. Perineal colostomy with appendicostomy as an alternative for an abdominal colostomy: symptoms, functional status, quality of life, and perceived health. Dis Colon Rectum. 2007;50:817–24.
65. Christensen P, Buntzen S, Krogh K, Laurberg S. Ileal neoappendicostomy for antegrade colonic irrigation. Br J Surg. 2001;88:1637–8.
66. Monti PR, Lara RC, Dutra MA, de Carvalho JR. New techniques

for construction of efferent conduits based on the Mitrofanoff principle. Urology. 1997;49:112–5.
67. Saunders JR, Williams NS, Eccersley AJP. The combination of electrically stimulated gracilis neoanal sphincter and continent colonic conduit: a step forward for total anorectal reconstruction? Dis Colon Rectum. 2004;47:354–66.
68. Farrugia MK, Malone PS. Educational article: the Mitrofanoff procedure. J Pediatr Urol. 2010;6:330–7.
69. Bar-Yosef Y, Castellan M, Joshi D, Labbie A, Gosalbez R. Total continence reconstruction using the artificial urinary sphincter and the Malone antegrade continence enema. J Urol. 2011;185(4):1444–7.
70. Cavina E, Seccia M, Banti P, Zocco G, Goletti O. Quality of life after total anorectal reconstruction: long-term results. Chir Ital. 2000;52:457–62.
71. Violi V, Boselli AS, De Bernardinis M, Costi R, Trivelli M, Roncoroni L, Working Party on Anal Sphincter Replacement. A patient-rated, surgeon-corrected scale for functional assessment after total anorectal reconstruction. An adaptation of the Working Party on Anal Sphincter Replacement scoring system. Int J Colorectal Dis. 2002;17:327–37.
72. Koch SM, Uludag Ö, Rongen M-J, Baeten CG, van Gemert W. Dynamic graciloplasty in patients born with an anorectal malformation. Dis Colon Rectum. 2004;47:1711–9.
73. Santoro E, Tirelli C, Scutari F, Garofalo A, Silecchia G, Scaccia M, Santoro E. Continent perineal colostomy by transposition of gracilis muscles. Dis Colon Rectum. 1994;37(Suppl):S73–80.
74. Pocard M, Sideris L, Zenasni F, Duvillard P, Boige V, Goéré D, Elias D, Malka D, Ducreux M, Lasser P. Functional results and quality of life for patients with very low rectal cancer undergoing coloanal anastomosis or perineal colostomy with colonic muscular graft. Eur J Surg Oncol. 2007;33:459–62.
75. Hirche C, Mrak K, Kneif S, Mohr Z, Slisow W, Hünerbein M, Gretschel S. Perineal colostomy with spiral smooth muscle graft for neosphincter reconstruction following abdominoperineal resection of very low rectal cancer: long-term outcome. Dis Colon Rectum. 2010;53:1272–9.
76. Lirici MM, Ishida Y, Di Paola M, et al. Dynamic graciloplasty versus implant of artificial sphincter for continent perineal colostomy after Miles' procedure: technique and early results. Minim Invasive Ther Allied Technol. 2004;13:347–61.
77. Ransley GP. The 'VQZ' plasty for catheterizable stomas. In: Frank DJ, Gearhart JP, Snyder III HM, editors. Operative pediatric urology. London/Edinburgh/New York/Philadelphia/St Louis/Sydney/Toronto: Churchill Livingstone; 2002. p. 109–14.
78. Levitt MA, Soffer SZ, Peña A. Continent appendicostomy in the bowel management of fecally incontinent children. J Pediatr Surg. 1997;32:1630–3.
79. Williams NS, Hughes SF, Stuchfield B. Continent colonic conduit for rectal evacuation in severe constipation. Lancet. 1994;343:1321–4.
80. De Ganck J, Everaert K, Van Laecke E, Oosterlinck W, Hoebeke P. A high easy-to-treat complication rate is the price for a continent stoma. BJU Int. 2002;90:240–3.
81. Bujko K, Nowacki MP, Oleddzki J, Sopyło R, Skoczylas J, Chwaliński M. Sphincter preservation after short-term preoperative radiotherapy for low rectal cancer- presentation of own data and a literature review. Acta Oncol. 2001;40:593–601.
82. Grumann MM, Noack EM, Hofmann IA, Schlag PM. Comparison of quality of life in patients undergoing abdominoperineal extirpation or anterior resection for rectal cancer. Ann Surg. 2001;233:149–56.
83. Minsky BD. Sphincter preservation for rectal cancer: fact or fiction? J Clin Oncol. 2002;20:1971–2.
84. Kerr J, Engel J, Holzel D. Colostomies may influence patient quality of life more than poor sphincter function. J Clin Oncol. 2002;20:3930–1.
85. Engel J, Kerr J, Schelesinger-Raab A, Eckel R, Sauer H, Hölzel D. Quality of life in rectal cancer patients: a four-year prospective study. Ann Surg. 2003;238:203–13.
86. Kirzin S, Lazhortes F, de Nouaille Gorce H, Rives M, Guimbaud R, Portier G. Benefits of perineal colostomy on perineal morbidity after abdominoperineal resection. Dis Colon Rectum. 2010;53:1265–71.

第 17 章 肛管上皮内瘤样变的医疗对策

Joel Palefsky

郑 阳 译　王西墨 审校

摘 要

虽然肛管癌在总人群中尚属于一种较为罕见的疾病，但是其在男性和女性中的发病率均以每年 2% 的速度递增。肛管癌在特定人群中的发病率依然处于较高的水平，特别是在那些有同性性行为的男性和免疫抑制的患者（包括人类免疫缺陷病毒感染者）中尤为显著。高级别的肛管上皮内瘤样变（high-grade anal intraepithelial neoplasia，HGAIN），即肛管上皮内瘤样变（anal intraepithelial neoplasia，AIN；2/3 级）是肛管癌的癌前病变，对 HGAIN 进行治疗有可能降低肛管癌的总体发病率。这是一个新兴的领域，许多地方的医疗卫生机构致力于开展针对高危人群的筛查项目，通过高分辨率的肛门镜检查和组织活检以确定 AIN 病变的级别，并排除肛管癌。肛肠科医师、普通外科医师和结直肠外科医师是 AIN 医疗团队的核心成员。HGAIN 的初治应主要在门诊机构开展，并可以由外科医师和非外科系统的医师开展。但是，通过在手术室实施有创操作，外科医师在其中承担了关键的角色，其中包括在麻醉状态下对那些因体积过大而无法在门诊得到允分评估的病变进行检查，以及那些不在门诊诊疗操作之内的广泛的局部切除或消融。外科支持在处理因门诊操作造成的并发症方面也同样重要，如出血或脓肿形成。

关键词

肛管癌；肛管上皮内瘤样变（anal intraepithelial neoplasia，AIN）；高级别肛管上皮内瘤样变（high-grade anal intraepithelial neoplasia，HGAIN）；人乳头瘤病毒（human papillomavirus，HPV）；宫颈上皮内瘤样变（cervical intraepithelial neoplasia，CIN）；人类免疫缺陷病毒（human immunodeficiency virus，HIV）。

引 言

肛管癌在生物学行为上与宫颈癌相似，二者都是由人乳头瘤病毒（HPV）诱发的[1-2]。高级别的宫颈上皮内瘤样变（CIN；2/3 级），特别是 CIN 3 级，属于宫颈癌的癌前病变。而最近几十年来，随着宫颈细胞学筛查的开展，并对 CIN 2/3 级的患者进行经阴道活检，确诊后进行相应的治疗，宫颈癌的患病率已经有所下降。同样，与 CIN 2/3 级相似，肛管上皮内瘤样变（AIN）2/3 级，被称为高级别肛管上皮内瘤样变（HGAIN），亦是肛管癌的癌前病变[3-5]。用于定位病变和确认病变的级别，从而筛查 HGAIN 的技术（肛管细胞学检查），高分辨率肛门镜检查（high-resolution anoscopy，HRA）和直视下活检是效仿了用于筛查 CIN 2/3 级的技术手段[6]。鉴于宫颈癌与肛管癌、CIN 与 AIN 之间的相似性，虽然尚未经证实，但通过切除 HGAIN 病变有可能降低发生肛管癌的风险，并且已有观察性研究提示了这一可能性[7]。目前，在宫颈癌最为高发的国家和地区尚未常规开展针对 CIN 2/3 级的细胞学筛查和治疗；并且值得注意的是，针对 AIN 的日常筛查对多数有患肛管癌风险的患者有极高价值，然而这一工作的开展却受到了诸多条件的局限，甚至根本没有办法开展。

肛管癌的高危人群

肛管癌在总人群中相对罕见，其患病率大约为 1/10 万。然而，肛管癌在男性和女性中的患病率都正以每年 2% 的速度逐年递增[8]。参考历史资料，女性较男性更易患肛管癌，但是肛管癌在有同性性行为的男性（men who have sex with men，MSM）中间更为高发；据估计，在人类免疫缺陷病毒流行之前，肛管癌在这组人群中的患病率已高达 37/10 万[10]。感染 HIV 的个体较 HIV 阴性的健康个体有更高的肛门生殖器 HPV 感染率[10]。与上述现象一致的是，与 HPV 感染相关的 CIN 和 AIN 的患病率在 HIV 阳性的男性和女性中更高[10-11]，包括宫颈癌和肛管癌在内的肛门生殖器恶性肿瘤的患病率亦呈现与之相似的趋势。不断有证据表明，进行高效抗逆转录病毒治疗尚不能在消除病变及清除 HPV 感染本身等方面发挥确实有益的效果[12]。鉴于目前多数 HIV 阳性患者未进行针对 HGAIN 病变的筛查及治疗，在进行高效抗逆转录病毒治疗延长了患者生存期的同时，HGAIN 病变也有了更加充足的时间进展为肛管癌。

人们已经预见到肛管癌在 HIV 阳性人群中的患病率会逐渐升高，并且目前有数个研究报道证实了这一预见。在这其中，Piketty 等[13]报道了法国自 1999 年以来，肛管癌在 HIV 阳性的有同性性行为的男性（MSM）中的登记年患病率达 75/10 万。同样，D'Souza 等研究表明[14]，在 1996 年进行的一项由 HIV 阳性的 MSM 患者参与的关于 AIDS 的多中心协作研究中，肛管癌在被调查者中的年患病率达 137/10 万。Patel 等从一项督导下的针对已登记的 HIV 阳性性伴侣流行病学终点事件研究项目中获得的数据显示[15]，肛管癌在 HIV 阳性的 MSM 人群中的年患病率为 78/10 万。值得注意的是，这些研究中报道的肛管癌的患病率超过了世界上一些宫颈癌高发地区宫颈癌的患病率。肛管癌患病风险上升的其他人群还包括 HIV 阳性的女性[16]、有宫颈癌或外阴癌病史的女性[17]，以及为防止实体器官移植后排斥而接受免疫移植治疗的患者，如接受肾移植的受体[18]。

开展针对 HGAIN 的筛查及治疗以降低肛管癌的患病率：证据的级别

虽然针对早期肛管癌进行的治疗（如放化疗）往往能取得比较好的疗效，但是治疗也确实常伴随着相关并发症的发生，如以疼痛和出血为表现的慢性直肠炎。针对晚期肛管癌的治疗疗效仍然欠佳。显然，针对癌症的预防措施才是识别和治疗进展期肛管癌的适宜方法。问题的焦点在于针对 HGAIN 的筛查及治疗是否能够达到这一目标。支持筛查的主要证据是，针对 CIN 的筛查及治疗能够较为成功地预防宫颈癌的发生。随着针对 HGAIN 的治疗经验在不断的积累，至少在短期内安全有效地切除病变的自信心也在不断增强。对于肛管癌筛查的主要不利证据包括：缺乏数据支持治疗 HGAIN 能降低肛管癌的患病率、缺乏关于肛管癌筛查方法的成本 – 效益分析数据，以及缺乏评价治疗 HGAIN 以消除病变的长期效果的数据。而且令人担忧的是，HGAIN 在 HIV 阳性人群中有较高的患病率[10]，因此需要在大量 HIV 阳性的 MSM 人群中开展相关治疗，以获得关于患者能从中获益的有统计学意义的结果。

而且，促使浸润性肛管癌进展的相关危险因素尚未知晓，并且许多 HGAIN 患者可能会经历非必要的治疗。显然，需要获得更多能够预测病变向肛管癌进展情况的生物学标志物的信息。要开展针对 HGAIN 的筛查及治疗，尚存在一些不利因素，如与 HGAIN 治疗相关的不利效应、因筛查与治疗而产生的花费及因需要门诊随访而给患者带来的不便。

基于上述原因，尚无全国性的指南推荐对 HIV 阳性的人群开展肛管细胞性筛查。美国结直肠外科医师协会公布的临床指南中以较低级别（C 级）建议"进行肛管巴氏涂片细胞学检查……以筛查和随访肛管上皮内瘤样变（AIN）"和进行针对 AIN 的各种治疗[19]。该指南以更高级别（B级）建议"应当对患有 AIN 的患者进行随访"以监测癌变的进展。尽管指南中提供了上述一些建议，但在美国和全世界范围内，有越来越多的临床医师相信，对于肛管癌的高危人群，开展针对 HGAIN 的筛查和治疗是防止肛管癌发生的有益方法；其结果是，这些临床医师正在接受 HRA 检查和治疗 HGAIN 的训练，而且专门针对肛管癌的预防项目正在建立起来。作为这些预防性措施的一部分，外科医生越来越有可能被召集到致力于开展 AIN 的筛查与治疗工作的多学科团队中。本章的目的在于，总结目前 HGAIN 筛查与治疗相关知识，并且阐释外科医师可能在其中发挥的作用。

目前针对 HGAIN 的筛查方法

目前，针对 HPV 相关疾病进行筛查的主要工具是细胞学检查，这项检查是通过对宫颈或肛管上皮细胞的刮取涂片进行细胞病理学检查来进行的。在美国，Besthesda 分级系统 2001 版是用来对进行宫颈细胞学分级的体系[20]，而且对肛管细胞学和组织学的分级命名也是类比宫颈疾病来进行的。治疗决策则是基于组织学检查而非细胞学分级而做出。

如果进行了筛查，肛管细胞学检查结果呈现异常的患者应当进一步接受 HRA 检查和肛管活检，而治疗决策是基于病变的组织学分级。人们描述过几种不同肛管细胞学检查方法，这些方法包括用涤纶拭子对肛管和结肠进行盲探，要尽可能伸入到直肠中，再将拭子浸在装有特殊液体的细胞学取样瓶中，用力搅动拭子以将其中的细胞甩出[21]。这种方法被进一步改进为通过肛门镜进行细胞的取样收集[22]。其他的取样方式还有"细胞刷取"，尽管可能成功取得样本，但这种方法较采用湿润拭子的取样方法，可能会给患者带来更多的不适感。在一些小样本的试验性研究中，患者自己取样也证明可行[10,23,24]。

与宫颈细胞学检查相似，肛管细胞学检查也有局限性。在筛查 CIN 2/3 级时，宫颈细胞学检查的敏感性尚有一定的变异度，而且宫颈细胞学的分级并不一定能真实反映病变的宫颈组织学分级。与之相似，肛管细胞学检查也表现出与宫颈细胞学检查类似的特性[6]。研究表明，肛管细胞学检查对于 HIV 阳性的患者较 HIV 阴性的患者表现出更好的灵敏度，可能是因为前者的病变更多或者更大，或者二者兼有之[10,21]。高级别的肛管细胞学检查结果对于高级别病变的肛管活检结果有很高的预测价值，但 HGAIN 病变常常与低级别的细胞学检查结果、诊断意义尚不明确的非典型的鳞状上皮细胞（atypical squamous cells of undetermined significance，ASCUS）、不能被判定为高级别病变的非典型的鳞状上皮细胞、甚至正常的细胞学检查结果相关。基于以上原因，我们建议，患者无论呈现出任何级别的肛管细胞学检查的异常结果，包括 ASCUS，都应当进一步接受 HRA 检查。HIV 阳性患者应每年都接受筛查，以降低出现假阴性结果的风险；HIV 阴性的高危患者可每 2~3 年接受一次筛查[25-26]。

在不同的临床背景下，肛管细胞学检查可被用于不同的目的。首先，这项检查可作为决定患者是否需要进一步接受 HRA 检查的筛检方法；其次，考虑到高级别的细胞学检查结果对 HGAIN 具有更高的预测价值，这项检查可在 HRA 检查前对患者进行筛检。在估计 AIN 患病率较高的地区，诸如在接诊患者中 HIV 阳性比例较高的诊所，在这样的临床背景下，鉴于缺乏经过 HRA 检查专门训练的临床医师，可能只有有限数量的患者能接受 HRA 检查专家的评估。那些细胞学检查结果表现为高级别鳞状上皮内病变，或不能被判定为高级别病变的非典型的鳞状上皮细胞的患者，可优先接受 HRA 检查；其次是那些表现为低级别鳞状上皮内病变的患者；再次是那些表现为 ASCUS 的患者。

肛管细胞学检查的第 3 个重要用途是作为一种进行质控的工具。在加利福尼亚旧金山大学（University of California San Francisco，UCSF）的肛管肿瘤诊所，对于初次接受评估的新患者，我们在进行 HRA 检查前,常规地重复进行肛管细胞学检查。因此，我们可在多次细胞学检查结果不一致的情况下进行 HRA 检查及 HRA 引导下的活检。表现为高级别鳞状上皮内病变而在活检中未检出 HGAIN 的细胞学检查结果，则强烈提示病变被漏检，我们就会要求患者返回诊所重复进行 HRA。对于已接受过治疗的 HGAIN 病变，应用肛管细胞学检查亦可提供独立证据，证明病变确实在 HRA 操作过程中被清除了。

与宫颈癌细胞学筛检项目类似，开展肛管癌细胞学筛检项目的主要目的是预防肛管癌，而非检出肛管癌。进行肛管细胞学检查及 HRA 引导下的活检的目的在于在病变进展癌变前识别和治疗 HGAIN 病变。然而，肛管癌的检出也十分重要，因此，除了进行肛管细胞学检查，我们还对高危患者常规进行每年一次的数字化肛门镜检查来筛检肛管癌，目的是在可治疗阶段就识别出这些癌肿。由于数字化肛门镜检查可识别出 HRA 检查漏检的癌肿，这一点就显得十分重要。

高分辨率肛门镜检查引导下的活检

与宫颈阴道镜检类似，医生要取得开展 HRA 操作的资质，需要经过一定时间的训练和相关机构的授权。在与美国宫颈阴道镜检查与病理学协会的合作下，UCSF 的工作组与其他机构开设了 HRA 相关训练课程，同时在 UCSF 的肛管肿瘤诊所提供现场观摩的机会作为补充。由于治疗决策的制定是基于组织学分级的结果，因此，进行肛管活检是评估病变的关键步骤。恰当的活检依赖于 HRA 检查医师肉眼辨别 HGAIN 病变的技能，包括 3% 的醋酸和卢戈氏碘液的使用。活检钳和钳取标本的尺寸不宜太大，以防止出血、感染等并发症的发生。如果操作得当，患者可在保证安全、较少发生并发症的前提下较好的耐受肛管活检操作。

在宫颈，病变的特征使得其更可能被判定为较高的级别；病变的一系列特性被描述为 Reid 评分。评分作为一种提供给临床医生在操作时能够参考的工具，充分考虑了病变的这些特征，包括颜色、局部解剖、血管分布等，使包含了进展最为活跃的病变区域被医生活检到的可能性达到最大。这对肛门部位的活检十分重要，因为此处的病变可能分布较为广泛，而医生又不可能对所有组织进行活检。位于肛管的高级别病变的特征类似于宫颈病变。

许多患者，特别那些免疫抑制的患者，其 AIN 病变与多型 HPV 感染相关，其 AIN 病变分布较为广泛或呈弥漫性分布。切缘完整地将整个 AIN 病变完全清除干净并不现实，因此通过广泛的活检来定位病变和确定高级别病变区域的轮廓就显得十分重要。这可以将最高级别 AIN 的区域作为治疗目标，而减少对低级别 AIN 区域的切除。

治疗 AIN 的目的

一旦在活检中识别出 HGAIN 病变，就要制定出相应的治疗计划。治疗的目的在于尽可能切除所有的 HGAIN 病变，以降低患者进展为肛管癌的风险。治疗的另一目的是消除患者的症状。HGAIN，特别是位于肛周的病变，可能导致出血、烧灼感或瘙痒，并且患者可能会因病变的外观而承受精神上的折磨。对病变的治疗可能对症状起到缓解作用。低级别的病变，包括乳头状瘤，也可能引起这些症状；而且，对低级别 AIN 进行治疗虽不会降低患癌的风险，但在不会导致并发症的前提下对患者进行治疗以缓解其症状同样也是值得的。

当最初尝试彻底清除病变失败时，或当病变反复复发时，需要重新审视治疗的目的。这些情况最有可能发生在 HIV 阳性的患者身上，并且，这些情况并不一定仅限于那些体内 CD4+T 细胞水平最低、HIV 病毒负荷最高或 AIN 病变呈弥漫性分布的患者。基于以上原因，对患者进行密切随访以期发现进展癌变，可能比继续尝试彻底清除病变显得更为恰当。

目前针对肛周 HGAIN 的治疗方法

针对 HGAIN 的治疗方法大致分为以下两类：①由临床医生或患者应用软膏或药液对病变进行局部治疗；②临床医生应用侵入性的手段，如电烧、激光、红外线热凝（infrared coagulation，IRC）及手术等进行治疗。这些方法应用于肛周病变和肛管内病变时的利弊已分别列于表 17.1 及表 17.2 中。医生可根据临床医生的偏好、临床条件、病变的大小和数量，以及病变的定位，对治疗方法进行选择。治疗的流程参见图 17.1。

在 UCSF，为了治疗局限性肛周 HGAIN，我们开始应用 85% 的三氯乙酸（trichloroacetic acid，TCA）或液氮。将上述两种方法进行联合可能更为有效，即首先用液氮冷冻病变，再应用 TCA。TCA 根据需要在 2 或 3 周内重复应用 4 次，如果疗效欠佳，应尝试改换方法。当不确定病变是否被清除干净时，可对治疗区域进行活检。如果有效，一些临床医生会在门诊进行透热治疗（低功率、高频、交

第 17 章 肛管上皮内瘤样变的医疗对策

表 17.1 肛周乳头状瘤和上皮内瘤样变（AIN）的治疗

治疗方式	肛周乳头状瘤	肛周 AIN 2/3 级	优点	缺点
医生应用				
液氮	×	×	廉价 门诊应用	疼痛 可导致瘢痕形成 需多次到门诊就诊 对局限性疾病更有效
85% 的三氯乙酸	×	×[a]	廉价 门诊应用	疼痛 可导致瘢痕形成 需多次到门诊就诊 对局限性病变更为有效
红外线热凝	×	×[a]	门诊应用 可用于治疗分布广泛的病变 相对廉价	疼痛 出血 感染
电灼烧	×	×	可门诊应用 廉价	疼痛 出血 感染
激光	×	×	可在一部分门诊条件下进行 可用于治疗分布广泛的病变	疼痛 出血 感染
冷刀切除	×	×	用于治疗分布广泛的病变	要求手术条件 疼痛 出血 感染
患者应用				
鬼臼素	×		患者可自行应用	疼痛/刺激性 需多次到门诊就诊 患者可能漏掉小的病变
赛儿茶素	×		患者可自行应用	疼痛/刺激性 需多次到门诊就诊 患者可能漏掉小的病变
咪喹莫特	×	×[a]	患者可自行应用	疼痛/刺激性 需多次到门诊就诊 患者可能漏掉小的病变 男性较女性可能更为有效 对 HIV 阳性患者可能疗效欠佳
5-氟尿嘧啶乳膏				

a：小样本的开放性试验或回顾性分析表明可能有效

流电脉冲治疗）或者红外线热凝（IRC）。如果患者知道在何部位进行使用，咪喹莫特软膏也可作为一种治疗手段。在欧洲开展的研究已经证实，咪喹莫特治疗 HGAIN 可取得一定的疗效[29-31]，但是我们在 UCSF 的肛管癌诊所应用时却只取得了相对有限的疗效。HIV 阳性患者对咪喹莫特疗效的反应可能不如 HIV 阴性患者，原因是咪喹莫特是通过 Toll 样受体介导的免疫反应起效的。当患者在接受标准剂量治疗后未引起疼痛及感染，同时未产生疗效时，一些医生会延长每周应用咪喹莫特的治疗时间，而标准的治疗时间是每周应用 3 天。当患者感觉极度不适时，应当中断治疗，而轻度的不适感应当被视

表 17.2 肛管内乳头状瘤和上皮内瘤样变（AIN）的治疗

治疗方式	肛管内乳头状瘤	肛管内 AIN 2/3 级	优点	缺点
医生应用				
液氮	×		廉价 门诊应用	疼痛 可导致瘢痕形成 需多次到门诊就诊 对局限性病变更为有效
85% 的三氯乙酸	×	×[a]	廉价 门诊应用	疼痛 可导致瘢痕形成 需多次到门诊就诊 对局限性病变更为有效
红外线热凝	×[a]	×[a]	门诊应用 可用于治疗分布广泛的病变 相对廉价	疼痛 出血 感染
电灼烧	×	×	可门诊应用 廉价	疼痛 出血 感染
激光	×	×	可在一部分门诊条件下进行 可用于治疗分布广泛的病变	疼痛 出血 感染
冷刀切除	×	×	用于治疗分布广泛的病变	要求手术条件 疼痛 出血 感染
患者应用				
咪喹莫特	×[a]	×[a]	患者可自行应用	疼痛/刺激性 需多次到门诊就诊 患者可能漏掉小的病变 男性较女性可能更为有效 对 HIV 阳性患者可能疗效欠佳
5-氟尿嘧啶乳膏				

a：小样本的开放性试验或回顾性分析表明可能有效

作治疗起效的征象。接受治疗的部位应当取样活检，以确定其对疗效的反应。和其他局部疗法类似，咪喹莫特尚未被美国食品药品监督管理局（U.S. Food and Drug Administration，FDA）批准应用于此项治疗目的。

对较大的肛周 HGAIN 病变往往需要应用更为强效的治疗手段。IRC 越来越为人们所接受，原因是 IRC 治疗能在门诊条件下开展，且不产生烟雾，也不需要排烟装置。那些在过去会被介绍到外科接受治疗的较大的病变，如今都可以用这种方法治疗。对统计数据进行的回顾性分析以及多中心的 I 期临床安全性试验的结果表明，IRC 在 1 年内治疗单例患者 HGAIN 病变的有效率约为 65%，与上述 3 种疗法的有效率处于同一水平[32-33]。激光和电灼术治疗肛周 HGAIN 的效果尚未被研究报道。

上面提到的每一种治疗方法都有其不良反应，多数表现为局部疼痛、炎症及溃疡。在多数时候，应用对乙酰氨基酚或非甾体抗炎药可有效缓解这种疼痛。有时可能需要应用含可待因成分的药物来缓解疼痛，但这肯会导致患者便秘，严重的出血或感

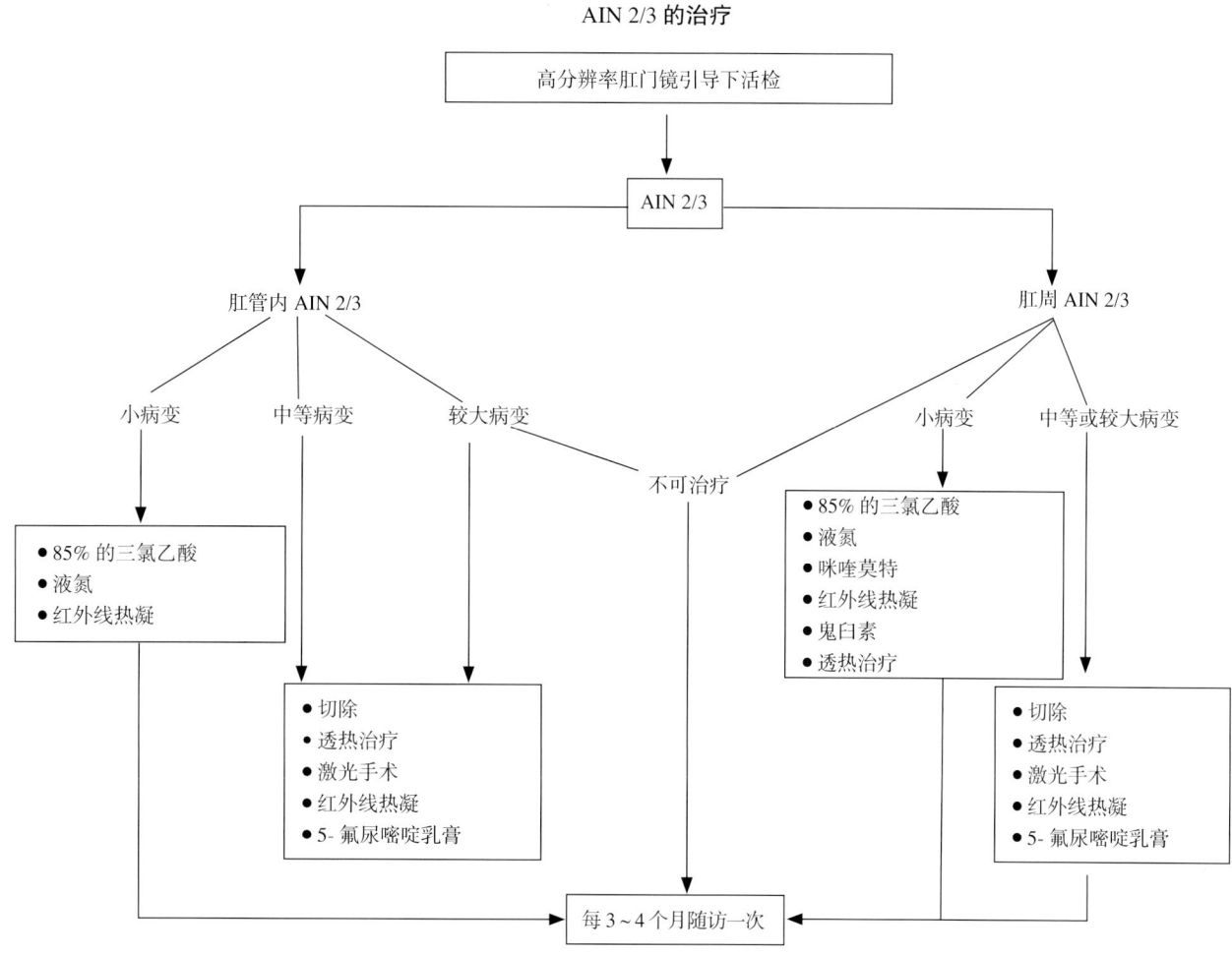

图17.1 肛管上皮内瘤样变（AIN）2/3 级的诊治流程

染也可发生，只是相对较为少见。对于分布广泛的肛周病变，应用 5-氟尿嘧啶（5-fluorouracil，5-FU）乳膏也是另一种治疗选择。5-FU 乳膏在治疗阴道上皮内瘤样变方面已经应用多年。其主要的不良反应是局部疼痛、炎症和溃疡，其严重程度可呈现轻度到重度不等[35]。在 UCSF，我们应用 5-FU 乳膏来尝试"压制"病变进展，同时治疗会保留病变区域，以期用其他更具靶向性的治疗手段发挥作用。但是，尚无前瞻性研究证实这种方法的疗效。

大体上说，手术治疗适用于大多数分布广泛、需要在麻醉下进行足够面积的活检取样以明确排除浸润性癌变的病变，或者极少数由门诊操作造成的并发症——最常见的是出血和感染。大面积切除肛管黏膜需要移植组织瓣，目前已经极少应用这项操作来治疗肛周 HGAIN 了，原因是这项操作伴随着较高的术后并发症发生率。

目前针对肛管内 HGAIN 的治疗方法

治疗肛管内 HGAIN 病变的方法类似于上述应用于肛周 HGAIN 的方法，但是可供选择的方法种类更少。较小的病变可应用 TCA 进行治疗[28]，但是多数需要行 IRC 或激光手术治疗。更多的分布广泛的病变可能需要行手术切除、电灼疗法或在手术室同时进行。类似于应用 5-FU 遏制肛周病变的方法，我们有时也会尝试先应用 5-FU 来"压制"位于肛管内的病变，以便随后进行靶向性治疗。其他方法还包括在肛管内应用咪喹莫特，可取得与在肛周应用时相似的疗效[29-31]。在一项回顾性研究中[34]，在联合应用 HRA 操作，特别是术后联合 IRC 以治疗残余病变或早期复发病变时，手术治疗 HGAIN 可收到一定的疗效。

同治疗肛周病变类似，针对肛管内 HGAIN 的治疗也可能带来不良反应，但如脓肿形成、大量出血等严重的并发症却较为少见。对于 IRC 疗法，多数严重出血常常发生于治疗后的 7～10 天时，其可能是由剧烈的肠蠕动导致刚刚愈合的组织被撕裂而造成的。

外科医生在 AIN 治疗团队中的作用

HGAIN 病变极为常见，并且当外科医生被要求处理所有这些患者时，他/她可能很快就会被繁重的任务所淹没。因此，在 UCSF，我们已经主张采取一种不同的工作模式，即让外科医生在处置这些患者的过程中发挥比较有限度、但仍然十分关键的作用。我们的目的在于，训练基本医疗提供者，让他们来开展针对高危人群的筛查，并更多地倾向于让基本医疗提供者在门诊承担 HRA、活检及门诊治疗工作。开展 HRA 项目的服务提供者可以有不同的背景，其中包括内科医师、病理医师、妇科医师、家庭医生以及其他人员，还可以是 MD、护理执业者，有些时候还可以是助理医师。当需要额外的协助或需要专门技术时，这些人员届时可请外科医生前来会诊。在 UCSF，我们目前倾向于只将不超过 5% 的患者介绍给外科的同事。然而，当发生与门诊活检或治疗相关的并发症时，外科医生将提供必要的外科后备支持，借此在这一模式中发挥着十分重要的作用。当病变范围过大以致不能在门诊行活检术，检查操作需在麻醉下进行以便更好的判定病变的浸润性，以及病变范围过大不能通过可移动式的门诊设备进行治疗时，外科医生同样扮演了十分重要的角色。

让外科医生具备 HRA 检查的技能是我们的理想，因为这项技术能够在手术室开展，并使外科医生在处理那些需要手术治疗的 HGAIN 病变时能够更好地观察病变。在门诊 HRA 项目的服务提供者可在手术室中与外科医生合作，以协助外科医生对病变进行定位，这也是一种可以选择的方案。

结　论

随着肛管癌的患病率不断上升，对 HGAIN 的治疗需求可能也会继续增加，特别是当随机对照试验证实了针对 HGAIN 的治疗能够有效降低肛管癌的患病率。外科医生在 HGAIN 的诊疗团队中发挥着十分重要的作用。由于目前几乎所有应用于 HGAIN 的治疗手段都未经过严谨的前瞻性临床试验的评估，因此外科医生尚有绝佳的机会在这一研究领域有所建树，其结果必将优化对肛管癌高危患者的医疗关怀。

参考文献

1. Hoots BE, Palefsky JM, Pimenta JM, Smith JS. Human papillomavirus type distribution in anal cancer and anal intraepithelial lesions. Int J Cancer. 2009;124(10):2375–83.
2. de Sanjose S, Quint WG, Alemany L, Geraets DT, Klaustermeier JE, Lloveras B, et al. Human papillomavirus genotype attribution in invasive cervical cancer: a retrospective cross-sectional worldwide study. Lancet Oncol. 2010;11(11):1048–56.
3. Palefsky JM. Anal cancer prevention in HIV-positive men and women. Curr Opin Oncol. 2009;21(5):433–8.
4. Scholefield JH, Castle MT, Watson NF. Malignant transformation of high-grade anal intraepithelial neoplasia. Br J Surg. 2005;92(9):1133–6.
5. Watson AJ, Smith BB, Whitehead MR, Sykes PH, Frizelle FA. Malignant progression of anal intra-epithelial neoplasia. ANZ J Surg. 2006;76(8):715–7.
6. Berry JM, Palefsky JM, Jay N, Cheng SC, Darragh TM, Chin-Hong PV. Performance characteristics of anal cytology and human papillomavirus testing in patients with high-resolution anoscopy-guided biopsy of high-grade anal intraepithelial neoplasia. Dis Colon Rectum. 2009;52(2):239–47.
7. Nathan M, Hickey N, Mayuranathan L, Vowler SL, Singh N. Treatment of anal human papillomavirus-associated disease: a long term outcome study. Int J STD AIDS. 2008;19(7):445–9.
8. Johnson LG, Madeleine MM, Newcomer LM, Schwartz SM, Daling JR. Anal cancer incidence and survival: the surveillance, epidemiology, and end results experience, 1973-2000. Cancer. 2004;101(2):281–8.
9. Daling JR, Weiss NS, Klopfenstein LL, Cochran LE, Chow WH, Daifuku R. Correlates of homosexual behavior and the incidence of anal cancer. JAMA. 1982;247(14):1988–90.
10. Chin-Hong PV, Berry JM, Cheng SC, Catania JA, Da Costa M, Darragh TM, et al. Comparison of patient- and clinician-collected anal cytology samples to screen for human papillomavirus-associated anal intraepithelial neoplasia in men who have sex with men. Ann Intern Med. 2008;149(5):300–6.
11. Harris TG, Burk RD, Palefsky JM, Massad LS, Bang JY, Anastos K, et al. Incidence of cervical squamous intraepithelial lesions associated with HIV serostatus, CD4 cell counts, and human papillomavirus test results. JAMA. 2005;293(12):1471–6.
12. Palefsky JM, Holly EA, Efirdc JT, Da Costa M, Jay N, Berry JM, et al. Anal intraepithelial neoplasia in the highly active antiretroviral therapy era among HIV-positive men who have sex with men. AIDS. 2005;19(13):1407–14.
13. Piketty C, Selinger-Leneman H, Grabar S, Duvivier C, Bonmarchand M, Abramowitz L, et al. Marked increase in the incidence of invasive anal cancer among HIV-infected patients despite treatment with combination antiretroviral therapy. AIDS. 2008;22(10):1203–11.
14. D'Souza G, Wiley DJ, Li X, Chmiel JS, Margolick JB, Cranston RD, et al. Incidence and epidemiology of anal cancer in the Multicenter AIDS Cohort Study. J Acquir Immune Defic Syndr. 2008;48(4):491–9.
15. Patel P, Hanson DL, Sullivan PS, Novak RM, Moorman AC, Tong TC, et al. Incidence of types of cancer among HIV-infected persons compared with the general population in the United States, 1992-

2003. Ann Intern Med. 2008;148(10):728–36.
16. Frisch M, Biggar RJ, Goedert JJ. Human papillomavirus-associated cancers in patients with human immunodeficiency virus infection and acquired immunodeficiency syndrome. J Natl Cancer Inst. 2000;92(18):1500–10.
17. Rabkin CS, Biggar RJ, Melbye M, Curtis RE. Second primary cancers following anal and cervical carcinoma: evidence of shared etiologic factors. Am J Epidemiol. 1992;136(1):54–8.
18. Patel HS, Silver AR, Northover JM. Anal cancer in renal transplant patients. Int J Colorectal Dis. 2005;22:1–5.
19. Fleshner PR, Chalasani S, Chang GJ, Levien DH, Hyman NH, Buie WD. Practice parameters for anal squamous neoplasms. Dis Colon Rectum. 2008;51(1):2–9.
20. Darragh TM, Winkler B. Anal cancer and cervical cancer screening: key differences. Cancer Cytopathol. 2011;119(1):5–19.
21. Palefsky JM, Holly EA, Hogeboom CJ, Jay N, Berry M, Darragh TM. Anal cytology as a screening tool for anal squamous intraepithelial lesions. J Acquir Immune Defic Syndr. 1997;14:415–22.
22. Vajdic CM, Anderson JS, Hillman RJ, Medley G, Grulich AE. Blind sampling is superior to anoscope guided sampling for screening for anal intraepithelial neoplasia. Sex Transm Infect. 2005;81(5):415–8.
23. Cranston RD, Darragh TM, Holly EA, Jay N, Berry JM, Costa MD, et al. Self-collected versus clinician-collected anal cytology specimens to diagnose anal intraepithelial neoplasia in HIV-positive men. J Acquir Immune Defic Syndr. 2004;36(4):915–20.
24. Lampinen TM, Miller ML, Chan K, Anema A, van Niekerk D, Schilder AJ, et al. Randomized clinical evaluation of self-screening for anal cancer precursors in men who have sex with men. Cytojournal. 2006;3:4.
25. Goldie SJ, Kuntz KM, Weinstein MC, Freedberg KA, Palefsky JM. Cost-effectiveness of screening for anal squamous intraepithelial lesions and anal cancer in human immunodeficiency virus-negative homosexual and bisexual men. Am J Med. 2000;108(8):634–41.
26. Goldie SJ, Kuntz KM, Weinstein MC, Freedberg KA, Welton ML, Palefsky JM. The clinical effectiveness and cost-effectiveness of screening for anal squamous intraepithelial lesions in homosexual and bisexual HIV-positive men. JAMA. 1999;281(19):1822–9.
27. Jay N, Holly EA, Berry M, Hogeboom CJ, Darragh TM, Palefsky JM. Colposcopic correlates of anal squamous intraepithelial lesions. Dis Colon Rectum. 1997;40:919–28.
28. Singh JC, Kuohung V, Palefsky JM. Efficacy of trichloroacetic acid in the treatment of anal intraepithelial neoplasia in HIV-positive and HIV-negative men who have sex with men. J Acquir Immune Defic Syndr. 2009;52(4):474–9.
29. Kreuter A, Brockmeyer NH, Altmeyer P, Wieland U. Anal intraepithelial neoplasia in HIV infection. German Competence Network HIV/AIDS. J Dtsch Dermatol Ges. 2008;6(11):925–34.
30. Kreuter A, Potthoff A, Brockmeyer NH, Gambichler T, Stucker M, Altmeyer P, et al. Imiquimod leads to a decrease of human papillomavirus DNA and to a sustained clearance of anal intraepithelial neoplasia in HIV-infected men. J Invest Dermatol. 2008;128(8):2078–83.
31. Fox PA, Nathan M, Francis N, Singh N, Weir J, Dixon G, et al. A double-blind, randomized controlled trial of the use of imiquimod cream for the treatment of anal canal high-grade anal intraepithelial neoplasia in HIV-positive MSM on HAART, with long-term follow-up data including the use of open-label imiquimod. AIDS. 2010;24(15):2331–5.
32. Goldstone SE, Hundert JS, Huyett JW. Infrared coagulator ablation of high-grade anal squamous intraepithelial lesions in HIV-negative males who have sex with males. Dis Colon Rectum. 2007;50(5):565–75.
33. Stier EA, Goldstone SE, Berry JM, Panther LA, Jay N, Krown SE, et al. Infrared coagulator treatment of high-grade anal dysplasia in HIV-infected individuals: an AIDS malignancy consortium pilot study. J Acquir Immune Defic Syndr. 2008;47(1):56–61.
34. Pineda CE, Berry JM, Jay N, Palefsky JM, Welton ML. High resolution anoscopy targeted surgical destruction of anal high-grade squamous intraepithelial lesions: a ten year experience. Dis Colon Rectum. 2008;51(6):829–35; discussion 835–7. Epub 2008 Mar 25.
35. Richel O, Wieland U, de Vries HJ, Brockmeyer NH, van Noesel C, Potthoff A, Prins JM, Kreuter A. Br J Dermatol. 2010;163(6):1301–7. doi:10.1111/j.1365.2010.09982.x. Epub 2010 Nov 4.

第 18 章 肛管癌复发后挽救性切除

James Hill · Malcolm Wilson
张 昭 译 王荫龙 审校

摘 要

本章重点讨论对于初始标准放化疗无效或复发的肛管癌的患者进行切除，以及肛门重建术的价值。对于患者的预后、生活质量以及这些患者采用的临床方法将作为重点介绍。

关键词

肛管癌；肛门上皮内瘤变（AIN）；人类乳头状瘤病毒（HPV）；人类免疫缺陷病毒（HIV）；挽救性切除；根治性腹会阴联合切除

引 言

在所有胃肠道肿瘤中，肛管癌的发病率占 1%。几乎所有的肛管癌都是上皮细胞来源，包括鳞癌、基底细胞癌、一穴肛原癌。肛管癌的发病率是肛门周围癌的两倍。肛管癌在女性多见，肛管周围癌在男性发病率高。来自英国的数据表明肛管癌的发病率逐年增加，尤其是女性患者（来自英国国家统计处）。从 1960 年 – 2004 年，女性患者肛门癌发生率增加 3 倍，男性患者发病率已经增加 1.5 倍。目前，肛管癌在女性患者发病率要高于男性患者[1]。

与来自美国的数据相比，在增加的人群中男性比例更高，尤其是在有过男性与男性肛交史和人类免疫缺陷病毒阳性者。增加人群中多合并人类乳头状瘤（HPV）感染、肛门上皮内瘤变、肛管癌，同时存在的患者占 70%～90%[2]。

HPV 感染是最常见的性传播疾病，HPV 有几种血清类型。与肛管癌发生密切相关的是 HPV16 和 HPV18。在北美，HIV 阴性的同性恋或双性恋患者约有 7% 存在肛门上皮内瘤变，HIV 阳性的同性恋或双性恋大概 1/3 存在肛门上皮内瘤变。HIV 阳性的患者对于治疗反应差，而且不良反应大。对 HPV 类型的检测有助于筛选出致癌高危人群[3]。从 AIN 进展到肛管癌的过程还不太清楚。对于可能从 AIN 进展到肛管癌的患者，早发现、早治疗是必要的，尽管这方面工作还比较欠缺。

近期即将出台的针对 HPV 的疫苗接种计划将影响到本病的发生率。加卫苗 (Gardasil) 是美国食品药物管理局最近批准的可以用于预防 HPV 6 型、11 型、16 型和 18 型的疫苗，针对 9～26 岁的人群。这种疫苗对于预防由于 HPV 的 16 型和 18 型感染导致的肛门上皮内瘤变，尤其是对于男性与男性之间性交感染患者的有效性为 78%。截至 2010 年 5 月，世界各地已经使用了 65 万剂加卫苗疫苗[4]。

目前，放化疗是表皮来源的肛管癌的标准治疗，同时结合 5-氟尿嘧啶（5-FU）、丝裂霉素 C 和总共 50.4Gy 的放射线照射。在一项针对肛管癌的 ACT Ⅱ期试验，从 2001 年 – 2008 年总共招募了 940 例患者，无间断地接受 28 次共 50Gy 的放射治疗。化学治疗使用 5-FU、丝裂霉素或顺铂。丝裂霉素 C

的完全缓解率是94%，顺铂的完全缓解率是95%[5]。ACT Ⅱ期研究得到了较高的完全缓解率（95%），完全可以与3个欧洲早期的试验报告结果相媲美，可能与放射治疗期间没有间隔有关[6-8]。此外，3年的无复发生存期是75%。丝裂霉素C和顺铂在完全缓解率方面无明显差异。研究表明综合治疗后的生活质量是可以接受的，但性功能减退比较常见[9]。

在没有得到切除标本的前提下，目前分期系统主要依赖原发肿瘤的大小、淋巴结转移情况的评估，还有一部分可通过影像学标准评估（表18.1和表18.2）。因为转移比较少见（<5%），治疗的首要目标仍是控制疾病本身。随后治疗失败会导致局部残留和肿瘤的复发。此时需要评估是否存在转移同时给予适当的治疗。

局部复发

肛管癌经过治疗后的复发率20%~25%。对于这些患者唯一可以延长生命的方法是进行抢救性治疗。可使5年生存率达到40%~60%，而如果不进行抢救性治疗3年生存率仅5%。

治疗失败的预测因素

在综合治疗(CMT)体系中，肿瘤的分期（表18.1和表18.2）与预后密切相关[10-12]。皮肤溃疡和淋巴结转移被证实是与局部复发[7]和癌症有关生存率有关的独立预后因素[7, 13]。

高危人群

放化疗的整体效果令人鼓舞，但是在一部分人群中仍存在较高的残留和局部复发的风险，这些患者需要接受更严格的综合治疗和密切的随访。

这些患者主要包括：

1. 肿瘤最大直径大于5cm或肿瘤侵犯周围组织(T4)
2. 肿瘤合并肛门瘘
3. 免疫力低下，包括艾滋病患者，尤其是存在高效抗逆转录病毒、治疗反应不佳或接受移植的患者
4. 无法接受综合治疗
5. 肛管的腺癌

综合治疗后的随访

临　床

综合治疗6~8周后可以观察完整的效果。局部治疗失败中相当多的比例发生在18个月以内，而且多数发生在开始治疗后的36个月内[14]。局部复发几乎都在肛管或肛缘[14]，并可能在出现症状前发现，对于高度怀疑的病例应门诊定期随访。在ACT Ⅱ期试验中对于随访第1年每2个月复查一次，第2年每3个月复查一次，从36~60个月每6个月复查一次。

区别放射治疗的辐射反应和早期复发是比较困难的，尤其是在经过综合治疗后仍有溃疡残留的患者（图18.1）。由于心脏疾病接受尼克地尔治疗的患者应该给予特殊护理，因为该药被公认为可以引起医源性的会阴溃疡，该溃疡与活动性肛管癌的溃疡相似。如果怀疑疾病复发，则必须在麻醉状态下进行活检。对活检切片的诊断应该由在多学科团队中专门的病理学家完成。对于女性直肠或肛管前壁进行穿刺一定要小心，避免造成直肠阴道瘘。

放射影像学

计算机断层扫描

虽然在坐骨直肠或肛周脂肪组织中发现肿块，可能预测肿瘤的复发或持续存在，但Cohan等[16]进行的一项研究表明，在19例患者中4例出现假阳性。这项研究也符合现在我们研究机构的观点，即对于盆腔内局部病变选择MRI更好。计算机断层扫描（CT）对于确定胸部、腹部、盆腔的转移仍是比较有效的方法，也可因为发现转移避免进行抢救性手术。

磁共振成像

现在关于磁共振成像（MRI）在检测盆腔疾病准确性方面的客观证据还比较少，但是它确实比CT观察盆腔和肛管更清晰，对于怀疑治疗失败的患者，可以常规应用磁共振来观察初始情况和以后的情况[17]。

术前MRI有助于判断肛管肿瘤侵犯肛管内外的程度，但是对于放化疗后患者的判断准确性下降。

表 18.1 美国癌症委员会（AJCC）关于肛管癌分期

原发肿瘤（T）			
Tx	原发肿瘤无法评价		
T0	没有原发肿瘤		
Tis	原位癌（Bowen 病、高级别上皮内瘤变、肛管上皮内瘤变）		
T1	肿瘤最大直径≤2cm		
T2	肿瘤最大直径≥2cm，但 <5cm		
T3	肿瘤的最大直径 >5cm		
T4	肿瘤侵犯邻近器官（阴道、尿道、膀胱[a]）		
淋巴结（N）			
Nx	区域淋巴结无法评价		
N0	区域淋巴结无转移		
N1	直肠周围淋巴结存在转移		
N2	存在单侧的髂内淋巴结转移和（或）腹股沟淋巴结转移		
N3	直肠周围淋巴结存在转移和腹股沟淋巴结转移和（或）双侧髂内淋巴结和（或）双侧腹股沟淋巴结转移		
远处转移（M）[b]			
M0	无远处转移		
M1	存在远处转移		
分期 / 预后			
0	Tis	N0	M0
Ⅰ	T1	N0	M0
Ⅱ	T2	N0	M0
	T3	N0	M0
Ⅲ A	T1	N1	M0
	T2	N1	M0
	T3	N1	M0
	T4	N0	M0
Ⅲ B	T4	N1	M0
	任何 T	N2	M0
	任何 T	N3	M0
Ⅳ	任何 T	任何 N	M1

转载于 AJCC 癌症分期分册纽约 7 版，发表于 2010 年斯普林格。

a：直接侵入直肠壁、直肠周围皮肤、直肠周围组织或直肠括约肌不属于 T4

b：Mx 意味无法判断远处转移

Reprinted with permission from AJCC Cancer Staging Manual, 7th edn, New York, Springer 2010

尽管 MRI 的检查结果可能不会改变最初的治疗方案（尽管它可以），但是对于后续治疗可以进行对比。同样在 T2 加权图像可以发现腹股沟或盆腔淋巴结转移，表现为高信号，并可以针对不能切除病变进行引导性穿刺活检。但是会阴成像仍是个问题。

正电子发射断层显像 /CT

在一项研究中[18]证明正电子发射断层扫描 /CT 可能是一个发现肛门癌的准确成像方法，可以发现残留和复发，敏感性和特异性可以达到 86% ~ 97%。它广泛应用于其他部位鳞状细胞癌的分期，也可以用于发现远处转移，但是在肛门癌的应用价值尚不明确，在英国也不是常规应用。

血清肿瘤标志物

对于肛管癌的诊断没有特异性的肿瘤标志物，测量癌胚抗原水平没有价值。患者应该在专科医院进行随后的后续治疗，那里有经验丰富的临床医师，

表 18.2　AJCC/UICC 的肛管癌分期

原发肿瘤			
Tx	原发肿瘤无法评价		
T0	没有原发肿瘤		
Tis	原位癌		
T1	肿瘤最大直径≤2cm		
T2	肿瘤最大直径≥2cm，但 <5cm		
T3	肿瘤的最大直径 >5cm		
淋巴结（N）			
Nx	无法判断淋巴结转移		
N1	无区域淋巴结转移		
N2	有区域淋巴结转移		
远处转移（M）			
Mx	无法判断远处转移		
M0	无远处转移		
M1	远处转移		
分期			
0	Tis	N0	M0
Ⅰ	T1	N0	M0
Ⅱ	T2	N0	M0
	T3	N0	M0
Ⅲ	T4	N1	M0
	任何 T	N1	M0
Ⅳ	任何 T	任何 N	M1

他们熟悉其中的难点，及时诊断并可以进行抢救性的治疗。由于肿瘤比较少见，因此建议肿瘤的初始和复发的治疗应去专科医院。

抢救性手术治疗

一旦确诊为复发，应该进行经腹会阴联合切除术的抢救性治疗。需要对患者身体情况进行评估，同时要通过 CT 排除胸部、腹部、盆腔的转移。如果发现可疑的淋巴结增大，要争取做组织活检。建议行切除活检而不是进行穿刺活检。对于存在腹股沟淋巴结或髂内淋巴结转移的患者再次进行手术的机会渺茫，只是在很少情况下可以对已经转移的疾病进行切除，这也只是作为一种姑息性措施。

辐射组织通常出现硬结、纤维化，对判断肿瘤复发范围造成难度。肛管癌切缘阳性的比例大约占 1/3，远远高于直肠癌[18]。治疗肛管癌的残留或复发时，其术中解剖与治疗低位直肠癌是不同的，可以总结为以下 3 点：

1. 切缘要尽可能宽，对于肛管癌，手术切除范围要超过肿瘤外 2cm。如果累及阴道后壁应该切除病变，约 70% 的女性患者进行抢救性治疗会累及阴道。

2. 病变累及坐骨直肠旁组织或直肠旁组织时，预后较差，应进行根治性手术，切除范围从肛提肌到骨盆侧壁。经过放射治疗后组织解剖很难辨认清楚。组织更脆，愈合不良，增加出血风险。抢救性手术中保证切缘阴性的关键是外侧缘要达到坐骨结节水平（相当于在直肠癌中的环周直肠系膜缘）。

3. 大剂量的照射会损害会阴周围的皮肤，表现为组织血供不佳，所以皮肤切除范围取决于放射后组织损伤范围。由于切除范围较大，往往需要进行重建，将正常组织游离至病变区域。

低位直肠癌经腹会阴联合切除被描述成"圆柱形"，肛管癌切除则是"口瓶状"（图 18.2）。

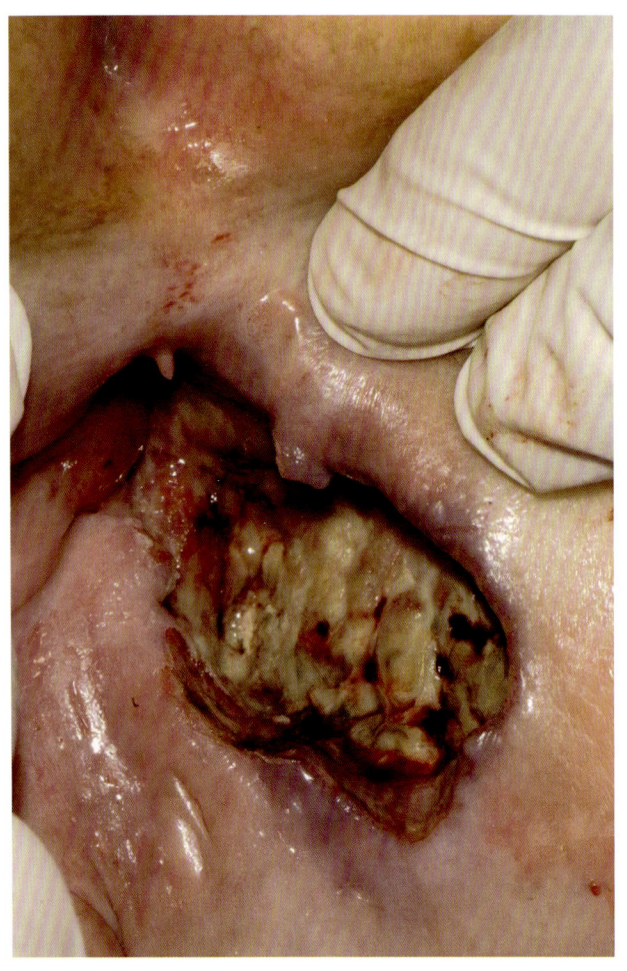

图18.1 肿瘤的溃疡。放射治疗造成的溃疡和肿瘤复发之间很难鉴别

修复组织缺损

大多数研究表明直接缝合创面出现延迟愈合和不愈合的概率高达70%。即使愈合也往往需要几个月的时间。随后还容易出现会阴疝,最高可达15%[19]。会阴皮肤广泛切除则往往需要皮瓣游离移植。下腹部腹直肌皮瓣是比较好的选择,腹直肌皮瓣较宽,可以为会阴和阴道提供足够的皮肤和血供。腹壁下动脉和皮肤下筋膜必须保留。皮肤下筋膜和肌肉从膀胱后方翻转。缝合皮瓣与会阴皮肤时应该避免张力(图18.3)。

Radice等[20]分别比较了局部晚期恶性肿瘤或局部复发的肛管癌的患者,采用一期缝合、一期大网膜移位覆盖骨盆及腹直肌肌皮瓣移植术后的并发症。总之,使用皮瓣移植治疗降低了严重的伤口并发症的发生率,同时并没有增加工作时间和住院时间。

两项研究特别关注了肛管癌进行抢救性手术治疗后会阴伤口的愈合情况。Sunesen等[21]报道了行垂直腹直肌肌皮瓣(VRAM)重建会阴组织损伤48例,未发现会阴伤口的感染及会阴伤口的裂开。Lefevre等[19]对比了VRAM瓣和大网膜成形术的使用,发现使用VRAM瓣的会阴部并发症显著减少(26.8% vs 48.9%),会阴疝同样如此(0% vs 15.4%)。腹部疝发生率无差异。某些患者需要第二伤口(即盆腔脏器切除术),或因既往手术腹壁有明显的疤痕。俯卧位时进行会阴解剖时比较困难,这是VRAM瓣的主要缺点。

在我们医院使用的替代皮瓣包括股薄肌(单侧或双侧;图18.4)和当地的"莲花瓣"lipocutaneous皮瓣(图18.5),这两种方法的优点都是避开腹壁,均能满足重建所需的体积和大小,除非缺口非常大。他们承受的张力比VRAM皮瓣弱,特别是股薄肌,供体位置可能遭受不良或延迟愈合。在我们的实践经验中,延迟愈合率(超过3个月愈合)已经从直接闭合的46%降低至应用多学科方法和重建观念后的24%。有足够的证据来支持皮瓣技术适用所有采用根治腹会阴联合切除术患者,并可常规使用。

挽救性手术的结果

研究表明,约50%的患者接受挽救性手术后可存活3～5年(表18.3)[14, 19, 22-30]。所有报告病例均描述局部复发率高。在纪念斯隆-凯特琳癌症中心,38例CMT后行挽救手术的回顾性报告表明[24],准确的生存率为44%,复发23例(60%)。腹股沟淋巴结肿大常为最初表现。肿瘤固定盆腔侧壁,侵犯直肠周围脂肪均影响生存率,但原发肿瘤的阶段和直肠周围淋巴结状态对生存率没有影响。

在1998年,Pocard等[26]报道了21例患者接受放射治疗失败行ARE的结果。在所有切除的标本中只有两例包含有淋巴结,除了1例其他都完整切除。尽管如此,38%的患者疾病有进一步发展。

在英国癌症研究试验中,577例患者被统筹委员会随机分配,比较单纯放射治疗与联合5-FU、丝裂霉素(CMT)的放射治疗的结果,其中有265例局部治疗失败(47%),143例接受了ARE[8]。手术组有44%发展为盆腔疾病,50%死于肛门癌[8]。大多数外科医生只对少数病例实施挽救性手术。1/3的手术治愈评估是不确定的,即使手术切除,

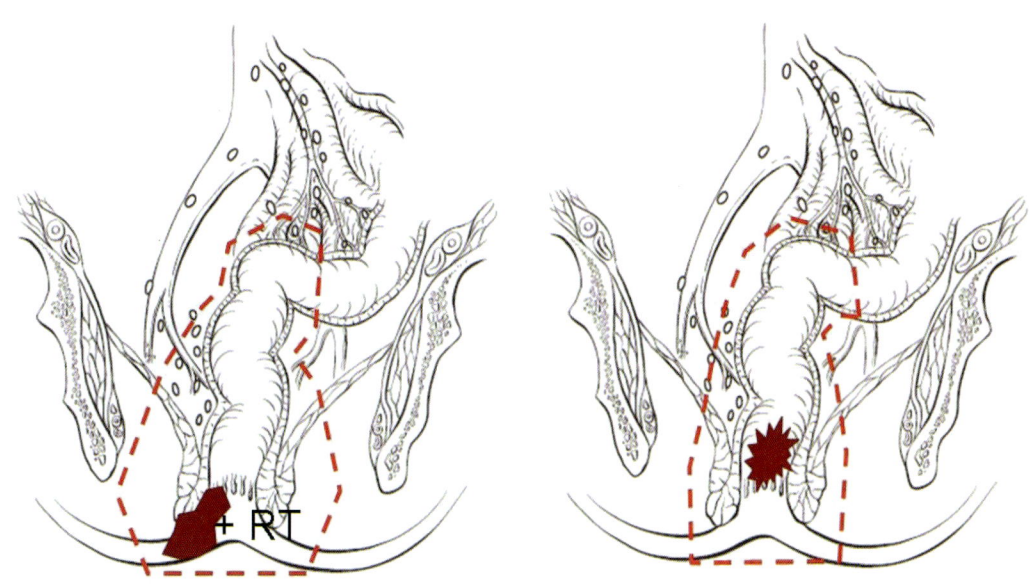

图 18.2　肛管癌切除为"口瓶状"（左图），直肠癌切除为"圆柱形"（右图）

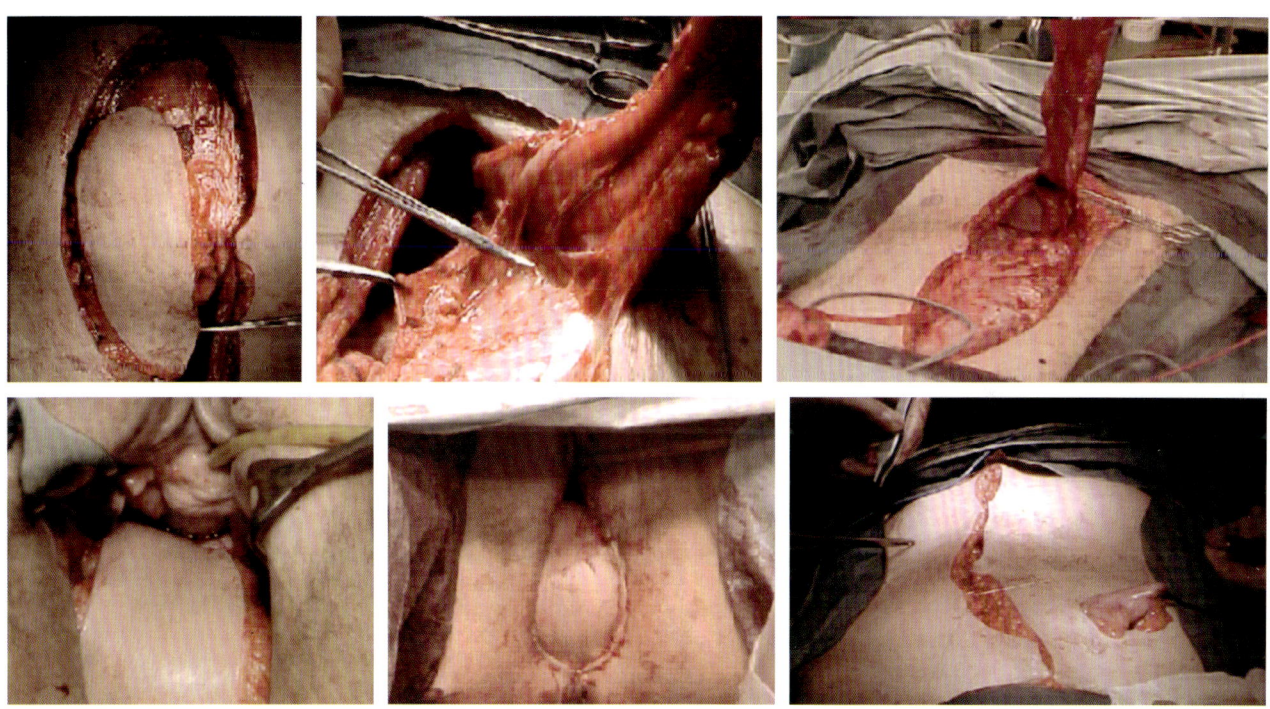

图 18.3　腹直肌肌皮瓣

28%以后仍会出现盆腔复发。69%的病例中环状边缘切除的结果与盆腔复发相关，疾病直接导致这些患者的死亡。相反，对于那些有明确的余量（>1mm）的病例，29%盆腔复发（癌特异性死亡率，39%）。当癌肿局限于肛门括约肌或直肠固有肌层时（一些放化学治疗后复发的是在直肠内），只有 19%的病例发生局部复发，16%的发生特定原因死亡。当疾病侵入坐骨直肠或直肠周围脂肪时，这些指标分别增加至 51%和 71%。当癌细胞已经侵入另一个器官，局部复发率增加至 78%，特定原因死亡率至 78%[14]。

Sunesen 等[21]报道，78%的病例切缘阴性（5

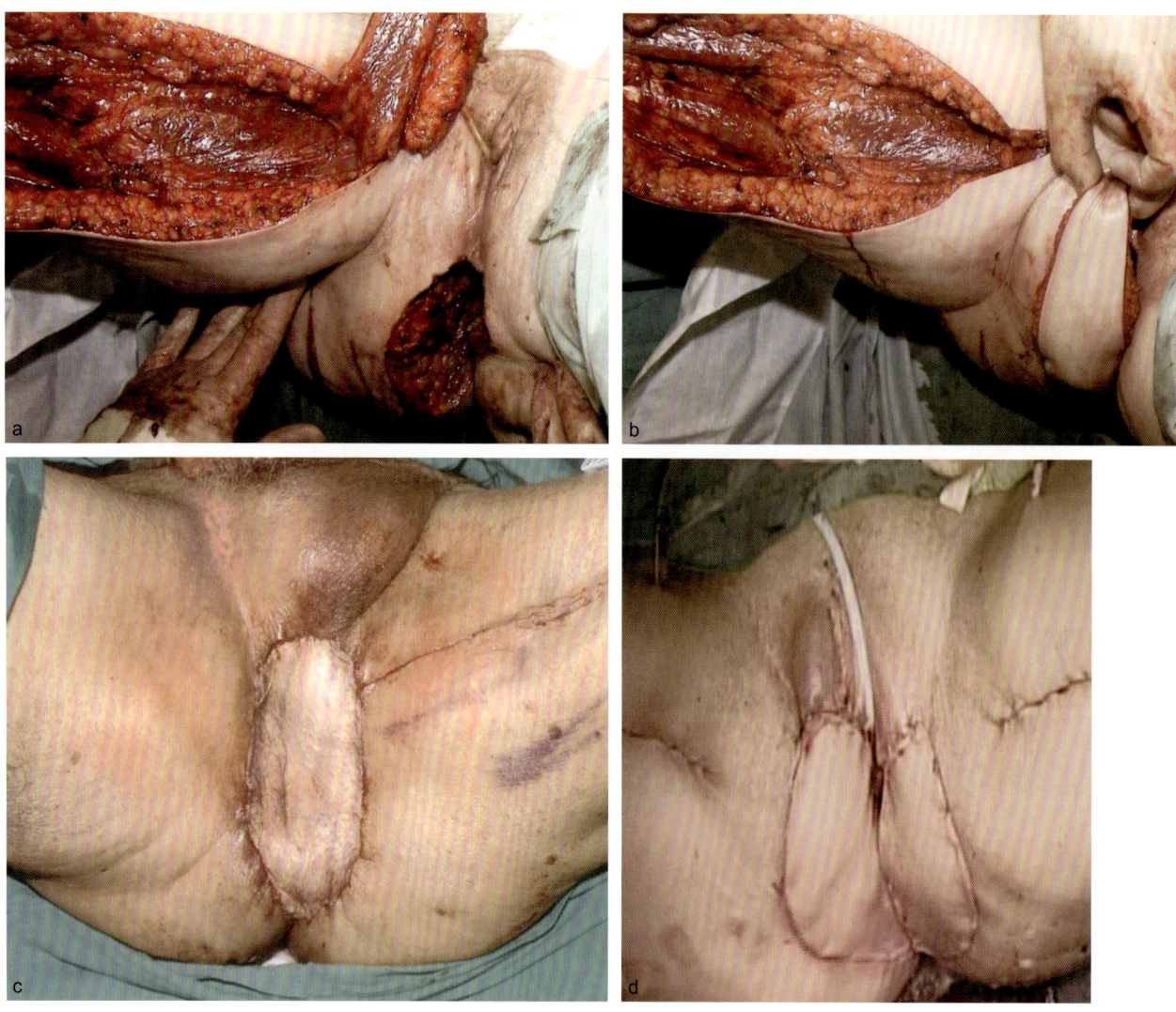

图 18.4　股薄肌肌皮瓣的使用见图（a，b），要分离至起始点，（c）为单侧应用，（d）为双侧应用

年生存率为 75%）；显微边缘（R1）和宏观边缘（R2）受到侵犯强烈预示着预后不良：根据年龄调整后的死亡率比（采用 95% 可信区间），R1∶R0 为 4.1（0.7~23.6），R2∶R0 为 10.9（2.2~54.2）。由 Rouquie 等[31]的进一步研究推断：对于肛管癌复发来说，完全（R0）切除术（76/95 例，80%）是唯一有效的预后因素。

实现切缘阴性似乎显得尤为重要。多数切缘阳性的患者在他们的手术后 2 年内死亡。侵犯坐骨直肠或直肠周围脂肪、固定在盆腔侧壁的肿瘤、侵犯邻近器官都提示预后不良，但原发肿瘤的 T 分期和肛门直肠系膜淋巴结状态似乎影响挽救性手术后的预后。当出现不良的组织学特征时，挽救性手术效果常欠佳，建议这些患者在挽救性手术之后进行化学治疗。

挽救性手术后随访

目前还没有令人信服的证据推荐使用何种随访策略。40%~50% 的病例发生在骨盆，几乎不可能进一步行挽救性手术。在检测全身性疾病方面 CT 是准确的，MRI 可被用于确定局部复发。局部复发症状通常是疼痛。对于不确定的病例，PET/CT 可能会有帮助。伴有肝或肺孤立远处转移的患者可能会受益于转移灶切除术，但适合这种方法的患者并不多见[32]。

对于单独采用放射治疗治疗存在一个公认的风险，即肿瘤"晚期治疗效果"。明显缓解后 >10 年

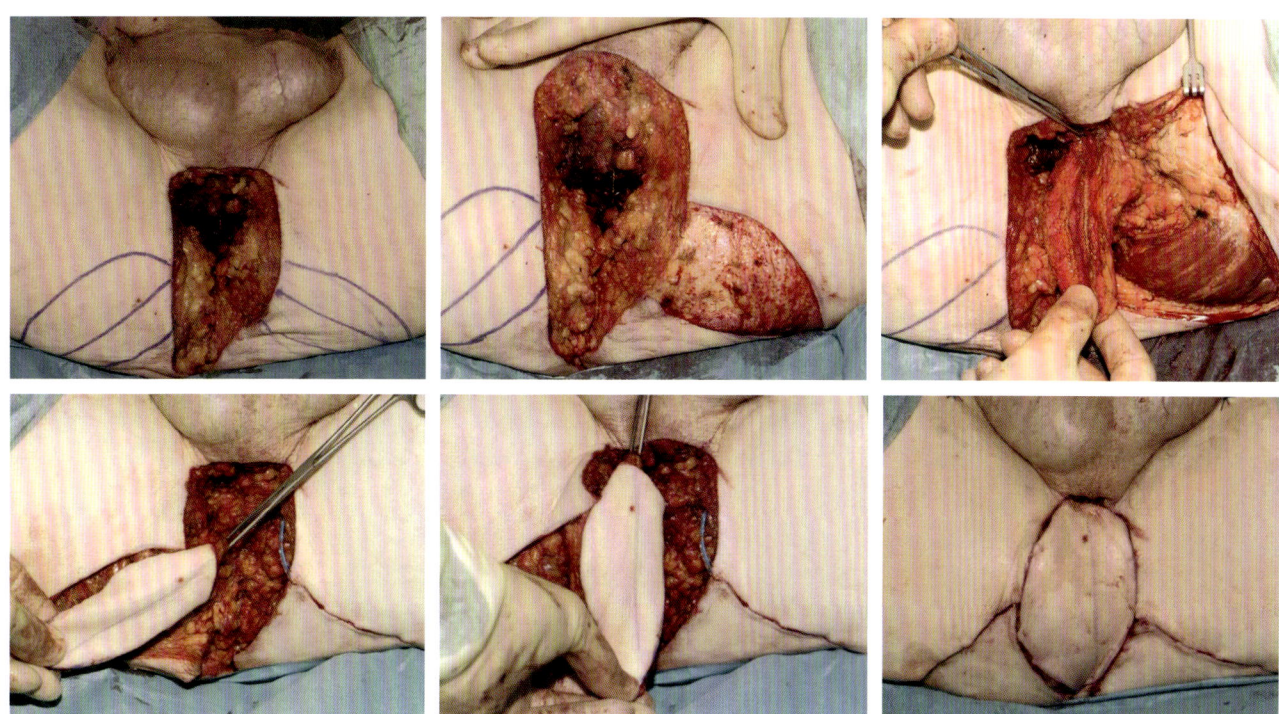

图 18.5　莲花皮瓣

表 18.3　已经发表的肛管癌放化疗治疗失败行抢救性手术的结果

研究者（年份）	数目	中位数随访（月）	生存率（%）
Zelnick 等（1992）[22]	25	20	29（3年）
Tanum 等（1993）[23]	9	36	67
Ellenhorn 等（1998）[24]	38	47	44（5年）
Longo 等（1994）[25]	14	18	57
Pocard 等（1998）[26]	21	-	58（3年）
UKCCCR（2003）[8]	133	3.3	50
Ghouti 等（2005）[27]	36	67	69（5年）
Papaconstantinou 等（2006）[28]	19	14	40
Schiller 等（2007）[29]	40	18	39（5年）
Mullen 等（2007）[30]	31	29	64（5年）
Lefevre 等（2009）[19]	95	60	56（5年）
Sunesen 等（2009）[21]	49	60	61（5年）

的患者属于这个组，尤其是当有持续的 HPV 感染的证据时。这提示在一部分患者中，长期随访是必要的[33]。

克罗恩病中的肛门癌

在肛门癌的患者中，有一个罕见的、但被详细描述的并发症——长期瘘，因为其症状类似于克罗恩瘘，所以诊断常被延迟。对于克罗恩病合并长期瘘的患者，持续和加重的疼痛、肿胀，以及肿物增长应该引起怀疑，并应在麻醉状态下进行活检。

结　论

肛门癌是一种罕见的疾病，但在过去的 30 年里发病率一直在增加。针对 HPV 的免疫接种计划，可能有助于降低其发病率。放化学治疗能使完全缓解率达到 95%，3 年无病生存率达到 75%。挽救性手术是对于残留和复发疾病的标准治疗方法。复发最可能发生在第一次治疗后2年，如果不切除是致命的。如果可以实现切缘阴性，手术是最好的治愈机会；并且若使用重建技术，会使会阴的愈合最好。多学科专家团队应在临床、病理、影像学评估和放射组织损伤疾病的外科治疗方面拥有足够的临床经验。

多学科小组

针对肛管癌行放化疗失败的患者应成立多学科小组，应该包括两名结直肠外科医生、一名整形外科医生、泌尿科医生、肿瘤科医生、影像科医生、胃肠道病理学专家、肠癌专科护士、造口治疗师。必要时需要专业的重症监护支持。如果疾病进一步发展则需要姑息治疗团队。为了推动这项工作，肛管癌的患者一旦进行放化疗，那么多学科小组一定要跟踪随访，而不是让其他的单位进行治疗。

评 定

手术前一定要进行标准的评定。

局部疾病

一定要在局麻下进行活检（复发的一定要进行组织学检查）、MRI。

转移性疾病

对临床可疑或通过胸部腹部CT发现的可疑淋巴结，应进行淋巴结细针穿刺活检、抽吸活检或组织活检。

治 疗

治疗的选择应根据疾病的程度。如果没有远处转移，ARE是标准的治疗。手术要求广泛切除肛管及周围组织，并保证盆腔的切除范围足够。无论是腹部区的操作还是会阴区的操作，都是比较困难的，两名结直肠外科医生同步进行手术具有优势。证据表明，即使侵犯周围组织，经过外科专家合作努力，也可将所累及的结构和组织一并切除。

重建术

鉴于会阴伤口裂开的发生率居高不下，所以使用腹直肌瓣或莲花瓣进行修复是非常必要的。

组织病理学报告

病理证实后所有的资料应该经过多学科小组讨论，以决定是否进行进一步辅助治疗。

参考文献

1. Robinson D, Coupland V, Moller H. An analysis of temporal and generational trends in anal and other HPV-related cancers in South East England. Br J Cancer. 2009;100:527–31.
2. Parkin DM. The global health burden of infection-associated cancers in the year 2002. Int J Cancer. 2006;118:3030–44.
3. Goldstone SE, Moshier E. Detection of oncogenic human papillomavirus impacts anal screening guidelines in men who have sex with men. Dis Colon Rectum. 2010;53:1135–42.
4. Statistical Review and Evaluation Anal Cancer - Gardasil, August 3, 2010. http://www.fda.gov.NewsEvents/Newsroom/PressAnnouncements/ucm237941.htm
5. James R, Wan S, Glynne-Jones R, Sebag-Montefiore D, Kadalayil L, Northover J, Cunningham D, Meadows H, Ledermann J. A randomized trial of chemoradiation using mitomycin or cisplatin, with or without maintenance cisplatin/5FU in squamous cell carcinoma of the anus (ACT II). J Clin Oncol. 2009;27:18s (suppl; abstr LBA4009).
6. Flam M, Madhu J, Pajak TF, et al. Role of mitomycin in combination with flourouracil and radiotherapy and of salvage chemoradiation in the definitive nonsurgical treatment of epidermoid carcinoma of the anal canal:results of a phase III randomized intergroup study. J Clin Oncol. 1996;14:2527–39.
7. Bartelink H, Roelofsen F, Eschwege R, et al. Concomitant radiotherapy and chemotherapy superior to radiotherapy alone in the treatment of locally advanced anal cancer:results of a phase III randomized trial of the EORTC Radiotherapy and Gastrointestinal Cooperative Groups. J Clin Oncol. 1997;15:1040–9.
8. UKCCCR Anal Cancer Trial Working Party. Epidermoid anal cancer: results from the UKCCCR randomised trial of radiotherapy alone versus radiotherapy, 5-flourouracil, and mitomycin. Lancet. 2003;348:1049–54.
9. Das P, Cantor SB, Zampieri JB, et al. Long term quality of life after radiotherapy for the treatment of anal cancer. Cancer. 2010;116:822–9.
10. Touboul E, Schlienger M, Buffat L, Lefkopoulos D, Pene F, Parc R, Tiret E, Gallot D, Malafosse M, Laugier A. Epidermoid carcinoma of the anal canal. Results of curative-intent radiation therapy in a series of 270 patients. Cancer. 1994;73:1569–79.
11. Myerson RJ, Karnell LH, Menck HR. The National Cancer Data Base report on carcinoma of the anus. Cancer. 1997;80:805–15.
12. Klas J, Rothenberger DA, Wong WD, Madoff RD. Malignant tumors of the anal canal: the spectrum of disease, treatment, and outcomes. Cancer. 1999;85:1686–93.
13. Grabenbauer GG, Matzel KE, Schneider IH, Meyer M, Wittekind C, Matsche B, Hohenberger W, Sauer R. sphincter preservation with chemoradiation in anal canal carcinoma: abdominperineal resection in selected cases. Dis Colon Rectum. 1998;41:441–50.
14. Hill J, Meadows H, et al. Pathological staging of epidermoid anal carcinoma for the new era. Colorectal Dis. 2003;5(3):206–13.
15. Tanum G, Tveit K, Karlsen KO. Diagnosis of anal carcinoma-Doctor's finger still the best? Oncology. 1991;48:383–6.
16. Cohan RH, Silverman PM, Thompson WM. Computed tomography of epithelial neoplasm of the anal canal. Am J Roentgenol. 1985;145:569–73.
17. Roach SC, Hulse PA, Moulding FJ, Wilson R, Carrington BM. Magnetic resonance imaging of anal cancer. Clin Radiol. 2005;60:1111–9.

18. Vercellino L, Montravers F, de Parades V, et al. Impact of FDG PET/CT in the staging and the follow-up of anal carcinoma. Int J Colorectal Dis. 2011;26(2):201–10.
19. Lefevre JH, Parc Y, Kerneis S, et al. Abdomino-perineal resection for anal cancer: impact of a primary vertical rectus abdominis myocutaneous flap on survival, recurrence, morbidity and wound healing. Ann Surg. 2009;250:707–11.
20. Radice E, Nelson H, Mercill S, Farouk R, Petty P, Gunderson L. Primary myocutaneous flap closure following resection of locally advanced pelvic malignancies. Br J Surg. 1999;86:349–54.
21. Sunesen KG, Buntzen S, Tei T. Perineal healing and survival after anal cancer salvage surgery: 10 year experience with primary perineal reconstruction using the vertical rectus abdominis myocutaneous (VRAM) flap. Ann Surg Oncol. 2009;16:68–77.
22. Zelnick RS, Haas PA, Ajlouni M, Szilagyi E, Fox TA. Results of abdominoperineal resections for failures after combination chemotherapy and radiation therapy for anal canal cancers. Dis Colon Rectum. 1992;35:574–8.
23. Tanum G. Treatment of relapsing anal carcinoma. Acta Oncol. 1993;32:33–5.
24. Ellenhorn JD, Enker WE, Quan SH. Salvage abdominoperineal resection following combined chemotherapy and radiotherapy for epidermoid carcinoma of the anus. Ann Surg Oncol. 1994;2:105–10.
25. Longo WE, Veranva III AM, Wade TP, Coplin MA, Virgo KS, Johnson FE. Recurrent squamus cell carcinoma of the anal canal. Predictors of initial treatment failure and results of salvage surgery. Ann Surg. 1994;220:40–9.
26. Pocard M, Tiret E, Nugent K, Dehni N, Parc R. Results of salvage abdominoperineal resection for anal cancer after radiotherapy. Dis Colon Rectum. 1998;4:1488–93.
27. Ghouti L, Houvenaeghel G, Moutardier V. Salvage abdominoperineal resection after failure of conservative treatment in anal epidermoid cancer. Dis Colon Rectum. 2005;48:16–22.
28. Papaconstantinou HT, Bullard K, Rothenberger DA, Madoff RD. Salvage abdominoperineal resection after failed Nigro protocol: modest success, major morbidity. Colorectal Dis. 2006;8(2):124–9.
29. Schiller DE, Cummings BJ, Rai S. Outcomes of salvage surgery for squamus cell carcinoma of the anal canal. Ann Surg Oncol. 2007;14:2780–9.
30. Mullen JT, Rodriquez-Bigas MA, Chang GJ. Results of surgical salvage after failed chemoradiation therapy for eidermoid carcinoma of the anal canal. Ann Surg Oncol. 2007;14:478–83.
31. Rouquie D, Lasser P, Castaing M, et al. Complete (R0) resection is the only valid prognostic factor in abdominoperineal resection for recurrent cancer of the anal canal (a consecutive series of 95 patients). J Chir (Paris). 2008;145:335–40.
32. Pawlik TM, Gleisner AL, Bauer TW, et al. Liver-directed surgery for metastatic squamous cell carcinoma to the liver: results of a multi-center analysis. Ann Surg Oncol. 2007;14:2807–16.
33. Chaturvedi AK, Engels EA, Gilbert ES, et al. Second cancers among 104,760 survivors of cervical cancer: evaluation of long-term risk. J Natl Cancer Inst. 2007;99:1634–43.

第三篇
炎性肠病的再次手术策略

引 言

Steven D. Wexner

对于结直肠外科医师来说，炎性肠病（IBD）的外科治疗充满挑战。炎症介质和免疫调节剂相结合的治疗方法与新的生物制剂引起了一系列独特的问题，从而造成了次优的愈合和术后感染。IBD患者的这些风险因术前的其他危险因素进一步加剧，包括低蛋白血症、营养不良和贫血。类固醇类药物的长期服用有发生糖尿病和肥胖症的风险。

对合并有上述提到的风险因素的IBD患者来说，再次手术增加了手术实施难度和术后感染性并发症的风险。此外，克罗恩病（CD）患者经常伴有1个或多个腹内脓肿或瘘管、肠管蜂窝织炎、增厚和质脆的肠系膜。溃疡性结肠炎患者经常伴有中毒性巨结肠和肠穿孔，并且他们在恢复性结直肠切除术后发生术后盆腔炎和吻合口愈合问题的风险要比其他结直肠手术高。克罗恩病（CD）患者术后有极高的复发率，特别是手术中进行吻合的患者，这个问题对再手术患者同样存在。对于住院患者来说，疾病复发不仅仅局限于回盲部克罗恩病（CD），也经常规律性地出现肛门部克罗恩病（CD）。

本质上，因为吻合口狭窄和复杂肛瘘行再次手术也许要比因疾病复发而再次手术要好。患者必须认识到，外科手术的意义本质是一种姑息治疗，而不是治愈；并且可以预测需要再次手术。这些导致再次手术的、特有的不利因素，也许能够解释为什么许多训练有素、经过认证的结直肠外科医生通常更喜欢将IBD患者转诊到专科中心。

本书第三篇是一个指南，帮助外科医师更有效地处理这些复杂的情况。本篇的一部分是由世界著名的IBD外科医师编写，他们每天的日常工作就是完成这些有特殊要求的手术操作。他们分享了手术技巧和细节。此外，术前准备期间有一个关键性的治疗方案，同时病理学家能够给我们提供一些线索，以确保取得手术成功。一个最重要的问题就是他们可以帮我们解释黏膜病变。非常幸运的是，本篇包含了世界著名的IBD病理学家的建议。

第 19 章 炎性肠病异型增生

Emil N. Salmo · Najib Y. Haboubi

李　毅译　李　宁审校

摘　要

本章讨论了炎性肠病的癌变风险，并提出了关于筛查、异型增生及异型增生相关病变或肿块的治疗等有争议问题的指南。此外，也将结肠炎相关损害与散发性结直肠癌进行了比较，对比了其特异的分子生物学表现。

关键词

溃疡性结肠炎；克罗恩病；异型增生；结直肠癌；炎性肠病（IBD）；原发性硬化性胆管炎（PSC）；结肠镜监测检查

引　言

鉴于 Crohn 和 Rosenburg 在 1925 年对溃疡性结肠炎（UC）[1,2]、Warren 和 Sommers 在 1948 年对克罗恩病（CD）[3,4]的报道，长期患有炎性肠病（IBD）的患者发生结直肠癌（CRC）的风险升高已成为共识。然而，这种风险的大小仍然值得商榷；以往的文献[3]报道患病 10 年后风险快速增加，然而更多新近的研究显示该风险较小[4-5]。总而言之，患病 10 年后，每年发生癌症的风险在 0.5%～1% 范围内[3,6-9]。最近一项基于荷兰全国人口的分析指出，溃疡性结肠炎相关的癌症 20% 发生在发病后的 8 年内[10]，这些研究者也建议应当比以往推荐更早开始筛查。

关于这些风险大小差异的研究还不多，可能原因是对照组疾病的改进、监测计划的实施和 IBD 伴发肿瘤病变的早期发现[11]。与非结肠炎相关 CRC 相比，结肠炎相关的肿瘤常常多发：约 20% 的患者初发灶为两个，10% 的患者初发灶为 3 个或以上[12]。这些肿瘤常表现为更高的等级及更多的印戒细胞类型[13]，通常起源于扁平黏膜而不是常见的腺癌。与散发性 CRC 相比，这些肿瘤发生人群也更加年轻[8]。有些意外的是，约 11% 的结肠炎相关的肿瘤由分化良好的腺体及最小粘连组成。这已经被命名为低级别管状腺癌，并且发现来源于低级别异型增生部位[14]。

IBD 基础上的肿瘤形成被认为是一个连续的过程，由无异型增生通过低级别异型增生（LGD）发展为非特异性异型增生，再由高级别异型增生（HGD）发展为肿瘤。然而，肿瘤形成可以不经过以上的所有这些步骤[15-16]。一些研究显示，淋巴结阳性的 CRC 发生过程不涉及 HGD，并且从监测检查结果为无异型增生到出现恶变的间隔小于一年[17-19]。

通过比较分期及病理亚型，结肠炎相关肿瘤患者的生存率与散发性肿瘤相比大致相当。与散发性肿瘤类似的是，结肠炎相关肿瘤最重要的预后因素是病理分期和分级[20-21]。最近一篇以摘要形式发表的文献显示，在长期患有 UC 的患者中，左侧 LGD 比右侧 LGD 更常见，并且更快的发展为进展期的 HGD 和肿瘤[22]。

IBD 中 CRC 发展的危险因素

溃疡性结肠炎

肿瘤发生的两个最重要的危险因素是疾病的持续时间和程度。重要的是要从症状发作的时间，而不是诊断成立之日起确定疾病的持续时间[23-24]。Eaden 等[3]确定了 CRC 风险在 UC 相关症状出现 8～10 年后上升，继而在疾病的后几十年里不断升高。在他们的研究中，CRC 在 10 年里的累计发病率是 2%，20 年里是 8%，30 年里是 18%。然而，Rutter 等[9]报道的 UC 患者 30 年监测结果显示，癌变风险更小——20 年里是 2.5%，30 年里是 7.6%，40 年里是 10.8%——并且在超过 40 年结肠炎病史时风险基本一致，提示在这样的随访后没有必要加强监测。

总之，绝大多数研究显示，在疾病前 10 年里肿瘤发生率较低，实际上可能比目前研究显示的更低[3,9,11]，因此在疾病前 8 年开始监测并不合理。广泛性结肠炎患者的肿瘤风险比正常人高 19 倍，左半结肠炎患者比正常人高 4 倍，而仅患有直肠炎者患癌风险并不增加[25-26]。大部分研究没有充分证据证明倒灌性回肠炎是 CRC 的风险因素[27]。

原发性硬化性胆管炎（PSC）是 UC 患者发生 CRC 的一个强大的独立危险因素[28]，高达 25% 的 UC 合并 PSC 患者产生异型增生；相较而言，仅患有 UC 的患者中只有 6% 产生异型增生[29]。重要的是，研究已经发现，即使针对 PSC 行肝移植后，这种上升的风险依旧很高[30]。这种关联非常高，没有确诊 IBD 的 PSC 患者也被推荐行诊断性结肠镜检查并取活检，以确定他们是否有亚临床结肠炎的证据[31]。

阳性的 CRC 家族史被认为是另一危险因素，特别是一级亲属在 50 岁之前被诊断 CRC，其 CRC 发生率增加两倍[32]。关于确诊年龄较轻及发病年龄较早是否是 IBD 患者发生 CRC 的危险因素的报道结论并不一致。因此目前的推荐是儿童患者和成人一样频繁地实施监测，并且应该基于病程而不是实际年龄[3]。

IBD 患者（除外 PSC）炎症的严重程度已经证明能够增加异型增生和 CRC 的风险[33]。疾病的组织学表现，而不是内镜（宏观）表现，能够更好地评估疾病的严重程度，从而评估癌症风险[27]。既往和持续的炎症宏观特征（炎症后的息肉、瘢痕和狭窄）提示风险增加，而宏观上结肠表现正常的患者与普通人群相比风险并不升高[34]。作为严重炎症标志的假息肉的出现，提示 CRC 的风险加倍[33]。狭窄也是 IBD 患者发生 CRC 的危险因素。一些研究已经显示 UC 合并狭窄的患者的癌变概率高于预期，在 24%～40%[37]。Gumaste 等[35]的一项研究显示，患有 UC 病史 20 年后出现的狭窄和位于脾曲近端并导致大肠梗阻症状的狭窄会增加癌变风险。他们也证明出现这些狭窄的癌变往往更具侵袭性。

克罗恩病

自 Warren 和 Barwick[38]在 1983 年首次报道 CD 患者出现 CRC 以来，已有明显证据表明 CD 能够增加小肠及大肠癌的风险，10 年 CRC 累计发病率为 2.9%[39]。结肠炎的程度也是一个重要因素；患有广泛性 CD 患者的患癌风险最高[40]。Ribeiro 等[41]发现发生 CRC 的 CD 患者大约 87% 发生在患病 20 年后。尽管资料有限，但结肠型 CD 患者癌变的风险可能仅在 8～10 年后变得明显，这点与 UC 相似[23]。Gillen 等[39]发现 CD 和 UC 患者 CRC 的发生率基本一致，20 年后分别是 8% 和 7%。他们也发现（与其他研究相似），在广泛性结肠炎 CD 患者中 CRC 风险增加了 18 倍，在广泛性溃疡性结肠炎患者中增加了 19 倍[42]。

有些研究已经显示，CD 患者发生 CRC 的相对风险在诊断年龄小于 30 岁的患者中更高[43]。进一步说，有证据显示结肠型 CD 狭窄的出现增加了 CRC 的发生率[44-45]，所以有必要进行活检排除癌变。也有报道指出 CD 旷置狭窄肠管的癌变率升高，而这种旁路手术现在已经很少实施[46]。

异型增生

定义和分类

异型增生是一种病理诊断，定义为一种局限在腺体基底膜内的、上皮内的明确的肿瘤变化[47]。异型增生被认为是 IBD 患者合并有 CRC 的一种前体和标志[17]。它在超过 90% 的 UC 合并癌变患者中出现，可发生在任一部位的结肠，常靠近肿瘤[15]。据报道 83%～100% 的 CD 合并癌变患者的异型增生临近回结肠肿瘤；相反，只有 2% 的 CD 未合并癌变患者的结肠切除标本包含轻度异型增生[18, 38]。在 1983 年一篇里程碑式的文章中，Riddell 等[47]建立了一种异型增生的标准分类法（表 19.1），基于上皮细胞及其细胞核将异型增生分为 HGD、LGD 和不确定异型增生（IND）（图 19.1）。

表 19.1 异型增生的分类

分类	建议随访时间
阴性	定期 1 年
不确定	
可能阴性	定期 1 年
未知	短间隔
可能阳性	短间隔
阳性	
低度	短间隔或有肿块时行结肠切除术
高度	结肠切除术

1. LGD（图 19.1a）的病变特征是大小相似的拥挤腺体，类似于结肠管状腺瘤。这些腺体由具有大的、梭状的、基底导向的核深染的异型增生细胞填充。几乎没有炎症。

2. HGD（图 19.1b）的大部分腺体结构异常，由大水泡样的核分层，伴或不伴有方向错乱的核深染的及有丝分裂异常的细胞一字排开。几乎没有炎症。

由 Riddell 等创建的异型增生原来的分类方法基本没有改变。2000 年，来自欧洲、日本和北美洲的一组胃肠病理学家们共聚于奥地利维也纳，提出了一个新的分类方法，用于将各自不同组织使用的术语联系在一起（表 19.2）[49-50]。但是，在患者的治疗方面，原来的分类方法和 2000 年创建的分类方法并无重大区别，推荐在必要时同时使用两者。

当初次结肠镜检查发现 IND 时，有 13%～26% 的病例进展至晚期肿瘤[9, 17]。纽约西奈山医院的一项研究显示，刚开始没有异型增生的患者、患有 IND

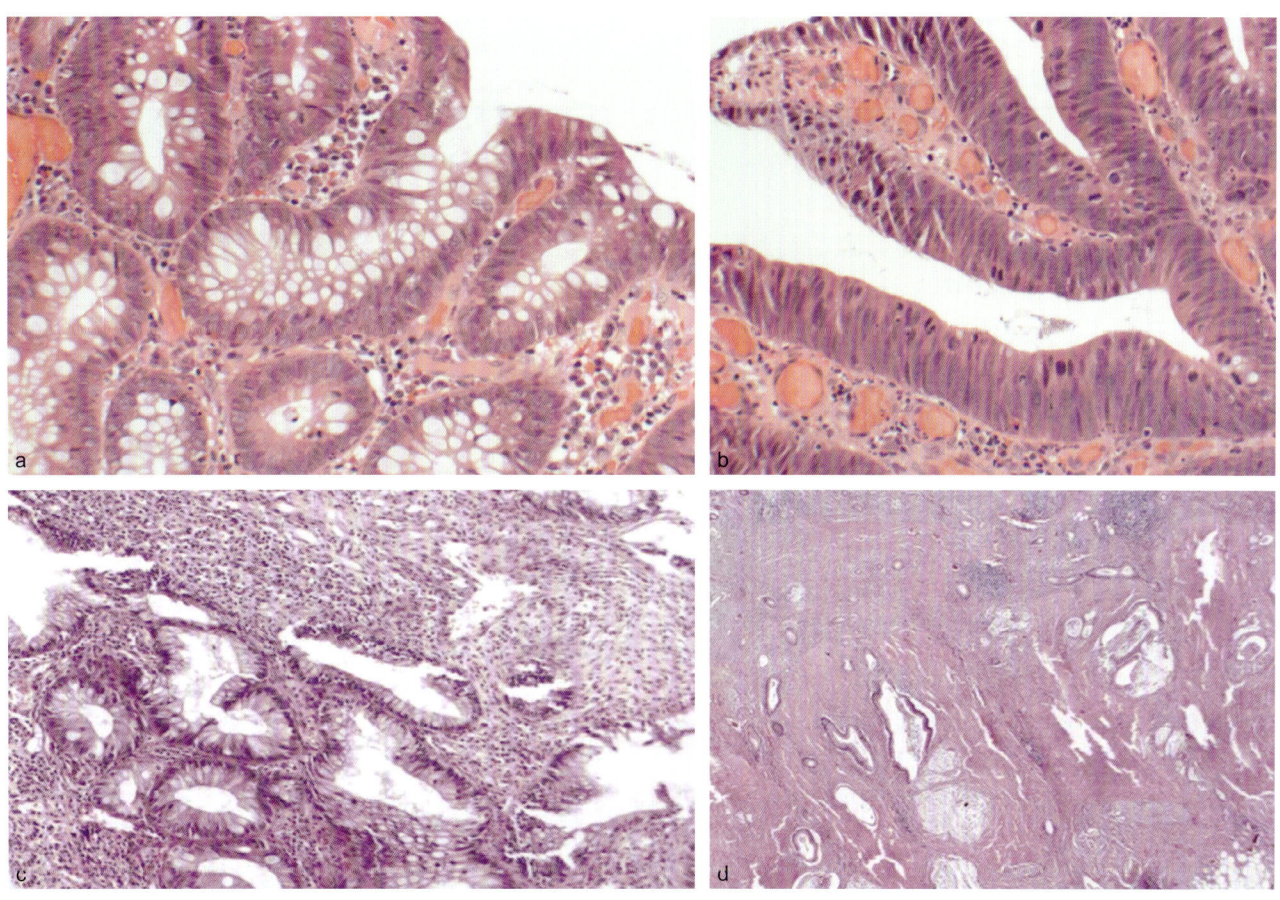

图 19.1 （a）低度异型增生有均匀、细长、拥挤、位于基部的细胞核和一些黏蛋白空泡；（b）高度异型增生有明显的核分层，细胞极性的损失和丰富的有丝分裂。（c, d）低度管状腺腺癌伴有高分化腺癌：（d）来源于低度异型增生，（c）浸润的腺体很少显示出异型性，不伴有或伴很少的纤维组织增生

表 19.2　胃肠道肿瘤的维也纳分型

1. 异型增生 / 肿瘤阴性
2. 异型增生 / 肿瘤不确定
3. 非侵袭性，低级别瘤变（低度腺瘤 / 异型增生）
4. 非侵袭性，高级别瘤变（高度腺瘤 / 异型增生，非浸润性癌，浸润可疑）
5. 浸润性癌（黏膜内癌，黏膜下癌或穿透）[a]

a：在修改后的维也纳分型中，黏膜内癌已经被移至分类 4 中

的患者和 LGD 的患者 5 年进展至 HGD 或 CRC 的概率分别为 1.1%、9% 和 45%[51]。一篇包含 10 项前瞻性研究的综述指出，当初次结肠镜监测检查发现 LGD 时，约有 29% 的患者进展至 HGD 或 CRC[17]。

观察者之间关于异型增生解读的不同

对于异型增生的病理诊断，在不同组织观察者之间及同一组织观察者内部存在显著差异。Collins 等[52] 发现当鉴定 HGD 时一致性最高，而鉴定 IND 和 LGD 则不那么准确。部分原因是对于术语"不确定异型增生"的理解存在差异，而该术语常用于描述标本的大小或方向不恰当，或存在严重的炎症和间接反应改变[24]。在这方面，经验不足的病理学家比经验丰富的病理学家更倾向于使用 IND。然而，即使在专家之间，差异也是存在的，总体的共识也远不是最佳[53]。这也导致了我们推荐应当有两位病理学家（其中一位是经验丰富的胃肠病理学家）协商一致后再报道这些异型增生的案例[54]。

最近，α-甲基酰基辅酶 A 消旋酶获得关注，该肽在前列腺上皮内瘤及前列腺癌中高表达，在 UC 病灶中不表达，被认为在异型增生中阴性，已经被证实在 LGD（96%）、HGD（80%）和腺癌（71%）病灶中明显增加。这种免疫组化染色已经作为一种辅助方法用于鉴别分类困难的病例。

检测异型增生所需的活检数量

第二个争议焦点是准确诊断或排除异型增生所需的活检数量。Itzkowitz 和 Harpaz[15] 认为一次典型的活检抽样率低于总结肠表面积的 0.05%。因此，普遍认为应采取相当数量的活检，但在目前临床实践中存在很大差异。Rubin 等[56] 认为至少需要 33 次活检才能对发现异型增生有 90% 的准确率，而需要 64 次活检才能将准确率提升至 95%。美国克罗恩病及结肠炎基金会[23]、美国胃肠病学会[57] 和英国胃肠病学会[58] 推荐的准确检测异型增生所需的确切活检次数及所需方法各有不同。但是，在临床实践中，采用的活检次数常常低于任何指南所推荐的次数[59-60]。可行的建议是沿着结肠每 10cm 采取 4 次随机活检，而额外的活检取自任何狭窄或异常部位。在 UC 患者中，推荐远端乙状结肠和直肠每 5cm 四象限取检[23, 58]。有必要行全结肠镜检查，因为大约有 1/3 的 UC 相关 CRC 发生在近端结肠[27, 61]。

新的检测异型增生的内镜技术

在检测 IBD 患者异型增生时，需要改善的是减少结肠镜检查的抽样误差，从而提高总体准确率。这可以通过针对性活检而不是随机结肠活检得到改善[27]。这方面的两个进步是在黏膜上喷涂染料（色素内镜）和高分辨率结肠镜的使用。色素内镜能发现更多的肿瘤病变[62-63]，却不会明显延长检查时间。英国胃肠病学会的新指南[61] 推荐内镜医师采用结肠黏膜喷涂染料作为技术选择。如果不使用色素内镜，就应该遵循 2002 年指南所强调的方案（即沿着结肠每 10cm 随机取检 2～4 次）[58, 61]。美国胃肠病学会正式同意由受过适当训练的内镜医师使用色素内镜[27]。借助色素内镜，可以通过评估坑纹对隐窝结构进行分类，进而便于区分瘤变和非瘤变，并且能够进行针对性活检[27]。此外，色素内镜被证明能够更加准确地评估疾病严重程度及炎症活动度[63]。

另一个有前景的领域是共聚焦激光显微内镜的使用，其允许在内镜检查同时进行体内组织学检查，当和色素内镜共同使用时，能显著减少 UC 患者监测癌变所需的活检数量，与用白光内镜随机活检相比，诊断率提高 4 倍[64]。

IBD 中 CRC 分子病理学

散发性 CRC 与结肠炎相关 CRC 之间的分子病理学之间存在一些差异。腺瘤性结肠息肉病基因功能的缺失是散发性 CRC 的一个常见早期事件，但在 UC 患者中并不多见，且通常发生在结肠炎相关 CRC 异型增生 - 癌序列的后期[15]。相反，p53 突变出现在散发性 CRC 的晚期，而在 IBD 中它们出现在早期并且可能具有重要作用。在这方面，Burmer

等[64]发现p53杂合性缺失与恶变有关,在被认为是IND的活检标本中发生率是9%,LGD活检标本中发生率是33%,HGD活检标本中发生率是63%,CRC活检标本中发生率是85%[65]。DPC4和K-ras基因突变在散发性CRC中常见,但在IBD伴癌症患者中不常见[66-67]。最终,Schulmann等[68]发现高水平的微卫星体突变的频率和数量在散发性结直肠癌及结肠炎CRC中存在显著差异。我们期待这些分子生物学特征提供关于IBD相关CRC风险分类的新概要,并继续成为未来研究的主要方向[69]。

异型增生的治疗

异型增生患者的治疗(图19.2)很多年来都是争议的焦点。异型增生被粗略分为扁平型(内镜检查不到)或突起型(内镜能检查到)。对于未检出异型增生的患者,应按照各国推荐的指南继续定期行随访和内镜监测检查。而对于IND患者,由于炎症,患者应进行结肠炎治疗,确保炎症在重复取检之前消退。如果仍存在核异常,就要保证改变诊断为扁平型LGD,如果级别仍保持在IND,就要更密集的进行定期随访和重复取检。

扁平型异型增生

扁平型LGD的治疗存在争议。大量研究表明50%的LGD超过5年会进展至HGD或CRC[19,53,70]。在因LGD行急诊结肠切除术的患者中,有16%~34%的标本中伴有CRC[17,70]。在这方面,Ullman等[70]发现进展概率与病灶多少无关,因为单发或多发扁平LGD的进展概率相似。该组研究人员也指出,扁平型LGD的出现是一个"进展期肿瘤的有力预测指标",并且相对于立即行结肠切除术,持续监测"充其量是一个冒险的策略"。伦敦圣马克医院30年的经验总结也得出类似的结论:行结肠切除术的LGD患者中,约有20%伴有CRC;此外随访发现,约有39.1%的LGD患者进展为HGD或CRC。

然而,关于这个问题还有其他的学派。Lim等[71]经10年随访发现,仅有10%的LGD患者发展为HGD或CRC,而无异型增生的UC患者中有4%发展为HGD或CRC。他们的结论是LGD的诊断不足以支持行结肠切除术。Befrits等[72]也有相似的报道。

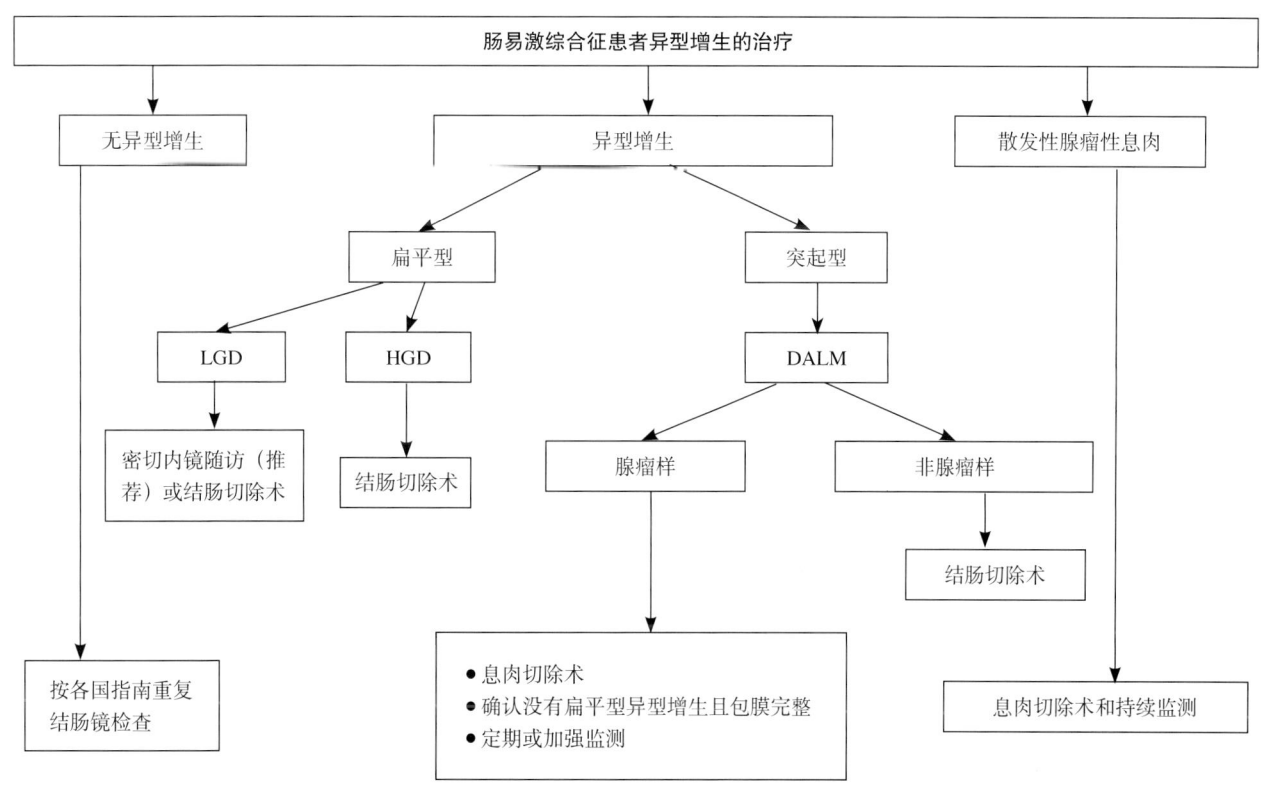

图19.2 肠易激综合征(IBD)患者异型增生的治疗。LGD:低度异型增生;HGD:高度异型增生;DALM:异型增生相关溃疡或肿块(Modified from reference.[24])

我们通过包含胃肠病学家、病理学家和结直肠外科医师的多学科团队会议讨论处理这些病例；应作出一个联合决定，并且患者应被告知出现结肠切除术失败、潜在死亡率和并发症的可能性或概率，以及手术治疗与等待观望方案的比较。如果不施行结肠切除术，那么应继续行密切的内镜及临床随访[24]。

对于扁平型 HGD 没有什么争议，因为这些患者的结肠切除标本中有 42%~45.5% 伴有 CRC[9, 17, 73]。因此，普遍认为 HGD 的出现提示行结肠切除术。LGD 肿块不像典型的散发性腺瘤性息肉，不能在内镜下切除，或有狭窄症状，内镜检查不能通过[35, 36, 75]，特别是长期患病者，通常提示伴发结肠癌，需行结肠切除术。

最近的一篇病理学文献鉴定出约有 11%IBD 相关腺癌的原因是低级别管状腺瘤（图 19.1c, d），并且表面的 LGD 与底层浸润性腺癌有关[14]。这一发现支持了对 LGD 患者行结肠切除术。Rodriguez 等[73] 的一项研究发现，约 60% 的美国胃肠病学家不建议 LGD 确诊病例立即行结肠切除术，更推荐行持续的进一步加强监测[27]。有趣的是，Siegel 等[76] 最近的一项研究显示，几乎所有回答问卷的患者都认为 UC 增加了他们患结肠癌的概率。该研究中，如果发现异型增生，60% 的患者会拒绝内科医师对选择性结肠切除术的建议，尽管被告知他们有 20% 的概率患结肠癌。平均而言，只有当这些患者的患结肠癌概率至少有 73% 时，他们才会同意行结肠切除术。

上皮的再生和修复，特别是在活动性炎症环境中，也许会导致异型性，而后者与真正的异型增生很难鉴别。这些病例被归类为 IND[77]。活检提示 IND 的患者在 IBD 患者中研究较少。Nugent 等[78] 在 1991 年的一篇报道中提到，20 例活检提示"不确定"的患者经过一段未指明时间的随访后，3 例发展为 HGD，1 例在行结肠切除术时发现存在腺癌。

突起型异型增生

结肠炎波及范围内的任意突起型损害称为异型增生相关病变或肿块（DALM）；这最早由 Blackstone 等在 1981 年描述[74]。在他们的原始文献中，这些病变中的 CRC 发病率很高。其他研究显示 DALMs 出现时 CRC 的发生率在 31%~65% 之间[9, 17, 52]。因此，开始出现 DALM 时增加了伴发 CRC 或进展为 CRC 的风险，所以强烈推荐结肠切除术。近年来的研究表明，并非所有 IBD 患者的息肉样病变都需要结肠切除术这样的根治性治疗。将 DALM 从散发性腺瘤性息肉病分离出来，这提出了新的问题，因为前者需要结肠切除术，而后者可以通过适当的息肉切除术和后续监测治疗[79]。

已有研究评估了免疫组化在区分 DALM 和散发性腺瘤性息肉病时的价值。在临床实践中，不管是组织学表现还是免疫组化都没有价值。目前两者的区别在患有这些疾病患者的治疗方面没有临床价值。最近有证据显示，在结肠炎波及范围之外的地方发现异型增生也许可以诊断为散发性腺瘤性息肉病，并行针对性治疗[80-81]。

最近有研究显示，DALM 能够粗略分为内镜下类似散发性腺瘤性息肉病者称为腺瘤样 DALMs（ALMs），和内镜下不像散发性腺瘤性息肉病者，称为非腺瘤样 DALMs（NALDs）[82-84]。ALM 内镜下表现为界限清楚、光滑或乳头状、无坏死、无柄或带蒂的息肉[82, 85]，而 NALD 损害表现为天鹅绒样的补丁、斑块、不规则的隆起或结节，或不适宜内镜切除的狭窄病变[86]。最近有研究[82-83] 显示，ALM 病变可以安全地经内镜切除，只要保证它们被完全切除，切除后柄的基底部及临近扁平黏膜处多点活检，且必须显示没有异型增生。如果实施了这样的内镜切除，就应当行密切的随访监测，以防近一步发生异型增生。事实表明，通过随访患 UC 及 ALM（62.5%）的患者、患 UC 及已知散发性腺瘤性息肉病（50%）的患者或这两组患者的亚组之间及不患有 UC 散发性腺瘤性息肉病的对照组患者（49%）发现，息肉形成的发生率无显著差异[84]。

但是，重要的是要意识到应在内镜下区别 ALM、NALD 和炎症息肉，而这是一项具有挑战性的任务。最近一篇 Farraye 等[87] 的文献总结道，即使是有经验的胃肠病学家在区分这些息肉时仍有困难。值得注意的是，当回顾性分析圣马克医院的病例时，Rutter 等[33] 发现绝大多数异型增生源于并归类为 ALM。在这方面，同样是该组研究者在伦敦圣马克医院主持的一项 14 年监测计划中评估了 56 例 UC 合并异型增生（扁平型或突起型）患者[86]。56 例患者中总共发现 110 个肿瘤区域，其中 77.3% 结肠镜下能够发现。更具体地说，可发现的病灶中有 74 个（87%）是"息肉状的"（腺瘤样），4 个被描述为有"不规则的"轮廓，1 个被描述为"斑块状的"。此外，6个被描述为肉眼可见的癌症。内镜下无法切除的 NALDs 与癌症之间有很强的关联，概率在 38%~83% 之间。因此，无论活检的异型增生分级如何，都推荐患有 UC 和内镜下无法切除的 NALD 患者行结肠切除术[88]。这些推荐适用于 UC 患者，不管他们的年龄或病程及结肠炎严重程度如何[82,88]。虽然结肠镜下切除术后的瘢痕也许能被发现，但最好是标记内镜下切除的任意可疑病变周围的黏膜，以便于今后的识别。从实用角度来看，重要的问题是确定病变能否完全内镜下切除且周围没有异型增生，以及剩余结肠是否有异型增生。

IBD 患者的监测

由于 IBD 中的肿瘤经历了一个慢性炎症 – 异型增生 – 肿瘤的途径，患者在肿瘤发生之前就开始进行监测计划，以便发现异型增生[31]。然而临床实践中的监测差别很大。最近一项 Rodriguez 等[73]进行的基于问卷调查的研究显示，回复的医师中有 80% 声称他们对于患有全结肠炎的患者，在 8~10 年病程时开始进行结肠镜监测检查，且有 54% 声称他们至少活检 31 次。然而，一项荷兰研究显示，受访者中仅有 53% 于正确的时间对全结肠炎患者开始监测，而在左半结肠炎时仅有 44% 胃肠病学家在正确时间开始筛查，且有 73% 受访者每次结肠镜检查取检次数少于 30 次[89]。患者对监测计划的依从性也是一个棘手的临床问题，并且差异很大。必须告诫患者进展为 CRC 的风险，以及如果他们退出监测计划发展为肿瘤的风险。也应告知患者，既往检查未见异型增生也有可能发展为肿瘤[15]。

溃疡性结肠炎监测的依据

Morson 和 Pang 报道在 9 例术前直肠活检确诊 HGD 的患者中，有 5 例的结肠切除标本伴有肿瘤[90]。这导致了采用多次活检检测异型增生的监测计划的进步。圣马克医院是世界上首个发起 UC 患者行这种结肠镜监测计划的组织[91]。从那时起，临床监测逐渐被广泛接受，即使关于其益处的证据仍有点局限。Rutter 等[9]报道了一项纳入 600 例长期广泛性 UC 患者的 30 年随访经验，得出的结论是他们的研究"显示结肠炎监测确有益处"。目前没有随机试验证明通过系统的结肠镜监测检查能够减少发展为 CRC 或病死于 CRC 的概率。通过比较监测与不监测的有效性能够得到有限的证据，但这很大程度上是因为伦理问题带来了可用的可判断的数据。

在一项包含 3 项研究的科克伦分析中，监测组的 110 例患者中有 8 例死于 CRC，而非监测组 117 例患者中有 13 例死于 CRC[95]。该科克伦分析结论如下："有证据表明，在进行监测的患者中肿瘤往往被早期发现，相应地这些患者的预后更好，……有间接证据表明，监测可能有效减少了死于 IBD 相关肿瘤的风险。"第 4 项由 Lutgens 等[96]进行的最近的研究显示，进行监测与未进行监测的患者相比，5 年肿瘤相关死亡率明显不同。

克罗恩病监测的依据

几乎没有数据说明克罗恩病结肠炎监测的有效性。一项随访了 259 例克罗恩病广泛性结肠炎（影响至少 1/3 的结肠）患者的研究发现，进行结肠镜检查的患者中有 7% 有异型增生或肿瘤，此外有 14% 的患者在后续监测中发现有异型增生或肿瘤[97]。在另一项 Friedman 等[98]的研究中，初始结肠镜检查阴性的克罗恩病结肠炎患者 3 次随访结肠镜检查后发现异型增生或肿瘤的累积概率为 22%。尽管缺乏数据，结肠镜监测检查目前仍被看做治疗的标准，并且克罗恩病结肠炎患者应当按照与 UC 患者类似的日程进行监测。新的美国胃肠病学会及英国胃肠病学会指南指出，"尽管缺乏随机对照试验，但是鉴于 IBD 患者发展为 CRC 风险增加，仍推荐行结肠镜监测。"广泛性 UC 及结肠 CD 患者最有可能从这个监测计划中获利[27,61]。

有回肠肛门贮袋患者监测的依据

复原性大肠直肠切除术最早在 1978 年被描述[99]。从那时起，回肠 – 肛管贮袋吻合术成为了需要手术的 UC 患者的选择性流程。这种情况下的异型增生虽然罕见，但能够发生在贮袋回肠黏膜或任何保留的肛管直肠黏膜上[61]。在两项包含了 2415 个病例的大型系列研究中[100-101]，没有报道贮袋内的肿瘤变化。虽然罕见，但很明显的是癌变确实有发生，似乎有一些危险因素，包括贮袋手术时有异型增生、结直肠癌、原发性硬化性胆管炎等[102-103]。几乎所有异型增生都发生在伴有严重炎症的回肠黏膜持续萎缩部位(所谓的 C 型黏膜)[104]。最近的英国胃肠病学会指南指出,"没有明确证据表明贮袋监测有益,因此不强烈推荐。但是,如果临床医师想提供监测,使用软式乙状结肠镜每年行贮袋监测,并于四个近端和四个远端取检似乎是合理的策略。"如果行大肠直肠切除术时没有结直肠癌,且目前不存在其他的危险因素,发生癌变是极为罕见的[105]。目前没有任何关于是否调查此类患者的数据存在,但每 5 年使用软式乙状结肠镜监测检查可能是合理的。

结论:应该如何进行乙状结肠镜监测检查?

2010 年,美国胃肠病学会及英国胃肠病学会都发表了关于 IBD 患者监测的新指南[27,61]。这类患者的危险因素的分层正变得越来越重要,而最近的监测指南采用了这种方法。这两个指南都指出,直肠炎患者的 IBD 相关 CRC 风险并不上升,因此可能在平均风险建议的基础上进行治疗。其他所有患者在出现症状 8~10 年后应当行结肠镜筛查,并通过全结肠多处取检获得准确的微观病变范围。当进行结肠镜监测检查时,任何时间点的疾病组织学上的最近端的严重程度应当能确定患者疾病的实际严重程度。理想情况下,每个解剖段的活检标本应在一个单独的容器中提交,以避免可能需要监测的异型增生部位的混淆。各个指南均推荐患者在临床缓解期行监测检查;但是,如果无法达到缓解期,监测检查不应拖延。

美国胃肠病学会推荐结肠镜筛查阴性的广泛性或左半结肠炎患者应在 1~2 年内开始常规结肠镜监测检查。对于结肠镜监测检查阴性的患者,后续的监测检查应每 1~2 年进行一次。对于两次检查结果阴性的患者,下次监测检查时间可在 1~3 年后,直到 UC 病程达到 20 年为止,接下来的检查应当每 1~2 年进行一次。各指南都指出,PSC 患者在他们初次诊断后就应该开始结肠镜监测检查,并每年进行 1 次。新的英国胃肠病学会指南允许经过适当训练的内镜医师使用色素内镜检查。自出现症状起有 8~10 年的 CD 患者及结肠大部病变(至少有 1/3 结肠受累)患者应当按照 UC 患者相同的规定行结肠镜筛查。

新的英国胃肠病学会指南根据患者危险因素的不同改变了监测检查的间隔,这些变化概括在图 19.3 中。推荐对全结肠行染料喷涂及异常部位的针对性活检,当无法施行该操作时,应当随机活检(沿结肠每 10cm 取 2~4 次活检)。新指南中,广泛性结肠炎定义为侵袭至脾区近端的溃疡性结肠炎或克罗恩病结肠炎按蒙特利尔分型,侵袭部位至少达到了结肠表面积的 50%[106]。

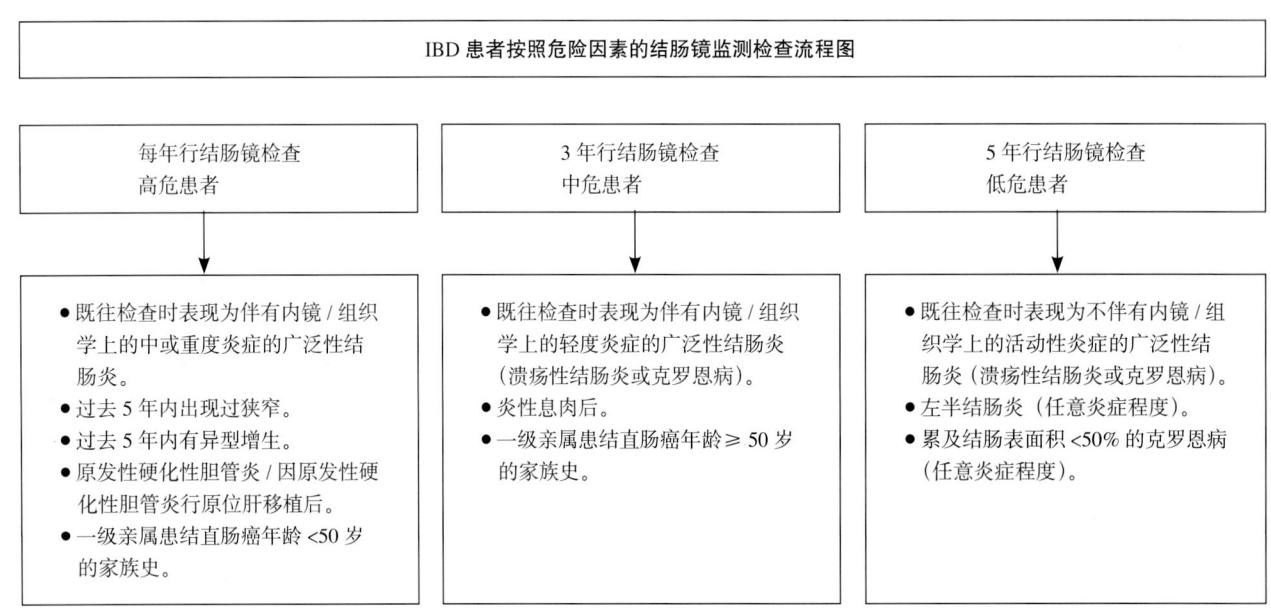

图 19.3 肠易激综合征(IBD)患者的监测指南。UC 溃疡性结肠炎,CD 克罗恩病,CRC 结直肠癌,PSC 原发性硬化性胆管炎(Modified from reference.[61])

参考文献

1. Crohn B, Rosenberg H. The sigmoidoscopic picture of chronic ulcerative colitis. Am J Med Sci. 1925;170:220–8.
2. Warren S, Sommers SC. Cicatrizing enteritis as a pathological entity. Am J Pathol. 1948;24:475–501.
3. Eaden JA, Abrams KR, Mayberry JF. The risk of colorectal cancer in ulcerative colitis: a meta-analysis. Gut. 2001;48:526–35.
4. Winther KV, Jess T, Langholz E, Munkholm P, Binder V. Long term risk of cancer in ulcerative colitis: a population-based cohort study from Copenhagen County. Clin Gastroenterol Hepatol. 2004;2:1088–95.
5. Lakatos L, Mester G, Erdelyi Z, David G, Pandur T, Balogh M, et al. Risk factors for ulcerative colitis-associated colorectal cancer in a Hungarian cohort of patients with ulcerative colitis: results of a population-based study. Inflamm Bowel Dis. 2006;12:205–11.
6. Greenstein AJ, Sachar DB, Smith H, Pucillo A, Papatestas AE, Kreel I, et al. Cancer in universal and left – sided ulcerative colitis: factors determining risk. Gastroenterology. 1979;77:290–4.
7. Gilat T, Fireman Z, Grossman A, Hacohen D, Kadish U, Ron E, Gilat T, Fireman Z, Grossman A, Hacohen D, Kadish U, Ron E. Colorectal cancer in patients with ulcerative colitis. A population study in central Israel. Gastroenterology. 1988;94:870–7.
8. Sugita A, Sachar DB, Bodian C, Ribeiro MB, Aufses Jr AH, Greenstein AJ. Colorectal cancer in ulcerative colitis. Influence of anatomical extent and age at onset on colitis – cancer interval. Gut. 1991;32:167–9.
9. Rutter M, Saunders B, Wilkinson K, Rumbles S, Schofield G, Kamm MA, et al. Thirty-year analysis of a colonoscopic surveillance program for neoplasia in ulcerative colitis. Gastroenterology. 2006;130:1030–8.
10. Lutgens MW, Vleggaar FP, Schipper ME, Stokkers PC, van der Woude CJ, Hommes DW, et al. High frequency of early colorectal cancer in inflammatory bowel disease. Gut. 2008;57:1246–51.
11. Loftus Jr EV. Epidemiology and risk factors for colorectal dysplasia and cancer in ulcerative colitis. Gastroenterol Clin North Am. 2006;35:517–31.
12. Greenstein AJ, Slater G, Heimann TM, Sachar DB, Aufses Jr AH. A comparison of multiple synchronous colorectal cancer in ulcerative colitis, familial polyposis coli, and de novo cancer. Ann Surg. 1986;203:123 8.
13. Ojeda VJ, Mitchell KM, Walters MN-I, Gibson MJ. Primary colorectal linitis plastica type of carcinoma: report of two cases and review of the literature. Pathology. 1982;14:181–9.
14. Levi GS, Harpaz N. Intestinal low-grade tubuloglandular adenocarcinoma in inflammatory bowel disease. Am J Surg Pathol. 2006;30:1022–9.
15. Itzkowitz SH, Harpaz N. Diagnosis and management of dysplasia in patients with inflammatory bowel disease. Gastroenterology. 2004;126:1634–48.
16. Itzkowtiz SH, Yio X. Colorectal cancer in inflammatory bowel disease: the role of inflammation. Am J Physiol Gastrointest Liver Physiol. 2004;287:G7–17.
17. Bernstein CN, Shanahan F, Weinstein WM. Are we telling patients the truth about surveillance colonoscopy in ulcerative colitis? Lancet. 1994;343:71–4.
18. Connell WR, Sheffield JP, Kamm MA, Ritchie JK, Hawley PR, Lennard-Jones JE. Lower gastrointestinal malignancy in Crohn's disease. Gut. 1994;35:347–52.
19. Ullman TA, Loftus Jr EV, Kakar S, Burgart LJ, Sandborn WJ, Tremaine WJ. The fate of low grade dysplasia in ulcerative colitis. Am J Gastroenterol. 2002;97:922–7.
20. Heimann TM, Oh SC, Martinelli G, Szporn A, Luppescu N, Lembo CA, et al. Colorectal carcinoma associated with ulcerative colitis: a study of prognostic indicators. Am J Surg. 1992;164:13–7.
21. Sugita A, Greenstein AJ, Ribeiro MB, Sachar DB, Bodian C, Panday AK, et al. Survival with colorectal cancer in ulcerative colitis: a study of 102 cases. Ann Surg. 1993;218:189–95.
22. Goldstone RN, Itzkowitz SH, Harpaz N, Ullman TA. Left-sided dysplasia progresses more rapidly than right-sided dysplasia to advanced neoplasia (AN) in patients with ulcerative colitis (UC). Gastroenterology. 2010;138:S1, S5, S112.
23. Itzkowitz SH, Present DH. Consensus conference: colorectal cancer screening and surveillance in inflammatory bowel disease. Inflamm Bowel Dis. 2005;11:314–21.
24. Mitchell PJ, Salmo E, Haboubi NY. Inflammatory bowel disease: the problems of dysplasia and surveillance. Tech Coloproctol. 2007;11:299–309.
25. Gyde SN, Prior P, MacCartney JC, Thompson H, Waterhouse JA, Allan RN. Malignancy in Crohn's disease. Gut. 1980;21:1024–9.
26. Rubin DT, Kavitt RT. Surveillance for cancer and dysplasia in inflammatory bowel disease. Gastroenterol Clin North Am. 2006;35:581–604.
27. Farraye FA, Odze RD, Eaden J, Itzkowitz SH, McCabe RP, Dassopoulos T, et al. AGA medical position statement on the diagnosis and management of colorectal neoplasia in inflammatory bowel disease. Gastroenterology. 2010;138:738–45.
28. Jayaram H, Satsangi J, Chapman RW. Increased colorectal neoplasia in chronic ulcerative colitis complicated by primary sclerosing cholangitis: fact or fiction? Gut. 2001;48:430–4.
29. Broome U, Lindberg G, Lofberg R. Primary sclerosing cholangitis in ulcerative colitis – a risk factor for the development of dysplasia and DNA aneuploidy? Gastroenterology. 1992;102:1877–80.
30. Vera A, Gunson BK, Ussatoff V, Nightingale P, Candinas D, Radley S, et al. Colorectal cancer in patients with inflammatory bowel disease after liver transplantation for primary sclerosing cholangitis. Transplantation. 2003;75:1983–8.
31. Ullman T, Odze R, Farraye FA. Diagnosis and management of dysplasia in patients with ulcerative colitis and Crohn's disease of the colon. Inflamm Bowel Dis. 2009;15:630–8.
32. Askling J, Dickman PW, Karlén P, Broström O, Lapidus A, Löfberg R, et al. Family history as a risk factor for colorectal cancer in inflammatory bowel disease. Gastroenterology. 2001;120:1356–62.
33. Rutter M, Saunders B, Wilkinson K, Rumbles S, Schofield G, Kamm M, et al. Severity of inflammation is a risk factor for colorectal neoplasia in ulcerative colitis. Gastroenterology. 2004;126:451–9.
34. Ekbom A, Helmick C, Zack M, Adami HO. Ulcerative colitis and colorectal cancer. A population based study. N Engl J Med. 1990;323:1228–33.
35. Gumaste V, Sachar DB, Greenstein AJ. Benign and malignant colorectal strictures in ulcerative colitis. Gut. 1992;33:938–41.
36. Reiser JR, Waye JD, Janowitz HD, Harpaz N. Adenocarcinoma in strictures of ulcerative colitis without antecedent dysplasia by colonoscopy. Am J Gastroenterol. 1994;89:119–22.
37. Lashner BA, Turner BC, Bostwick DG, Frank PH, Hanauer SB. Dysplasia and cancer complicating strictures in ulcerative colitis. Dig Dis Sci. 1990;35:349–52.
38. Warren R, Barwick KW. Crohn's colitis with adenocarcinoma and dysplasia. Am J Surg Pathol. 1983;7:151–9.
39. Gillen CD, Andrews HA, Prior P, Allan RN. Crohn's disease and colorectal cancer. Gut. 1994;35:651–6.
40. Friedman S. Cancer in Crohn's disease. Gastroenterol Clin North Am. 2006;35:621–39.
41. Ribeiro MB, Greenstein AJ, Sachar DB, Barth J, Balasubramanian S, Harpaz N, et al. Colorectal adenocarcinoma in Crohn's disease. Ann Surg. 1996;223:186–93.
42. Van Assche G. The second European evidence-based consensus on the diagnosis and management of Crohn's disease: special situations. J Crohn's Colitis. 2010;4:63–101.
43. Ekbom A, Helmick C, Zack M, Adami HO. Increased risk of large-bowel cancer in Crohn's disease with colonic involvement. Lancet. 1990;336:357–9.
44. Yamazaki Y, Ribeiro MB, Sachar DB, Aufses Jr AH, Greenstein AJ. Malignant colorectal strictures in Crohn's disease. Am J Gastroenterol. 1991;86:882–5.
45. Stahl TJ, Schoetz DJ, Roberts PL, Coller JA, Murray JJ, Silverman

ML, et al. Crohn's disease and carcinoma: increasing justification for surveillance? Dis Colon Rectum. 1992;35:850–6.
46. Greenstein AJ, Sachar DB, Pucillo A, Kreel I, Geller S, Janowitz HD, et al. Cancer in Crohn's disease after diversionary surgery: a report of seven carcinomas occurring in excluded bowel. Am J Surg. 1978;135:86–90.
47. Riddell RH, Goldman H, Ransohoff DF, Appelman HD, Fenoglio CM, Haggitt RC, et al. Dysplasia in inflammatory bowel disease: standardized classification with provisional clinical applications. Hum Pathol. 1983;14:931–68.
48. Schlemper RJ, Riddell RH, Kato Y, Borchard F, Cooper HS, Dawsey SM, et al. The Vienna classification of gastrointestinal epithelial neoplasia. Gut. 2000;47:251–5.
49. Schlemper RJ, Kato Y, Stolte M. Diagnostic criteria for gastrointestinal carcinomas in Japan and western countries: proposal for a new classification system of gastrointestinal epithelial neoplasia. J Gastroenterol Hepatol. 2000;15:49–57.
50. Schlemper RJ, Iwashita I. Classification of gastrointestinal epithelial neoplasia. Curr Diagn Pathol. 2004;10:128–39.
51. Ullman T, Croog V, Harpaz N, Hossain S, Kornbluth A, Bodian C, et al. Progression to colorectal neoplasia in ulcerative colitis: effect of 5-aminosalicylic acid. Clin Gastroenterol Hepatol. 2008;6:1225–30.
52. Collins RH, Feldman M, Fordman JS. Colon cancer, dysplasia, and surveillance in patients with ulcerative colitis: a critical review. N Engl J Med. 1987;316:1654–8.
53. Connell WR, Lennard-Jones JE, Williams CB, Talbot IC, Price AB, Wilkinson KH. Factors affecting the outcome of endoscopic surveillance for cancer in ulcerative colitis. Gastroenterology. 1994;107:934–44.
54. Dixon NF, Brown LJR, Gilmour HM, Price AB, Smeeton NC, Talbot IC, et al. Observer variation in the assessment of dysplasia of ulcerative colitis. Histopathology. 1988;13:385–98.
55. Dorer R, Odze RD. AMACR immunostaining is useful in detecting dysplastic epithelium in Barrett's esophagus, ulcerative colitis, and Crohn's disease. Am J Surg Pathol. 2006;30:871–7.
56. Rubin CE, Haggitt RC, Burmer GC, Brentnall TA, Stevens AC, Levine DS, et al. DNA aneuploidy in colonic biopsies predicts future development of dysplasia in ulcerative colitis. Gastroenterology. 1992;103:1611–20.
57. Kornbluth A, Sachar DB. Ulcerative colitis practice guidelines in adults (update): American College of Gastroenterology, Practice Parameters Committee. Am J Gastroenterol. 2004;99:1371–85.
58. Eaden JA, Mayberry JF. Guidelines for the screening and surveillance of asymptomatic colorectal cancer in patients with inflammatory bowel disease. Gut. 2002;51:10–2.
59. Bernstein CN, Weinstein WM, Levine DS, Shanahan F. Physicians' perceptions of dysplasia and approaches to surveillance colonoscopy in ulcerative colitis. Am J Gastroenterol. 1995;90:2106–14.
60. Eaden JA, Ward BA, Mayberry JF. How gastroenterologists screen for colonic cancer in ulcerative colitis: an analysis of performance. Gastrointest Endosc. 2000;51:123–8.
61. Cairns SR, Scholefield JH, Steele RJ, Dunlop MG, Thomas HJ, Evans GD. British Society of Gastroenterology; Association of Coloproctology for Great Britain and Ireland. Guidelines for colorectal cancer screening and surveillance in moderate and high risk groups (update from 2002). Gut. 2010;59:666–89.
62. Rutter MD, Saunders BP, Schofield G, Forbes A, Price AB, Talbot IC. Pancolonic indigo carmine dye spraying for the detection of dysplasia in ulcerative colitis. Gut. 2004;53:256–60.
63. Kiesslich R, Fritsch J, Holtmann M, Koehler HH, Stolte M, Kanzler S, et al. Methylene blue-aided chromoendoscopy for the detection of intraepithelial neoplasia and colon cancer in ulcerative colitis. Gastroenterology. 2003;124:880–8.
64. Kiesslich R, Goetz M, Vieth M, Galle PR, Neurath MF. Technology insight: confocal laser endoscopy for in vivo diagnosis of colorectal Cancer. Nat Clin Pract Oncol. 2007;4:480–90.
65. Burmer GC, Rabinovitch PS, Haggitt RC, Crispin DA, Brentnall TA, Kolli VR, et al. Neoplastic progression in ulcerative colitis: histology, DNA content and loss of p53 allele. Gastroenterology. 1992;103:1602–10.
66. Hoque AT, Hahn SA, Schutte M, Kern SE. DPC4 gene mutation in colitis associated neoplasia. Gut. 1997;40:120–2.
67. Umetani N, Sasaki S, Watanabe T, Shinozaki M, Matsuda K, Ishigami H, et al. Genetic alterations in ulcerative colitis-associated neoplasia focusing on APC, K-ras gene and microsatellite instability. Jpn J Cancer Res. 1999;90:1081–7.
68. Schulmann K, Mori Y, Croog V, Yin J, Olaru A, Sterian A, et al. Molecular phenotype of inflammatory bowel disease-associated neoplasms with microsatellite instability. Gastroenterology. 2005;129:74.
69. Herszenyi L, Miheller P, Tulassay Z. Carcinogenesis in inflammatory bowel disease. Dig Dis. 2007;25:267–9.
70. Ullman T, Croog V, Harpaz N, Sachar D, Itzkowitz S. Progression of flat low grade dysplasia to advanced neoplasia in patients with ulcerative colitis. Gastroenterology. 2003;125:1311–9.
71. Lim CH, Dixon MF, Vail A, Forman D, Lynch DA, Axon AT. Ten-year follow-up of ulcerative colitis patients with and without low grade dysplasia. Gut. 2003;52:1127–32.
72. Befrits R, Ljung T, Jaramillo E, Rubio C. Low grade dysplasia in extensive long standing inflammatory bowel disease: a follow up study. Dis Colon Rectum. 2003;45:615–20.
73. Rodriguez SA, Collins JM, Knigge KL, Eisen GM. Surveillance and management of dysplasia in ulcerative colitis. Gastrointest Endosc. 2007;65:432–9.
74. Blackstone MO, Riddell RH, Rogers BH, Levin B. Dysplasia-associated lesion or mass (DALM) detected by colonoscopy in long-standing ulcerative colitis: an indication for colectomy. Gastroenterology. 1981;80:366–74.
75. Rutter M, Saunders B, Wilkinson KH, Rumbles S, Schofield G, Kamm MA, et al. Cancer surveillance in longstanding ulcerative colitis: endoscopic appearances help predict cancer risk. Gut. 2004;53:1813–6.
76. Siegel CA, Schwartz LM, Woloshin S, Cole EB, Rubin DT, Vay T, et al. When should ulcerative colitis patients undergo colectomy for dysplasia? Mismatch between patient preferences and physician recommendations. Inflamm Bowel Dis. 2010;16:1658–62.
77. Odze RD. Pathology of dysplasia and cancer in inflammatory bowel disease. Gastroenterol Clin North Am. 2006;35:533–52.
78. Nugent FW, Haggitt RC, Gilpin PA. Cancer surveillance in ulcerative colitis. Gastroenterology. 1991;100:1241–8.
79. Ludeman L, Shephard NA. Problem areas in the pathology of chronic inflammatory bowel disease. Curr Diagn Pathol. 2006;12:248–60.
80. Goldblum JR. The histologic diagnosis of dysplasia associated lesion or mass, and adenoma. A pathologists' perspective. J Clin Gastroenterol. 2003;36:S63–9.
81. Torres C, Antonioli D, Odze RD. Polypoid dysplasia and adenomas in inflammatory bowel disease; a clinical, pathologic and follow-up study of 89 polyps from 50 patients. Am J Surg Pathol. 1998;22:275–84.
82. Odze RD, Farraye FA, Hecht JL, Hornick JL. Long-term follow-up after polypectomy treatment for adenoma-like dysplastic lesions in ulcerative colitis. Clin Gastroenterol Hepatol. 2004;2:534–41.
83. Rubin PH, Friedman S, Harpaz N, Goldstein E, Weiser J, Schiller J, Present DH. Colonoscopic polypectomy in chronic colitis: conservative management after endoscopic resection of dysplastic polyps. Gastroenterology. 1999;117:1295–300.
84. Engelsgjerd M, Farraye FA, Odze RD. Polypectomy may be adequate treatment for adenoma-like dysplastic lesions in chronic ulcerative colitis. Gastroenterology. 1999;117:1288–94.
85. Odze RD. Adenomas and adenoma-like DALMs in chronic ulcerative colitis: a clinical, pathological, and molecular review. Am J Gastroenterol. 1999;94:1746–50.
86. Rutter CE, Saunders DP, Wilkinson KH, Kamm MA, Williams CB, Forbes A. Most dysplasia in ulcerative colitis is visible at colonoscopy. Gastrointest Endosc. 2004;103:1611–20.
87. Farraye FA, Waye JD, Moscandrew M, Heeren TC, Odze RD. Variability in the diagnosis and management of adenoma-like and non-adenoma-like dysplasia-associated lesions o masses in inflammatory bowel disease: an internet based study. Gastrointest Endosc. 2007;66:519–29.

88. Friedman S, Odze RD, Farraye FA. Management of neoplastic polyps in inflammatory bowel disease. Inflamm Bowel Dis. 2003;9:260–6.
89. van Rijn AF, Fockens P, Siersema PD, Oldenburg B. Adherence to surveillance guidelines for dysplasia and colorectal carcinoma in ulcerative and Crohn's colitis patients in the Netherlands. World J Gastroenterol. 2009;15:226–30.
90. Morson BC, Pang LSC. Rectal biopsy as an aid to cancer control in ulcerative colitis. Gut. 1967;8:423–34.
91. Lennard-Jones JE, Morson BC, Ritchie JK, Williams CB. Cancer surveillance in ulcerative colitis. Experience over 15 years. Lancet. 1983;2:149–52.
92. Choi PM, Nugent FW, Schoetz Jr DJ, Silverman ML, Haggitt RC. Colonoscopic surveillance reduces mortality from colorectal cancer in ulcerative colitis. Gastroenterology. 1993;105:418–24.
93. Karlen P, Kornfeld D, Brostrom O, Löfberg R, Persson PG, Ekbom A. Is colonoscopic surveillance reducing colorectal cancer mortality in ulcerative colitis? A population based case control study. Gut. 1998;42:711–4.
94. Lashner BA, Kane SV, Hanauer SB. Colon cancer surveillance in chronic ulcerative colitis: historical cohort study. Am J Gastroenterol. 1990;85:1083–7.
95. Collins PD, Mpofu C, Watson AJ, Rhodes JM. Strategies for detecting colon cancer and/or dysplasia in patients with inflammatory bowel disease. Cochrane Database Syst Rev. 2006:CD000279.
96. Lutgens MW, Oldenburg B, Siersema PD, van Bodegraven AA, Dijkstra G, Hommes DW, et al. Colonoscopic surveillance improves survival after colorectal cancer diagnosis in inflammatory bowel disease. Br J Cancer. 2009;17(101):1671–5.
97. Friedman S, Rubin PH, Bodian C, Harpaz N, Present DH. Screening and surveillance colonoscopy in chronic Crohn's colitis: results of a surveillance program spanning 25 years. Clin Gastroenterol Hepatol. 2008;6:993–8.
98. Friedman S, Rubin PH, Bodian C, Goldstein E, Harpaz N, Present DH. Screening and surveillance colonoscopy in chronic Crohn's colitis. Gastroenterology. 2001;120:820–6.
99. Parks AG, Nicholls RJ. Proctocolectomy without ileostomy for ulcerative colitis. Br Med J. 1978;2:85–8.
100. Fazio VW, Ziv Y, Church JM, Oakley JR, Lavery IC, Milsom JW, et al. Ileal pouch-anal anastomoses complications and function in 1005 patients. Ann Surg. 1995;222:120–7.
101. Meagher AP, Farouk R, Dozois RR, Kelly KA, Pemberton JH. J ileal pouch-anal anastomosis for chronic ulcerative colitis: complications and long-term outcome in 1310 patients. Br J Surg. 1998;85:800–3.
102. O'Riordan MG, Fazio VW, Lavery IC, Remzi F, Fabbri N, Meneu J, et al. Incidence and natural history of dysplasia of the anal transitional zone after ileal pouch-anal anastomosis: results of a five-year to ten-year follow-up. Dis Colon Rectum. 2000;43:1660–5.
103. Gorgun E, Remzi FH, Feza H, Preen M, Shen B, Fazio VW. Surgical outcome in patients with primary sclerosing cholangitis undergoing ileal pouch-anal anastomosis: a case–control study. Surgery. 2005;138:631–7.
104. Gullberg K, Stahlberg D, Liljeqvist L, Tribukait B, Reinholt FP, Veress B. Neoplastic transformation of the pelvic pouch mucosa in patients with ulcerative colitis. Gastroenterology. 1997;112:1487–92.
105. Duff SE, O'Dwyer ST, Hultén L, Willén R, Haboubi NY. Dysplasia in the ileo-anal pouch. Colorectal Dis. 2002;4:420–9.
106. Silverberg M, Satsangi J, Ahmad T, Arnott ID, Bernstein CN, Brant SR. Toward an integrated clinical, molecular and serological classification of inflammatory bowel disease: report of a working party of the 2005 Montreal World Congress of Gastroenterology. Can J Gastroenterol. 2005;19(Suppl A):1A–32.

第 20 章　再次手术行贮袋肛管吻合术的手术注意事项

Feza H. Remzi · Hasan T. Kirat
李　毅译　李　宁审校

摘　要

复原性结肠直肠切除伴回肠贮袋肛管吻合术对于溃疡性结肠炎患者和大多数家族性腺瘤性息肉病患者来说是首选的手术方式。回肠贮袋肛管吻合术后最常见的并发症包括盆腔脓毒症、贮袋炎和肠梗阻，其中任何一种都有可能导致贮袋坏死。累计贮袋坏死率介于 1 年 2% 至 10 年 9% 之间。然而，一个"失败的"贮袋能够通过再次手术挽救，这包括了经肛、经腹或两者相结合的方法。这些挽救过程与可接受的结果有关，我们也讨论了其适应征和相关的治疗决策。

关键词

再次手术；复原性结肠直肠切除术；回肠贮袋肛管吻合术（IPAA）；溃疡性结肠炎；家族性腺瘤性息肉病

引　言

克利夫兰诊所的方法

复原性结肠直肠切除伴回肠贮袋肛管吻合术（IPAA）对于溃疡性结肠炎患者和需要手术的家族性腺瘤性息肉病患者来说是常选择的术式（图 20.1）[1-2]。J 形贮袋吻合的 IPAA 是首选技术（图 20.2）[2-3]。在我们机构里，当 J 形贮袋不能无张力地进入骨盆时，我们常选择 S 形贮袋（图 20.3）。对于那些有异型增生、低位直肠癌或吻合器吻合失败的患者，我们常选择手工缝合（图 20.4）。据报道，绝大多数行 IPAA 的患者有良好的功能预后和生活质量（QOL）评分[4]。这种方法的早期和晚期并发症发生率分别为 27% 和 50%[4]。

感染性并发症是最常见的短期问题，而贮袋炎和小肠梗阻是最常遇到的长期问题[4-5]。虽然随着治疗策略的改进，并发症发生率已经有所下降[5]，这些并发症仍有可能导致贮袋坏死。盆腔脓毒症和克罗恩病被认为是贮袋坏死的主要独立预测指标[6]，并且已经有人设计出一种特殊的回肠贮袋坏死模型来预测失败的总体风险[7]。据报道，贮袋坏死的累积概率在 1 年时为 2%，5 年时为 5%，10 年时为 9%[5]。失败的贮袋可以通过切除或不切除贮袋的再次手术进行挽救，从而避免永久性回肠造口[8-31]。这些手术方式带来的结果令人鼓舞：大多数患者能够获得与初次行 IPAA 相似的贮袋功能和生活质量。

IPAA 失败后的再次手术

IPAA 失败后的再次手术包括经肛、经腹或两者联合的方式。报道中最常见的经腹方式的成功结果显示在表 20.1 中。脓毒症是修正性贮袋手术的主要适应证，因为这是贮袋阴道瘘的一个可怕的并

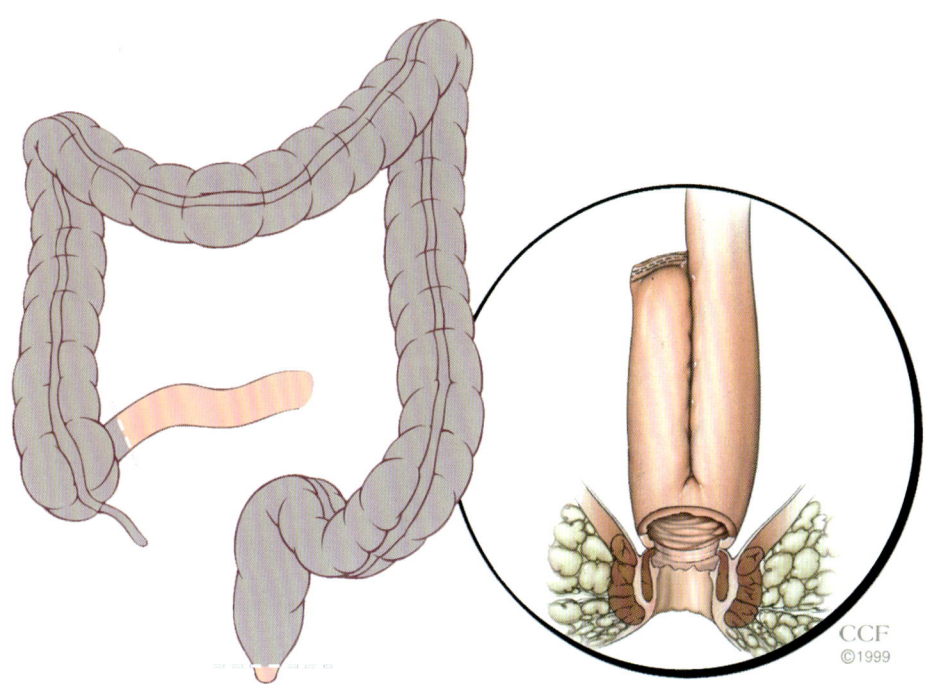

图 20.1 复原性结肠直肠切除伴回肠贮袋肛管吻合术（Copyright CCF. Reprinted by permission of Cleveland Clinic Foundation）

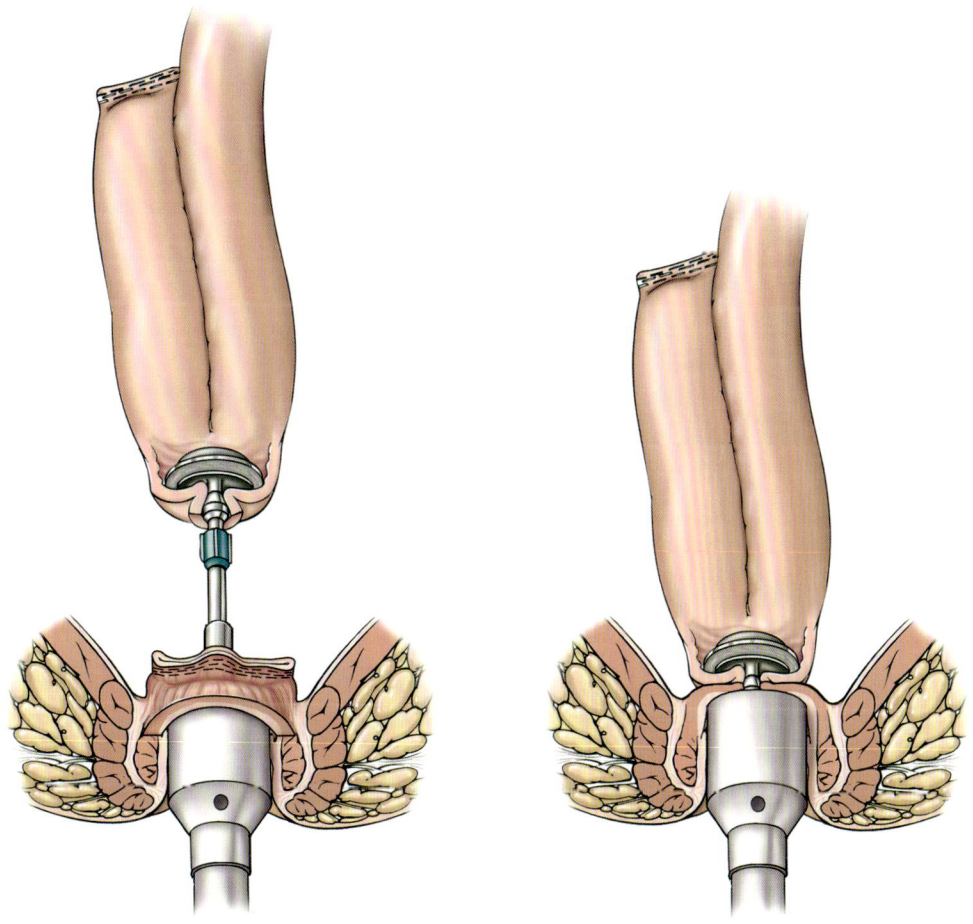

图 20.2 吻合器吻合的 J 形贮袋回肠贮袋肛管吻合术（Copyright CCF. Reprinted by permission of Cleveland Clinic Foundation）

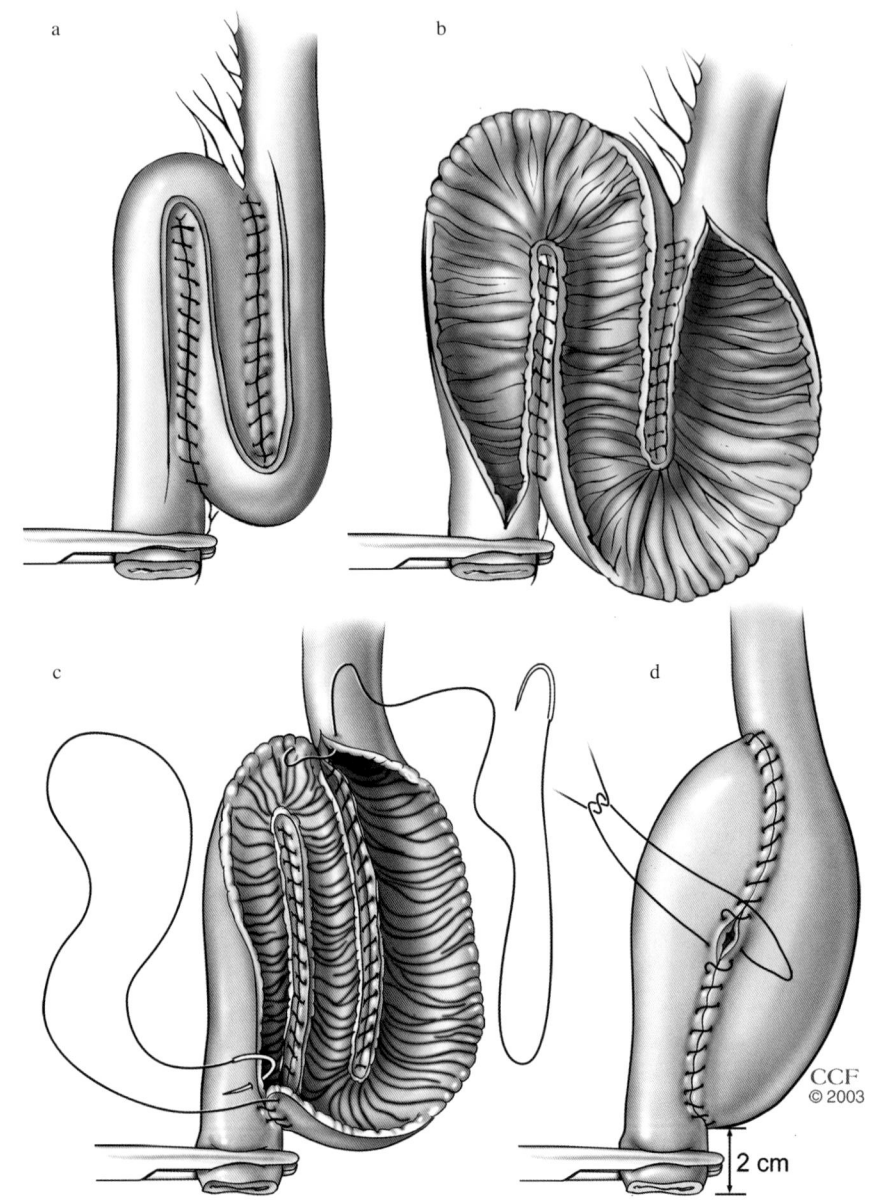

图 20.3 S 形贮袋的建立（a 和 b）通过近似环形的连续浆肌层缝合构建 S 形的贮袋，然后行 S 形的肠切开术。（c 和 d）从袋内连续缝合关闭两个后吻合口，接着通过连续浆肌层缝合关闭前壁（Copyright CCF. Reprinted by permission of Cleveland Clinic Foundation）

发症，即使许多研究显示这伴随着通过贮袋挽回及可接受的长期功能结果和生活质量的精心挑选的病例。

在一系列包含有 114 例 IPAA 术后需要再次手术患者中，Galandiuk 等[9]使用了包括肛门局部技术在内的多种方法来治疗感染性并发症，如挂线引流术治疗肛周脓肿，剖腹探查腹腔脓肿引流术或正式的贮袋重建术。2/3 的患者获得了贮袋功能的恢复，其中 70% 最终有"优秀的临床和功能预后"。这组研究中 20% 患者最终需要贮袋切除，最常见原因是持续的盆腔脓毒症。在另一项 Johnson 等[24]的加拿大报道中，在 22 例因贮袋 - 阴道瘘需行贮袋修复术的患者中，50% 在再次术后痊愈。经腹手术方法的成功率应用于这种瘘修补时似乎高于应用于后会阴修补时。在这方面，Shah 等[22]也报道了 60 例因贮袋阴道瘘需再次手术患者的结果，其中有 28% 有持续的盆腔脓毒症。手术方式包括局部修复，如回肠推进皮瓣（39 例）和腹部再次手术 / 再次吻合术。在中位数为 49 个月的随访之后，整体治愈率为 52%，而在 16 例再次行 IPAA 手术的患者中，成

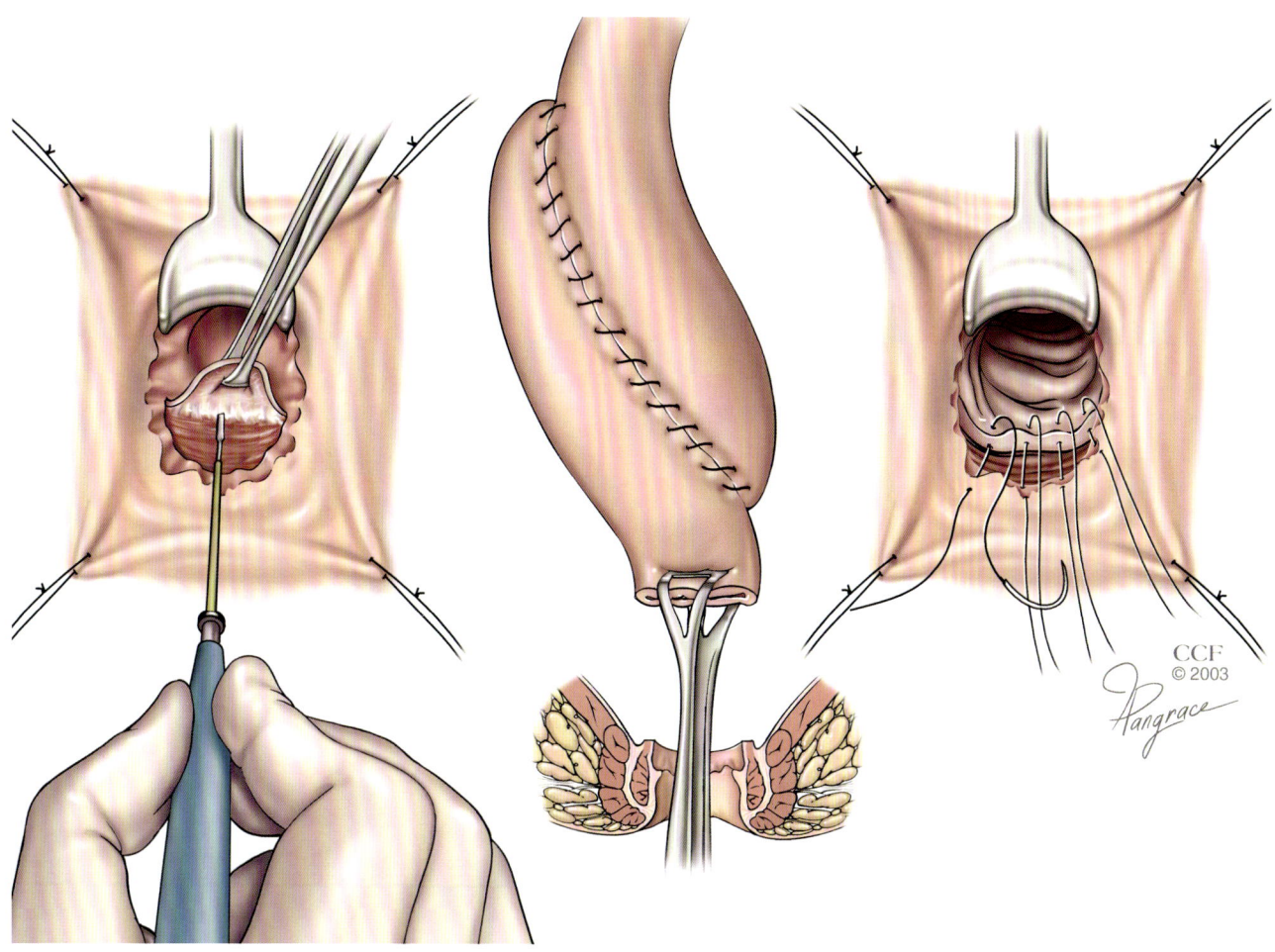

图 20.4 手工缝合回肠贮袋肛管吻合术（Copyright CCF. Reprinted by permission of Cleveland Clinic Foundation）

表 20.1 经腹再次贮袋手术的成功报道

研究者	年份	患者（数量）	成功率（%）
Liljeqvist 和 Lindquist[8]	1985	7	86
Nicholls 和 Gilbert[10]	1990	5	100
Fazio 等[15]	1998	35	86
Cohen 等[14]	1998	24	79
Fonkalsrud 和 Bustorff-Silva[16]	1999	90	95
Dayton[17]	2000	16	100
MacLean 等[20]	2002	57	74
Heuschen 等[21]	2002	39	未列出
Shah 等[22]	2003	16	62
Dehni 等[25]	2005	45	93
Baixauli 等[23]	2004	100	75
Tekkis 等[26]	2006	112	79
Mathis 等[30]	2009	51	89
Shawki 等[28]	2009	23	69
Remzi 等[27]	2009	241	85

功率为62%。24例患者最终修正诊断为克罗恩病，他们的治愈率也相对较低。类似的是，Zmora等[18]也报道在延误诊断为克罗恩病的患者中，再次手术行贮袋切除的概率很高。

在Cohen等报道[14]的包含有24例行再次手术患者的研究中，一半是因为贮袋阴道瘘。虽然该研究中的患者在再次手术前平均接受了2.9次局部拯救手术，超过75%的再次手术病例最终获得了良好的预后。Cohen等因此总结，对于局部手术失败的患者，可以行根治性的重建手术，这能带来可接受的结果。在另一项包含了27例接受贮袋拯救手术病例的英国文献中，盆腔脓毒症是修补术后失败的主要原因。有人建议拯救手术最好用于没有伴发不可控盆腔脓毒症的病例。这一结论得到了由Tekkis等报道的含有112例腹部再次手术病例的支持[26]，该研究提示5年成功率与非脓毒症适应证而不是脓毒症并发症有关。相反，Fazio等[15]报道因脓毒症并发症行再次IPAA手术的患者6个月后成功率为95%。这些结论与Dehni等[25]报道的含有64例再次手术者的结果相似，他们使用了经肛或经腹会阴的手术方式；绝大多数（47例）因脓毒症问题行修补术，尽管如此，94%的患者在最近一次随访时有具功能性的贮袋。普遍认为脓毒症具有高风险，是手术修补贮袋的主要适应证，并且我们最近一篇含有241例患者的报道确定了因感染性并发症行腹部再次手术的患者与因非感染性并发症行修补术的患者相比，成功率相似。

在以术后脓毒症为主要适应证的再次手术病例中，贮袋存活率约为3/4[20]，在由IPAA阴道瘘造成的贮袋坏死患者中，推荐首先采用腹会阴重建方法。然而这依赖于一部分需要修补术的患者；也有报道采用较小的手术会带来相对低的贮袋坏死率（6.1%），而较大的手术修补术后贮袋切除率较高（10.8%）。

对于因IPAA术后机械性梗阻或保留直肠残端引起的贮袋功能障碍，再次手术也能带来好的预后。在一个包含7例因S形贮袋有长的、扭曲的输出袢造成位置不正，进而引起贮袋坏死的报道中[8]（图20.5），患者表现为显著的排便困难。在腹会阴修补手术时，贮袋及其输出肠管被松解，输出袢被截短。然后贮袋被放置在靠近肛门的位置，一个正式的重建IPAA就成形了。6例患者（86%）手术获得成功。类似的，Nicholls和Gilbert[10]鉴定

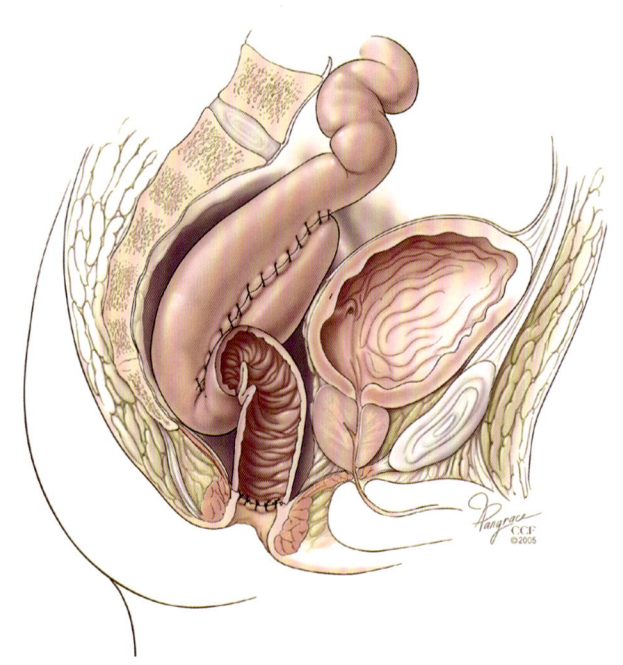

图20.5 输出袢梗阻（Copyright CCF. Reprinted by permission of Cleveland Clinic Foundation）

了41例因输出袢过长引起症状的患者。其中6例需要修补手术。在所有需要手术的患者中输出袢长度至少8cm。他们切除了这一输出袢并再次实施了吻合术。在3例行经肛手术的患者中，2例失败，这2例加上另3例行经腹会阴再次手术。所有6例患者最终控制和排便功能都得到了改善。在这方面，Herbst等[11]描述了16例IPAA后机械性梗阻的患者，其中11例输出袢过长、肛门直肠袖套过长或两者兼有，另5例IPAA吻合术后存在持续性狭窄。在他们的报道中，贮袋被松解并从吻合口拆除，并经腹手术再次行IPAA成形术。12例患者（75%）的出口梗阻明显改善。在另一Fonkalsrud和Bustorff-Silva的研究中[16]，164例回肠贮袋慢性功能不全的患者施行了经肛切除术、腹会阴重建术或新贮袋成形术，各自成功率分别为98%、92%和86%。

IPAA术后输入袢梗阻的患者也可能出现贮袋功能障碍并需要手术治疗（图20.6）。Read等[13]报道了6例因输入袢梗阻进而引起无法解决的梗阻而施行剖腹探查术的患者。在这些患者中，从回肠末端到贮袋行梗阻节段的旁路手术是有效的，但推荐再行一个额外的"贮袋固定术"，因为存在输入袢再次成角的风险。在我们机构的18例输入袢梗阻的患者中，主要表现为间断性的梗阻症状[31]。9例

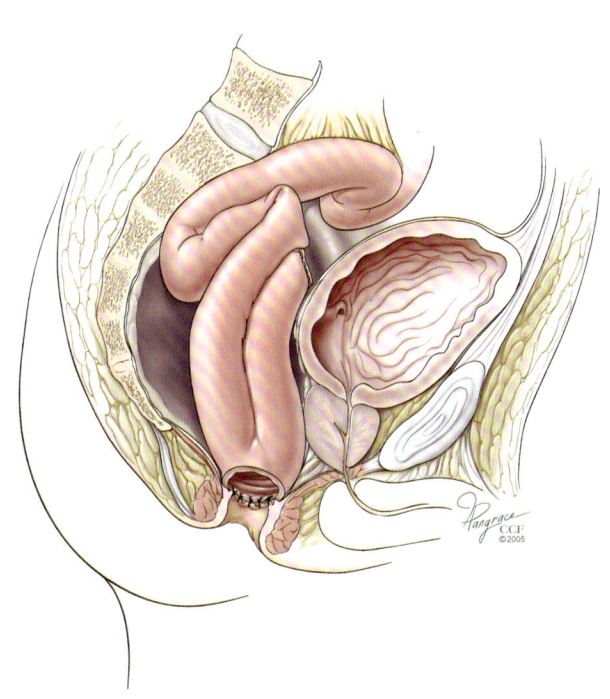

图 20.6 输入袢梗阻（Copyright CCF. Reprinted by permission of Cleveland Clinic Foundation）

行输入袢经验性球囊扩张，另 8 例行修复手术。1 例未采取任何干预。我们认为输入袢梗阻患者通常需要治疗，这与整体良好的预后有关。

初次吻合器吻合的 IPAA 术后保留的直肠残端也许会造成持续的症状，通常需要修复手术。在这方面，Tulchinsky 等[19]鉴别了 22 例因 IPAA 术后保留直肠残端行经腹会阴再次手术的患者。15 例患者（68%）术后的贮袋功能和生活质量有了主观改善，虽然在中位数为 22.5 个月的随访后发现，5 例患者最终需要切除贮袋并行永久性造口。

克利夫兰诊所的经验

我们机构的最近一篇大样本研究包含了自 1983 年－2007 年 241 例行再次贮袋手术的患者[27]。经腹或经腹会阴手术方式都有使用。如果拆除了贮袋，我们通常采用手工缝合重建吻合，经常行分流回肠造口术或在原位留一个造口。59% 的研究对象是女性，67% 因初次 IPAA 术后并发症由其他机构转至我们这里。初次 IPAA 距再次贮袋手术的中位时间是 4.4 年。132 例患者再次手术的适应证是脓毒症，109 例是非感染性并发症。拯救性手术后，172 例（71%）的最终诊断是溃疡性结肠炎，其中 71 例（29%）作为修复手术的一部分有了新的贮袋。在 170 例患者中，已存在的贮袋通过贮袋修复 / 修改 / 扩张能够挽救。6 例再次行修改手术，另有 20 例因为初次挽救手术失败而行贮袋切除术。中位数为 5 年的随访显示整体贮袋挽救率为 85%。贮袋有功能的患者平均排便次数是 7.9 次，63% 的患者从来没有或很少反映失禁。绝大多数患者称如有必要，他们愿意行再次手术，并且愿意推荐给其他患者。

该研究中患者的功能预后和生活质量与初次行 IPAA 的患者做了比较。与初次行 IPAA 的患者相比，这些患者在白天和夜间渗液更多，白天使用垫子的比例更高。两组患者的排便次数、里急后重或失禁的比例、手术后的身体限制及所有的生活质量评分都相似。我们总结认为，使用经腹再次手术方式是一合适的替换，因为它有良好的临床及功能结果。

吻合口瘘是再次行贮袋手术的一种常见适应证。对于转流的患者，我们的方法是在麻醉下（EUA）进行检查，并经缺损部位用一个小蘑菇头导管行经肛 / 经吻合口盆腔脓肿引流。然后我们在接下来的 6 ～ 12 个月里每 8 ～ 10 周定期行麻醉下检查和泛影葡胺灌肠，以检查瘘口及盆腔涉及部位的愈合情况。蘑菇头导管通常在急性发作期消退后或脓腔缩小到不再需要，或无法使用导管引流后拔除。在这 6 ～ 12 个月的阶段之后，如果病理治愈了（图 20.7a-d），我们再行回肠造口封闭。当无法完全愈合时，如果有小的骶前窦道，我们在告知患者有再发感染可能后封闭回肠造口。有小的骶前窦道和大的引流腔道且脓腔清楚，患者往往预后较好，并且转流性回肠造口可以关闭。更进一步的，脓腔被黏膜上皮覆盖的患者常常预后较好，可以关闭造口。然而，如果引流 9 ～ 12 个月后，仍有大脓腔及大的骶前窦道持续存在，我们会行经腹再次手术。

图 20.8 显示的是基于克利夫兰诊所经验推荐的对 IPAA 术后伴有盆腔脓毒症的吻合口瘘的治疗方法。修复手术治疗慢性吻合口瘘 / 窦道的成功关键是在经腹会阴分离 IPAA 后清除慢性蜂窝组织炎 / 脓腔（图 20.9）。重要的是要注意外科医师要做好再次贮袋手术的术中和术后面对意外情况的准备。在行这种大手术之前，患者应当同意有行永久性回肠造口术或套叠乳头法手术的可能[32-33]。对于一个有修复手术经验的积极的外科医师治疗下的积极的患者来说，经腹会阴再次手术可能是个好的选择。

手术时，应当使用输尿管支架，并预备血制品。

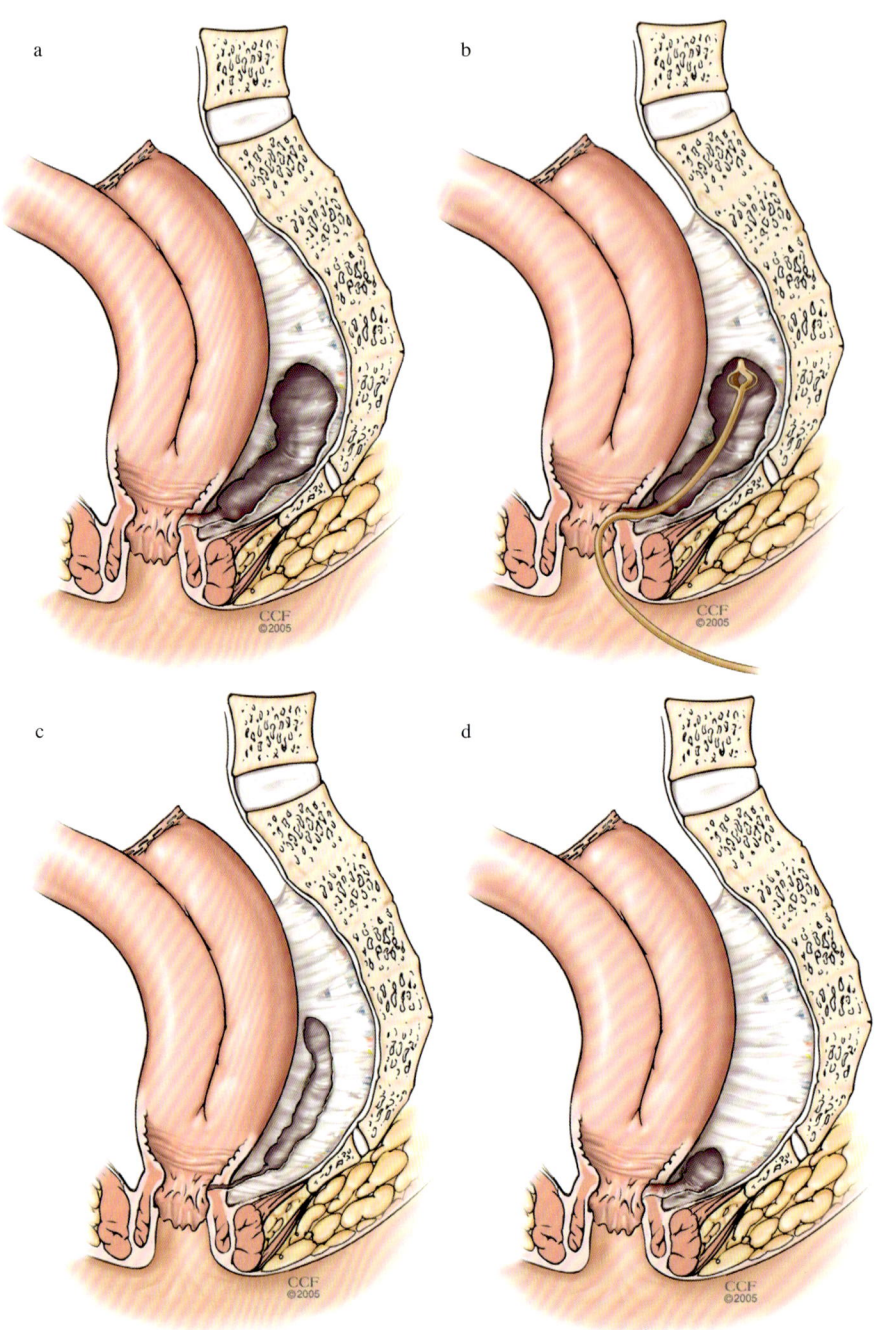

图 20.7 （a–d）经过 6～12 个月后吻合口瘘伴骶前脓肿的愈合过程。（b）经缺损部位用一个小蘑菇头导管行经肛/经吻合口引流；（c）急性发作期消退后撤除蘑菇头导管；（d）脓腔大小缩小到不再需要到管引流（Copyright CCF. Reprinted by permission of Cleveland Clinic Foundation）

如果患者在初次行 IPAA 时没有行转流术，在考虑行修复手术以最小的死亡率获得最优的预后机会之前，施行 3～6 个月的转流回肠造口术也许有益。由于局部挽救手术与经腹再次手术相比两者的成功率存在争议，因此首先尝试局部手术是可以接受的；然而，重复局部手术的滥用对确定性经腹会阴手术的预后有不利影响。

有些在初次 IPAA 术后出现技术性并发症的患者也许会被误诊为克罗恩病。我们机构的一项研究[29]调查了变更诊断为克罗恩病并行再次贮袋手术的患者的结果[32]。值得注意的是所有患者在修复手术之前都接受了针对克罗恩病的治疗。再次手术的适应证包括内瘘、盆腔脓毒症、外瘘、狭窄、憩室炎、输出袢过长和保留了直肠残端。在中位数为

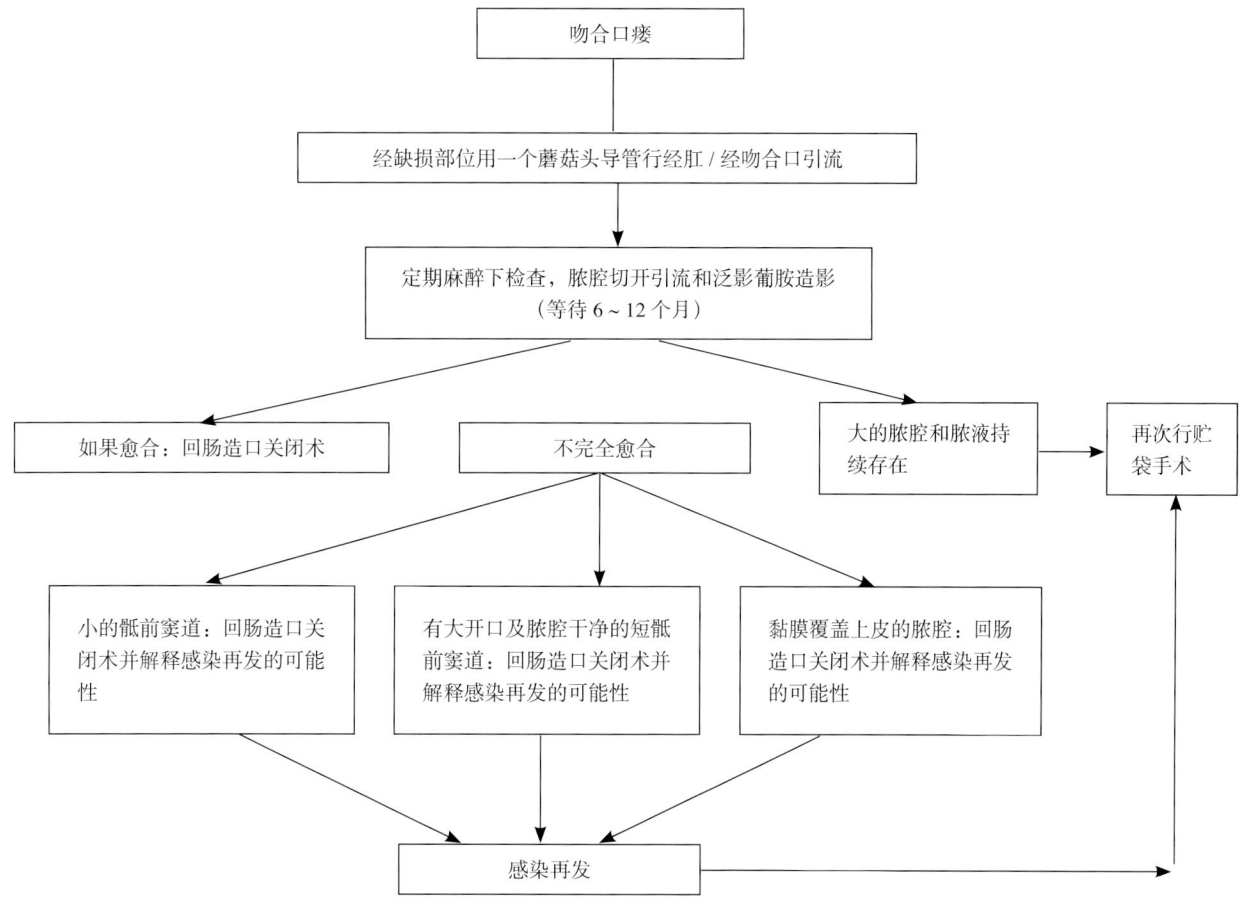

图 20.8　回肠贮袋肛管吻合术后吻合口瘘的推荐治疗流程。EUA：麻醉下检查，I&D 切开引流，GGE：泛影葡胺造影

1.7 年随访中，总体贮袋存活率为 84.8%。只有 7 例最终病理诊断为克罗恩病，其中两例发展为贮袋坏死。因此得出的结论是，IPAA 术后变更诊断为克罗恩病的患者应当再次评估，因为他们常常不是克罗恩病，并会从再次贮袋手术中获益[34]。

J 形贮袋尖端瘘很罕见（图 20.10）；但是，有报道认为这是贮袋坏死的一个原因[35]。我们机构最近的一篇报道[36]包括了 27 例 J 形贮袋尖端瘘的患者。这些病例中，14 例为男性，10 例在外院行初次 IPAA。22 例最终病理诊断为溃疡性结肠炎；21 例在术前被诊断瘘。25 例患者行再次手术治疗，一部分（23 例）直接从 J 形贮袋尖端行修补术（图 20.11 和图 20.12），另一部分（2 例）建立了新的贮袋。1 例在 CT 引导下引流成功，另 1 例需要行贮袋切除和永久造口。在平均 3.2 年的随访后，24 例患者贮袋有功能。这 24 例患者与初次 IPAA 术后没有并发症并获得功能性预后和生活质量参数的患者相一致。两组患者的贮袋功能和所有生活质量评分都相似。我们因此总结，对于 J 形贮袋尖端瘘的患者，剖腹探查术修补瘘口是有必要的，并且这种方式能够保留贮袋，带来好的预后。

伴或不伴回肠肛管贮袋切除的永久性回肠造口术

伴或不伴贮袋切除的永久性回肠造口术是重建手术的一种选择。当实施永久性回肠造口术时，面临的问题是贮袋是否应被切除或留在原位。我们机构最近的一项研究[33]旨在比较贮袋切除和贮袋留在原位（LI）的永久转流术患者的手术预后和长期生活质量。纳入了贮袋留在原位（31 例）和贮袋切除（105 例）的 136 例贮袋坏死的患者。两组患者的一般情况、病程、诊断和随访时间一致。贮袋坏死最常见的原因是感染性并发症；贮袋留在原位组有 15 例（48%）发生，而贮袋切除组有 39 例（33%）发生。

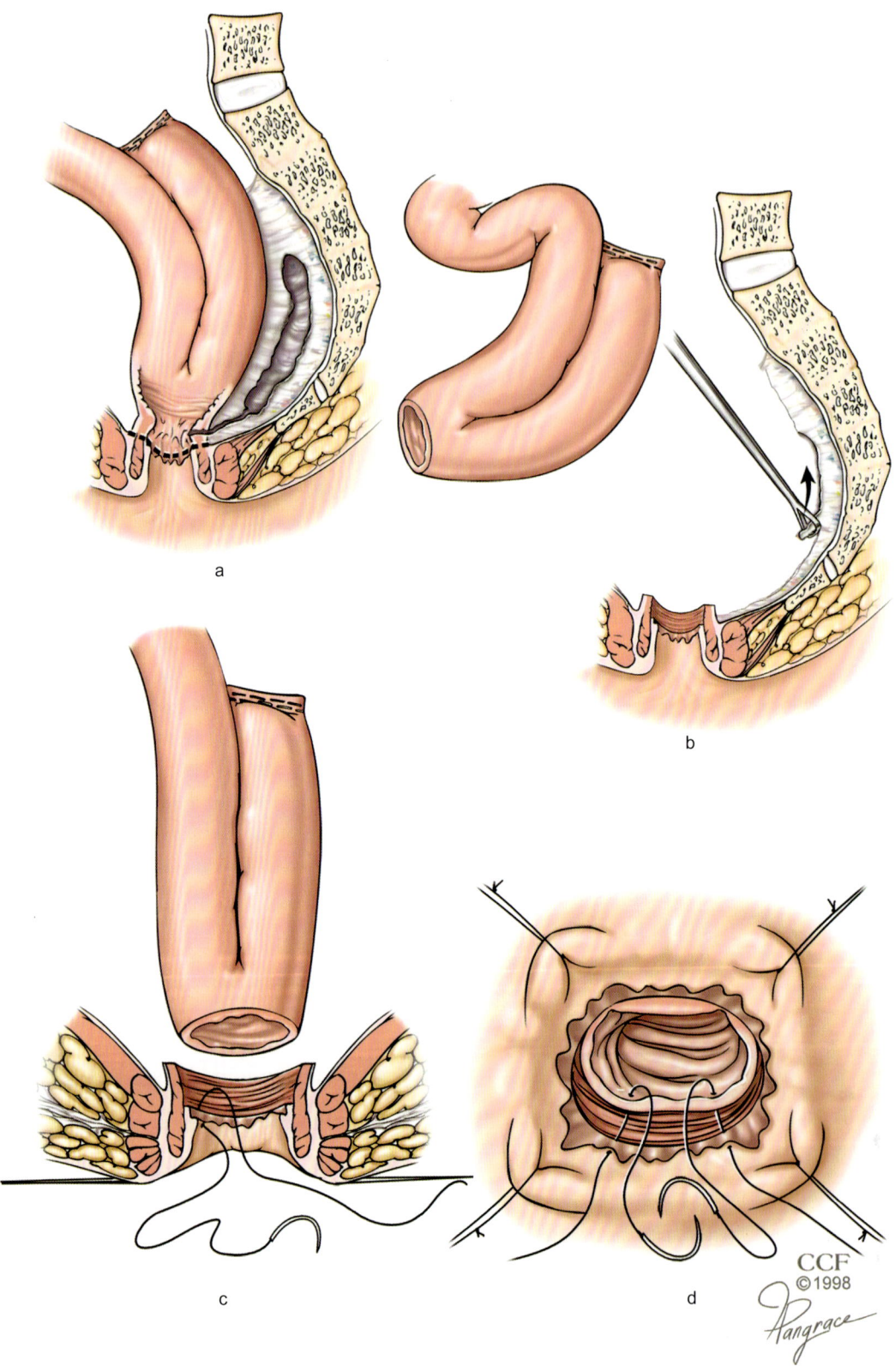

图20.9 对于慢性吻合口瘘/窦道行贮袋松解，慢性蜂窝组织炎/脓腔清创以及手工缝合再造回肠贮袋肛管吻合术。（a）慢性吻合口瘘/窦道；（b）贮袋松解，慢性蜂窝组织炎/脓腔清创；（c和d）手工缝合再造回肠贮袋肛管吻合术（Copyright CCF. Reprinted by permission of Cleveland Clinic Foundation）

第 20 章 再次手术行贮袋肛管吻合术的手术注意事项

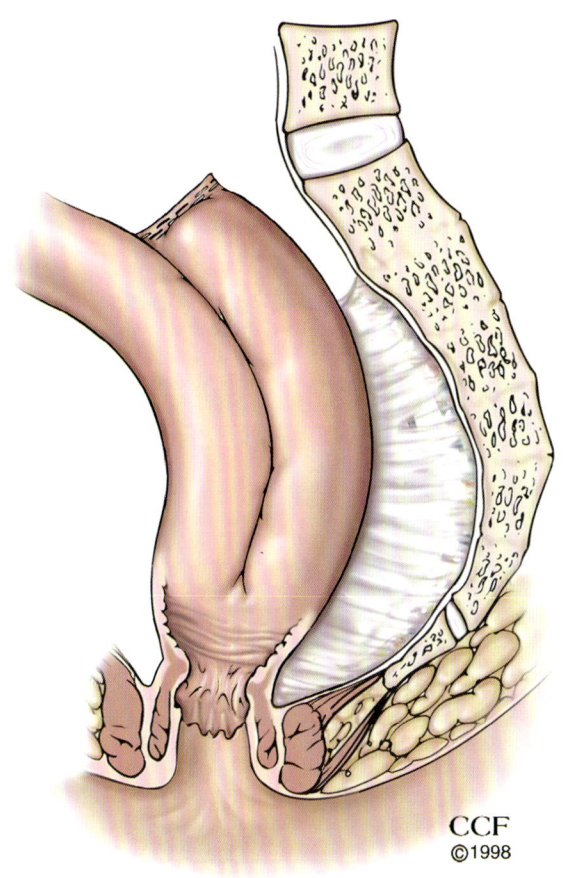

图 20.10　J 形贮袋尖端瘘（Copyright CCF. Reprinted by permission of Cleveland Clinic Foundation）

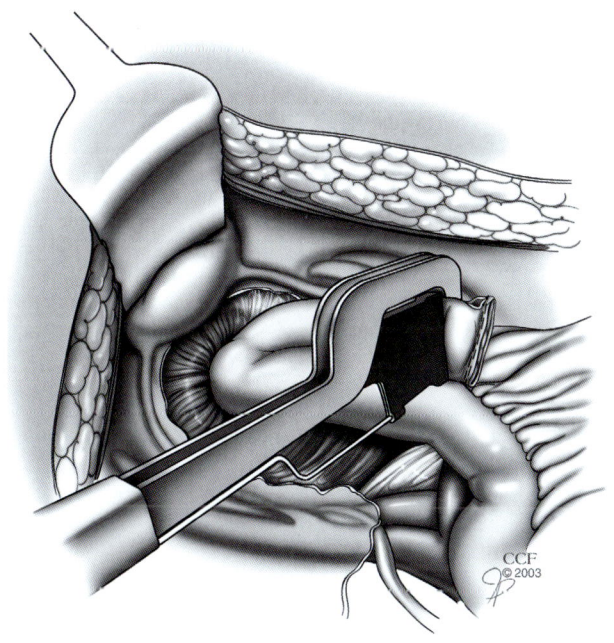

图 20.11　吻合器修复 J 形贮袋尖端瘘（Copyright CCF. Reprinted by permission of Cleveland Clinic Foundation）

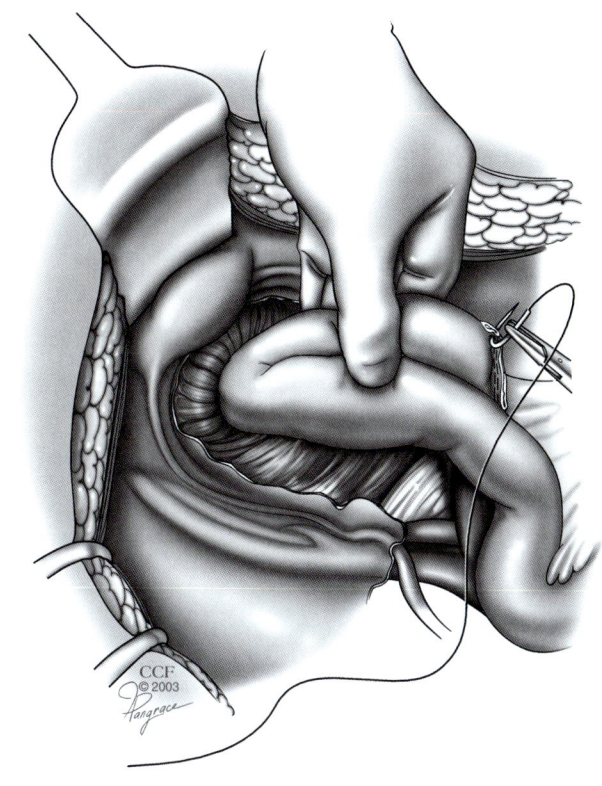

图 20.12　手工缝合修复 J 形贮袋尖端瘘（Copyright CCF. Reprinted by permission of Cleveland Clinic Foundation）

两组术后 30 天死亡率相似。在行贮袋和肛门移行区（ATZ）监测检查的 18 例贮袋保留组患者中未见异型增生或肿瘤。在中位数为 9.9 年的随访后发现，贮袋切除组患者的生活质量和健康状况，包括目前能量代谢水平、克利夫兰整体生活质量评分和 12 项短形式的身体心理组成参数都要显著高于贮袋保留组。此外，贮袋保留组有些患者在长期随访中反馈肛门疼痛（4 例）和使用防渗垫（8 例）。我们因此认为贮袋切除比贮袋保留在手术技术上更具挑战性；但是，如果患者在 IPAA 术后出现贮袋坏死时不再追求肠道连续性的修复，贮袋切除是更好的选择，因为其长期生活质量比贮袋保留更好。

结　论

贮袋坏死对于 IPAA 术后患者来说是个可怕的问题。但是，选择性的贮袋坏死修复手术可能会带来较好的预后。当在局部挽救尝试后并发症仍持续存在时，不管手术适应证是感染性或非感染性并发症，经腹会阴手术方式都是一个可行的选择。

参考文献

1. Parks AG, Nicholls RJ. Proctocolectomy without ileostomy for ulcerative colitis. Br Med J. 1978;2:85–8.
2. Fazio VW, O'Riordain MG, Lavery IC, Church JM, Lau P, Strong SA, Hull T. Long-term functional outcome and quality of life after stapled restorative proctocolectomy. Ann Surg. 1999;230:575–84.
3. Kirat HT, Remzi FH, Kiran RP, Fazio VW. Comparison of outcomes after hand-sewn versus stapled ileal pouch-anal anastomosis in 3,109 patients. Surgery. 2009;146:723–9.
4. Fazio VW, Ziv Y, Church JM, Oakley JR, Lavery IC, Milsom JW, et al. Ileal pouch-anal anastomosis: complications and function in 1005 patients. Ann Surg. 1995;222:120–7.
5. Meagher AP, Farouk R, Dozois RR, Kelly KA, Pemberton JH. J ileal pouch-anal anastomosis for chronic ulcerative colitis: complications and long-term outcome in 1310 patients. Br J Surg. 1998;85:800–3.
6. Forbes SS, O'Connor BI, Victor JC, Cohen Z, McLeod RS. Sepsis is a major predictor of failure after ileal pouch-anal anastomosis. Dis Colon Rectum. 2009;52:1975–81.
7. Fazio VW, Tekkis PP, Remzi F, Lavery IC, Manilich E, Connor J, et al. Quantification of risk for pouch failure after ileal pouch anal anastomosis surgery. Ann Surg. 2003;238:605–17.
8. Liljeqvist L, Lindquist K. A reconstructive operation on malfunctioning S-shaped pelvic reservoirs. Dis Colon Rectum. 1985;28:506–11.
9. Galandiuk S, Scott NA, Dozois RR, Kelly KA, Ilstrup DM, Beart Jr RW. Ileal pouch-anal anastomosis. Reoperation for pouch-related complications. Ann Surg. 1990;212:446–54.
10. Nicholls RJ, Gilbert JM. Surgical correction of the efferent ileal limb for disordered defaecation following restorative proctocolectomy with the S ileal reservoir. Br J Surg. 1990;77:152–4.
11. Herbst F, Sielezneff I, Nicholls RJ. Salvage surgery for ileal pouch outlet obstruction. Br J Surg. 1996;83:368–71.
12. Ogunbiyi OA, Korsgen S, Keighley MR. Pouch salvage. Long-term outcome. Dis Colon Rectum. 1997;40:548–52.
13. Read TE, Schoetz Jr DJ, Marcello PW, Roberts PL, Coller JA, Murray JJ, et al. Afferent limb obstruction complicating ileal pouch-anal anastomosis. Dis Colon Rectum. 1997;40:566–9.
14. Cohen Z, Smith D, McLeod R. Reconstructive surgery for pelvic pouches. World J Surg. 1998;22:342–6.
15. Fazio VW, Wu JS, Lavery IC. Repeat ileal pouch-anal anastomosis to salvage septic complications of pelvic pouches: clinical outcome and quality of life assessment. Ann Surg. 1998;228:588–97.
16. Fonkalsrud EW, Bustorff-Silva J. Reconstruction for chronic dysfunction of ileoanal pouches. Ann Surg. 1999;229:197–204.
17. Dayton MT. Redo ileal pouch-anal anastomosis for malfunctioning pouches-acceptable alternative to permanent ileostomy? Am J Surg. 2000;180:561–5.
18. Zmora O, Efron JE, Nogueras JJ, Weiss EG, Wexner SD. Reoperative abdominal and perineal surgery in ileoanal pouch patients. Dis Colon Rectum. 2001;44:1310–4.
19. Tulchinsky H, McCourtney JS, Rao KV, Chambers W, Williams J, Wilkinson KH, et al. Salvage abdominal surgery in patients with a retained rectal stump after restorative proctocolectomy and stapled anastomosis. Br J Surg. 2001;88(12):1602–6.
20. MacLean AR, O'Connor B, Parkes R, Cohen Z, McLeod RS. Reconstructive surgery for failed ileal pouch-anal anastomosis: a viable surgical option with acceptable results. Dis Colon Rectum. 2002;45:880–6.
21. Heuschen UA, Allemeyer EH, Hinz U, Lucas M, Herfarth C, Heuschen G. Outcome after septic complications in J pouch procedures. Br J Surg. 2002;89:194–200.
22. Shah NS, Remzi FH, Massmann A, Baixauli J, Fazio VW. Management and treatment outcome of pouch-vaginal fistulas following restorative proctocolectomy. Dis Colon Rectum. 2003;46:911–7.
23. Baixauli J, Delaney CP, Wu JS, Remzi FH, Lavery IC, Fazio VW. Functional outcome and quality of life after repeat ileal pouch-anal anastomosis for complications of ileoanal surgery. Dis Colon Rectum. 2004;47:2–11.
24. Johnson PM, O'Connor BI, Cohen Z, McLeod RS. Pouch-vaginal fistula after ileal pouch-anal anastomosis: treatment and outcomes. Dis Colon Rectum. 2005;48:1249–53.
25. Dehni N, Remacle G, Dozois RR, Banchini F, Tiret E, Parc R. Salvage reoperation for complications after ileal pouch-anal anastomosis. Br J Surg. 2005;92:748–53.
26. Tekkis PP, Heriot AG, Smith JJ, Das P, Canero A, Nicholls RJ. Long-term results of abdominal salvage surgery following restorative proctocolectomy. Br J Surg. 2006;93:231–7.
27. Remzi FH, Fazio VW, Kirat HT, Wu JS, Lavery IC, Kiran RP. Repeat pouch surgery by the abdominal approach safely salvages failed ileal pelvic pouch. Dis Colon Rectum. 2009;52:198–204.
28. Shawki S, Belizon A, Person B, Weiss EG, Sands DR, Wexner SD. What are the outcomes of reoperative restorative proctocolectomy and ileal pouch-anal anastomosis surgery? Dis Colon Rectum. 2009;52:884–90.
29. Garrett KA, Remzi FH, Kirat HT, Fazio VW, Shen B, Kiran RP. Outcome of salvage surgery for ileal pouches referred with a diagnosis of Crohn's disease. Dis Colon Rectum. 2009;52:1967–74.
30. Mathis KL, Dozois EJ, Larson DW, Cima RR, Wolff BG, Pemberton JH. Outcomes in patients with ulcerative colitis undergoing partial or complete reconstructive surgery for failing ileal pouch-anal anastomosis. Ann Surg. 2009;249:409–13.
31. Kirat HT, Kiran RP, Remzi FH, Fazio VW, Shen B. Diagnosis and management of afferent limb syndrome in patients with ileal pouch-anal anastomosis. Inflamm Bowel Dis. 2011;17(6):1287–90.
32. Börjesson L, Oresland T, Hultén L. The failed pelvic pouch: conversion to a continent ileostomy. Tech Coloproctol. 2004;8:102–5.
33. Kiran RP, Kirat HT, Rottoli M, Remzi FH, Fazio VW. Permanent ostomy after ileoanal pouch failure: pouch in situ or pouch excision? Dis Colon Rectum. 2012;55(1):4–9.
34. Martínez-Ramos D, Gibert-Gerez J, Escrig-Sos J, Alcalde-Sánchez M, Salvador-Sanchis JL. Ileal pouch-anal anastomosis for Crohn's disease. Current status. Cir Esp. 2009;85:69–75.
35. MacRae HM, McLeod RS, Cohen Z, O'Connor BI, Ton EN. Risk factors for pelvic pouch failure. Dis Colon Rectum. 1997;40:257–62.
36. Kirat HT, Kiran RP, Oncel M, Shen B, Fazio VW, Remzi FH. Management of leak from the tip of the "j" in ileal pouch-anal anastomosis. Dis Colon Rectum. 2011;54:454–9.

第 21 章 结肠克罗恩病的再手术

Hagit Tulchinsky·Micha Rabau
龚剑锋 译　龚剑锋 审校

摘　要

尽管炎性肠病的医疗管理有了巨大进步，估计有 50%～74% 的克罗恩病患者在诊断 10 年后需要手术治疗。其中，许多人需要多次手术，同时该领域的结直肠专家会因为对这些复杂患者超专业的手术治疗建立起自己的声望。本章讨论了需要行再次手术的流行病及临床危险因素，以及可选的手术方式及报道的预后及并发症。

关键词

切除术；克罗恩病（CD）；结肠；回结肠疾病；结直肠切除术；并发症；肠保留；回肠切除术；结肠切除术；低位哈特曼手术

引　言

克罗恩病（CD）会累及胃肠道的任何部分或多个节段。Farmer 等[1] 在一项对 615 例新诊断为 CD 的患者的研究发现，40.9% 有回结肠病变，28.6% 病变局限于小肠，30.4% 病变仅累及结肠或直肠肛管区域。病变局限于结肠和直肠的 CD 患者中有 25% 无直肠或乙状结肠直肠病变，但是病变局限于结肠的患者中，仅 25% 有炎症累及整个结肠。其余 75% 的患者会累及结肠的任何部分，以远端结肠受累及最多见[2]。

虽然 CD 患者在医疗管理上有了巨大进步，但是手术治疗仍然常用于该病的并发症。然而，由于该病的性质，手术治疗的目的在于减轻症状而不是治愈疾病。据估计有 50%～74% 的克罗恩病患者在诊断 10 年后需要手术治疗[3-5]。很多因素都与初次手术的风险有关。疾病解剖部位是一个主要因素。与病变累及结肠和直肠的患者相比，回结肠或回肠的患者手术治疗的风险增加[6]。病变累及回结肠的患者相比病变局限于其他解剖部位的手术率增加。实际上结直肠病变患者手术治疗的概率是最低的[1,3]。建议早期手术的其他因素包括狭窄、穿透性临床表型、肛周疾病及确诊疾病时年龄小于 40 岁[1,3,7,8]。

CD 患者治疗的最大挑战之一是术后疾病高频复发。接受肠切除手术的患者，有近 50% 会在 10 年内出现复发[9-10]。复发的确切原因仍旧未能确定。药物治疗失败的情况下如果出现复发，可能会需要附加手术治疗，一期切除术后有 9.5%～43% 的患者在 5 年内会需要重复手术[9,11]。据调查，以下几个预后因素会潜在影响复发率和重复手术率，即吸烟习惯、疾病发生年龄、解剖部位及累及程度、肠外表现、手术指征、吻合技术、狭窄成形术、术后并发症和药物治疗的类型[3,12-15]。

然而，CD 复发的重复手术是一个复杂问题。与初次手术相比，术中及术后并发症的发生率较高，包括小肠损伤、腹腔脓肿和住院时间较长，常见原因有粘连、复杂的术前药物治疗和疾病严重程度[16-17]。Brouquer等[17]观察到总体发病率为38%。与手术期间的关联率很高（23%），小肠损伤率也是如此（5%）。

结直肠克罗恩病的手术治疗

结直肠克罗恩病在世界范围内发病率大幅增加：一半的患者在最初10年内会接受手术切除治疗。结直肠克罗恩病的手术指征通常取决于其并发症，包括结肠出血、狭窄、梗阻、异型增生或癌症。肛周疾病影响功能及药物治疗失败，会造成患者反复住院或对与健康相关的生活质量产生不利影响。在儿童中，学龄期儿童反复住院的影响，类固醇药物依赖对生长发育迟缓的破坏性作用或其他节制激素疗法药物的不良反应也需要考虑在内[18]。虽然尽可能保留小肠是小肠克罗恩病的治疗标准，克罗恩结肠炎的切除程度仍受争议。对累及结直肠的患者可采用几种不同的手术方法。手术方式取决于病变部位及持续时间、累及节段的程度、手术指征、干预的紧迫性、存在的不良反应，以及患者的年龄、一般状况、直肠顺应性及粪便控制的预期功能结局。

手术方式可以分成3种主要类型：①一期大肠切除加及时恢复肠道连续性；②阶段性大肠切除加回肠造口、恢复或不恢复肠道连续性；③大肠切除加括约肌消融、经腹会阴直肠切除、永久回肠或结肠造口术。大肠切除包括节段性结肠切除、结肠次全切除、经腹结肠全切除和结直肠切除。节段性结肠切除或经腹结肠全切除加回直肠吻合术（IRA）已应用于保肛患者。两种术式都有相当大的风险出现直肠或小肠复发，这时会需要再次手术。在接受手术治疗的结直CD患者中，相当比例的患者终会接受回肠造口术。Lapidus等[19]发现，在确诊5年、10年和25年的患者需要行永久回肠造口的绝对累积风险分别是16%、25%和38%。

回肠造口术

对注定要接受结直肠切除手术的患者，为行粪便转流以控制盆腔感染，通常把回肠造口术作为阶段性手术治疗的第1步；对同时接受重建手术的患者，回肠造口术起到了保护作用，如IRA或恢复性结直肠切除术（回肠贮袋肛管吻合术），或者在结肠切除时把回肠与其余的结肠或直肠在后期吻合。在很多情况下，回肠造口术会减轻远期病变，包括严重的肛周疾病。这个问题在本书这一部分的第22章曾已提及；造成永久性回肠造口的因素超出了本章的范围[20]。

经腹结肠切除及回肠造口术

经腹结肠切除、哈特曼远端封闭或黏膜瘘管成形及回肠造口术可能是阶段性治疗过程中的初次手术。该术式多用于紧急情况（暴发性中毒性巨结肠、穿孔），以及计划随后行结肠切除的广泛结肠炎患者，但是应除外太过虚弱以致不能承受如此大型手术、有严重肛周感染或诊断不明确的患者。在不同的研究中，10年复发率在13%~35%之间不等，经腹结肠切除或结直肠切除术后同样如此[21]。然而，一些患者在结肠切除术后不会再行IRA手术，同时因为严重的结肠或肛周疾病会留下永久性回肠造口。Lock等[22]发现，结肠切除和回肠造口术后直肠保留患者有45%可能会因持续严重的结肠炎或肛周疾病随后行直肠切除。

分段性结肠切除加结肠吻合

节段性结肠切除在克罗恩结肠炎中的作用一直备受争议。直到最近，经腹结肠全切加IRA一直是标准手术方式；然而，节段性结肠切除在某些特定患者中承担的作用日益增长，其中约10%会在结肠和直肠剩余的正常部分发生节段性疾病（10~20cm）。文章表明，与结肠次全切除加回肠-乙状结肠吻合或结肠全切除加回肠-直肠吻合相比，节段性结肠切除后在剩余大肠早期复发的风险及再手术率有所增加。Prabhakar等[23]报道指出，在随访14年后，节段性结肠切除术后有59%的患者病情反复发作，以结直肠最多见；这些患者中有44%需重复手术或者长期药物治疗。Andersson等[24]报道指出，结肠次全切除与节段性结肠切除相比，10年再切除率分别是41%和55%。虽然结直肠复发更常见于节段性结肠切除术，但两者造口率无区别[25-26]。

结肠次全切或全切除加回肠-乙状结肠吻合/回肠-直肠吻合

经腹结肠全切除加IRA或结肠次全切除加回

肠－乙状结肠吻合可有效地使克罗恩结肠炎的慢性患者恢复健康。患有广泛克罗恩结肠炎的年轻患者，因其在回肠贮袋或接近回肠贮袋处的高复发风险禁忌做 IPAA 手术，因此该术式尤其困难，且是唯一的括约肌保留手术。该术式的其他优点包括由盆腔分离引起的性功能和膀胱功能障碍较小、避免了会阴创伤愈合问题和避免永久性造口。为减少失败率，应谨慎选择患者。保留可扩张的远端乙状结肠或直肠、肛周累及较轻和可接受的括约肌功能是该术式成功的关键。当乙状结肠因其功能性优势得到保留，人们更偏爱结肠次全切除（即保留乙状结肠）加回肠－乙状结肠吻合术。因为即使结肠炎症局限于几个节段，节段性结肠切除相比结肠全切除手术更易导致结直肠复发，一些研究者也更支持结肠全切除加 IRA[21, 27, 28]。在超过 10 年的随访后，约 40% 的患者获得了满意性的效果而不需要进一步手术。Ambrose 等[29] 报道指出，在这些患者中，10 年累积复发率是 64%，而累积再手术率是 48%。Cattan 等[30] 的一项最新研究报道指出，IRA 术后 5 年和 10 年的累积复发率分别是 58% 和 83%。尽管临床复发率很高，患病 10 年得以保留直肠的患者达到 86%。

结直肠全切加回肠造口术

从患者的角度，保护肛门功能避免造口和优化生活质量极其重要。因为 CD 是一种在患者年轻时发生的疾病，恢复肠道连续性或作为阶段性治疗计划的一部分，通过节段性切除、结肠切除术、IRA 或 IPAA 后实施。常规性结直肠切除加远端回肠造口术适用于有广泛结肠疾病的患者，特别是当存在明显结肠和肛门累及时，包括做或不做结肠切除的回肠造口术，或完成直肠切除后哈特曼袋/黏膜瘘管成形术。

在克罗恩结肠炎的治疗中，结直肠全切及回肠造口术的复发率和再手术率最低。10%～25% 的复发率相比其他手术方式 50% 的复发率明显占优势[21]。然而，该术式带给患者永久的回肠造口。很多并发症与结肠直肠切除术相关，包括性功能障碍（尤其是男性阳痿和射精功能障碍）、会阴伤口愈合不完全和针对盆腔和会阴部分的手术并发症。会阴伤口愈合问题在很多报告中提及。采用肌周或括约肌间切除显著减少了这些并发症[31]；60%～90% 的会阴伤口会在 6 个月内愈合[32]。

恢复性结肠直肠切除术（IPAA）

从历史来看，IPAA 因其不良预后一直认为是克罗恩病患者的禁忌。一些研究已经公布，其中列举了 CD 患者行 IPAA 手术相关的不良结局[33-37]。Brown 等[36] 报道指出，贮袋并发症在 CD 患者（64%）中比 UC 患者（22%）更为常见。在平均近 7 年随访后，56% 的患者切除了贮袋或贮袋失去功能，而 UC 患者仅为 6%。贮袋患有 CD 与难治性憩室炎、袋周脓肿、瘘管形成、贮袋狭窄及贮袋最终失败有关。在一项由 10 篇文章包含 3103 例炎性肠病患者的 meta 分析中，Reese 等[37] 研究了 CD 患者行恢复性结直肠切除术后的效果。CD 患者相比非 CD 患者更易发生回肠贮袋失败、膀胱脓肿、贮袋相关瘘及吻合口狭窄。关于功能性结果，贮袋炎、尿急及尿失禁在 CD 患者中较常见。

然而，Panis 等[38] 表明，某些特定 CD 患者 IPAA 术后效果可能较好。在 5 年的随访后，行 IAA 手术的 CD 和 UC 患者间在贮袋功能上没有显著区别。这些结果得到 Regimbeau 等[39] 的印证，他们证明在选择的合适患者中贮袋失败率仅 10%。目前，对 CD 患者行 IPAA 手术仍极受争议，而且该术式常用于误诊的 UC 患者。如果外科医生打算对存在 CD 的患者行 IPAA 手术，其先决条件应包括孤立性结直肠疾病、无小肠累及、无肛周病史且括约肌功能良好[38, 40]。一些研究表明，结直肠切除及回肠造口术后患者生活质量的改善可媲美 IPAA[41-42]；这个问题应该在术前与患者详细讨论，这点很重要。

克罗恩结肠炎的重复手术

肠道切除术后 CD 复发似乎是其自然史的一部分。通过免疫调节药物硫唑嘌呤/6-巯基嘌呤或 IFX 的治疗可能会使复发率降低[43-44]。尽管一期切除手术后，药物可预防复发的进展，5 年内仍然有近 50% 的患者临床复发，同时这一预期值在较长随访期后会有增加[3]。10 年内二期手术的风险为 25%～45%[10, 45]。人们做出许多尝试，试图去定义孤立性克罗恩结肠炎一期术后复发的危险因素。吸烟是引起初次肠切除最广泛认同的危险因素[13]。此外，一些研究总结指出，CD吸烟者可能更需要手术治疗复发[46-47]。大多数的研究表明，性别对复发率无影响[48-49]；然而一些报告显示，女性比男性复发风险增加明显[3, 50]。一些研究对解剖程度是否可以预测复发进行了调查，其中大多数研究显示克罗恩结肠炎比回结肠或孤立性回肠疾病复发率要低[1, 3, 51-53]，因此在结肠切除时回肠疾病的存在对复发有影响[22]。有肛周瘘管的患者相比，无肛周瘘管的患者风险也有增加[24, 50, 54]。在这方面，Polle等[50]报道指出，有肛周病史的患者2/3有造口，而无肛周病史者为20%。一些报告发现年轻患者的复发率增加[32, 55]。此外，有肠外表现患者的复发风险可能有增加，直肠保留的机会也较低[30]。

正如前面提及的，手术类型对疾病复发率和重复手术率有重要影响。人们关注的一个问题是：当与结肠全切除术相比，节段性结肠切除术后复发是否更早，复发率是否更高。研究此问题的报告指出，节段性结肠切除术与复发和重复手术的风险增加有关[23, 28]；然而，其他的研究也报道了一个类似的风险[24, 56-58]。由Tekkis等[57]作出的一份荟萃分析显示，结肠全切除加IRA和节段性结肠切除在复发上无显著差异；虽然这项研究在其评估上有点缺陷，因其未能根据疾病程度随机化。他们指出节段性结肠切除组术后复发时间缩短4.4年。在一项前瞻性研究中，Fichera等[28]对因原发性结肠疾病行手术治疗的179例CD患者进行了报道。总体上有31例患者（24.4%）在随访期间有CD复发的需要手术治疗：节段性结肠切除组占38.8%，经腹结肠全切除组占22.9%，结直肠全切除组占9.3%；节段性结肠切除患者比结直肠全切除患者初次复发时间明显较短。在按照疾病程度进行纠正后，节段性结肠切除组比结直肠全切组术后复发风险明显较高。此外，行结直肠全切除患者比结肠全切除或节段性结肠切除患者术后1年仍然服用药物的患者数显著减少。复发部位可能包括结肠、直肠和小肠。第二个关注的问题是吻合口的存在促使炎症复发。吻合口的数目同样是术后症状复发重要的预后指标。

各种研究表明，结直肠切除加回肠造口术的复发率约为30%[20, 59]，但是由其他非随机化研究报告指出，结肠全切除或节段性结肠切除一期吻合复发率可增加到50%~70%[22, 23, 60-62]。由Bernell等[54]作出的一项基于群体的研究表明，发生在结肠次全切除加回肠造口术后的10年累积症状复发可能性最低（24%），其次是结直肠切除加回肠造口术，总当量率为37%。相比而言，结肠切除术和结肠全切除加IRA术后患者复发率分别是47%和58%。回肠造口分流的形成应该在术前考虑每一位患者，因为与一期切除相比时，CD复发的重复手术与回肠造口率较高有关[45]。当然，术前与造口师商议及标记造口位置应该常规进行。

节段性结肠切除术后的重复手术

只有在出现外科并发症后才考虑手术，且尽可能切除最少肠段。在这方面，虽然备受争议，节段性结肠切除可能会在讨论的情况下进行。手术方式的安全性相对并发症的风险在一些研究中已经得到表明[56-57]。二期手术的指征包括有症状的瘘管、出血、狭窄、吻合口复发、脓肿和难治性疾病。虽然有可能施行另一种限制性结肠切除手术（在二期手术时保护胃肠道的连续性），推荐的有效术式包括完全结直肠切除加永久回肠造口术、结肠全切除加IRA或恢复性结直肠切除[62]。当直肠残端在结肠部分或全切除术后看似仍正常时，回肠贮袋直肠吻合术也是一种替代永久回肠造口的术式。以肉眼观察的正常肠段作为术中评估来切断直肠，包括直肠的外在表现和术中结肠镜观察。虽然回肠J形贮袋常常制作得较短，但是回肠J形贮袋是为IPAA而创作的。利用管状吻合器或手工吻合把贮袋吻合到直肠残端。虽然直肠残端保留过长会出现功能性症状，相比直行IRA术后，这些患者获得一个可接受的功能性效果和生活质量[63]。

结肠全切除及IRA术后的重复手术

结肠切除及IRA术后疾病复发通常发生于直肠或肛周，而不是小肠或吻合口。因此，多数患者最终将施行直肠切除及回肠造口术。仅有少数患者最终会通过行IPAA恢复胃肠道[51]。最新的报道表明，超过75%的患者在IRA术后10年内维持功能性吻合，这为直肠相对保留患者提供了一个可行选择[30, 54, 64]。Cattan等[30]报道指出，尽管IRA术后5年和10年的临床复发率分别为58%和83%，术后5年和10年直肠保留的可能性为86%，疾病复发不会必然需要重复手术。以前的报道表明，25%~60%直肠保留患者会因严重直肠炎症或肛周疾病随后行直肠切除手术[22]。

完全直肠切除加肌周分离和括约肌间切除

完全直肠切除加永久回肠造口的指征通常是因为渐重的直肠肛管疾病及并发症，比如直肠阴道瘘管、直肠纤维化和进展性肛周化脓感染。很多年来，CD患者盆腔和直肠肛周解剖同直肠癌的解剖一样，都广泛采用经腹会阴直肠周围组织和括约肌分离。然而，由广泛组织切除和淋巴管中断所造成的会阴伤口不愈合、排尿中断及性功能疾病的发生促使手术分离更加保守。自20世纪70年代后期，人们开始施行直肠肌周组织和括约肌间切除，取得了良好的效果[65]，且并发症较低[66]。Lee和Dowling[67]于1972年初次发表了肌周分离技术；Lyttle和Parks[68]于1977年描述了括约肌间直肠切除术。自那以后，以括约肌间直肠切除同肌周分离技术治疗炎性肠病得到了很好的描述[31,65,66,69]。在括约肌间平面行分离手术（在内括约肌和外括约肌之间）减小了会阴伤口的大小，降低了会阴伤口不愈合的发生率。保留外括约肌和肛提肌，将其用于安全闭合伤口。在有广泛肛周疾病的患者中，行直肠切除术的同时进行清创术、刮宫术及暴露肛周受累皮肤。一个成功的括约肌间直肠切除术也包括控制促成术后伤口愈合不良的其他技术因素。细致止血、使用封闭负压引流、去除所有直肠黏膜岛状物及避免粪便污染都是获得成功愈合的术中技术因素。

低位哈特曼手术

在会阴脓肿存在情况下行直肠切除面临的一个问题是：会阴伤口愈合不良或会阴瘘管是其常见并发症，而且会引起比术前更严重的症状。直肠切除术后6~12个月会阴伤口不愈合的发生率从12%~80%不等[70-71]。正是因为这个原因，低位哈特曼手术受到推荐（如封闭直肠下端或肛管上端切除直肠、保留括约肌的直肠全切除）。因为仅保留有短的直肠袖口，无需采用经腹切除；如果需要，以后可采用经会阴括约肌间途径。在低位哈特曼术后，直肠残端开始萎缩，同时会阴肛管疾病消退，因此需要随后在炎症较轻组织行经会阴直肠切除术。Sher等[71]报道了25例患有严重直肠肛管CD及会阴瘘管而有必要行手术切除的患者，他们接受了低位哈特曼手术代替标准直肠切除术。60%的患者会阴伤口完全愈合，而不需要进一步手术治疗。会阴疾病持续存在于其余10例患者，他们的会阴状况较初期治疗时大为改善。有3例患者在报道时仍然有会阴不愈合，随后进行了经会阴直肠切除手术，总体而言，88%的患者在平均69.1个月随访期后会阴伤口完全愈合。

低位哈特曼手术的益处（如上所述）值得商榷。部分经转流手术仍有症状性疾病的肛周CD患者，需要进一步手术治疗，以切除残留直肠残端病变。同样，虽然低位哈特曼术后残留组织量很少，但是剩余的肛管会因排便、血肿和脓毒症继续成为发病的源头[72-74]。

IPAA

如前所述，虽然IPAA是CD的相对禁忌证[32,35,75]，但是一些研究者认为IPAA可能会适用于无回肠、肛管或肛周累及的选择性CD患者[37-38]。CD患者行IPAA的并发症发生率和失败率接近UC患者行IPAA的3倍[32,35,36,76]；CD的复发过程较长，往往导致小肠狭窄和瘘管。Mylonakis等[76]报道指出，在IPAA术后平均10.2年的随访后，贮袋切除占47.8%，近端造口占4.3%。然而，贮袋保留患者的功能性结局与成功进行IRA的患者相同。IPAA在CD患者手术治疗中的作用仍未能定义。

我们认为结直肠切除和回肠造口术应该仍然是累及结肠和直肠克罗恩结肠炎患者的标准术式。如果建议CD患者行IPAA，需强制进行细心咨询，以列出功能结局不良和贮袋失败的风险。

IPAA术后的重复手术

重建术后发展为反复发作复杂性CD的患者，其重复手术的选择术式相当有限。疾病复发通常是由于回肠肛管贮袋的炎症、贮袋近端的回肠血液循环或肛管周围部位贮袋外的瘘管疾病。当药物治疗失败时，很多手术方式可供选择。补救手术大致可分为经会阴修复、经腹恢复性手术或经腹会阴联合恢复性手术。贮袋入口或出口的狭窄症状可用内镜指导下球囊扩张术治疗[77]。贮袋狭窄成形术是长期纤维性狭窄患者的选择术式[78]。药物难治性瘘管患者可行挂线引流治疗或通常用于非 CD 瘘管修复的其他手术方法。然而，CD 患者的补救率仅 30%~35%，而 UC 患者为 70%~75%[79-81]。最后，如果这些手术失败，需要行重复手术。这些患者可适用两种手术方式：在不能明确失去功能的贮袋之上行分流性回肠造口或者切除回肠贮袋行永久性回肠造口。

IPAA 切除术

盆腔贮袋切除有潜在的显著的并发症发生率，包括小肠长度损失、盆腔神经损伤和常见慢性窦道形成术后会阴感染的发生率高[79, 82]。持久性会阴窦道可能会引起相当高的并发症发生率，且难于治疗。在这种情况下，Karoui 等[82] 报道了 68 例贮袋切除的患者。总体并发症发生率为 62.3%，其中 53.7% 的患者因晚期并发症再次入院。贮袋切除后 1 年和 5 年再次入院的风险分别为 38% 和 58%，多数在再次入院期间需要手术治疗。对这些患者，持续性会阴窦道是最常见的晚期并发症，40% 患者会阴伤口在 6 个月后仍未愈合，12 个月仍未愈合的概率为 10%。7% 的患者抱怨有阳痿，其他的患者有短肠综合征及需要永久肠外营养。

永久性造口

因为贮袋切除术后发病率相当高，可考虑把贮袋留在原位仅行永久性回肠造口，该手术较小，短期和长期并发症较少。Bengtsson 等[83] 研究了随访 10 年的 13 例不明确贮袋分流的患者：85% 患者无贮袋相关症状，且没有随后发生不典型增生或癌变的病例。

结 论

CD 复发仍是一个主要问题，无论采用何种手术策略，再次手术干预率都很高。CD 复发的重复手术对技术要求较高，且复杂。这与比初次手术并发症发生率较高、住院时间较长和造口率较高有关。根据其性质，结肠 CD 是一种常见的复发情况，重复手术需求高；尤其是当初次行节段性结肠切除并同时合并有，或随后发生难治性肛周疾病时。meta 分析（尽管有其局限性）显示在这些患者中，结肠次全切除相对节段性结肠切除会发挥较大的作用。已知患有 CD 的患者行 IPAA 的机会可能有限，因其围术期和术后并发症发生率高，且后期手术多为永久分流，这比贮袋切除更简单。结直肠切除术在减轻会阴伤口大小上仍占有一定地位，但会阴窦道愈合不良发生率高。需要考虑在选择性病例中行超低位哈特曼手术（并非没有其固有并发症发生率）和更常规应用括约肌间直肠切除术。小肠疾病、吸烟和低龄的合并存在更可能预测重复手术患者因为术后并发症或对药物无效的复发疾病行永久回肠造口。

参考文献

1. Farmer RG, Whelan G, Fazio VW. Long-term follow-up of patients with Crohn's disease. Relationship between the clinical pattern and prognosis. Gastroenterology. 1985;88:1818–25.
2. Sands BE. Crohn's disease. In: Feldman M, Friedman LS, Sleisenger MH, editors. Sleisenger and Fordtran's gastrointestinal and liver disease, vol. 2. Philadelphia: WB Saunders; 2002. p. 2005–38.
3. Binder V, Hendriksen C, Kreiner S. Prognosis in Crohn's disease – based on results from a regional patient group from the county of Copenhagen. Gut. 1985;26:146–50.
4. Goldberg PA, Wright JP, Gerber M, Claassen R. Incidence of surgical resection for Crohn's disease. Dis Colon Rectum. 1993;36:736–9.
5. Bernell O, Lapidus A, Hellers G. Risk factors for surgery and postoperative recurrence in Crohn's disease. Ann Surg. 2000;231:38–45.
6. Basilisco G, Campanini M, Cesana B, Ranzi T, Bianchi P. Risk factors for first operation in Crohn's disease. Am J Gastroenterol. 1989;84:749–52.
7. Polito II JM, Childs B, Mellits ED, Tokayer AZ, Harris ML, Bayless TM. Crohn's disease: influence of age at diagnosis on site and clinical type of disease. Gastroenterology. 1996;111:580–6.
8. Ramadas AV, Gunesh S, Thomas GA, Williams GT, Hawthorne AB. Natural history of Crohn's disease in a population-based cohort from Cardiff (1986–2003): a study of changes in medical treatment and surgical resection rates. Gut. 2010;59:1200–6.
9. Greenstein AJ, Sachar DB, Pasternack BS, Janowitz HD. Reoperation and recurrence in Crohn's colitis and ileocolitis Crude and cumulative rates. N Engl J Med. 1975;293:685–90.
10. Wettergren A, Christiansen J. Risk of recurrence and reoperation after resection for ileocolic Crohn's disease. Scand J Gastroenterol. 1991;26:1319–22.
11. Simillis C, Yamamoto T, Reese GE, Umegae S, Matsumoto K, Darzi AW, et al. A meta-analysis comparing incidence of recurrence and indication for reoperation after surgery for perforating versus nonperforating Crohn's disease. Am J Gastroenterol. 2008;103:196–205.
12. Lock MR, Farmer RG, Fazio VW, Jagelman DG, Lavery IC, Weakley FL. Recurrence and reoperation for Crohn's disease: the role of disease location in prognosis. N Engl J Med. 1981;304:1586–8.
13. Cottone M, Rosselli M, Orlando A, Oliva L, Puleo A, Cappello M, et al. Smoking habits and recurrence in Crohn's disease. Gastroenterology. 1994;106:643–8.
14. Caprilli R, Corrao G, Taddei G, Tonelli F, Torchio P, Viscido A. Prognostic factors for postoperative recurrence of Crohn's disease. Gruppo Italiano per lo Studio del Colon e del Retto (GISC). Dis Colon Rectum. 1996;39:335–41.
15. Borley NR, Mortensen NJ, Jewell DP. Preventing postoperative recurrence of Crohn's disease. Br J Surg. 1997;84:1493–502.
16. Michelassi F, Balestracci T, Chappell R, Block GE. Primary and

recurrent Crohn's disease. Experience with 1379 patients. Ann Surg. 1991;214:230–8.
17. Brouquet A, Blanc B, Bretagnol F, Valleur P, Bouhnik Y, Panis Y. Surgery for intestinal Crohn's disease recurrence. Surgery. 2010;148:936–46.
18. Leonor R, Jacobson K, Pinsk V, Webber E, Lemberg DA. Surgical intervention in children with Crohn's disease. Int J Colorectal Dis. 2007;22:1037–41.
19. Lapidus A, Bernell O, Hellers G, Löfberg R. Clinical course of colorectal Crohn's disease: a 35-year follow-up study of 507 patients. Gastroenterology. 1998;114:1151–60.
20. Galandiuk S, Kimberling J, Al-Mishlab TG, Stromberg AJ. Perianal Crohn's disease: predictors of need for permanent diversion. Ann Surg. 2005;241:796–802.
21. Yamamoto T, Allan RN, Keighley MR. Audit of single-stage proctocolectomy for Crohn's disease: postoperative complications and recurrence. Dis Colon Rectum. 2000;43:249–56.
22. Lock MR, Fazio VW, Farmer RG, Jagelman DG, Lavery IC, Weakley FL. Proximal recurrence and the fate of the rectum following excisional surgery for Crohn's disease of the large bowel. Ann Surg. 1981;194:754–60.
23. Prabhakar LP, Laramee C, Nelson H, Dozois RR. Avoiding a stoma: role for segmental or abdominal colectomy in Crohn's colitis. Dis Colon Rectum. 1997;40:71–8.
24. Andersson P, Olaison G, Hallböök O, Sjödahl R. Segmental resection or subtotal colectomy in Crohn's colitis? Dis Colon Rectum. 2002;45:47–53.
25. Sanfey H, Bayless TM, Cameron JL. Crohn's disease of the colon. Is there a role for limited resection? Am J Surg. 1984;147:38–42.
26. Longo WE, Ballantyne GH, Cahow CE. Treatment of Crohn's colitis. Segmental or total colectomy? Arch Surg. 1988;123:588–90.
27. Fazio VW, Wu JS. Surgical therapy for Crohn's disease of the colon and rectum. Surg Clin North Am. 1997;77:197–210.
28. Fichera A, McCormack R, Rubin MA, Hurst RD, Michelassi F. Long-term outcome of surgically treated Crohn's colitis: a prospective study. Dis Colon Rectum. 2005;48:963–9.
29. Ambrose NS, Keighley MR, Alexander-Williams J, Allan RN. Clinical impact of colectomy and ileorectal anastomosis in the management of Crohn's disease. Gut. 1984;25:223–7.
30. Cattan P, Bonhomme N, Panis Y, Lémann M, Coffin B, Bouhnik Y, et al. Fate of the rectum in patients undergoing total colectomy for Crohn's disease. Br J Surg. 2002;89:454–9.
31. Bauer JJ, Gelernt IM, Salk B, Kreel I. Proctectomy for inflammatory bowel disease. Am J Surg. 1986;151:157–62.
32. Hurst RD, Gottlieb LJ, Crucitti P, Melis M, Rubin M, Michelassi F. Primary closure of complicated perineal wounds with myocutaneous and fasciocutaneous flaps after proctectomy for Crohn's disease. Surgery. 2001;130:767–73.
33. Hyman NH, Fazio VW, Tuckson WB, Lavery IC. Consequences of ileal pouch-anal anastomosis for Crohn's colitis. Dis Colon Rectum. 1991;34:653–7.
34. Sagar PM, Dozois RR, Wolff BG. Long-term results of ileal pouch-anal anastomosis in patients with Crohn's disease. Dis Colon Rectum. 1996;39:893–8.
35. Braveman JM, Schoetz Jr DJ, Marcello PW, Roberts PL, Coller JA, Murray JJ, et al. The fate of the ileal pouch in patients developing Crohn's disease. Dis Colon Rectum. 2004;47:1613–9.
36. Brown CJ, Maclean AR, Cohen Z, Macrae HM, O'Connor BI, McLeod RS. Crohn's disease and indeterminate colitis and the ileal pouch-anal anastomosis: outcomes and patterns of failure. Dis Colon Rectum. 2005;48:1542–9.
37. Reese GE, Lovegrove RE, Tilney HS, Yamamoto T, Heriot AG, Fazio VW, et al. The effect of Crohn's disease on outcomes after restorative proctocolectomy. Dis Colon Rectum. 2007;50:239–50.
38. Panis Y, Poupard B, Nemeth J, Lavergne A, Hautefeuille P, Valleur P. Ileal pouch/anal anastomosis for Crohn's disease. Lancet. 1996;347:854–7.
39. Regimbeau JM, Panis Y, Pocard M, Bouhnik Y, Lavergne-Slove A, Rufat P, et al. Long-term results of ileal pouch-anal anastomosis for colorectal Crohn's disease. Dis Colon Rectum. 2001;44:769–78.
40. Morpurgo E, Petras R, Kimberling J, Ziegler C, Galandiuk S. Characterization and clinical behavior of Crohn's disease initially presenting predominantly as colitis. Dis Colon Rectum. 2003;46:918–24.
41. Seidel SA, Newman M, Sharp KW. Ileoanal pouch versus ileostomy: is there a difference in quality of life? Am Surg. 2000;66:540–6.
42. Camilleri-Brennan J, Munro A, Steele RJ. Does an ileoanal pouch offer a better quality of life than a permanent ileostomy for patients with ulcerative colitis? J Gastrointest Surg. 2003;7:814–9.
43. Hanauer SB, Korelitz BI, Rutgeerts P, Peppercorn MA, Thisted RA, Cohen RD, et al. Postoperative maintenance of Crohn's disease remission with 6-mercaptopurine, mesalamine, or placebo: a 2-year trial. Gastroenterology. 2004;127:723–9.
44. Doherty G, Bennet G, Patil S, Cheifettz A, Moss AC. Interventions for prevention of post operative recurrence of Crohn's disease. Cochrane Database Syst Rev. 2009;7(4):CD006873.
45. Heimann TM, Greenstein AJ, Lewis B, Kaufman D, Heimann DM, Aufses Jr AH. Comparison of primary and reoperative surgery in patients with Crohns disease. Ann Surg. 1998;227:492–5.
46. Lindberg E, Järnerot G, Huitfeldt B. Smoking in Crohn's disease: effect on localisation and clinical course. Gut. 1992;33:779–82.
47. Breuer-Katschinski BD, Holländer N, Goebell H. Effect of cigarette smoking on the course of Crohn's disease. Eur J Gastroenterol Hepatol. 1996;8:225–8.
48. Trnka YM, Glotzer DJ, Kasdon EJ, Goldman H, Steer ML, Goldman LD. The long-term outcome of restorative operation in Crohn's disease: influence of location, prognostic factors and surgical guidelines. Ann Surg. 1982;196:345–55.
49. Chardavoyne R, Flint GW, Pollack S, Wise L. Factors affecting recurrence following resection for Crohn's disease. Dis Colon Rectum. 1986;29:495–502.
50. Polle SW, Slors JF, Weverling GJ, Gouma DJ, Hommes DW, Bemelman WA. Recurrence after segmental resection for colonic Crohn's disease. Br J Surg. 2005;92:1143–9.
51. Mekhjian HS, Switz DM, Watts HD, Deren JJ, Katon RM, Beman FM. National Cooperative Crohn's Disease Study: factors determining recurrence of Crohn's disease after surgery. Gastroenterology. 1979;77:907–13.
52. Whelan G, Farmer RG, Fazio VW, Goormastic M. Recurrence after surgery in Crohn's disease. Relationship to location of disease (clinical pattern) and surgical indication. Gastroenterology. 1985;88:1826–33.
53. Borley NR, Mortensen NJ, Chaudry MA, Mohammed S, Warren BF, George BD, Clark T, Jewell DP, Kettlewell MG. Recurrence after abdominal surgery for Crohn's disease: relationship to disease site and surgical procedure. Dis Colon Rectum. 2002;45:377–83.
54. Bernell O, Lapidus A, Hellers G. Recurrence after colectomy in Crohn's colitis. Dis Colon Rectum. 2001;44:647–54.
55. Frikker MJ, Segall MM. The resectional reoperation rate for Crohn's disease in a general community hospital. Dis Colon Rectum. 1983;26:305–9.
56. Martel P, Betton PO, Gallot D, Malafosse M. Crohn's colitis: experience with segmental resections; results in a series of 84 patients. J Am Coll Surg. 2002;194:448–53.
57. Tekkis PP, Purkayastha S, Lanitis S, Athanasiou T, Heriot AG, Orchard TR, Nicholls RJ, Darzi AW. A comparison of segmental vs subtotal/total colectomy for colonic Crohn's disease: a meta-analysis. Colorectal Dis. 2006;8:82–90.
58. Kiran RP, Nisar PJ, Church JM, Fazio VW. The role of primary surgical procedure in maintaining intestinal continuity for patients with Crohn's colitis. Ann Surg. 2011;253:1130–5.
59. Heimann TM, Greenstein AJ, Lewis B, Kaufman D, Heimann DM, Aufses Jr AH. Prediction of early symptomatic recurrence after intestinal resection in Crohn's disease. Ann Surg. 1993;218:294–8.
60. Scammell B, Ambrose NS, Alexander-Williams J, Allan RN, Keighley MR. Recurrent small bowel Crohn's disease is more frequent after subtotal colectomy and ileorectal anastomosis than proctocolectomy. Dis Colon Rectum. 1985;28:770–1.
61. Longo WE, Oakley JR, Lavery IC, Church JM, Fazio VW. Outcome

of ileorectal anastomosis for Crohn's colitis. Dis Colon Rectum 1992;35:1066–71.
62. Kariv Y, Remzi FH, Strong SA, Hammel JP, Preen M, Fazio VW. Ileal pouch rectal anastomosis: a viable alternative to permanent ileostomy in Crohn's proctocolitis patients. J Am Coll Surg. 2009;208:390–9.
63. Tulchinsky H, McCourtney JS, Rao KV, Chambers W, Williams J, Wilkinson KH, et al. Salvage abdominal surgery in patients with a retained rectal stump after restorative proctocolectomy and stapled anastomosis. Br J Surg. 2001;88:1602–6.
64. Yamamoto T, Keighley MR. Fate of the rectum and ileal recurrence rates after total colectomy for Crohn's disease. World J Surg. 2000;24:125–9.
65. Zeitels JR, Fiddian-Green RG, Dent TL. Intersphincteric proctectomy. Surgery. 1984;96:617–23.
66. Leicester RJ, Ritchie JK, Wadsworth J, Thomson JPS, Hawley PR. Sexual function and perineal wound healing after intersphincteric excision of the rectum for inflammatory bowel disease. Dis Colon Rectum. 1984;27:244–8.
67. Lee ECG, Dowling BL. Perimuscular excision of the rectum for Crohn's disease and ulcerative colitis. Br J Surg. 1972;59:29–32.
68. Lyttle JA, Parks AG. Intersphincteric excision of the rectum. Br J Surg. 1977;64:413–6.
69. Lubbers EJC. Healing of the perineal wound after proctectomy for nonmalignant conditions. Dis Colon Rectum. 1982;25:351–7.
70. Scammell BE, Keighley MRB. Delayed perineal wound healing after proctectomy for Crohn's colitis. Br J Surg. 1986;73:150–2.
71. Sher ME, Bauer JJ, Gorphine S, Gelernt I. Low Hartmann's procedure for severe anorectal Crohn's disease. Dis Colon Rectum. 1992;35:975–80.
72. Guillem JG, Roberts PL, Murray JJ, Coller JA, Viedenheimer MC, Schoetz Jr DJ. Factors predictive of persistent or recurrent Crohn's disease in excluded rectal segments. Dis Colon Rectum. 1992;35:768–72.
73. Frizelle FA, Pemberton JH. For debate: removal of the anus during proctectomy. Br J Surg. 1997;84:68.
74. Windsor AC, Northover JM. Removal of the anus during proctectomy. Br J Surg. 1997;84:1176.
75. Penner RM, Madsen KL, Fedorak RN. Postoperative Crohn's disease. Inflamm Bowel Dis. 2005;11:765–77.
76. Mylonakis E, Allan RN, Keighley MR. How does pouch construction for a final diagnosis of Crohn's disease compare with ileoproctostomy for established Crohn's proctocolitis? Dis Colon Rectum. 2001;44:1137–42.
77. Shen B, Fazio VW, Remzi FH, Delaney CP, Achkar JP, Bennett A, et al. Endoscopic balloon dilation of ileal pouch strictures. Am J Gastroenterol. 2004;99:2340–7.
78. Matzke GM, Kang AS, Dozois EJ, Sandborn WJ. Mid pouch strictureplasty for Crohn's disease after ileal pouch-anal anastomosis: an alternative to pouch excision. Dis Colon Rectum. 2004;47:782–6.
79. Breen EM, Schoetz Jr DJ, Marcello PW, Roberts PL, Coller JA, Murray JJ, et al. Functional results after perineal complications of ileal pouch-anal anastomosis. Dis Colon Rectum. 1998;41:691–5.
80. Prudhomme M, Dehni N, Dozois RR, Tiret E, Parc R. Causes and outcomes of pouch excision after restorative proctocolectomy. Br J Surg. 2006;93:82–6.
81. Shawki S, Belizon A, Person B, Weiss EG, Sands DR, Wexner SD. What are the outcomes of reoperative restorative proctocolectomy and ileal pouch-anal anastomosis surgery? Dis Colon Rectum. 2009;52:884–90.
82. Karoui M, Cohen R, Nicholls J. Results of surgical removal of the pouch after failed restorative proctocolectomy. Dis Colon Rectum. 2004;47:869–75.
83. Bengtsson J, Börjesson L, Willén R, Oresland T, Hultén L. Can a failed ileal pouch anal anastomosis be left in situ? Colorectal Dis. 2007;9:503–8.

第 22 章 肛周克罗恩病的治疗

Dana R. Sands

龚剑锋 译　龚剑锋 审校

摘 要

克罗恩病是一种病因不明合并肛周表现的慢性、反复发作和使人衰弱的炎性肠病。肛周活动性病变常与腹部疾病活动同时出现，偶尔可能为病变的原发部位，且严重损害患者的生活质量。手术对治疗这些患者起到关键的作用。详细的病史和完善的临床检查为主治医师提供宝贵的信息，并可作为进一步的学术研究和治疗方案的依据。除了脓肿引流，通过药物治疗来控制近端疾病往往优于手术治疗。一个涉及患者、外科医生、肠胃病专家、病理学家、营养学家等专家共同参与的多学科方法使肛周克罗恩病的成功治疗成为可能。

关键词

肛周克罗恩病；炎性肠病（IBD）；透壁性炎症；脓肿；瘘管；损害；肛周疾病活动指数（PDAI）；英夫利昔单抗；瘘道切开术；瘘道切除术

引 言

克罗恩病是一种局限性、节段性的透壁性炎症，可累及消化道任何部位。透壁性炎症破坏肠黏膜的完整性，有利于脓肿和瘘道的形成。Penner 和 Crohn[1] 在 1938 年描述了第 1 例局限性肠炎患者患有肛瘘，后来通过队列研究发现 14% 的患者患有肛周病变。现已确立，克罗恩病常并发各种肛周病变。症状可多变，从疼痛和脓性分泌物到出血和大小便失禁，伴有显著的并发症发生率和生活质量受损。这些病变使经治医师面临一个临床挑战。因此，对病因的充分了解和潜在的治疗方案是成功的关键。

流行病学

关于克罗恩病患者合并肛周病变的流行报告差异显著，而最新的基于人群的系列报告（从瑞典到明尼苏达州）发现 14%～38% 的患者可见累及肛肠[2-4]，孤立的肛周疾病只占 5%[5]。这种差异的原因部分是由于对肛周克罗恩病定义的不同引起。一些报告样本只采用手术后的患者，而另外一些则包含了所有合并肛周表现的患者。随着疾病进展至晚期，肛周表现的发病率也不断增高。

年龄、种族和病变部位是克罗恩病肛周并发症的发生率和模式的相关因素。性别是不确定因素。

年 龄

年龄小于 40 岁的克罗恩病患者更容易合并肛周病变[6]。年轻时就出现肛周并发症的患者或以出现肠瘘为肛周疾病首发表现的患者，更可能需要采用直肠切除术[7-9]。

种 族

一项纳入 1126 例克罗恩病患者的研究发现近端疾病在白人患者中更常见（比值比为 1.8），且白人患者比西班牙裔和非裔美国人患者更少合并肛周表现（比值比为 0.58）[10]。在红十字会等的报告中也有类似的结果[11]。

病变部位

在回结肠克罗恩病患者中，只有 15% 出现瘘，而 92% 的结肠和直肠的克罗恩病患者出现瘘[4]。大多数病例肠段受累早于肛周疾病的出现[12]，但是多达 4/10 的患者出现肛周症状早于肠受累症状的出现。

肛周疾病的存在和无效的自然病史[9]、肠外表现发病率的增长[14]和激素抵抗的增强[15]相关联。肛周克罗恩病易复发，35%～39% 的患者在 2 年内复发[16]。超过 80% 的患者需要手术，且多达 20% 的患者需要行直肠切除术[2-4]。此外，已知克罗恩病患者有更易患结肠癌的风险[17]。大量的研究发现直肠癌的发病率无明显增加[18-19]，但肛门直肠受累的患者患肛门鳞状细胞癌和腺癌的概率有所增加[20-21]。

病 因

肛瘘疾病的病因尚不清楚。以往这些病变被认为是感染性病变（根据 Parks 的隐窝腺学说）。1978年，Hughes[22]把克罗恩病的肛门直肠病变分为原发性和继发性病变；原发性病变包括溃疡和肛裂，这些病变在机械性影响下会形成狭窄和上皮化的瘘道（继发性病变）。他提出由向外张开的近端疾病引起的深部肛裂为粪便通过形成了一个口袋。随着向外张开的近端疾病的解决和在排便的压力下，这个口袋就会越来越深入到皮下组织，最后就形成了脓肿。

已有人提出克罗恩病和定位于 5 号染色体的基因易感性的关联已经提出过[23-24]。在 5q31(IBD5) 上，左旋肉碱/有机阳离子转运蛋白与克罗恩病相关，特别是有机阳离子转运蛋白变体与肛周疾病相关。最近，已经提出另一个定位于染色体 5q33.1 的基因易感性[23-26]。肛周克罗恩病的一个理论认为隐窝腺感染导致脓肿再形成瘘管，随后瘘管在手术切口、引流或者脓肿自发性破裂后从肛周皮肤流出。排泄物改道促使肛瘘长期好转，而抗生素作为治疗手段，暗示了肠道微生物在克罗恩病肛瘘的发病机理的作用。关于肛周克罗恩病肛瘘在免疫细胞的数量和质量上改变的影响的数据很少。Bataille 等[27]曾检验克罗恩病患者患有瘘道的本质，从瘘道的根源上"控制"，而不是炎性肠病。他们能够证明在两组中，T 细胞、B 细胞及巨噬细胞在位置和数量上的不同。现在我们相信，和管腔克罗恩病一样，肛周克罗恩病的病因涉及微生物学、免疫学和遗传学因素的相互作用。

肛周解剖

克罗恩病的治疗需要对肛门周围的解剖结构有详细的了解。对于疾病的程度的解剖定义和与不同结构之间的关系是了解肛瘘和其他肛周病变的病因和分类的基本条件。肛管是大肠的末端，包括两组括约肌：肛门内括约肌和肛门外括约肌。肛门内括约肌由直肠壁环形肌层的增厚形成，为不随意肌，而肛门外括约肌为盆腔肌肉（耻骨直肠肌和肛提肌）向下增厚形成，属于骨骼肌。齿状线距肛缘约 2cm，接近于肛管的中点，是从头端的直肠柱状上皮到尾端的肛门鳞状上皮的转变点。下段直肠的黏膜皱襞进入肛管形成肛柱，肛柱终止于齿状线。肛隐窝位于肛柱的底部。肛腺开口于肛隐窝底部。通常，每个人有 6 个肛腺，多见于前象限。

分 类

根据克罗恩病的肛周表现，有很多分类方法。在解剖上最精确的分类是 Parks 等[28]提出的将肛门外括约肌作为参考点，描述了肛瘘的 5 种基本类型，即表浅型、括约肌间型、经括约肌型、括约肌上型和括约肌外型（图 22.1）[29]。

1992 年，Hughes[30]提出了一个基于解剖和病理方面的临床分类，这得益于一项在英国加的夫进行的关于肛周克罗恩病的 20 年的前瞻性研究。主要通过数值反映严重性的分类方法明确了溃疡、瘘或脓肿的存在和狭窄的程度：0= 不存在，1= 有限的临床影响，2= 严重。辅助的分类方法明确了相关的情况（如痔疮和伴随癌症）、近端肠管受累（小

第 22 章 肛周克罗恩病的治疗

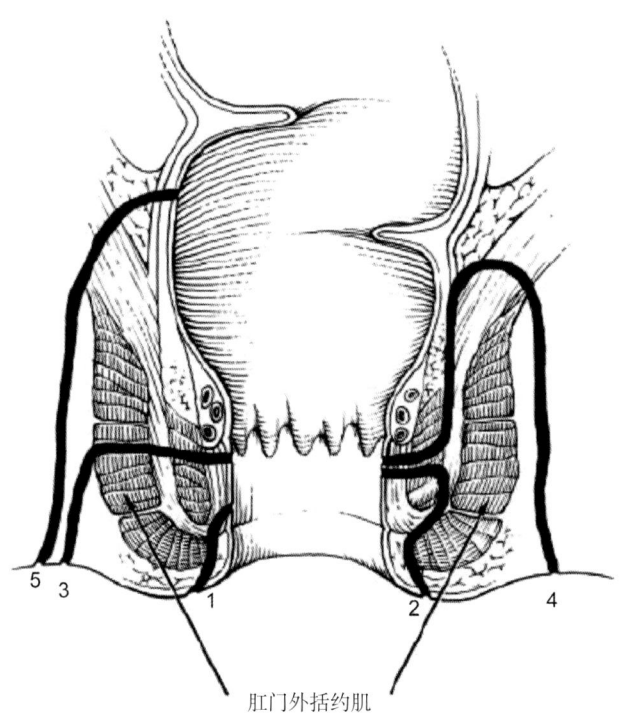

图 22.1 肛瘘的 5 种基本类型，即表浅型（1）、括约肌间型（2）、经括约肌型（3）、括约肌上型（4）和括约肌外型（5）（Reprinted with permission from Hughes.[30]）

肠和结肠）以及疾病活动性（不活跃和活跃）（表 22.1 和表 22.2）。

美国胃肠病协会在 2003 年的技术审查中提出一个有两大类的分类方法[31]：单纯性和复杂性肛

表 22.1 Hughes-Cardiff 分类

溃疡（U）	瘘/脓肿（F）	狭窄（S）
0 不存在	*0 不存在*	*0 不存在*
1 表浅肛裂	*1 低位表浅型*	*1 膜状的*
肉质皮垂	Anovulval/ 阴囊	
	经括约肌型	
	肛门阴道的	
2 空洞的溃疡	*2 高位表浅型*	*2 不可逆狭窄*
肛管	Blind supralevator	肛门狭窄
直肠	直肠阴道	
融合的皮肤溃疡	肛门直肠回肠	
相关的肛门疾病（A）	*近端疾病（P）*	
痔疮	0 无	
恶性肿瘤	1 邻近的直肠疾病	
	2 结肠（直肠不受累）	
	3 小肠	

表 22.2 简单的 Hughes 分类

溃疡（U）	瘘/脓肿（F）	狭窄（S）
0 不存在	0 不存在	0 不存在
1 表浅肛裂	1 低位	1 膜状的
2 空洞性的	2 高位	2 纤维化的

瘘。单纯性肛瘘为低位的（如表浅型、低位括约肌间型和低位经括约肌型），只有一个外口，并且无肛周脓肿、直肠狭窄和巨结肠炎，不累及阴道或膀胱。相反，复杂性肛瘘为高位的（如高位括约肌间型、高位经括约肌型、括约肌上型和括约肌外型），可以有数个外口，且可能合并肛周脓肿、直肠狭窄或巨结肠炎，可累及阴道或膀胱。

Irvine[32] 提出用肛周克罗恩病活动指数（PDAI）去计算肛周疾病的发病率。这个指数评估肛瘘的 5 项指标，包括排泄物、疼痛、对性生活的限制、肛周疾病的类型和硬化程度。PDAI 评估对肛周疾病患者的生活质量影响最大的各个方面。表 22.3 是一个改良过的 Irvine 分类法。

诊断 / 评估

肛周克罗恩病的大多数表现在彻底的体格检查中很容易发现。在决定任何治疗措施前，肠道病变程度的完整评估和肛周的病理结果是必要的，而组织活检证明出肉芽肿只有在某些情况下是必要的。诊断时常着重确定受累的肛周的类型、位置和性质。这个评估常常需要详细的病史、体格检查和联合肛管内超声检查（EAUS）、骨盆的磁共振影像（MRI）和麻醉状态下手术探查（EUA），或者 3 者都需要。传统上，麻醉状态下探查（EUA）是金标准。在 Schwartz 等采用 34 例患者的前瞻性研究中发现，与 EUA 联合肛管内超声检查（EAUS）和骨盆 MRI 相比，单独采用 EUA 的准确率只有 90%。同样的研究发现当采用 3 种检查的任何两种的诊断准确率是 100%。

EAUS 使肛门括约肌更清晰直观。在普通超声中，内括约肌、括约肌间的空间和外括约肌看起来就像一个同心圆图层。内括约肌是低回声，2～3mm 宽。括约肌间的空间是等回声的，而肛门外括约肌是混合回声模式。这容易使正常解剖形态受到干扰，看到一个低回声的线型结构，尽管在某

表 22.3 改良的肛周克罗恩病 Irvine 分类法 [32]

Irvine 分类法				
排出物	无	最小量的黏液	化脓的	粪便的
疼痛	无	轻微的	中等的	严重的
对性生活的限制	无	轻微的	中等的	严重的
肛周疾病的类型				
无		肛裂	有 3 个瘘以上	有 3 个瘘以上	溃疡
硬化程度	无	轻微的	中等的	广泛性脓肿

些时候等回声气泡也能出现。对瘘道分类的准确率在 86.5%～95%[34-35] 之间。在更大量的患者队列中发现内口的比例在 62.5%～94%[36-37]。这和文献中关于 EAUS 检测肛瘘的准确性不一致，这可以部分地解释为是由于那些报告使用了过氧化氢装置，以及在某些情况下当声影穿过括约肌间脓肿时，可能过多地诊断为肛瘘。过氧化氢能改善肛瘘的可视化效果是大家公认的[34,35,38-43]。随着对二维影像的三维重建的使用，有些调查显示 EAUS 的效果可以和 MRI 相媲美，而且使用起来患者能很好耐受[44-45]。在这方面，最近的数据提示 EAUS 三维影像的再处理改变了影像的透明度、亮度、射线穿透厚度和图像过滤，通过从数据集除去低强度像素，提高术前对脓肿和内口的明确[46]。这个容积呈现模式建议采用低厚度、低滤过、中度光亮和中－低透明度参数。有一个小试验将便携式经会阴超声和非克罗恩病的肛瘘患者的手术结果对比，结果显示经会阴超声对于确定肛瘘类型和内口的位置有很高的准确度，尽管如果有显著的马蹄形状或相关的含气体的脓肿[47]将降低准确度。过氧化氢滴注则没有益处。

骨盆 MRI 已被证明对肛瘘分类的准确率为 90%，描述复杂性脓肿的准确率为 97%[48-49]。此外，由于 MRI 和 EUA 的使用，10%～20% 的患者的手术治疗方案可能改变，而在克罗恩病患者中将增加至 40%[50-51]。由于伴随直肠炎症，因此在复杂的肛周克罗恩病患者中联合骨盆 MRI、EUA 和直肠镜检查去评估是常用的方案。肛管内 MRI 是利用一种连接外部磁石的半缩醛聚合物的直肠探条，对于靠近探条的内口的描述具有高度的准确性，即使只有克罗恩病的有限信息[52-53]。这个装置还没有广泛使用，并具有所有腔内技术的局限性，如一侧的括约肌外肛瘘超出探条的焦距，以及耻骨直肠肌与探条不能够充分连接，这些都没有很好地证明。动态对比增强 MRI 在测定肛周克罗恩病的疾病活动度的使用是最近的一个发展。使用这个技术，执行二维 T1 加权扫描和得到对比增强的时间强度曲线，所以能够测量瘘的"活动"。活跃的肛瘘患者增强像素的量比不活跃的肛瘘患者更高[54]。

瘘管造影术被证实有 16%～50%[55-56] 的准确率，但不是常规推荐的检查。尽管很多报道描述它对内口勾画的准确性，但也是苦痛的，这可能和严重的菌血症相关，瘘管造影术还能够推测出瘘道和主要的括约肌复合体的关系。同样，计算机断层扫描（CT）被证明用于评估肛周疾病不可靠；准确率为 24%～60%[57-63]，部分因为这个技术的平均容积效应没有提供足够的分辨率来分辨粪便瘘道和坐骨直肠的脂肪。

只要肛肠疾病能够描绘出来，就可以考虑对近端克罗恩病的内窥镜检查和小肠的放射学检查的评估。一项 5491 例克罗恩病患者的研究发现近端肠瘘疾病和肛瘘之间有关联[64]。有些研究者发现近端疾病的治疗可能促进肛肠症状的消退[2,65]；可是，另外一些研究者没有观察到这些方面的改善[66-67]。大多数专家没有仅仅为了改善肛肠疾病的症状而采用近端小肠的手术干预[68-69]。

治 疗

鉴于肛周病变和相关症状的多样化，治疗也常常是多变和个性化的。一个多学科的方法对于成功治疗患有复杂疾病的患者很有必要，而对于肛周克罗恩病患者的治疗需要外科医师和胃肠科医师的密切合作。由于症状严重程度不同，治疗也可能不同。还包括患者的营养状态、胃肠道病变的范围和严重性等其他注意事项。在决策过程中必须考虑患者的担忧和期望。在一些只有很少症状的患者中，即使可能是严重的肛周疾病，目标也应该是使症状减少到最低限度或缓解，而不是根治疾病；并且要避免采用直肠切除术，尽管在 20% 的患者中直肠切除术不可避免[10]。在个别患者特定病变的治疗可能不同，而某些一般措施对大多数患者有益，如改善营养状态、近端疾病的治疗，以及包括坐浴、淋浴、使用局部防护脂等局部皮肤措施。

疾病谱

肛周克罗恩病包含不成瘘病变和成瘘病变。不成瘘病变主要有皮垂、痔疮、溃疡、狭窄和癌症；而成瘘病变包括肛瘘、脓肿和直肠阴道瘘。

皮 垂

在对联合药物和手术治疗的克罗恩病的随访中，Keighley 和 Allan[70] 报道在 375 例克罗恩病患者中，患有肛门皮垂的患者在克罗恩病和肛周疾病的分组患者中占 68%。尽管克罗恩病患者中常常发现皮垂局限于结肠，大约 36.7% 患有肛门皮垂的患者累及回肠[71]。这里描述了两种类型的皮垂[72]。第 1 种是典型的克罗恩病皮垂，外形巨大、水肿、坚硬及发绀，这种皮垂由于淋巴水肿导致淋巴回流受阻产生，常合并肠炎。第 2 种类型是扁平、宽基或窄基的病变，通常被称为"象耳"皮垂，这种皮垂柔软而无痛。

皮垂一般持久存在，为良性。它们常常变大，合并肠炎时形成水肿。只有 1 例恶性转变曾在文献中报道过[73]。一个医疗中心提及的 109 例患者中 68% 的患者在诊断时患有皮垂，直到 10 年后仍然存在[74]。这些患者中 86% 是没有症状的[75]。皮垂在大小和厚度上可能增加，而且在突然发作的活跃的克罗恩病可能变得更坚硬[76]。

治 疗

肛门皮垂是良性的，人们希望治疗是因为它们影响卫生，或由于症状持续存在会增加伤口延迟愈合的风险。

痔 疮

克罗恩病患者很少患有痔疮，患者中发病率只有 7%[70]，低于一般人群的估计发病率 24%[77]。尽管常常无症状，可是由于克罗恩病相关的严重腹泻，症状也可能恶化。

治 疗

由于伤口延迟愈合、炎症、感染和狭窄的显著发生率，一般避免采用手术干预[78]。克罗恩病患者有症状的痔疮的保守治疗来自 St. Mark 小组在 1977 年对一小部分病例所做的回顾性研究报道称发现切口愈合不良导致一半患者要进行直肠切除术。这个报道延续了相当长的一段时期，因此对痔疮切除术的实施和本质应该给予一些怀疑，而且对于随后的直肠切除指征没有明确的评估标准。在没有任何直肠克罗恩病证据的患者中，痔疮切除术在高达 88% 的有症状的患者中安全有效[79]。其他治疗痔疮的小范围的手术方法，包括橡皮带结扎法、多普勒超声引导下的痔动脉结扎术、脱肛的吻合器手术以及吻合器痔固定术，这些手术的作用目前尚不明确。

肛裂和溃疡

根据简化的卡的夫分类，溃疡在克罗恩病中可分为肛裂和溃疡。报道的克罗恩病肛门溃疡的发病率是 43%[12, 80-83]。浅表肛裂在所有克罗恩病的肛门肛裂中占 21%～35%[80, 84]，空洞溃疡的发病率是 5%～10%[12, 70, 85]。

溃 疡

虽然权威上认为克罗恩病相关的肛门溃疡不痛，可是有报道高达 70% 的患者感觉疼痛[82, 86, 87]。其他症状包括有排出物、皮肤瘙痒和出血。空洞性溃疡更可能形成主要的瘘道。溃疡的边缘常常是水肿的、不规则、被破坏的和剥脱的。空洞性溃疡可能出现在肛管上部或邻近直肠黏膜。溃疡扩大至肛管外和肛周皮肤很罕见，但可能以激烈的侵蚀性的发病形式出现[29]。在 75%～96% 的病例中伴随直肠炎[85, 88]。14%～33% 的溃疡患者观察到患有多个溃疡[81-83]。溃疡有两种不同的演化模式：大多数自然痊愈，而部分病例会形成肛瘘、脓肿或肛门狭窄。空洞型溃疡的远期疗效常常不理想，报道高达 83% 的患者有采用直肠切除术的风险[70]。在图 22.2 中可以看到扩大的溃疡的例子。

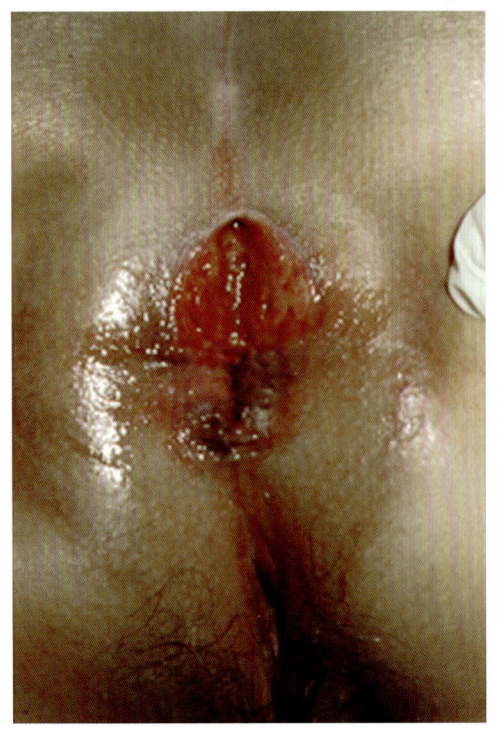

图 22.2　肛周溃疡

肛　裂

克罗恩病的肛裂一般认为是由于疾病进展中的溃疡导致，与肛门内括约肌抽搐可能没有必然的关系，原发性肛裂就是如此。与原发性肛裂几乎常位于中线的情况相反，高达 20% 的克罗恩病患者的肛裂位于偏离中线的地方，而且常多发。在图 22.3 中可见与克罗恩病相关的肛裂扩大至肛周皮肤，与原发性肛裂的外形相比有显著的差异。

药物治疗

外用药物可用于减轻症状，但不能促进损伤愈合。甲硝唑（10%）软膏对于降低肛周疾病活动指数（PDAI）得分无效，但是对于一些次要指标如疼痛和排出物具有改善的治疗效果[89]。两项分别包括 5 例患者的小样本研究和 7 例患者的随机对照试验显示，他克莫司（0.5～1mg/g）虽然不能治愈溃疡，但是可以迅速改善患者的溃疡深度、表面积、硬结和疼痛[90]。局部病灶的激素治疗在某些患者也是有效的。

全身中毒性毒剂也曾用于肛门溃疡的治疗，虽然有部分疗效，但是其不良反应妨碍了它们的使用。在最近的一项 99 例患者的回顾性研究中发现英夫利昔单抗治疗可以很好地被患者耐受，并能有效地使肛门溃疡诱导和维持临床完全缓解状态[91]。经过英夫利昔诱导治疗后，42.5% 患者的溃疡得到完全缓解。175 周的中期随访后的远期疗效显示，72% 的溃疡患者得到了完全缓解，而浅表肛裂和空洞性溃疡等症状也有明显相似的结果。英夫利昔具有快速消除症状和长期维持的优点。总之，最近有证据支持使用肿瘤坏死因子（TNF）疗法治疗症状性溃疡。一些报道提出，高压氧和要素饮食可以促进肛门溃疡和肛裂的愈合[92-95]。外用硝酸甘油、钙通道阻滞剂和肉毒杆菌毒素这些曾在治疗克罗恩病原发性肛裂被证明有效的药物治疗的作用还不明确[96]。

手术治疗

幸运的是，肛裂在克罗恩病患者中主要表现出自限性进展：在一个小组的 53 例患者中，只有 10 例 (19%) 在 10 年的随访后仍然患有肛裂[96]。伴有疼痛的难治性肛裂的患者在排除了脓毒症的情况下可行侧方内括约肌切开术。手术后的治愈率高，且并发症发生率低。持续存在的肛裂有进展成肛周脓肿、肛瘘或者两者同时存在的倾向，最终常常需要行直肠切除术。在不愿意采取保守治疗的患者应该慎重选用局部肛肠手术，特别是侧方内括约肌切开术。如果选用括约肌切开术，应该考虑采取闭式手术来减小潜在的不愈合伤口的大小[83]。继发的巨大空洞性溃疡的症状常可以用对突出边缘清创术和病灶内类固醇注射来控制。虽然如此，由于持续的疼痛、脓毒症或大便失禁，部分患者可能最终仍需行直肠切除术。

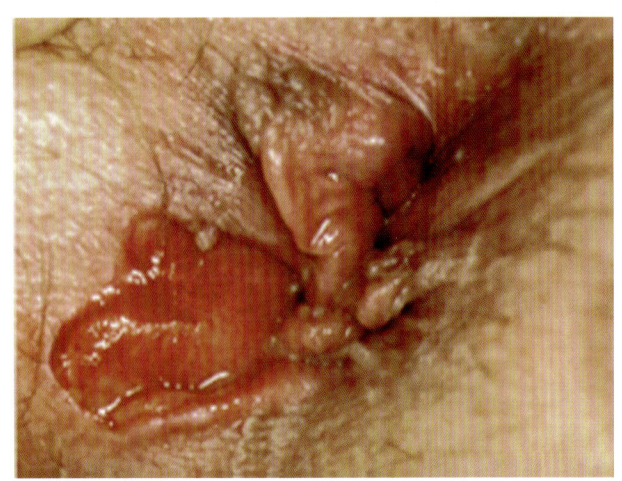

图 22.3　与克罗恩病相关的肛裂

狭　窄

肛门或直肠狭窄可能作为肛管或直肠溃疡、肛周脓肿和肛瘘的并发症出现，而且常伴随正在进行的直肠炎症、复杂性肛瘘和阴道直肠肛瘘。克罗恩病患者常患有低度的肛管狭窄。转诊中心报道了肛门狭窄的不同的发病率，从9%～22%[97-98]。在肛周克罗恩病的肛门狭窄中区分肛门和直肠下端的狭窄的病理结果，各占34%和50%。根据直肠的长度不同，狭窄可分为短肛门狭窄和长管状狭窄。结肠疾病和肛门狭窄的存在与永久性人造瘘的需要具有显著的相关性[99]。

治　疗

肛管扩张术常用来治疗症状性肛门狭窄，通过轻柔的扩张术或使用同轴球囊技术[87]。刚开始必须在麻醉下非常轻柔地进行。由于存在脓毒症的风险，选用扩张术必须慎重：严重的直肠炎或手术中发生的脓毒症会增加风险。反复扩肛而无效的患有严重狭窄的患者可能需要行直肠切除术[96]。

脓肿和肛瘘

肛周克罗恩病患者常出现化脓的并发症，常以脓肿或肛瘘的形式出现。克罗恩病肛瘘的发生率据报道占克罗恩病患者数的17%～43%[100]。肛瘘的复杂性取决于脓肿引流的种类。脓肿患者常表现为急性发作的疼痛，往往需要紧急手术干预。肛瘘可表现为再发脓肿伴随或不伴随自发破溃，持续的排出物和疼痛，偶有失禁。克罗恩病肛瘘的发病机理尚未完全了解，但一般认为是由于排泄物对肛周溃疡的逐渐损害、侵袭作用或脓肿形成的结果。血纤蛋白的生成和基质金属蛋白酶表达的缺陷也被认为促进克罗恩病肛瘘的形成[101]。

肛周克罗恩病无法通过药物或手术治愈。治疗目的在于减轻症状和治疗疾病并发症来改善患者生活质量。引导治疗的原则包括清除脓毒症区域的能力、避免损害肛门括约肌和药物治疗辅助最终手术治疗的成效。

脓肿 / 肛周脓毒症

脓肿可出现在任何平面（浅表的、括约肌间、坐骨直肠和盆腔直肠），但不管在什么位置，都需要尽快手术切除和引流及选用广谱抗生素治疗全身症状。疼痛、肿胀和发热是患有脓肿的标志。患盆腔直肠脓肿的患者可能主诉臀部肌肉疼痛的症状。也有报道直肠出血。严重的直肠疼痛伴有无法避免的泌尿系统症状如排尿困难和尿潴留，可能提示患有括约肌间或盆腔直肠脓肿。

患有肛周或坐骨直肠脓肿的患者检查发现红斑、肿胀和可能的波动感。对于括约肌间或盆腔直肠脓肿的患者，必须认识到，尽管患者诉有剧烈的疼痛，却没有可见的外在表现。患有盆腔直肠脓肿的患者，可能在直肠或阴道检查中触诊到柔软的包块。如果有黑斑可能提示存在坏死性感染的扩散。

治　疗

对于浅表性脓肿，简单的切开和引流手术就有效，切口（椭圆形或十字形的）选在表皮的内侧。肛瘘的炎症消除时，手术应该尽可能减少切开组织。大多数坐骨直肠脓肿可以用类似的方式来切开和引流，但是马蹄形脓肿应该在局麻、最好是全麻的条件下引流。在后正中线和内括约肌的下半部的分离处做一个开口，从一般认为是感染灶的肛后空间中引流。在每个坐骨直肠窝开一个小切口就可以引流脓肿的前部，不需要宽切口。当一个患者表现出的疼痛与其阳性体征不对称时，需要考虑诊断为括约肌间脓肿，因此通过麻醉状态下探查（EUA）对疼痛原因的彻底评估是必须的。确诊后，沿着脓腔的范围分开肛门内括约肌。

盆腔直肠脓肿在引流前，须先弄清起因：可能由括约肌间脓肿或坐骨直肠脓肿向上扩大引起；也可能是盆腔脓肿向下扩大引起。如果是由括约肌间脓肿引起，应该通过直肠引流而不通过坐骨直肠窝，因为后者将会导致括约肌上型肛瘘。可是，如果是由坐骨直肠引起，就应该通过坐骨直肠窝来引流，而不是直肠，因为通过直肠引流会形成括约肌外型肛瘘。如果脓肿是从盆腔产生，则可以根据它的指向通过直肠、坐骨直肠窝或腹壁来引流，尽管有可能形成难以有效治疗的括约肌外型肛瘘的风险。对于深位或高位脓肿（位于盆腔直肠或坐骨直肠），瘘道或手术切口的引流很可能阻塞，需要放置蘑菇头导管或无切口挂线来保证持续充分的引流。在由原发的坐骨直肠脓肿扩散至盆腔直肠脓肿中使用缩短的护理引流管有效。导管的外露部分缩短至只留

2~3cm在皮肤外，而吸头放在脓腔的深部。这减少了在某些情况下导管滑出脓腔外或进入脓腔里的概率，而且这可能是复杂性肛瘘的长期解决方案，特别是如果还存在活动性直肠炎的情况。

是否需要在初次脓肿引流时确定内口是值得争议的。许多研究建议不应过分地检查。对于复发，在解决活动性炎症后，对于伴随的肛瘘的检查是必需的。一个简单的方法是在麻醉状态下检查（EUA）时将过氧化氢或稀释亚甲蓝注射进蕈头导管或通过外口注射。通过初次脓肿引流，患者仍然患有顽固性脓毒症或疾病恶化时，暂时性的转移性造口有效，制造一个利于肛周局部修复的有利环境。在这方面，选择腔镜更好，因为其损害小，且能够检查相关近端肠道疾病的存在。

肛　瘘

图 22.4 示联合肛管内超声检查时的经括约肌型肛瘘瘘道。

药物治疗
抗生素

理论上，细菌对于肛瘘疾病的外观和顽固性有影响。因此，抗生素在治疗肛瘘有时会选择作为一线药物。在其他情况，鉴于抗生素对于感染和脓肿的预防作用，也会用于辅助性（过渡性）治疗。大多数使用抗生素治疗肛瘘疾病的研究没有对照，而且样本数量太小。在这些研究中，甲硝唑[102-104]、环丙沙星[105]及联合两种药物[106]在治疗肛瘘时表现出最初的有益作用。疗效一般在 6~8 周的疗程后出现，常表现为引流物减少。肛瘘闭合的情况罕见，但是在治疗暂停后症状有复发的倾向[104]。

甲硝唑一般起始量按体重每天20mg/kg的剂量，分3次服用，每天共1000~1500mg。不良反应包括恶心、口中金属味和以感觉异常为表现形式的周围神经病变。不良反应常严重至必须减量甚至停止用药。Bernstein 等[102]报道过 21 例肛周克罗恩病患者使用甲硝唑治疗的研究，所有患者都有疼痛减轻和变柔软的临床反应。56% 的患者肛周疾病完全治愈。临床疗效一般发生在治疗后的 6~8 周。对同一人群[103]的随访研究发现，50% 的患者由于剂量减少而恶化，以及出现感觉异常的症状。

环丙沙星一般每天用量 1000mg（每片 500mg），可单独用药，也可与甲硝唑联合用药。类似的研究已有报道[104]。West 等[105]最近在 22 例患者中联合使用英夫利昔与环丙沙星或安慰剂的对照试验。18周的短期随访发现患者中使用环丙沙星组比安慰剂组（1/4，2.4）效果更好。疗效通过临床（引流的肛瘘数量下降了 50%）和影像学检查（使用三维联合肛管内超声检查或过氧化氢注射）检测。环丙沙星的不良反应很少，包括头痛、恶心、腹泻和皮疹[106]。Solomon 等[107]所做的类似的研究发现无英夫利昔的联合用药治疗具有相似的优点。

硫嘌呤类药物

咪唑硫嘌呤 (AZA) 和 6-硫基嘌呤 (6-MP) 证实对治疗克罗恩病肛瘘有效。5 组对照试验的荟萃分析发现，在使用 AZA 或 6-MP 的患者中有 54% 有疗效（定义为瘘道完全闭合或引流量减少），而安慰剂组只有 21% 患者有疗效（比值比为 4.44；95% 可信区间为 1.50~13.2）[108]。这个荟萃分析所包含的所有研究都存在局限，它们的肛瘘的疗效均是次要结果指标而不是主要结果指标。硫嘌呤类药物在克罗恩病患者中封闭瘘道的疗效评估中的次要指标没有进行对照试验。AZA 的初始剂量为每天按体重 2.0~3.0mg/kg，6-MP 的初始剂量为每天按体重 1.0~1.5mg/kg。开始用药后必须监测全血血细胞和检测肝功酶。由于这类药物药效起效时间较长，开始常常需要联合其他药物如抗生素或英夫利昔。

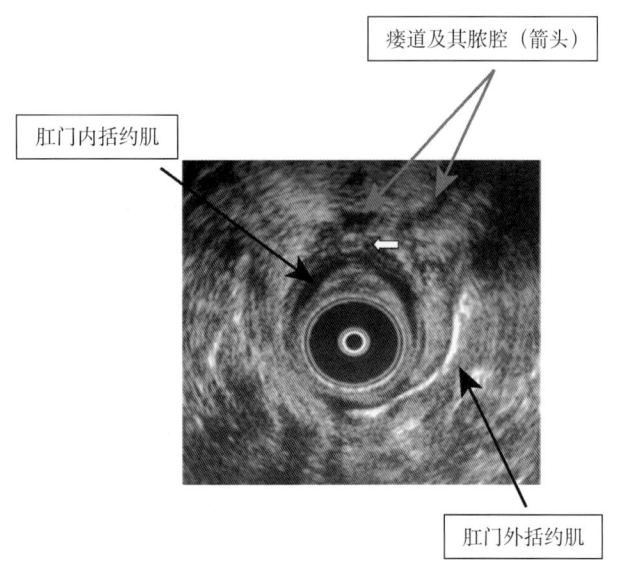

图 22.4　经括约肌型肛瘘瘘道的肛管内超声图

免疫抑制剂疗法

环孢素和他克莫司是一种钙调神经磷酸酶抑制剂，消除T细胞活性和白介素（IL）-2的产物。两种药都有潜在的免疫调节的功能，成功用于实质器官排斥的预防已有数十年。许多非对照试验已经证明环孢素治疗肛周疾病的有效性，瘘道闭合率约90%，且作用快速持久。在Present和Lichtiger[109]的研究中，先以每天4mg/kg的药量通过静脉注射环孢素，再换成每天口服6~8mg/kg的药量。治疗暂停后复发率很高。由Sandborn等[110]进行的随机安慰剂对照试验中，20例肛瘘患者每天服用他克莫司0.2mg/kg。服用10周，结果50%的患者瘘道闭合，而且闭合至少维持4周以上。他克莫司（经口服）能有效地促进肛瘘引流（43% vs 8%），但无法消除肛瘘（10% vs 8%）。两种药物都有明显的不良反应，特别是肾损害。患者需要经常监测血药浓度和肾功能。

单克隆抗体治疗

肿瘤坏死因子（TNF）-a是克罗恩病发病机理中非常关键的炎症介质。不同的抗TNF-a抗体疗法对于治疗克罗恩病有效，包括妥珠单抗（赛妥珠单抗，优时比制药公司，佐治亚州士麦那）、阿达木单抗（修美乐，雅培制药，艾伯特公园，伊利诺伊州）和英夫利昔（类克，山淘克公司，马尔文迪，宾夕法尼亚州）。近期，英夫利昔仍然是治疗克罗恩病使用最广泛的抗TNF-a抗体疗法。英夫利昔一般是指导嵌合型的单克隆免疫球蛋白直接对抗可溶性的穿膜的人类TNF-a。TNF-a是促炎症细胞因子，主要由单核细胞、巨噬细胞和T淋巴细胞产生。它具有重要的促进炎症和免疫刺激的功能，包括白细胞激活、中性粒细胞趋化性、抑制炎症细胞凋亡及对其他促炎症因子的诱导，如白细胞介素-1、白细胞介素-6和白细胞介素-8。在克罗恩病，TNF-a及其产物的水平在有炎症的肠道里是增加的，以维持炎症反应。英夫利昔的作用还未完全清楚，除了中和可溶性、穿膜的TNF-a外，英夫利昔可能还有其他重要的功能，如在抗体与穿膜的TNF-a结合后诱导单核细胞和固有层T细胞凋亡和抑制中性粒细胞趋化性。最近，英夫利昔被证实有刺激肌成纤维细胞转移的作用，这个作用对于治愈肛瘘有重大作用。

在一个双盲随机对照试验，Present等[111]将服用0周、2周、6周的不同剂量（5mg和10mg）的英夫利昔的患者与服用同样时间的安慰剂组的患者对比。首要目标是以在连续两次甚至多次的考察注意到50%肛瘘闭合为基线，而次要目标是所有肛瘘都闭合。接受5mg/kg剂量的患者中68%患者达成了首要目标，55%的患者达成了次要目标，而接受安慰剂的小组达成首要目标的只有26%，次要目标只有13%。接受10mg/kg剂量的患者没有比5mg/kg剂量的患者有更好的疗效，而且服用2周时都出现了中值响应时间。服用英夫利昔的患者中有11%在治疗过程中出现了肛周胀肿，而安慰剂组则只有3%。推测是由于在瘘道的闭合前外口的过快闭合导致这种并发症。ACCENT试验检测英夫利昔维持治疗的作用，通过研究306例患克罗恩病肛瘘的患者服用0周、2周和6周的英夫利昔。195例响应者（69%）被随机分配至服用每8周5mg/kg剂量的安慰剂或英夫利昔。安慰剂组无效的中值时间是14周，显著不同的是英夫利昔组超过40周。联合英夫利昔和咪唑硫嘌呤（AZA）或6-硫基嘌呤（6-MP）可能导致持续更长时间的缓解和更易耐药[112]。一般来说，只要肛瘘确诊及脓毒症控制后，英夫利昔可按5mg/kg的剂量开始服用。这可以在医院的门诊治疗中按0、2和6周疗程实施。建议在2~6周（在第2次和第3次剂量之间）时肛瘘引流停止后取出挂线。如果患者在前两次用药后症状没有改善，以后也不可能有效，应该停止治疗。此外，尽管报道的服用英夫利昔的临床治愈率惊人，完全的影像学闭合却不一定发生[106, 113, 114]，问题是当治疗停止后这些肛瘘最后会不会再次张开。包括头痛、恶心、上呼吸道感染、腹痛和疲乏等大多数报道的不良反应都是轻微的，而且不一定与英夫利昔有关。主要的不良反应很少，包括肺炎、发热和呼吸苦难。粟粒性肺结核、脓毒症和卡氏肺孢子肺炎的机会性感染的风险增加。还有报告淋巴瘤和心衰的风险增加。

最近，有提议英夫利昔局部给药用于治疗克罗恩病肛瘘，具有增加治疗的有效性、同时减少全身治疗相关的不良反应的优点。两项评估使用英夫利昔局部注射入瘘道的安全和有效性的小研究有令人鼓舞的结果。Lichtiger[115]报道9例患者中有4例在4周里肛瘘完全治愈，还有3例患者有部分疗效，无不良反应报道，6个月后没有检测自身抗体。同样，Poggioli等[116]报道15例患者中的10例治愈，且无主要的不良反应。这些最初的调查结果需要更多的确证来检测局部给药途径的有效性。尽管有药物治疗后肛瘘闭合的临床表现，但 MRI 和直肠腔内超声分析发现主要的瘘道仍然存在。这解释了在某些情况下药物停止后肛瘘复发的原因，提示需要长期使用药物保持瘘道的畅通。但由于许多药物的不良反应和高成本，长期药物治疗不可行。

其他治疗

一个开放性试点研究提供的数据表示，粒细胞巨噬细胞集落刺激因子（GM-CSF）是活动性肛周克罗恩病安全且潜在的有效治疗方法[117]。GM-CSF 曾用于管腔克罗恩病患者的安慰剂对照试验，部分患者有肛瘘引流史的研究记录。在 6 个月时，GM-CSF 小组的 8 例患者中有 4 例肛瘘完全闭合，而安慰剂对照组的 5 例患者中有 2 例肛瘘完全闭合[118]。没有足够的数据支持素膳和口服球面吸附碳[119]在肛周克罗恩病患者中的作用。

药物治疗的总结

在美国胃肠病协会的技术评估中[30]，英夫利昔是治疗复杂性肛周疾病的推荐药物，在诱导期还能联合咪唑硫嘌呤（AZA）、6-硫基嘌呤（6-MP）和抗生素。维持治疗则推荐选用咪唑硫嘌呤（AZA）、6-硫基嘌呤（6-MP），在某些情况还可联合英夫利昔。

手术治疗

克罗恩病患者肛瘘的手术治疗是基于是否存在全结肠炎及肛瘘的位置和类型。手术对每个患者应该在外科医师的经验和判断的基础上个体化治疗。直肠组织的状态及是否存在全结肠炎常常决定合适的手术治疗方式。

用于治疗肛瘘的手术方式基本没有变化，仍然可以导致再次发病。如高位经括约肌型和括约肌上型肛瘘等复杂性肛瘘的手术治疗更可能导致术后并发症，特别是大便失禁或肛管狭窄。打开复杂性肛瘘的方法在超过 50% 的病例中导致大便失禁[120]。保留括约肌技术包括除芯瘘管切开术、永久挂线治疗和推移皮瓣技术用于治疗复杂性肛瘘，然而这些手术仍然有很高的复发率。

瘘管切开术/瘘管切除术

瘘管切开术，也称为肛瘘切除缝合术，是目前最常使用的肛瘘治疗手术。通过在瘘道中开一个切口，然后打开瘘道，再与肛管结合起来，因此使肛瘘可以从内到外愈合。没有累及肛门外括约肌的括约肌间型肛瘘和低位经括约肌型肛瘘相对容易治疗，常选用瘘道切开术治疗，大便失禁的风险低[121]。将切开的瘘道内侧缝合至切口的皮肤边缘，这种切开术切口的袋形缝合术可能促进愈合[122]。确定内口是瘘道切开术治疗成功的关键。如果疏忽会导致形成假的瘘道。真正脓毒症的来源没有根除。影像学可能帮助引导外科医师定位内口。首先插入肛门牵开器（一般是 Hill-Ferguson），然后通过伸入探条或探条从外口伸到内口（相反也可），试着精确定位内口。注入过氧化氢可能在内口产生气泡，有助于定位。

另外一个常用于治疗括约肌间型或低位经括约肌型肛瘘的手术是瘘道切除术，这种手术是将整个瘘道完全切除。复发率与瘘道切开术类似，但瘘道切除术的切口更大。同切开术相似，瘘道切除术的袋形缝合术也有助于减小切口和促进愈合[122]。

挂线疗法

由于瘘道切开术和切除术可能导致切口的不愈合，选用无切口的（引流）的挂线疗法更好。最早的挂线由马鬃制成，后来还用过丝绸、尼龙、聚酯、橡胶、硅橡胶、乳胶、塑料、电线等，最近使用新材料如自锁式尼龙扎带。挂线用于防止瘘道外口的闭合，而且可以引流肛周脓肿，对于引流的连续性只有轻微的影响。事实上，很少有关于使用切口挂线后对引流连续性的影响的资料，最近的证据显示形成多个近端内口的损伤率大约为 12%[123]。用这种方式，挂线可预防脓肿复发，尽管这种效果在克罗恩病中不是普遍成功。宽松的挂线常用于治疗克罗恩病患者的高位肛瘘。尽管长期挂线引流治疗克罗恩病高位肛瘘具有保留肛门括约肌功能的作用，但是 39% 的患者脱除挂线后导致肛瘘的复发[124]，在某些情况下，可能建议需要放置永久性挂线。此外，发现 5% 使用这种方法的患者发生大便失禁[124]。

切口挂线用于缓慢地切开括约肌却又不损害肌肉。这种疼痛的手术可能需要几个月的时间去完成，也可能需要行瘘道切开术，高达 50% 的患者排便的控制受到影响[125-128]。

图 22.5 示挂线在肛周克罗恩病患者的使用。

推移皮瓣技术

直肠黏膜的推移皮瓣技术最早描述于 1912 年，

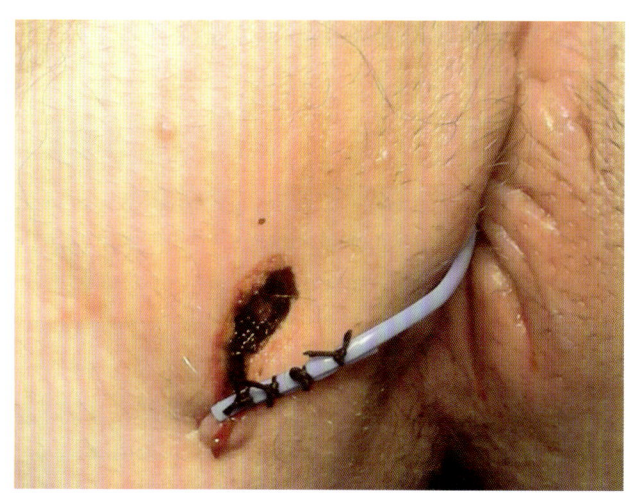

图 22.5 在继发高位肛瘘的肛周克罗恩病患者使用长期挂线

是一种通用的手术,不会危及排便的控制,也没有直肠切除术的风险。当没有活动性直肠炎时,推移皮瓣技术是一个手术选择。手术在经过化学和生物的肠道准备后在全麻下进行。需要仔细确认瘘道的位置及用刮匙刮干净肉芽组织。用含或不含肾上腺素的生理盐水注射入黏膜下有助于明确解剖层次。在直肠黏膜至包含内口的最远端上做一个菱形的门状或弧形切口,菱形皮瓣的基底部是顶端的两倍宽。弧形切口弧度在 120~180 度之间。注意止血,否则皮瓣的黏膜会和底部的肛门内括约肌的一小部分形成降起,尽管这一步值得争议。在皮瓣广泛松动后,切除位于瘘道的括约肌部分,并缝合关闭,再切除瘘道的黏膜部分。皮瓣通过正闭合的肌肉开口的远端排出血肿,无需牵拉远端的位于齿状线尾部的黏膜边缘就已牢固。外部的瘘道用蘑菇头导管引流,直到皮瓣成活和瘘道收缩。除非患者正在进行多次皮瓣推移手术或者在皮瓣松动时大量纤维化,否则不需要进行临时的粪便转流。在复发且有大量的黏膜纤维化的病例中,一个选择是皮肤推移的肛门成形术[130]。肛周克罗恩病肛瘘选用皮瓣推移技术治疗的成功率在表 22.4 中可见。甚至对于肛瘘复发的患者,这个相对简单的手术也能保证症状的短期改善。

LIFT 和 BioLIFT

最新增加的治疗复杂性经括约肌型肛瘘的保留括约肌手术是括约肌间型瘘管结扎术——LIFT 手术。这个手术的最初的研究是由 Rojanasakul 等[137-138]在 18 例患者 3 个月的随访后,报道 94% 患者的肛瘘治愈。随后对这技术的研究报道 57%~89% 患者的肛瘘成功治愈[139],大多数只是作为摘要发表。手术需要进入括约肌间沟或瘘道所在的平面,再分辨和结扎瘘道。手术的优点是安全、无显著的临床并发症发生率及相对容易操作。通过将生物瓣放置在括约肌间水平来加强瘘道的闭合(BioLIFT)是 LIFT 手术的变化,由 Ellis[140] 通过对 27 例患有直肠阴道瘘的患者长达 12 个月的随访后报道。在这项研究中,81% 的患者直肠阴道瘘成功闭合,可是 27 例患者中只有 4 例是继发于克罗恩病的肛瘘。这个手术在括约肌间水平涉及大量的清扫和放置生物瓣移植物。经过外括约肌的瘘道留下的开口有助于从伤口中引流。这两种手术入选的都是不同病因的患者,克罗恩病患者只占很少一部分。仍需要更多研究去证明这些手术在肛周克罗恩病中的作用。

生物胶

早在 1990 年,纤维蛋白凝胶就常用作肛瘘的密封剂。纤维蛋白凝胶是一种组织黏合剂,由纤维蛋白和凝血酶成分组成。把这两种成分同时注射入瘘道,纤维蛋白被凝血酶激活形成纤维蛋白凝块,然后封闭瘘道。这种纤维蛋白凝块据报道有助于促

表 22.4 肛周克罗恩病肛瘘选用皮瓣推移技术治疗的成功率

研究者	隐窝腺(N)	节段性肠炎(N)	随访(mo)	研究类型	成功率(%)
Jones 等[131]	6	6	25	R	66.7
Makowiec 等[132]	0	20	19.5	P	75
Joo 等[133]	0	8	17.3	R	73.1
Marchesa 等[134]	0	9	15	R	61.5
Hyman 等[135]	6	14	39	P	75
Van der Hagen 等[136]	29	12	72	R	36.6

R:回顾性的;P:前瞻性的

进伤口愈合及促进止血和血管再生。自体的和商业的纤维蛋白凝胶都可以使用。不像自体纤维蛋白凝胶，商业纤维蛋白凝胶不需要自体献血，所以准备时间更少[141]。此外，商业纤维蛋白凝胶在体外结合的能力是自体纤维蛋白凝胶的10倍。可是两种类型的凝胶在治愈肛瘘上没有明显差异[141]。

至今为止，很少有研究评估纤维蛋白凝胶对克罗恩病肛瘘患者的治疗，研究结果显示成功率很低，尽管大多数的研究报道纤维蛋白凝胶治疗克罗恩病相关的肛瘘的成功率在31%～60%[141-145]。Singer等[146]最近的研究发现用纤维蛋白凝胶治疗克罗恩病患者的肛瘘均以失败告终。此外，尽管Vitton等[147]报道在治疗后的3个月71%的克罗恩病患者的肛瘘闭合，可是直肠内超声检查确定只有14%的患者的瘘道完全闭合。纤维蛋白凝胶与其他手术和药物治疗方法联合起到促进肛瘘愈合的作用。如在两步法中引流挂线在使用纤维蛋白凝胶前放置，然而最初的成功率只有29%，再治疗后提升到69%[148-150]。在克利夫兰诊所弗罗里达分院的Zmora等[150]发现当纤维蛋白凝胶作为主要治疗材料时，12.1个月的随访后的治愈率是33%，而当联合直肠内的皮瓣推移技术时是54%。Ellis和Clark[151]报道了类似的结果，发现尽管纤维蛋白凝胶和皮瓣推移联合比单独使用纤维蛋白凝胶效果好，却没有比单独用皮瓣推移的治愈率更高（联合时为54%，单独使用纤维蛋白凝胶为33%）。这可能是因为纤维蛋白凝胶填充了瘘道，阻止了引流，而引流是皮瓣推移技术所需要的[152]。

第二种生物黏合剂是生物胶（由纯化的牛血清白蛋白和戊二醛组成的外科黏合剂），曾广泛用于粘合软组织，最近才用于瘘道治疗。少量研究得出的数据令人失望，有研究报道生物胶及脓血在术后第1周就被排出体外，因此需要手术清创[153]。

胶原材料

至今为止，治疗肛瘘的最成功、且经常研究的胶原材料是小肠黏膜下组织。这是从猪的肠道黏膜下组织分离的自然存在的可降解的生物材料，在处理时呈现出无细胞和免疫原性（百得塞肛瘘栓[AFP]，库克医疗，布卢明顿）。百得塞肛瘘栓由冻干的猪黏膜下组织制成，呈圆锥形，能够更容易地插入瘘道。不像纤维蛋白凝胶是半固体的稠度，肛瘘栓是固体结构，能够缝合至瘘道的两端。百得塞肛瘘栓在闭合肛瘘的作用比纤维蛋白凝胶好，闭合率达87%，而经纤维蛋白凝胶治疗后只有40%[154]，可与皮瓣推移技术的结果相比。

百得塞肛瘘栓的成功使肛瘘闭合的报道具有差异性，治愈率从14%～87%[143, 155-159]。然而，有报道发现肛瘘栓的治愈率随着时间推移递减，而且重复肛瘘栓手术成功的可能性变小[156, 158]。此外，由于研究有限的可用性和相互矛盾的结果，百得塞肛瘘栓在治疗克罗恩病肛瘘的有效性目前尚不清楚。2008年的消化疾病周会议报道了一项最近的回顾性研究结果，肛瘘栓的使用比之前报道的成功率低：22例克罗恩病相关的肛瘘患者只有2例患者治愈。报道的百得塞肛瘘栓治疗克罗恩病肛瘘的成功率见表22.5[155-157, 160]。

其他治疗
自体细胞联合生物材料

最近，研究者们热衷于使用自体细胞联合生物材料的方法。Garcia-Olmo等[161-162]引进从脂肪组织分离自体干细胞联合纤维蛋白凝胶治疗肛瘘的方法。脂肪组织分离处的干细胞具有诱导复杂性肛瘘愈合，比单独使用纤维蛋白凝胶的治愈率更高。至今为止，这些研究的结果是有保证的，尽管这项工作现在处于二期临床试验。这个方法安全，不影响排便控制，而且使用自体细胞避免了受体免疫反应；可是，这个方法的一个缺陷就是寻找细胞来源和扩增细胞所花费的时间很多。此外，还有细胞污染的风险和细胞活力的问题。

微球体

利用微球体组成的支架是使用生物材料治疗肛瘘的新方法。Blaker等[163]最近制成的多孔聚乳酸-羟基乙酸共聚物微粒体包含抗菌、可释放银、可降解的磷酸盐玻璃或甲硝唑。这两种微粒体具有抑制细菌生长的作用，因此可能适用于肛瘘治疗。

直肠阴道瘘/肛门阴道瘘

这个问题将在第38章介绍，接下来讨论与克罗恩病相关的肛门阴道瘘和直肠阴道瘘的治疗。5.9%～10%的患者患有直肠阴道瘘/肛门阴道瘘[164]。这些瘘根据它们和直肠括约肌复合体的关系来分类。当内口在肛管上时，称为肛门阴道瘘，而当出现在括约肌复合体上面时则称为直肠阴道瘘。病因

表 22.5 肛瘘栓治疗肛周克罗恩病肛瘘的成功率

O'Connor 等[155]	肛瘘栓在 20 例不愿接受瘘道切开术的克罗恩病肛瘘患者的非对照试验	成功率为 80%；在复杂性肛瘘的成功率更低
Schwandner 等[157]	19 例患有经括约肌型肛瘘患者（7 例患克罗恩病）的非对照试验	7 例克罗恩病患者中有 6 例治疗成功（86%）
Ky 等[156]	对 45 例患者（20 例为复杂性肛瘘，14 例为克罗恩病）的前瞻性研究	在经过 6.5 个月的中位随访后 14 例克罗恩病患者中有 4 例患者治愈（29%）
Safar 等[160]	对 35 例复杂性肛瘘的患者（4 例为克罗恩病）的回顾性研究	成功率为 13.9%；4 例克罗恩病患者中有 1 例治愈

与诊断类似于病因不明的肛瘘。药物治疗效果不好，长期症状的控制率低，复发率高[164]。

手术治疗

尽管通过打开或切除低位的表浅的（肛门阴道的）肛瘘[165-166]能成功治愈，引起肛管畸形可能导致轻微的粪便污染。直肠阴道瘘瘘道经过肛门外括约肌或在肛门外括约肌上方，行瘘道切开术总是导致肛门控便能力严重受损。在这种情况，初始治疗是引流所有的继发性瘘道和脓肿，常在完全修复前[167-168]使用长期挂线治疗。可行的手术选择包括经肛门或阴道进行的皮瓣推移技术。直肠套筒皮瓣推移也可选用，描述的闭合率在 54%~87% 之间，尽管大多数的观察研究来自于专业中心的少数患者[133, 169-171]。

直肠的皮瓣推移技术最适用于无大便失禁和侵犯括约肌的低位瘘道患者。Crim 等[172] 和 Makowiec 等[173] 分别报道了他们研究的 14 例肛瘘患者中有 10 例患者治愈和 12 例肛瘘患者有 5 例治愈。Hull 和 Fazio[170] 描述的使用多种外科手术治疗克罗恩病肛瘘，总成功率为 70%。分流回肠造口术选择性地用于这些患者。Joo 等[133] 报道使用直肠内皮瓣推移技术的直肠阴道瘘患者中有 75% 达到根除，而 Alabaz 和 Weiss[174] 使用经阴道的方法能够在 93% 的患者中获得成功。大多数研究者认为最好的治疗是采用经直肠路径，因为修复是从高到低压分流的高压侧开始进行，然后切除瘘道的主要来源，插入一层完整的健康组织[175]。股薄肌介植治疗和重叠的括约肌成形术连同皮瓣推移技术共同使用取得了不同程度的成功[96]。

肿 瘤

尽管罕见，恶性变应该考虑与慢性不愈合的肛瘘进行鉴别诊断。恶性变发病率很低，大约 0.7%[20-21]。鳞状细胞癌和腺癌都曾有报告。一旦下了这个令人意外的诊断，治疗必须遵循标准的肿瘤学指南[176]。

参考文献

1. Penner A, Crohn BB. Perianal fistulae as a complication of regional ileitis. Ann Surg. 1938;108:867–73.
2. Hellers G, Bergstrand O, Ewerth S, Holmström B. Occurrence and outcome after primary treatment of anal fistulae in Crohn's disease. Gut. 1980;21:525–7.
3. Sandborn WJ, Fazio VW, Feagan BG, Hanauer SB, American Gastroenterological Association Clinical Practice Committee. AGA technical review on perianal Crohn's disease. Gastroenterology. 2003;125:1508–30.
4. Schwartz DA, Loftus Jr EV, Tremaine WJ, Panaccione R, Harmsen WS, Zinsmeister AR, et al. The natural history of fistulising Crohn's disease in Olmsted County, Minnesota. Gastroenterology. 2002;122:875–80.
5. Lockhart-Mummery HE. Symposium. Crohn's disease: anal lesions. Dis Colon Rectum. 1975;18:200–2.
6. Cosnes J, Cattan S, Blain A, Beaugerie L, Carbonnel F, Parc R, et al. Long-term evolution of disease behavior of Crohn's disease. Inflamm Bowel Dis. 2002;8:244–50.
7. Regimbeau JM, Panis Y, Marteau P, Benoist S, Valleur P. Surgical treatment of anoperineal Crohn's disease: can abdominoperineal resection be predicted? J Am Coll Surg. 1999;189:171.
8. Lapidus A, Bernell O, Hellers G, Lofberg R. Clinical course of colorectal Crohn's disease: a 35-year follow-up study of 507 patients. Gastroenterology. 1998;189:171.
9. Beaugerie L, Seksik P, Nion-Larmurier I, Gendre JP, Cosnes J. Predictors of Crohn's disease. Gastroenterology. 2006;130:650–6.
10. Lewis R, Maron D. Anorectal Crohn's disease. Surg Clin North Am. 2010;90:83–97.
11. Cross RK, Jung C, Wasan S, Joshi G, Sawyer R, Roghmann MC. Racial differences in disease phenotypes in patients with Crohn's disease. Inflamm Bowel Dis. 2006;12:192–8.
12. Williams DR, Coller JA, Corman ML, Nugent FW, Veidenheimer MC. Anal complications in Crohn's disease. Dis Colon Rectum.

1981;24:22–4.
13. Gray BK, Lockhart-Mummery HE, Morson BC. Crohn's disease of the anal region. Gut. 1965;6:515–24.
14. Rankin GB, Watts HD, Melnyk CS, Kelley Jr ML. National Cooperative Crohn's Disease Study: extraintestinal manifestations and perianal complications. Gastroenterology. 1979;77:914–20.
15. Gelbmann CM, Rogler G, Gross V, Gierend M, Bregenzer N, Andus T, et al. Prior bowel resections, perianal disease, and a high initial Crohn's disease activity index are associated with corticosteroid resistance in active Crohn's disease. Am J Gastroenterol. 2002;97:1438–45.
16. Makowiec F, Jehle EC, Starlinger M. Clinical course of perianal fistulas in Crohn's disease. Gut. 1995;37:696–701.
17. Mahmoud N, Rombeau JL, Ross HM. Colon and rectum. PA. In: Townsend CM, Beauchamp RD, Evers BM, editors. Sabiston textbook of surgery. Philadelphia: Saunders; 2004. p. 1401.
18. Gillen CD, Walmsley RS, Prior P, Andrews HA, Allan RN. Ulcerative colitis and Crohn's disease: a comparison of the colorectal cancer risk in extensive colitis. Gut. 1994;35:1590–2.
19. Ekbom A, Helmick C, Zack M, Adami HO. Increased risk of large-bowel cancer in Crohn's disease with colonic involvement. Lancet. 1990;336(8711):357–9.
20. Sjodahl RI, Myrelid P, Soderholm JD. Anal and rectal cancer in Crohn's disease. Colorectal Dis. 2003;5:490–5.
21. Ky A, Sohn N, Weinstein MA, Korelitz BI. Carcinoma arising in anorectal fistulas of Crohn's disease. Dis Colon Rectum. 1998;41:992–6.
22. Hughes LE. Surgical pathology and management of anorectal Crohn's disease. J R Soc Med. 1978;71:644–51.
23. Armuzzi A, Ahmad T, Ling KL, de Silva A, Cullen S, van Heel D, et al. Genotype-phenotype analysis of the Crohn's disease susceptibility haplotype on chromosome 5q31. Gut. 2003;52:1133–9.
24. Onnie CM, Fisher SA, Prescott NJ, Mirza MM, Green P, Sanderson J, et al. Diverse effects of the CARD15 and IBD5 loci on clinical phenotype in 630 patients with Crohn's disease. Eur J Gastroenterol Hepatol. 2008;20:37–45.
25. Palmieri O, Latiano A, Valvano R, D'Incà R, Vecchi M, Sturniolo GC, et al. Variants of OCTN1–2 cation transporter genes are associated with both Crohn's disease and ulcera- tive colitis. Aliment Pharmacol Ther. 2006;23:497–506.
26. Vermeire S, Pierik M, Hlavaty T, Claessens G, van Schuerbeeck N, Joossens S, et al. Association of organic cation transporter risk haplotype with perianal penetrating Crohn's disease but not with susceptibility to IBD. Gastroenterology. 2005;129:1845–53.
27. Bataille F, Klebl F, Rummele P, Schroeder J, Farkas S, Wild PJ, et al. Morphological characterisation of Crohn's disease fistulae. Gut. 2004;53:1314–21.
28. Parks AG, Gordon PH, Hardcastle JD. A classification of fistula-in-ano. Br J Surg. 1976;63:1–12.
29. Vermiere S, Van Aasche G, Rutgeerts P. Perianal Crohn's disease: classification and clinical evaluation. Dig Liver Dis. 2007;39:959–62.
30. Hughes LE. Clinical classification of perianal Crohn's disease. Dis Colon Rectum. 1992;35:928–32.
31. American Gastroenterological Association Clinical Practice Committee. American Gastroenterological Association medical position statement: perianal Crohn's disease. Gastroenterology. 2003;125:1503–7.
32. Irvine EJ. Usual therapy improves perianal Crohn's diseaseas measured by a new disease activity index. McMaster IBD. Study Group. J Clin Gastroenterol. 1995;20:27–32.
33. Schwartz DA, Wiersema MJ, Dudiak KM, Fletcher JG, Clain JE, Tremaine WJ, et al. A comparison of endoscopic ultrasound, magnetic resonance imaging, and exam under anesthesia for evaluation of Crohn's perianal fistulas. Gastroenterology. 2001;121:1064–72.
34. Sudol-Szopinska I, Gelsa J, Jakubowski W, Noszczyk W, Szczepkowsi M, Sarti D. Reliability of endosonography in evaluation of anal fistulae and abscesses. Acta Radiol. 2002;43:599–602.
35. Poen AC, Felt-Bersma RJ, Eijsbouts QA, Cuesta MA, Meuwissen SG. Hydrogen peroxide-enhanced transanal ultrasound in the assessment of fistula-in-ano. Dis Colon Rectum. 1998;41:1147–52.
36. Cho DY. Endosonographic criteria for an internal opening of fistula-in-ano. Dis Colon Rectum. 1999;42:515–8.
37. Ortiz H, Marzo J, Jimenez G, DeMiguel M. Accuracy of hydrogen peroxide-enhanced ultrasound in the identification of internal openings of anal fistulas. Colorectal Dis. 2002;4:280–3.
38. Cheong DM, Nogueras JJ, Wexner SD, Jagelman DG. Anal endosonography for recurrent anal fistulas: image enhancement with hydrogen peroxide. Dis Colon Rectum. 1993;36:1158–60.
39. Maor Y, Chowers Y, Koller M, Zmora O, Bar-Meir S, Avidan B. Endosonographic evaluation of perianal fistulas and abscesses: comparison of two instruments and assessment of the role of hydrogen peroxide injection. J Clin Ultrasound. 2005;33:226–32.
40. Navarro-Luna A, Garcia-Domingo MI, Rius-Marcias J, Marco-Molina C. Ultrasound study of anal fistulas with hydrogen peroxide enhancement. Dis Colon Rectum. 2004;47:108–14.
41. Ratto C, Grillo E, Parello A, Costamagna G, Doglietto GB. Endoanal ultrasound guided surgery for anal fistula. Endoscopy. 2005;37:722–8.
42. Sudol-Szopinska I, Jakubowski W, Szczepkowski M. Contrast enhanced endosonography for the diagnosis of anal and anovaginal fistulas. J Clin Ultrasound. 2002;30:145–50.
43. Tsankov T, Tankova L, Deredjan H, Kovatchki D. Contrast enhanced endoanal and transperineal sonography in perianal fistulas. Hepatogastroenterology. 2008;55:13–6.
44. West RL, Dwarkasing S, Felt-Bersma RJ, Schouten WR, Hop WC, Hussain SM, et al. Hydrogen peroxide-enhanced three-dimensional endoanal ultrasonography and endoanal magnetic resonance imaging in evaluating perianal fistulas: agreement and patient preference. Eur J Gastroenterol Hepatol. 2004;16:1319–24.
45. West RL, Zimmerman DD, Dwarkasing S, Hussain SM, Hop WC, Schouten WR, et al. Prospective comparison of hydrogen peroxide-enhanced three-dimensional endoanal ultrasonography and endoanal magnetic resonance imaging of perianal fistulas. Dis Colon Rectum. 2003;46:1407–15.
46. Sudoł-Szopińska I, Kolodziejczak M, Szopiński TR. The accuracy of a postprocessing technique – volume render mode – in three dimensional endoanal ultrasonography of anal abscesses and fistulas. Dis Colon Rectum. 2011;54:238–44.
47. Zbar AP, Oyetunji RO, Gill R. Transperineal versus hydrogen peroxide-enhanced endoanal ultrasonography in never operated and recurrent cryptogenic fistula-in-ano: a pilot study. Tech Coloproctol. 2006;10:297–302.
48. Buchanan GN, Halligan S, Bartram CI, Williams AB, Tarroni D, Cohen CR. Clinical examination, endosonography, and MR imaging in preoperative assessment of fistula in ano: comparison with outcome-based reference standard. Radiology. 2004;233:674–81.
49. Schaefer O, Lohrmann C, Langer M. Assessment of anal fistulas with high-resolution subtraction MR-fistulography: comparison with surgical findings. J Magn Reson Imaging. 2004;19:91–8.
50. Beets-Tan RG, Beets GL, van der Hoop AG, Kessels AG, Vliegen RF, Baeten CG, et al. Preoperative MR imaging of anal fistulas: does it really help the surgeon? Radiology. 2001;218:75–84.
51. Buchanan GN, Halligan S, Williams AB, Cohen CR, Tarroni D, Phillips RK, et al. Magnetic resonance imaging for primary fistula in ano. Br J Surg. 2003;90:877–81.
52. Zbar AP, de Souza NM, Puni R, Kmiot WA. Comparison of endoanal magnetic resonance imaging with surgical findings in perirectal sepsis. Br J Surg. 1998;85:111–4.
53. Sun MR, Smith MP, Kane RA. Current techniques in imaging of fistula in ano: three-dimensional endoanal ultrasound and magnetic resonance imaging. Semin Ultrasound CT MR. 2008;29:454–71.
54. Horsthuis K, Lavini C, Bipat S, Stokkers PC, Stoker J. Perianal Crohn's disease: evaluation of dynamic contrast MR imaging as an indicator of disease activity. Radiology. 2009;251:380.
55. Kuijpers HC, Schulpen T. Fistulography for fistula-in-ano. Is it useful? Dis Colon Rectum. 1985;28:103–4.
56. Weisman RI, Orsay CP, Pearl RK, Abcarian H. The role of fistulography in fistula-in-ano. Report of five cases. Dis Colon Rectum. 1991;34:181–4.
57. Berliner L, Redmond P, Purow E, Megna D, Sottile V. Computed

tomography in Crohn's disease. Am J Gastroenterol. 1982;77:548–53.
58. Goldberg HI, Gore RM, Margulis AR, Moss AA, Baker EL. Computed tomography in the evaluation of Crohn's disease. AJR Am J Roentgenol. 1983;140:277–82.
59. Kerber GW, Greenberg M, Rubin JM. Computed tomography evaluation of local and extraintestinal complications of Crohn's disease. Gastrointest Radiol. 1984;9:143–8.
60. Fishman EK, Wolf EJ, Jones B, Bayless TM, Siegelman SS. CT evaluation of Crohn's disease: effect on patient management. AJR Am J Roentgenol. 1987;148:537–40.
61. Yousem DM, Fishman EK, Jones B. Crohn's disease: perirectal and perianal findings at CT. Radiology. 1988;167:331–4.
62. Van Outryve MJ, Pelckmans PA, Michielsen PP, Van Maercke YM. Value of transrectal ultrasonography in Crohn's disease. Gastroenterology. 1991;101:1171–7.
63. Schratter-Sehn AU, Lochs H, Vogelsang H, Schurawitzki H, Herold C, Schratter M. Endoscopic ultrasonography versus computed tomography in the differential diagnosis of perianorectal complications in Crohn's disease. Endoscopy. 1993;25:582–6.
64. Sachar DB, Bodian CA, Goldstein ES, Present DH, Bayless TM, Picco M, Task Force on Clinical Phenotyping of the IOIBD. Is perianal Crohn's disease associated with intestinal fistulization? Am J Gastroenterol. 2005;100:1547–9.
65. Heuman R, Bolin T, Sjödahl R, Tagesson C. The incidence and course of perianal complications and arthralgia after intestinal resection with restoration of continuity for Crohn's disease. Br J Surg. 1981;68:528–30.
66. Marks CG, Ritchie JK, Lockhart-Mummery HE. Anal fistulas in Crohn's disease. Br J Surg. 1981;68(8):525–7.
67. Orkin BA, Telander RL. The effect of intra-abdominal resection or fecal diversion on perianal disease in pediatric Crohn's disease. J Pediatr Surg. 1985;20:343–7.
68. Singh B, McC Mortensen NJ, Jewell DP, George B. Perianal Crohn's disease. Br J Surg. 2004;91:801–14.
69. Strong SA. Perianal Crohn's disease. Semin Pediatr Surg. 2007;16:185–93.
70. Keighley MR, Allan RN. Current status and influence of operation on perianal Crohn's disease. Int J Colorectal Dis. 1986;1:104–7.
71. Bonheur JL, Braunstein J, Korelitz BI, Panagopoulos G. Anal skin tags in inflammatory bowel disease: new observations and a clinical review. Inflamm Bowel Dis. 2008;14:1236–9.
72. Sandborn WJ, Fazio VW, Feagan BG, Hanauer SB, American Gastroenterological Association Clinical Practice Committee. AGA technical review on perianal Crohn's disease. Gastroenterology. 2003;125:1508–30.
73. Somerville KW, Langman MJ, Da Cruz DJ, Balfour TW, Sully L. Malignant transformation of anal skin tags in Crohn's disease. Gut. 1984;25:1124–5.
74. Buchmann P, Keighley MR, Allan RN, Thompson H, Alexander-Williams J. Natural history of perianal Crohn's disease. Ten year follow-up: a plea for conservatism. Am J Surg. 1980;140: 642–4.
75. Peyrin-Biroulet L, Loftus Jr EV, Tremaine WJ, Harmsen WS, Zinsmeister AR, Sandborn WJ. Perianal Crohn's disease findings other than fistulas in a population-based cohort. Inflamm Bowel Dis. 2011. doi:10.1002/ibd.21674.
76. Alexander-Williams J, Buchmann P. Perianal Crohn's disease. World J Surg. 1980;4:203–8.
77. Nelson RL, Abcarian H, Davis FG, Persky V. Prevalence of benign anorectal disease in a randomly selected population. Dis Colon Rectum. 1995;38:341–4.
78. Jeffery PJ, Parks AG, Ritchie JK. Treatment of haemorrhoids in patients with inflammatory bowel disease. Lancet. 1977;1(8021): 1084–5.
79. Wolkomir AF, Luchtefeld MA. Surgery for symptomatic hemorrhoids and anal fissures in Crohn's disease. Dis Colon Rectum. 1993;36:545–7.
80. Wolff BG, Culp CE, Beart Jr RW, Ilstrup DM, Ready RL. Anorectal Crohn's disease. A long-term perspective. Dis Colon Rectum. 1985;28:709–11.
81. Bernard D, Morgan S, Tasse D. Selective surgical management of Crohn's disease of the anus. Can J Surg. 1986;29:318–21.
82. Sweeney JL, Ritchie JK, Nicholls RJ. Anal fissure in Crohn's disease. Br J Surg. 1988;75:56–7.
83. Fleshner PR, Schoetz Jr DJ, Roberts PL, Murray JJ, Coller JA, Veidenheimer MC. Anal fissure in Crohn's disease: a plea for aggressive management. Dis Colon Rectum. 1995;38:1137–43.
84. Sangwan YP, Schoetz Jr DJ, Murray JJ, Roberts PL, Coller JA. Perianal Crohn's disease. Results of local surgical treatment. Dis Colon Rectum. 1996;39:529–35.
85. Siproudhis L, Mortaji A, Mary JY, Juguet F, Bretagne JF, Gosselin M. Anal lesions: any significant prognosis in Crohn's disease? Eur J Gastroenterol Hepatol. 1997;9:239–43.
86. Ingle SB, Loftus Jr EV. The natural history of perianal Crohn's disease. Dig Liver Dis. 2007;39:963–9.
87. Bougen G, Siproudhis L, Bretagne JF, Bigard MA, Peyrin-Biroulet L. Nonfistulizing perianal Crohn's disease:clinical features, epidemiology, and treatment. Inflamm Bowel Dis. 2010;16:1431–42.
88. Bergstrand O, Ewerth S, Hellers G, Holmström B, Ullman J, Wallberg P. Outcome following treatment of anal fistulae in Crohn's disease. Acta Chir Scand Suppl. 1980;500:43–4.
89. Maeda Y, Ng SC, Durdey P, Burt C, Torkington J, Rao PK, Topical Metronidazole in Perianal Crohn's Study Group. Randomized clinical trial of metronidazole ointment versus placebo in perianal Crohn's disease. Br J Surg. 2010;97:1340–7.
90. Hughes LE, Donaldson DR, Williams JG, Taylor BA, Young HL. Local depot methylprednisolone injection for painful anal Crohn's disease. Gastroenterology. 1988;94:709–11.
91. Bouguen G, Trouilloud I, Siproudhis L, Oussalah A, Bigard MA, Bretagne JF, et al. Long-term outcome of non-fistulizing (ulceration, stricture) perianal Crohn's disease in patients treated with infliximab. Aliment Pharmacol Ther. 2009;30:749–56.
92. Russell RI, Hall MJ. Elemental diet therapy in the management of complicated Crohn's disease. Scott Med J. 1979;24:291–5.
93. Brady 3rd CE, Cooley BJ, Davis JC. Healing of severe perineal and cutaneous Crohn's disease with hyperbaric oxygen. Gastroenterology. 1989;97:756–60.
94. Teahon K, Bjarnason I, Pearson M, Levi AJ. Ten years' experience with an elemental diet in the management of Crohn's disease. Gut. 1990;31:1133–7.
95. Colombel JF, Mathieu D, Bouault JM, Lesage X, Zavadil P, Quandalle P, et al. Hyperbaric oxygenation in severe perineal Crohn's disease. Dis Colon Rectum. 1995;38:609–14.
96. Safar B, Sands D. Perianal Crohn's disease. Clin Colon Rect Surg. 2007;20:282–93.
97. Linares L, Moreira LF, Andrews H, Allan RN, Alexander-Williams J, Keighley MR. Natural history and treatment of anorectal strictures complicating Crohn's disease. Br J Surg. 1988;75: 653–5.
98. Hamlyn E, Taylor C. Sexually transmitted proctitis. Postgrad Med J. 2006;82:733–6.
99. Fields S, Rosainz L, Korelitz BI, Panagopoulos G, Schneider J. Rectal strictures in Crohn's disease and coexisting perirectal complications. Inflamm Bowel Dis. 2008;14:29–31.
100. Schwartz DA, Pemberton JH, Sandborn WJ. Diagnosis and treatment of perianal fistulas in Crohn disease. Ann Intern Med. 2001;135:906–18.
101. Schuppan D, Freitag T. Fistulising Crohn's disease: MMPs gone awry. Gut. 2004;53:622–4.
102. Bernstein LH, Frank MS, Brandt LJ, Boley SJ. Healing of perineal Crohn's disease with metronidazole. Gastroenterology. 1980;79: 357–65.
103. Brandt LJ, Bernstein LH, Boley SJ, Frank MS. Metronidazole therapy for perineal Crohn's disease: a follow-up study. Gastroenterology. 1982;83:383–7.
104. Jakobovits J, Schuster MM. Metronidazole therapy for Crohn's disease and associated fistulae. Am J Gastroenterol. 1984;79:533–40.
105. West RL, Van der Woude CJ, Hansen BE, Felt-Bersma RJ, van Tilburg AJ, Drapers JA, et al. Clinical and endosonographic effect of ciprofloxacin on treatment of perianal fistulae in Crohn's dis-

106. Turunen U, Farkkila M, Seppala K. Long term treatment of perianal or fistulous Crohn's disease with ciprofloxacin. Scand J Gastroenterol. 1989;24(Suppl):144.
107. Solomon MJ, McLeod RS, O'Connor BI, et al. Combination ciprofloxacin and metronidazole in severe perianal Crohn's disease. Can J Gastroenterol. 1993;7:571–3.
108. Pearson DC, May GR, Fick GH, Sutherland LR. Azathioprine and 6-mercaptopurine in Crohn disease. A meta-analysis. Ann Intern Med. 1995;123:132–42.
109. Present DH, Lichtiger S. Efficacy of cyclosporine in treatment of fistula of Crohn's disease. Dig Dis Sci. 1994;39:374–80.
110. Sandborn WJ, Present DH, Isaacs KL, Wolf DC, Greenberg E, Hanauer SB, et al. Tacrolimus for the treatment of fistulae in patients with Crohn's disease: a randomized, placebo-controlled trial. Gastroenterology. 2003;125:380–8.
111. Present DH, Rutgeerts P, Targan S, Hanauer SB, Mayer L, van Hogezand RA, et al. Infliximab for the treatment of fistulae in patients with Crohn's disease. N Engl J Med. 1999;340:1398–405.
112. Ochsenkuhn T, Goke B, Sackmann M. Combining infliximab with 6 mercaptopurine/azathiprine for fistula therapy in Crohn's disease. Am J Gastroenterol. 2002;97:2022–5.
113. Van Assche G, Vanbeckevoort D, Bielen D, Coremans G, Aerden I, Noman M, et al. Magnetic resonance imaging of the effect of infliximab on perianal fistulizing Crohn's disease. Am J Gastroenterol. 2003;98:332–9.
114. Rasul I, Wilson SR, MacRae H, Irwin S, Greenberg GR. Clinical and radiological responses after infliximab treatment for perianal fistulizing Crohn's disease. Am J Gastroenterol. 2004;99:82–8.
115. Lichtiger SI. Healing of perianal fistulae by local injection of antibody to TNF. Gastroenterology. 2008;120(Suppl):A3154.
116. Poggioli G, Laureti S, Pierangeli F, Rizzello F, Ugolini F, Gionchetti P, et al. Local injection of Infliximab for the treatment of perianal Crohn's disease. Dis Colon Rectum. 2005;48:768–74.
117. Korzenik JR, Dieckgraefe BK. An open-labelled study of granulocyte colony-stimulating factor in the treatment of active Crohn's disease. Aliment Pharmacol Ther. 2005;21:391–400.
118. Korzenik JR, Dieckgraefe BK, Valentine JF, Hausman DF, Gilbert MJ. Sargramostim for active Crohn's disease. N Engl J Med. 2005;352:2193–201.
119. Fukuda Y, Takazoe M, Sugita A, Kosaka T, Kinjo F, Otani Y, et al. Oral spherical adsorptive carbon for the treatment of intractable anal fistulas in Crohn's disease: a multicenter, randomized, double-blind, placebo-controlled trial. Am J Gastroenterol. 2008;103:1721–9.
120. Lunniss PJ, Kamm MA, Phillips RK. Factors affecting continence after surgery for anal fistula. Br J Surg. 1994;81:1382–5.
121. Morris J, Spencer JA, Ambrose NS. MR imaging classification of perianal fistulas and its implications for patient management. Radiographics. 2000;20:623–35.
122. Pescatori M, Ayabaca SM, Cafaro D, Iannello A, Magrini S. Marsupialization of fistulotomy and fistulectomy wounds improves healing and decreases bleeding: a randomized controlled trial. Colorectal Dis. 2006;8:11–4.
123. Ritchie RD, Sackier JM, Hodde JP. Incontinence rates after cutting seton treatment for anal fistula. Colorectal Dis. 2009;11:564–71.
124. Faucheron JL, Saint-Marc O, Guibert L, Parc R. Long-term seton drainage or high anal fistulas in Crohn's disease – a sphincter-saving operation? Dis Colon Rectum. 1996;39:208–11.
125. Parks AG, Stitz RW. The treatment of high fistula-in-ano. Dis Colon Rectum. 1976;19:487–99.
126. Kennedy HL, Zegarra JP. Fistulotomy without external sphincter division for high anal fistulas. Br J Surg. 1990;77:898–901.
127. Van Tets WF, Kuijpers JH. Seton treatment of perianal fistula with high anal or rectal opening. Br J Surg. 1995;82:895–7.
128. McCourtney JS, Finlay IG. Cutting seton without preliminary internal sphincterotomy in management of complex high fistula-in-ano. Dis Colon Rectum. 1996;39:55–8.
129. Elting AW. The treatment of fistula in ano: with especial reference to the Whitehead operation. Ann Surg. 1912;56:744–52.
130. Hossack T, Solomon MJ, Young JM. Ano-cutaneous flap repair for complex and recurrent supra-sphincteric anal fistula. Colorectal Dis. 2005;7:187–92.
131. Jones IT, Fazio VW, Jagelman DG. The use of transanal rectal advancement flaps in the management of fistulas involving the anorectum. Dis Colon Rectum. 1987;30:919–23.
132. Makowiec F, Jehle EC, Becker HD, Starlinger M. Clinical course after transanal advancement flap repair of perianal fistula in patients with Crohn's disease. Br J Surg. 1995;82:603–6.
133. Joo JS, Weiss EG, Nogueras JJ, Wexner SD. Endorectal advancement flap in perianal Crohn's disease. Am Surg. 1998;64:147–50.
134. Marchesa P, Hull TL, Fazio VW. Advancement sleeve flaps for treatment of severe perianal Crohn's disease. Br J Surg. 1998;85:1695–8.
135. Hyman N. Endoanal advancement flap repair for complex anorectal fistulas. Am J Surg. 1999;178:337–40.
136. Van der Hagen SJ, Baeten CG, Soeters PB, Beets-Tan RG, Russel MG, van Gemert WG. Staged mucosal advancement flap for the treatment of complex anal fistulas: pretreatment with noncutting Setons and in case of recurrent multiple abscesses a diverting stoma. Colorectal Dis. 2005;7:513–8.
137. Rojanasakul A, Pattanaarun J, Sahakitrungruang C, Tantiphlachiva K. Total anal sphincter saving technique for fistula-in-ano: the ligation of intersphincteric fistula tract. J Med Assoc Thai. 2007;90:581–6.
138. Rojanasakul A. LIFT procedure: a simplified technique for fistula-in-ano. Tech Coloproctol. 2009;13:237–40.
139. Shanwani A, Nor AM, Amri N. Ligation of the intersphincteric fistula tract (LIFT): a sphincter-saving technique for fistula-in-ano. Dis Colon Rectum. 2010;53:39–42.
140. Ellis N. Outcomes with the use of bioprosthetic grafts to reinforce the ligation of the intersphincteric fistula tract (BioLIFT Procedure) for the management of complex anal fistulas. Dis Colon Rectum. 2010;53:1361–4.
141. Cintron JR, Park JJ, Orsay CP, Pearl RK, Nelson RL, Sone JH, et al. Repair of fistulas-in-ano using fibrin adhesive: long-term follow-up. Dis Colon Rectum. 2000;43:944–9.
142. Abel ME, Chiu YS, Russell TR, Volpe PA. Autologous fibrin glue in the treatment of rectovaginal and complex fistulas. Dis Colon Rectum. 1993;36:447–9.
143. Venkatesh KS, Ramanujam P. Fibrin glue application in the treatment of recurrent anorectal fistulas. Dis Colon Rectum. 1999;42:1136–9.
144. Park JJ, Cintron JR, Orsay CP, Pearl RK, Nelson RL, Sone J, et al. Repair of chronic anorectal fistulae using commercial fibrin sealant. Arch Surg. 2000;135:166–9.
145. Loungnarath R, Dietz DW, Mutch MG, Birnbaum EH, Kodner IJ, Fleshman JW. Fibrin glue treatment of complex anal fistulas has low success rate. Dis Colon Rectum. 2004;47:432–6.
146. Singer M, Cintron J, Nelson R, Orsay C, Bastawrous A, Pearl R, et al. Treatment of fistulas-in-ano with fibrin sealant in combination with intra-adhesive antibiotics and/ or surgical closure of the internal fistula opening. Dis Colon Rectum. 2005;48:799–808.
147. Vitton V, Gasmi M, Barthet M, Desjeux A, Orsoni P, Grimaud JC. Long-term healing of Crohn's anal fistulas with fibrin glue injection. Aliment Pharmacol Ther. 2005;21:1453–7.
148. Sentovich SM. Fibrin glue for all anal fistulas. J Gastrointest Surg. 2001;5:158–61.
149. Sentovich SM. Fibrin glue for anal fistulas: long-term results. Dis Colon Rectum. 2003;46:498–502.
150. Zmora O, Mizrahi N, Rotholtz N, Pikarsky AJ, Weiss EG, Nogueras JJ, et al. Fibrin glue sealing in the treatment of perianal fistulas. Dis Colon Rectum. 2003;46:584–9.
151. Ellis CN, Clark S. Fibrin glue as an adjunct to flap repair of anal fistulas: a randomized, controlled study. Dis Colon Rectum. 2006;49:1736–40.

152. Johnson EK, Gaw JU, Armstrong DN. Efficacy of anal fistula plug vs. fibrin glue in closure of anorectal fistulas. Dis Colon Rectum. 2006;49:371–6.
153. de la Portilla F, Rada R, Vega J, Cisneros N, Maldonado VH, Sánchez-Gil JM. Long-term results change conclusions on BioGlue in the treatment of high transsphincteric anal fistulas. Dis Colon Rectum. 2010;53:1220–1.
154. Lawes DA, Efron JE, Abbas M, Heppell J, Young-Fadok TM. Early experience with the bioabsorbable anal fistula plug. World J Surg. 2008;32:1157–9.
155. O'Connor L, Champagne BJ, Ferguson MA, Orangio GR, Schertzer ME, Armstrong DN. Efficacy of anal fistula plug in closure of Crohn's anorectal fistulas. Dis Colon Rectum. 2006;49:1569–73.
156. Ky AJ, Sylla P, Steinhagen R, Khaitov S, Ly EK. Collagen fistula plug for the treatment of anal fistulas. Dis Colon Rectum. 2008;51:838–43.
157. Schwandner O, Stadler F, Wirsching RP, Wirsching RP, Fuerst A. Initial experience on efficacy in closure of cryptoglandular and Crohn's transsphincteric fistulas by the use of the anal fistula plug. Int J Colorectal Dis. 2008;23:319–24.
158. Christoforidis D, Etzioni DA, Goldberg SM, Madoff RD, Mellgren A. Treatment of complex anal fistulas with the collagen fistula plug. Dis Colon Rectum. 2008;51:1482–7.
159. El-Gazzaz GS, Zutshi M, Hull TL. Plugging away at the anal fistula: an exercise in futility? Gastroenterology. 2008;134:A862.
160. Safar B, Jobanputra S, Sands D, Weiss EG, Nogueras JJ, Wexner SD. Anal fistula plug: initial experience and outcomes. Dis Colon Rectum. 2009;52:248–52.
161. Garcia-Olmo D, Garcia-Arranz M, Herreros D. Expanded adipose derived stem cells for the treatment of complex perianal fistula including Crohn's disease. Expert Opin Biol Ther. 2008;9:1417–23.
162. Garcia-Olmo D, Herreros D, Pascual I, Pascual JA, Del-Valle E, Zorrilla J, et al. Expanded adipose derived stem cells for the treatment of complex perianal fistula: a phase II clinical trial. Dis Colon Rectum. 2009;52:79–86.
163. Blaker JJ, Pratten J, Ready D, Knowles JC, Forbes A, Day RM. Assessment of antimicrobial microspheres as a prospective novel treatment targeted towards the repair of perianal fistulae. Aliment Pharmacol Ther. 2008;28:614–22.
164. Andreani SM, Dang HH, Grondona P, Khan AZ, Edwards DP. Rectovaginal fistula in Crohn's disease. Dis Colon Rectum. 2007;50:2215–22.
165. Scott NA, Nair A, Hughes LE. Anovaginal and rectovaginal fistula in patients with Crohn's disease. Br J Surg. 1992;79:1379–80.
166. Levy C, Tremaine WJ. Management of internal fistulas in Crohn's disease. Inflamm Bowel Dis. 2002;8:106–11.
167. Fry RD, Shemesh EI, Kodner IJ, Timmcke A. Techniques and results in the management of anal and perianal Crohn's disease. Surg Gynecol Obstet. 1989;168:42–8.
168. Lichtenstein GR. Treatment of fistulizing Crohn's disease. Gastroenterology. 2000;119:1132–47.
169. Cohen JL, Stricker JW, Schoetz DJ, Coller JA, Veidenheimer MC. Rectovaginal fistula in Crohn's disease. Dis Colon Rectum. 1989;32:825–8.
170. Hull TL, Fazio VW. Surgical approaches to low anovaginal fistula in Crohn's disease. Am J Surg. 1997;173:95–8.
171. Simmang CL, Lacey SW, Huber PJ. Rectal sleeve advancement: repair of rectovaginal fistula associated with anorectal stricture in Crohn's disease. Dis Colon Rectum. 1998;41:787–9.
172. Crim RW, Fazio VW, Laveri IC. Rectal advancement flap repair in Crohn's disease. Factors predictive of failure. Dis Colon Rectum. 1990;33:P3.
173. Makowiec F, Jehle EC, Becker HD, Starlinger M. Clinical course after transanal advancement flap repair of perianal fistula in patients with Crohn's disease. Br J Surg. 1999;82:603–6.
174. Alabaz O, Weiss EG. Anorectal Crohn's disease. In: Beck D, Wexner SD, editors. Fundamentals of anorectal surgery. 2nd ed. Philadelphia: WB Saunders; 1999. p. 498–509.
175. Greenwald JC, Hoexter B. Repair of rectovaginal fistulas. Surg Gynecol Obstet. 1978;146:443–5.
176. Iesalnieks I, Gaertner WB, Glass H, Strauch U, Hipp M, Agha A, et al. Fistula-associated anal adenocarcinoma in Crohn's disease. Inflamm Bowel Dis. 2010;16:1643–8.

第四篇
功能性便秘和排便困难的再次手术

引 言

Steven D. Wexner

　　功能性疾病是一个棘手的问题。尽管有大量该症状和病痛的患者，但是我们对本疾病的病因和病理生理学的认知有限。此外，我们用来诊断该疾病的检查通常发生在疾病的晚期。在这方面，直肠脱垂至少在理论上是一个例外，因为它的病因是解剖学问题。

　　在过去的几十年里，尽管生理学检查已经得到极大地应用和推广，但我们对该病的治疗和治愈能力却没有同样的进步。更讽刺的说法是，生理学检查的指数化增长，导致了更多的外科医师在进行外科手术时，根本没有足够的经验来评估和处理这些复杂的问题或者没有接受过必要、相关、专业化的训练。

　　不管首次手术是何时何地完成，只要手术未能达到最理想的效果，患者总是会千篇一律地咨询结直肠外科医师有关该疾病比较成熟的评估、解释和处理这些问题的方法。因此，因便秘（不管是巨结肠、巨直肠还是结肠运输异常）或盆腔出口梗阻进行首次手术，比因直肠内套叠、肠疝或直肠前突而进行手术的手术效果更难以令人满意，即使是经专家之手。

　　第四篇包括了一系列针对因初次手术失败造成的解剖异常而进行再手术的方法。这部分由6个临床上高度相关的章节组成，由本领域世界著名的专家编写。每个部分详述怎样最佳地评估和管理这些复杂的患者，以及如何协调患者和医生在这个复杂问题上的期望值。

第 23 章　慢性便秘行回肠/盲肠直肠吻合失败后再手术

Urban Karlbom · Lars Påhlman

冯啸波　译　冯啸波　审校

摘　要

众所周知，结肠次全或全切除后腹泻、排便紧迫感和肛门失禁是常见的并发症，发生率超过 30%。最近的非随机对照研究表明，结肠次全切除后盲肠直肠吻合较结肠全切除后回直肠吻合术后便秘复发率更高，需继续服用泻药或灌肠治疗，且腹泻和肛门失禁发生率无明显区别。本章主要讨论手术适应证明确的顽固性便秘行结肠次全或全切除后临床预后不佳的原因，阐明手术失败后的处理原则和方法。

关键词

回直肠吻合；盲直肠吻合；慢性便秘；肠易激综合征；假性肠梗阻；失禁；胃肠道出血；粘连

引　言

便秘是一种常见的消化道症状，各个不同标准的调查显示，西方国家便秘的发生率在 2%～20% 之间，多见于女性，随着年龄的增长，发病率也会增加[1]。

目前，对功能性便秘的定义和严重程度评估多依据 Roma Ⅲ 标准[2]。临床上，根据症状和检查发现，将功能性便秘分为 3 种类型：慢运输型便秘、出口梗阻型便秘和混合型便秘，近来的研究发现这些患者中很多应诊断为肠易激综合征[3-4]。长期以来，许多因盆底问题就诊的患者被诊断为功能性便秘出口梗阻型，实际上应归为肠易激综合征[5-6]，这类患者如针对盆底问题如直肠前突进行手术后，仍会有持续症状。

正规的便秘治疗应起始于饮食调理或膳食纤维，对轻度的慢运输型便秘多数有效。对于保守治疗无效者，考虑手术治疗。经术前严格检查明确为慢运输型便秘的患者，可行结肠全切除、回直肠吻合。有巨结肠或巨直肠的患者，必须手术治疗，但处理起来较为困难，这部分内容在第 25 章详细介绍。文献报道中，结肠全切除、回直肠吻合术的成功率在 50%～90% 之间[7-11]。特别是中期随访结果显示患者腹痛、腹胀症状明显缓解，排便改善，生活质量亦令人满意[12]。腹腔镜或手助腹腔镜结肠切除技术应用于结肠慢运输型便秘在缓解腹痛、改善生活质量方面也有成功的报道[13-15]。但随着随访时间延长，手术疗效也逐渐降低，很多患者便秘症状复发。而且腹泻、排便紧迫感和肛门失禁等症状发生率超过 30%[7, 10, 16, 17]。

结肠次全切除、盲肠直肠吻合也常应用于慢运输型便秘，其疗效与结肠全切除、回直肠吻合接近，选择合适的患者亦能获得较好的生活质量[18-20]。也有根据结肠节段性运输检测结果行部分结肠切除的方法，报道的早期结果也令人满意，但目前尚无大宗病例的结果支持[21]。一项非随机对照研究显示结肠次全切除、盲肠直肠吻合术后便秘症状复发率要高于结肠全切除、回直肠吻合术，需继续使用泻剂或灌肠[22]，而且在比较了34例盲肠直肠吻合术和45例回直肠吻合术后的结果显示，腹泻、排便紧迫感和肛门失禁等症状发生率无明显差异。

因结肠次全切除、盲肠直肠吻合术长期预后不佳，Sarli等[23]采用结肠次全切除、盲肠直肠逆蠕动吻合的方式，后来又将腹腔镜技术运用其中[24]。近期的多项研究报道了该术式应用于合适的患者取得了较好的中期随访结果[25-27]。尽管如此，文献中报道的较差的预后使得结肠切除术在顽固性便秘中的应用日益谨慎。新的技术如骶神经刺激取得了良好的临床结果，一些中心甚至已将骶神经刺激作为标准化治疗[28-29]。Malone术式尽管有需插管造口和再手术率高的缺点，仍被使用[30-31]。药物治疗亦有进展，如高选择5-HT$_4$受体拮抗剂改善粪便性状和排便频率[31-33]，促进肠道蠕动[34]。其缺点在于潜在的对心脏功能长期的不良反应。

本章重点讨论顽固性便秘行结肠次全切除、盲肠直肠吻合或结肠全切除、回直肠吻合术后疗效不佳时的处理途径。

手术失败的原因

顽固性便秘手术失败的主要原因在于医师过度相信主观判定或术前检查不精确。不透X线标记法虽然精确度不及放射性核素闪烁扫描法[35-36]，但可对胃、小肠动力进行评估，很多术后效果不佳的患者术前即存在胃、小肠动力的障碍[37]。拟手术治疗的结肠慢运输型便秘患者，对直肠肛门功能进行评估十分关键，术前需明确肛门括约肌功能正常（平均静息压和收缩压）。还需要行排粪造影检查以评估直肠排空和盆底的解剖异常。先天性巨结肠患者需明确排除各种表现的假性肠梗阻，可通过直肠肛门抑制反射或组织活检明确[38]，如有怀疑，应进一步行小肠测压。

术后最常见的并发症有便秘症状持续或复发、假性肠梗阻、严重腹泻、肛门失禁、消化道出血以及粘连性肠梗阻。

持续便秘或假性肠梗阻

如手术方式为结肠次全切除、回肠-乙状结肠吻合，需考虑结肠剩余长度是否过长。应重新评估患者术前检查结果，确定慢运输便秘还是出口梗阻型便秘是关键。巨直肠患者要与普通慢运输型便秘区分，其处理原则不同，需行顺行灌肠或结肠全切除、回肠肛管吻合术，具体根据个体情况来选择。

另一种情况是术前存在直肠低敏感性而高度扩张[39-41]，术前就应行小肠测压[42-43]。术前应明确告知患者，即使通过手术，缓解排便困难，腹痛、腹胀等症状仍将持续。术前的心理和精神情况也可能是术后疗效不佳的重要原因[44]。

肛门失禁

肛门失禁是结肠全切除、回直肠吻合的常见并发症。需排除直肠功能障碍或肛门括约肌失功。术前直肠肛管测压可评估直肠的功能、测定肛门括约肌压力、检查肛管的长度和完整度，这些结果有助于对术后出现肛门失禁的原因进行分析。另外，粪便的性状与肛门失禁也有一定的关系，水样便常引起肛门失禁[45-46]。

消化道出血

结肠全切除、回直肠吻合口术后吻合口发生溃疡，可导致贫血。发生率不高，其发病机理尚不清楚，可能与排便过程中腹内压增高形成肠套叠、吻合口受损有关。

粘连性肠梗阻

一般而言，手术创伤越大，腹腔内粘连越重，粘连性肠梗阻发生率越高。但原因不明的是，便秘患者行结肠切除术后肠梗阻的发生率高于同样术式的溃疡性结肠炎或克罗恩病患者。

并发症的处理

持续的便秘和假性肠梗阻

如小肠测压未提示有假性肠梗阻，视残留的直肠或结肠长度，可考虑行直肠或结肠切除[47]。如留有乙状结肠，可行乙状结肠切除、回直肠吻合。但上述手术缺乏依据，其效果也不明确。如首次手术为标准的结肠全切除、回直肠吻合，检查明确括约肌功能良好，可试行直肠切除、回肠贮袋肛管吻合[42, 48]。同样，该手术也缺乏文献报道支持，试行前需全面考虑患者的一般情况、并存病、术后生活质量等因素。

如小肠测压提示为假性肠梗阻，则不宜再手术切除剩余直肠或乙状结肠[49]，最好的选择是回肠造口。在患者未能接受永久性 Brook 造口前，可先行回肠襻式造口，让患者获取造口护理经验，体会造口的功能和造口后的生活质量。或可在造口前行灌肠治疗，观察患者能否获得满意的生活质量[50]。亦可尝试生物反馈治疗[51]。

肛门失禁

虽然肛门失禁的程度可决定治疗的方向，可通过直肠肛门测压、直肠内超声、阴部神经诱发电位研究、肌电图对失禁原因进行分析。但如果肛门失禁已成为影响患者生活治疗的主要因素时，则缺乏恰当的治疗手段。如肛门失禁漏出为气体或偶有疏松粪便，可尝试应用膳食纤维或洛哌丁胺治疗，如为稀便或直肠肛门测压明确为括约肌功能障碍，上述治疗无效。

当肛门失禁保守治疗无效时，可行暂时性骶前神经刺激，观察是否能有所改善[52]，如无改善则应行回肠造口。直肠残端可先予保留，或可先行回肠襻式造口，为患者提供一段适应期，后再关闭远端回肠。如残留直肠内分泌物引起肛门污粪，影响患者生活质量，可考虑切除剩余直肠及肛管。这类问题文献中很少提及，亦缺乏有效客观数据。

消化道出血

对有吻合口溃疡引起贫血的患者，应先行保守治疗，如内镜下注射硬化剂或氩激光束治疗等。如保守治疗无效，而贫血严重，可考虑切除吻合口重建。我们进行回直肠吻合术治疗便秘的经验显示，吻合口区域再切除是必要的，出血问题的中短期缓解率较高。

粘连性肠梗阻

尽管粘连的形成有各种原因，在处理复杂情况时，必须采用同样严格的手术规则。当出现腹痛、肠腔扩张等机械性梗阻症状时，应及时手术治疗。但文献中明确指出，因腹痛而缺乏其他梗阻表现时，手术效果不佳[53-55]。重复探索疼痛起因并不合理。

结 论

当决定对顽固性便秘患者施行结肠手术时，应详细告知患者术后可能存在的持续或复发的消化道症状，必要时需再手术治疗或行回肠造口。只有充分取得患者理解的情况下，方可手术。

参考文献

1. Walter S, Hallböök O, Gotthard R, Bergmark M, Sjödahl R. A population-based study on bowel habits in a Swedish community: prevalence of faecal incontinence and constipation. Scand J Gastroenterol. 2002;37:911–6.
2. Thompson WG, Longstreth GF, Drossman DA, Heaton KW, Irvine EJ, Müller-Lissner SA. Functional bowel disorders and functional abdominal pain. Gut. 1999;45 Suppl 2:43–7.
3. Nyam DC, Pemberton JH, Ilstrup DM, Rath DM. Long-term results of surgery for chronic constipation. Dis Colon Rectum. 1997;40:273–9.
4. Glia A, Lindberg G, Nilsson LH, Mihocsa L, Åkerlund JE. Constipation assessed on the basis of colorectal physiology. Scand J Gastroenterol. 1998;33:1273–9.
5. Wong RK, Palsson OS, Turner MJ, Levy RL, Feld AD, von Korff M, et al. Inability of the Rome III criteria to distinguish functional constipation from constipation-subtype irritable bowel syndrome. Am J Gastroenterol. 2010;105:2228–34.
6. Suttor V, Prott GM, Hansen RD, Kellow JE, Malcolm A. Evidence for pelvic floor dyssynergia in patients with irritable bowel syndrome. Dis Colon Rectum. 2010;53:156–60.
7. Kamm MA, Hawley PR, Lennard-Jones JE. Outcome of colectomy for severe idiopathic constipation. Gut. 1988;29:969–73.
8. Yoshioka K, Keighley MR. Clinical results of colectomy for severe constipation. Br J Surg. 1989;76:600–4.
9. Wexner SD, Daniel N, Jagelman DG. Colectomy for constipation: physiologic investigation is the key to success. Dis Colon Rectum. 1991;34:851–6.
10. Lubowski DZ, Chen FC, Kennedy ML, King DW. Results of colectomy for severe slow transit constipation. Dis Colon Rectum. 1996;39:23–9.
11. Raahave D, Loud FB, Christensen E, Knudsen LL. Colectomy for refractory constipation. Scand J Gastroenterol. 2010;45:592–602.
12. Marchesi F, Sarli L, Percalli L, Sansebastiano GE, Veronesi L, Di Mauro D, et al. Subtotal colectomy with antiperistaltic cecorectal anastomosis in the treatment of slow-transit constipation: long-term impact on quality of life. World J Surg. 2007;31:1658–64.
13. Iannelli A, Fabiani P, Mouiel J, Gugenheim J. Laparoscopic subtotal colectomy with cecorectal anastomosis for slow-transit constipation. Surg Endosc. 2006;20:171–3.
14. Hsiao KC, Jao SW, Wu CC, Lee TY, Lai HJ, Kang JC. Hand-assisted laparoscopic total colectomy for slow transit constipation. Int J Colorectal Dis. 2008;23:419–24.
15. Conzo G, Stanzione F, Celsi S, Palazzo A, Della Pietra C, Candilio G, et al. Videolaparo-assisted subtotal colectomy with cecorectal anastomosis in the treatment of chronic slow transit constipation. G Chir. 2010;31:487–90.
16. Redmond JM, Smith GW, Barofsky I, Ratych RE, Goldsborough DC, Schuster MM. Physiological tests to predict long-term outcome of total abdominal colectomy for intractable constipation. Am J Gastroenterol. 1995;90:748–53.

17. Christiansen J, Rasmussen OO. Colectomy for severe slow-transit constipation in strictly selected patients. Scand J Gastroenterol. 1996;31:770–3.
18. Kamm MA, van der Sijp JR, Hawley PR, Phillips RK, Lennard-Jones JE. Left hemicolectomy with rectal excision for severe idiopathic constipation. Int J Colorectal Dis. 1991;6:49–51.
19. De Graaf EJ, Gilberts EC, Schouten WR. Role of segmental colonic transit time studies to select patients with slow transit constipation for partial left or subtotal colectomy. Br J Surg. 1996;83:648–51.
20. You YT, Wang JY, Changchien CR, Chen JS, Hsu KC, Tang R, et al. Segmental colectomy in the management of colonic inertia. Am Surg. 1998;64:775–7.
21. Lundin E, Karlbom U, Påhlman L, Graf W. Outcome of segmental colonic resection for slow-transit constipation. Br J Surg. 2002;89:1270–4.
22. Feng Y, Jianjiang L. Functional outcomes of two types of subtotal colectomy for slow-transit constipation: ileosigmoidal anastomosis and cecorectal anastomosis. Am J Surg. 2008;195:73–7.
23. Sarli L, Costi R, Sarli D, Roncoroni L. Pilot study of subtotal colectomy with antiperistaltic cecoproctostomy for the treatment of chronic slow-transit constipation. Dis Colon Rectum. 2001;44:1514–20.
24. Sarli L, Costi R, Violi V, Roncoroni L. Intracorporeal laparoscopic cecorectal anastomosis. Surg Laparosc Endosc Percutan Tech. 2007;17:190–2.
25. Sarli L, Costi R, Iusco D, Roncoroni L. Long-term results of subtotal colectomy with antiperistaltic cecoproctostomy. Surg Today. 2003;33:823–7.
26. Jiang CQ, Qian Q, Liu ZS, Bangoura G, Zheng KY, Wu YH. Subtotal colectomy with antiperistaltic cecoproctostomy for selected patients with slow transit constipation-from Chinese report. Int J Colorectal Dis. 2008;23:1251–6.
27. Wang Y, Zhai C, Niu L, Tian L, Yang J, Hu Z. Retrospective series of subtotal colonic bypass and antiperistaltic cecoproctostomy for the treatment of slow-transit constipation. Int J Colorectal Dis. 2010;25:613–8.
28. Kenefick NJ, Nicholls RJ, Cohen RG, Kamm MA. Permanent sacral nerve stimulation for treatment of idiopathic constipation. Br J Surg. 2002;89:882–8.
29. Naldini G, Martellucci J, Moraldi L, Balestri R, Rossi M. Treatment of slow-transit constipation with sacral nerve modulation. Colorectal Dis. 2010;12:1149–52. doi:10.1111/j.1463-1318.2009.02067.x.
30. Malone PS, Ransley PG, Kiely EM. Preliminary report: the antegrade continence enema. Lancet. 1990;336:1217–89.
31. Lees NP, Hodson P, Hill J, Pearson RC, MacLennan I. Long-term results of the antegrade continent enema procedure for constipation in adults. Colorectal Dis. 2004;6:362–8.
32. Sloots CE, Poen AC, Kerstens R, Stevens M, De Pauw M, Van Oene JC, et al. Effects of prucalopride on colonic transit, anorectal function and bowel habits in patients with chronic constipation. Aliment Pharmacol Ther. 2002;16:759–67.
33. Coremans G, Kerstens R, De Pauw M, Stevens M. Prucalopride is effective in patients with severe chronic constipation in whom laxatives fail to provide adequate relief. Results of a double-blind, placebo-controlled clinical trial. Digestion. 2003;67:82–9.
34. Johanson JF. Review article: tegaserod for chronic constipation. Aliment Pharmacol Ther. 2004;20 Suppl 7:20–4.
35. Emmanuel AV, Roy AJ, Nicholls TJ, Kamm MA. Prucalopride, a systemic enterokinetic, for the treatment of constipation. Aliment Pharmacol Ther. 2002;16:1347–56.
36. Southwell BR, Clarke MC, Sutcliffe J, Hutson JM. Colonic transit studies: normal values for adults and children with comparison of radiological and scintigraphic methods. Pediatr Surg Int. 2009;25:559–72.
37. Rao SS, Camilleri M, Hasler WL, Maurer AH, Parkman HP, Saad R, et al. Evaluation of gastrointestinal transit in clinical practice: position paper of the American and European Neurogastroenterology and Motility Societies. Neurogastroenterol Motil. 2011;23:8–23. doi:10.1111/j.1365-2982.2010.01612.x.
38. Vorobyov GI, Achkasov SI, Biryukov OM. Clinical features' diagnostics and treatment of Hirschsprung's disease in adults. Colorectal Dis. 2010;12:1242–8. doi:10.1111/j.1463-1318.2009.02031.x.
39. Åkervall S, Fasth S, Nordgren S, Öresland T, Hultén L. The functional results after colectomy and ileorectal anastomosis for severe constipation (Arbuthnot Lane's disease) as related to rectal sensory function. Int J Colorectal Dis. 1988;3:96–101.
40. Pluta H, Bowes KL, Jewell LD. Long-term results of total abdominal colectomy for chronic idiopathic constipation. Value of preoperative assessment. Dis Colon Rectum. 1996;39:160–6.
41. Nylund G, Öresland T, Fasth S, Nordgren S. Long-term outcome after colectomy in severe idiopathic constipation. Colorectal Dis. 2001;3:253–8.
42. Glia A, Akerlund JE, Lindberg G. Outcome of colectomy for slow-transit constipation in relation to presence of small-bowel dysmotility. Dis Colon Rectum. 2004;47:96–102.
43. Lindberg G, Iwarzon M, Törnblom H. Clinical features and long-term survival in chronic intestinal pseudo-obstruction and enteric dysmotility. Scand J Gastroenterol. 2009;44:692–9.
44. Dykes S, Smilgin-Humphreys S, Bass C. Chronic idiopathic constipation: a psychological enquiry. Eur J Gastroenterol Hepatol. 2001;13:39–44.
45. FitzHarris GP, Garcia-Aguilar J, Parker SC, Bullard KM, Madoff RD, Goldberg SM, et al. Quality of life after subtotal colectomy for slow-transit constipation: both quality and quantity count. Dis Colon Rectum. 2003;46:433–40.
46. bin Mohd Zam NA, Tan KY, Ng C, Chen CM, Wong SK, Chng HC, et al. Mortality, morbidity and functional outcome after total or subtotal abdominal colectomy in the Asian population. ANZ J Surg. 2005;75:840–3.
47. Ozuner G, Strong SA, Fazio VW. Effect of rectosigmoid stump length on restorative proctocolectomy after subtotal colectomy. Dis Colon Rectum. 1995;38:1039–42.
48. Hosie K, Kmiot WA, Keighley MRB. Functional bowel disorders: further indications for restorative proctocolectomy. Paper presented at the British Society of Gastroenterology. Dublin; 1989. p. 47.
49. Hasegawa H, Fatah C, Radley S, Keighley MRB. Long term results of colorectal resection for chronic constipation. Colorectal Dis. 1999;1:137–40.
50. Iwarzon M, Gardulf A, Lindberg G. Functional status, health-related quality of life and symptom severity in patients with chronic intestinal pseudo-obstruction and enteric dysmotility. Scand J Gastroenterol. 2009;44:700–7.
51. Sloots CE, Felt-Bersma RJ. Effect of bowel cleansing on colonic transit in constipation due to slow transit or evacuation disorder. Neurogastroenterol Motil. 2002;14:55–61.
52. Holzer B, Rosen HR, Zaglmaier W, Klug R, Beer B, Novi G, et al. Sacral nerve stimulation in patients after rectal resection – preliminary report. J Gastrointest Surg. 2008;12:921–5.
53. Ivarsson M-L, Holmdahl L, Franzén G, Risberg B. Cost of bowel obstruction resulting from adhesions. Eur J Surg. 1997;163:679–84.
54. Matter I, Khalemsky L, Abrahamson J, Nash E, Sabo E, Eldar S. Does the index operation influence the course and outcome of adhesive intestinal obstruction. Eur J Surg. 1997;163:767–72.
55. Emmanuel AV, Kamm MA. Response to a behavioural treatment, biofeedback, in constipated patients is associated with improved gut transit and autonomic innervation. Gut. 2001;49:214–9.

第 24 章 Malone 治疗方法及其衍生治疗方式

Peter Christensen · Søren Laurberg
姜　军译　姜　军审校

摘　要

随着如经皮内镜下结肠造口、威廉姆斯控制大便结肠导管或回肠部位导管化等外科方式的改变，本章将讨论顺行控制大便灌肠（Malone方法）的部位。这些方法已用于动态股薄肌成形术和先天性肛门直肠畸形治疗失败后的治疗。本章重点讨论Malone顺行灌肠的治疗和并发症的处理。

关键词

顺行控制排便灌肠（ACE）；Malone方法；回肠导管；逐渐变细的末端回肠；阑尾造口术；痛神经安定镇痛阑尾造口术；V-Y成形术；经皮内镜结肠造口术；威廉姆斯导管；顺行结肠灌肠；结肠造口灌肠；盲肠瓣；自体中毒；便秘；大便失禁；出口梗阻；神经源性小肠功能障碍；经肛门灌肠；腹腔镜手术；结肠造口术；灌肠；灌肠液骶神经刺激

引　言

根据古埃及人的信仰，尸体防腐者发现人类的气魄流淌于脉管网络结构之中[1-2]。心脏是这些网络的中心，但认为最终连接于肛门周围。它不仅输送全身的体液，同时也接收来自于粪便和全身产生疾病和疼痛的有害物质。人们认为肠道有规律的清洁能让气魄自由流淌，从而保持健康。重要的是，通过祛除有害物质，所有疾病将得到治愈[2-3]。在公元1500年的埃伯斯草纸[4]和公元1200年的切斯特比蒂VI纸莎草纸[5]等最古老的医学文献上可以看到灌肠剂的使用。

在1905年，有人提出在阑尾中形成瘘管，通过进行灌肠来治疗便秘[6]。虽然因操作带来的死亡率高达20%，但在随后的10年中，该方法得到广泛的应用[7]。在那段时期，自体排毒成为了医学中的教条[8-9]。人们痴迷于调节肠道运动，在中产阶级人群中，清洗肠道备受推崇[10-11]。

根据当时的医学专业来说，由于受材料的限制导致治疗失败，同时其他如药理学和外科治疗的革新导致灌肠成为了一种难以信服的治疗方式[8]。自体排毒的概念从此失宠，顺行灌肠也消失在了医学界中，直到Malone等在1990年利用Mvitrofanoff创新使用的可控性尿流改道技术[13]重新提出该概念，他们建议使用阑尾造口进行顺行灌肠，治疗儿童脊裂和肛门畸形导致的大便失禁和便秘。Malone等简单推测，计划性的灌肠可能预防在冲洗和重新建立排便时间之间和排便地点的粪便漏出，从而既能规律地进行充分排便，也能预防便秘。此后，该手术方式被命名为Malone治疗方法。

Malone 治疗方法

起初的Malone术是通过阑尾建立一个连续的

导管化的腹部造口。基于可控性尿流改道技术的原理，将阑尾翻转后固定于盲肠闭合的盲肠浆肌层的黏膜下隧道，从而形成一非反流性管道[13]。一个简单的方法无需反转[14-16]，需或不需浆肌层盲肠重叠构造作为抗反流机制[17-18]在随后被采用。

一直以来，Malone 术主要为开腹手术，但它非常适合腹腔镜手术，因为具有微创手术的所有优点，且与开腹手术有相同的功能效果和并发症发生率[19-22]。通过游离阑尾，可将它外置于选择的位点，通常选择右侧腹股沟与皮肤形成 V-Y 形状。将一个 10# 的硅胶导管置入阑尾并填充气囊。然后将盲肠缝合到前腹壁的背面，并关闭腹中线切口。阑尾造口最终通过 V-Y 成形完成，通过 4-0 可吸收线交替的将皮瓣的顶端缝入阑尾中（图 24.1a，b）。在手术后，导管留在原位 2 周。最终目标是实现一个简易的导管化和可控的管道。

对于萎缩的阑尾或已行阑尾切除术，可通过其他一些衍生的技术来建立一个新的阑尾。如导管可以从盲肠瓣[23]、末端回肠[24-25]、节段的回肠[15, 26]或者是盲肠造口[27]形成。逐渐变细的末端回肠被认为是首选的方式[25]。通过 80mm 胃肠切割闭合器将末端回肠切开，将一个 12# 带气囊导管置入远端回肠并通过回盲瓣，同时将气囊充气用于鉴别回盲瓣。远端回肠的管径直径的大小通过切除部分对系膜缘肠壁进行重建，并保留回盲瓣（图 24.2a,b）。将近端回肠和升结肠进行吻合。

随访护理引导的重要性

术后，开始给予灌肠剂，并在术后 1 周逐渐达到 1000ml/ 天，灌肠的最终频率和灌肠剂的剂量最终通过第 1 个月的反复试验和矫正后确定。通常，每天或隔日进行灌肠，灌肠剂平均给予量为 1300ml。每次灌肠的时间平均为 50min[28]。

Malone 治疗方法取得成功的基础是敬业，依靠专业的门诊护士的不断支持和帮助，尤其是在治疗的起始阶段。该治疗方法通常非常麻烦且耗时，它需要不断调整灌肠的频率和灌肠剂的剂量。通常需要辅助口服泻剂，管道的局部并发症非常常见。因此，Malone 技术也需要敢于挑战的积极患者。

功能结果

自从 Malone 治疗方法得以应用，被认为对于儿童脊裂和肛门畸形导致的大便失禁和慢性便秘安全且有效[14, 15, 17, 18, 29-31]。在儿童中获得的结果已经被长期和更庞大的病例中所证实[31-37]。

近期，顺行结肠灌肠已经开始应用于成人。虽然目前它的效果仅基于几项单中心的患者研究中（表 24.1），但目前既无循证医学证据也无系统分析。总之，成人严重结肠自发的便秘、出口梗阻或大便失禁可通过顺行灌肠而有所改善。不包括已知的重复发表的，评估了共 277 例顺行结肠灌洗患者，发现发现 204（74%）例患者有效。但需强调的是，长期效果并不明显，在一项研究中评估了时间依赖的顺行灌肠，发现长时间的顺行灌肠是有害的[44]。

有一种趋势，即于神经源性的肠道功能障碍的患者获益更为明显[28, 29, 40, 43, 48]。一项决策性的分析表明，对于通过保守治疗无效的神经源性的肠道功能衰竭的患者来说，顺行灌肠是最有效的治疗方法[52]。但是，该研究并未考虑更为简便的经肛灌肠方法[41]。现有的经肛灌肠的研究中，大部分为回顾性的分析，且没有使用肠道功能评分。但是，

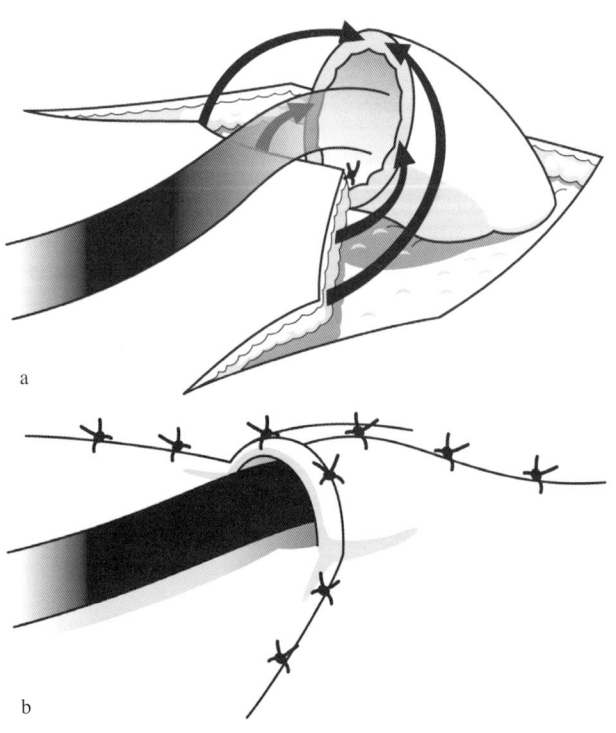

图 24.1　V-Y 成形。(a) 将皮肤的顶端与缩短的阑尾缝合或使用 4-0 可吸收线将回肠的导管与皮瓣顶端的皮肤缝合；(b) 随后皮肤隧道形成并遮盖造口

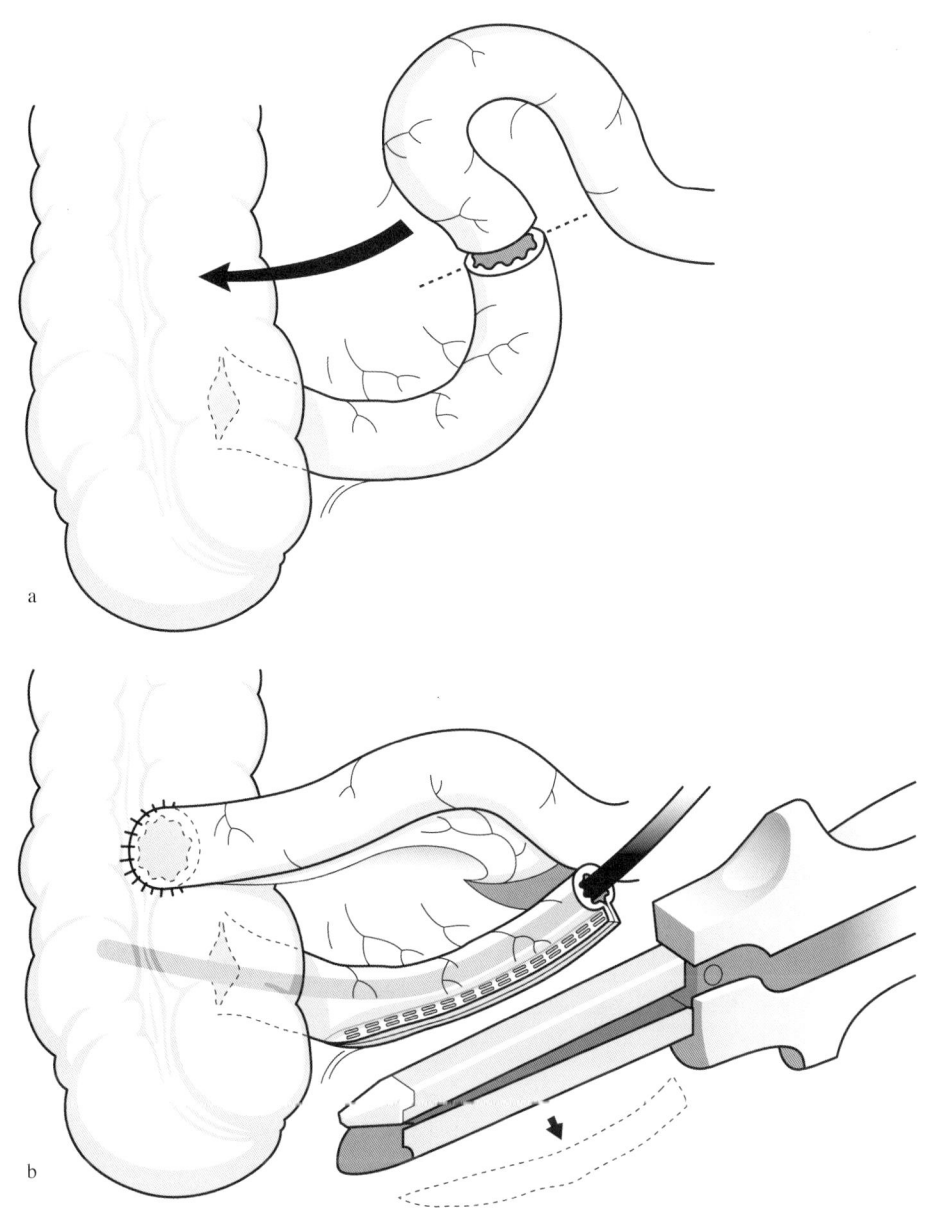

图 24.2 逐渐变细的回肠。(a) 近端回肠与升结肠性回结肠吻合；(b) 通过切除对系膜缘，降低远端回肠的直径，并保留回盲瓣

一些使用肠道功能评分和前瞻性的研究中表明经肛灌肠能明显改善症状[35, 42, 45, 47, 49]。尽管这些研究对于改善社会关系和生活质量并无明显的效果。

Malone 治疗的局部并发症

虽然顺行灌肠治疗对于功能和患者的满意度是明显的，但治疗过程中仍然有一些并发症，尤其是局部的造口部位的并发症，这些并发症可能会掩盖了治疗效果。在这些方面，23%～55% 的患者存在造口狭窄[28, 31, 35, 37, 44, 53]。对于大部分的患者来说，该并发症可通过简单的扩张治疗，少部分患者需经外科手术的矫正。此外，53% 的患者通过管道反流黏液或粪液[28]，这能通过简单的创口带治疗，严重的患者可置入胃造口管治疗[40, 46, 54, 55]，造口的狭窄和黏液或粪液的反流均可在去除原先的导管后置入硅胶气囊管避免[56]。总体上来说，并发症的发生率可高达 88%。局部并发症的发生与管道的形成方式无关[28]；但是，其他研究发现逐渐变细的回肠新阑尾造口是最为优良的方式[46, 47, 57]。

管道穿孔（盲肠穿孔）是潜在的并发症，需要及时诊断和早期干预[58-59]。在一项对 187 名患儿历

表 24.1　成人顺行灌肠

参考文献[a]	病因	随访时间（月）	总病人数 N	成功率	不良反应	并发症
Hill 等[38]	慢传输	NR	6	6	NR	50%
Krogh[16]	混合型	17	16	12	25%	25%
Yang[39]	神经源性	3	1	1	NR	NR
Christensen 等[40]	混合型	38	8	7	38%	38%
Christensen 等[41]	混合型	10	9	8	50%	78%
Rongen 等[42]	慢传输	18	12	8	NR	83%
Teichman 等[43]	神经源性	54	6	5	NR	67%
Lees 等[44]	慢传输	36	32	15	NR	88%
Hirst 等[45]	梗阻型	6	20	13	NR	85%
Portier 等[46]	混合型	NR	28	28	NR	50%
Lefévre 等[47]	混合型	26	22	18	NR	20%
Poirier 等[48]	混合型	19	18	14	NR	56%
Altomare 等[49]	混合型	44	11	8	NR	0%
Koivusalo 等[35]	混合型	25	27	24	NR	63%
Worsoe 等[28]	混合型	75	69	51	63%	38%
Meurette[50]	慢传输	55	25	13	NR	NR

NR：尚无报道
a：参考文献根据时间编排

经 13 年顺行灌肠的研究发现，7 例患儿（3.7%）发生了管道穿孔。其中 2 例患儿需要剖腹，5 例需要通过内镜置入导管治疗[58]。在我们的研究所，发生 1 例患者因暴力取出导管发生穿孔，该患者通过内镜置入 Mic-key 钮扣治愈[28]。

如果患者不再需要顺行灌肠，或者出现无法接受的并发症时，那么需停止使用造口；并常需要关闭造口，以免患者在手术之前状态变差。一旦无功能的阑尾造口持续分泌液体，则需进行阑尾切除术。

其他结肠灌肠的新外科技术

一项新的顺行结肠灌肠技术是经皮内镜结肠造瘘（PEC）。该方法是在经皮内镜下放置胃管进行营养支持衍生而来，经皮将人工管放入左半或右半结肠。起初，PEC 是用于再发性乙状结肠扭转或假性肠梗阻的减压[60-61]。但是，置入的导管也可进行肠道到肛门的冲洗。这种方法的好处可能是顺行灌肠可能比逆行灌肠效果更好。另一个优点是通过微创的方式放置导管，这通常是在局部麻醉清醒状态下进行的。该治疗方法指南已发表于《英国国家健康与临床优化》杂志[62]。

PEC 对于功能性的结果是令人鼓舞的。对于儿童顽固性便秘的患者，90% 可控制症状[63]；对于严重便秘或神经源性的肠道功能衰竭的成年人，这些获益的结果也被证实[64-66]，一项最近的单中心回顾性研究发现，PEC 对于 81% 的患者有效[67]。但是，由于并发症的因素，长期的结果是有害的。在这项研究中，2 例患者死于并发症，27 例中的 18 例出现局部的脓肿和频繁的导管相关并发症。最终在随访中，仅有 2 例患者（2/28）管道保持原位。其他的研究也报道了 PEC 后期的并发症[68]和高失败率[64]。尽管起初 PEC 可控制症状，但仍不能推荐 PEC 的普及。

在大部分的病例中，右侧结肠顺行灌肠（从盲肠形成管道）具有满意的效果。但在另一些的病例中，病原在左半结肠或直肠。因此，从生理学角度来说，靠近病灶进行灌肠可能更为有效。作为 PEC 的替代方式治疗左半结肠疾病，几种新的外科术式已经被提出。威廉姆等创新了一种可控性的结肠管道[69]。它提供一个自皮肤到结肠的导管化的通道。结肠导管可置入降结肠和乙状结肠的任何位置。该手术更为复杂，且技术相关的并发症与其他类型的新阑尾造口术相似。有 Monti 等描述的一个再导管化的回肠段[71]或由胃大弯形成的导管也能吻合至乙状结肠。最终，一个导管化的降结肠被推荐使用[73-74]。通常文献报道的左侧顺行控制粪便灌肠主要用于肠道功能衰竭的脊裂[75]、自发性便秘、巨结肠或者肛门直肠畸形的儿童患者。最近的 meta 分析发现，控制粪便的成功率可达 94%（87/93）[76]。它也用于治疗顽固性便秘或动态股薄肌成形术后肠功能衰竭后的大便失禁[77]。这些结果与右侧顺行控制粪便灌肠相一致。左侧顺行控制粪便灌肠和控制粪便结肠管道是否比右侧顺行粪便灌肠有明显优势，需要进一步的研究[78]。

目前已经证明，顺行结肠灌肠较逆行结肠灌肠效果更为明显[79-80]，阑尾造口联合结肠造口已经被推荐用于择期手术的结直肠癌患者顺行结肠灌肠的结肠造口护理[81]。在灌肠期间，患者通过阑尾造口冲洗结肠，并通过灌肠袖套置入便池进行肠道排空（图 24.3）。在近期发表的关于应用该方法的文章显示，25 例患者其中 14 例为神经源性肠功能衰竭，有效率高达 72%，表明该方法相比逆行灌肠对残存无功能的结肠更为有效。

顺行灌肠的不良反应

便秘相关的并发症如腹痛、腹胀和反胃，仍无法通过灌肠解决[42]，且灌肠暂时性的不良反应如轻度的腹部痉挛、疼痛、反胃、寒战和疲劳的发生率可高达 50%～63%[16, 28, 40]。灌肠的目的是通过短时间、大剂量的灌肠液突然灌入引起顺行的蠕动。研究已经表明，结肠较大的运动可通过灌肠[82]、比沙可啶[83]和气囊扩张[84]诱导，轻度的腹部痉挛可能是由于灌肠引起。

采用核素双同位素技术研究发现，3 例回肠阑尾新造口患者可通过回结肠吻合口反流至回肠。反流也发现在通过回盲瓣形成的新阑尾造口患者的末端回肠。但与无反流患者相比，轻度和短暂的不良反应并无明显的差异。此外，在其他的研究中，通

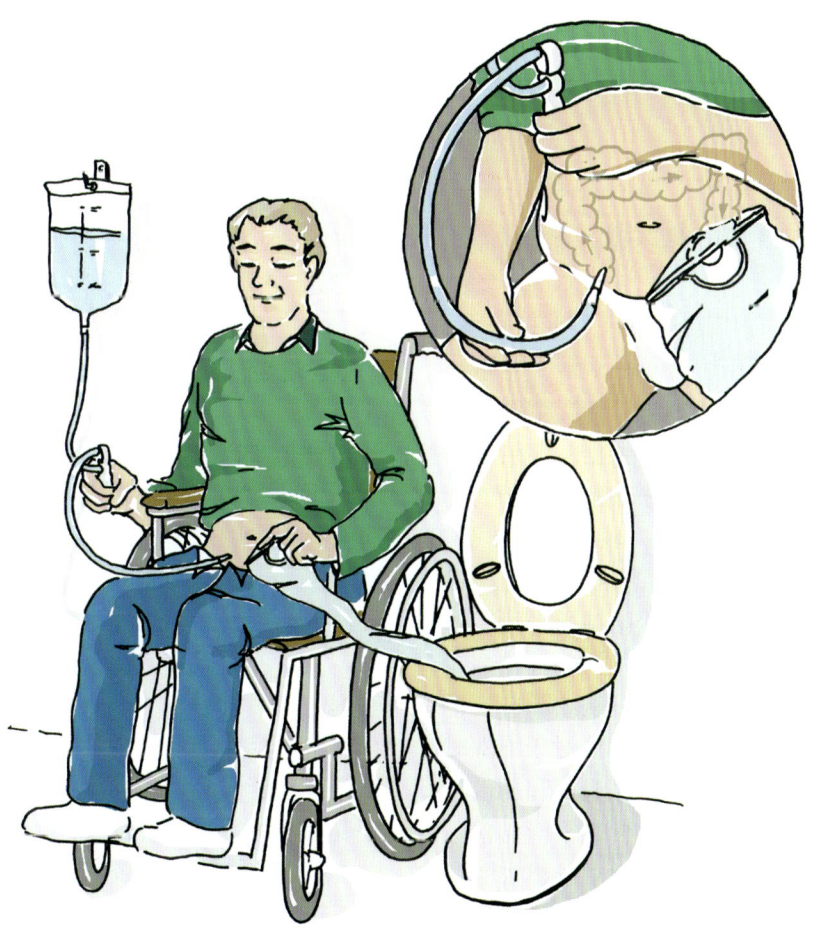

图 24.3　阑尾造口和结肠造口患者的顺行灌肠。当进行灌肠时，需置入 10# 的导管至阑尾造口并给予灌肠剂。结肠常可以排空，且粪便通过袖套排入便池。当患者残存结肠无功能，尤其是神经源性肠道功能衰竭的患者可考虑进行双造口

过氢呼吸实验并未发现新回肠末端细菌过度繁殖[49]。在一些相似的研究中发现，与基础水平相比，胆囊排空、胃的排空、口-盲肠的运输时间维持不变，无症状的回肠末端细菌过度繁殖可能影响胆汁酸和维生素的吸收。

作用机理

逆行经肛门灌肠对于解决便秘疗效较差[85-87]。正如以前研究结果显示，便秘患者肠壁动力差，且对于推进刺激无明显反应[88]。然而，通过闪烁扫描研究发现，8例便秘患者中的7例有大段顺行运输和通过顺行结肠灌肠引起结肠和直肠的显著排空。这些更为有效的结果表明，顺行结肠灌肠较经肛灌肠更为有效，它灌肠液的初始流动是高振幅传播收缩，且与肠运动的方向相反有关。通过猪的动物实验证实顺行结肠灌肠优于逆行结肠造口灌肠[80]。且一小部分的临床研究也表明，顺行结肠灌肠在改进结肠管理和生活质量上优于逆行造口灌肠[81]。因此，对于结肠动力异常的患者，顺行结肠灌肠可能获益更为明显。

灌肠剂

Malone起初建议进行顺行结肠灌肠的灌肠液首选为磷酸盐[89]，其他的研究提提出其他不同种类的灌肠液[29, 31, 65, 90]。联合使用如自来水、生理盐水、磷酸盐、磷酸钠、聚乙二醇、甘草根溶液、花生油和在灌肠前使用解痉药，并根据患者情况个体化进行。但是使用这些药物仍缺乏科学依据。但结肠造口灌肠的经验教训可提供有意义的经验。

在一项猪的灌肠模型研究中，较自来水灌肠，聚乙二醇或1.5%的甘氨酸注入灌肠液能明显增加结肠的排空，且加入硝酸甘油可松弛结肠平滑肌和改善排空[80]。一项临床研究显示，使用甘油栓剂能促进结肠造口排空，这是由于栓剂可从结肠造口排出[91]。另一些研究证实，硝酸甘油溶液对于冲洗时间和瘘的发生方面均优于自来水，且头疼和肠道痉挛等不良反应也较低[92]，这可能是促进平滑肌松弛后允许灌肠液更快速地进入结肠，随后肠道排泄物的排出与结肠运动无关。其他的一些临床研究显示，聚乙二醇较自来水能减少灌肠时间，获得更低的粪便漏出的发生率、更高的满意度评分和更低的造口袋使用率；相反，另一些临床研究显示，加入比沙可啶、前列腺素E_2[93]、前列腺素F_{2a}[94]和肥皂水[95]进行结肠造口灌肠并不能改善肠道排空。因此，如何选择最佳灌肠剂需要进一步的研究。

电解质紊乱

温自来水作为灌肠液[16, 40, 96, 97]，费用低且易获取，通常可保证足够的肠道灌洗[65]。建议避免使用过度氯化的自来水和不能饮用的自来水。自来水灌肠因进入肠腔的量较少，因此不会导致电解质紊乱，且低渗透压也不会导致黏膜损伤，因此长期使用是安全的。

一些儿科中的研究已经证实，自来水灌肠对血浆中钠离子并无明显的影响[98]，且一项纳入71例儿科患者的研究显示，在术后8个月的顺行结肠灌肠中，患者电解质并无明显的变化[99]。正常结肠能吸收大约每天6L的液体[100]，因此结肠能快速吸收存储于结肠中的液体。但在某种条件下也需谨慎使用。从日常时间中我们已经观察到，对于处在脱水边缘的患者使用大剂量的灌肠液，将导致排空效果变差。使用自来水灌肠，唯一的影响是灌洗不充分，因此常规的调整方法是加入磷酸盐或盐制剂药片进行灌肠。如果灌肠需要持续进行，磷酸盐或磷酸钠盐可能导致高磷[101]或高钠血症[102]。因此，对于儿童、疲劳的老年人或慢性肾衰竭的患者需谨慎使用[103]。

肠道功能疾病的治疗措施

对于肠道功能疾病的治疗，不同的治疗模式反映了不同的病理生理特点，在本书中广泛讨论。目前只有很少的对照试验，治疗主要基于临床经验和短期随访[104]。因此，由于一些偏见和错误的治疗方法导致临床医师在治疗过程中存在相当大的矛盾，需要不断研究使每个治疗模式成为恰当和有理有据的。只有得到更多有用的客观结果后，使用这种方法治疗功能性肠道疾病才是合理的，同时还应与患者进行充分沟通。保守治疗应该加以利用，且经肛灌肠的治疗方法通常就足够了[87]。

顺行结肠灌肠较经肛灌肠往往更为有效，Malone治疗方法对2/3的患者效果明显，且与疾病的病理生理无关。如果患者发现效果差，那么他们可以中断使用导管。大部分患者将关闭导管，且在手术前对患者无明显损害。但这种治疗方法的缺陷是需要一个能力精干的护理团队。

骶神经刺激对于大便失禁的患者已取得了良好的效果[105]，且该治疗方式已经应用于自发性便秘[106-107]和继发于马尾神经功能不全综合征的大便失禁[108-110]患者。这一局限的治疗方式将引起广大医务工作者的兴趣，虽然它的作用机理目前并不清楚，可能于它诱导刺激传入中枢神经系统和中枢活动有关[111]。目前研究表明，在进行Malone治疗前进行经皮针评估（PNE）是有意义的。如果PEN测试阳性，那么患者需进行骶神经刺激治疗；相反，如果是阴性，需进行Malone治疗。

虽然结肠造口某种程度上是一种治疗良性功能性肠道疾病的根治性方法，但它常可明显改善生活质量、降低腹痛、降低肠道护理时间和改善个体的独立能力，最终具有更好的社会和自我认同感[112-113]。许多患者经常直接质疑，他们应该进行更早的结肠造口手术[51]。结肠次全切除和直肠回肠吻合是慢性便秘患者的手术方式，有许多并发症，且功能问题是多样性的[114-116]，且很少有明显的指标。

结　论

Malone治疗方法及其衍生治疗方式在本章中已经讨论。基于儿童的成功治疗，该治疗方法已经用于成年人。对于成年人的治疗，随着外科技术的进步，瘘和狭窄的发生率已经明显降低，且可保持患者相对清洁[117]。Malone治疗方法可联合人工泌尿括约肌进行粪便控制重建[118]，且可作为一种治疗严重便秘的永久性治疗方法，并可达到长期的成功，还可作为连接其他手术或非手术治疗的桥梁[50]。如患者能很好地调节肠道功能，那么生活质量可明显提高[119-120]。可能对于先天性肛门畸形的患者进行确定性外科术后仍残存大便失禁的特殊人群具有特殊的定位。

参考文献

1. Nunn JF. Concept of anatomy, physiology and pathology. Ancient Egyptian medicine. London: The British Museum Press; 1996. p. 61–2.
2. Chen TS, Chen PS. Intestinal autointoxication: a medical leitmotif. J Clin Gastroenterol. 1989;11:434–41.
3. Gotfredsen E. Medicinens historie. 2nd ed. Copenhagen: Nyt Nordisk Forlag Arnold Busck; 1964.
4. Ebbel B. The papyrus ebers. Copenhagen: Levin & Munksgaard; 1937.
5. Nunn JF. The medical papyri. Ancient Egyptian medicine. London: The British Museum Press; 1996. p. 24–41.
6. Keighley MR, Willams NS. Constipation. In: Keighley MR, Willams NS, editors. Surgery of the anus, the rectum and colon. 2nd ed. London: W.B.Saunders; 1999. p. 701–55.
7. Corbett RS. A review of the surgical treatment of chronic ulcerative colitis. Proc R Soc Med. 1945;38:277–90.
8. Whorton J. Civilization and the colon. Constipation as "the disease of diseases". West J Med. 2000;173:424–7.
9. Ernst E. Colonic irrigation and the theory of autointoxication: a triumph of ignorance over science. J Clin Gastroenterol. 1997;24:196–8.
10. Doyle D. Per rectum: a history of enemata. J R Coll Physicians Edinb. 2005;35:367–70.
11. Kravetz RE. The enema. Am J Gastroenterol. 2001;96:2486.
12. Malone PS, Ransley PG, Kiely EM. Preliminary report: the antegrade continence enema. Lancet. 1990;336(8725):1217–8.
13. Mitrofanoff P. Cystostomie continente trans-appendiculire dans le traitement des vessies neurologiques. Chir Pediatr. 1980;21:297–305.
14. Griffiths DM, Malone PS. The Malone antegrade continence enema. J Pediatr Surg. 1995;30:68–71.
15. Squire R, Kiely EM, Carr B, Ransley PG, Duffy PG. The clinical application of the Malone antegrade colonic enema. J Pediatr Surg. 1993;28:1012–5.
16. Krogh K, Laurberg S. Malone antegrade continence enema for faecal incontinence and constipation in adults. Br J Surg. 1998;85:974–7.
17. Koyle MA, Kaji DM, Duque M, Wild J, Galansky SH. The Malone antegrade continence enema for neurogenic and structural fecal incontinence and constipation. J Urol. 1995;154:759–61.
18. Ellsworth PI, Webb HW, Crump JM, Barraza MA, Stevens PS, Mesrobian HG. The Malone antegrade colonic enema enhances the quality of life in children undergoing urological incontinence procedures. J Urol. 1996;155:1416–8.
19. Casale P, Grady RW, Feng WC, Joyner BD, Mitchell ME. A novel approach to the laparoscopic antegrade continence enema procedure: intracorporeal and extracorporeal techniques. J Urol. 2004;171:817–9.
20. Antao B, Ng J, Roberts J. Laparoscopic antegrade continence enema using a two-port technique. J Laparoendosc Adv Surg Tech A. 2006;16:168–73.
21. Lynch AC, Beasley SW, Robertson RW, Morreau PN. Comparison of results of laparoscopic and open antegrade continence enema procedures. Pediatr Surg Int. 1999;15:343–6.
22. Kim J, Beasley SW, Maoate K. Appendicostomy stomas and antegrade colonic irrigation after laparoscopic antegrade continence enema. J Laparoendosc Adv Surg Tech A. 2006;16:400–3.
23. Kiely EM, Ade-Ajayi N, Wheeler RA. Caecal flap conduit for antegrade continence enemas. Br J Surg. 1994;81:1215.
24. Marsh PJ, Kiff ES. Ileocaecostomy: an alternative surgical procedure for antegrade colonic enema. Br J Surg. 1996;83:507–8.
25. Christensen P, Buntzen S, Krogh K, Laurberg S. Ileal neoappendicostomy for antegrade colonic irrigation. Br J Surg. 2001;88:1637–8.
26. Yang WH. Yang needle tunneling technique in creating antireflux and continent mechanisms. J Urol. 1993;150:830–4.
27. Shandling B, Chait PG, Richards HF. Percutaneous cecostomy: a new technique in the management of fecal incontinence. J Pediatr Surg. 1996;31:534–7.
28. Worsoe J, Christensen P, Krogh K, Buntzen S, Laurberg S. Long-term results of antegrade colonic enema in adult patients: assessment of functional results. Dis Colon Rectum. 2008;51:1523–8.
29. Malone PS, Curry JI, Osborne A. The antegrade continence enema procedure why, when and how? World J Urol. 1998;16:274–8.
30. Sheldon CA, Minevich E, Wacksman J, Lewis AG. Role of the antegrade continence enema in the management of the most debilitating childhood recto-urogenital anomalies. J Urol. 1997;158:1277–9.
31. Curry JI, Osborne A, Malone PS. The MACE procedure: experience in the United Kingdom. J Pediatr Surg. 1999;34:338–40.
32. Clark T, Pope JC, Adams C, Wells N, Brock III JW. Factors that

influence outcomes of the Mitrofanoff and Malone antegrade continence enema reconstructive procedures in children. J Urol. 2002; 168:1537–40.
33. Dey R, Ferguson C, Kenny SE, Shankar KR, Coldicutt P, Baillie CT, et al. After the honeymoon – medium-term outcome of antegrade continence enema procedure. J Pediatr Surg. 2003;38:65–8.
34. Krogsgaard SM, Milling MD, Qvist N. Appendicostomy in the treatment of severe defecation disorders in children. Ugeskr Laeger. 2006;168:692–4.
35. Koivusalo AI, Pakarinen MP, Pauniaho SL, Rintala RJ. Antegrade continence enema in the treatment of congenital fecal incontinence beyond childhood. Dis Colon Rectum. 2008;51:1605–10.
36. Bani-Hani AH, Cain MP, Kaefer M, Meldrum KK, King S, Johnson CS, et al. The Malone antegrade continence enema: single institutional review. J Urol. 2008;180:1106–10.
37. Curry JI, Osborne A, Malone PS. How to achieve a successful Malone antegrade continence enema. J Pediatr Surg. 1998;33:138–41.
38. Hill J, Stott S, MacLennan I. Antegrade enemas for the treatment of severe idiopathic constipation. Br J Surg. 1994;81:1490–1.
39. Yang CC, Stiens SA. Antegrade continence enema for the treatment of neurogenic constipation and fecal incontinence after spinal cord injury. Arch Phys Med Rehabil. 2000;81:683–5.
40. Christensen P, Kvitzau B, Krogh K, Buntzen S, Laurberg S. Neurogenic colorectal dysfunction – use of new antegrade and retrograde colonic wash-out methods. Spinal Cord. 2000;38:255–61.
41. Christensen P, Bazzocchi G, Coggrave M, Abel R, Hultling C, Krogh K, et al. A randomized, controlled trial of transanal irrigation versus conservative bowel management in spinal cord-injured patients. Gastroenterology. 2006;131:738–47.
42. Rongen MJ, van der Hoop AG, Baeten CG. Cecal access for antegrade colon enemas in medically refractory slow-transit constipation: a prospective study. Dis Colon Rectum. 2001;44:1644–9.
43. Teichman JM, Zabihi N, Kraus SR, Harris JM, Barber DB. Long-term results for Malone antegrade continence enema for adults with neurogenic bowel disease. Urology. 2003;61:502–6.
44. Lees NP, Hodson P, Hill J, Pearson RC, MacLennan I. Long-term results of the antegrade continent enema procedure for constipation in adults. Colorectal Dis. 2004;6:362–8.
45. Hirst GR, Arumugam PJ, Watkins AJ, Mackey P, Morgan AR, Carr ND, et al. Antegrade continence enema in the treatment of obstructed defecation with or without faecal incontinence. Tech Coloproctol. 2005;9:217–21.
46. Portier G, Ghouti L, Kirzin S, Chauffour M, Lazorthes F. Malone antegrade colonic irrigation: ileal neoappendicostomy is the preferred procedure in adults. Int J Colorectal Dis. 2006;21:458–60.
47. Lefevre JH, Parc Y, Giraudo G, Bell S, Parc R, Tiret E. Outcome of antegrade continence enema procedures for faecal incontinence in adults. Br J Surg. 2006;93:1265–9.
48. Poirier M, Abcarian H, Nelson R. Malone antegrade continent enema: an alternative to resection in severe defecation disorders. Dis Colon Rectum. 2007;50:22–8.
49. Altomare DF, Rinaldi M, Rubini D, Rubini G, Portincasa P, Vacca M, et al. Long-term functional assessment of antegrade colonic enema for combined incontinence and constipation using a modified Marsh and Kiff technique. Dis Colon Rectum. 2007;50:1023–31.
50. Meurette G, Lehur PA, Coron E, Regenet N. Long-term results of Malone's procedure with antegrade irrigation for severe chronic constipation. Gastroenterol Clin Biol. 2010;34:209–12.
51. Branagan G, Tromans A, Finnis D. Effect of stoma formation on bowel care and quality of life in patients with spinal cord injury. Spinal Cord. 2003;41:680–3.
52. Furlan JC, Urbach DR, Fehlings MG. Optimal treatment for severe neurogenic bowel dysfunction after chronic spinal cord injury: a decision analysis. Br J Surg. 2007;94:1139–50.
53. Driver CP, Barrow C, Fishwick J, Gough DC, Bianchi A, Dickson AP. The Malone antegrade colonic enema procedure: outcome and lessons of 6 years' experience. Pediatr Surg Int. 1998;13:370–2.
54. Byrne CM, Pager CK, Rex J, Roberts R, Solomon MJ. Assessment of quality of life in the treatment of patients with neuropathic fecal incontinence. Dis Colon Rectum. 2002;45:1431–6.
55. Heshmat S, Defoor W, Minevich E, Reddy P, Reeves D, Sheldon C. Use of customized MIC-KEY gastrostomy button for management of MACE stomal complications. Urology. 2008;72(5):1026–9.
56. Lopez PJ, Ashrafian H, Clarke SA, Johnson H, Kiely EM. Early experience with the antegrade colonic enema stopper to reduce stomal stenosis. J Pediatr Surg. 2007;42(3):522–4.
57. Tackett LD, Minevich E, Benedict JF, Wacksman J, Sheldon CA. Appendiceal versus ileal segment for antegrade continence enema. J Urol. 2002;167:683–6.
58. Defoor W, Minevich E, Reddy P, Barqawi A, Kitchens D, Sheldon C, et al. Perforation of Malone antegrade continence enema: diagnosis and management. J Urol. 2005;174:1644–6.
59. Meier DE, Foster ME, Guzzetta PC, Coln D. Antegrade continent enema management of chronic fecal incontinence in children. J Pediatr Surg. 1998;33:1149–51.
60. Thompson AR, Pearson T, Ellul J, Simson JN. Percutaneous endoscopic colostomy in patients with chronic intestinal pseudo-obstruction. Gastrointest Endosc. 2004;59:113–5.
61. Lynch CR, Jones RG, Hilden K, Wills JC, Fang JC. Percutaneous endoscopic cecostomy in adults: a case series. Gastrointest Endosc. 2006;64:279–82.
62. National Institute for Health and Clinical Excellence. Percutaneus endoscopic colostomy: interventional procedure guidance (IPG161). http://guidance.nice.org.uk/IPG161/Guidance/pdf/English.
63. Rawat DJ, Haddad M, Geoghegan N, Clarke S, Fell JM. Percutaneous endoscopic colostomy of the left colon: a new technique for management of intractable constipation in children. Gastrointest Endosc. 2004;60:39–43.
64. Baraza W, Brown S, McAlindon M, Hurlstone P. Prospective analysis of percutaneous endoscopic colostomy at a tertiary referral centre. Br J Surg. 2007;94:1415–20.
65. Bani-Hani AH, Cain MP, King S, Rink RC. Tap water irrigation and additives to optimize success with the Malone antegrade continence enema: the Indiana University algorithm. J Urol. 2008;180(4 Suppl):1757–60.
66. Rivera MT, Kugathasan S, Berger W, Werlin SL. Percutaneous colonoscopic cecostomy for management of chronic constipation in children. Gastrointest Endosc. 2001;53:225–8.
67. Cowlam S, Watson C, Elltringham M, Bain I, Barrett P, Green S, et al. Percutaneous endoscopic colostomy of the left side of the colon. Gastrointest Endosc. 2007;65:1007–14.
68. Bertolini D, De Saussure P, Chilcott M, Girardin M, Dumonceau JM. Severe delayed complication after percutaneous endoscopic colostomy for chronic intestinal pseudo-obstruction: a case report and review of the literature. World J Gastroenterol. 2007;13:2255–7.
69. Williams NS, Hughes SF, Stuchfield B. Continent colonic conduit for rectal evacuation in severe constipation. Lancet 1994 May 28;343(8909):1321–4.
70. Kock NG. Intra-abdominal "reservoir" in patients with permanent ileostomy. Preliminary observations on a procedure resulting in fecal "continence" in five ileostomy patients. Arch Surg. 1969;99:223–31.
71. Monti PR, Lara RC, Dutra MA, de Carvalho JR. New techniques for construction of efferent conduits based on the Mitrofanoff principle. Urology. 1997;49:112–5.
72. Bruce RG, el Galley RE, Wells J, Galloway NT. Antegrade continence enema for the treatment of fecal incontinence in adults: use of gastric tube for catheterizable access to the descending colon. J Urol. 1999;161:1813–6.
73. Calado AA, Macedo Jr A, Barroso Jr U, Netto JM, Liguori R, Hachul M, et al. The Macedo-Malone antegrade continence enema procedure: early experience. J Urol. 2005;173:1340–4.
74. Liloku RB, Mure PY, Braga L, Basset T, Mouriquand PD. The left Monti-Malone procedure: preliminary results in seven cases. J Pediatr Surg. 2002;37:228–31.
75. Kim SM, Han SW, Choi SH. Left colonic antegrade continence enema: experience gained from 19 cases. J Pediatr Surg. 2006;41:1750–4.
76. Sinha CK, Butler C, Haddad M. Left antegrade continent enema

(LACE): review of the literature. Eur J Pediatr Surg. 2008;18:215–8.
77. Saunders JR, Williams NS, Eccersley AJ. The combination of electrically stimulated gracilis neoanal sphincter and continent colonic conduit: a step forward for total anorectal reconstruction? Dis Colon Rectum. 2004;47:354–63.
78. Eccersley AJ, Maw A, Williams NS. Comparative study of two sites of colonic conduit placement in the treatment of constipation due to rectal evacuatory disorders. Br J Surg. 1999;86:647–50.
79. Christensen P, Olsen N, Krogh K, Laurberg S. Scintigraphic assessment of antegrade colonic irrigation through an appendicostomy or a neoappendicostomy. Br J Surg. 2002;89:1275–80.
80. O'Bichere A, Sibbons P, Dore C, Green C, Phillips RK. Experimental study of faecal continence and colostomy irrigation. Br J Surg. 2000;87:902–8.
81. Kotanagi H, Koyama K, Sato Y, Takahashi K. Appendicostomy irrigation for facilitating colonic evacuation in colostomy patients. Preliminary report. Dis Colon Rectum. 1998;41:1050–2.
82. Gattuso JM, Kamm MA, Myers C, Saunders B, Roy A. Effect of different infusion regimens on colonic motility and efficacy of colostomy irrigation. Br J Surg. 1996;83:1459–62.
83. Hardcastle JD, Mann CV. Physical factors in the stimulation of colonic peristalsis. Gut. 1970;11:41–6.
84. Narducci F, Bassotti G, Gaburri M, Speakman CT, Morelli A. Distension stimulated motoractivity of the human transverse, descending and sigmoid colon. Gastroenterology. 1985;88:1515.
85. Christensen P, Olsen N, Krogh K, Bacher T, Laurberg S. Scintigraphic assessment of retrograde colonic washout in fecal incontinence and constipation. Dis Colon Rectum. 2003;46:68–76.
86. Koch SM, Melenhorst J, van Gemert WG, Baeten CG. Prospective study of colonic irrigation for the treatment of defecation disorders. Br J Surg. 2008;95:1273–9.
87. Christensen P, Krogh K, Buntzen S, Payandeh F, Laurberg S. Long-term outcome and safety of transanal irrigation for constipation and fecal incontinence. Dis Colon Rectum. 2009;52:286–92.
88. Waldron DJ, Kumar D, Hallan RI, Wingate DL, Williams NS. Evidence for motor neuropathy and reduced filling of the rectum in chronic intractable constipation. Gut. 1990;31:1284–8.
89. Shandling B, Gilmour RF. The enema continence catheter in spina bifida: successful bowel management. J Pediatr Surg. 1987;22:271–3.
90. Graf JL, Strear C, Bratton B, Housley HT, Jennings RW, Harrison MR, et al. The antegrade continence enema procedure: a review of the literature. J Pediatr Surg. 1998;33:1294–6.
91. McClees N, Mikolaj EL, Carlson SL, Pryor-McCann J. A pilot study assessing the effectiveness of a glycerin suppository in controlled colostomy emptying. J Wound Ostomy Continence Nurs. 2004;31:123–9.
92. Karadag A, Ayaz S, Mentes BB. The effect of glyceryl trinitrate on irrigation time and patient satisfaction. ANZ J Surg. 2007;77:917–8.
93. Kjaergaard J, Christensen U, Stadil F, Anderson B. Colostomy irrigation with prostaglandin E2 and bisacodyl. A double- blind cross-over study. Br J Surg. 1984;71:556–7.
94. Christensen U, Kjaergaard J, Stadil F. Colostomy irrigation with prostaglandin F 2 alpha. Dis Colon Rectum. 1982;25:429–30.
95. Doran J, Hardcastle JD. A controlled trial of colostomy management by natural evacuation, irrigation and foam enema. Br J Surg. 1981;68:731–3.
96. Krogh K, Kvitzau B, Jørgensen T, Laurberg S. Behandling af anal inkontinens og obstipation ved hjælp af transanal irrigation. Ugeskr Laeger. 1999;161:253–6.
97. Johanson JF, Sonnenberg A, Koch TR. Clinical epidemiology of chronic constipation [see comments]. J Clin Gastroenterol. 1989;11:525–36.
98. Mattsson S, Gladh G. Tap-water enema for children with myelomeningocele and neurogenic bowel dysfunction. Acta Paediatr. 2006;95:369–74.
99. Yerkes EB, Rink RC, King S, Cain MP, Kaefer M, Casale AJ. Tap water and the Malone antegrade continence enema: a safe combination? J Urol. 2001;166:1476–8.
100. Debongnie JC, Phillips SF. Capacity of the human colon to absorb fluid. Gastroenterology. 1978;74:698–703.
101. Biebl A, Grillenberger A, Schmitt K. Enema-induced severe hyperphosphatemia in children. Eur J Pediatr. 2009;168:111–2.
102. Schreiber CK, Stone AR. Fatal hypernatremia associated with the antegrade continence enema procedure. J Urol. 1999;162:1433–4.
103. Mendoza J, Legido J, Rubio S, Gisbert JP. Systematic review: the adverse effects of sodium phosphate enema. Aliment Pharmacol Ther. 2007;26:9–20.
104. Coggrave M, Wiesel PH, Norton C. Management of faecal incontinence and constipation in adults with central neurological diseases. Cochrane Database Syst Rev. 2006:CD002115.
105. Kenefick NJ, Vaizey CJ, Cohen RC, Nicholls RJ, Kamm MA. Medium-term results of permanent sacral nerve stimulation for faecal incontinence. Br J Surg. 2002;89:896–901.
106. Kenefick NJ, Nicholls RJ, Cohen RG, Kamm MA. Permanent sacral nerve stimulation for treatment of idiopathic constipation. Br J Surg. 2002;89:882–8.
107. Holzer B, Rosen HR, Novi G, Ausch C, Holbling N, Hofmann M, et al. Sacral nerve stimulation in patients with severe constipation. Dis Colon Rectum. 2008;51:524–9.
108. Holzer B, Rosen HR, Novi G, Ausch C, Holbling N, Schiessel R. Sacral nerve stimulation for neurogenic faecal incontinence. Br J Surg. 2007;94:749–53.
109. Jarrett ME, Matzel KE, Christiansen J, Baeten CG, Rosen H, Bittorf B, et al. Sacral nerve stimulation for faecal incontinence in patients with previous partial spinal injury including disc prolapse. Br J Surg. 2005;92:734–9.
110. Gstaltner K, Rosen H, Hufgard J, Mark R, Schrei K. Sacral nerve stimulation as an option for the treatment of faecal incontinence in patients suffering from cauda equina syndrome. Spinal Cord. 2008;46:644–7.
111. Hull TL. Sacral neuromodulation stimulation in fecal incontinence. Int Urogynecol J. 2010;21:1565–8.
112. Colquhoun P, Kaiser Jr R, Efron J, Weiss EG, Nogueras JJ, Vernava III AM, et al. Is the quality of life better in patients with colostomy than in patients with fecal incontinence? World J Surg. 2006;30:1925–8.
113. Randell N, Lynch AC, Anthony A, Dobbs BR, Roake JA, Frizelle FA. Does a colostomy alter quality of life in patients with spinal cord injury? A controlled study. Spinal Cord. 2001;39:279–82.
114. Kamm MA, Hawley PR, Lennard-Jones JE. Outcome of colectomy for severe idiopathic constipation. Gut. 1988;29:969–73.
115. Bernini A, Madoff RD, Lowry AC, Spencer MP, Gemlo BT, Jensen LL, et al. Should patients with combined colonic inertia and nonrelaxing pelvic floor undergo subtotal colectomy? Dis Colon Rectum. 1998;41:1363–6.
116. Yoshioka K, Keighley MR. Clinical results of colectomy for severe constipation. Br J Surg. 1989;76:600–4.
117. Lawal TA, Rangel SJ, Bischoff A, Pena A, Levitt MA. Laparoscopic-assisted Malone appendicostomy in the management of fecal incontinence in children. J Laparoendosc Adv Surg Tech A. 2011;21(5):455–9.
118. Bar-Yosef Y, Castellan M, Joshi D, Labbie A, Gosalbez R. Total continence reconstruction using the artificial urinary sphincter and the Malone antegrade continence enema. J Urol. 2011;185(4):1444–7.
119. Bischoff A, Levitt MA, Bauer C, Jackson L, Holder M, Pena A. Treatment of fecal incontinence with a comprehensive bowel management program. J Pediatr Surg. 2009;44:1278–84.
120. Tiryaki S, Ergun O, Celik A, Ulman I, Avanoglu A. Success of Malone's antegrade continence enema (MACE) from the patient's perspective. Eur J Pediatr Surg. 2010;20:405–7.
121. Ardelean MA, Bauer J, Schimke C, Ludwikowski B, Schimpl G. Improvement of continence with reoperation in selected patients after surgery for anorectal malformation. Dis Colon Rectum. 2009;52:112–8.

第 25 章 巨直肠的处理

Marc A. Gladman · Norman S. Williams
丁威威 译　姜　军 审校

摘　要

本章讨论诊断和治疗巨直肠的外科方法，重点强调直肠缩减成形术的应用和临床预后，其发病机理、病理生理学改变、外科切除和重建的方式选择也一并叙述。

关键词

巨直肠；慢性结直肠扩张；巨结直肠；巨结肠；顽固性便秘；成人先天性巨结肠

引　言

在急诊情况下，下消化道扩张的发生可能由机械性梗阻、假性梗阻和严重的炎症（如中毒性巨结肠）引起。而对临床医生来说，更难处理的是那些慢性结肠扩张合并顽固性便秘的患者。本章节将重点讨论如何识别和处理此类患者。关于处理的原则，必须将此类结肠扩张的患者与结肠直径正常的便秘（如结肠慢传输型便秘或直肠排空功能障碍型便秘）相区别，因为两者外科治疗的原则和策略是不同的[1]。本文将着重强调巨直肠特殊的发病机制、病理生理学改变、外科切除和重建的术式选择。

在儿童，慢性结直肠扩张的最重要原因是Hirschsprung病（即先天性巨结肠），其主要的病理学改变是肌间神经丛先天性缺如。关于此疾病的专科化治疗，包括外科术式的评价，并不在本文的讨论范畴。然而，在鉴别诊断成人巨直肠时，需要排除先天性巨结肠的可能。

巨直肠的定义和流行病学资料

巨直肠通常定义为"直肠持续性增粗、直径超过正常"的疾病[2]。然而，人们更希望有客观诊断标准应用于临床实践（参见"巨直肠的确诊"部分）。在此类患者当中，虽然病变仅局限于直肠，但巨直肠通常伴有不同程度近端肠管的扩张[3]。因此，扩张可引起单纯的直肠扩张（巨直肠）或合并结肠扩张(巨结直肠)。单独结肠扩张而直肠直径正常者(特发性巨结肠)也可发生，但发生率不超过总人数的5%[4]。

巨直肠精确的发病率尚不清楚。实际上，关于结肠的任一部分扩张的流行病学资料都是缺乏的。但是，此疾病并不是一种常见病[5]。从位于伦敦的圣马可医院（每年从7家三级大医院的转诊而来）[6]的资料来看，10年时间有1600例顽固性便秘中，仅20例合并影像学确诊的巨直肠[7]。然而，值得注意的是，很多轻型的患者并未得到诊断和治疗[6,8]。根据不同诊断标准，这种轻型巨直肠患者在顽固性便秘人群中的比例可高达11%[9-10]。此疾病可影响所有年龄段[6]，发病年龄可从1~83岁[11-12]。巨结肠的发病在男女之间均可发生，在巨结肠中男女比例为1:2，在巨直肠中比例为2:1[12]。

巨直肠的病因学

巨直肠的发生可由于先天性或继发性原因（表25.1）。从临床角度看，巨直肠通常在顽固性便秘的患者当中多见，但有一部分患者可无明显原因持续性地发生直肠扩张。这是评价便秘患者的重要区别点，因为巨直肠通常由于表25.1中列举的原因而发生。

表 25.1　巨直肠的原因

先天性	神经节细胞缺乏症（如先天性巨结肠）
	肛门直肠畸形
继发性	神经元降解症（Chagas病）
	梗阻性疾病
	内分泌疾病
	中枢神经系统疾病
	精神心理性疾病
	特发性

在没有明确器质性因素的条件下，单纯直肠扩张被定义为特发性巨直肠[13]，此部分患者的临床处理最具有挑战性。

特发性巨直肠可能的病因学

在一些功能性直肠疾病或者是其他消化系统疾病中，为何会发生肠管的扩张，这个有趣的问题尚不能完全回答。虽然研究发现此类患者存在神经生理学、行为学和生理学的异常，特发性巨直肠的病理生理学机理和病因尚未完全清楚[5]。通常认为在特发性巨直肠的发病过程中，即使同一例患者，也不止一个病理生理机制参与其过程。目前提出两种理论假说。第一个假说认为特发性巨直肠继发于排便的行为障碍[14-15]，伴发如厕训练失败、不能控制大便等，使得直肠扩张，最终导致直肠控便能力丧失、功能下降[5, 16]。另外一个假说认为主要的异常存在于直肠本身[17]，因此，内在的神经肌肉异常（如直肠感觉功能缺失、扩约功能下降）导致大便的慢性蓄积和直肠扩张[17-19]。但此类原发性功能异常在文献中很少提及，因此上述改变是原发还是继发，尚不清楚[20]。

特发性巨直肠的病理改变

特发性巨直肠是一种界于功能性和器质性胃肠道疾病之间的异常。因此，虽然它存在功能和显著的宏观异常（脏器扩张），但目前仍缺乏具有诊断意义的组织形态学异常。组织病理学可发现三种末梢感受器（肠神经系统、平滑肌、肠间质Cajal细胞）均有异常，并且已有文献总结出他们的共同点[20]。关于神经元的研究提示，在常规和银染时形态学的异常是缺失的[12, 21-23]，但各种神经化学的改变存在[24]。平滑肌细胞的研究发现存在明显的细胞肥大和不同程度的纤维化。目前尚无关于特发性巨直肠的肠间质Cajal细胞研究，但两项巨结肠的研究中提到存在不同程度Cajal细胞的下降[25-26]，其中一项研究提示神经传递长度减少[25]。但这两项研究并不能明确疾病发生过程中的因果关系，因此需要谨慎采纳[20, 27]。

巨直肠患者的临床处理

IMR患者多合并严重的顽固性便秘，因此有必要针对此类慢性便秘的IMR患者选择合适的临床治疗方法，特别在合并结肠或直肠扩张的情况下。通过详细评估病情、病史回顾、体格检查和相关辅助检查等手段，以达到以下几个目的：

1. 明确临床症状的严重程度和影响；
2. 鉴别慢性便秘的患者有无合并巨直肠；
3. 排除其他合并症或其他原因导致的巨直肠（如先天性巨结肠）；
4. 推测可能的发病机理（神经生理学因素或心理行为学因素）；
5. 确定外科手术的适应证。

临床评价

仔细详尽地询问病史可揭示一下几个重要的问题：①便秘严重程度；②临床症状对生活质量的影响；③同时合并的其他症状：如遗粪、大便失禁等；④可能的发病原因。评价症状的严重程度可询问大便频率、排便是否费力等。需要明确症状的起病时间、持续时间等，因为在婴幼儿或青少年起病的患者都有遗粪的病史，而成人后起病的患者并无此类症状[6, 28]。同时，还需要了解大便的黏稠度、费力大便的次数、是否合并需要用力解大便、直肠肛门出口梗阻、排便不尽感、用力大便不成功等情况。排便时间、是否需要手助排便（经直肠或阴道）等情况也需要记录。腹痛、腹胀、应用泻剂/栓剂/灌肠等情况存在大多数患者当中[6, 22, 28]，也应记录在案。

建议应用客观的量表来记录患者的症状和严重程度，如克利夫兰便秘评分系统[29]。在做科学研究时，罗马Ⅲ便秘评分标准也应该详细记录[30]。同样，为评估症状对日常生活和社会活动的影响，建议应用标准化的便秘患者自评生活质量问卷调查表来评估病情[31]。

为本章讨论方便，假定可引起巨直肠的其他下消化道器质性疾病已通过相关检查排除，详细询问下消化道的相关症状有利于排除上述疾患。同时，与巨直肠密切相关的症状，如遗粪和大便失禁的情况、频率、遗漏的量和性状，均需详尽记录，并通过客观的量化表格，如克利夫兰评分系统[32]等作为评估依据。盆底器官相关的症状，直肠脱垂等也应了解。

详细的病史回顾可帮助医生排除其他引起巨直肠的疾病，如心理因素、内分泌紊乱、中枢神经系统疾病，包括心理行为学改变（如儿童时期功能性粪便潴留、成人时期的厕所厌恶）。与患者的良好沟通也可使医生了解患者既往接受非外科治疗的情况。

全面的系统和腹部体格检查应在所有患者中实施。在粪石嵌顿的患者中，可发现腹胀、腹部触及肿大粪块等情况，触诊时发现自盆腔往上的大包块。与 IMR 特别相关的是神经系统和直肠肛门的检查。神经系统的检查应着重于躯体腰骶脊神经束的功能，包括步态测试和双下肢的神经功能。若上述检查提示有神经系统的疾病，应安排神经科相关的进一步检查。

检查直肠肛门时，患者通常取双下肢弯曲、左侧卧位，另外也可取折刀位。检查从肛门和肛门周围开始，任何先天性异常需要记录。记录肛周皮肤颜色和周围组织的情况，以确认遗粪、黏液或脓液渗出、表皮剥脱等情况。皮肤赘生物、外痔、瘘等需要详细记载。上述发现可在 IMR 患者中常见，需要单独列出记录。

静息状态下肛门通常处于闭合状态，张力松弛提示可能存在括约肌功能障碍（参见"IMR 病理生理检查"章节）。肛门检查由直肠指诊开始，虽然不一定准确，但可初步了解静息和用力排便状态下的肛门张力。直肠的检查需要排除有无异常肿块、嵌顿粪块等情况，同时直肠的容积也能通过肛门指诊来感知。乙状结肠直肠内镜检查可排除远端结肠是否存在局部机械性或功能性病变（内痔脱垂、直肠黏膜内套叠）。直肠孤立性溃疡的发现常常提示可能存在排便功能障碍。从我们的经验看，硬制乙状结肠直肠镜检查可以给外科医生提供评估直肠容积、扩张能力等有用信息，因为在 IMR 直肠空虚状态下镜子可容易地深入直肠的最大长度。

虽然仅根据患者的病史和体格检查结果，就可以确诊严重的巨直肠（如极少频次排便、反复粪石嵌顿和遗粪、腹部触及较大粪块，直肠指诊发现巨大粪石、乙状结肠直肠镜发现明显的直肠扩张和变长等），但很多症状较轻的便秘患者并未被及时确诊、治疗。

怀疑巨直肠患者的检查

从临床角度出发，鉴别巨直肠通常是比较困难的。同前文所述，必须认识到目前尚无可预测、可靠的临床征象来提醒临床医生诊断巨直肠。部分原因归咎于胃肠道症状的非特异性，此类症状不能准确反映内在的病理改变。这一原则可能适用于所有的功能性胃肠病，都需要正规的检查来鉴别表面看起来一致的疾病分类，如巨直肠。

因此，此部分关于检查的章节，以下内容会重点介绍：

1. 鉴别便秘合并巨直肠患者的检查策略；
2. 巨直肠诊断的确诊方法，如何评价结肠口径；
3. 排除其他引起巨直肠的疾病，如成人 HSCR，明确 IMR 的诊断；
4. 考虑对 IMR 进一步诊断和分类的新检查方法。

鉴别便秘合并巨直肠的检查策略

显而易见，对所有慢性便秘的患者进行检查是不可能，也是不合适的。因为在西方国家，慢性便秘的发生率高达 10%[33]。因此，针对此类患者的检查应该优化、有选择性。从我们的经验看，我们推荐在严重的、顽固性、慢性的便秘患者中进行进一步检查，因为便秘已严重影响生活质量，且简单的处理不能缓解症状，尤其是那些转诊到内外科综合治疗实力较强的三级医院的患者。在排除潜在的器质性疾病后，我们根据目前的推荐[34]进行相应的检查。需要对血清钙、甲状腺功能进行测定，虽然其诊断意义有限。然后，便秘的患者需进一步接受关于结直肠生理功能的详细检查。我们常规对转诊的便秘患者进行以下生理学检查：

直肠肛管压力测定：评估肛门括约肌功能、直肠敏感度和直肠肛管反射[35]；

神经生理学测定：通过检测阴部神经末梢的运动潜伏期评估盆底神经分布[35]；

超声学检查：评价肛门括约肌的形态性完整性；

排粪造影（有些研究者喜欢气囊排出实验）：评估直肠排便功能，明确有无合并的影像学异常（如直肠黏膜脱垂或内套叠）；

结肠运输实验：评估结肠运输时间，明确有无结肠慢运输。我们应用不透 X 线标记物实验进行筛查，而在确诊慢传输患者当中选用结肠闪烁扫描技术。

MRI：在部分患者当中用此技术评价直肠容积、直径和直肠排便能力。

IMR 患者的生理学检查结果

虽然病因学不明，IMR 患者的直肠肛管功能测定的结果通常提示直肠过度松弛[37-39]和感觉障碍[6,38]。同时，患者也合并直肠排便功能障碍[6,37]、继发性结肠运输减慢[39]。

IMR 患者直肠肛管测压的结果通常也有异常。肛管压力方面，有报道指出静息压力而不是收缩压力有所下降[3,6]。这可能与长期粪石存在、继发慢性松弛有关，而在外科切除扩张的结肠后，肛门括约肌的功能是可逆的[40]。然而，在全麻下抠出嵌顿的粪石后内括约肌的功能可能受到损伤，因此经肛超声学检查括约肌形态在此类患者是提倡的。

在 IMR 患者当中，肛门的感觉运动功能也受损，值得特别关注。首先，结肠慢运输通常并存于 IMR[38,42,43]，尤其在那些结肠扩张的肠管[3,38]。其次，无法感知扩张肠管，几乎存在于所有 IMR 患者中。这一点可由直肠肛管测压时，感觉阈值容积的上升方可引出肛管反射来证实[6,42,43]。

同样，若发现患者存在无法自我感知扩张的肠管，临床医生应高度警惕可能存在的巨直肠诊断，同时应进行一系列相关细化的检查（详见"巨直肠的诊断"章节）。然而，虽然直肠感觉下降广泛存在于巨直肠患者，但此结果是非特异性的，同样可存在于一些传输神经功能障碍而直肠直径正常的患者当中。[44]

巨直肠诊断的确定、结肠直径的测定

巨直肠的概念通常被任意使用。在临床检查、剖腹探查（图 25.1）、腹部 X 线平片（图 25.2）均可以看到明显扩张的直肠，然而这种肉眼所见的诊断有点主观性，尚无明确的诊断标准。传统上，有两种方法可以用作诊断巨直肠。

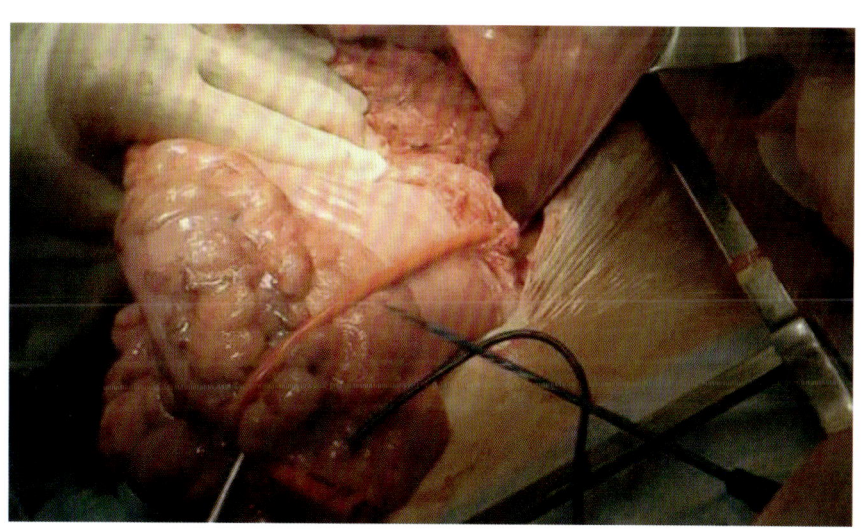

图 25.1　开腹手术中遇到的巨直肠病例

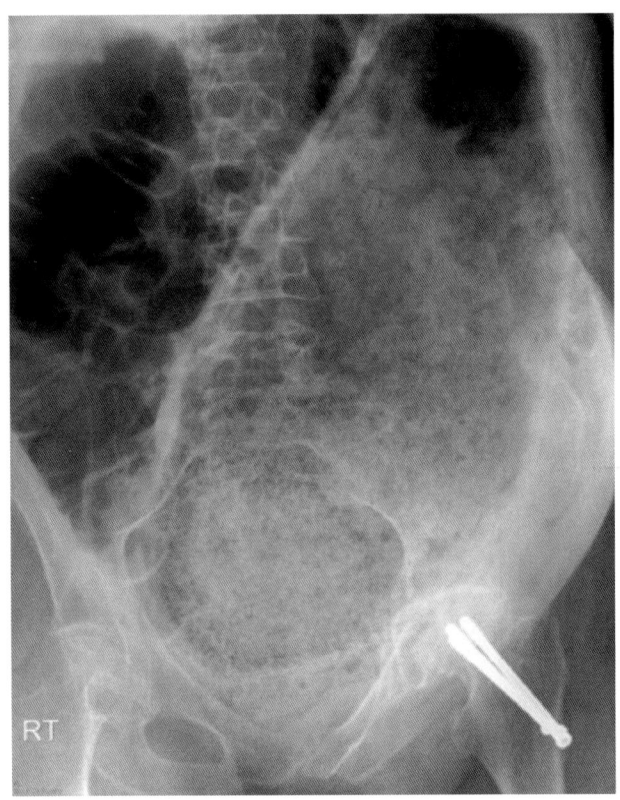

图 25.2 巨结肠患者的腹部平片显示，受粪便影响，严重扩张的巨结肠超出骨盆，延伸到左上腹

第一种方法通常在双重对比钡剂灌肠侧位片显示直肠骨盆边缘直径大于 6.5cm 时作出诊断[45]。近几年排粪造影已被用于便秘患者的评估，对该项检查结果，上述定义是否适用尚未得到证实。我们需要充分认识到，对比造影检查对于便秘患者可能无法准确地反应或者分析直肠管径[46-47]，原因在于这类检查依赖于直肠体积的扩张，但不同便秘患者直肠的原始体积或扩张度难以控制[48-49]。加上近端对比剂进展到乙状结肠以及可能发生的对比剂漏出导致的不完全扩张，使得整体直肠的直径被低估[8]。

第二种方法依据肛门测压诊断巨直肠，通过简单的"乳胶"球囊扩张可以检测直肠最大的耐受体积[37, 50]从而反应直肠的扩张能力[51-53]。然而，直肠容受体积的增加并不等同于直肠直径的增加（巨直肠诊断要点），因为同时受到直肠传入神经敏感度的影响[49]，这条通道出现神经信号问题时，直肠传入神经敏感度会升高（如盆腔神经或脊神经受损）[44]。此外，直肠球囊的轴向膨胀以及吻端延伸至乙状结肠会影响感觉阈值[54]。直肠球囊吻端的挤压和其固有塑形性会影响直肠的测量以及直肠固有的几何形状，而直肠的固有几何形状本来就已受到巨结肠的影响。新技术如阻抗平面和恒压器（稍后讨论）可以使标准化的直肠扩张等同于直肠的推定截面面积，这种新技术的应用很有必要。

鉴于上述技术的局限性，我们团队已经研究出诊断巨结肠的新技术[8]。这项技术涉及恒压器的使用，这是一个计算机化的装置，能够通过改变吹入空气的体积获得内脏内恒定的扩张压力，同时这项技术是现在直肠各个组成部分功能评估的可选方法[57-59]。在透视检查中使用恒压器进行直肠的恒压扩张，能够使直肠直径得到一致而准确的评估。当扩张压力最小（吹入的气体刚好能够防止肠壁塌陷而不引起扩张），直肠的最大直径超过 6.3cm 时，就可以诊断巨结肠[8]。巨结肠患者和直肠管径正常的便秘患者的影像学图片如图 25.3a,b 所示。这种技术似乎能很好地耐受，使用者之间表现出高度的一致性，并且具有诊断的标准（通过对无症状对照组的观察得到直肠管径的范围）[8]。此外，使用恒压将直肠扩张到一个特定的、预定的"阈值"，保证了个体之间方法学的标准化[8]。

综合考虑各种诊断技术，最近提出了当代巨直肠的诊断策略（图 25.4）[20]。巨直肠的诊断需要符合以下一条客观标准：

1. 在双重对比钡剂灌肠侧位片显示直肠骨盆边缘直径大于 6.5cm；

2. 排粪造影侧位片的最宽直肠直径大于 8.3cm[8]；

3. 在透视检查中使用恒压器进行直肠的恒压扩张，当扩张压力最小时（压力依赖），直肠的最大直径超过 6.3cm[8]。

当决定合适的手术策略（如有临床指征）时，判断是否伴随近端结肠扩张（巨结肠）的存在是至关重要的；不过，上面提到的 3 种成像方法，只有双重对比钡剂灌肠的研究可以排除近端肠管扩张，因此该项检查手术前是必须进行的。然而，应当指出，这种技术用于诊断巨直肠并不总是敏感的，而且会低估扩张度。因此，如果临床高度怀疑巨结肠时，也需要采用其他技术。与此相反，不能够依据在肛门直肠测压中提高的敏感阈值体积做出诊断，因为这并不充分，而且还会过度诊断。

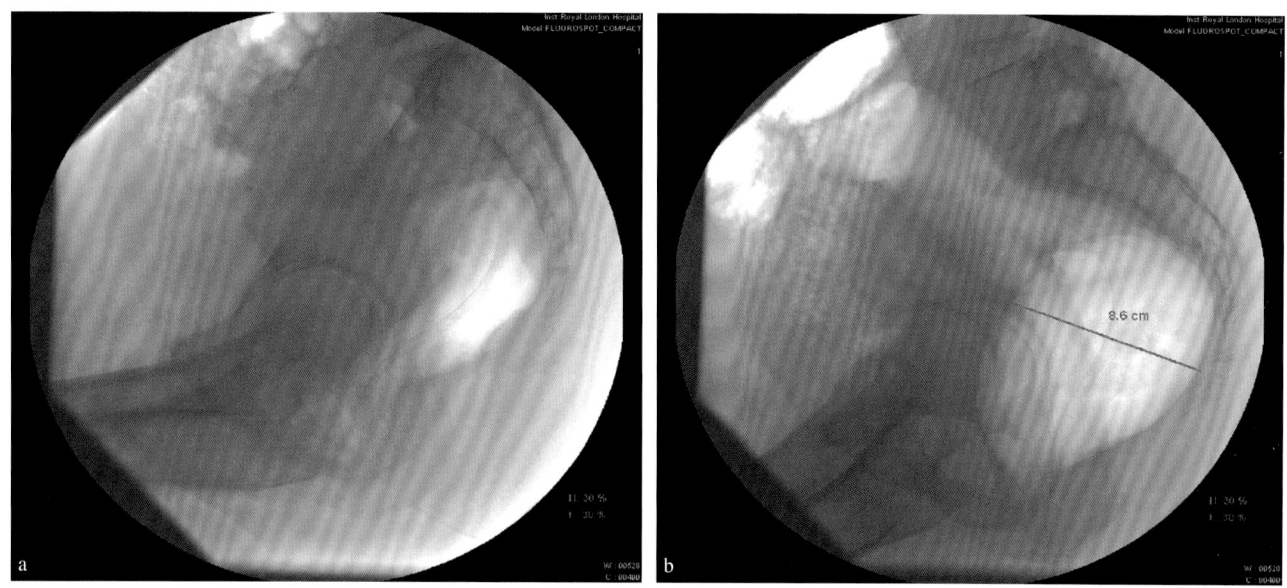

图 25.3 便秘患者使用恒压器进行直肠扩张时的直肠管径。慢性便秘患者使用最小的扩张压力得到的透视图像显示。(a)正常的直肠管径;(b)巨结肠

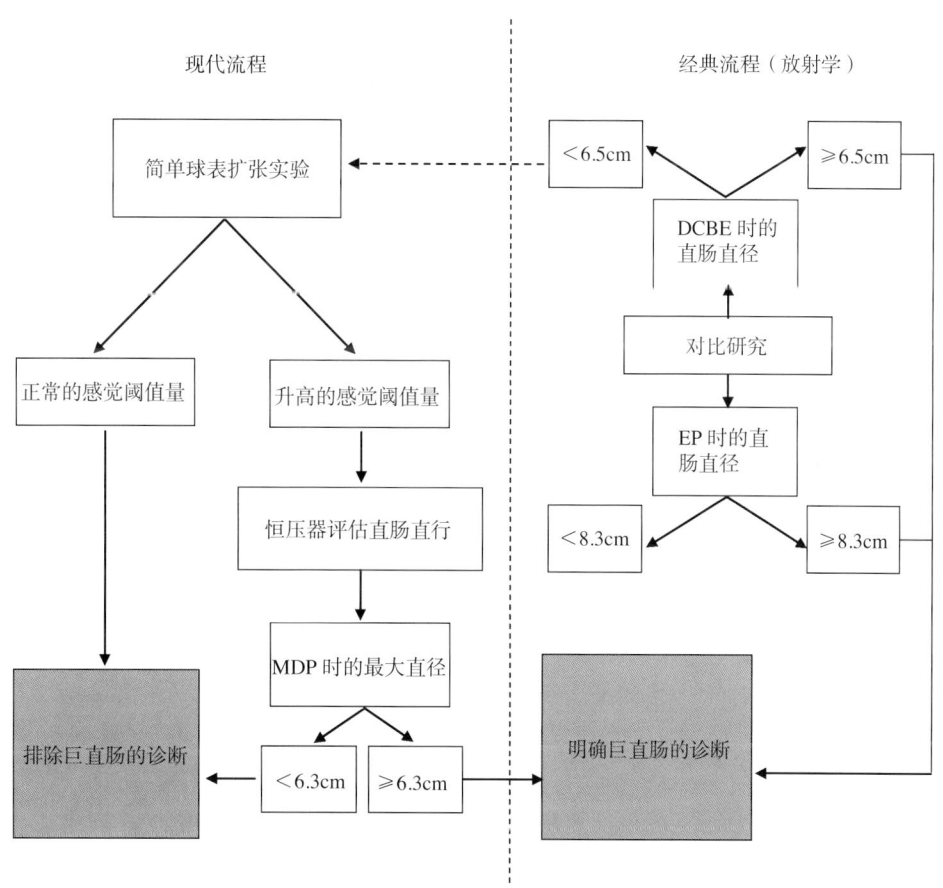

图 25.4 可疑巨结肠患者的诊断流程。可疑巨结肠患者的最初诊断最好选择是乳胶气球扩张实验,因为可以避免健康人电离辐射。** 除非在直肠没有粪便时,简单的球囊扩张实验正常的感觉阈值才能够拍出巨结肠的存在。DCBE:双重对比钡剂灌肠,EP:排粪造影,MDP:最小的直肠扩张压力(Reprinted with permission from Gladman and Knowles.[20])

排除其他导致巨直肠的潜在原因（包括成人 HSCR），确立 IMR 的诊断

正如前面所提及的，应该通过恰当的评估来排除导致直肠扩张的其他原因，其中最重要的就是要排除成人 HSCR。

成人 HSCR 的排除

IMR 和成人 HSCR 的区别一直是诊断上的一个难点。尽管在教科书里已经做了相当多的讨论，但事实上，至少在发达国家，成人 HSCR 非常罕见，仅有约 300 例病案的疾病。即使在最大的医疗机构（包括 Mayo Clinic 和 St. Mark's Hospital），1950 年之前，每年也只能看到 1 例这样的疾病。在西方的经验中，大部分典型的 HSCR 都是在新生儿或婴儿期（甚至在宫内）便被诊断出来，这些患者直肠乙状结肠可变区通常会受累。因此，对于成人的短节段或超短节段的病变都应当仔细检查。临床上，污粪污染的肛门常在 IMR 的患者中见到，而非常干净的肛门往往提示 HSCR。典型 HSCR 的诊断是建立在钡餐观察到直肠肛门抑制反射（RAIR）的缺失和直肠活检，而短节段或超短节段的病变在诊断上则存在很多问题。在前者中，RAIR 缺失但活检明确；然而在后者中，这两项都不太可靠，尤其是肛门移行区有超短节段的病变时，更可能是神经节细胞减少症的表现。

用 RAIR 来作为诊断的标准时还存在一些问题。即使在接受较大的直肠扩张刺激后，有 30%~50% 的 IMR 患者（用活检排除了 HSCR）仍然会有 RAIR 的缺失。这有可能是由于：①球囊对直肠壁的刺激不够；②由于粪便的嵌顿导致直肠内括约肌慢性松弛；③之前在全麻下实施粪便排出时对内括约肌的损伤。根据我们的经验，在直肠肛门测压法中发现 RAIR 缺失的患者中，要证实神经节细胞减少症，做直肠全层活检很有必要，可以确诊或者排除 HSCR。

IMR 的最新研究及其分类亚群

在肠功能紊乱的患者中，对结直肠和肛门生理功能的评估越来越细，出现了一些比较新的方法，尤其是对怀疑 IMR 的患者进行直肠感觉及顺应性的细致而全面的评估。

如前所述，在 IMR 患者中，引出直肠反射的感觉阈值普遍升高，事实上，这是一个诊断巨直肠的最有用的指标。传统观念中，"直肠低敏感性"反映了传入神经功能的受损。然而，由于直肠直径的增加，刺激直肠产生直肠反射所需的球囊体积也相应增大[44, 54]。因此，可以想象的是，在巨直肠患者中，感知受损仅仅反映直肠直径的增加和刺激不足，而不是直肠传入神经的功能不全[44]。

直肠感觉功能测试，如直肠黏膜电刺激，理论上可以更准确地反应"真"的直肠传入神经功能，因为它完全依赖于黏膜的触觉反射，而不会受直肠本身特质的影响[65]。在一些 IMR 患者中电刺激敏感性的阈值会升高，提示直肠传入神经功能受损，但这种功能障碍的定位（外周或中枢）尚未明确。

IMR 患者的治疗

内科治疗

因为治疗特发性巨结肠的最初目标是通过促进和维持直肠的排空，来防止粪便的堵塞，所以起初并不需要外科干预[4]。研究证实，只要直肠可以排空，就能保证结肠功能的正常[67]，大多数患者可以通过利用渗透性泻药（通常是硫酸镁）使粪便保持半流质状态，从而解除粪便阻塞，防止复发[6]。因为小肠的肌张力低下，因此应该避免使用大剂量的泻药来维持结直肠的排空[4]。另一种方法是避免使用可能使大量粪便进入已排空的直肠的泻药。而改用定期进行逆行直肠灌肠的方法（有时可以在住院时进行）来保持直肠的通畅[67]。

内科治疗的有效性并未完全清楚。在有些研究中观察到了很好的结果，68%~93% 的患者用泻药、灌肠剂或两者合用治疗获得了成功[6, 68]。但是这些患者并不能被称为正常，因为后期常常会有大量软便存在于直肠当中[68]。Barnes 等[28]报道了在儿童期就发病的患者中，内科治疗具有更高的成功率。在其他研究中，有 55%~70% 的患者不能通过内科治疗缓解症状[4]。另外，泻药的耐受性较差，而且需要长期使用。此外，内科治疗并不能恢复直肠的正常直径，即使治疗了几年之后[17]。这也就不奇怪为什么在肠道完全失去功能或者近段造口的情况下，直肠依然是扩张的[70]。尽管有研究表明，如果症状出现的时间短，内科治疗成功率高[4]；

而如果直肠存在巨大的扩张，则内科治疗的成功率低[69]。但是现在还没有标准可以预测哪些患者适合内科治疗。

行为再训练技术与生物反馈

Mimura 等[5]追溯了 6 例通过影像学诊断的 IMR 患者，他们完成了一个周期这个疗法的生物反馈，每 2～3 周进行 4～5 次治疗，包括：①有关排便行动和动态的指令；②尝试不用泻药；③生物反馈，其中两名患者利用盆底肌肉活动的视觉反馈[5]。患者在接受干预之前经过了临床、放射及生理治疗。完成生物反馈治疗 18 个月以后，将进行后续治疗，包括电话采访去评价治疗对小肠功能的影响及对患者整体的影响。

所有患者都认为治疗对症状改善有积极的影响，两例患者的症状完全缓解，其余 4 例患者仍然有一定的症状，但其中两例可以不再继续使用泻药[5]。只有两例患者在干预之后有生理和放射治疗，所有人都仍然存在严重的直肠扩张。一例患者的感官检测阈值下降，但其他人都上升[5]。这种单一的小案例是唯一可以说明这种治疗特发性巨结肠病的方法的疗效的证明。尽管支持这种方法的数据是有限的，研究者建议患者在进行外科治疗之前，可先试验一下生物反馈治疗：一方面希望可以避免外科治疗；另一方面也可以证实排便动力学的优化，增加手术治疗的成功率。很显然，行为再训练很重要，尤其是术前存在心理问题的患者。

外科干预

如果保守治疗无效或者患者不能耐受，则应寻求外科干预[69]。此外，如果患者出现特发性巨结肠的并发症，如复发性乙状结肠扭转[2, 71]，也需要进行外科干预。而且这些患者需要有经验的外科医生进行治疗，因为他们需要全面的临床、生理和心理的评估。

关于巨结肠和巨直肠的手术操作有许多文献报道。简单地说，结肠手术或者解除相关巨结肠病例中扩张的肠管，或者根据他们的理论使大便变稀，手术本身并没有得到解决（结肠次全切除术）。这些手术的低死亡率使得它们具有吸引力，但是功能效果很差。直肠手术具有较高的成功率，但是发病率与死亡率也比较高（如下）。现在盆底手术在很大程度上被废除，因为效果不佳以及可能会导致失禁，并且粪便分流是一种可选方法，尽管在年轻患者中并不受欢迎[72]。

直肠严重扩张的患者，手术操作具有很大的挑战性和潜在的风险，因为骨盆内正常解剖结构的严重扩张以及扩张的结肠血管在手术中比较容易碰触。因此，IMR 患者的外科治疗具有导致盆底出血和脓毒症的风险，所致的死亡率为 5%[72]。从长远角度来看，还有盆底神经损伤和肠管梗阻[72]。垂直减少直肠切除术（VRR）（图 25.5a,b），最近设计的一种新颖的创伤较小的手术，可以避免/减少手术风险[42]。而且，VRR 被特异性地用来处理 IMR 患者的生理异常，依据前提是减少直肠储备能力和顺从性，恢复直肠胀满的感觉，并提高直肠敏感性和排泄功能[42]。

VRR 已被证明在适应证患者中的安全性和有效性。在中期（5 年）随访中，VRR 在大部分患者中都获得了成功，能够维持直肠的管径、顺从性和敏感性，并且可以给 70% 的患者带来临床获益[43]。而且，传统手术造成肠道梗阻、盆底神经损伤等远期并发症也没有在 VRR 手术中被报道。

我们团队系统回顾了近期巨结肠或巨直肠手术的结果，并归纳为表 25.2。报道的数据结果必须仔细解读；然而，因为所有的证据质量都比较低，并且没有比较外科或者内科治疗，以及不治疗的研究[72]。而且,这些研究通常包含的患者数量较少(平均 12 例)，并且没有进行长期随访研究（平均 3 年）。此外，成功率、死亡率和功能性结果的报道也具有很大的差异性[72]。除了数据质量的局限性之外，这些结果的解读还受到了数据不完整的阻碍。另外一个重要的局限性是缺少巨结肠的准确定义。

这些局限性意味着不同手术之间的比较存在问题，所以就不能给患者推荐最合适的手术干预方法[72-73]。然而，当伴或不伴近端结肠扩张的 IMR 患者考虑外科干预时，可以做出下面尝试性的推荐：

- 伴有近端结肠扩张，导致直肠和结肠的扩张（巨肠管）：最佳的手术可能是治愈性结直肠切除，并进行回肠贮袋重建。成功率在 70%～80% 之间。但是手术复杂，而且患者还有发生储袋功能次优的风险，以排便频繁和夜间活动性排便为特点。

- 远端肠管扩张（巨直肠伴或不伴巨乙状结肠）：若只考虑手术的成功率（70%～80%），VRR 和直肠切除后结肠肛管吻合术似乎没有区别。然而，

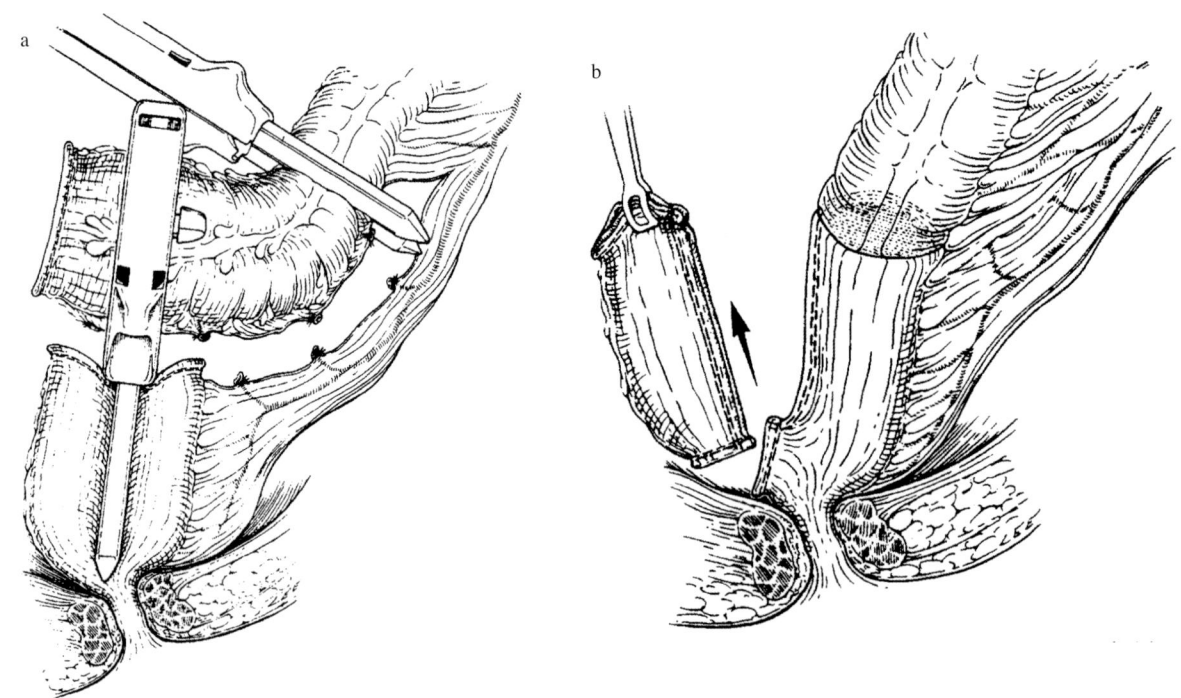

图 25.5 垂直减少直肠切除术。使用直线吻合器进行垂直减少直肠和冗长的乙状结肠。（a）直肠前半部分于远端分离后被移走；（b）垂直减少的直肠与近端降结肠吻合（Reprinted from Williams et al. [42] © 2000 British Journal of Surgery Society Limited, with permission from John Wiley and Sons Ltd. On behalf of the British Journal of Surgery Society Limited）

表 25.2 其他治疗 IMR 的手术方案的结果

手 术	研究数量	患者数量	成 功	死亡率	发病率	进一步外科干预
直肠手术						
前切除术	1	8	6/8(75%)	0	4/8(50%)	0
直肠切除	3	31	22/31(71%)	2/31(6%)	2/31(6%)	3/31(10%)
范 围			67%~72%	0~14%	0~29%	0~17%
拉 通	1	4	3/4(75%)	1/4(25%)	2/4(50%)	0
Duhamel 手术	4	107	93/107(87%)	3/107(3%)	30/104(29%)	5/70(7%)
范 围			50%~98%	0~6%	9%~60%	0~9%
VRR	1	6	5/6(83%)	0	2/6(33%)	0
直肠切除	3	22	16/22(73%)	0	2/22(9%)	4/22(18%)
范 围			57%~100%	0	0~40%	0~18%
盆底手术						
括约肌切开术	2	8	3/8(38%)	无法确定	无法确定	无法确定
范 围			33%~40%	无法确定	无法确定	无法确定
耻骨直肠肌	1	3	1/3(33%)	无法确定	无法确定	无法确定
粪便改道						
造 口	3	20	13/20(65%)	无法确定	无法确定	无法确定
范 围			40%~100%	无法确定	无法确定	无法确定

Reprinted with permission from Gladman et al. [72]

VRR 由于对盆底的创伤小，所以表现得更安全，所以在特定适应证的患者中是一个更安全的选择。虽然这个手术目前还缺少足够的患者和随访。

结 论

巨结肠患者的治疗对于结肠外科医生而言仍然是一个挑战。在评估患有严重的慢性顽固性便秘的患者时，临床医生应积极寻求患者肠道扩张的原因。因为不同的原因，治疗方案是不同。图 25.6 介绍了确定肠道扩张的病因的方法。在临床、放射和生理检查的基础上，患者应当进行直肠功能的客观评估。那些发现有巨结肠的患者应将基础原因（尤其是成人 HSCR）排除在外。在可以进行这些检查的医院，更多更详细的关于直肠功能的检查可以将患者进行更细致地分类，但是这种分类是否具有临床意义仍不清楚。大部分有巨结肠的患者需要进行干预来减轻症状。有效的内科、行为和外科治疗并没有充分建立起来。此外，由于外科手术治疗相对较少，患者应该理解预后的不可预测性，并可能面临肠道永久扩张的风险。

考虑到治疗的复杂性，巨结肠患者应该在专门的中心进行治疗。他们的治疗经常涉及儿科医生、胃肠病学家、精神病医生和外科医生。考虑到巨直肠的病理生理和病因的几个方面仍不清楚，因此，有进一步的理由将患者集中在这些中心，由对肠动

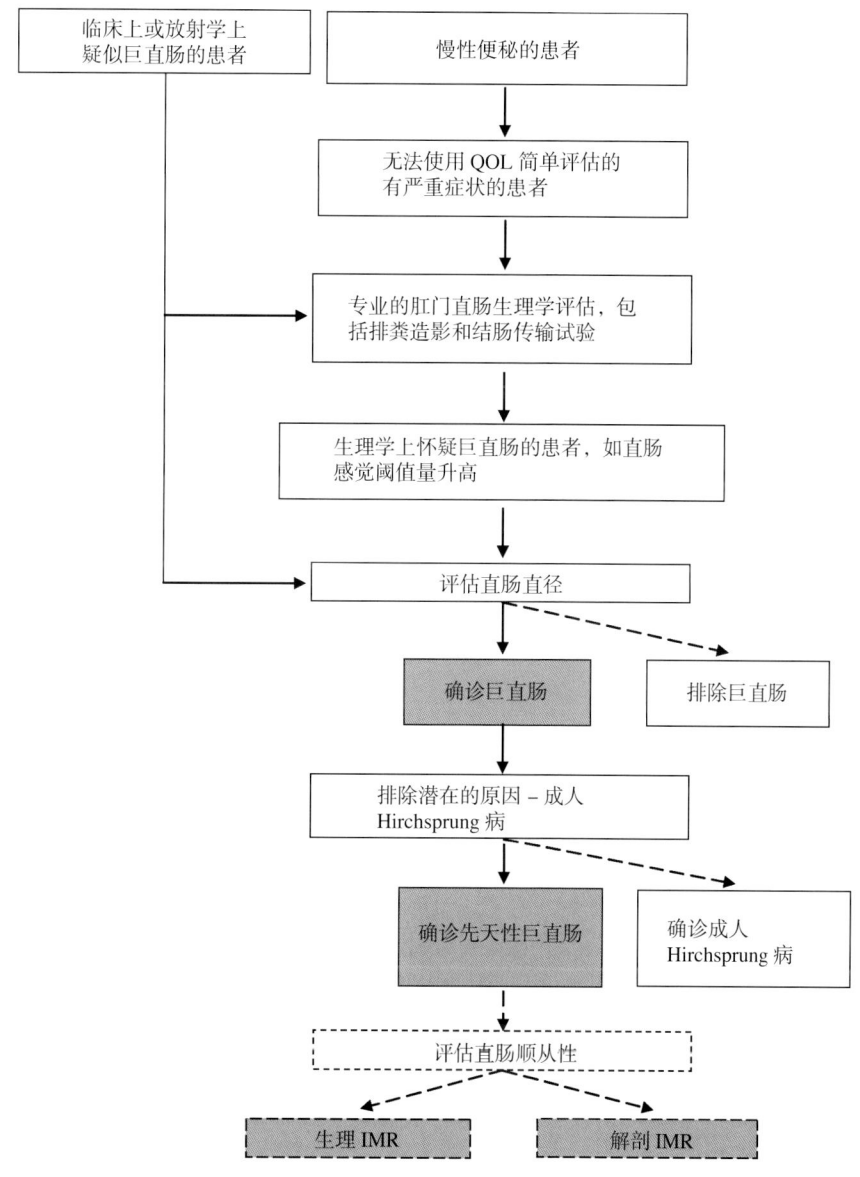

图 25.6　确定 IMR 患者亚群的检查策略

力障碍科学有兴趣的医生照顾。因为手术治疗的稀有，这将有利于不同中心综合他们治疗的经验，并讨论他们的发现。这无疑将促使 IMR 诊断和治疗的规范性，并整合目前对 IMR 零散的理解。

参考文献

1. Gladman MA, Knowles CH. Surgical treatment of constipation and fecal incontinence. Gastroenterol Clin North Am. 2008;37:605–25.
2. Todd IP. Discussion on megacolon and megarectum with the emphasis on conditions other than Hirschsprung's disease. Proc R Soc Med. 1961;54:1035–40.
3. Stewart J, Kumar D, Keighley MR. Results of anal or low rectal anastomosis and pouch construction for megarectum and megacolon. Br J Surg. 1994;81:1051–3.
4. Lane RH, Todd IP. Idiopathic megacolon: a review of 42 cases. Br J Surg. 1977;64:307–10.
5. Mimura T, Nicholls T, Storrie JB, Kamm MA. Treatment of constipation in adults associated with idiopathic megarectum by behavioral retraining including biofeedback. Colorectal Dis. 2002;4:477–82.
6. Gattuso JM, Kamm MA. Clinical features of idiopathic megarectum and idiopathic megacolon. Gut. 1997;41:93–9.
7. Knowles CH, Scott SM, Rayner C, Glia A, Lindberg G, Kamm MA, et al. Idiopathic slow-transit constipation: an almost exclusively female disorder. Dis Colon Rectum. 2003;46:1716–7.
8. Gladman MA, Dvorkin LS, Scott SM, Lunniss PJ, Williams NS. A novel technique to identify patients with megarectum. Dis Colon Rectum. 2007;50:621–9.
9. Varma JS, Smith AN. Neurophysiological dysfunction in young women with intractable constipation. Gut. 1988;29:963–8.
10. Waldron D, Bowes KL, Kingma YJ, Cote KR. Colonic and anorectal motility in young women with severe idiopathic constipation. Gastroenterology. 1988;95:1388–94.
11. Parc R, Berrod JL, Tussiot J, Loygue J. Megacolon in adults. Apropos of 76 cases. Ann Gastroenterol Hepatol. 1984;20:133–41.
12. Belliveau P, Goldberg SM, Rothenberger DA, Nivatvongs S. Idiopathic acquired megacolon: the value of subtotal colectomy. Dis Colon Rectum. 1982;25:118–21.
13. Ehrenpreis T. Megacolon and megarectum in older children and young adults. Classification and terminology. Proc R Soc Med. 1967;60:799–801.
14. Kamm MA. Constipation and its management. BMJ. 2003;327:459–60.
15. van der Plas RN, Benninga MA, Staalman CR, Akkermans LM, Redekop WK, Taminiau JA, et al. Megarectum in constipation. Arch Dis Child. 2000;83:52–8.
16. Nixon HH. Megarectum in the older child. Proc R Soc Med. 1967;60:801–3.
17. Goligher J. Discussion on megacolon and megarectum with the emphasis on conditions other than Hirschsprung's disease. Proc R Soc Med. 1961;54:1053–5.
18. Devadhar DS. Surgical correction of rectal procidentia. Surgery. 1967;62:847–52.
19. Rao SS. Pathophysiology of adult fecal incontinence. Gastroenterology. 2004;126(1 Suppl 1):S14–22.
20. Gladman MA, Knowles CH. Novel concepts in the diagnosis, pathophysiology and management of idiopathic megabowel. Colorectal Dis. 2008;10:531–8.
21. Smith B, Grace RH, Todd IP. Organic constipation in adults. Br J Surg. 1977;64:313–4.
22. Stabile G, Kamm MA, Hawley PR, Lennard-Jones JE. Colectomy for idiopathic megarectum and megacolon. Gut. 1991;32:1538–40.
23. Stabile G, Kamm MA, Phillips RK, Hawley PR, Lennard-Jones JE. Partial colectomy and coloanal anastomosis for idiopathic megarectum and megacolon. Dis Colon Rectum. 1992;35:158–62.
24. Gattuso JM, Hoyle CH, Milner P, Kamm MA, Burnstock G. Enteric innervation in idiopathic megarectum and megacolon. Int J Colorectal Dis. 1996;11:264–71.
25. Wedel T, Spiegler J, Soellner S, Roblick UJ, Schiedeck TH, Bruch HP, et al. Enteric nerves and interstitial cells of Cajal are altered in patients with slow-transit constipation and megacolon. Gastroenterology. 2002;123:1459–67.
26. Lee JI, Park H, Kamm MA, Talbot IC. Decreased density of interstitial cells of Cajal and neuronal cells in patients with slow transit constipation and acquired megacolon. J Gastroenterol Hepatol. 2005;20:1292.
27. van den Berg MM, Di Lorenzo C, Mousa HM, Benninga MA, Boeckxstaens GE, Luquette M. Morphological changes of the enteric nervous system, interstitial cells of Cajal, and smooth muscle in children with colonic motility disorders. J Pediatr Gastroenterol Nutr. 2009;48:22–9.
28. Barnes PR, Lennard-Jones JE, Hawley PR, Todd IP. Hirschsprung's disease and idiopathic megacolon in adults and adolescents. Gut. 1986;27:534–41.
29. Agachan F, Chen T, Pfeifer J, Reissman P, Wexner SD. A constipation scoring system to simplify evaluation and management of constipated patients. Dis Colon Rectum. 1996;39:681–5.
30. Longstreth GF, Longstreth GF, Thompson WG, Chey WD, Houghton LA, Mearin F, et al. Functional bowel disorders. Gastroenterology. 2006;130:1480–91.
31. Marquis P, De La Loge C, Dubois D, McDermott A, Chassany O. Development and validation of the patient assessment of constipation quality of life questionnaire. Scand J Gastroenterol. 2005;40:540–51.
32. Jorge JM, Wexner SD. Etiology and management of fecal incontinence. Dis Colon Rectum. 1993;36:77–97.
33. Higgins PD, Johanson JF. Epidemiology of constipation in North America: a systematic review. Am J Gastroenterol. 2004;99:750–9.
34. Diamant NE, Kamm MA, Wald A, Whitehead WE. AGA technical review on anorectal testing techniques. Gastroenterology. 1999;116:735–60.
35. Scott SM, Gladman MA. Manometric, sensorimotor and neurophysiological evaluation of anorectal function. Gastroenterol Clin North Am. 2008;37:511–38.
36. Camilleri M. New imaging in neurogastroenterology. Neurogastroenterol Motil. 2006;18:805–12.
37. Verduron A, Devroede G, Bouchoucha M, Arhan P, Schang JC, Poisson J, et al. Megarectum. Dig Dis Sci. 1988;33:1164–74.
38. Chiarioni G, Bassotti G, Germani U, Brunori P, Brentegani MT, Minniti GH, et al. Idiopathic megarectum in adults. An assessment of manometric and radiologic variables. Dig Dis Sci. 1995;40:2286–92.
39. Gattuso JM, Kamm MA, Morris G, Britton KE. Gastrointestinal transit in patients with idiopathic megarectum. Dis Colon Rectum. 1996;39:1044–50.
40. Brown SR, Shorthouse AJ. Restorative proctocolectomy for idiopathic megarectum: postoperative recovery of hypotonic anal sphincters. Report of two cases. Dis Colon Rectum. 1997;40:625–7.
41. Gattuso JM, Kamm MA, Halligan SM, Bartram CI. The anal sphincter in idiopathic megarectum: effects of manual disimpaction under general anesthetic. Dis Colon Rectum. 1996;39:435–9.
42. Williams NS, Fajobi OA, Lunniss PJ, Scott SM, Eccersley AJP, Ogunbiyi OA. Vertical reduction rectoplasty: a new treatment for idiopathic megarectum. Br J Surg. 2000;87:1203–8.
43. Gladman MA, Williams NS, Ogunbiyi OA, Scott SM, Lunniss PJ. Medium-term results of vertical reduction rectoplasty and sigmoid colectomy for idiopathic megarectum. Br J Surg. 2005;92:624–30.
44. Gladman MA, Lunniss PJ, Scott SM, Swash M. Rectal hyposensitivity. Am J Gastroenterol. 2006;101:1140–51.
45. Preston DM, Lennard-Jones JE, Thomas BM. Towards a radiologic definition of idiopathic megacolon. Gastrointest Radiol. 1985;10:167–9.

46. Connell AM. Colonic motility in megacolon. Proc R Soc Med. 1961;54:1040–3.
47. Shouler P, Keighley MR. Changes in colorectal function in severe idiopathic chronic constipation. Gastroenterology. 1986;90:414–20.
48. Felt-Bersma RJ, Sloots CE, Poen AC, Cuesta MA, Meuwissen SG. Rectal compliance as a routine measurement: extreme volumes have direct clinical impact and normal volumes exclude rectum as a problem. Dis Colon Rectum. 2000;43:1732–8.
49. Gladman MA, Dvorkin LS, Lunniss PJ, Williams NS, Scott SM. Rectal hyposensitivity: a disorder of the rectal wall or the afferent pathway? An assessment using the barostat. Am J Gastroenterol. 2005;100:106–14.
50. Siproudhis L, Le Gall R, Ropert A, Reignier A, Heresbach D, Raoul JL, et al. Does manometric megarectum have a symptomatic role in patients complaining of dyschezia? Gastroenterol Clin Biol. 1993;17:162–7.
51. Felt-Bersma RJ, Klinkenberg-Knol EC, Meuwissen SG. Anorectal function investigations in incontinent and continent patients. Differences and discriminatory value. Dis Colon Rectum. 1990;33:479–85.
52. Miller R. The measurement of anorectal sensation. In: Kumra D, Waldron DR, Williams NS, editors. Clinical measurement in coloproctology. London: Springer; 1991. p. 60–6.
53. Broens PM, Penninckx FM, Lestar B, Kerremans RP. The trigger for rectal filling sensation. Int J Colorectal Dis. 1994;9:1–4.
54. Madoff RD, Orrom WJ, Rothenberger DA, Goldberg SM. Rectal compliance: a critical reappraisal. Int J Colorectal Dis. 1990;5:37–40.
55. Dall FH, Jørgensen CS, Houe D, Gregersen H, Djurhuus JC. Biomechanical wall properties of the human rectum. A study with impedance planimetry. Gut. 1993;34:1581–6.
56. Zbar AP. Compliance and capacity of the normal human rectum – physical considerations and measurement pitfalls. Acta Chir Iugosl. 2007;54:49–57.
57. Azpiroz F, Enck P, Whitehead WE. Anorectal functional testing: review of collective experience. Am J Gastroenterol. 2002;97:232–40.
58. Whitehead WE, Delvaux M. Standardization of barostat procedures for testing smooth muscle tone and sensory thresholds in the gastrointestinal tract. Dig Dis Sci. 1997;42:223–41.
59. Scott SM, Gladman MA. Rectal barostat for sensory testing. In: Parkman HP, McCallum RW, Rao SSC, editors. Gastrointestinal motility testing: laboratory and office handbook. Thorofare: Slack; 2011. p. 209–22.
60. Todd IP. Adult Hirschsprung's disease. Br J Surg. 1977;64:311–2.
61. McCready RA, Beart Jr RW. Adult Hirschsprung's disease: results of surgical treatment at Mayo Clinic. Dis Colon Rectum. 1980;23:401–7.
62. Bashiri A, Burstein E, Hershkowitz R, Maor E, Landau D, Mazor M. Fetal echogenic bowel at 17 weeks' gestational age as the early and only sign of a very long segment of Hirschsprung disease. J Ultrasound Med. 2008;27:1125–6.
63. Poisson J, Devroede G. Severe chronic constipation as a surgical problem. Surg Clin North Am. 1983;63:193–217.
64. Taylor I, Hammond P, Darby C. An assessment of anorectal motility in the management of adult megacolon. Br J Surg. 1980;67:754–6.
65. Kamm MA, Lennard-Jones JE. Rectal mucosal electrosensory testing-evidence for a rectal sensory neuropathy in idiopathic constipation. Dis Colon Rectum. 1990;33:419–23.
66. Gladman MA, Aziz Q, Scott SM, Williams NS, Lunniss PJ. Rectal hyposensitivity: pathophysiologic mechanisms. Neurogastroenterol Motil. 2009;21:508–16.
67. Browne D. Discussion on megacolon and megarectum with the emphasis on conditions other than Hirschsprung's disease. Proc R Soc Med. 1961;54:1055–6.
68. Jennings PJ. Megarectum and megacolon in adolescents and young adults: results of treatment at St. Mark's Hospital. Proc R Soc Med. 1967;60:805–6.
69. Kamm MA, Stabile G. Management of idiopathic megarectum and megacolon. Br J Surg. 1991;78:899–900.
70. Walsh PV, Peebles-Brown DA, Watkinson G. Colectomy for slow transit constipation. Ann R Coll Surg Engl. 1987;69:71–5.
71. Chung YF, Eu KW, Nyam DC, Leong AF, Ho YH, Seow-Choen F. Minimizing recurrence after sigmoid volvulus. Br J Surg. 1999;86:231–3.
72. Gladman MA, Scott SM, Lunniss PJ, Williams NS. Systematic review of surgical options for idiopathic megarectum and megacolon. Ann Surg. 2005;241:562–74.
73. Suilleabhain CB, Anderson JH, McKee RF, Finlay IG. Strategy for the surgical management of patients with idiopathic megarectum and megacolon. Br J Surg. 2001;88:1392–6.

第 26 章 直肠前突修补失败的处理

Donato F. Altomare · Giovanni Milito · Federica Cadeddu · Filippo Pucciani

冯啸波 译　冯啸波 审校

摘　要

本章针对直肠前突修补术失败的问题，提出了全面的评估和处理方法。分别就经肛门、经会阴/阴道、经腹路径进行阐述，并总结了经肛吻合器手术的结果。阐明了初次手术适应证、禁忌证，修补失败后再次手术的途径和方法。

关键词

直肠前突；直肠前突修补失败；经会阴再手术；直肠前突复发；经阴道、会阴、直肠修补；经会阴修补、肛提肌成形术（TPR-L）；补片

出口梗阻的原因之一：直肠前突

直肠前突是一种多发于女性的盆底解剖异常，因直肠阴道隔薄弱导致阴道后壁在用力排便时向前膨出形成阴道后壁疝（图 26.1），当前突位置较低时，阴道后壁直接疝入会阴则形成会阴疝。这种解剖的移位使排便过程中直肠推进力方向分散，直肠前壁向前膨出，导致粪便潴留[1]。排粪造影检查时常可见直肠前突、直肠肛门脱垂、会阴下降、盆底失迟缓、直肠黏膜脱垂等解剖改变并存，直肠前突是最突出的原因，占出口梗阻病因的 30%，可单因素引起出口梗阻症状。当前突超过 3cm、排便结束后粪便潴留显著、需经阴道手助排便时，需行直肠前突修补手术以改善患者排便困难[2]，术后经阴道手助排便症状缓解最为显著[3]。关于前突的类型、相关的盆底解剖异常如何处理，本章不作进一步讨论。

直肠前突修补的途径：经阴道和肛门

直肠前突的治疗缺乏统一标准。主要原因有：对 Denonvilliers 筋膜扩张和直肠阴道隔膨出的解剖意义存在争议；直肠前突的尺度与症状的严重程度缺乏关联性；相关的盆底解剖异常对直肠前突的影响尚不明确；众多专科中心分散完成的小样本病例的手术方式选择不标准，影响了临床数据的可信度[1]。仅有极少数设计良好的临床试验针对不同类型患者施行了相应的手术方式[4-5]。

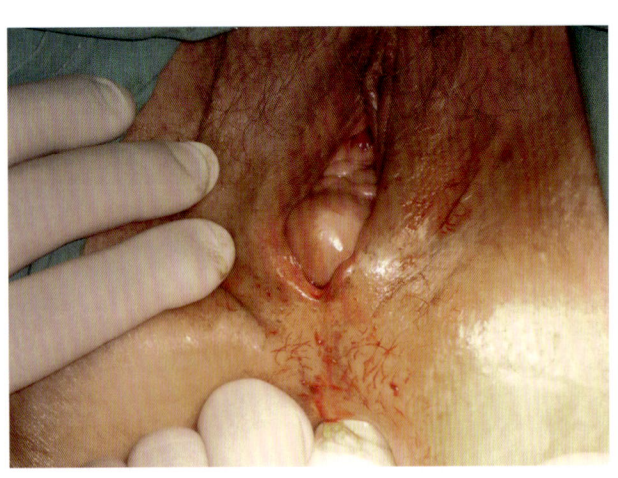

图 26.1　直肠前突

19世纪80年代以前，直肠前突手术治疗的适应证为阴道膨出、脱垂，很少关注其消化道症状，主要由妇科医生施行，手术方式以传统的阴道后穹隆修补术为主[6-7]，常同时行肛提肌成形术以缩窄阴道，也有伴行阴道荐骨后壁固定术或后穹隆成形术以预防阴道后穹窿脱垂和肠疝[8-10]。

直肠前突补修引起的消化道症状逐渐被结直肠病专家所认识并开展治疗，手术的方法为加强直肠阴道隔。手术路径主要有经直肠、经阴道、经会阴和腹腔镜辅经腹4种。应用最多的是经直肠开放式修补法，对确定的直肠阴道隔薄弱处进行修补或直肠前壁的黏膜切除肌层折叠缝合术（相当于完成 Delorme 术的前壁部分）[11-14]。各治疗中心手术方法大同小异，均为切除冗余黏膜、折叠缝合肌层、缝合剩余黏膜[15-16]（图 26.2）。

Block 法[17]是闭式修补法的代表，不切除黏膜，全层折叠缝合直肠前壁，此法术后可能会有无症状的轻度直肠前突，但不影响其预后。新近发展的新型手术方式有 STARR（吻合器经肛直肠切除术）和 trans-STARR 技术，近几年在欧洲应用尤为广泛，文献报道了较高的成功率[18-19]。同时也存在一些争议和手术禁忌证：一些治疗中心报道术后约 1/3 的患者会出现长期的肛门失禁和里急后重等不适症状，且药物和手术治疗效果不佳[20]；当直肠前突合并有肠疝时不能应用上述技术，或需要在腹腔镜辅助下完成[21]，关于该术式更深入的内容在本书第 27 章中将有详细的介绍。

经会阴路径的步骤是经阴道与直肠间皮肤切开，沿直肠阴道间隙分离至直肠前突顶部，将直肠前壁肌层折叠缝合。如放置合成或非合成材料补片进行修补，需自直肠外括约肌与阴道后壁间隙游离至阴道尖，充分暴露直肠前突、直肠筋膜、提肌板内侧缘，植入补片后，自阴道尖至会阴中心腱，间断缝合两侧肛提肌边缘 4~5 针加强直肠前壁。经阴道路径已较少应用，多是伴有阴道后穹隆或膀胱脱垂等妇科相关疾病时，由妇科医师完成。经阴道后壁中线纵行切开，将阴道后壁自直肠阴道隔分离，折叠缝合直肠阴道隔，或放置补片后将阴道后壁黏膜缝合固定于补片上，是否同时行肛提肌成形术尚存在争议。同时行会阴缝补术时，经会阴皮肤做横向菱形切口，切除冗余组织后做缝合[22-23]。为防止复发，一些单位进一步经直肠、阴道后壁修补。

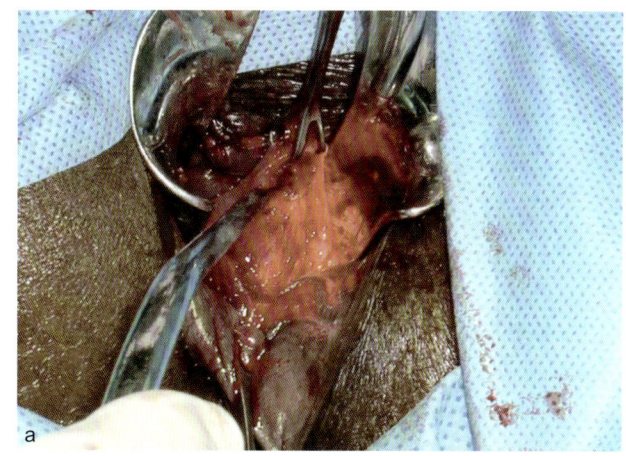
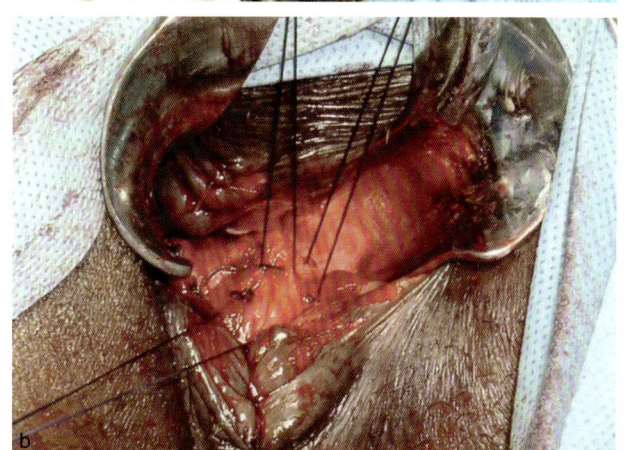
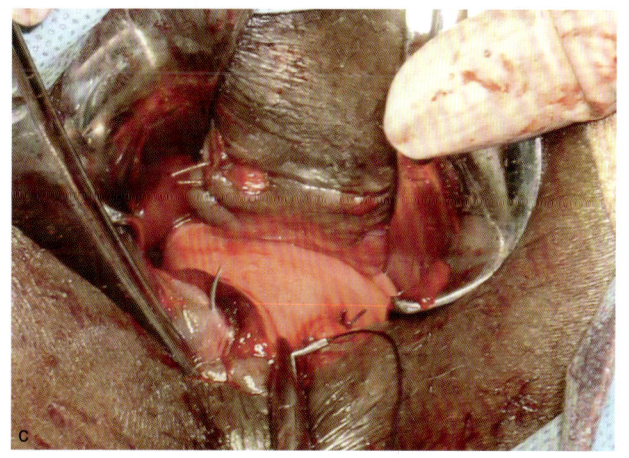

图 26.2 直肠内直肠前突修补。(a) 黏膜切除；(b) 直肠阴道隔修补和加强；(c) 黏膜缝合

随着腹腔镜技术的发展，近年来，腹腔镜辅助直肠固定术广泛应用，该路径在腔镜下经 Douglas 窝分离直肠与阴道间隙[24]，由于视野清晰，可有效保护直肠、阴道的支配神经，同时完成放置会阴补片、直肠/肛提肌固定、肛提肌成形或补片骶骨固

定等手术[25-26]。到目前为止，虽然文献报道中各组病例选择存在差异性，早期临床结果均较好，此路径对合并有直肠肛管病变时操作更为方便，但对于缓解便秘、失禁、精神性性交困难症状较传统方法则无显著优势。

对于手术治疗失败的患者，采用何种路径则取决于前次手术的方式、复发的程度、患者接受再次手术的意愿。二次手术风险较大，难点在于前次手术不可吸收材料的存在，如直肠阴道间隙放置的补片和肠壁遗留的吻合钉。

直肠前突修补失败的原因

文献中关于直肠前突外科治疗失败后再次手术效果的报道很少，需要区分是为解剖性失败还是功能性失败。解剖性的失败多因手术技术应用不当，多见于子宫切除后前突面积较大者。功能性失败则可能是因为术前未发现合并有直肠套叠或其他的盆底解剖异常，如乙状结肠疝、会阴下降、直肠敏感性下降等。通过排粪造影或直肠肛管测压常可发现这些失败的原因[28]。

尽管前突的面积、钡截留、需手助排便作为手术的指征，但缺乏证据证明这些因素与手术疗效有相关性[29]。Infantino等[30]的研究认为解剖的纠正不代表功能的恢复。对这些患者，术前需进行详细的检查评估，包括心理测试，收集详细的回忆数据，甚至包含是否有幼年受虐史。次要原因在于手术技术的应用不当，如修补不完全、缝线早期断裂等亦会造成手术的失败。

第三种情况是术后直肠造影、排便频率均正常，但可能并存有盆底、结肠、直肠的功能异常而引起的症状，导致患者对手术不满意[31]。比如很多直肠前突患者同时诊断有肠易激综合征，对于这类病例，单纯的直肠修补并不能获得排便功能的改善[32-33]。既往认为，需要经阴道或直肠手助排便者，手术疗效明显[34]，但部分患者通过饮食调整或生物反馈资料，甚至心理治疗也能获得缓解。有些患者存在直肠前突、乙状结肠疝和直肠套叠，尽管客观检查显示直肠已排空，但患者仍有排便不尽感[35]。有些会阴下降综合征的女性患者，实际没有直肠前突，也会有排便障碍。从这方面来说，手术成功的标准很难定义[36-38]。

直肠前突修补术失败后处理指南

直肠前突修补失败后再手术的处理取决于前次手术的方式。具体处理路径见图26.3。

经直肠路径修补失败

前次手术切除黏膜后折叠直肠修补，如为手工缝合，较易处理，可再次手工或使用吻合器进行手术，切除原手术疤痕，完成前突修补，如无其他盆底功能异常，可缓解复发的直肠前突症状。或可应

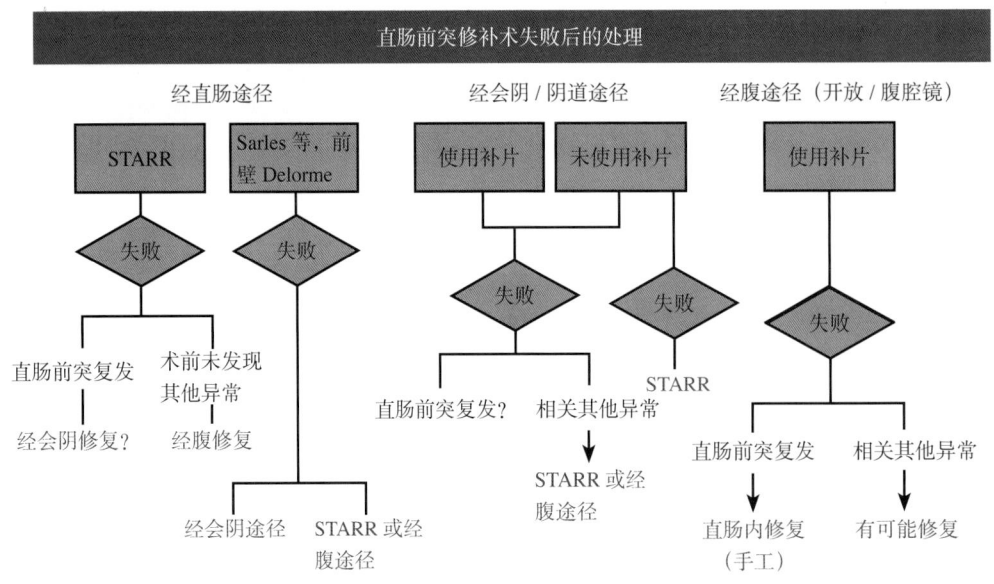

图26.3 直肠前突修补失败后的处理原则，基于初次手术的类型。STARR：经肛吻合器直肠切除术

用腹腔镜经腹技术，也可简便完成，取决于医师的选择[31]。而 STARR 术后复发，处理就相对困难，因前次手术的疤痕和遗留的吻合钉增加了再次手术的风险[18]。分离阴道直肠间隙时较为困难、易出血。此类情况下，经会阴路径优于经直肠路径。

经阴道/会阴路径修补失败

经会阴或阴道路径修补如果复发，再次经会阴/阴道路径手术难度极大，阴道直肠间隙分离困难，易引起直肠阴道瘘，如前次植入有不可吸收性补片，则操作更困难[31]。这种情况下需先考虑是否是其他并存盆底异常引起的"复发"症状，是否可通过纠正这些异常来缓解症状。如前次手术仅为单纯直肠前壁折叠缝合，可考虑经直肠路径进行前突修补或行 STARR 手术。

经腹路径修补失败

经腹（腹腔镜或开腹）路径通常使用补片加强直肠阴道隔，同时游离直肠完成直肠骶骨前固定。如复发，经腹手术风险较大，分离直肠周围的粘连可引起直肠穿孔或骶前出血，可尝试经直肠路径进行再次修补。使用生物补片或可吸收补片可减少这些风险，但长期效果不能确定[39]。

附：文献一篇

直肠前突修补后再手术（经会阴途径）
Filippo Pucciani

直肠前突修补失败多因为复发或修补不彻底而导致术前症状复发。有些则是并存的其他结直肠解剖病理改变如结肠慢运输、直肠内套叠、肛门括约肌功能障碍等影响了手术疗效[1]。

直肠前突的修补途径有：经阴道阴道会阴修补术、直肠内黏膜切除术、经阴道特定薄弱部分修补术、经会阴修补术和腹腔镜下修补术。这些手术都有一定的复发率，多因患者或手术方式选择不恰当引起。文献报道为小宗病例或前瞻性的对照研究，直肠前突修补术是连同其他并存病同时完成手术，文献数据可用度不高，影响了对直肠前突手术效果的有效评估。有文献报道，经肛门行 STARR 术后，便秘持续或复发率为 13%~35%[2-3]，术后排粪造影显示术后 6%~7% 的患者仍存在直肠前突[2,4]。Zbar 等[5]总结相关文献显示，经肛门路径行直肠前突修补术后肛门失禁发生率为 17.9%~23.3%，经阴道途径发生率为 11.5%~16.8%。近年来，仅两项前瞻性随机试验比较了经直肠途径和阴道途径的效果。经阴道途径的 39 例单纯直肠前突的女性中 2 例术后复发，经直肠途径的 48 例中 7 例术后复发，两者复发率有差异但不显著[6-7]。一项循证医学的综述显示，关于直肠前途修补使用补片的数据太少而不能说明问题，无法确定使用补片是否能减少直肠前突修补后的复发率[8]。最近的一项随机试验也显示，使用补片和不使用补片直肠前突修补术后复发率分别为 7.5% 和 8.7%[9]，无显著差异。

对于直肠前突修补后复发的治疗策略并无统一标准，只有经过进一步检查，排除其他并存盆底异常引起类似症状，且明确直肠前突与症状相关后，方可考虑再次手术治疗。此时，手术的选择主要取决于前次手术的方法、复发后的重新检查明确的解剖或功能性病理改变。经直肠修补失败后再次手术多选择经会阴途径。经会阴或阴道修补失败后再次手术难度较大，因直肠阴道间隙存在粘连，分离困难，容易出现并发症或修补不完全导致再次复发。因此首次经经会阴手术应再修补的基础上同时行肛提肌成形或放置补片以减少复发率。

经会阴直肠前突修补术和肛提肌成形术

经直肠阴道平面分离，2-0 可吸收缝线折叠缝合直肠阴道隔，再使用 2-0 可吸收缝线将两侧肛提肌间断缝合，使直肠前突的薄弱区消失。

补 片

步骤同前，仅在完成修补后，于直肠阴道间隙置入补片以加强直肠阴道隔。迄今为止，尚无明确证据提示应该使用何种补片（不可吸收合成补片、可吸收合成补片、可吸收生物补片）。经会阴的直肠前突再次手术文献中仅有个别病例报道[1, 10]，病例数量极少，预后情况缺乏科学性。因此在选择进行前突修补手术时应该谨慎。

参考文献

1. Hirst GR, Hughes RJ, Morgan AR, Carr ND, Patel B, Beynon J. The role of rectocele repair in targeted patients with obstructed defecation. Colorectal Dis. 2005;7:159–63.
2. Madbouly KM, Abbas KS, Hussein AM. Disappointing long-term outcomes after stapled transanal rectal resection for obstructed defecation. World J Surg. 2010;34:2191–96.
3. Gagliardi G, Pescatori M, Altomare DF, Binda GA, Bottini C, Dodi G, et al. Results, outcome predictors, and complications after stapled transanal rectal resection for obstructed defecation. Dis Colon Rectum. 2008;51:186–95.
4. Ommer A, Rolfs TM, Walz MK. Long-term results of stapled transanal rectal resection for obstructive defecation syndrome. Int J Colorectal Dis. 2010;25:1287–92.
5. Zbar AP, Lienemann A, Fritsch H, Beer-Gabel M, Pescatori M. Rectocele: pathogenesis and surgical management. Int J Colorectal Dis. 2003;18:369–84.
6. Kahn MA, Stanton SL, Kumar D, et al. Posterior colporrhaphy is superior to the transanal repair for treatment of posterior vaginal wall prolapse. Neurourol Urodyn. 1999;18:329–30.
7. Nieminen K, Hiltunen K, Laitinen J, Oksala J, Heinonen PK. Transanal or vaginal approach to rectocele repair: a prospective, randomized pilot study. Dis Colon Rectum. 2004;47:1636–42.
8. Maher C, Feiner B, Baessler K, Adams EJ, Hagen S, Glazener CM. Surgical management of pelvic organ prolapse in women. Cochrane Database Syst Rev. 2010;(4):CD004014.
9. Sand PK, Koduri S, Lobel RW, Winkler HA, Tomezsko J, Culligan PJ, et al. Prospective randomized trial of polyglactin 910 mesh to prevent recurrence of cystoceles and rectoceles. Am J Obstet Gynecol. 2001;184:1357–64.
10. Sardeli C, Axelsen SM, Bek KM. Use of porcine small intestinal submucosa in the surgical treatment of recurrent rectocele in a patient with Ehlers-Danlos syndrome type III. Int Urogynecol J Pelvic Floor Dysfunct. 2005;16:504–5.

参考文献

1. Lefevre R, Davila GW. Functional disorders: rectocele. Clin Colon Rectal Surg. 2008;21:129–37.
2. Goh JTW, Tjandra JJ, Carey MP. How could management of rectocele be optimized? ANZ J Surg. 2002;72:896–901.
3. Stojkovic SG, Balfour L, Burke D, Finan PJ, Sagar PM. Does the need to self-digitate or the presence of a large or nonemptying rectocele on proctography influence the outcome of transanal rectocoele repair? Colorectal Dis. 2003;5:169–72.
4. Arnold MW, Stewart WR, Aguilar PS. Rectocele repair. Four years' experience. Dis Colon Rectum. 1990;33:684–7.
5. Harris MA, Ferrara A, Gallagher J, DeJesus S, Williamson P, Larach S. Stapled transanal rectal resection vs. transvaginal rectocele repair for treatment of obstructive defecation syndrome. Dis Colon Rectum. 2009;52:592–7.
6. Kahn MA, Stanton SL. Posterior colporrhaphy: its effects on bowel and sexual function. BJOG. 1997;104:82–6.
7. Maher C, Baessler K, Glazener CM, Adams EJ, Hagen S. Surgical management of pelvic organ prolapse in women. Cochrane Database Syst Rev. 2004;4:CD004014.
8. Lamah M, Ho J, Leicester RJ. Results of anterior levatorplasty for rectocele. Colorectal Dis. 2001;3:412–6.
9. Montella JM, Morrill MY. Effectiveness of the McCall culdeplasty in maintaining support after vaginal hysterectomy. Int Urogynecol J Pelvic Floor Dysfunct. 2005;16:226–9.
10. Akladios CY, Dautun D, Saussine C, Baldauf JJ, Mathelin C, Wattiez A. Laparoscopic sacrocolpopexy for female genital organ prolapse: establishment of a learning curve. Eur J Obstet Gynecol Reprod Biol. 2010;149:218–21.
11. Sarles JC, Arnaud A, Selezneff I, Olivier S. Endo-rectal repair of rectocele. Int J Colorectal Dis. 1989;4:167–71.
12. Khubchandani IT, Sheets JA, Stasik JJ, Hakki AR. Endorectal repair of rectocele. Dis Colon Rectum. 1983;26:792–6.
13. Tjandra JJ, Ooi BS, Tang CL, Dwyer P, Carey M. Transanal repair of rectocele corrects obstructed defecation if it is not associated with anismus. Dis Colon Rectum. 1999;42:1554–50.
14. Dippolito A, Esser S, Reed 3rd J. Anterior modification of Delorme procedure provides equivalent results to Delorme procedure in treatment of rectal outlet obstruction. Curr Surg. 2005;62:609–12.
15. Khubchandani IT, Clancy JP, Rosen L, Reither RD, Stasik JJ. Endorectal repair of rectocele revisited. Br J Surg. 1997;84:89–91.
16. Trompetto M, Clerico G, Realis Luc A, Marino F, Giani I, Ganio E. Transanal Delorme procedure for treatment of rectocele associated with rectal intussusception. Tech Coloproctol. 2006;10:389.
17. Block IR. Transrectal repair of rectocele using obliterative suture. Dis Colon Rectum. 1986;29:707–11.
18. Gagliardi G, Pescatori M, Altomare DF, Binda GA, Bottini C, Dodi G, et al. Italian Society of Colo-Rectal Surgery (SICCR): Results, outcome predictors, and complications after stapled transanal rectal resection for obstructed defecation. Dis Colon Rectum. 2008;51:186–95.
19. Pescatori M, Zbar AP. Reinterventions after complicated or failed STARR procedure. Int J Colorectal Dis. 2009;24:87–95.
20. Meurette G, Lehur PA. Commentary: STARR and Transtar proce-

dures. Colorectal Dis. 2009;11:828–30.
21. Carriero A, Picchio M, Martellucci J, Talento P, Palimento D, Spaziani E. Laparoscopic correction of enterocele associated to stapled transanal rectal resection for obstructed defecation syndrome. Int J Colorectal Dis. 2010;25:381–7.
22. Leventoğlu S, Menteş BB, Akin M, Karen M, Karamercan A, Oğuz M. Transperineal rectocele repair with polyglycolic acid mesh: a case series. Dis Colon Rectum. 2007;50:2085–92.
23. Milito G, Cadeddu F, Grande M, Selvaggio I, Farinon AM. Advances in treatment of obstructed defecation: Biomesh transperineal repair. Dis Colon Rectum. 2009;52:2051.
24. D'Hoore A, Penninckx F. Laparoscopic ventral recto(colpo)pexy for rectal prolapse: surgical technique and outcome for 109 patients. Surg Endosc. 2006;20:1919–23.
25. D'Hoore A, Vanbeckevoort D, Penninckx F. Clinical, physiological and radiological assessment of rectovaginal septum reinforcement with mesh for complex rectocele. Br J Surg. 2008;95:1264–72.
26. Slawik S, Soulsby R, Carter H, Payne H, Dixon AR. Laparoscopic ventral rectopexy, posterior colporrhaphy and vaginal sacrocolpopexy for the treatment of recto-genital prolapse and mechanical outlet obstruction. Colorectal Dis. 2008;10:138–43.
27. Watson SJ, Loder PB, Halligan S, Bartram CI, Kamm MA, Phillips RK. Transperineal repair of symptomatic rectocele with Marlex mesh: A clinical, physiological and radiologic assessment of treatment. J Am Coll Surg. 1996;183:257–61.
28. Halligan S, Bartram CI, Hall C, Wingate J. Enterocele revealed by simultaneous evacuation proctography and peritoneography: does defecation block exist? Am J Roetngenol. 1996;167:461–6.
29. Murthy VK, Orkin BA, Smith LE, Glassman LM. Excellent outcome using selective criteria for rectocele repair. Dis Colon Rectum. 1996;39:374–8.
30. Infantino A, Masin A, Melega E, Dodi G, Lise M. Does surgery resolve outlet obstruction. Int J Colorectal Dis. 1995;10:97–100.
31. Pescatori M, Milito G, Fiorino M, Cadeddu F. Complications and reinterventions after surgery for obstructed defecation. Int J Colorectal Dis. 2009;24:951–9.
32. Wong RK, Palsson OS, Turner MJ, Levy RL, Feld AD, von Korff M, et al. Inability of the Rome III criteria to distinguish functional constipation from constipation-subtype irritable bowel syndrome. Am J Gastroenterol. 2010;105:2228–34.
33. Suttor V, Prott GM, Hansen RD, Kellow JE, Malcolm A. Evidence for pelvic floor dyssynergia in patients with irritable bowel syndrome. Dis Colon Rectum. 2010;53:156–60.
34. Lehur PA, Stuto A, Fantoli M, Queralto M, Lazorthes F, Hershman M, ODS II Study Group. Outcomes of stapled transanal rectal resection vs. biofeedback for the treatment of outlet obstruction associated with rectal intussusception and rectocele: a multicenter, randomized, controlled trial. Dis Colon Rectum. 2008;51:1611–8.
35. Cundiff GW, Weidner AC, Visco AG, Addison WA, Bump RC. An anatomic and functional assessment of the discrete defect rectocele repair. Am J Obstet Gynecol. 1998;179:1451–7.
36. Mellgren A, Anzen B, Nilsson BY, Johansson C, Dolk A, Gillgren P, et al. Results of rectocele repair- a prospective study. Dis Colon Rectum. 1995;38:7–13.
37. Porter WE, Steele A, Walsh P, Kohli N, Karram MM. The anatomic and functional outcomes of defect-specific rectocele repairs. Am J Obstet Gynecol. 1999;181:1353–9.
38. Lopez A, Anzen B, Bremmer S, Mellgren A, Nilsson BY, Zetterström J, et al. Durability of success after rectocele repair. Int Urogynecol J. 2001;12:97–103.
39. Smart NJ, Mercer-Jones MA. Functional outcome after transperineal rectocele Repair with porcine dermal collagen implant. Dis Colon Rectum. 2007;50:1422–7.

第 27 章　STARR 术式的利与弊

Mario Pescatori

丁威威 译　姜　军 审校

摘　要

在排便障碍综合征的患者中，一些特殊的形态学改变包括直肠前突、直肠肛门肠套叠、直肠黏膜内脱垂及直肠膨出等均提示患有"冰山综合征"可能。在这些患者中，一些较轻的因素就可以引起显著的排便功能障碍，如耻骨直肠肌综合征、肠道易激综合征及心理因素等。这些因素可能也是导致患者 STARR 术后仍存在排便障碍的重要原因。约超过 90% 的排便障碍患者有多种骨盆及会阴部软组织的异常，这些异常仅凭直肠前突修复等无法得到彻底解决。STARR 术式在此类患者中的适应证和禁忌证仍无定论，既往研究对该类患者行 STARR 术式的疗效也存在争议：有研究认为 STARR 术式可以取得预期的手术效果；另一部分研究却指出 STARR 术式会导致严重的术后并发症，部分患者甚至难以进行二次手术。因此从医学法律角度讲，患者有权被告知 STARR 术存在的风险，常见的包括大便失禁、里急后重及反复发作的排便困难等。

STARR 和 trans-STARR 术式：优势和劣势

10 年前，在佛罗里达克利夫兰诊所的年会上 Antonio Longo 首次描述了经肛吻合器直肠切除术（STARR 术）的过程。该手术可以矫正排便障碍患者的直肠形态异常。该术式的提出主要基于直肠肛门肠套叠、直肠内膜脱垂及直肠前突等是排便障碍综合征患者主要病因的理论观点。

来源于 Pescatori[1] 等首次描述的直肠黏膜切除术，该手术需要用一个环形吻合器经肛门进行直肠前部和后部的切除，所用吻合器与直肠脱垂及痔疮手术中所使用的相同 (PPH, Ethicon 内镜显微外科，Cincinnati, OH)。STARR 是一个新型的手术，同样存在术后并发症和手术失败的风险[2-4]。基于以上问题，最近提出的 trans-STARR 术式旨在使用新设备 Contour 缝合器（Ethicon 内镜显微外科）改善疗效。这是一种能够目视下同时进行冗余组织"切割和缝合"的弯型缝合器[5]。与 PPH-01 缝合器相比，trans-STARR 的 multifire 技术最主要的优势是术中缝合可见性提高并且有效避免黏膜瓣残留。

不少随机试验证明两种手术的效果没有显著差异[6-8]，但与早期的 STARR 术式相比，trans-STARR 痛苦相对少，大便失禁发生率低，可操作性更好。在 Lenisa 等报道的手术案例中，仅 0.5% 受慢性肛部痛的影响[7]。此研究中，所有患者均由擅长经肛门吻合的手术医师行 trans-STARR 手术。但因为这些手术医师同时也是器械公司的顾问，并且报道案例缺乏深入讨论，病案报道的主观导向性很难避免。Corman 等[9] 已在一篇对在功能性肠病中使用缝合器技术共识的分析文章中提出，这种手术只应由专门的结直肠外科医生操作。由于目前所报道的仅是

STARR 术后效果不良或失败而转入三级护理中心的少数病例。这种病例选择的偏倚也可能导致两种术式疗效比较的偏差。STARR 和 trans-STARR 术式各自的支持者以及擅长处理 STARR 术后并发症的三级分送小组对目前的研究结果仍存在较大分歧。

排便障碍的经肛吻合治疗：结直肠医师的争论

随着新手术器械不断出现，一些支持者开始进一步强调 STARR 和 trans-STARR 术式的优点。既往该术式使用率约 14%，主要原因是排便困难被认为是一种功能性障碍，应按照指南要求严格把握手术适应证。随着新指南的制定实施，该术式的使用率增加到 77%，积极行该术式的外科医生也成为该术式的推动者[10-12]，甚至有医生推荐常规使用 STARR 术式。但是目前外科医生在 STARR 术式的适应证和禁忌证的选择上尚未达成共识，实际盆底操作训练水平也参差不齐。

2008 年 9 月发表在意大利《M. Pappagalloof Corriere della sera》杂志上的一篇关于 STARR 术式发明人的综述宣称该术式是无需缝合的，进一步引起了学术界关于该术式的争论。因 STARR 术式常规包括 52 针的缝合，Ira Kodner（美国结直肠外科医师协会副主席）在一篇评论中认为，临床医师和器械公司之间的联系使得该术式的适应证被夸大了[13]。我们的团队多年以前就一直坚持一个原则，即尽管器械公司宣传产品最终目的是为了盈利，但是临床医师的根本宗旨只是为了治愈患者[14]。信息、宣传及营销之间的重叠使得在遇到 STARR 术后并发症及复发性的排便障碍时，STARR 术式的应用成了一个颇具争议的话题。然而，10 年内超过 50 篇文献表示的对该技术的兴趣不可否认。我们已经关注到市场营销宣传对临床上手术方案决定的影响，这在目前尚未得到重视。

术后并发症及复发率：常规术式和 STARR 术式的差异

既往文献报道的长期随访中，常规术式和 STARR 术式的远期排便困难复发及症状持续的发生率均在 32%~50% 之间[15-17]。根据我们的临床经验，STARR 术后需再次手术干预的并发症发生率约为常规术式的 2 倍左右（4.6% vs 8%）[18-20]。

我们目前已在文献中报道的术后严重并发症包括严重直肠出血、直肠阴道瘘、大便失禁、直肠狭窄、结直肠血肿、盆腔脓肿及慢性肛部痛等，这些并发症均需要再次手术干预[10, 21-24]。一系列并发症的处理方法也被提出，包括出血点的缝合、再次 STARR 手术、直肠乙状结肠切除及结肠造口术等[4]。目前文献报道 STARR 术后 18 个月内并发症的再次手术率约为 8%。

STARR 术后排便障碍症状持续存在及复发的可能原因是同时存在的肠疝及直肠脱垂[25-26]，并常常需要二次鉴别诊断。总之，过去的 8 年里，我大约见到了 50 例失败或者严重术后并发症的 STARR 患者。其中大部分在其他地方做过治疗，大约有 1/3 需再次手术。相比于其他手术 2% 的并发症发生率，记录在 Observatory for Emerging Colorectal Technologies Section of the Italian Society of Colorectal Surgery 数据库里的 STARR 术后并发症发生率高达 44%。

STARR 和 trans-STARR 术式的早期和晚期疗效：冰山综合征

STARR 术式的早期疗效令人欣喜。2004 年发表的首篇有关的多中心前瞻性研究发现 STARR 术后短期内无严重的并发症发生，90% 的患者短期内有较好疗效[8]，仅 20% 患者术后 1 年中出现排便疼痛。但术后 18 个月超过一半的患者出现至少 3 种排便困难的症状[19]，长期随访 44% 患者有排便困难复发症状[16, 28]。这些症状可能是由于以下因素造成：①手术切除不完全；②未能严格把握手术适应证；③持续被忽视的功能异常或多种其他潜在因素。肛门痉挛、肠道易激惹综合征、精神压力及直肠低感等共同构成排便障碍的易忽视因素，这些因素被称为"冰山综合征"，是大部分 STARR 手术失败的主要原因[10]。这些患者手术失败后处理非常复杂，需行腹会阴联合手术。再次手术患者术后 4 年治愈率可达 90%[29]。

trans-STARR 术式发明的第 3 年，Boccasanta 等[8]报道 trans-STARR 术式的结直肠套叠矫正率可达 100%。然而，正常结构的恢复并不代表正常功能的恢复[30]。目前仅有上述唯一的研究报道了100%的手术成功率。尽管trans-STARR术式的中期疗效相当有前景，但新技术的高费用仍然是一个问题，在作者所在地区，每个患者大约需要耗费1650欧元进行一次trans-STARR手术[7]。

STARR术后的并发症及复发

既往文献报道的STARR术后并发症见表27.1

STARR术后并发症及复发的干预

STARR术后因并发症（直肠出血及肛管直肠狭窄）再干预率见表27.2。

美国的STARR术式的引入晚于欧洲和其他一些国家，FDA已经报道了一系列直肠穿孔的案例，部分案例因STARR术中钉的不恰当使用导致[37]。表27.3总结并更新了既往研究中[25]报道的关于STARR术后因并发症再次手术的结果[图27.1 a–c]。

另一项系列研究报道了STARR术后18个月再次手术的发生率为19%；大部分再次手术是因为术后并发症及持续存在的或复发的排便功能障碍[19]。

Miliacca等[38]研究发现，仅有一半的再次手术患者症状得到缓解或治愈；值得注意的是，再次手术后未缓解的患者经心理科医师或自测量表评估后发现，他们中的大部分都有明显的焦虑及抑郁症状，且大部分患者在服用抗抑郁药或镇定药。正如前面所述，精神状态的改变对排便困难患者术后疗效有不良影响[39]，因而对此类患者术前有必要进行心理评估。在术前进行心理因素的排查可以显著减少术后并发症的发生，然而文献中关于术前进行此类评估的报道很少[40]。尽管该问题比较复杂，已有的文献报道也很少，但术前的心理评估结果应该纳入手术的适应证及禁忌证中[41]。

STARR术后并发症及复发的病因学

STARR和trans-STARR术式是两种非常有潜力的术式，其共同的原理都是切除多余及嵌顿的直肠组织，以使排便困难的患者获得正常的排便功能。然而，STARR术式似乎不适合于广口型的脱肛患者[19]，因其不能加强直肠阴道隔的力量，而薄弱的直肠阴道隔被认为是导致该症状的主要原因，因为运用补片或肛提肌成形术可以解决该问题。另外，

表27.1 排便梗阻患者经肛吻合器直肠切除术后并发症

术后并发症	发生率（%）	参考文献	研究者	年份
直肠出血	4.4	[31]	Stuto 等	2007
	3.1	[32]	Lehur	2008
	4.0	[7]	Boccasanta 等	2011
肛门直肠狭窄	3.0	[33]	Pechlivanides 等	2007
	3.7	[34]	Ellis	2007
	1.2	[31]	Stuto 等	2007
	1.5	[32]	Lehur	2008
肛门和盆腔痛	20.0	[8]	Boccasanta 等	2004
	9.5	[31]	Stuto 等	2007
	11.0	[19]	Gagliardi 等	2007
	23.0	[17]	Meurette 等	2011
里急后重	22.0	[35]	Nicolas 等	2004
	23.0	[31]	Stuto 等	2007
	44.0	[6]	Wadhavan 等	2010
	34.0	[8]	Boccasanta 等	2011
肛门失禁	14.0	[35]	Nicolas 等	2004
	3.0	[8]	Boccasanta 等	2004
	16.0	[33]	Pechlivanides 等	2007
	27.0	[28]	Jongen 等	2010

表 27.2　严重直肠出血和狭窄后再干预率

手术适应证	再手术患者（%）	参考文献	研究者	年　份
直肠出血	2.7	[36]	Arroyo 等	2007
	4.0	[20]	Scarcliff 和 Parker	2010
	2.0	[8]	Boccasanta	2011
肛门直肠狭窄	4.0	[20]	Scarcliff 和 Parker	2010

表 27.3　经肛吻合器直肠切除术后再干预的适应证和结果相关并发症 [a]

适应证	干预方式	结　果
严重直肠出血	经肛吻合口缝合	术后 8 年排便困难
肛门痛，大小便失禁，焦虑/抑郁	前路肛提肌成形术	未改善
阴道瘘，便秘，焦虑/抑郁	黏膜切除术，阴道修补，结肠造口术	术后 4 年排便困难
肛部痛，焦虑/抑郁	Agraphectomy	未改善
直肠憩室，肛部痛	切开	好转
失败（排便障碍复发）		
直肠乙状结肠狭窄，憩室病	乙状结肠切除术	好转
肠疝	道格拉斯网袋修复	好转
直肠套叠，焦虑/抑郁	直肠切除固定术	未改善
直肠憩室，肛部痛	直肠成形术，Agraphectomy	治愈
里急后重，肛部痛，焦虑/抑郁	直肠烧灼术/折叠术	未改善
急救，肛部痛	Agraphectomy	改善
直肠脱垂，肛部痛	Altemeier 术式，Agraphectomy	治愈
大便失禁	膨胀剂注射	治愈
大便失禁，肛部痛，焦虑/抑郁	前路肛提肌成形术	未改善
肠疝，盆底失迟缓	道格拉斯窝修复，生理反馈训练	改善
直肠狭窄，焦虑/抑郁 [b]	Agraphectomy，肛门扩张术	失随访

Reprinted with permission from Pescatori and Zbar[25]
a：16 例患者，平均随访 23 个月（2～96 个月），15 例患者外院行 STARR
b：此病例详见图 27.1

STARR 术式需要在无法获得清晰的周围组织如直肠系膜和道格拉斯窝的视野条件下切除两处直肠组织，这无疑增加了并发症的风险。最后，并不是所有的排便障碍手术都能矫正神经肌肉的病因[42]，吻合技术可能加重已经存在的盆底失迟缓症状。现已证明[26,43]，耻骨直肠肌可能部分参与钉旁机化组织的形成，从而使其变得更加僵硬且无法松弛，造成顽固性疼痛，且即使拔除钉子仍无法缓解。与肛管再次手术和重建有关的医学法律问题，在本书的最后一章将会阐述。然而，术前向患者明确说明该术式的优缺点，使其明确可能的并发症风险，让患者自由选择是否需要承受该手术风险，以排除不愿承受风险的患者，是非常必要的。向患者说明该术式的适应证及禁忌证等，可以减少医患双方对于术后疗效判定的分歧。

trans-STARR 术式在此方面有所改进：术者能更好地操作，有更清晰的术中视野。有关此方面的前瞻性随机试验有待进行，如凯途吻合器在对耻骨直肠肌功能及形态的影响。期待无金钱利益的有关研究团队做此类研究。

STARR 术后并发症处理指南

在严重的直肠出血、对肛门扩张无反应的肛门直肠狭窄、有大的进展性活动性直肠或直肠后血肿、可导致生命危险的盆腔感染的患者中，唯一的机会

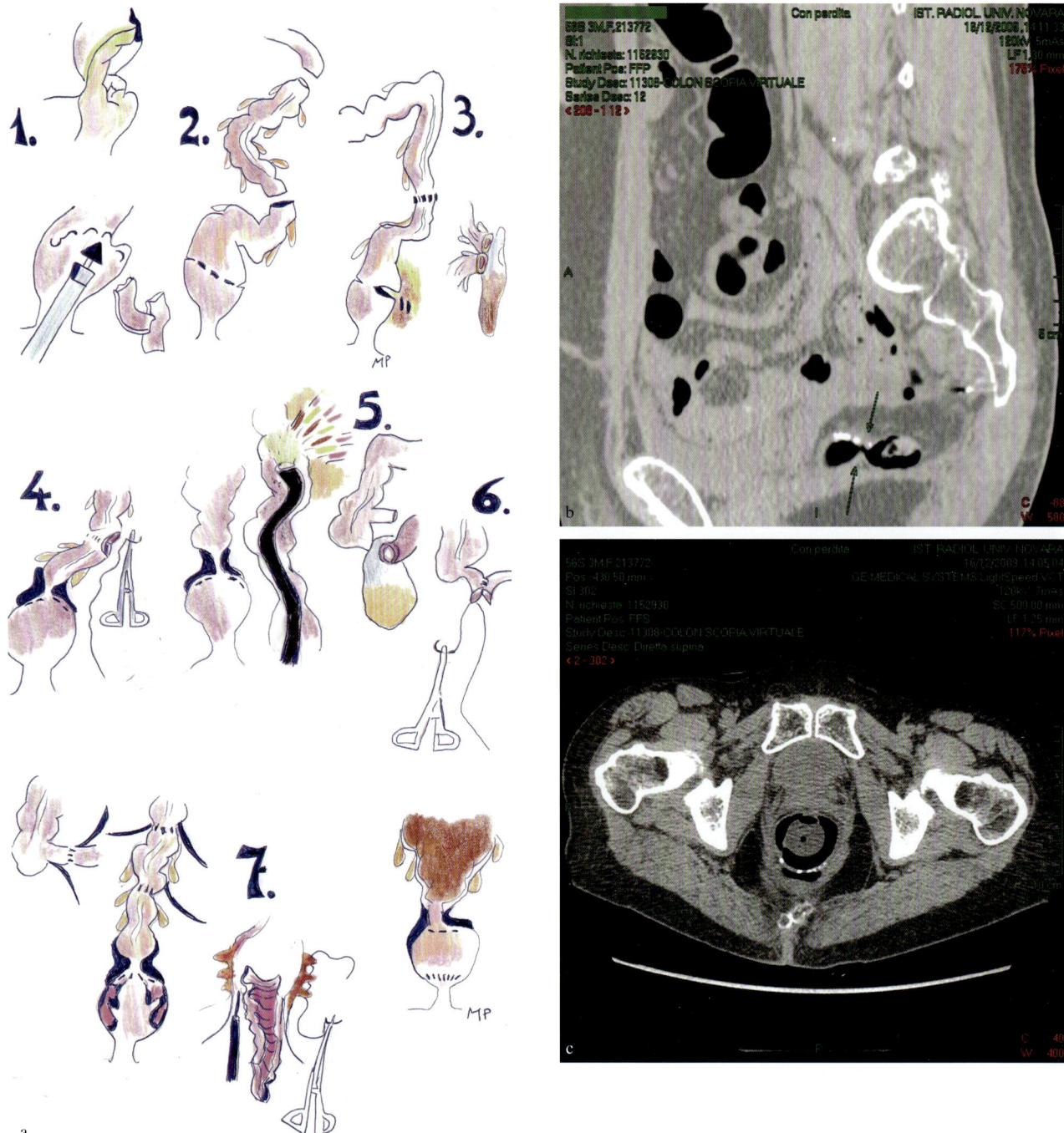

图 27.1 (a) 一例复杂的经肛吻合器直肠切除术后示意图。33 岁男性（表 27.3 最后一例患者），经肛吻合器直肠切除术后 1 年内行 5 次翻修，并发钉线裂开。因直肠内脱垂而行经肛缝合，患者情绪焦虑，轻度便秘，有肠易激惹综合征，并且有厌食病史。(1~3) 乙状结肠过长被认为是引起症状的原因，因此 STARR 的同时行腹腔镜下乙状结肠部分切除术，未行术前肠道运输时间的研究。STARR 术式吻合口裂开导致腹膜炎，后转院行肠造口术后造口还纳。(4~5) 同时，患者在吻合口裂开处并发直肠狭窄，自诉腹痛、排便困难。行一个疗程的肛肠扩张术，初次接诊医师建议患者行结肠镜检查，检查期间发生穿孔(6)。行第二次造口，3 个月后造口还纳。患者由于粘连仍感觉剧烈腹痛，另因直肠狭窄造成排便困难，患者出现抑郁症状。一名结直肠外科医生诊断其直肠内脱垂复发，随即进行了内部 Delorme 术。一段时间后，患者再次出现相同的症状，遂来到 Ars 医院肛肠科。患者精神焦虑，极度消瘦，生活质量极差。直肠下段距肛门边缘 7cm 处严重狭窄（图 b、c 中 CT 示），门诊局麻下第 1 次肛门扩张时去除两个钉子(7)。1 周后在手术室全麻下进行第 2 次扩张，最多达 23mm。患者未作第 3 次扩张。(b) 矢状面和 (c) 轴向的扫描显示 STARR 术的钉线及低位狭窄

就是再次手术。手术必须由专业的结直肠外科医生进行，必须对盆底的结构和功能熟知。直肠阴道瘘，与 PPH 术后的直肠阴道瘘相似，如果位置很低有症状，可以通过保守治疗的方法治愈[44]。手术修复常常是需要的[10, 22-23]，直肠阴道瘘修补术在此书的其他部分详述。STARR 术后肛门不适的原因很多，如术中的括约肌撑开牵引及 STARR 术后直肠依从性降低等。术后盆底运动恢复及患者能适应术后的变化后，依从性可能随着时间推移而得到缓解。局部病变括约肌内注射大剂量的药物可能有效[45]，这在 33 章中有描述。肛门不适的第一步治疗就是盆底康复治疗，需谨记任何腔内的钉子都是经肛门电刺激术的禁忌证，因为有局部灼伤的风险。胫骨后神经的外部电刺激术可能是更安全、更廉价的替代疗法[46]，近期已在类似病例中选择性使用。

严重的慢性肛门痛和排便痛感：STARR 术后麻烦的慢性并发症

经验表明，严重的慢性肛门痛是 STARR 术后麻烦的严重慢性并发症，因为它可能严重影响患者的生活质量，且很难治愈。当认定疼痛是由可触及疼痛的吻合钉导致时，切开术被认为是理想的治疗方法。然而，在我的经验中，很少有患者可以得到完全缓解。与 STARR 术后 20% 的发生率相比，报道称凯途吻合器仅有 0.5% 的术后肛门痛可能[7-8]；trans-STARR 吻合钉钉旁纤维化的风险更小。钉旁纤维化可能是导致术后患者会阴部及最后一根骶神经根支配区顽固性外周神经痛的重要机制。Phillips 教授[47]关于 PPH 术后痛的理论已经从宏观和组织学角度进行研究，这篇文章中报道了一例 STARR 术后两个吻合钉与耻骨直肠肌发生粘连的病例[26]（图 27.2）。

关键在于，如果只是切除吻合钉，纤维化已经存在。因此，扩大性切除更可取，包括纤维化部分、吻合钉以及一部分黏膜和平滑肌。当类似的问题出现在 PPH 术后时，一些专业人士已经成功地使用了这种方法：来自维也纳的 Wunderlich 等成功地治疗了 37 例中的 26 例由于吻合钉残留导致 PPH 和 STARR 术后肛门痛的患者。与其他报道结果相似

（Rabau M, personal communication）。

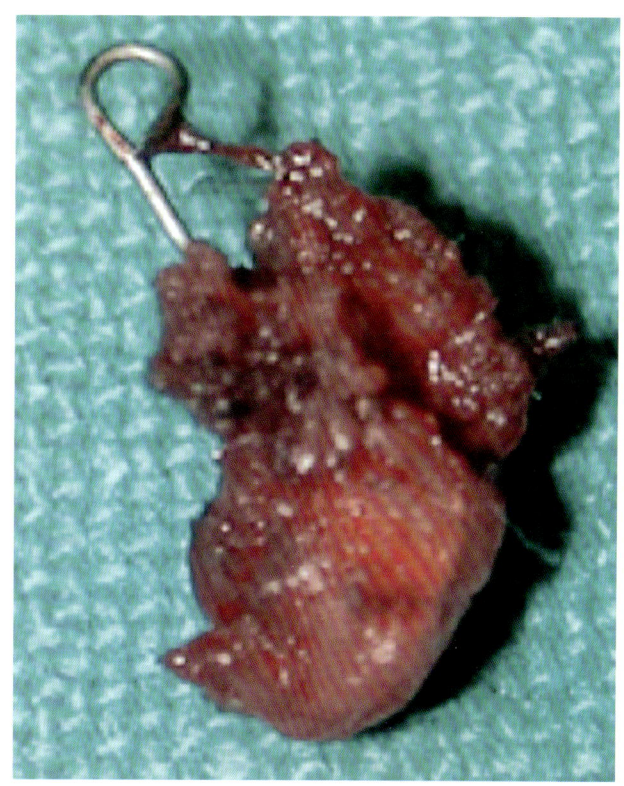

图 27.2　附着于耻骨直肠肌上的一个钉子，该患者在其他医院进行 STARR 术式，在我科再手术。该患者呈现严重的肛门痛和直肠脱垂。疼痛可能由钉旁纤维化引起，刺激耻骨直肠肌上的躯体神经受体，经病理检查证实（Reprinted with permission from De Nardi et al.[26]）

STARR 术后复发排便困难：安全保守的策略似乎比风险干预更好

STARR 术后持续或复发的排便障碍患者，对其干预应是包含心理学在内的系统的方法，因为这些患者可能有手术无法治愈的相关问题。经验表明，精神性神经官能症预示着术后干预的效果不佳，会阴和骨盆的软组织更易出血，PPH 术后干预对此已有证实。约 1/4 的患者出现术后括约肌乏力和直肠不适；并且需要吻合的患者中，因局部缺血吻合口裂开的现象更易发生[25, 28, 49]。

正如 Vermeulen 等[30]研究中表明的在复发性直

肠内脱垂或直肠前突患者中，恢复了解剖结构并不代表患者可以获得满意的排泄功能。相反，更多并发症和失败的风险增加，表明这些干预措施是最后的考虑，这些信息需要传递给患者；患者的期望值与外科医生所能达到的效果必须一致。

已有的简单替代疗法具有安全且部分免费的优点，包括温水坐浴、催眠、瑜伽、康复治疗、心理支持疗法和hydrocolon疗法等；还有昂贵且较少使用的骶神经调节术。这些替代疗法旨在放松盆底，让患者理解正确的排便机制，协助清空结肠，改善生态失调。但阴部的神经病变会增加直肠敏感性，增加直肠和乙状结肠的推进动力，需在手术前予以排除[50]。

结 论

与其他治疗排便障碍综合征的手术相比，STARR术式产生术后并发症的风险更高，并且复发率随时间延长而增加（长期复发率高达44%）。术后肛门失禁、里急后重和慢性疼痛的发生率分别为27%、44%和23%。目前报道中18个月内19%患者需再干预治疗。术后出现直肠出血及狭窄的患者约2%~4%需再次手术，直肠穿孔及骨盆感染患者则可能需行结肠造口术。排便时加重的慢性肛部疼痛严重影响一些患者的生活质量，且难以治疗。这些严重并发症的风险必须提前告知行STARR术式的患者。2/3排便障碍综合征的患者有精神性神经官能症，这是STARR术失败后再干预效果不佳的重要因素。新的凯途设备依然十分昂贵，但是新型的trans-STARR术式提供更好的手术视野，避免了术中黏膜瓣的形成。但目前仅1例前瞻性随机研究报道了trans-STARR术式相对于STARR术式的优越性。Trans-STARR术式在疼痛、便频和复发等问题上是否能有优势，需要更多的研究证实。这两种术式都不是微创，均可引起严重并发症。trans-STARR术式会引起严重的直肠系膜出血[51]。因此，两种术式都应由直肠手术方面的专家进行，排便障碍综合征的患者治疗成功的关键是必须包含一个多学科整体性的治疗方案。作为直肠肛门吻合术的指征的直肠前突，直肠内脱垂的患者仅仅只是排便障碍综合征患者的"冰山一角"。更多的原因如肛门痉挛、精神性神经官能症、直肠感觉减退及会阴部神经病变均属于功能性紊乱，不能通过手术治愈，应该通过康复及其他辅助方法治疗。STARR术后失败和复发大多是由于术前评估不完整，尤其忽视心理评估所致。

参考文献

1. Pescatori M, Favetta U, Dedola S, Orsini S. Transanal stapled excision of rectal mucosal prolapse. Tech Coloproctol. 1997;1:96–8.
2. Jayne DG, Finan PJ. Stapled transanal rectal resection for obstructed defaecation and evidence-based practice. Br J Surg. 2005;92:793–4.
3. Binda GA, Pescatori M, Romano G. The dark side of double-stapled transanal rectal resection. Dis Colon Rectum. 2005;48:1830–1.
4. Pescatori M, Gagliardi G. Postoperative complications after procedure for prolapsed hemorrhoids (PPH) and stapled transanal rectal resection (STARR) procedures. Tech Coloproctol. 2008;12:7–19.
5. Renzi A, Talento P, Giardiello C, Angelone G, Izzo D, Di Sarno G. Stapled trans-anal rectal resection (STARR) by a new dedicated device for the surgical treatment of obstructed defaecation syndrome caused by rectal intussusception and rectocele: early results of a multicenter prospective study. Int J Colorectal Dis. 2008;23:999–1005.
6. Wadhavan H, Shorthouse AJ, Brown SR. Surgery for obstructed defaecation: does the use of the Contour device (Trans-STARR) improve results? Colorectal Dis. 2010;12:885–90.
7. Lenisa L, Schwandner O, Stuto A, Jayne D, Pigot F, Tuech JJ, et al. STARR with Contour Transtar: prospective multicentre European study. Colorectal Dis. 2009;11:821–7.
8. Boccasanta P, Venturi M, Stuto A, Bottini C, Caviglia A, Carriero A, et al. Stapled transanal rectal resection for outlet obstruction: a prospective, multicenter trial. Dis Colon Rectum. 2004;47:1285–96.
9. Corman ML, Carriero A, Hager T, Herold A, Jayne DG, Lehur PA, et al. Consensus conference on the stapled transanal rectal resection (STARR) for disordered defaecation. Colorectal Dis. 2006;8:98–101.
10. Pescatori M, Spyrou M, Pulvirenti d'Urso A. A prospective evaluation of occult disorders in obstructed defecation using the 'iceberg diagram'. Colorectal Dis. 2006;8:785–9.
11. Schwandner O, Stuto A, Jayne D, Lenisa L, Pigot F, Tuech JJ, et al. Decision-making algorithm for the STARR procedure in obstructed defecation syndrome: position statement of the group of STARR Pioneers. Surg Innov. 2008;15:105–9.
12. Boccasanta P, Venturi M, Roviaro G. What is the benefit of a new stapler device in the surgical treatment of obstructed defecation? Three-year outcomes from a randomized controlled trial. Dis Colon Rectum. 2011;54:77–84.
13. Kodner IJ. Innovations in colorectal surgery. Tech Coloproctol. 2009;13:167–8.
14. Pescatori M, Seow Choen F. Use and abuse of new technologies in colorectal surgery. Tech Coloproctol. 2003;7:1–2.
15. Brown AJ, Anderson JH, McKee RF, Finlay IG. Surgery for occult rectal prolapse. Colorectal Dis. 2004;6:176–9.
16. Madbouly KM, Abbas KS, Hussein AM. Disappointing long-term outcomes after stapled transanal rectal resection for obstructed defecation. World J Surg. 2010;34:2191–6.
17. Meurette G, Wong M, Frampas E, Regenet N, Lehur PA. Anatomical and functional results after stapled transanal rectal resection (STARR) for obstructed defaecation syndrome. Colorectal Dis. 2011;13:e6–e11.
18. Pescatori M, Milito G, Fiorino M, Cadeddu F. Complications and reinterventions after surgery for obstructed defecation. Int J Colorectal Dis. 2009;24:951–9.

19. Gagliardi G, Pescatori M, Altomare DF, Binda GA, Bottini C, Dodi G, Italian Society of Colo-Rectal Surgery (SICCR), et al. Results, outcome predictors, and complications after stapled transanal rectal resection for obstructed defecation. Dis Colon Rectum. 2008;51:186–95.
20. Scarcliff SD, Parker MA, Birmingham AL. Efficacy of stapled transanal rectal resection for the treatment of obstructive defecation syndrome. In: The ASCRS annual meeting, Dis Colon Rectum 2010. Poster presentation P64.
21. Dodi G, Pietroletti R, Milito G, Binda G, Pescatori M. Bleeding, incontinence, pain and constipation after STARR transanal double stapling rectotomy for obstructed defecation. Tech Coloproctol. 2003;7:148–53.
22. Pescatori M, Dodi G, Salafia C, Zbar AP. Rectovaginal fistula after double-stapled transanal rectotomy (STARR) for obstructed defaecation. Int J Colorectal Dis. 2005;20:83–5.
23. Naldini G. Serious unconventional complications of surgery with stapler for haemorrhoidal prolapse and obstructed defaecation because of rectocoele and rectal intussusception. Colorectal Dis. 2009;13:323–7.
24. Stolfi VM, Micossi C, Sileri P, Venza M, Gaspari A. Retroperitoneal sepsis with mediastinal and subcutaneous emphysema complicating stapled transanal rectal resection (STARR). Tech Coloproctol. 2009;13:69–71.
25. Pescatori M, Zbar AP. Reinterventions after complicated or failed STARR procedure. Int J Colorectal Dis. 2009;24:87–95.
26. De Nardi P, Bottini C, Faticanti Scucchi L, Palazzi A, Pescatori M. Proctalgia in a patient with staples retained in the puborectalis muscle after STARR operation. Tech Coloproctol. 2007;11:353–6.
27. Basso L. Observatory of the adverse events after emerging technologies. In: Proceedings of biennial meeting of the SICCR, Catania, 2009.
28. Jongen JH, Eberstein A, Peleikis H, Kahlke V. Complaints and patient's satisfaction after STARR/TransSTARR operation for obstructed defecation. In: The ASCRS meeting. Dis Colon Rectum 2010. Poster presentation P65.
29. Pescatori M. Long-term follow-up of simultaneous abdominoperineal repair of enterorectocele and internal mucosal prolapse. Dis Colon Rectum. 2009;52:327–35.
30. Vermeulen J, Lange JF, Sikkenk AC, van der Harst E. Anterolateral rectopexy for correction of rectoceles leads to good anatomical but poor functional results. Tech Coloproctol. 2005;9:35–41.
31. Stuto A, Renzi A, Carnero A, Gabrielli F, Gianfreda V, Villani RD, et al. Stapled trans-anal rectal resection (STARR) in the surgical treatment of the obstructed defecation syndrome: results of STARR Italian Registry. Surg Innov. 2011;18(3):248–53.
32. Lehur PA, Stuto A, Fantoli M, Villani RD, Queralto M, Lazorthes F, ODS II Study Group, et al. Outcomes of stapled transanal rectal resection vs. biofeedback for the treatment of outlet obstruction associated with rectal intussusception and rectocele: a multicenter, randomized, controlled trial. Dis Colon Rectum. 2008;51:1611–8.
33. Pechlivanides G, Tsiaoussis J, Athanasakis E, Zervakis N, Gouvas N, Zacharioudakis G, et al. Stapled transanal rectal resection (STARR) to reverse the anatomic disorders of pelvic floor dyssynergia. World J Surg. 2007;31:1329–35.
34. Ellis CN. Stapled transanal rectal resection (STARR) for rectocele. J Gastrointest Surg. 2007;11:153–4.
35. Nicolas R, Meurette G, Frampas E, Mirallie E, Coat K, Leborgne J, Lehur P-A. Stapled transanal rectal resection is efficient to correct obstructed defecation but could compromise anal continence. Colorectal Dis. 2004;6:35.
36. Arroyo A, González-Argenté FX, García-Domingo M, et al. Prospective multicentre clinical trial of stapled transanal rectal resection for obstructive defaecation syndrome. Br J Surg. 2008;95:1521–7.
37. http://www.accessdata.fda.gov/scripts/cdhr. Accessed 2 Oct 2007.
38. Miliacca C, Gagliardi G, Pescatori M. The 'Draw-the-Family Test' in the preoperative assessment of patients with anorectal diseases and psychological distress: a prospective controlled study. Colorectal Dis. 2010;12:792–8.
39. Pescatori M, Boffi F, Russo A, Zbar AP. Complications and recurrence after excision of rectal internal mucosal prolapse for obstructed defaecation. Int J Colorectal Dis. 2006;21:160–5.
40. Schwandner O. Conversion in transanal stapling techniques for haemorrhoids and anorectal prolapse. Colorectal Dis. 2011;13:87–93.
41. Russo A, Pescatori M. Psychological assessment of patients with proctological disorders. In: Wexner SD, Zbar A, Pescatori M, editors. Complex anorectal disorders: investigation and management. London: Springer; 2005. p. 747–60.
42. Farid M, Youseff T, Mahdy T, Omar W, Moneim HA, El-Nakeeb A, et al. Comparative study between botulinum toxin injection and partial division of puborectalis for treating anismus. Int J Colorectal Dis. 2010;24:327–34.
43. Pucciani F, Ringressi MN, Giani I. Persistent dyschezia after double stapled transanal rectal resection for outlet obstruction: four case reports. Pelviperineology. 2007;26:132–5.
44. McDonald PJ, Bona R, Cohen CR. Rectovaginal fistula after stapled haemorrhoidopexy. Colorectal Dis. 2004;6:64–5.
45. Spyrou M, De Nardi P. The last images. Fecal incontinence after stapled transanal rectotomy managed with Durasphere injection. Tech Coloproctol. 2005;9:87.
46. Eléouet M, Siproudhis L, Guillou N, Le Couedic J, Bouguen G, Bretagne JF. Chronic posterior tibial nerve transcutaneous electrical nerve stimulation (TENS) to treat fecal incontinence (FI). Int J Colorectal Dis. 2010;25:1127–32.
47. Cheetham MJ, Mortensen NJ, Nystrom PO, Kamm MA, Phillips RK. Persistent pain and faecal urgency after stapled haemorrhoidectomy. Lancet. 2000;356:730–3.
48. Wunderlich M, Freitas A, Langmayr J, Tentschert G. Agraffectomy for complications after PPH and STARR. Proktologia. 2006;(Suppl 1):83.
49. Brusciano L, Ayabaca SM, Pescatori M, Accarpio GM, Dodi G, Cavallari F, et al. Reinterventions after complicated or failed stapled hemorrhoidopexy. Dis Colon Rectum. 2004;47:1846–51.
50. Pescatori M. Spinal cord stimulation for constipated patients. Dis Colon Rectum. 2009;52:1196.
51. Gelos M, Frommhold K, Mann B. Severe mesorectal bleeding after transanal rectal resection (STARR-operation) using the "Contour TransSTARR curved stapler". Colorectal Dis. 2010;12:265–6.

第 28 章 直肠前突与直肠疝：妇科医生的处理方式

Hans Peter Dietz

管 群 译 管 群 审校

摘 要

直肠前突和直肠疝常导致阴道后壁膨出，因此首诊常接受妇科医生的诊治，即使其临床表现属于胃肠病和结直肠外科领域。由于我们对病因学、病理生理学及基本肛直肠解剖的理解有限，因此我们在选择最佳治疗方案上存在分歧，并缺乏相关可用的盆底功能及解剖学知识。本章旨在阐明已知的直肠前突和直肠疝的病因及病理生理，介绍最新的功能成像技术的进展，介绍妇科医师对此类疾病的手术处理。理解妇科医师的处理方式，有利于肛肠外科医师管理这类已行妇科手术的患者，这是多学科管理合作的一部分。

关键词

直肠前突；直肠疝；妇科手术；远端消化道；疝气；阴道；后壁阴道修补；荷包缝合；骶棘阴道固定术；排便造影术；磁共振成像；磁共振排粪造影；超声

引 言

尽管直肠前突和直肠疝主要是远端消化道疾病，应当属于结直肠外科医师治疗的领域，但很多女性患者还是很传统地就诊于妇产科。因为其多伴有阴道后壁的膨出或肿块。妇科医师和结直肠外科医师对此病有截然不同的观点：前者注重解剖治疗而后者更关注功能方面的治疗；对于妇科医生而言，肠疝或者直肠前突表现为阴道后壁膨出，主要原因是因为肛提肌断裂损伤或者外阴损伤。传统观点认为这种损伤是由于分娩引起，因此妇科医生基于此观点进行治疗。最终，女性盆底功能失调导致一系列的盆腔器官功能紊乱，因此，会引发一系列的健康问题。

直到最近，妇科医生对直肠前突和直肠疝的治疗仅行经阴道手术。经典手术为阴道后壁修补术。手术矫正异常的解剖位置并将疝囊行荷包缝合包埋入道格拉斯窝。该手术最早由 Richter 和 Albrich[1] 在 1960s 提出，并由 Miyazaki[2] 于 20 世纪 70 年代改良为骶棘阴道固定术，该手术方式沿用至今。后来开展了经腹或经腹腔镜的手术方式；然而需要修复的部位往往离腹部较远[3]。最终，在 20 世纪 80 年代早期，Richardson 开展了 defect-specific 方法[4]。

这些方法和对患者的评估都有一个主要缺点，就是诊断不足。"直肠前突"从影像学上的描述为，由于腹压和大气压差，直肠前壁形成囊型结构突进阴道。妇科医生简单将其定义为由于各种原因导致阴道后壁膨出。阴道后壁膨出可以继发于一个"真"直肠前突、肠疝气、会阴损伤、会阴缺陷，甚至可能是肠套叠。另外，对引起"直肠前突"的原因也没有统一的认识。似乎最合理的解释是直肠阴道隔的缺损（无论是先天性的，还是后发性的），而目前针对直肠阴道纵隔的解剖还存在争议。目前认为它是自会阴体至后穹窿阴道间的一层结缔组织，但这一观点没有被普遍接受。大多数直肠前突修补手术中也没有对这一层解剖结构进行仔细解剖。但是目前我们仍将直肠前突的主要原因归结于直肠阴道隔的缺损。这类缺损可以是先天性的，也可以是继发性的，有多种表现形式但主要是横向缺损（图28.1）[6]。缺损在正确的平面可以充分暴露，并得到有效的手术封闭。

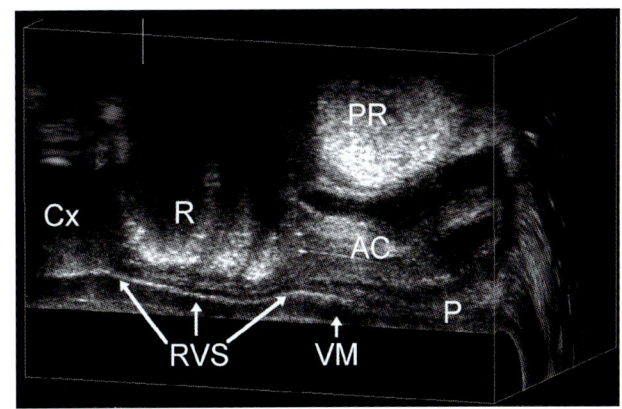

图 28.2 由三维彩超展示的阴道静息状态下直肠隔（RVS）结构：自会阴体（P）延伸至宫颈（Cx）的线形高回声影将阴道肌层（VM）和直肠壶腹部（R）、肛管（AC）分离开

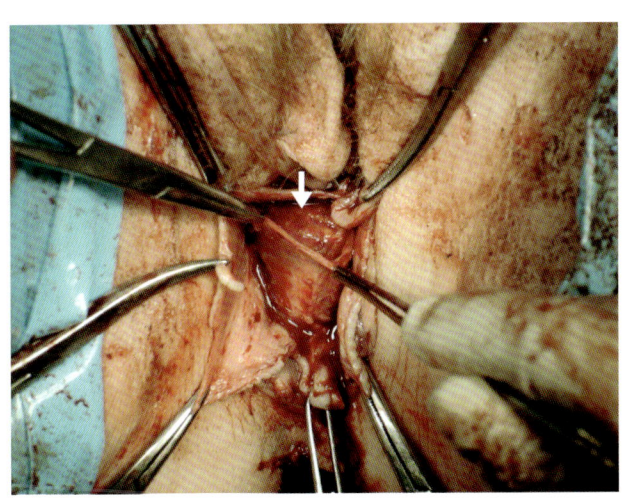

图 28.1 治疗直肠前突、便秘患者的手术中暴露阴道直肠隔的缺损，图中由镊子夹持出（箭头所指）

病 因

目前对直肠前突和直肠疝这一病症的定义仍存在争议，导致在直肠前突和直肠疝的病因学研究上更是少有进展。如果将直肠前突定义为直肠突入阴道内的疝气或憩室，那么必须有某处的解剖结构薄弱环节与之对应。换句话说，正常人需要某种屏障结构来维持阴道和直肠（腹内压）间的压力差，即耻骨直肠肌所维持的阴道内高压力区域[7]。很难理解这样的压力维持系统中居然没有一个强有力的筋膜组织，而仅仅是依靠阴道直肠膈或称为Denonvilliers筋膜。由于直肠阴道隔的缺损能引起直肠前突，因此其病因也应当归结于直肠阴道隔[6]。

阴道直肠膈很难进行检查，尽管似乎可以应用超声检查[8-9]，但首先这需要使用腔内探头（图28.2），这就不能进行功能评估，因为某些直肠前突和直肠疝症状需要负荷压力（如持续闭气用力）的情况下才能表现出来。我们可以通过尸体解剖[10-11]或经阴道手术时暴露显现直肠阴道隔的缺损（图28.1）。这类解剖需要非常谨慎，阴道直肠膈在阴道后壁纵行切开时往往会和阴道壁一起切开，而被忽视。这也许解释了为何这个解剖结构的重要性得不到关注。

因此，研究直肠前突的病因需要特殊的影像学检查。通过这些检查可能可以解释 10% 的年轻未生育女性患直肠前突的病因[12]，目前认为这类人群的体重指数和患病率相关。阴道分娩也是直肠前突的诱因和加重因素[13]。然而肛提肌裂隙的大小和肛提肌损伤的程度与直肠前突无明显相关性。[14-15]

慢性便秘、慢性腹压增加、肥胖都是直肠前突的诱因，有些特殊体质如（深盆腔）也认为能诱发直肠前突[6]。

直肠疝增加了直肠前突病因研究的复杂性。全子宫切除术是引起直肠疝的危险因素，因为术后引起的深盆腔结构[16]。有时，直肠疝气可以是先天性的，由于肛提肌裂隙引起，这种发生情况明显多于直肠前突[16]。然而，可以明确的是存在一个完整的直肠阴道纵隔防止直肠疝突入阴道内。这提示我们，任何肠疝修补术最重要的部分是重建阴道直肠膈。最后，会阴体在该病的发病机理中的作用尚不明确。几十年来，盆腔外科医生均表示成功的脱垂修补手术需要进行会阴体重建术，但没有试验来验证这一说法。

诊 断

对于妇科医师，诊断直肠前突和直肠疝往往是通过临床，虽然两者具体的区分需要通过手术。一般情况下，阴道后壁脱出（根据国际脱垂协会制定的标准测量）[17]往往暗示直肠前突而且不需要进一步诊断措施[6]。我相信，这样的理解是不全面的。临床上，将后壁组织脱出诊断为"直肠前突"，这忽视了至少5种情况能实际诊断为阴道后壁脱垂。一个Ⅱ度的直肠前突可能由于真正的直肠前突（如直肠阴道隔的缺陷），最常见的特征表现为脱垂、排便不全和不尽[18]。然而，如果肠管膨胀不全，而且有完整的直肠阴道隔，那么往往仅表现为脱垂。另一种情况是合并直肠疝气，这很少发生，比如孤立的直肠疝或者会阴缺损，但这给人一个"膨胀"的印象[19]。偶尔，直肠前突是直肠/肛门套叠的早期表现：在Valsalva方法中直肠壁反转进入肛管。很显然，光凭临床检查来诊断直肠前突是不够的[20]。

近20年来，对于直肠外科医师和放射科医生，直肠排便造影（DP）是诊断女性直肠前突的金标准，该技术的应用大幅提高了对该病的诊治[6]。然而，DP检查结果和临床检查结果、临床症状之间的关联很少[21]，因此限制了这项技术的应用推广。最近，动态磁共振显像和磁共振排便造影取得了很大的进步，尽管这个检查很贵、不方便、缺乏对胃肠道功能的评估。争论主要围绕磁共振检查下仰卧位排便方式能否反应生理状态下的排便方式，即使是取坐位造影或磁共振检查也同样面临这样的质疑。另外一个检查方法是超声，经肛门[22]或者经阴道[23]的超声检查。超声检查能最大程度的模拟排便的过程，同时又不需要过多的检查前准备，这简化了诊疗程序又缩减了费用和减轻了患者的痛苦[19]。这项技术最早由妇科医师为患者行腹部超声检查时应用[24-25]。直肠外科医生在检查时于肛门或者阴道内使用超声凝胶以形成对比，尽管粪便已经可以足够区分肠管和阴道。

超声检查方法比较容易被患者接受，但通过超声检查所测得的直肠前突面积要比通过DP检查的要大[28-29]。经阴道超声检查最大的优势是操作容易，并能同时评估阴道其他情况，比如尿道和其他盆底结构[30]。因此，该方法对诊断直肠前突是十分有必要的，因为很多女性患者排便障碍是由于合并其他盆底脏器的脱垂[31]。

在泌尿妇产科方面，患有直肠前突或者直肠疝的女性患者，很大一部分合并有尿失禁、脱垂等并发症。同时，阴道悬吊术最常见的远期并发症就是阴道后壁脱垂直肠膨出[32-33]。直肠前突往往没有症状，而仅仅表现为大便习性改变而造成梗阻症状[34]。然而，直肠前突患者往往会有表现为阴道出现包块，进而出现排便受阻症状，比如排便不尽、排便费劲、指压阴道包块以帮助排便等症状[18, 34]。妇科医生需要考虑、评估排便梗阻症状，而直肠外科医生需要注意阴道脱垂和膀胱功能障碍。因此两个学科需要沟通、合作共同治疗盆底功能障碍[31]。

直肠前突

直肠前突最典型的B超检查影像为直肠壶腹进入阴道后壁的憩室，该征象需要患者行Valsalva动作而不是在静息状态下（图28.3）。图28.4展现了一个典型的直肠前突患者行透视和超声检查的对比。成年女性很少患直肠前突，更多情况是某种形式的肠套叠（图28.5）。直肠前突通常包含有等回声或高回声的分辨，且通常会有肠管积气导致的反射回声。一些偶然情况下，壶腹部并没有粪便，而是被推进到直肠前突部位，从而使得它结构较小且被直肠黏液所填充。直肠前突的扩张度通常取决于粪便的存在及性质，它今天和明天的形态可能会大不相同。直肠前突的严重性可通过测量其疝囊向内突出的角度，并测量疝囊形成的最大深度进行量化（见图28.4，比较了一个直肠前突患者的超声影像和放射影像）。

图28.6和图28.7从三维和剖面（断层或多层）超声图像清晰显示直肠前突最常发生于直肠壶腹部，如前所述，前突没有"高"和"低"的区别。

直肠疝

直肠疝通常被描述为腹内容物下移形成阴道或者肛管膨出。这个现象在膀胱或者肠管充盈的情况下比较容易观察，因此临床上检查脱垂需要排空小便及大便。有时，患者不能排空则需要重复检查。小肠可以通过蠕动来辨别，有时腹腔内积液可以指示肠疝的顶端。肠疝很少有远侧的声影，往往表现为不规则的等回声区域或者片状区域（图28.8）。

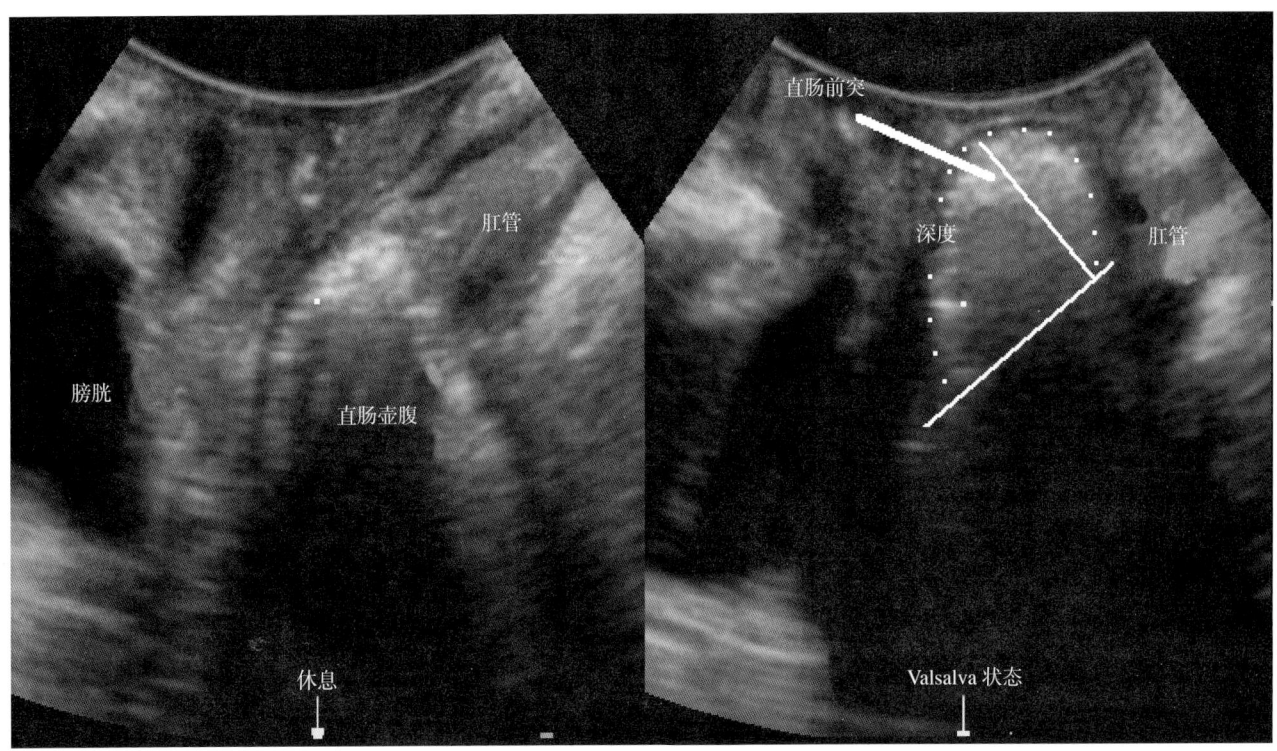

图 28.3 经阴道彩超显示了在休息和 Valsalva 状态下的盆底结构。两条垂直线显示了如何测量脱肛的深度：一条为肛管轮廓，垂直线测量深度，白点显示直肠前突的轮廓

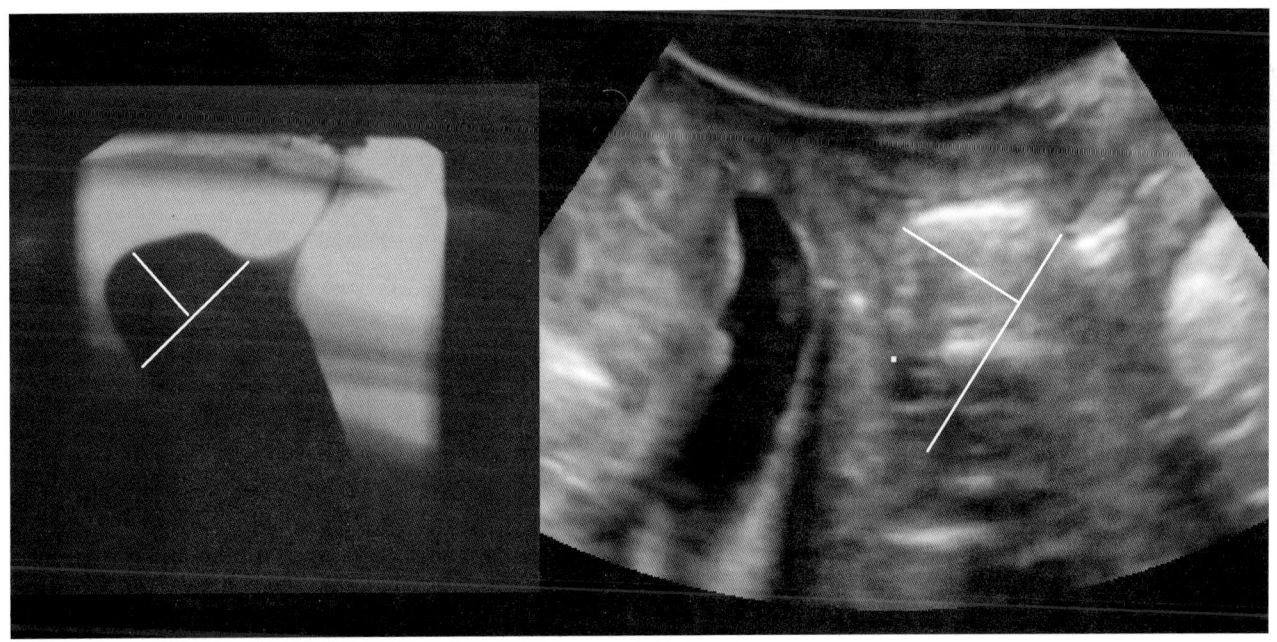

图 28.4 通过排便成像（左）和经阴道超声（右）显示的典型的直肠前突影像。成像质量很大程度受粪便质量影响，而且很多具有典型影像的患者是无症状的（Reprinted with permission from Perniola et al.[28]）。该阴道超声还显示了一个Ⅲ度的膀胱膨出

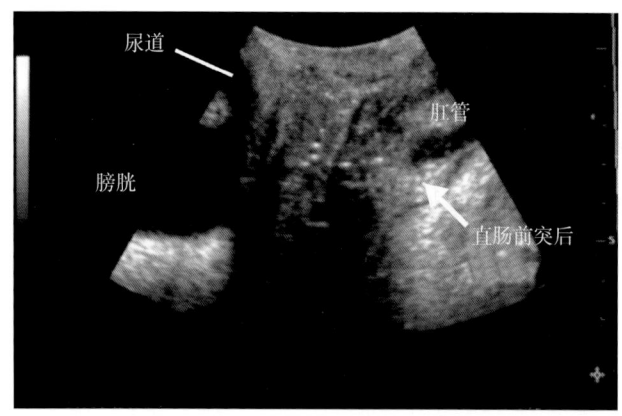

图 28.5 直肠前突（箭头所指）患者表现出排便梗阻症状，这种表现在成人中罕见

乙状结肠疝在超声检查中显示为不均质回声，易与直肠内容物相混淆（图 28.9）。一个特殊情况是直肠套叠，表现为直肠壶腹部前壁翻转突向肛管，致使肛管扩张。图 28.9 展现了直肠套叠患者的影像学检查和超声检查。通常，直肠套叠是由于小肠向下推进形成直肠疝，但是其他腹腔内容物如乙状结肠（图 28.9）、腹膜、子宫也可以由此方式形成直肠疝。最终，直肠黏膜和肌层完全从肛管内脱出，往往此时患者不会再求助于妇产科医生。

当直肠前突或者直肠疝经通过影像学检查进行诊断时，我们往往需要更好的成像效果，比如患者使劲时大便没有进入肛管而是进入阴道，或者小肠进入肛管，这都有助于诊断。最近几个研究显示，

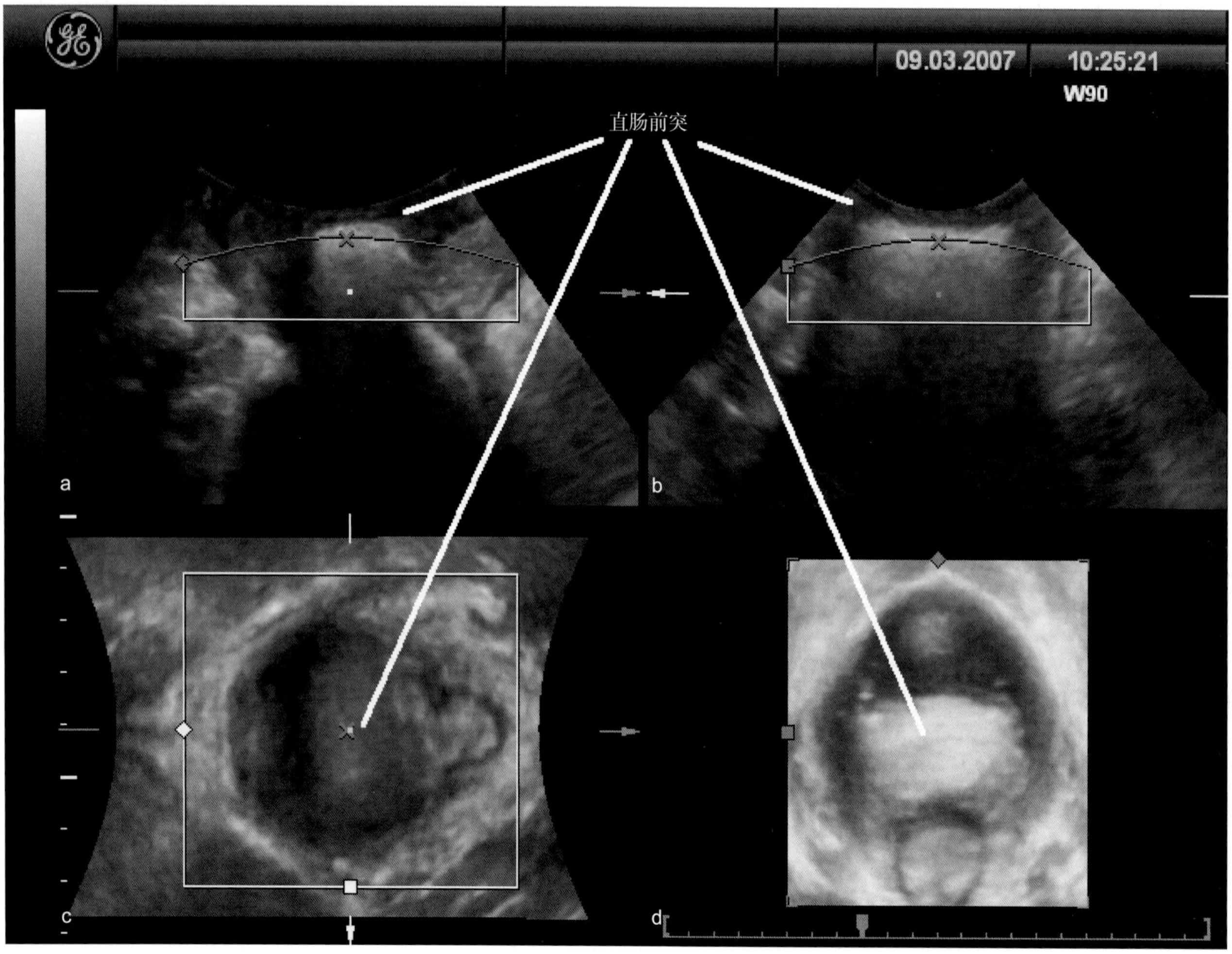

图 28.6 直肠前突的三维超声成像，显示壶腹部的憩室完全对称。(a) 矢状位图；(b) 冠状位图；(c) 水平位图；(d) 水平位图上显示容积

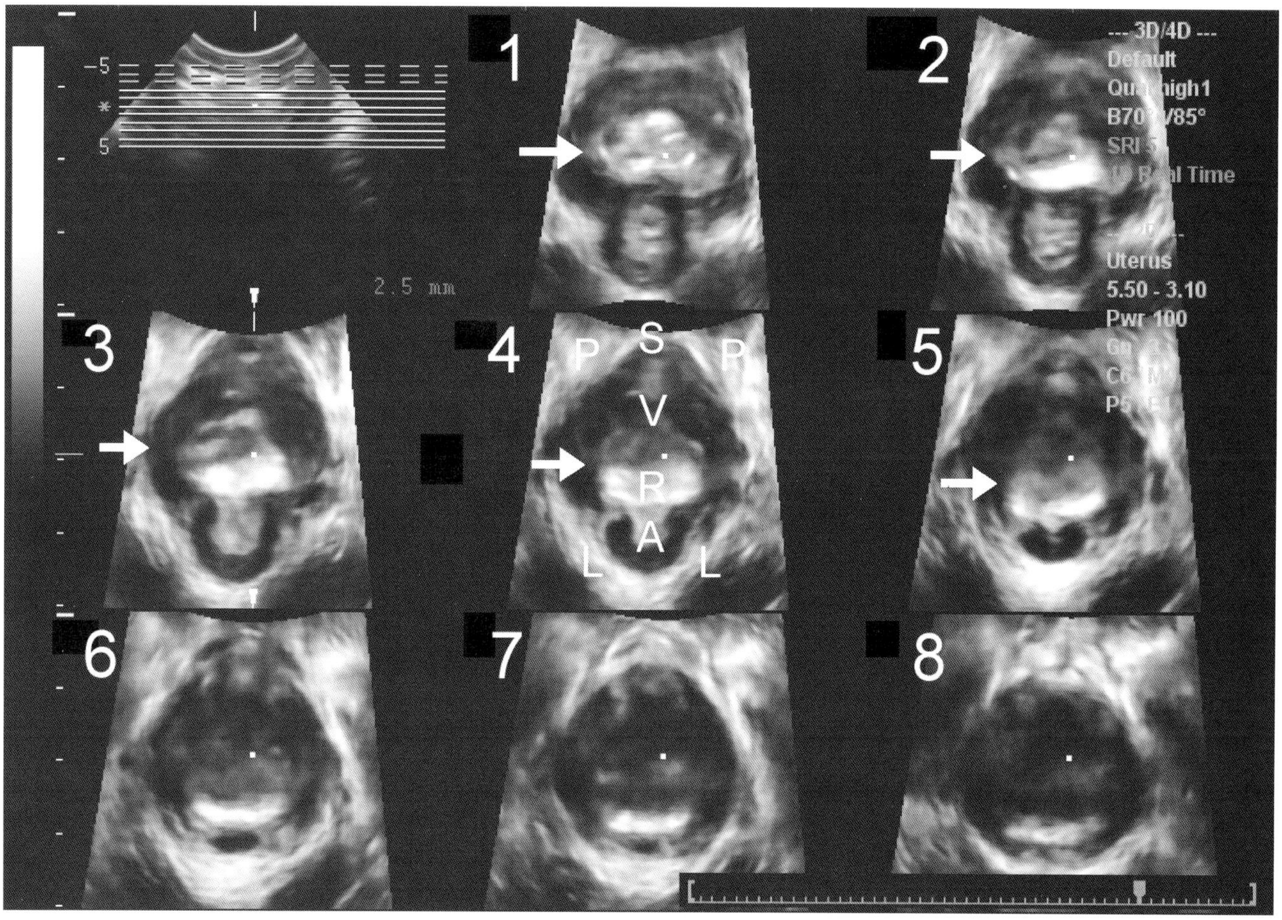

第 28 章 直肠前突与直肠疝：妇科医生的处理方式

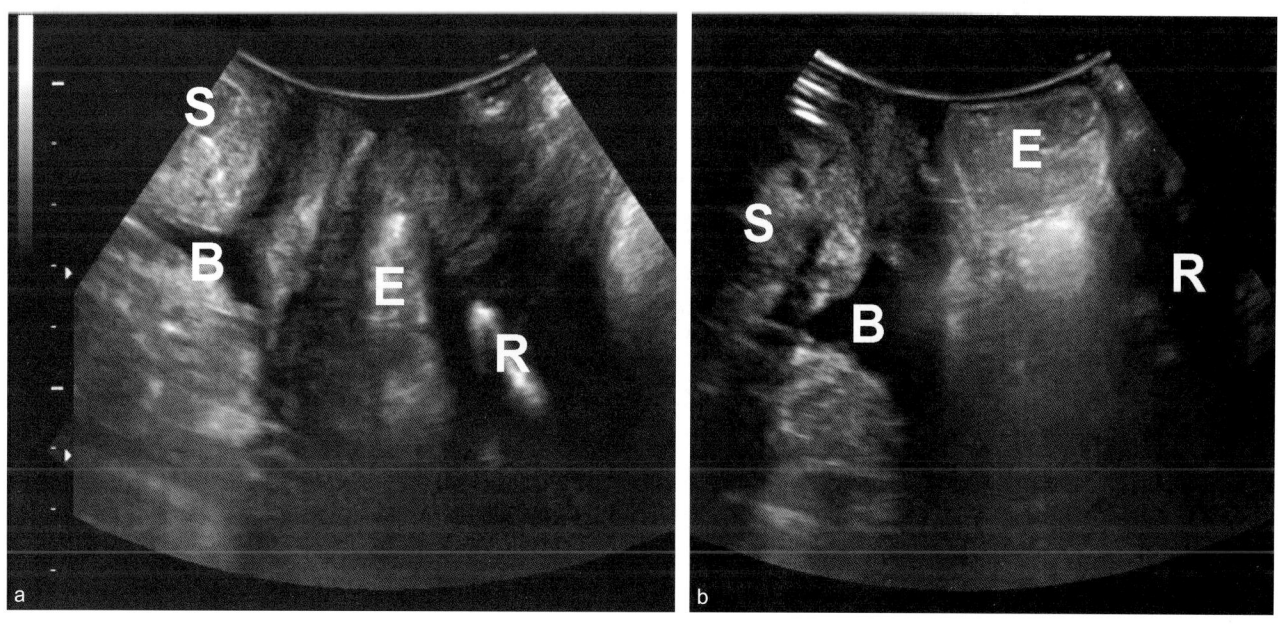

图 28.7 通过断层成像显示典型的直肠前突（R），显示前突部具有对称性，逐渐填满整个肛提肌裂孔。断层超声在最大 Valsalva 状态时观察测量，断层观察范围由 5mm 以下（1）至 12.5mm 以上（8）[55]，裂孔显示在断层 3，箭头所指为直肠前突。S：耻骨联合；P：耻骨支；V：阴道；R：直肠膨出；A：肛管；L：肛提肌

图 28.8 肠疝内容物为小肠，在矢状位平面所得图像，(a) 休息状态下 (b) Valsalva。S：耻骨联合；B：膀胱；R：直肠；E：肠体腔

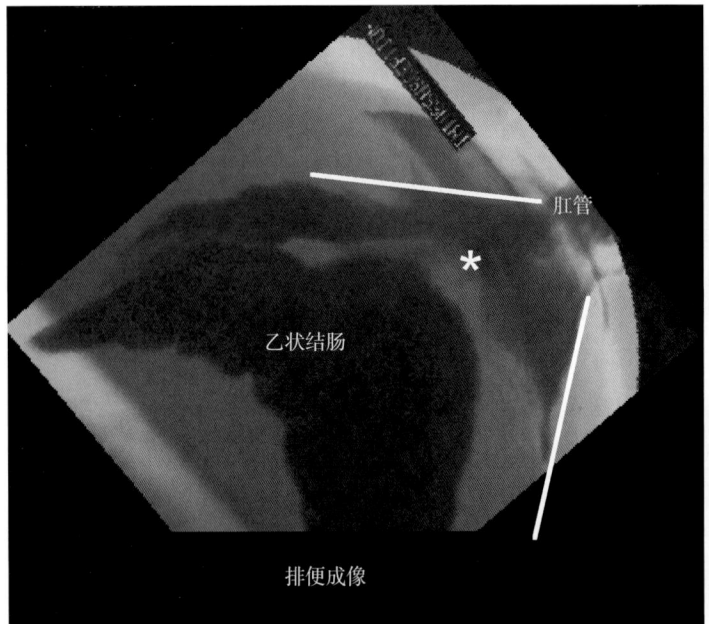
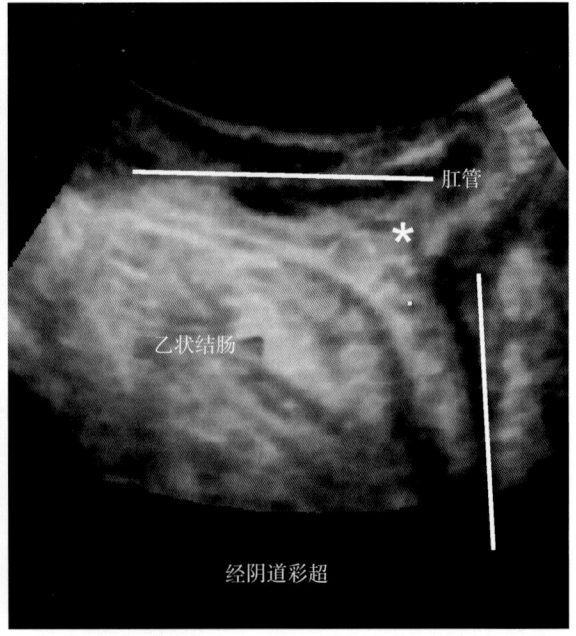

图 28.9 直肠肠套叠由于乙状结肠疝引起（*所指处），通过排便成像（左）和经阴道彩超（右）显示。一般很难分清小肠还是结肠引起了肠疝，从而促进肠套叠的形成，尽管该部位的疝囊较小肠明显粗大很多（Reprinted with permission from Perniola et al.[28]）

使用超声检查较 DP[28] 检查更容易被患者接受，由于其廉价、易操作，因此，超声检查将替代 DP 检查，尤其是盆底功能障碍的女性患者首次接受检查时，如果直肠前突或者肠套叠可以从超声检查判断，那么使用 X 线检查也能发现[28-29]。另外，肛门痉挛的患者（无法放松肛提肌）在测量直肠肛管角的过程中，也可因为排便而混淆了诊断。

治 疗

手术治疗直肠前突与直肠疝的目的在于恢复正常的解剖结构以缓解患者脱垂、便秘的症状。这两个目的与固定直肠盆底结构密切相关，包括缓解排便梗阻，尤其是排便不尽、难以排空的症状，还包括纠正阴道脱垂。纵向数据显示，肠道症状在接受直肠前壁修补和盆底结构重建后将会明显改善[35]。

阴道后壁修补术

阴道后壁修补术是治疗阴道后壁膨出的传统手术方式[36]，可追溯到 19 世纪末。该手术暴露会阴体及直肠壶腹部末端，通过压低肛门直肠后暴露肛提肌内侧面。将分离的两侧肛提肌通过缝合向中心区域集中[6]。最终在直肠阴道间建立一个隔板，不管是否存在阴道直肠隔缺陷，这都将能有效防止脱垂的发生。这个方法似乎对治疗临床上表现为明显脱垂的患者十分有效[37]，但这不能有效地治疗排便梗阻的症状[38-39]，并且会导致少数患者出现性交疼痛[38]。因此很多患者术后再行影像学检查时直肠前突的症状依旧存在，只是较术前略有减小[40]。

缺陷特异性修补术

该方法最早由 Richardson 发表[4,41]，使用阴道直肠膈来纠正直肠前突。2001 年该作者去世后，这个方法没有被广泛地推广，他的观点由于缺乏影像学的支持也没有得到广泛认可。该方法另一个难点在于需要极为仔细地解剖来使缺损结构移位，这个方法最适用于中心缺损的情况，但有时我们术中会发现两侧的缺损。不管它是两侧或是横向缺损，我们都需要通过手术将其修补。另外我们术中需要足够面积的隔来进行折叠缝合。

我认为缺陷特异性方法是现代功能影像所支持

的唯一的外科技术。当然，有很多患有阴道后壁脱垂的女性患者不适于使用直肠阴道隔缺陷重建：只有大约1/2到2/3的临床有"脱肛"的患者具有真正意义的直肠前突，也就是直肠阴道隔缺陷[19]。一般手术中发现阴道后壁脱垂的可能性不大，除非在术前已经经影像学证实了缺陷的存在。图28.1是典型的术中所见的直肠前突；图20.10则是手术封闭缺陷之前及术后的图像；图28.11显示了术前及术后的超声影像。虽然手术并非总是成功的，但是缺陷特异性方法很显然具有重组出完全正常的阴道直肠间结构的潜力。这对于直肠疝也同样适用，只要穿窿结构是完整的。如果不是这种情况，则该方法应该与骶阴道固定术结合[1]，使得直肠阴道隔完全封闭，指导骶缝线被束缚，或通过直肠阴道隔的侧缘融入穿窿悬浮缝合。该技术也可与穿窿与宫骶韧带[42]，或与骶棘韧带[43]的悬挂相结合，但我对这种方法并没有多少个人经验。

网 片

在过去10年中，阴道后壁脱垂的手术治疗多应用网片技术。首次应用于Peter Papa Petros所应用的阴道后路悬吊成形术，现在该技术已过时了。自此以后，网片技术就得到了广泛应用，可固定至坐骨直肠窝（例如Apogee™，美国医学系统，Minnetonka，MN）或固定至骶棘韧带（如posterior Elevate™，美国医学系统）。这大大增加了潜在的操作成本，在生物网片技术如猪异种移植中尤其是如此。目前尚无关于这些手术方法的预后数据，所以我们对于这些方法对直肠前突的治愈率并没有确切的结论。另一方面，这些手术具有潜在的网片侵蚀（4%～10%）、慢性疼痛、性交痛的风险[44]。正因为这些额外的并发症，这些技术在本章将不进行进一步的讨论。我认为，真正的直肠前突是不会被植入的网片或移植物所治愈的。最可能的结果是直肠前突突入隐性阴道的后方，且仍然带来显性或隐性的临床症状（图28.12）。也正是因为这样的原因，组织修复技术目前也未能得到广泛认可。

腹腔镜技术

腹腔镜技术并不适用于直肠前突的修复[3]，因为它难以关闭直肠阴道隔的缺陷，同样不适用于直肠疝的治疗。孤立肠疝，特别是穿窿脱垂所导致的孤立肠疝，可能通过腹腔镜技术进行治疗，但这一技术并非本章节介绍的范围。

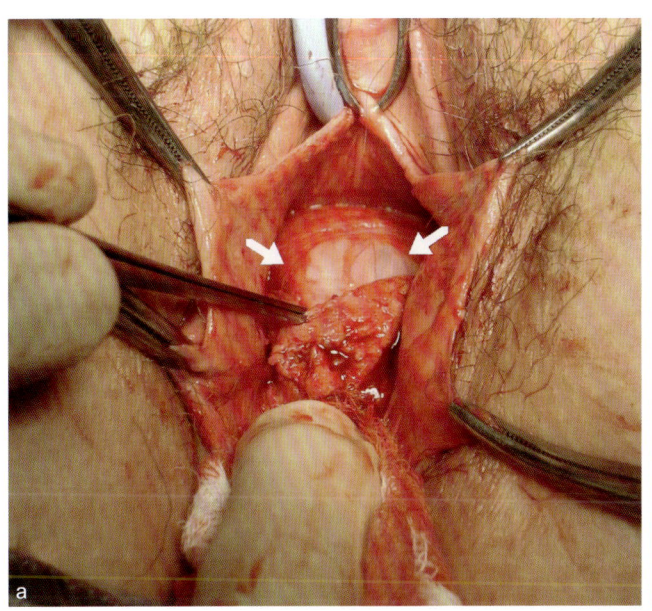 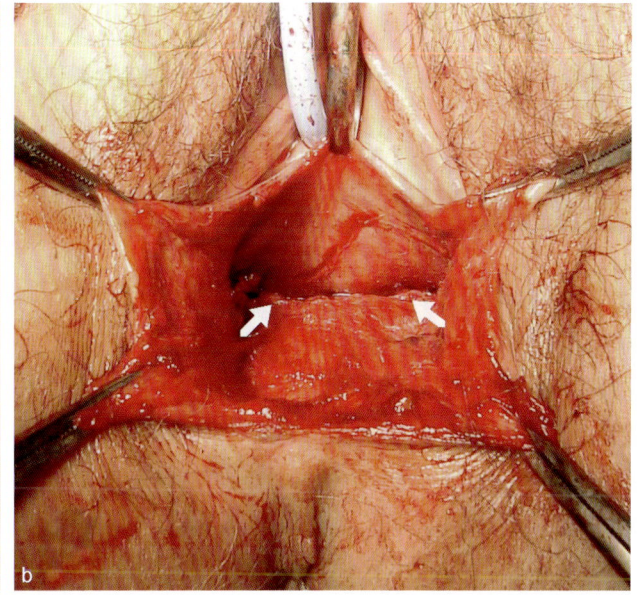

图28.10 缺陷特异性修补术。（a）显示修补术前，箭头所指为缺陷处；（b）为修补术后，箭头所指为缝线，实际缝线是不可见的。直肠阴道隔的缺损常见为横向、中心性的，如图所示

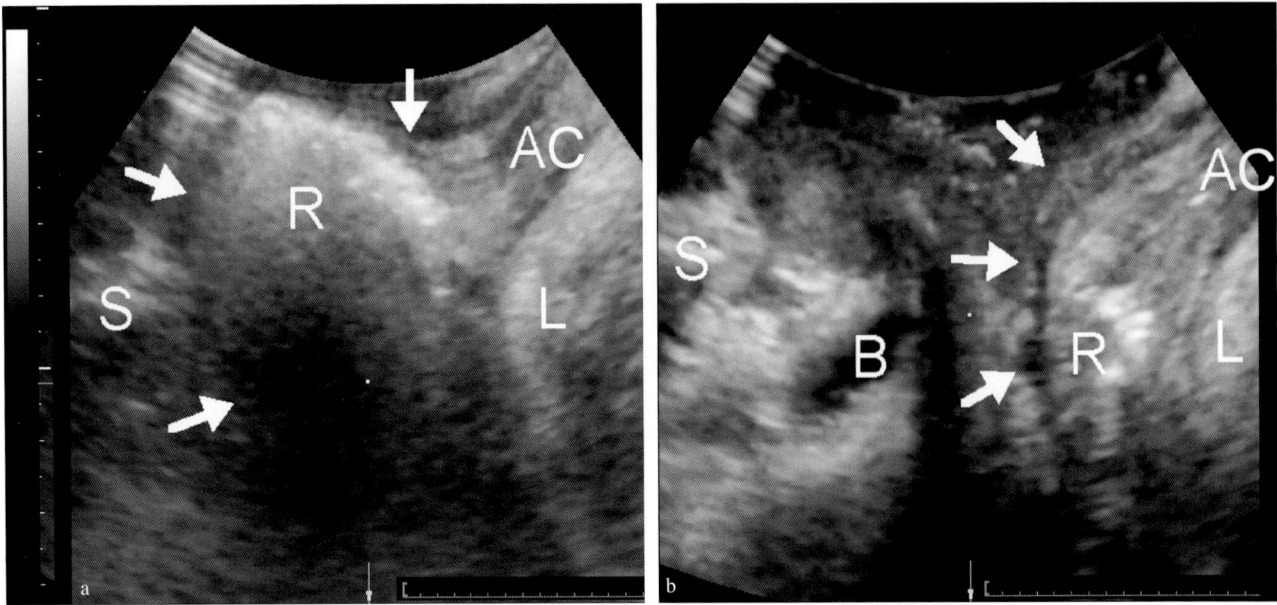

图 28.11 （a）为经典直肠前突的图像；（b）为行缺陷特异性修补术术后 3 个月的图像。S：耻骨联合，AC：肛管，R：左图代表直肠前突在，右图代表直肠壶腹部。缺陷特异性修补术如图 28.10 所示，后壁修补使用纤维网片加固，使用可吸收线缝合缺损部位。左图箭头所指为直肠前突，右图箭头所指为恢复正常形态的直肠壶腹部。B：膀胱；L：肛提肌

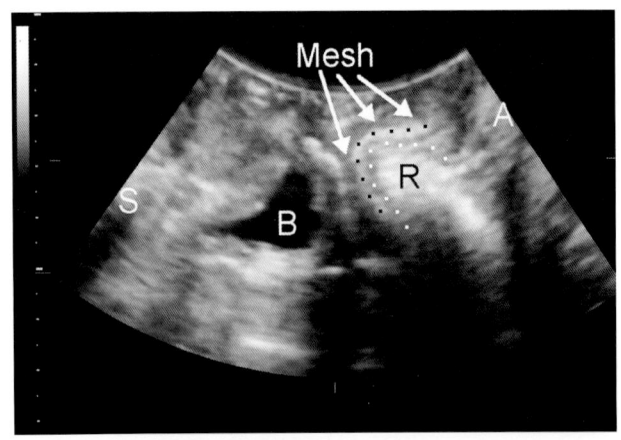

图 28.12 网片植入后形成的临床隐匿性直肠前突（箭头所指）。S：耻骨联合；B：膀胱；R：直肠前突（白点所示）；A：膀胱，黑点所指为网片的轮廓

临床证据

与不同直肠前突手术有关的临床证据有哪些呢？目前仅有极少的小型的随机对照试验（RCTs），其中两项研究指出肛门修复术要逊色于后壁修补术[36, 46]。另一项小型临床研究比较了后壁修补术、缺陷特异性修补术及移植术，发现后壁修补术及缺陷修补术在解剖学及功能学预后方面都是类似的。在术中增加一个猪源性移植物也并不能改善解剖学预后[47]。在许多文献中，手术技术并未得到充分的描述，而在部分研究中，所介绍的缺陷特异性修补术并不能修补影像学中所发现的所有缺陷。另外，通常看不到术后的图像，也并没有 RCT 使用影像资料作为前瞻性的研究结果。

在一个泌尿-妇科单位开展了一项非随机的回顾性临床研究，Abramov 等比较了缺陷特异性修补术、后壁修补术及中线筋膜折叠术，证实使用后壁修补术，临床复发及经常性脱垂的出现概率较低，而在性交痛及肠功能紊乱的发生率则无明显差异[48]。尽管如此，该研究在术前并未得到影像学证实，也就是说明在术前可能并非是一个真正的直肠前突。这是该类研究需面临的一个共同的问题[49-52]。另外，所用的描述方法与本章节所应用的影像学结果并不一致，研究结果更容易被混淆[50-53]。

最近的关于女性盆腔脏器脱垂的 Cochrane 评价（2010 更新）并未对后壁修补术及缺陷修补术进行比较。研究者指出经阴道手术与经肛手术相比，直肠前突或肠疝的发生率均较低（相对危险比为 0.24；95% 可信区间 0.09～0.64）。目前没有关于聚丙烯网片在后阴道隔修补术疗效的数据[54]。

结 论

现代影像学技术正逐步改变着我们看待盆底功能障碍的方式。这不仅适用于失禁和脱垂,对于肛门和直肠的功能学和形态学异常同样适用。最近,妇科医生将阴道后壁脱垂定义为"直肠前突"。现在已经清楚的是,阴道后壁脱垂至少由 5 种解剖结构异常导致,其中两种(直肠前突和直肠疝)很可能是因为直肠阴道隔或 Denonvilliers 筋膜的缺陷。这种缺陷可在术前经过影像学(超声、DP 或动态磁共振)进行诊断。考虑到成本、软组织分辨率、依从性及可获得性等多个因素,我认为在临床应用过程中,超声是最为方便的一种方式。

妇科医生通常使用 3 种方法来治疗直肠前突和直肠疝:后壁修补术,缺陷修补术及网片修补技术(合成物或异种移植物,如变性猪胶原蛋白)。从目前来看,没有一种方法能在解剖学上治愈,改善临床症状或者减少并发症等方面胜过另外两种方法。而达成一致的是缺陷修补术术后发生性交痛的概率较低。网片技术通常较贵,且常会伴随有网片侵蚀或疼痛综合征。从一个病理生理学家的角度看,基于影像学经验,缺陷修补技术稍好,因为一个真正的直肠前突也就是直肠阴道隔的缺陷,而缺陷修补技术很可能更好地关闭这类缺陷。遗憾的是,关于缺陷修补术的几项研究并没有术前及术后的影像学证实。我们期待着未来的临床研究能够克服这些瓶颈,从而为患者选择恰当的手术方式提供更多临床证据。

参考文献

1. Richter K, Albrich W. Long-term results following fixation of the vagina on the sacrospinal ligament by the vaginal route (vaginaefixatio sacrospinalis vaginalis). Am J Obstet Gynecol. 1981;141:811–6.
2. Miyazaki FS. Miya Hook ligature carrier for sacrospinous ligament suspension. Obstet Gynecol. 1987;70:286–8.
3. Kim D, Ghoniem G. The abdominal approach to urogenital prolapse. In: Santoro GA, Wieczorek AP, Bartram C, editors. Pelvic floor disorders. Milan: Springer Italia; 2010. p. 457–66.
4. Richardson AC. The rectovaginal septum revisited: its relationship to rectocele and its importance in rectocele repair. Clin Obstet Gynecol. 1980;36:976–83.
5. DeLancey J, Shobeiri SA. State of the art pelvic floor anatomy. In: Santoro GA, Wieczorek AP, Bartram CI, editors. Pelvic floor disorders. Milan: Springer Italia; 2010. p. 3–15.
6. Silva W, Karram M. Rectocele- anatomic and functional repair. In: Cardozo L, Staskin D, editors. Textbook of female urology and urogynecology. London: Informa Healthcare; 2006. p. 1036–51.
7. Jung S, Pretorius D, Padda B, Weinstein M, Nager C, den Boer D, et al. Vaginal high-pressure zone assessed by dynamic 3-dimensional ultrasound images of the pelvic floor. Am J Obstet Gynecol. 2007;197:52.e51–57.
8. Bignardi T, Condous G. Sonorectovaginography: a new sonographic technique for imaging of the posterior compartment of the pelvis. J Ultrasound Med. 2008;27:1479–83.
9. Dietz HP. Can the rectovaginal septum be visualised by transvaginal 3D ultrasound? Ultrasound Obstet Gynecol. 2011;37(3):348–52. doi:10.1002/uog.8896. Epub 2011 Jan 10.
10. Milley P, Nichols D. A correlative investigation of the human rectovaginal septum. Anat Rec. 1969;163:443–52.
11. Leffler KS, Thompson JR, Cundiff GW, Buller JL, Burrows LJ, Schon Ybarra MA. Attachment of the rectovaginal septum to the pelvic sidewall. Am J Obstet Gynecol. 2001;185:41–3.
12. Dietz H, Clarke B. The prevalence of rectocele in young nulliparous women. Aust N Z J Obstet Gynaecol. 2005;45:391–4.
13. Dietz HP, Steensma AB. The role of childbirth in the etiology of rectocele. Br J Obstet Gynaecol. 2006;113:264–7.
14. Dietz H, De Leon J, Shek K. Ballooning of the levator hiatus. Ultrasound Obstet Gynecol. 2008;31:676–80.
15. Dietz H, Simpson J. Levator trauma is associated with pelvic organ prolapse. Br J Obstet Gynaecol. 2008;115:979–84.
16. Baessler K, Schuessler B. Enterocele. In: Cardozo L, Staskin D, editors. Textbook of female urology and urogynecology. London: Informa Healthcare; 2006. p. 1023–34.
17. Bump RC, Mattiasson A, Bo K, Brubaker LP, DeLancey JO, Klarskov P, et al. The standardization of terminology of female pelvic organ prolapse and pelvic floor dysfunction. Am J Obstet Gynecol. 1996;175:10–7.
18. Dietz HP, Korda A. Which bowel symptoms are most strongly associated with a true rectocele? Aust N Z J Obstet Gynaecol. 2005;45:505–8.
19. Dietz HP, Steensma AB. Posterior compartment prolapse on two-dimensional and three- dimensional pelvic floor ultrasound: the distinction between true rectocele, perineal hypermobility and enterocele. Ultrasound Obstet Gynecol. 2005;26:73–7.
20. Burrows L, Sewell C, Leffler K, Cundiff GW. The accuracy of clinical evaluation of posterior vaginal wall defects. Int Urogynecol J Pelvic Floor Dysfunct. 2003;14:160–3.
21. Kenton K, Shott S, Brubaker L. The anatomic and functional variability of rectoceles in women. Int Urogynecol J Pelvic Floor Dysfunct. 1999;10:96–9.
22. Dietz H. Ultrasound imaging of the pelvic floor: part 1: 2D aspects. Ultrasound Obstet Gynecol. 2004;23:80–92.
23. Santoro GA, Wieczorek AP, Dietz HP, Mellgren A, Sultan A, Shobeiri SA, et al. State of the art: an integrated approach to pelvic floor ultrasonography. Ultrasound Obstet Gynecol. 2010. doi:10.1002/uog.8816.
24. Creighton SM, Pearce JM, Stanton SL. Perineal video-ultrasonography in the assessment of vaginal prolapse: early observations. Br J Obstet Gynaecol. 1992;99:310–3.
25. Dietz HP, Haylen BT, Broome J. Ultrasound in the quantification of female pelvic organ prolapse. Ultrasound Obstet Gynecol. 2001;18:511–4.
26. Beer-Gabel M, Teshler M, Barzilai N, Lurie Y, Malnick S, Bass D, et al. Dynamic transperineal ultrasound in the diagnosis of pelvic floor disorders: pilot study. Dis Colon Rectum. 2002;45:239–45.
27. Beer-Gabel M, Teshler M, Schechtman E, Zbar AP. Dynamic transperineal ultrasound vs. defecography in patients with evacuatory difficulty: a pilot study. Int J Colorectal Dis. 2004;19:60–7.
28. Perniola G, Shek K, Chong C, Chew S, Cartmill J, Dietz H. Defecation proctography and translabial ultrasound in the investigation of defecatory disorders. Ultrasound Obstet Gynecol. 2008;31:567–71.
29. Steensma AB, Oom DMJ, Burger C, Schouten W. Assessment of posterior compartment prolapse: a comparison of evacuation proctography and 3D transperineal ultrasound. Colorectal Dis. 2010;12:533–9.

30. Dietz H. Ultrasound imaging of the pelvic floor: 3D aspects. Ultrasound Obstet Gynecol. 2004;23:615–25.
31. Dietz HP. The elephant's other bits. Tech Coloproctol. 2009;13:285–6.
32. Wiskind AK, Creighton SM, Stanton SL. The incidence of genital prolapse after the Burch colposuspension. Am J Obstet Gynecol. 1992;167:399–404, discussion 404–5.
33. Dietz HP, Wilson PD. Colposuspension success and failure: a long-term objective follow-up study. Int Urogynecol J Pelvic Floor Dysfunct. 2000;11:346–51.
34. Dietz H. Rectocele or stool quality: what matters more for symptoms of obstructed defecation? Tech Coloproctol. 2009;13:265–8.
35. Gustilo-Ashby A, Paraiso M, Jelovsek J, Walters M, Barber M. Bowel symptoms 1 year after surgery for prolapse: further analysis of a randomized trial of rectocele repair. Am J Obstet Gynecol. 2007;197:76e1–5.
36. Nichols DH, Randall CL. Posterior colporrhaphy and perineorrhaphy. In: Nichols DH, Randall CL, editors. Vaginal surgery. Baltimore: Williams & Wilkins; 1996. p. 257–89.
37. Kahn MA, Stanton SL, Kumar D, Fox SD. Posterior colporrhaphy is superior to the transanal repair for treatment of posterior vaginal wall prolapse. Neurourol Urodyn. 1999;18:329–30.
38. Kahn MA, Stanton SL. Posterior vaginal wall prolapse and its management. Contemp Rev Obstet Gynaecol. 1997;9:303–10.
39. Kahn MA, Stanton SL. Posterior colporrhaphy: its effects on bowel and sexual function [see comments]. Br J Obstet Gynaecol. 1997;104:82–6.
40. Qatawneh AM, Maher CF, Schluter PL. Posterior colporrhaphy for rectocele and obstructed defecation. Obstet Gynecol. 2002;13:S38.
41. Richardson AC. The anatomic defects in rectocele and enterocele. J Pelvic Surg. 1996;1:214–21.
42. Raz S, Nitti VW, Bregg KJ. Transvaginal repair of enterocele. J Urol. 1993;149:724–30.
43. Maher CF, Murray CJ, Carey MP, Dwyer PL, Ugoni AM. Iliococcygeus or sacrospinous fixation for vaginal vault prolapse. Obstet Gynecol. 2001;98:40–4.
44. Feiner B, Jelovsek J, Maher C. Efficacy and safety of transvaginal mesh kits in the treatment of prolapse of the vaginal apex: a systematic review. Br J Obstet Gynaecol. 2009;116:15–24.
45. Petros P. Total pelvic floor reconstruction. In: Santoro GA, Wieczorek AP, Bartram C, editors. Pelvic floor disorders. Milan: Springer Italia; 2010. p. 485–91.
46. Farid M, Madbouly K, Hussein A, Mahdy T, Moneim H, Omar W. Randomized controlled trial between perineal and anal repairs of rectocele in obstructed defecation. World J Surg. 2010;34:822–9.
47. Paraiso M, Barber M, Muir T, Walters M. Rectocele repair: a randomized trial of three surgical techniques including graft augmentation. Am J Obstet Gynecol. 2006;195:1762–71.
48. Abramov Y, Gandhi S, Goldberg RP, Botros SM, Kwon C, Sand PK. Site-specific rectocele repair compared with standard posterior colporrhaphy. Obstet Gynecol. 2005;105:314–8.
49. Cundiff GW, Weidner AC, Visco AG, Addison WA, Bump RC. An anatomic and functional assessment of the discrete defect rectocele repair. Am J Obstet Gynecol. 1998;179:1451–6.
50. Singh K, Cortes E, Reid W. Evaluation of the fascial technique for surgical repair of isolated posterior vaginal wall prolapse. Obstet Gynecol. 2003;101:320–4.
51. Porter W, Steele A, Walsh P, Kohli N, Karram M. The anatomic and functional outcomes of defect-specific rectocele repairs. Am J Obstet Gynecol. 1999;181:1353–8.
52. Glavind K, Madsen H. A prospective study of the discrete fascial defect rectocele repair. Acta Obstet Gynecol Scand. 2000;79:145–7.
53. Kenton K, Shott S, Brubaker L. Outcome after rectovaginal fascia reattachment for rectocele repair. Am J Obstet Gynecol. 1999;181:1360–3.
54. Maher C, Feiner B, Baessler K, Adams EJ, Hagen S, Glazener CM. Surgical management of pelvic organ prolapse in women. Cochrane Database Syst Rev. 2007:CD004014;PMID: 17636742.
55. Dietz H, Shek K, Clarke B. Biometry of the pubovisceral muscle and levator hiatus by three-dimensional pelvic floor ultrasound. Ultrasound Obstet Gynecol. 2005;25:580–5.

第五篇
大便失禁的再手术

引 言

Steven D. Wexner

仅仅在 20 余年前，大便失禁患者的外科治疗还仍局限于直接或折叠的括约肌成形术、Parks 直肠后修补术和造口重建等有限的术式。虽然相关报道中，这些传统的括约肌修补术的早期成功率能够达到 85%，甚至更高；但是，在研究周期更长的相关报道中，成功率却都不理想，通常在 15% 左右。而直肠后修补的成功率则更会降至 30% 左右。

由于年轻的患者及一些女性患者迫切需要能替代造口的方法，促进了大便失禁的手术治疗在近些年得到了全面的进步。对于括约肌功能的治疗，除了传统的修补和改道之外，目前主要有 3 大类新的治疗方式：替代、增加及刺激。在过去的 20 年中，臀大肌和股薄肌都被用于移植到肛管周围，而后者的应用受到了更多的认可。此外，一些新的人工合成材料，包括近几年来发展起来的磁性肛门括约肌，也被应用于肛门括约肌功能欠佳的患者。

第二类改善肛门括约肌功能的方法是通过黏膜下或括约肌间注射各种填充剂，同时能够释放射频能量，以支持肛门的收缩机制以及肛门黏膜下悬吊系统。

最后一类治疗措施包括骶神经刺激，以及近些年发展起来的胫后神经刺激。尽管现在的功能性中枢系统成像似乎表明，可以通过调节大脑中枢与棘上神经间的功能性反射，达到神经活动的可控性，但这种神经刺激方法的具体机制仍不是很清楚。此外，包括结肠顺行灌洗术（malone antegrade continent enema，MACE）在内的肠管改道术式也被用于治疗大便失禁。

随着我们对这些新术式经验的不断增长，我们评估和处理治疗失败的知识也越来越丰富。本篇共包括 7 章，撰写这 7 章的专家及他们的团队在文中分享了他们在实际工作中的成功经验及失败的情况，增加了我们对这些新术式的理解。我们可以通过这些经验制定更好的诊断和治疗大便失禁的临床策略。

第 29 章 重复括约肌成形术

Brooke H. Gurland · Massarat Zutshi
张　林 译　　王荫龙 审校

摘　要

在出现骶神经调节的时代，肛门外括约肌有显而易见的缺陷、甚至出现肛门失禁的患者可能是合适的人选。括约肌修补的最终位置不断发展，但重复进行此过程的作用存有争议。在美国，重叠肛门括约肌修复虽然已经取得了与直接修补受损伤肌肉两端类似的结果，但仍是肛门外括约肌断裂的失禁的女性患者的手术选择。重复括约肌成形术，既不需要专门的设备，也不需高级的训练，是一个可行的选择。通过经验丰富的结直肠外科医生的一期修补，获得最好的结果，肛门持久良好功能，超声检测括约肌没有缺陷。本章将详细介绍肛门失禁患者括约肌修补的位置及其技术。

关键词

重复括约肌成形术；大便失禁；括约肌创伤；神经性损伤；直肠内超声；重复重叠肛门括约肌修复

引　言

既往健康的年轻女性，阴道分娩导致的直接括约肌创伤或神经损伤，是大便失禁发展过程中的主要致病因素[1]。在美国，重叠肛门括约肌修复虽然已经取得了与直接修补受损伤肌肉两端类似的结果，但仍是肛门外括约肌解剖结构上断裂的失禁的女性患者的手术选择[2]。重叠肛门括约肌修复适合于任何类型的创伤性肛门括约肌损伤的修补，但最常用于产科创伤后的修复。重叠括约肌修复后的持续性大便失禁的患者可能有残留的肛门括约肌前壁缺损[3]，特别是在它的前端范围[4]。重复括约肌成形术，既不需要专门的设备，也不需高级的训练，显然是一个可行的选择，通过经验丰富的结直肠外科医生的一期修补，获得肛门持久良好功能，超声检测括约肌没有缺陷[5]。特定的患者中，一个持久的肛门外括约肌缺损患者，重复括约肌修复功能的结果等同于那些一期修补结果[6-7]。

患者的确定

当患者在括约肌修补后又出现持续性大便失禁，以下是确定最佳治疗方案的重要考虑因素：

1. 排便习惯
2. 患者年龄
3. 肥胖
4. 复发的时间
5. 症状的轻重
6. 局部的体格检查
7. 直肠内超声检查

排便习惯

当括约肌功能减弱时，稀便或水样便可能会导致大便失禁。膨胀剂和止泻药旨在增加肠液的浓度和减少排便次数，仍然是括约肌成形术后的第一线疗法。直到排便习惯达到医学上的调节前，不应采用重复修补。

患者年龄

随着时间的推移，衰老的组织不太可能恢复和保持其质量。一些回顾性的分析表明，老年妇女有肛门直肠功能障碍，并随着时间的推移而恶化[8-9]。随着年龄的增长，可伴有其他盆底缺陷，包括纤维化增加和胶原沉积[10]。然而，文献中关于年龄的影响是相互矛盾的，一些研究表明，年龄并没有影响一期括约肌修复的结果[11-12]。每个案例都应单独考虑，需考虑如组织的质量和肛门肌肉收缩等因素是否是重复外科修补的禁忌证，而不仅仅是实际年龄。

肥　胖

高体重指数常伴随着较差的括约肌成形术后的预后[8]。肥胖妇女可能有其他因素促使她们发生失禁，如过度下降的盆底和糖尿病。虽然肥胖不是重复修复的禁忌，但病态肥胖患者可能无法达到与其他患者相同的成功率。在对这些患者考虑进行修复时，患者和医生的期望值均应该调整。

复发的时间

括约肌成形术后不久出现的持续性或复发性大便失禁，可能是由于肛门括约肌断裂造成的，在这种情况下，直肠内超声证明括约肌缺损征象是重复括约肌成形术的最佳适应证。直肠内超声提示已经完整修复的患者，不可能受益于重复括约肌成形术，其大便失禁应考虑其他治疗方式。成功修复后1年（或以上）复发的大便失禁，往往有多方面的原因，最可能的有括约肌及括约肌周围组织纤维化或萎缩，排便习惯改变，或进行性神经功能障碍（阴部神经病变及骶前神经丛病变）。直肠内超声提示存在括约肌缺损是重复括约肌成形术的指征。

症状的轻重

即使成功修复括约肌后，仍可能存在轻度大便失禁症状或仅气体失禁，尽管不完美，患者也认为比术前得到了很大的改善。最初成功的一期括约肌修复术，也会随着时间的推移，出现术后复发恶化的症状，这一潜在风险，术前应在手术期望值方面告知患者[13]。严重的大便失禁症状不排除重复括约肌成形术，Nikiteas 等[8]研究发现，症状严重的患者，进行一期修复实际上结果更好。这个结论并没有在重复括约肌成形术后的相关文献中检索到。

局部的体格检查

肛门括约肌肌肉松懈或肛门扩张可能与直肠黏膜或全层脱垂有关。体格检查时发现肛门括约肌收缩力降低（或消失），对括约肌修复术来说是预后不良的标志，因为它代表了肛门括约肌功能整体缺乏。为了取得最好的功能，Vaizey 等[6]报道良好的肌肉体积是一个重要的选择标准。

直肠内超声检查

直肠内超声显示残留的括约肌前壁缺损，同时临床检查时提示肛门外括约肌功能良好，是重复重叠肛门括约肌修复术的主要适应证。虽然目前还没有可用的文献或随机数据，但出现某些超声征象时，不应行重复外科修复，这包括混杂回声的肛门外括约肌（表示萎缩的肌肉）、非常薄的肛门内括约肌或大的（超过120°）肛门外括约肌缺损。

外科病例

接受过重复括约肌成形术的患者可能有更广泛的瘢痕组织，整块重叠的外部和内部肛门括约肌修复比层状修复效果更好。在一期修复中，已经表明，当肛门内括约肌基本完好时会获得更好的持久的结果[14]，最近的证据表明，独立的外部和内部肛门括约肌的缝合可改善肛门功能[15]。在一期修复中，我们建议避免涉及大范围的肛门外括约肌，以避免进一步的阻断血运和肌肉去神经化。

结 果

无论是术前或在游离括约肌时，括约肌修复的成功依赖于组织的质量、完整性和邻近范围的修复，以及神经是否损伤。事实上几乎没有关于重复括约肌成形术效果的文献。Giordano 等[7]进行回顾性评价来确定重叠括约肌成形术后的结果是否受前次手术影响，重复括约肌修复术是否是一个明智的选择。他们比较了接受一期括约肌修复术的 115 例患者和 36 例之前至少经历了 1 次修复术（1~7 次手术）的患者。残余前壁缺损的患者中，有 62% 成功地接受了重复括约肌成形术。这项研究并没有找到年龄、阴道分娩次数、会阴切开术、术前阴部神经末端运动潜伏期与临床效果的相关性。然而，增加重复修复的次数会导致功能变差的结果。

Vaizey 等[6]评估进行重复括约肌修复的患者：在 20 个月到 60 个月中，21 例患者中有 14 例患者出现了 50%（甚至更高）的症状改善，其中 60% 在 5 年的随访中症状持续改善。这些结果可以和一期修复的结果相媲美。在一项类似研究中，Pinedo 等[16]对 23 例患者进行了 3 年的随访。依据他们的 Wexner 评分和推迟排便能力，其中 15 例改善了 50%。以前修复的次数、患者的年龄或是预防性结肠造口术，都没有影响成功率。直肠肛门压力测定提示直肠静息和排便压力没有改善的患者，总体的结果较差，那些未能改善的患者，超声检查会明显提示一个永久的括约肌缺陷。目前没有数据显示一期或二期括约肌修复中，前壁上提成形术的优势，往往这个过程和患者的年龄独立相关，因为它的易用性和经会阴入路上提的相近性[17-19]。重复前括约肌成形术和上提成形术的手术照片见图 29.1a-f。

其他方案

当括约肌成形术失败，其他治疗大便失禁的方案包括骶神经刺激、植入人工肛门括约肌、肛门后修复、电刺激股薄肌成形术或结肠造口术。骶神经刺激已经被用于治疗大便失禁超过 10 年，对于有或无括约肌缺陷的患者，均具有良好的效果[20-23]。骶神经刺激的长期结果令人满意（长达 7 年）[24-25]；然而在美国，这种方法仍然没有批准作为大便失禁的主要适应证，因为合并粪便和尿失禁的患者是被限制使用的。

在欧洲，骶神经调节在有明确的肛门外括约肌缺损患者中的成功，使研究者们对正式肛门括约肌成形术的作用提出了疑问。有限的数据显示[26]，大多数此类患者临时刺激成功后，向着永久性地植入，并伴随着生活质量的显著改善，因为骶神经刺激影响了生活方式、应对行为、抑郁、自我认知得分和困境得分[27]。英国赫尔的 Brouwer 和 Duthie[27]研究，随访了 37 个月（15~41 个月）。尽管研究者改善了所有患者的控便得分，而直肠内超声看到括约肌缺损的患者、阴部神经病变的患者、经历过括约肌修复术的患者，均在随访期间恢复到治疗前的控便得分。

最近，Ratto 等[28]从罗马报道了类似的数据。他们的小样本随机试验对比经过完整的括约肌成形术（如直肠内超声确认）和肛门外括约肌缺损接受骶神经调节的患者，中位随访 60 个月后，结果无显著差异。骶神经调节的持久性获得成功，其适应证为出现大便失禁和明确的肛门外括约肌缺损的亚组患者，它将会对此条件下简单的正规的括约肌成形术产生显著的影响，包括一期和再次手术的制定。目前，在美国相对缺乏可用性的骶神经刺激并局限于某些特定的中心，缺乏更广泛的认可，骶神经调节的成本也或多或少阻碍它在临床的扩展应用。重复括约肌成形术的初步效果是能改善大多数患者功能（尽管随着时间的推移，功能逐渐降低），使其仍能在较小的中心，由有经验的结直肠病专家实施可接受的治疗。骶神经刺激可获得良好、长期的疗效，并使专家更好地了解亚群，当出现糟糕的长期结局时对其进行评估，解决这一重要问题。当括约肌缺陷时，可决定行括约肌成形术[29]。

人工肛门括约肌仍然是可行的，能得到可接受的结果，虽然这种技术的使用在减少，因为即使专家手术，报道的感染率仍为 33%[30-31]。人工肛门括约肌再手术率比较高，在许多情况下导致设备故障或挤压，不是特别适用于括约肌成形术失败后大便失禁复发的患者。肛管后修复被用于神经性失禁，但因为无法复制其先前的结果并不流行。报道中最多只有约 30% 的患者有持续改善[32-35]，虽然一些长期研究已显示良好的功能结局[36-37]。目前还不清楚正规盆底修复（即重叠肛门前括约肌成形术加肛管后修复）对神经性失禁复发的病例能否提供任何显著的功能优势[38]。在肛门外括约肌的质量较差、游离困难的病例中，可选择肌肉瓦状重叠（无分离）联合其他盆底修复操作，本组病例有相对少的数据[39]。

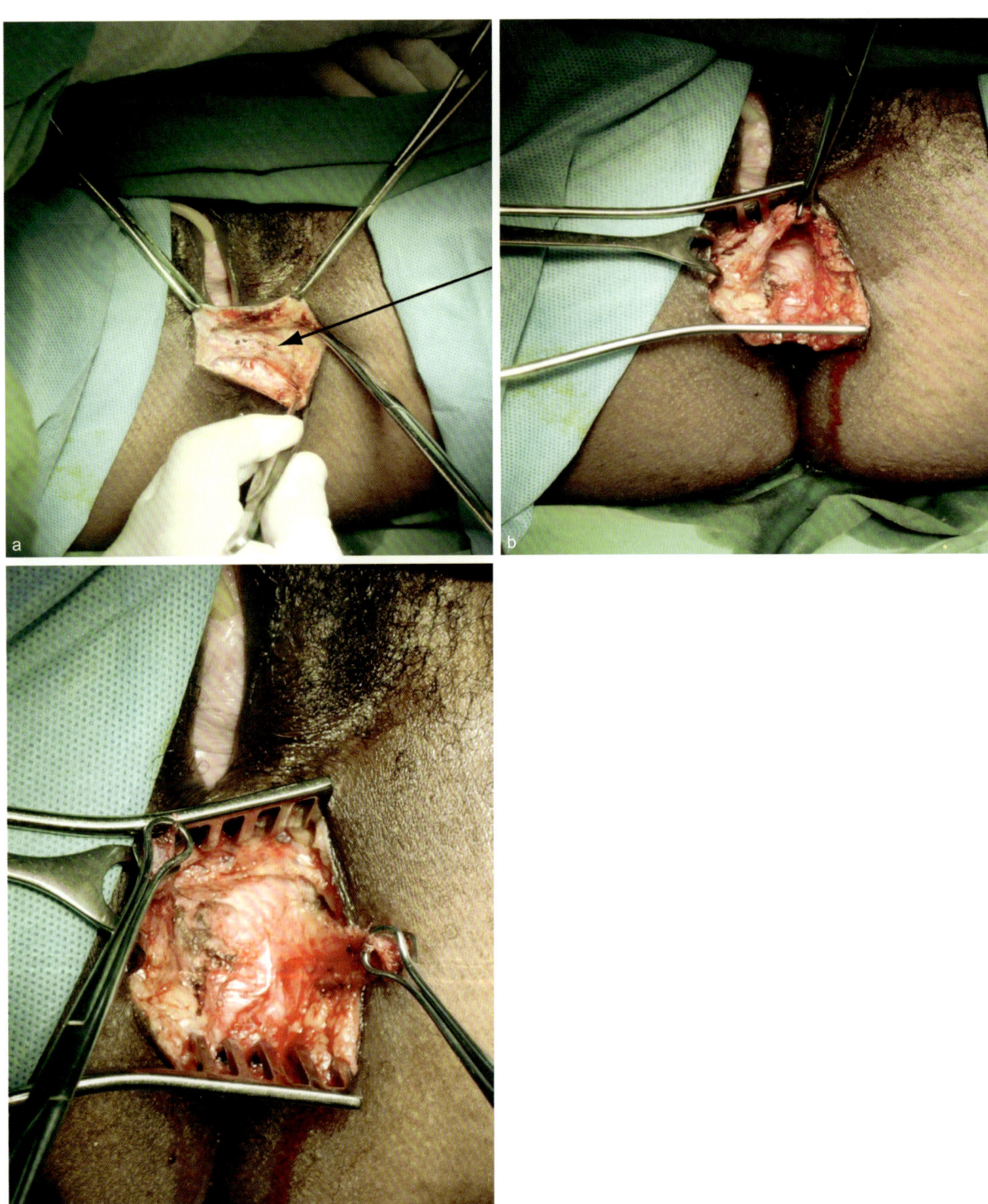

图 29.1 (a) 会阴解剖薄弱的肛门外括约肌（箭头）。(b)Babcock 手术钳夹持的修复前的萎缩组织。(c) 重复重叠修复中分离和游离肛门外括约肌。(d) 重叠肛门外括约肌成形术。(e) 完成重叠肛门外括约肌成形术。(f) 伴随的前壁上提成形术（解开缝合）（Photos courtesy of A. P. Zbar）

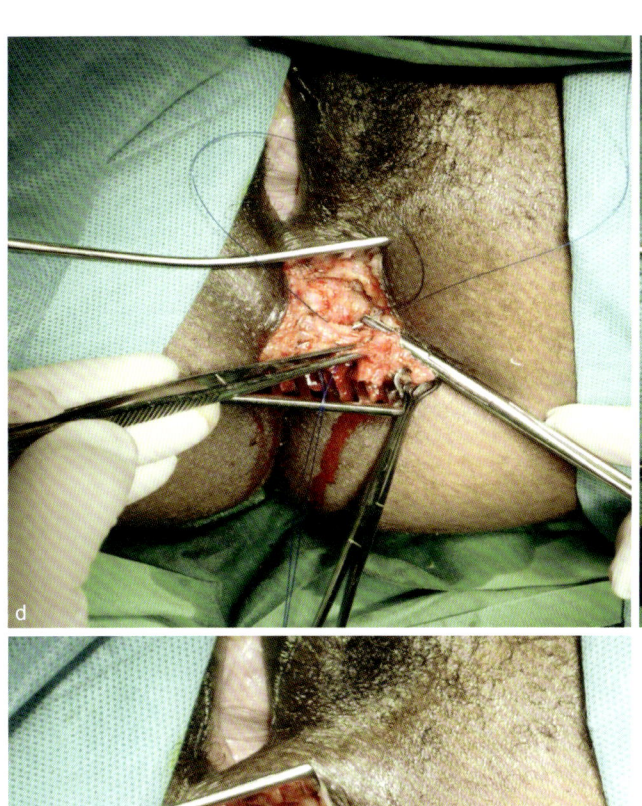
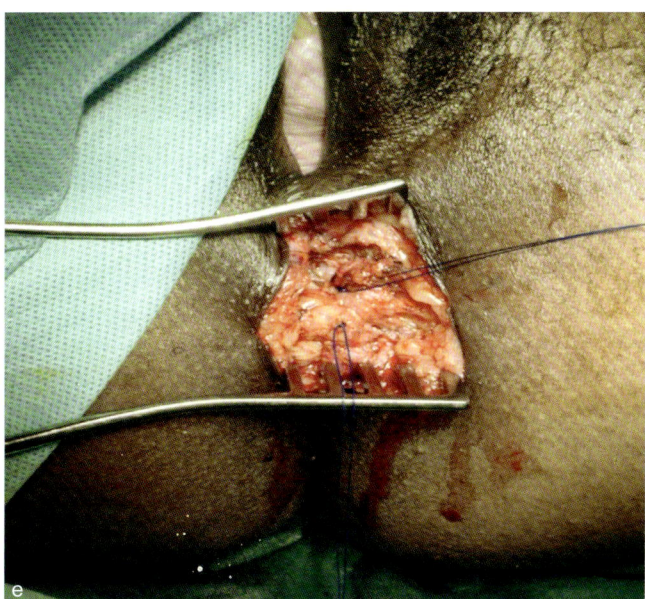
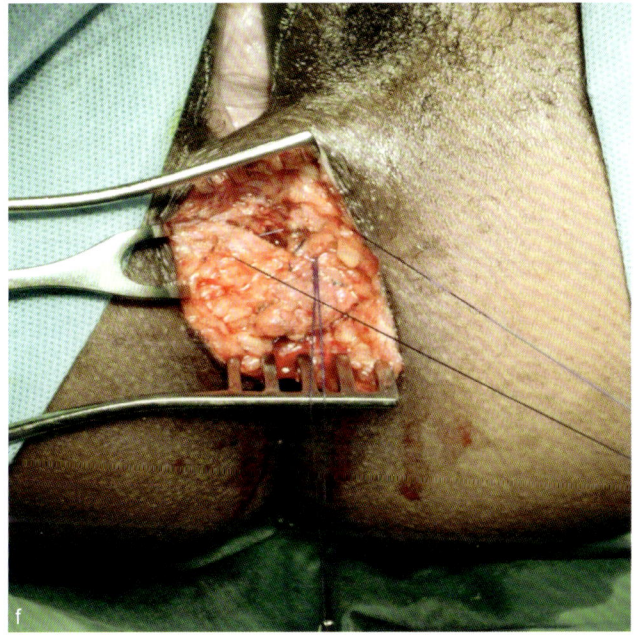

图 29.1 续

电刺激股薄肌成形术（第 30 章）是一个复杂的过程，需要特殊的专门技术，它价格昂贵，并往往伴有大量的并发症发生率和适度的手术返修率[40-46]。目前在美国，将肌肉纤维变成慢收缩肌肉的刺激，不能供临床使用。用于生物扩展制剂的可注射的填充剂被用来修补断裂的肛门内括约肌，在一些研究中证明有效，但目前在美国并未获得批准治疗大便失禁[47-50]，此内容见第 33 章。在这个年龄组的复发患者还有其他供选方案，包括使用直肠经闭孔吊带（在美国进行试验）[51]和一些新的使用肌肉祖细胞自体移植动物研究，研究已经表明，随着增强括约肌肌电活动，能加速兔受损括约肌的肌纤维修复[52]。

结 论

重复括约肌成形术对大便失禁的患者是一个可行的选择。重复括约肌修复的接受率与一期修补相同，因此，对于某些特定的一期修补失败的患者可考虑使用重复括约肌修复。结直肠病专家可以告诉他们的患者（尽管有广泛可用的数据），类似一期括约肌修复的经验，大多数患者有可能改善，虽然随着时间的推移疗效会自然恶化。虽然许多患者不知道对他们来说什么是"正常"（与对照组相比，控便仍然显著减弱），这种控便改进可以改善相关的社会功能和性功能[53]。在骶神经调节时代，重复括约肌成形术的特定作用是即使有明确的肛门外括约肌缺损，尽管还不确定，但在治疗复发性严重大便失禁中，当神经刺激无效或未经批准时，它可能是最廉价和最简单的方案。

参考文献

1. Sultan AH, Kamm MA, Bartram CI, Hudson CN. Anal sphincter trauma during instrumental delivery. Int J Gynaecol Obstet. 1993;43:263–70.
2. Rygh AB, Körner H. The overlap technique versus end-to-end approximation technique for primary repair of obstetric anal sphincter rupture: a randomized, controlled study. Acta Obstet Gynecol Scand. 2010;89:1256–62.
3. Engel AF, Kamm MA, Sultan AH, Bartram CI, Nicholls RJ. Anterior anal sphincter repair in patients with obstetric trauma. Br J Surg. 1994;81:1231–4.
4. Gold DM, Bartram CI, Halligan S, Humphries KN, Kamm MA, Kmiot WA. Three-dimensional endoanal sonography in assessing anal canal injury. Br J Surg. 1999;86:365–70.
5. McNicol FJ, Bruce CA, Chaudhri S, Francombe J, Kozman E, Taylor BA, et al. Management of obstetric anal sphincter injuries – a role for the colorectal surgeon. Colorectal Dis. 2010;12:927–30.
6. Vaizey CJ, Norton C, Thornton MJ, Nicholls RJ, Kamm MA. Long-term results of repeat anterior anal sphincter repair. Dis Colon Rectum. 2004;47:858–63.
7. Giordano P, Renzi A, Efron J, Gervaz P, Weiss EG, Nogueras JJ, et al. Previous sphincter repair does not affect the outcome of repeat repair. Dis Colon Rectum. 2002;45:635–40.
8. Nikiteas N, Korsgen S, Kumar D, Keighley MR. Audit of sphincter repair. Factors associated with poor outcome. Dis Colon Rectum. 1996;39:1164–70.
9. Zutshi M, Tracey TH, Bast J, Halverson A, Na J. Ten-year outcome after anal sphincter repair for fecal incontinence. Dis Colon Rectum. 2009;52:1089–94.
10. Keighley MR, Williams N, editors. Fecal incontinence. Surgery of the anus, colon and rectum, vol. 1. London: W. B. Saunders; 2001. p. 592–700.
11. Simmang C, Birnbaum EH, Kodner IJ, Fry RD, Fleshman JW. Anal sphincter reconstruction in the elderly: does advancing age affect outcome? Dis Colon Rectum. 1994;37:1065–9.
12. Evans C, Davis K, Kumar D. Overlapping anal sphincter repair and anterior levatorplasty: effect of patient's age and duration of follow-up. Int J Colorectal Dis. 2006;21:795–801.
13. Mevik K, Norderval S, Kileng H, Johansen M, Vonen B. Long-term results after anterior sphincteroplasty for anal incontinence. Scand J Surg. 2009;98:234–8.
14. Mahony R, Behan M, Daly L, Kirwan C, O'Herlihy C, O'Connell PR. Internal anal sphincter defect influences continence outcome following obstetric anal sphincter injury. Am J Obstet Gynecol. 2007;196:217.e1–5.
15. Lindqvist PG, Jernetz M. A modified surgical approach to women with obstetric anal sphincter tears by separate suturing of external and internal anal sphincter. A modified approach to obstetric anal sphincter injury. BMC Pregnancy Childbirth. 2010;10:51.
16. Pinedo G, Vaizey CJ, Nicholls RJ, Roach R, Halligan S, Kamm MA. Results of repeat anal sphincter repair. Br J Surg. 1999;86:66–9.
17. Osterberg A, Graf W, Homberg A, Pahlman L, Ljung A, Hakelius L. Long-term results of anterior levatorplasty for fecal incontinence. A retrospective study. Dis Colon Rectum. 1996;39:671–5.
18. Aitola P, Hiltunen KM, Matikainen M. Functional results of anterior levatorplasty and external sphincter plication for fecal incontinence. Ann Chir Gynaecol. 2000;89:29–32.
19. Evans C, Davis K, Kumar D. Overlapping anal sphincter repair and anterior levatorplasty: effect of patient's age and duration of follow-up. Int J Colorectal Dis. 2006;21:795–801.
20. Leroi AM, Parc Y, Lehur PA, Mion F, Barth X, Rullier E, Study Group, et al. Efficacy of sacral nerve stimulation for fecal incontinence: results of a multicenter double-blind crossover study. Ann Surg. 2005;242:662–9.
21. Jarrett ME, Dudding TC, Nicholls RJ, Vaizey CJ, Cohen CR, Kamm MA. Sacral nerve stimulation for fecal incontinence related to obstetric anal sphincter damage. Dis Colon Rectum. 2008;51:531–7.
22. Chan MK, Tjandra JJ. Sacral nerve stimulation for fecal incontinence: external anal sphincter defect vs. intact anal sphincter. Dis Colon Rectum. 2008;51:1015–25.
23. Wexner SD, Coller JA, Devroede G, Hull T, McCallum R, Chan M, et al. Sacral nerve stimulation for fecal incontinence: results of a 120-patient prospective multicenter study. Ann Surg. 2010;251:441–9.
24. Altomare DF, Ratto C, Ganio E, Lolli P, Masin A, Villani RD. Long-term outcome of sacral nerve stimulation for fecal incontinence. Dis Colon Rectum. 2009;52:11–7.
25. Matzel KE, Lux P, Heuer S, Besendörfer M, Zhang W. Sacral stimulation for fecal incontinence: long-term outcome. Colorectal Dis. 2009;11:636–41.
26. Boyle DJ, Knowles CH, Lunniss PJ, Scott SM, Williams NS, Gill KA. Efficacy of sacral nerve stimulation for fecal incontinence in patients with anal sphincter defects. Dis Colon Rectum. 2009;52:1234–9.
27. Brouwer R, Duthie G. Sacral nerve neuromodulation is effective treatment for fecal incontinence in the presence of a sphincter defect, pudendal neuropathy, or previous repair. Dis Colon Rectum. 2010;53:273–8.
28. Ratto C, Litta F, Parello A, Donisi L, Doglietto GB. Sacral nerve stimulation is a valid approach in fecal incontinence due to sphincter lesions when compared to sphincter repair. Dis Colon Rectum. 2010;53:264–72.
29. Altomare DF, DeFazio M, Giuliani RT, Catalano G, Cuccia F. Sphincteroplasty for fecal incontinence in the era of sacral nerve modulation. World J Gastroenterol. 2010;16:5267–71.
30. Wong WD, Jensen LL, Bartolo DC, Rothenberger DA. Artificial anal sphincter. Dis Colon Rectum. 1996;39:1345–51.
31. Christiansen JO, Rasmussen O, Lindorf-Larsen K. Long-term results of artificial anal sphincter implantation for severe anal incontinence. Ann Surg. 1999;230:45–8.
32. Engel AF, van Baal SJ, Brummelkamp W. Late results of postanal repair for idiopathic fecal incontinence. Eur J Surg. 1994;160:637–40.
33. Jameson JS, Speakman CT, Darzi A, Chia YW, Henry MM. Audit of postanal repair in the treatment of fecal incontinence. Dis Colon Rectum. 1994;37:369–72.
34. Setti-Carraro P, Kamm MA, Nicholls RJ. Long-term results of postanal repair for neurogenic fecal incontinence. Br J Surg. 1994;81:140–4.
35. Matsuoka H, Mavrantonis C, Wexner SD, Oliveira L, Gilliland R, Pikarsky A. Postanal repair for fecal incontinence–is it worthwhile? Dis Colon Rectum. 2000;43:1561–7.
36. Abbas SM, Bissett I, Neill ME, Barry BR. Long-term outcome of postanal repair in the treatment of fecal incontinence. ANZ J Surg. 2005;75:783–6.
37. Mackey P, Mackey L, Kennedy ML, King DW, Newstead GL, Douglas PR, et al. Postanal repair–do the long-term results justify the procedure? Colorectal Dis. 2010;12:367–72.
38. Steele SR, Lee P, Mullenix PS, Martin MJ, Sullivan ES. Is there a role for concomitant pelvic floor repair in patients with sphincter defects in the treatment of fecal incontinence? Int J Colorectal Dis.

2006;21:508–14.
39. Oberwalder M, Dinnewitzer A, Nogueras JJ, Weiss EG, Wexner SD. Imbrication of the external anal sphincter may yield similar functional results as overlapping repair in selected patients. Colorectal Dis. 2008;10:800–4.
40. Baeten C, Geerdes BP, Adang EM, Heineman E, Konsten J, Engel GL, et al. Anal dynamic graciloplasty in the treatment of intractable fecal incontinence. N Engl J Med. 1995;332:1600–5.
41. Eccersley AJ, Williams NS. Dynamic graciloplasty for severe anal incontinence. Br J Surg. 1998;85:1158–9.
42. Rosen HR, Novi G, Zoech G, Feil W, Urbarz C, Schiessel R. Restoration of anal sphincter function by single-stage dynamic graciloplasty with a modified (split sling) technique. Am J Surg. 1998;175:187–93.
43. Christiansen J, Rasmussen OO, Lindorff-Larsen K. Dynamic graciloplasty for severe anal incontinence. Br J Surg. 1998;85:88–91.
44. Mander BJ, Wexner SD, Williams NS, Bartolo DC, Lubowski DZ, Oresland T, et al. Preliminary results of a multicentre trial of the electrically stimulated gracilis neoanal sphincter. Br J Surg. 1999;86:1543–8.
45. Sielezneff I, Malouf AJ, Bartolo DC, Pryde A, Douglas S. Dynamic graciloplasty in the treatment of patients with fecal incontinence. Br J Surg. 1999;86:61–5.
46. Baeten CG, Bailey HR, Bakka A, Belliveau P, Berg E, Buie WD, et al. Safety and efficacy of dynamic graciloplasty for fecal incontinence: report of a prospective, multicenter trial. Dynamic Graciloplasty Therapy Study Group. Dis Colon Rectum. 2000;43:743–51.
47. Davis KD, Kumar D, Poloniecki J. Preliminary evaluation of an injectable anal sphincter bulking agent (Durasphere) in the management of fecal incontinence. Aliment Pharmacol Ther. 2003;18:237–43.
48. Vaizey C, Kamm MA. Injectable bulking agents for treating fecal incontinence. Br J Surg. 2005;92:521–7.
49. Chan MK, Tjandra JJ. Injectable silicone biomaterial (PTQ) to treat fecal incontinence after hemorrhoidectomy. Dis Colon Rectum. 2006;49:433–9.
50. Kenefick N, Vaizey CJ, Malouf AJ, Norton CS, Marshall M, Kamm MA. Injectable silicone biomaterial for fecal incontinence due to internal sphincter dysfunction. Gut. 2007;51:225–8.
51. Yamana T, Takahashi T, Iwadare J. Perineal puborectalis sling operation for fecal incontinence: preliminary report. Dis Colon Rectum. 2004;47:1982–9.
52. Kajbafzadeh AM, Elmi A, Talab SS, Esfahani SA, Tourchi A. Functional external anal sphincter reconstruction for treatment of anal incontinence using muscle progenitor cell auto-grafting. Dis Colon Rectum. 2010;53:1415–21.
53. Riss S, Stift A, Teleky B, Rieder E, Mittlböck M, Maier A, et al. Long-term anorectal and sexual function after overlapping anterior anal sphincter repair: a case-match study. Dis Colon Rectum. 2009;52:1095–100.

第 30 章　电刺激股薄肌成形术失败后治疗策略

Cornelius G.M.I. Baeten · Stephanie O. Breukink
许　晨 译　王国逊 审校

摘　要

电刺激股薄肌成形术（DGP）是治疗部分大便失禁患者的一种特殊的重建方法，但此治疗方法的应用在逐渐减少。电刺激股薄肌成形术是通过植入自体肌肉组织来维持控便功能，这种肌肉组织可自主控制或通过电刺激控制。虽然有证据显示股薄肌的固有特性决定了其并不是控便的最理想选择，但其补充植入电刺激器可以提供长期的、"自主的"收缩。这种股薄肌的动态化导致了特殊条件下，使易疲劳的（Ⅱ类）肌纤维和慢收缩的（Ⅰ类）纤维更适合达到这个目的。本章针对电刺激股薄肌成形术治疗失败进行了专业描述，其失败原因主要是由于肌肉或是电刺激的过程。DGP 的患者其并发症和复发率非常高，包括感染、硬件故障和术后排便功能障碍。特殊的并发症包括纤维化、大腿皮下积液、刺激器侵蚀和暴露、粪便嵌塞、肛瘘形成、刺激器扭转、过早的电池放电、骨折、会阴部纤维化和电极移位。DGP 在腹会阴联合根治术后肛门直肠完全重建中具有特殊地位，在儿童期存在先天性肛门直肠畸形的治疗中具有补充作用。

关键词

电刺激股薄肌成形术；失败的电刺激股薄肌成形术；股薄肌；肛门括约肌；大便失禁；失神经支配；灌肠；人工括约肌；骶神经调节；结肠造瘘术

引　言

电刺激股薄肌成形术是一种原位肛门括约肌替换的外科手术，并用于修复最严重的大便失禁。在大部分顽固的大便失禁的患者中，既存在功能的障碍，也存在括约肌组织的缺失。而 DGP 是通过移植同时具备自主收缩和电刺激收缩的同类肌肉来达到控便的效果。股薄肌是一种正常的骨骼肌，其并不具备长时间保持收缩的特性；作为内收肌，其特性是短期、有力和自主收缩。从这方面看，股薄肌的遗传特性使其并不是的用于控便的最佳选择，因为控便需要长期的自主收缩，而不是有意识的控制。

在 DGP 中，使股薄肌环绕肛门括约肌，同时提供一个植入的电刺激器用于长期的收缩[1]。这种股薄肌的动态化的现象导致肌纤维从快速收缩、易疲劳的纤维（Ⅱ类）变为慢收缩的纤维（Ⅰ类）[2-3]。

无法满足控制排便标准的 DGP 被认为手术失败。失败的 DGP 可能是由于肌肉或电刺激的过程造成。对于植入电刺激器的患者而言，并发症和复发的几率很高，包括感染，硬件问题和术后排便功能障碍。特殊的并发症包括纤维化、大腿皮下积液、刺激器侵蚀和暴露、粪便嵌塞、肛瘘形成、刺激器旋转、过早的电池放电、骨折、会阴部纤维化和电极移位[4-5]。

股薄肌和肌腱的治疗失败

股薄肌是由股薄肌神经（闭孔神经）支配，其包括感觉和运动纤维。通常，每一个控制肌肉的神经都与一块或更多的肌肉纤维相连；一个运动神经纤维和与其相连的肌肉纤维被定义为一个运动单位。股薄肌的刺激意味着神经的刺激带动许多运动单位同时发生作用。股薄肌成形术可以因为损害肌肉的神经支配而失败；股薄肌神经的主要成分出现损害会导致肌肉萎缩和收缩乏力。因此，去神经化的肌肉与神经支配良好的肌肉相比，并不能很好的受到刺激，此类肌肉是通过直接刺激肌肉纤维产生收缩，不是运动单位中的运动神经元。直接刺激肌肉纤维需要更高的电压，通常会导致疼痛。虽然股薄肌在解剖学上填补了括约肌的缺损，但肌肉的萎缩会导致最初的括约肌缺口的重新出现。

在许多病例中，肌肉收缩的力量随着时间的推移逐渐减弱，可能会发生在股薄肌肌腱出现分离、破裂或拉长时[6]。在肌腱分离或破裂的情况下，肌腱必须重新缝合。应用不可吸收线缩短肌腱可以帮助拉长肌腱，提供更高的肌肉张力。随着时间的发展，股薄肌易于伸长，而与之相伴的血管和神经也会伸长和调整。在此过程中，股薄肌的反折点移向腹股沟，同时环绕肛门的股薄肌部分逐渐变大，所以随着时间的发展，肛门的闭合力量逐渐减弱。股薄肌的刺激收缩并不能代偿股薄肌的拉长，这就导致 DGP 失败。

刺激失败

当收缩失败的时候，可以很容易的区分是肌肉问题还是刺激机制的功能障碍[7]。当肌肉仍然具备提供自主收缩的能力时，刺激器打开仍无自主收缩，这意味着刺激存在问题。相反，自主收缩的缺失意味着肌肉问题。最大的收缩力量可以通过刺激获得。当问题肯定出自刺激器时，有很多原因与硬件相关。收缩的缺失象征着刺激器的工作结束，这个现象通常出现在 7.5 年后。解决的办法仅需更换电池。在一些情况下，刺激器可以工作，但是电极的漏电会阻止肌肉的收缩。处理的办法可通过重新连接电极和刺激器解决。若电极出现破坏或损伤，需要重新更换。电极完全破坏会导致所有收缩的停止，电极的损坏或绝缘可能导致线路的短路，会导致收缩缺失或减少。电极与肌肉的连接不佳，阻止了有效的收缩；在一些病例中，需要重新插入电极，但是这么做很困难，因为电极的原位缝合已经不存在。通常，随着时间的发展，需要更高的电压来保持相同的收缩力量。植入肌肉内的电极被周围的纤维组织包裹很常见，需要更高的电压以抵抗电极与神经之间纤维组织的阻断作用[8]。这导致阻抗增加可能减弱信号。这种阻抗增加可能导致信号被减弱。

检查的原则

DGP 治疗的失败意味着大便失禁患者最终治疗手段的失败，因为其他很多的治疗选择已经被尝试过。为了评估患者，需要一套诊断实验的方案，包括肛门测压、腔内超声、结肠镜、排粪造影或直肠容量法。MRI 是显影股薄肌的最好方法；然而，由于刺激器的原因，MRI 无法开展检查，所以有时需要在 MRI 评估之前移除刺激器。在一些病例中，消毒后的刺激器是允许重新植入的。CT 扫描和超声诊断均可以显示股薄肌，但在某些情况下其分辨率不如 MRI。在一些特殊病例中，排粪造影可以提供直肠排便和容量的动态评估信息，这可用于 Hirschprung 病患者术后排便困难的评估。

电刺激股薄肌成形术后重新编程

刺激器可以由患者通过遥控器或医生通过编程器进行非手术重新编程。医生的编程器与患者的手控遥控器相比，其选择的范围要更广。编程的指标包括频次、电压、脉冲宽度和开始是柔和或是猛烈的脉冲。更高的频率和更高的脉冲宽度可以改善治疗效果，但患者无法修改这两项指标。患者可以在一定范围内增加振幅，电压的增加会调动更多的运动单位，从而导致股薄肌的更强有力的收缩。然而，这种力量的增加是有限度的。电压的进一步增加会触发感觉纤维，从而导致过度的疼痛。

电刺激股薄肌成形术失败后的肠道灌洗

当对失效的股薄肌进行进一步编程，并不能提供任何改善时，还有一些其他的治疗选择。大便失禁可以通过逆行结肠灌洗来治疗。通常情况下，这种净化治疗是应用 DGP 治疗前常用的保守治疗；然而，股薄肌成形术为肛门提供了更好的控便功能，使得液体能停留在直肠内而不漏出。Koch 等描述了这一类患者[9]。这种方法可以通过药物和食物的改变来调节大便的形状；对于失败的 DGP 来说，更紧密的大便要优于疏松的大便。由于这种治疗的失败，植入的刺激器已没有任何使用价值，可以移除；然而成形的股薄肌通常已经与周围的软组织相融合，无法移除，只能留在原位。有证据显示，灌洗之后排便可控只是表面上的假象，对于一些患者这种生活质量是可以接受的。在少数病例中，肌腱的远端可以被切除，同时肛门可以通过扩张变宽。肠道灌洗是很好的选择，但由于诸多原因无法接受，其他的治疗包括顺行节制灌肠，其可通过盲肠造口手术或阑尾造口术实现。

电刺激股薄肌成形术失败后的人工肠道括约肌手术（ABS）

对于部分患者而言，一个现实的选择是人工肠道括约肌（第 31 章）。在肛门植入人工肠道括约肌比想象的要简单得多：肛门周围新的手术切口可以经过旧的瘢痕组织。对于肛门残端的处理，肛门可以被股薄肌环绕，但是直肠前壁的处理需要特别小心，因为阴道后壁的会阴体会变薄。即使准备充分，不经意的阴道损伤会导致人工肠道括约肌不能正常工作，在 Michot 的研究中[10]，经阴道植入人工肠道括约肌并不增加感染风险。在一项 75 例人工肠道括约肌植入病例的研究中，8 例曾是 DGP 患者。在这些病例中，在以往股薄肌移植术的窦道处可以建立新的通道，而且 ABS 可以确保比 DGP 有更好的控便功能[11]。在这组患者中，虽然治疗的功能效果令人满意，但并发症的风险更高。

电刺激股薄肌成形术失败后的二次手术

几乎无法查找到电刺激股薄肌成形术失败后的二次手术的相关文献。第一次的报道来自 Cavina 等[12]，在他们的研究中，这项治疗用于第 16 章中讨论的腹会阴联合根治术后全肛门直肠重建术治疗的一部分。这组患者治疗的原理是应用一块股薄肌替换括约肌，另一块股薄肌用于替代耻骨直肠悬带。最初是用外括约肌给予补充，随后开始使用电刺激器。有研究也提到这种方法[13]。二次股薄肌成形术的临床经验有限，但却是一种可行的选择。

电刺激股薄肌成形术失败后的骶神经调节

骶神经调节是最近开始的能有效治疗大便失禁的新的治疗方法，而且，作为一种干预手段，它看起来比 DGP 更加安全和可靠，很少需要校正[14]。正常情况下，DGP 是治疗大便失禁的手段中比较靠后的治疗选择，虽然一些治疗失败的 DGP 患者在随后的骶神经调节的治疗中获得了成功，这些患者适合刺激治疗。作为一种有效的治疗手段，骶神经调节的患者可以重新使用股薄肌刺激器，并将其植入臀部。

电刺激股薄肌成形术失败后的结肠造瘘术

严重的肛门失禁的最终的治疗方法当然是结肠造瘘术。在这种情况下控便功能无法恢复，但这种方法使得患者能维持一种可接受的生活质量。

总 结

虽然复发率很高，但如果具备足够的专业知识，DGP 也是一种有效治疗大便失禁的手段。与仪器有关的并发症包括硬件感染、仪器故障和移位，在一些病例中会出现与刺激器相关的明显的疼痛和肌肉分离。虽然发病率高，但专业的调整常常有效。随着时间的推移，治疗过程的不断的调整会降低并发症发生率，其中包括肌肉内部分神经周围的导线布局，这样可以减少神经周围的纤维化和刺激问题[15]。对于一些术前存在直肠高敏感、严重的便急迫感和直肠顺应性低的患者，其随后出现的排便功能障碍可能导致处理困难，这些问题随着时间的推移已经有了一些改善。DGP 可能在腹会阴联合根治术后全肛门直肠重建术中有特殊的作用[12, 16]，而且是罹患先天性肛门直肠畸形患儿治疗的重要补充手段[17-18]，在这两组病例中，有一半获得了可接受的控便功能。其中部分病例的控便功能良好，而且不需要使用刺激器。研究的数据显示，在谨慎选择的病例中，虽然与保守治疗相比，终身使用 DGP 的治疗费用昂贵，但使用 DGP 能有更好的生活质量[19]。

参考文献

1. Baeten CG, Geerdes BP, Adang EM, Heineman E, Konsten J, Engel GL, et al. Anal dynamic graciloplasty in the treatment of intractable fecal incontinence. N Engl J Med. 1995;332:1600–5.
2. Salmons S, Henriksson J. The adaptive response of skeletal muscle to increased use. Muscle Nerve. 1981;4:94–105.
3. Baeten CGMI, Rongen MJ. Managing functional problems following dynamic graciloplasty. In: Wexner SD, Zbar A, Pescatori M, editors. Complex anorectal disorders: investigation and management. New York: Springer; 2010. p. 706–14.
4. Wexner SD, Gonzalez-Padron A, Ruis J, Teoh TA, Cheong DM, Nogueras JJ, et al. Stimulated gracilis neosphincter operation. Initial experience, pitfalls and complications. Dis Colon Rectum. 1996;39:957–64.
5. Cera SM, Wexner SD. Muscle transposition: does it still have a role? Clin Colon Rectal Surg. 2005;18:46–54.
6. Matzel KE, Madoff RD, LaFontaine LJ, Baeten CG, Buie WD, Christiansen J, Dynamic Graciloplasty Therapy Study Group, et al. Complications of dynamic graciloplasty: incidence, management and impact of outcome. Dis Colon Rectum. 2001;44:1427–35.
7. Geerdes BP, Heineman E, Konsten J, Soeters PB, Baeten CG. Dynamic graciloplasty. Complications and management. Dis Colon Rectum. 1996;39:912–7.
8. Lanmuller H, Bijak M, Mayr W, Rafolt D, Sauermann S, Thoma H. Useful applications and limits of battery powered implants in functional electrical stimulations. Artif Organs. 1997;21:210–2.
9. Koch SM, Uludağ O, El Naggar K, van Gemert WG, Baeten CG. Colonic irrigation for defecation disorders after dynamic graciloplasty. Int J Colorectal Dis. 2008;23:195–200.
10. Michot F, Lefebure B, Bridoux V, Gourcerol G, Kianifard B, Leroi AM, et al. Artificial anal sphincter for severe fecal incontinence implanted by a transvaginal approach: experience with 32 patients treated at one institution. Dis Colon Rectum. 2010;53:1155–60.
11. Melenhorst J, Koch SM, van Gemert WG, Baeten CG. The artificial bowel sphincter for fecal incontinence: a single centre study. Int J Colorectal Dis. 2008;23:107–11.
12. Cavina E, Seccia M, Evangelista G. Neosphincter and neostomy [new surgical techniques as a function of the prospects of electro-stimulation for continence. Clinical experience. Preliminary reports]. Minerva Chir. 1981;36:389–92.
13. Geerdes B, Konsten J, Baeten CG. Bilateral gracilis neosphincter construction for treatment of fecal incontinence. Br J Surg. 1996;83:1015–6.
14. Edden Y, Wexner SD. Therapeutic devices for fecal incontinence: dynamic graciloplasty, artificial bowel sphincter and sacral nerve stimulation. Expert Rev Med Devices. 2009;6:307–12.
15. Konsten J, Rongen MJ, Ogunbiyi OA, Darakhshan A, Baeten CG, Williams NS. Comparison of epineural or intramuscular nerve electrodes for stimulated graciloplasty. Dis Colon Rectum. 2001;44:581–6.
16. Ho KS, Seow-Choen F. Dynamic graciloplasty for total anorectal reconstruction after abdominoperineal resection for rectal tumour. Int J Colorectal Dis. 2005;20:38–41.
17. Baeten CG, Konsten J, Heineman E, Soeters PB. Dynamic graciloplasty for anal atresia. J Pediatr Surg. 1994;29:922–5.
18. Koch SM, Uludağ O, Rongen MJ, Baeten CG, van Gemert W. Dynamic graciloplasty in patients born with an anorectal malformation. Dis Colon Rectum. 2004;47:1711–9.
19. Adang EMM, Engel GL, Rutten FH, Geerdes BP, Baeten CG. Cost-effectiveness of dynamic graciloplasty in patients with fecal incontinence. Dis Colon Rectum. 1998;41:725–34.

第 31 章 人工肛门括约肌植入术后并发症的处理

Valérie Bridoux · Francis Michot · Anne-Marie Leroi

陈建军 译　王西墨 审校

摘 要

随着其他治疗方式的发展，人工肛门括约肌（AAS）植入术的使用逐渐减少，尤其是骶神经调节治疗的出现，其术后并发症更少，且极少需要再次手术。传统认为人工肛门括约肌是治疗失禁患者的最后的一种手段，类似于其在尿失禁患者中的应用。本章首先着重介绍人工肛门括约肌植入术的技术；然后评估人工肛门括约肌植入术治疗大便失禁的安全性和有效性；最后描述了如何选择合适的患者，并讨论了此技术在大便失禁患者的治疗中所占的地位。

关键词

人工肛门括约肌（AAS）；人工肛门括约肌植入术；大便失禁；移除

引 言

难治性大便失禁是肛肠疾病中最具有挑战性的问题之一。当保守治疗、括约肌修补及骶神经刺激治疗失败，没有其他合适的治疗手段的时候，传统上认为人工括约肌植入是这种患者最后的选择。最早的人工括约肌是由 Christensen 和 Lorentzen[1] 在 1987 年植入的尿道假体（AMS 800, American Medical Systems, Minneapolis, MN）。他们对尿道括约肌进行了改造，使其能用于替代大便失禁患者的肛门括约肌（Acticon®, American Medical Systems）。之后报道了 400 多例，并对其中大部分患者进行了短期的随访[2]。所有的研究指出在植入人工括约肌后，平均大便失禁评分有了明显的降低。但是这种治疗有着较高的并发症发生率，并经常需要再次手术[2]。

此章首先着重介绍人工肛门括约肌植入技术，然后总结了一篇综述，此综述评价了采用人工肛门括约肌植入治疗大便失禁的安全性和有效性，最后介绍了如何选择最合适患者，讨论了其治疗策略。

人工肛门括约肌技术

人工肛门括约肌的介绍

Acticon® neosphincter（American Medical System）是目前唯一可以有效治疗大便失禁的可植入的括约肌。由三部分组成：一个压力调节球囊，一个可膨胀的硅制束带，一个控制泵，通过皮下的管道连接（图 31.1）。

压力调节球囊

压力调节球囊植入在膀胱前的腹膜下间隙，能控制放置于肛管的闭合束带的压力，使其在 7 个压力范围内变化。最常用的压力范围是 91~100cmH$_2$O 和 101~110cmH$_2$O。通过组织厚度和完整性，以及

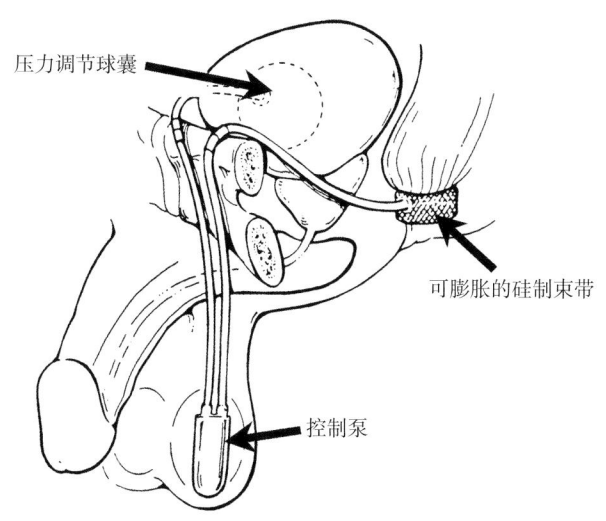

图31.1 用于治疗严重大便失禁的人工肛门括约肌

束带的紧密程度来选择合适的压力[3]。

可膨胀的硅制束带

束带置于肛管的上部，当束带膨胀的时候，束带通过环向压力闭合肛管。American Medical Systems 公司为 Acticon® neosphincter 提供了 12 种束带的规格，束带的长度从 9～14cm，宽度有 2.0cm 和 2.9cm 两种。术中我们通过束带筛选器来为每个患者选择合适的束带。

控制泵

控制泵植入在阴囊或大阴唇的皮下。控制泵包括电阻器和将液体从束带注入和排出的阀门。控制泵较硬的上半部特别设有一个灭活选项，使束带在较长时间内处于排空的状态。而较软的下半部会被反复的挤压来转运液体，其底部还设计了一个隔，可以无需手术添加液体。控制泵只有一种规格，他能满足各种型号的束带和球囊。

人工肛门括约肌的运作

人工肛门括约肌是半自动的，束带使肛门自动关闭，并维持近似于生理状态下的肛门静息压。患者自己控制排便，激活控制泵后，束带中的液体流向球囊，使束带排空，就可以开始排便。随后，束带在 5～8min 内自动再次膨胀，并维持到下一次排便[4]。

植入技术

手术首先植入肛周的闭合束带，可以通过采用横穿会阴体的前横切口，或是在肛管的两侧采取两个曲线切口。单个前切口常用于会阴体有瘢痕或较薄的女性患者。建立肛周的腔道以后，采用束带筛选器来测量束带合适的长度和宽度。合适的束带长度要比筛选器的测量值长 1cm。当束带放置好后，与束带连接的管道经皮下到达腹部切口。还要分离腹直肌来建立到达膀胱侧面腹膜上间隙的通道，并在此建立一个囊腔，置入未膨胀的储存球囊，之后在球囊中注入不透射线的液体。然后通过金属扩张器经腹部切口建立一个皮下的通道，将控制泵置入阴囊或大阴唇。并将闭合束带和压力调节球囊与控制泵连接起来。在确保整个通路正确连接后，将切口关闭，不放置引流管。最后应关闭这个设备。

对于会阴被破坏或有严重瘢痕存在的女性患者，我们推荐采用经阴道路径[5]。在阴道口上方 2cm 处的阴道后壁做一横切口。并将直肠壁和直肠阴道结缔组织与阴道壁分离开来。经任意一侧进入坐骨直肠窝，并建立环绕肛管的腔道，再置入束带筛选器选择合适的束带长度。其他的植入步骤与刚才描述的方法类似。

围术期护理

术前、围术期和术后的治疗，对于人工肛门括约肌置入术来说十分的关键，尤其可以预防早期的并发症的发生。根据我们的经验，有以下几个关键点[5-6]：

- 在整个过程中要重视消毒。这包括术前，从手术区向肛门用消毒液的清洗，术中使用抗生素，并充分及反复使用消毒液进行消毒[7]。此外，如同其他假体植入术一样，术中不允许进出手术室，且手术室人数应控制在 10 人以下[6]。

- 在术后，良好的卫生和护理人员是十分重要的。常规一天两次以及每次排便后均要进行会阴的清洁。女性患者在术后 7d 内使用导尿管，防止排尿后污染会阴及阴道，尤其是对于经阴道通路的患者[6]。

- 人工括约肌应在术后 8 周后激活，此时控制泵周围的水肿及疼痛已消退[7]。
- 术后排便对此手术十分的重要，尤其是避免便秘和粪便嵌塞。人工肛门括约肌植入术后，应指导患者进行合理的饮食，口服通便药，并采用直肠冲洗预防粪便嵌塞。

临床效果

在效果方面，所有的研究都指出进行人工肛门括约肌植入术后，患者的平均便失禁指数有了显著的降低，生活质量得到了改善[2]。手术成功的患者均能恢复排便功能[6, 8, 9]。我们最近的研究连续调查了 32 例接受经阴道植入的患者，并随访超过了 41 个月；在人工括约肌仍有功能的患者中，有 23 例（72%）患者的克利夫兰临床失禁程度评分显著的降低，从 18.4 降至 6.8[6]。在所有人工括约肌仍有功能的患者中，有 82.6% 的患者可以自己控制固体样便的排出，82.6% 的患者可以控制液体样便的排出，47.8% 的患者可自己控制排气。

但是在已发表的研究中，仍存在许多方法上的不足[2]。首先，我们没有在意向性治疗的基础上对结果进行分析，这样会导致此手术的有效性与实际存在差异。其次，大部分研究均为病例报告，只有一篇随机对照研究，此研究的手术组包含了 14 例随机行人工括约肌置入术患者，而对照组的患者采用支持治疗，治疗 6 个月后，对照组的症状没有明显改变，而手术组患者的克利夫兰临床评分从 19.1 降至 4.8[7]，得到了明显的改善。患者的生活质量也发生了类似的变化。第三，只有当长期随访患者的数量足够时，数据才是有效的，而这些数据十分有限。Parker 等[8] 报道，一旦手术成功，人工肛门括约肌能长期的改善排便功能和生活质量。但其他研究的远期疗效却不理想，一篇中位随访期为 6 年的研究指出，对于那些人工肛门括约肌有功能的患者，他们的排便自制评分并没有明显的改善[10]。

并发症

目前，在植入和移除人工肛门括约肌的过程中没有死亡病例的报道，但是植入人工肛门括约肌的并发症发生率较高。目前已经发现的两个主要问题：①人工肛门括约肌的移除率；②便秘及粪便嵌塞。

设备的移除

目前已报道的人工肛门括约肌永久移除的发生率为 17%～41%，随访期为 10～58 个月[2, 9, 11]。移除的原因包括感染、伤口无法愈合、设备导致皮肤破损而外露、由于束带或球囊的破裂导致设备故障。Lehur 等[11-13] 报道了 1998－2002 年 3 组连续的患者资料，其每组的手术植入/修复率在 31%、29%、31%。Wexner[14] 证实，移除率随着时间增长。人工肛门括约肌存在的时间越长，并发症发生率及设备移除率均会增加，5 年后移除率会达到 57%。

感 染

尽管严格的执行消毒流程，但是人工肛门括约肌植入术的感染率仍较高（4%～38%）[2]，而感染的人工肛门括约肌必须要移除。由于相关数据太少，无法评估感染的危险因素。Wexner 等[14] 报道第一次排便的时间是早期人工肛门括约肌感染的独立危险因素。术后第二天或更早发生排便的患者发生术后感染的风险较高，这一结论支持术后给予患者肠外营养[15]。Wexner 等还指出肛周感染病史也是其危险因素。

由于此手术是在肛门直肠区植入异物，所以其术后感染的发生率要高于其他手术。为了降低术后感染的风险，Finlay 等[16] 发明了一种新的人工括约肌，通过开腹手术放置在盆底肌肉组织上，他们认为这个位置的括约肌可以如同耻骨直肠悬带发挥功能。但是最初 12 例患者的结果令人失望：3 例（25%）患者由于感染进行了移除，之后又有 5 例（41.7%）患者出现了技术问题[16]。本希望经阴道手术能降低感染的发生率，但是到目前，这项新技术未能降低感染发生率[6]。

技术故障

设备失灵、束带破裂、球囊和泵泄漏是后期移除最常见的原因（46.1%）[14]。大部分研究指出人工肛门括约肌在激活后能在技术和功能上均达到满意的效果，但是随着时间其功能逐渐减退[17]。Christiansen等[17]的研究随访时间最长，他们指出术后超过5年的8例患者中，有5例（63%）因技术故障需再次手术修复。

糜烂

直肠黏膜、肛膜、皮肤的糜烂是移除人工肛门括约肌第二常见的原因[14]。Devesa等[18]研究了与糜烂发生的相关危险因素，发现预先存在的纤维化、会阴伤口的缝合方式、伤口张力以及排便时发生的污染或损伤与糜烂的发生无关。

束带应尽量放置在靠近肛提肌的位置，而不是靠近皮肤，因为这可能会引起极度不适和皮肤糜烂[19]。虽然阴道壁裂开是经阴道手术最常见的并发症[6]，但目前没有发现相关的危险因素。

便秘伴粪便嵌塞

术后高达一半的患者会发生排便困难[3,20]，虽然能通过服用通便药或灌肠解决，但会显著增加发生持续便失禁的风险[21]，我们仍不清楚其原因。一些术前的因素会增加患者发生出口梗阻型便秘的发生率（如术前便秘、直肠固定术、神经系统疾病、肛门闭锁、盆底失弛缓征、肛门超慢波）[21]，当束带过紧也会发生这种情况[12]。有学者认为束带在重新膨胀前开放的时间过短也会导致排便困难[22]。

人工肛门括约肌植入术后持续性大便失禁

如果患者在人工肛门括约肌植入术后再次发生大便失禁，我们不能排除存在肠道传输障碍。伴或不伴出口梗阻的便秘及慢性腹泻，并不能通过改变饮食和药物治愈的患者会更容易发生植入失败[21]。因此应努力治疗肠道传输障碍，来提高植入成功率。

可以通过肛门测压来弄清失败的原因。弄清3个压力指标十分重要（图31.2）。第1个指标是基础压力，提示人工肛门括约肌重建一个被动的高压力区域的能力，这个高压力区有助于恢复肛门控便功

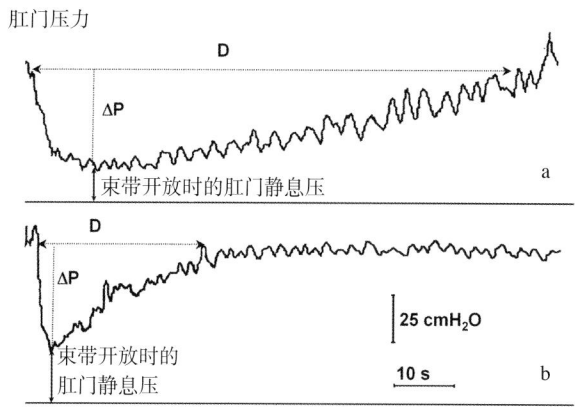

图31.2 人工肛门括约肌的运作。(a) 没有排泄障碍的患者，人工肛门括约肌运行正常。(b) 排泄障碍的患者（人工肛门括约肌开放后关闭的时间要短于无排泄障碍的患者）。ΔP：束带关闭与开放时肛门静息压力的差值。D：人工肛门括约肌开放后关闭所需的时间

能。如果出现压力不足，可对束带进行再次增压。第2个指标是人工肛门括约肌开放时的基础压力，反映了残余压力，高残余压力可能会导致术后排便困难。第3个指标是人工肛门括约肌开放后再次关闭所需的时间，反映了直肠排空的效果（一般至少3min），开放时间过短会导致排便困难[22]。肛门测压也可用于检测患者是否正确的使用人工肛门括约肌。

患者的选择

一篇系统回顾中，Mundy等[2]指出人工肛门括约肌对于特定人群的排便控制和生活质量均有积极作用，但是我们仍不知道通过哪些术前的特征来明确这些人群。我们提出了一份标准，帮助我们为人工肛门括约肌植入术选择合适的患者（下表）。根据我们的经验，最适合行人工括约肌植入术的指征是肛门括约肌广泛的损伤，并不伴有直肠脱垂，没有神经系统疾病，没有肛门闭锁，没有肛管超慢波和盆底失弛缓症，没有长期服用泻药治疗便秘的病史，没有出口梗阻性便秘，没有通过调节饮食和药物无法控制的便秘，术前没有行直肠固定术[15,21]（下表）。对于其他的病例，我们应术前对患者进行全面的评估。对于那些通过直肠固定术治疗慢运输型

表 31.1 人工肛门括约肌的患者选择标准

选择标准	基础排便习惯记录评估中，每周有 1 次或更多的固体粪便失禁
	保守治疗无效（包括生物反馈）
	引起大便失禁的主要原因是自主收缩受限或消失
	克利夫兰临床大便失禁评分 >10
	严重影响生活质量
禁忌证	会阴及肠道的放射性损伤
	克罗恩病
	活动期的盆腔脓肿
	怀孕
	肛交
可能的禁忌证，应具体病例具体分析	
合并直肠或会阴病变	直肠最大耐受容积 <100ml
	直肠内脱垂
合并运输障碍	饮食和药物治疗无效的慢性腹泻
	需要每天服用泻药的慢性便秘
	因结肠慢运输而采用直肠固定术的患者
	对术前直肠灌洗缺少顺从性的神经系统疾病患者，肛门闭锁，超慢波，盆底失弛缓患者
会阴脓肿史	

便秘的患者，植入术前应考虑行乙状结肠切除术。植入术前还应评估和治疗患者的直肠内脱垂[23]。这是由于结肠运输障碍会严重影响人工肛门括约肌的功能，资料提示，对于那些顽固性腹泻的患者或是伴有或不伴有出口梗阻的便秘患者，应谨慎的考虑是否行植入术[21]。专科护士应重新评估那些不能按要求进行肛门冲洗的患者，尤其是那些伴有神经性疾病或肛门闭锁的患者。生物反馈能成功的治疗肛门失弛缓症的患者。最后，只有那些术前进行挑选的患者才适合进行人工肛门括约肌植入术，他们必须有能力操作控制泵，并能理解人工肛门括约肌的功能。

人工肛门括约肌在便失禁的治疗中所处的地位

国际尿控协会最近提出了一个治疗规范，其中包括人工肛门括约肌的植入（图 31.3）[24]，被认为是外科常规治疗无效的顽固性大便失禁的指南，这些治疗是基于患者是否存在括约肌缺陷以及其严重程度。那些括约肌缺陷超过 180°或是主要的会阴组织缺损的患者都考虑进行人工肛门括约肌植入术。对于括约肌明显缺陷小于 50% 的患者，括约肌成形术长期以来一直是其常规治疗。但由于括约肌成形术的长期疗效随着时间减退，同时骶神经刺激被证明对很多伴有括约肌缺陷的患者有效，所以目前的发展趋势是采用经皮神经评估进行初步评价。如果评估成功，就可以采用骶神经刺激治疗。对于没有括约肌缺陷或缺陷小于 30% 的患者，也应进行经皮神经评估，如果评估成功，应该采用骶神经刺激治疗。对于那些尽管成功进行了括约肌成形术，但仍存在大便失禁的患者，应推荐行骶神经刺激治疗，倘若治疗不成功，则可以考虑行人工肛门括约肌植入术。

结 论

人工肛门括约肌对控制严重大便失禁是有效的，并不会引起全身性并发症。对于 2/3 的患者，人工肛门括约肌使用方便，并能明显改善生活质量。人工肛门括约肌应该只用于保守治疗无效的严重大便失禁患者，以及不适合进行括约肌修复或骶神经刺激或治疗无效的患者。人工肛门括约肌植入术并不是没有并发症，但是此手术成功率较高，尤其适用于那些不愿意行永久结肠造口的患者。但是，更高的植入率仍需要仔细的患者筛选和设备不断的改进。

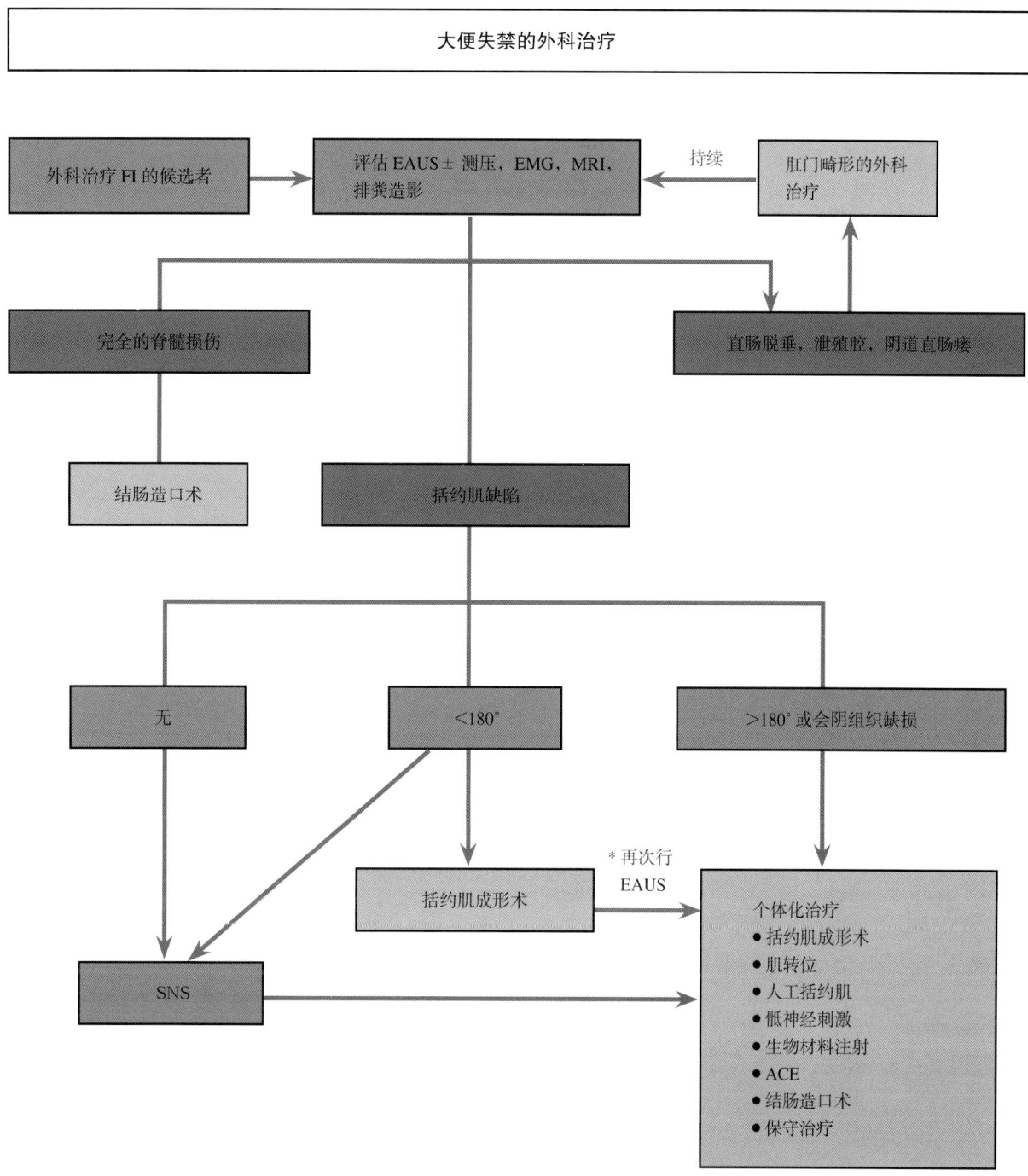

图 31.3　国际尿控协会提出的治疗规范,其中包括人工肛门括约肌。* 症状缓解不充分;FI:大便失禁;ACE:顺行性失禁灌肠法;EAUS:肛门内超声;EMG:肌电图;MRI:磁共振;SNS:骶神经刺激

参考文献

1. Christiansen J, Lorentzen M. Implantation of artificial sphincter for anal incontinence. Lancet. 1987;2:244–5.
2. Mundy L, Merlin TL, Maddern GJ, Hiller JE. Systematic review of safety and effectiveness of an artificial bowel sphincter for faecal incontinence. Br J Surg. 2004;91:665–72.
3. Wong WD, Congliosi SM, Spencer MP, Corman ML, Tan P, Opelka FG, et al. The safety and efficacy of the artificial bowel sphincter for fecal incontinence. Dis Colon Rectum. 2002;45:1139–53.
4. Lehur PA, Meurette G. The artificial bowel sphincter in the treatment of severe fecal incontinence in adults. In: Ratto C, Doglietto G, editors. Fecal incontinence. Diagnosis and treatment. Milan: Springer; 2007.
5. Michot F, Tuech JJ, Lefebure B, Bridoux V, Denis P. A new implantation procedure of artificial sphincter for anal incontinence: the transvaginal approach. Dis Colon Rectum. 2007;50:1401–4.
6. Michot F, Lefebure B, Bridoux V, Gourcerol G, Kianifard B, Leroi AM, et al. Artificial anal sphincter for severe fecal incontinence implanted by a transvaginal approach: experience with 32 patients treated at one institution. Dis Colon Rectum. 2010;53:1155–60.
7. O'Brien PE, Dixon JB, Skinner S, Laurie C, Khera A, Fonda D. A prospective, randomized, controlled clinical trial of placement of the artificial bowel sphincter (Acticon Neosphincter) for the control of fecal incontinence. Dis Colon Rectum. 2004;47:1852–60.
8. Parker SC, Spencer MP, Madoff RD, Jensen LL, Wong WD, Rothenberger DA. Artificial bowel sphincter. Long-term experience at a single institution. Dis Colon Rectum. 2003;46:722–9.
9. Melenhorst J, Koch SM, van Gemert WG, Baeten CG. The artificial bowel sphincter for faecal incontinence: a single centre study. Int J Colorectal Dis. 2008;23:107–11.
10. Carmona MDR, Company RA, Vila JVR, Bueno AS, Marti VP. Long-term results of artificial bowel sphincter for the treatment of severe faecal incontinence. Are they what we hoped for? Colorectal Dis. 2009;11:831–7.
11. Lehur PA, Glemain P, Bruley des Varannes S, Buzelin JM, Leborgne J. Outcome of patients with an implanted artificial anal sphincter for severe faecal incontinence. A single institution report. Int J Colorectal Dis. 1998;13:88–92.
12. Lehur PA, Roig JV, Duinslaeger M. Artificial anal sphincter: prospective clinical and manometric evaluation. Dis Colon Rectum. 2000;43:1100–6.
13. Lehur PA, Zerbib F, Neunlist M, Glemain P, Bruley des Varannes S. Comparison of quality of life and anorectal function after artificial sphincter implantation. Dis Colon Rectum. 2002;45:508–13.
14. Wexner SD, Jin HY, Weiss EG, Nogueras JJ, Li VK. Factors associated with failure of the artificial bowel sphincter: a study of over 50 cases from Cleveland Clinic Florida. Dis Colon Rectum. 2009;52:1550–7.
15. Michot F, Costaglioli B, Leroi AM, Denis P. Artificial anal sphincter in severe fecal incontinence: outcome of prospective experience with 37 patients in one institution. Ann Surg. 2003;237:52–6.
16. Finlay IG, Richardson W, Hajivassiliou CA. Outcome after implantation of a novel prosthetic anal sphincter in humans. Br J Surg. 2004;91:1485–92.
17. Christiansen J, Rasmussen O, Lindorff-Larsen K. Long-term results of artificial anal sphincter implantation for severe anal incontinence. Ann Surg. 1999;230:45–8.
18. Devesa JM, Rey A, Hervas PL, et al. Artificial anal sphincter: complications and functional results of a large personal series. Dis Colon Rectum. 2002;45:1154–63.
19. O'Brien PE, Skinner S. Restoring control. The Acticon Neosphincter artificial bowel sphincter in the treatment of anal incontinence. Dis Colon Rectum. 2000;43:1213–6.
20. Altomare DF, Dodi G, La Torre F, Romano G, Melega E, Rinaldi M. Multicentre retrospective analysis of the outcome of artificial anal sphincter implantation for severe faecal incontinence. Br J Surg. 2001;88:1481–6.
21. Gallas S, Leroi AM, Bridoux V, Lefebure B, Tuech JJ, Michot F. Constipation in 44 patients implanted with an artificial bowel sphincter. Int J Colorectal Dis. 2009;24:969–74.
22. Savoye G, Leroi AM, Denis P, Michot F. Manometric assessment of an artificial bowel sphincter. Br J Surg. 2000;87:586–9.
23. Benoist S, Panis Y, Michot F, Coffin B, Messing B, Valleur P. Artificial sphincter with colonic reservoir for severe anal incontinence because of imperforate anus and short-bowel syndrome: report of a case. Dis Colon Rectum. 2005;48:1978–82.
24. Abrams P, Andersson KE, Birder L, Brubaker L, Cardozo L, Chapple C, Members of Committees; Fourth International Consultation on Incontinence. Fourth International Consultation on Incontinence Recommendations of the International Scientific Committee, et al. Evaluation and treatment of urinary incontinence, pelvic organ prolapse, and fecal incontinence. Neurourol Urodyn. 2010;29(1):213–40.

第 32 章 肛门括约肌重建的手术方式

David A. Etzioni · Michael J. Stamos
徐 彬 译 王荫龙 审校

摘 要

本章概括了大便失禁患者的手术治疗方式，详细阐述了股薄肌（电刺激和免刺激方式）和臀大肌转位治疗的效果。文献报道肌肉转位治疗肛门失禁是有效的。该技术具有挑战性会有一定的并发症，尽管有文献报道结肠造瘘患者的生活质量与括约肌重建术后肛门功能不全患者相当。结直肠科医生必须能够选择适宜的患者来实施肌肉转位的外科治疗。

关键词

肛门括约肌；大便失禁；大便失禁严重程度评分；大便失禁患者生活质量量表；克利夫兰临床评分系统；股薄肌成形术；电刺激股薄肌成形术；臀大肌转位术

引 言

大便失禁在成人中很常见，发病率至少为 2%～18%[1-2]。由于界定标准不同，很难准确估计该病的流行病学因素。罹患大便失禁的危险因素包括高龄、女性、多产。多种病因导致的肛门失禁可以通过相似的疗法处理。本章介绍了传统疗法无效的患者应用手术治疗的过程。

诊 断

在大便失禁患者诊断和治疗的初始阶段一般不会考虑肌肉转位的手术治疗方案。Madoff 等于 2004 年出版了治疗开始阶段的评估方案[3]，我们依照该方案进行评估。评估的要素之一是要应用标准的量表，同时记录下大便失禁的严重程度，从而更客观的判定疗效。用于大便失禁的程度分级的标准量表有好几种，包括大便失禁严重程度量表[4]、大便失禁患者生活质量量表[5]、克利夫兰临床评分系统[6]。表 32.1 列出了克利夫兰临床评分系统。除了大便失禁严重程度外，还要记录是否出现过便急、内衣污粪及明显的大便或气体失控。另外，还要记录患者是稀便失禁还是成形便失禁，因为这一点对选择止泻剂使大便量正常还是增加纤维素饮食治疗来治疗大便失禁有指导作用。

通常，适合接受肌肉转位手术治疗的患者包括：

表 32.1 克利夫兰临床评分系统 a

	从不	很少	有时	通常	一直
成形便	0	1	2	3	4
稀便	0	1	2	3	4
气体	0	1	2	3	4
应用护垫	0	1	2	3	4
生活方式改变	0	1	2	3	4

Reprinted with permission from Jorge and Wexner.[6]
a：由每行的分数计算出总得分，范围为 0～20

①一次或多次括约肌成形失败的患者；②因特定先天性疾病（如脊柱裂或先天肛门闭锁）或后天疾患（如创伤）导致括约肌复合体缺失的患者；③外科切除肛门（如腹会阴切除术）。手术效果满意与否取决于手术医生的操作和患者的期望值。手术前，应彻底控制盆腔/肛门周围的感染。可以选择粪便转流手术，而且通常是推荐的术式。供体肌肉的游离对手术至关重要，这有赖于手术者的操作技能。

股薄肌成形术

股薄肌的解剖和生理

股薄肌是大腿内侧一条菲薄的肌肉，平均长度41cm，平均直径4.4cm（前后径）和1.1cm（左右径）[7]。近端固定于耻骨支，远端穿入胫骨近端，它由闭孔神经支配（L2~L3）动脉供应来源于股动脉旋支。该肌肉没有重要的功能，是转位手术的理想供体，可以带蒂游离，也可带皮瓣游离。1952年Pickrelldeng[8]首次报道应用股薄肌转位治疗大便失禁，他们治疗4名脊柱裂的儿童，取得了成功。该术式出现半个世纪以来有了改进，现就该手术的操作过程进行讨论。

手术过程

股薄肌成形术需要将该肌肉从原来的解剖位置游离至肛门周围。游离时可以采用1个或多个纵行切口，并精心保护近端的血液供应和神经支配。肌腱的离段部位应在膝盖以下。然后在肛门两侧行对口切开，分离肛门周围软组织，沿大腿上方（供肌肉侧）隧道将肌肉环形植入肛门周围。根据股薄肌的血液供应特点，有学者应用腔镜进行肌肉游离[9-10]：在膝盖附近做横行切口暴露出股薄肌肌腱，置入腔镜，沿筋膜下间隙逆行至大腿内侧切口附近。该操作可以有效减小瘢痕的长度，降低并发症。如果应用刺激电极可以将其放置在神经血管束远端，电极经皮下与同侧的刺激器相连。患者的局部解剖条件和瘢痕的范围决定了肌肉环的形状。阿尔法型的肌肉呈环形，远端固定在同侧坐骨结节处。伽马型和伊普西隆型肌肉完全环绕直肠，远端固定于对侧坐骨结节。伽马型（图32.1）肌环从前向后走行，而伊普西隆型肌肉从后向前走行。

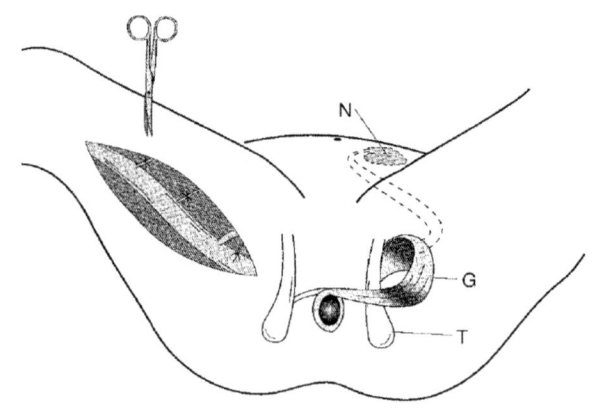

图32.1 结扎小的神经血管束后对右侧股薄肌进行游离。大的血管束和闭孔神经位于近端。在左侧显示了肌肉转为后置入电刺激装置行电刺激股薄肌成形的示意图。N：神经刺激器；G：股薄肌；T：坐骨嵴（Reprinted with permission from Chapman et al. [11]）

电刺激股薄肌成形术的疗效

到目前为止，有关电刺激股薄肌成形术疗效的文献还不是很多，但都有意义。Chapman等于2002年分析了当时的17项研究（383例患者）[11]，其成功率达42%~85%，其余的评价指标还包括术前术后肛管压力和控便的时间，这些指标和生活质量的改善都进行了记录。该研究入组严格，不同研究组内各指标改善的效果很有限。

自Chapman后有几篇文献是值得关注的。截至目前，关于电刺激股薄肌成形术成功的最大规模研究为2002年由Wexner[12]等实施的一项国际多中心研究，包括了115例患者。该研究的患者包括造瘘和未造瘘患者，在2年的随访期内有55%的患者取得成功（定义为大便失禁减少50%）。患者术后生活质量较术前有明显改善。Thornton等[13]报道了38例电刺激股薄肌成形术患者的疗效，发现无论是控便能力还是患者满意度均良好。但从专业角度讲，长期的疗效尚存在不足，手术后5年只有15%的患者能够控制成形大便。Penninckx[14]报道了来自比利时的60例因获得性或先天性肛门失禁进行电刺激股薄肌成形术的患者，其中27例失败（45%）。

取得成功的病例也会有并发症。Chapman等[11]报道该手术死亡率为4%，并发症发生率为100%。表32.2列出了各并发症的发生情况。在Wexner等[12]的多中心研究中没有报道并发症的发生率，至今还尚未公布该组大样本病例的远期疗效。在比利时的研究中，Penninckx[14] 报道在 60 例患者中出现了 61 次需全麻下处理的并发症，但未发生患者死亡。Thornton 等[13] 也发现，几乎每例患者都会出现并发症，但无死亡患者。

表 32.2 电刺激股薄肌成形术的并发症（$n=383$）

感染	106（28%）
刺激器和电极脱落	59（15%）
腿疼	54（13%）
股薄肌或结肠损伤	31（8%）
电池耗尽	29（8%）
便秘	28（7%）
肛门疼痛	30（7%）
躯干疼	24（6%）
刺激器相关疼痛	15（4%）
肛门狭窄	16（4%）
深静脉血栓形成	6（2%）
肌腱错位或断裂	9（2%）
无效或股薄肌不能收缩	6（2%）
肺栓塞	2（1%）
腿部水肿、血肿或血清肿	3（1%）
神经失用症	2（1%）
结肠瘘	3（1%）

Adapted from Chapman et al [11].

对于肛门功能不良（失禁或便秘）的患者来说，通过顺行（结肠、盲肠造口或阑尾造口）或逆行（经肛）结肠灌洗来挽救结肠功能是合理的。Koch 等[15] 进行了这方面的工作，报道了 46 例股薄肌成形术后患者，应用了结肠灌洗治疗（42 例逆行，4 例顺行），术后满意率为 81%。对于电刺激股薄肌成形术后仍有控便功能异常患者，Ho 和 Seow-Choen[16] 应用新肛门灌洗作为一种辅助治疗手段，并取得成功。Saunders 等[17] 给 14 例患者通过结肠导管进行顺行灌肠，并有 57% 的患者取得成功。

由于手术相关并发症较高但疗效一般，因此对患者的选择存在争议。但遗憾的是，截至目前还没有强有力的证据来支持哪些指标可用来判断患者术后会取得成功或失败。Wexner 等[12] 对患者症状出现的时间和术后效果进行了研究，但未发现二者之间的联系。在没有明确指南的情况下，一些原则可以用来指导该手术的临床应用。①患者应能够耐受手术后并发症并知晓有再手术的可能；②患者有强烈的手术意愿，并就手术的选择、手术的风险和并发症进行了广泛咨询。

无刺激和电刺激股薄肌成形术

是否应用电刺激来提高术后的疗效是股薄肌成形术需要考虑的重要问题。应用电刺激治疗的理由充分，值得探讨。通常，骨骼肌由 I 型和 II 型纤维混合而成，每种纤维都有各自的特性。I 型纤维适于提供张力，耐疲劳，而 II 型纤维对短时间收缩更为有效。肛门外括约肌主要由 I 型纤维组成，能够提供肛管静息压力[18]。但是，股薄肌主要由 II 型纤维组成，不适合长期收缩。电刺激后，从组织形态学上可以发现肌肉纤维从 II 型向 I 型转化。

一些学者质疑是否必须通过神经刺激才能取得股薄肌成形术成功[19-22]。Shatari 等[22] 指出成功控制大便有赖于：①患者感知直肠内粪便的存在；②产生暂时的足够大的张力来控制粪便。他们报道一例没有应用电刺激治疗的股薄肌成形术患者可以随意控制其股薄肌产生压力，这提示神经传导通路可以改变，位置可能在大脑皮层。目前尚无对电刺激必须性的相关研究。一些常见的感觉可用来决定是否应用电刺激治疗。对于股薄肌成形术后收缩功能良好的患者来说，加用电刺激理论上是有害的。同样，如果出现肛门口梗阻，就有理由终止刺激治疗。

臀大肌转位术

解剖和生理学

臀大肌不作为用肌肉转位手段治疗肛门失禁的首选，1902 年 Chetwood[23] 首次将该术式应用于小儿临床。1929 年 Wreden[24] 改进了这一术式，他将游离的筋膜围绕在肛周，并与对侧缝合，来产生自主收缩的效应。自从应用更为表浅的股薄肌治疗后，该术式的应用受到一定限制，且这种方法需要游离两侧臀大肌。臀大肌的解剖特点及临近肛门的位置使其成为肛门括约肌重建的次选材料。它起始于髂嵴沿髂胫束到达股骨，由臀下神经支配（L5，S1，S2 神经根），血液供应来源于臀下动脉和髂内动脉前支。通过对尸体的研究表明，与股薄肌成形术相比，臀大肌转位术后收缩力减弱，但一般情况下臀大肌纤维量远超过行肛门括约肌成形术的要求[25]。

手术过程

臀大肌转位有几种不同的术式。肌肉可以单侧也可双侧游离，然后将肌肉环绕或从一侧挤压肛门（图32.2）。我们推荐读者参考Sato[26]、Devesa[27]和Meehan等[28]的著作来完善手术的细节。

肌肉可以自远端也可以自近端游离。通过对12具尸体进行研究，Pak-art等[29]发现自近端游离可以使肌肉更容易到达肛门处，提倡该手术操作。可以游离一侧肌肉，也可以游离两侧，游离时要严格保护神经血管束，该结构位于坐骨结节外上侧[29]。

臀大肌转位术的疗效

臀大肌成形术疗效的相关文献很少。1992年Devesa等[27]报道了10例患者结果，9例症状有改善，其中6例效果明显。2005年，Sato[26]报道了19例患者，结果显示患者术后肛门功能无改善与回肠造瘘相关，有些患者可以应用单侧臀大肌转位术作为肛门成形术的补充[30]。

结论

肌肉转位是治疗肛门失禁的有效手段。该手术可以提高患者控制成形大便的能力，大部分患者对该手术效果满意[31]。对患者和医生来说肌肉转位手术都不是非做不可的。该手术技术上有挑战性，并会带来一定的并发症。手术前，医生应完全取得患者的知情同意，并对术式选择进行充分讨论。有文献报道保留括约肌手术后肛门功能不完善患者的生活质量与结肠造瘘患者相当，这一点在病情会商时应加以考虑[32]。股薄肌成形术比末端肠造瘘或人工肛门花费高很多[33]；对很多患者来说，选择结肠造瘘术可以省很多花费。结直肠医生必须在这组患者中有选择的实施肌肉成形手术，作为完整治疗的一部分[34]。

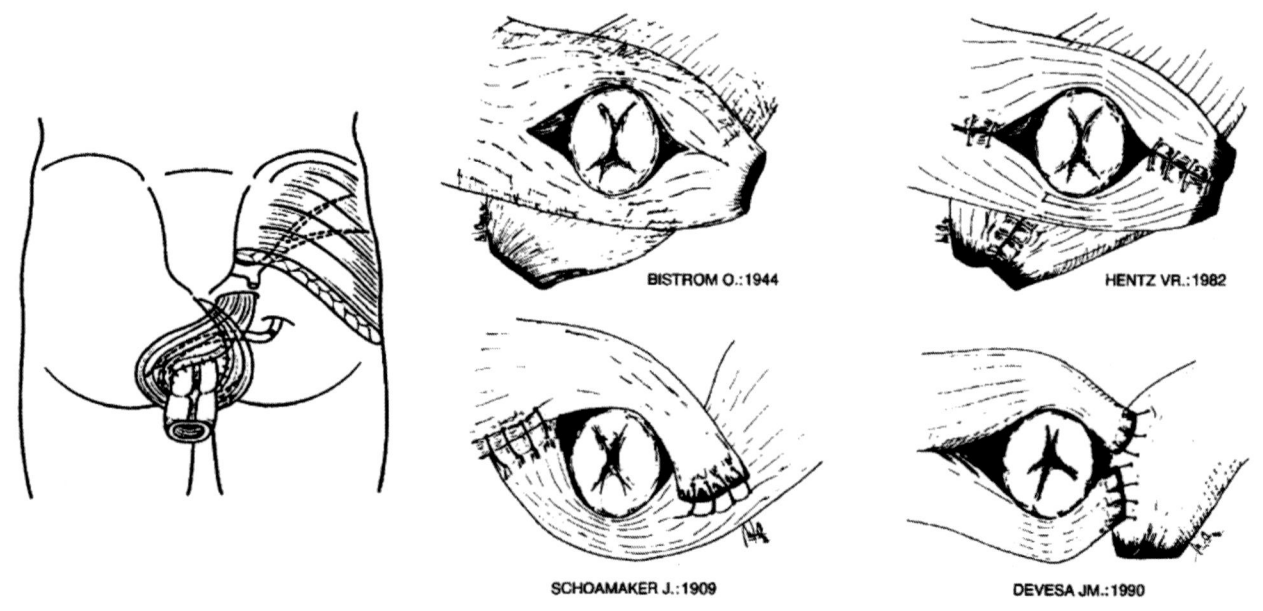

图32.2 左侧：腹会阴联合直肠切除术后行肌肉重建的折刀位肛门示意图。行阴部神经吻合后，臀大肌被转位至会阴伤口处的乙状结肠周围，该肌肉从骨盆起始部拉出至会阴部（Reprinted with permission from Sato et al[26].）。右侧：为获得闭合无张力的肛门可以采用多种术式（Biström, Hentz, Schoamaker），1990年Devesa等[27]的术式效果最好（Reprinted with permission from Devesa et al.[27]）

参考文献

1. Nelson R, Norton N, Cautley E, Furner S. Community-based prevalence of anal incontinence. JAMA. 1995;274:559–61.
2. Macmillan AK, Merrie AE, Marshall RJ, Parry BR. The prevalence of fecal incontinence in community-dwelling adults: a systematic review of the literature. Dis Colon Rectum. 2004;47:1341–9.
3. Madoff RD, Parker SC, Varma MG, Lowry AC. Fecal incontinence in adults. Lancet. 2004;364(9434):621–32.
4. Rockwood TH, Church JM, Fleshman JW, Kane RL, Mavrantonis C, Thorson AG, et al. Patient and surgeon ranking of the severity of symptoms associated with fecal incontinence: the fecal incontinence severity index. Dis Colon Rectum. 1999;42:1525–32.
5. Rockwood TH, Church JM, Fleshman JW, Kane RL, Mavrantonis C, Thorson AG, et al. Fecal incontinence quality of life scale: quality of life instrument for patients with fecal incontinence. Dis Colon Rectum. 2000;43:9–17.
6. Jorge JM, Wexner SD. Etiology and management of fecal incontinence. Dis Colon Rectum. 1993;36:77–97.
7. Macchi V, Vigato E, Porzionato A, Tiengo C, Stecco C, Parenti A, et al. The gracilis muscle and its use in clinical reconstruction: an anatomical, embryological, and radiological study. Clin Anat. 2008;21:696–704.
8. Pickrell KL, Broadbent TR, Masters FW, Metzger JT. Construction of a rectal sphincter and restoration of anal continence by transplanting the gracilis muscle; a report of four cases in children. Ann Surg. 1952;135:853–62.
9. Spiegel JH, Lee C, Trabulsy PP, Coughlin RR. Endoscopic harvest of the gracilis muscle flap. Ann Plast Surg. 1998;41:384–9.
10. Hallock GG. Minimally invasive harvest of the gracilis muscle. Plast Reconstr Surg. 1999;104:801–5.
11. Chapman AE, Geerdes B, Hewett P, Young J, Eyers T, Kiroff G, et al. Systematic review of dynamic graciloplasty in the treatment of fecal incontinence. Br J Surg. 2002;89:138–53.
12. Wexner SD, Baeten C, Bailey R, Bakka A, Belin B, Belliveau P, et al. Long-term efficacy of dynamic graciloplasty for fecal incontinence. Dis Colon Rectum. 2002;45:809–18.
13. Thornton MJ, Kennedy ML, Lubowski DZ, King DW. Long-term follow-up of dynamic graciloplasty for fecal incontinence. Colorectal Dis. 2004;6:470–6.
14. Penninckx F. Belgian experience with dynamic graciloplasty for fecal incontinence. Br J Surg. 2004;91:872–8.
15. Koch SM, Uludağ O, El Naggar K, van Gemert WG, Baeten CG. Colonic irrigation for defecation disorders after dynamic graciloplasty. Int J Colorectal Dis. 2008;23:195–200.
16. Ho KS, Seow-Choen F. Dynamic graciloplasty for total anorectal reconstruction after abdominoperineal resection for rectal tumour. Int J Colorectal Dis. 2005;20:38–41.
17. Saunders JR, Williams NS, Eccersley AJ. The combination of electrically stimulated gracilis neoanal sphincter and continent colonic conduit: a step forward for total anorectal reconstruction? Dis Colon Rectum. 2004;47:354–66.
18. Konsten J, Baeten CG, Havenith MG, Soeters PB. Morphology of dynamic graciloplasty compared with the anal sphincter. Dis Colon Rectum. 1993;36:559–63.
19. Christiansen J, Sorensen M, Rasmussen OO. Gracilis muscle transposition for fecal incontinence. Br J Surg. 1990;77:1039–40.
20. Sielezneff I, Bauer S, Bulgare JC, Sarles JC. Gracilis muscle transposition in the treatment of fecal incontinence. Int J Colorectal Dis. 1996;11:15–8.
21. Niriella DA, Deen KI. Neosphincters in the management of fecal incontinence. Br J Surg. 2000;87:1617–28.
22. Shatari T, Fujita M, Kodaira S. Dynamic graciloplasty resulting fecal continence without electrical stimulation: report of a case. Surg Today. 2004;34:463–5.
23. Chetwood CH. Plastic operation of the sphincter ani with report of a case. Med Rec. 1902;61:529.
24. Wreden RR. A method of constructing a voluntary sphincter ani. Arch Surg. 1929;18:841.
25. Guelinckx PJ, Sinsel NK, Gruwez JA. Anal sphincter reconstruction with the gluteus maximus muscle: anatomic and physiologic considerations concerning conventional and dynamic gluteoplasty. Plast Reconstr Surg. 1996;98:293–304.
26. Sato T, Konishi F, Endoh N, Uda H, Sugawara Y, Nagai H. Long-term outcomes of a neo-anus with a pudendal nerve anastomosis contemporaneously reconstructed with an abdominoperineal excision of the rectum. Surgery. 2005;137:8–15.
27. Devesa JM, Vicente E, Enriquez JM, Nuño J, Bucheli P, de Blas G, et al. Total fecal incontinence – a new method of gluteus maximus transposition: preliminary results and report of previous experience with similar procedures. Dis Colon Rectum. 1992;35:339–49.
28. Meehan JJ, Hardin Jr WD, Georgeson KE. Gluteus maximus augmentation for the treatment of fecal incontinence. J Pediatr Surg. 1997;32:1045–8.
29. Pak-Art R, Silapunt P, Bunaprasert T, Tansatit T, Vajrabukka T. Prospective, randomized, controlled trial of proximally based vs. distally based gluteus maximus flap for anal incontinence in cadavers. Dis Colon Rectum. 2002;45:1100–3.
30. Enriquez-Navascues JM, Devesa-Mugica JM. Traumatic anal incontinence. Role of unilateral gluteus maximus transposition supplementing and supporting direct anal sphincteroplasty. Dis Colon Rectum. 1994;37:766–9.
31. Tillin T, Chambers M, Feldman R. Outcomes of electrically stimulated gracilis neosphincter surgery. Health Technol Assess 2005;9(28):iii, ix–xi, 1–102.
32. Cornish JA, Tilney HS, Heriot AG, Lavery IC, Fazio VW, Tekkis PP. A meta-analysis of quality of life for abdominoperineal excision of rectum versus anterior resection for rectal cancer. Ann Surg Oncol. 2007;14:2056–68.
33. Tan EK, Vaizey C, Cornish J, Darzi A, Tekkis PP. Surgical strategies for fecal incontinence – a decision analysis between dynamic graciloplasty, artificial bowel sphincter and end stoma. Colorectal Dis. 2008;10:577–86.
34. Cera SM, Wexner SD. Muscle transposition: does it still have a role? Clin Colon Rectal Surg. 2005;18:46–54.

第 33 章 肛门内括约肌增强方法

Fernando de la Portilla

张春泽 译　李国逊 审校

摘　要

外科手术改善肛门外括约肌功能的结果不尽如人意，而对于肛门内括约肌功能的疗效更糟。种类多样的技术旨在治疗肛门外括约肌缺陷，这些技术包括直接修复、折叠修复、电刺激股薄肌成形术、臀大肌移植括约肌成形术、人造肠括约肌和骶神经刺激。人们已经试图直接修复肛门内括约肌，但是所有结果均令人失望。肛门内括约肌的肌肉薄，不易于固定手术缝线，肌肉难于获得较好的愈合。修复的替代疗法是肛门后修补术，但是这种手术只有约 35% 的长期成功率，因此基本上成为了历史，而不能被大家所接受。在过去的几年中，可注射的材料得到了开发和评估。虽然没有哪种药单独使用被证明是灵丹妙药，但仅仅是括约肌能被增强的概念也很有趣。除了可以注射材料，射频能量也获得一些成功。各种材料的详细讨论以及对结果的回顾均列于本章中。在以后的几年中，我们希望能为肛门内括约肌缺陷的患者成功开发一种或多种供选择的、并发症较少的治疗方法。

关键词

肛门内括约肌（IAS）增强；大便失禁；填充剂；聚四氟乙烯；自体脂肪；硅酮；用戊二醛处理的牛胶原；GAX 胶原；碳珠；羟磷灰石陶器微球体；聚糖酐；非动物的稳定透明质酸；交联的猪真皮胶原；交联的聚丙烯酰胺；微球；间质干细胞（MSCs）

引　言

据估计有 2% 的人受到大便失禁的影响，其患病率随着年龄增大而增加，50 岁以上的男性和女性发病率分别为 11% 和 26%[1-2]。如果肛门括约肌出现断裂，大多数的患者可以进行保守治疗或手术修复。失禁通常由多种原因造成。肛门内括约肌（IAS）对肛门静止压力贡献较大，但是肛门黏膜和黏膜下层的脉管组织对促进肛门导管的关闭也很重要[3-4]。

肛门内括约肌功能减弱或被破坏、肛门黏膜或黏膜下层的损伤都可能导致被动性大便失禁。

被动性大便失禁是无意识的情况下的不随意排便，主要与肛门内括约肌功能障碍有关。肛门内括约肌功能障碍的原因，可分为两大类。一类是形态完整，但肛门内括约肌的功能减弱；另一类是肛门内括约肌结构上的损坏，结构完整。但功能弱的肛门内括约肌可能是由于原发性功能减退（随着年龄增长）或全身性疾病，如系统性硬化病[5]。放射线疗法也能损伤肌间神经丛，导致肛门内括约肌功能减弱[6]。肛门手术可致内括约肌破坏或结构损坏，例如肛门扩张、括约肌切开术、肛瘘手术或痔切除术[7]和产科损伤。

一些患者大便失禁主要是肛门内括约肌损伤造成的，用止泻药例如洛哌丁胺和可待因，以及经生物反馈治疗会有效，不过对此类大便失禁的效果可能仅仅是暂时性的。其他可能的、更复杂的治疗方法包括：直接手术修复[8]、岛状肛门成形术[9]、射频能量（Secca 手术）[10]、动力股薄肌成形术、人造肠括约肌的植入、骶神经刺激[11]与经皮胫后神经刺激[12]。由于这些技术的经验有限，使得这些新技术都有并发症。

泌尿科医师使用注射填充剂较为成功地改善了膀胱颈的闭合，为其最终用于治疗肛门内括约肌功能障碍导致的大便失禁开辟了途径[13]。在使用填充剂持久关闭膀胱颈成功之后，在肛门内括约肌功能障碍的患者中，试验填充剂就是顺其自然的进展。证据表明，随着该病进行肛门成形术获得成功[9]，使用这样的试剂治疗孤立的内括约肌缺陷可能会有效。然而，填充剂的作用机制不确定。填充沟状畸形或抬高肛垫保持肛管的闭合，防止粪便泄漏，似乎可能是纯粹的机械作用。或者，当肛门内括约肌强直收缩时，可以提供充足的体积够大的肛门衬料，能塞住肛门口。尽管存在这些假设，但没有研究显示在其放置后，静止或挤压时肛压增加（图 33.1）。

材料的类型

理想的充填材料应该具有生物不相容、无免疫原性，应该导致极少的炎症和纤维化反应[14]。材料颗粒应足够大，以免从注射部位漏出（直径大于 80mm）；也应该持久耐用，能用到最后。动物研究显示，在淋巴结和肺、肾、脾和脑[15]中发现直径为 4~80mm 的粒子远距离移动。更为严重的是，由于移动耐久性差，在移动部位可能形成慢性肉芽肿。通常，大多数的电流材料由悬浮在赋形剂中的粒子组成（无活性的载体），其通常是一种可生物降解的凝胶。

理想试剂包括以下特性：
- 生物相容性
- 不移动
- 不会引起过敏
- 无免疫原性
- 无致癌性
- 容易注射
- 产生持久的效果

已在动物中检查过植入的修复材料的潜在致癌

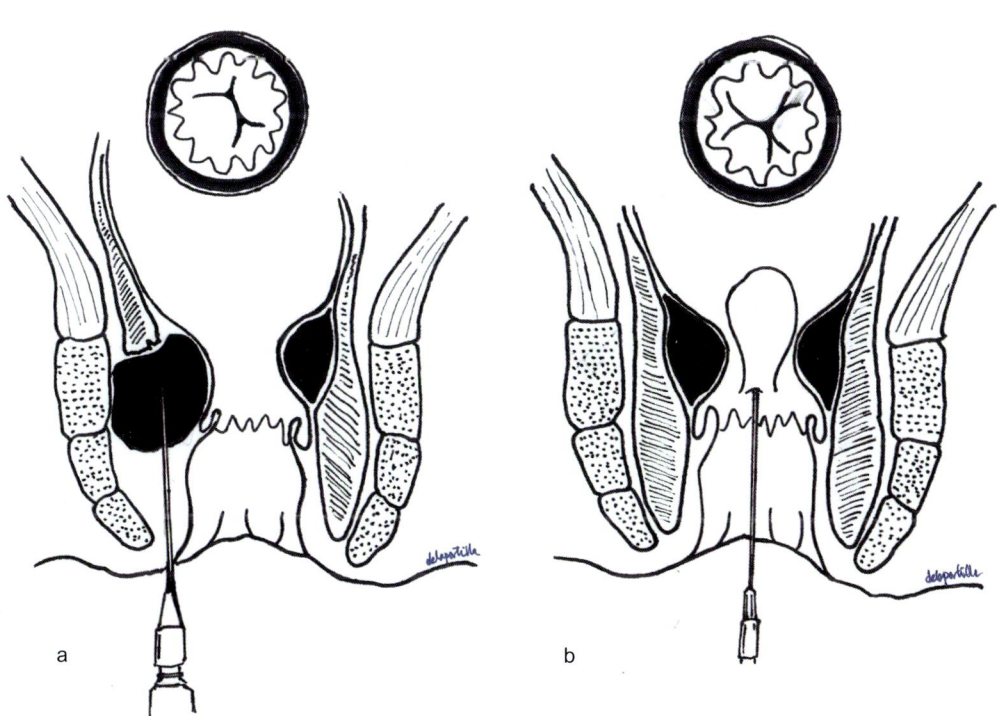

图 33.1 填充剂的作用机制。（a）在肛门内括约肌缺陷中注射；（b）象限注射

性，但还没有在人类[16-17]中证实。

现肺内脂肪组织和脂滴栓子。

聚四氟乙烯

在 Shafik[18] 报道聚四氟乙烯注射剂（Polytef 或特氟纶；杜邦，威尔明顿、DE）用于大便失禁约 20 年以前，早在 1964 年，由泌尿科医师 Politano[19] 开始的一项研究，发表了其首个报告。聚四氟乙烯是特氟纶经高温分解（在高温、缺氧的情况下，有机材料的热化学分解）产生。聚四氟乙烯颗粒的大小范围为 4~100mm，90% 为 4~40mm。用于注射疗法的充填材料是一种由聚四氟乙烯、甘油和聚异山梨醇[20]组成的软膏。因为可能移动，本产品在临床上已经停止使用[21]。

自体脂肪

对于固有的免疫原性减少，使用取自患者的材料是一个有吸引力的方案。从腹壁抽吸的脂肪中提取细胞。随后将细胞纯化并悬浮于盐溶液中，之后将其注入肛管。不过，该材料有迅速溶解和移动的可能性，所以已经停止了此方案的进一步开发[22]，不过，Shafik[23] 最初发表了一份其成功治疗大便失禁的报告。尿道周围注射填充剂后，唯一的死亡报告发生于泌尿科中自体脂肪的注射[24]，尸检时，发

硅酮颗粒

到目前为止，硅酮是目前治疗大便失禁使用最广泛的容积增大剂。泌尿科医师所熟知的名称为 Macroplastique，其与报道的大便失禁填充剂是相同的物质，不过其商品名为 Bioplastique[25-26]。后来改名为 PTP 植入物和 PTQ 植入物（Uroplasty BV, Geleen，荷兰）。

PTQ 植入物产品是一种可注射的异质性材料，由悬浮于可生物排泄的载体中的聚二甲基硅氧烷颗粒、聚乙烯－吡咯烷酮的水凝胶（聚维酮，PVP）组成。固体颗粒含量约占材料容积的 1/3，颗粒大小一般为 100~450μm，但是在凝胶[27]内颗粒较小。颗粒的灵活性和结构使胶原以不规则的方式环绕和穿过植入物。全方位的沉积至少在理论上防止植入物被压缩成硬化软膏。在适当的位置也保持其容积不变（图 33.2）。

动物研究产生的不同结果取决于颗粒的大小，已经报道[28-29]较小颗粒有移动的可能性，这增加了肉芽肿形成的可能。在这方面，用 Bioplastique（硅胶 + PVP）注射大鼠的研究显示，局部的反应最小，缺乏远处转移[30]。最近 de la Portilla 等[31] 通过成像证明，硅酮植入物可能移动或甚至丢失；然而，在

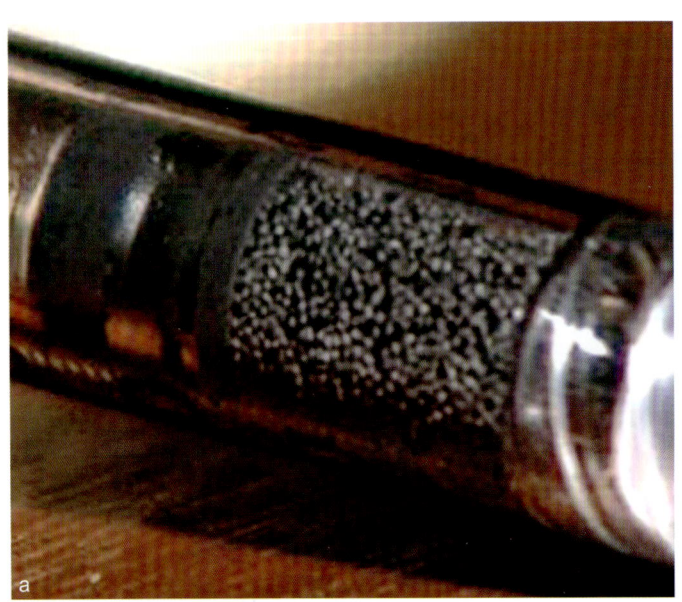
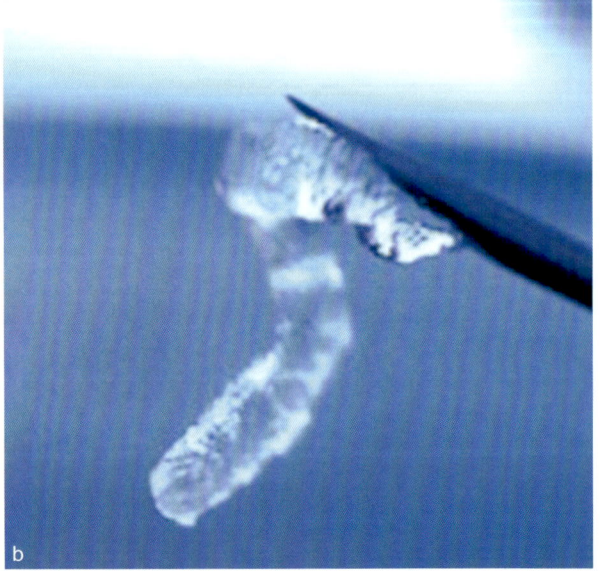

图 33.2 两个填充剂的详细情况。（a）PTQ 植入物；（b）矽胶颗粒悬浮液

一些患者中，仍然怀疑植入物无显影是否是由于植入物断裂成小颗粒，经内镜超声没有检测到。我们进一步关注硅酮和自身免疫病之间可能的联系，但是近期的数据似乎表明不可能存在这种联系[32-33]。

用戊二醛处理牛胶原后交联的胶原（GAX胶原）

用戊二醛处理的牛胶原（Contigen；Bard，Covington，GA），由真皮牛胶原与戊二醛交联构成，分散在浸磷酸盐的生理盐水溶液中[34]。至少95%的GAX胶原是Ⅰ型胶原，1%和5%之间是Ⅲ型胶原[20]。肉芽肿形成或移动没问题，具有生物相容性，注射后约12周，没有开始降解。在注射后9～19个月，GAX胶原的持久性在组织学上得到证实[35-36]。虽然没有不利影响，不过3%的患者发生变态反应，报道了临床症状不明显的血清阳性[37]。在注射GAX胶原之前，必须完成皮肤测试，以检测超敏反应。

碳珠

此填充剂（矽胶颗粒悬浮液，碳医疗技术股份有限公司，保罗街，MN）由固体、热解的、碳涂层的小珠构成，悬浮于黏性载体凝胶中。载体凝胶由水和β-葡聚糖组成。碳涂层的小珠约比移动阈值80mm大3倍，不能被吸收[38]。在生物学上热解碳不反应。有一定的流动阻力，注射需要18G的针头。小珠是不可生物降解的，因此可能具有的优点是，相对于易于随时间分解的材料，更具耐久性。在泌尿学的研究中提到，显著移动到局部和远处的淋巴结以及尿道黏膜[39]（图33.2）。

羟磷灰石陶瓷微球

此填充剂（团块剂，Bioform，Franksville，WI）由羟磷灰石陶瓷的微球悬浮在羧甲基纤维素钠、甘油和水的载体凝胶中组成。制造的颗粒大小为75～125mm，以避免移动。填充物是无抗原性和非炎性的。注射后，填充物陷入未封装的、稳定的软胶原基质内，即使在固体颗粒缓慢降解和吸收后，都会维持容积。两个主要的使用优势包括：①用21G针头减轻注射及其射线不能透过；②在平

片上可见[40]。

聚糖酐/透明质酸共聚物

此容积增大材料（Solesta，QMED，Uppsala，瑞典）包括聚糖酐微珠和非动物的、直径为120mm稳定的透明质酸凝胶[41]。在微球之间，聚糖酐促进成纤维细胞向内生长和胶原的生成，降解透明质酸，以便用内源组织稳固推注、稳定其容积，以便持续长期反应。本产品在凝胶中对治疗大便失禁的生物学评价，是基于用最后的聚糖酐和非动物的稳定透明质酸产品进行的生物相容性测试。

临床前研究最重要的发现是该产品的耐受性良好，并没有表现出任何迹象的细胞毒性、致畸性、遗传不稳定性或一般毒性[42-43]。同样已证明其在体内的生物相容性良好；2年以来，植入物似乎没有移动到其他组织[44]。

交联猪真皮胶原

这种生物材料（Permacol，组织科学实验室PLC，Aldershot，英国）含交联猪真皮胶原的大颗粒；在过去的6年中，在75 000多例患者的各种修复术中以片状形式植入。现在正在介绍的交联猪真皮胶原，作为具有天然生物相容性、无过敏性胶原的替代品，其耐用性得到改善，这是血运重建和细胞向内生长的结果。其较易于注入[45]。

交联聚丙烯酰胺

这是一种合成的、非颗粒的水凝胶（Bulkamid，Contura国际的A/S，Soeborg，丹麦），由97.5%的水和2.5%交联聚丙烯酰胺组成。其具有生物相容性，但不能生物降解。其不能被吸收、耐移动，并对周围组织几乎不产生作用。没有颗粒的均匀的水凝胶，据说会保持弹性，不会造成硬组织纤维化。因此，它实际上不会引起过敏反应[45]。

微球

可膨胀微球（Urosurge公司 Corallville，IA）是由硅酮制成，填充物由一种聚N-乙烯基吡咯烷酮形成的生物相容性水凝胶组成。输送系统由不锈

钢制成的套针样的针、外壳、输送导管和连接到末端的微球组成。该填充剂的经验只限于一项研究，因此，目前不能得出其安全性的结论[46]。

干细胞

近年来，一些试验已经研究了体外或体内的间质干细胞（MSCs）分化成许多组织成熟细胞的能力，描述了在不同的器官损伤并注入干细胞后，组织修复得到特别的改善。尤其是在肌肉组织中，注入的干细胞可以成活并形成多核肌管，有效参与损伤后再生[47]。已有人报道干细胞注射可能可以治疗尿失禁，在动物实验中已经取得成功。干细胞注入能使受损伤的排尿肌和尿道括约肌的再生作用增强和收缩性改善[48]。因此，MSCs 注射可能是括约肌病变造成的肛门失禁的新疗法[49]。最近已迈出了动物实验的第一步，实验性损伤后，通过临床、组织学、肌电图评价，肛门括约肌功能再生成功[50-51]。

用填充剂治疗的适应证和禁忌证

适应证

这种疗法的适应证包括被动性固体或液体大便失禁，每周 1 次或更多次，因为肛门内括约肌功能障碍或相关的单一或复合的肛门内括约肌缺陷，以及保守治疗失败（图 33.3）。

禁忌证

直肠疾病

- 只是排气失禁
- 肛门外括约肌缺损
- 显著的直肠或黏膜脱垂

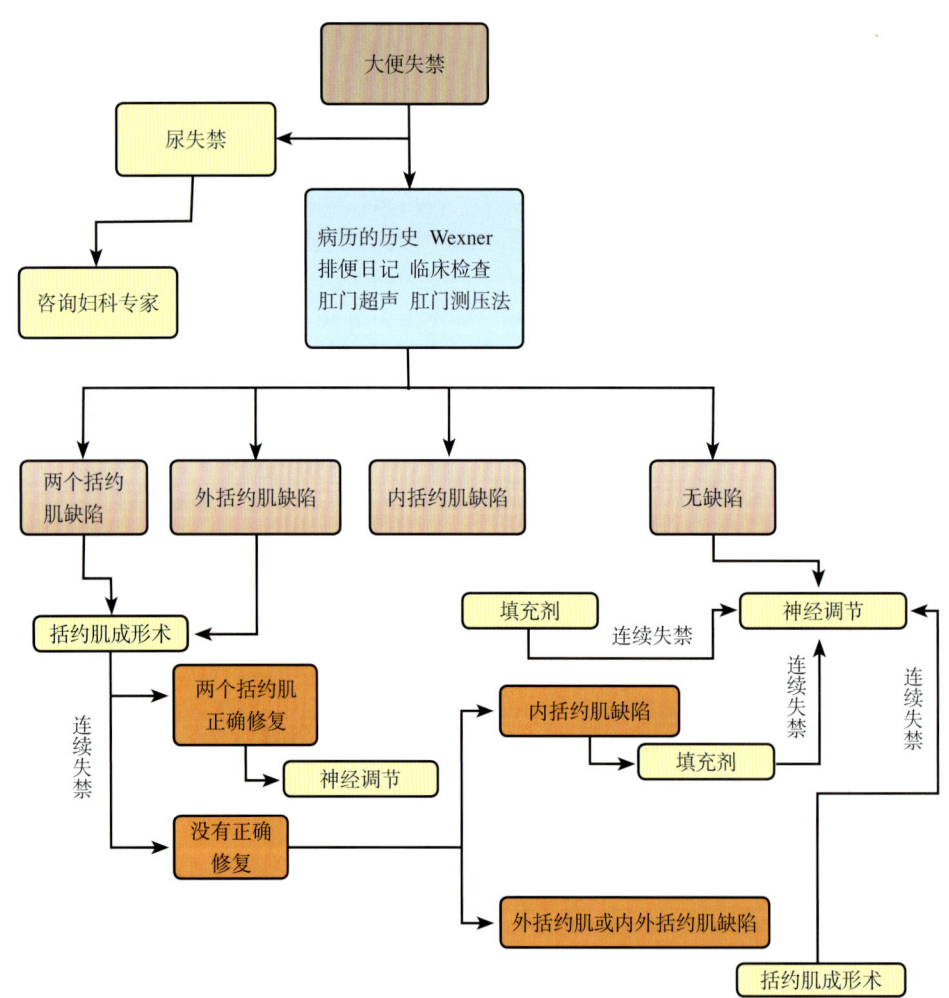

图 33.3　大便失禁治疗算法中容积增大物的位置

- 活性的肛肠败血症
- 当前肛肠肿瘤
- 当前肛裂
- 在距肛门缘 <10cm 进行直肠吻合术
- 活动性直肠炎
- 自发性肛门直肠出血、直肠静脉曲张或血管畸形
- 肛门直肠狭窄
- 慢性肛门直肠或骨盆的显著疼痛
- Ⅲ~Ⅳ级痔疮病
- 肛门直肠畸形

并发症/合并用药

- 炎性肠病
- 药物治疗无效的慢性腹泻
- 人类免疫缺陷病毒感染的病史、任何严重的免疫功能低下状态或免疫抑制治疗的给药
- 出血素质或正在接受抗凝疗法，例如华法林、肝素、肝素类似物

一般适用对象

- 怀孕或产后前 6 个月内
- 年龄小于 18 岁或大于 80 岁

用填充剂治疗的常规实践方面

注射准备

在一般情况下，无论选取何处注射部位（内括约肌或黏膜下层），所有填充剂都需要至少术前 2h 为直肠进行简单的磷酸盐灌肠。虽然一些方案建议至少术前 2 天使用泻药治疗以软化大便，有研究者认为其对于治疗成功并不重要。与此相反，其会加重失禁，造成肛门周围的皮肤过敏、皮炎和污染的风险。目前公认在术前应预防性使用抗生素，采用第一代头孢菌素（覆盖皮肤菌群）和甲硝唑（厌氧菌群）[25-26]。

注射技术

不同的试剂可选不同的方式注射，通过肛周肌肉复合体或只能通过肛门内括约肌以及黏膜下层注射（图 33.4）。黏膜下层注射发生糜烂和败血症的风险较高[52]。植入物可放置在括约肌间平面或在黏膜下层的平面中，但总应在齿状线以上。植入物放在齿状线下会导致术后显著的疼痛（图 33.5）。植入物可被注射到 4 个或更少的象限中，或仅仅在肛门内括约肌缺陷位置以增进肛管的对称。注射可以用数字化引导（通过直接显影）或经肛门超声引导。最近有研究者认为超声引导与短期失禁的改善有关[53]，以前认为使用超声会分散植入物[26]。通常门诊患者进行手术，可以在局部麻醉下镇静处理；然而，一些患者不需要任何镇静，所以，作为非卧床的手术，可以在医生的办公室中进行（图 33.6）。

注射量取决于使用的试剂和选择的注射法（表 33.1）。到目前为止，尚无研究比较植入物的数目和位置以及不同治疗方案的效力[54]。

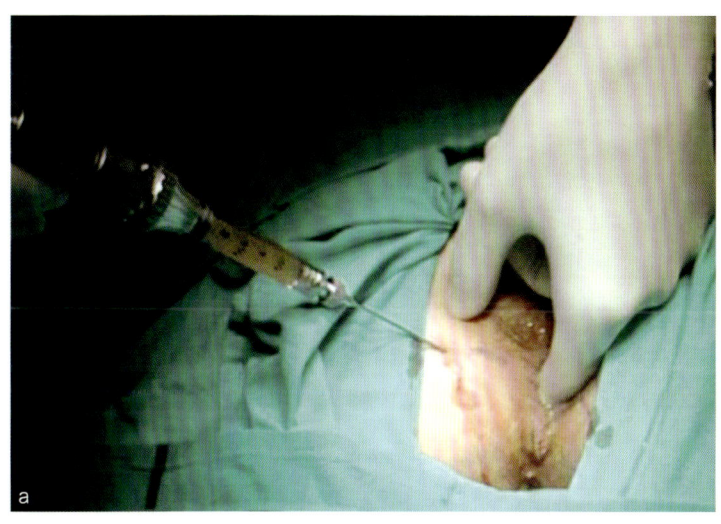 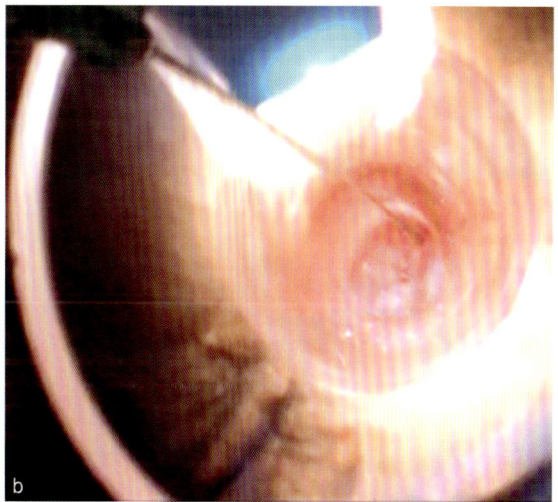

图 33.4 填充剂注射方式。(a)肛周注射；(b)黏膜下层注射

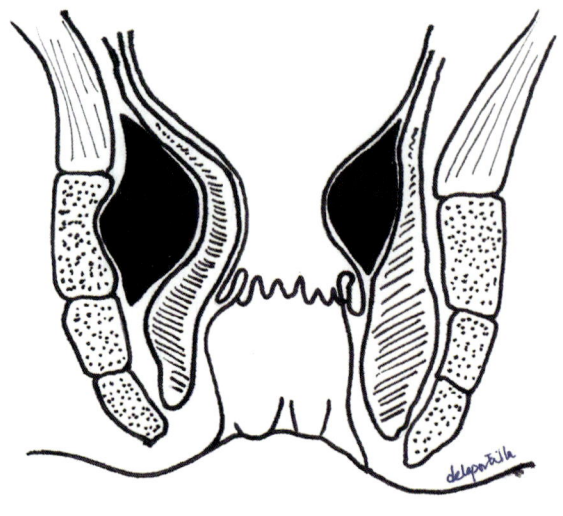

图33.5 植入物的位置，注射试剂的右半球黏膜下层和左半球括约肌间

表33.1 目前销售的植入物的注入方式、位置和主要填充剂的容积

试 剂	注入路径	植入物的位置	总容积
Teflon	黏膜下层	黏膜下层	10 mL
自体脂肪	黏膜下层	黏膜下层	15～20 mL
PTQ 植入物	肛门周围	黏膜下层或括约肌间	7.5 mL
Contigen	黏膜下层	黏膜下层	2～5 mL
矽胶颗粒悬浮液	黏膜下层或肛门周围	黏膜下层的或括约肌间	8～10 mL
Coaptite	肛门周围	黏膜下层	4 mL
Solesta	黏膜下层	黏膜下层	4 mL
Permacol	肛门周围	黏膜下层	15 mL
Bulkamid	肛门周围	黏膜下层	9 mL
Urosurge	黏膜下层	黏膜下层	到5气囊

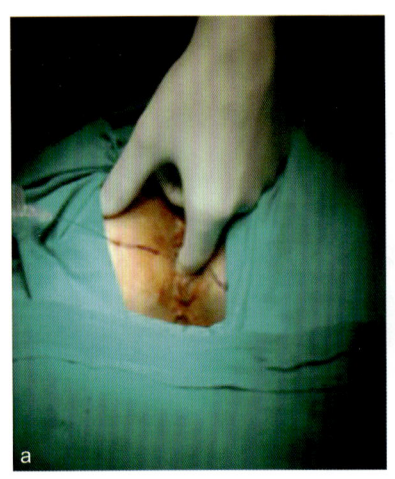
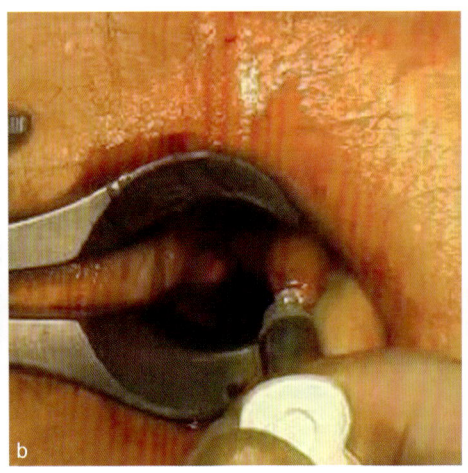
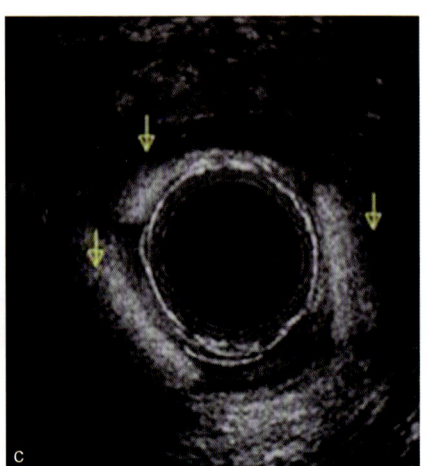

图33.6 不同的注射法。(a)数字化引导；(b)通过直接显影；(c)肛门内超声引导

手术后的测量

手术以后，患者接受7～10d日程的抗生素治疗[25-26]。一些方案建议患者使用轻泻药软化粪便以避免植入物压缩；也有建议用轻度镇痛药，因为疼痛通常轻微。

结 果

最近发表的旨在评估容积扩增效力的循证医学系统性回顾分析表明，缺乏设计完善的随机比对临床试验。4项选定的随机比对临床试验中，仅1个有充足的样品量，而其他的试验样品量不充分、缺乏对照、缺乏盲法评估，或患者随访通知不正确[53]。

有多种观察研究显示短期改善有显著的统计学差异，不过使用的试剂和技术有许多变化。评估全球发表的研究似乎表明，大多数试剂比较安全；不过并发症常见，对于大多数试剂，并发症相对不显著，是暂时的。然而，鉴于目前信息的质量和可用性较低，这些结论只是临时的。

虽然许多已发表的研究比较了不同的试剂，得出了一些成果，不过一些材料，例如硅酮，似乎比其他试剂至少在短期内更有效[55]。硅酮（PTQ植入物）是使用最广泛的材料，可以认为是目前治疗的金标准。不过在这方面，与矽胶颗粒悬浮液比较效力时，仅一个对照试验显示出PTQ植入物的优势，伴有的并发症较少[55]。仅安慰剂对照试验可以在患者队列之间，比较生理盐水治疗与 PTQ 植入物治疗，没有显示任何统计学显著差异[56]。仍然缺乏关于试剂应该注射的容积、精确位置，以及植入方式的准确信息。一项在 6 例患者中评价长期效力的研究[57]，在 61 个月的随访中，1 例患者做过结肠造口术以治疗大便失禁，其余 5 例患者的失禁得分基本没变，但是 36 项简表得分表明，身体和社会功能有实质的改善，满意得分高。主观上，3 例患者有改善：其中 1 例进行再次注射，1 例在生物反馈治疗一个疗程后改善。随访周期后，5 例患者中有 1 例由于相关的直肠阴道瘘而做了结肠造口术。该研究的结论是，用 PTQ 植入物治疗被动性大便失禁的效力随着时间的推移而变化，大多数患者或许将需要再次注入以保持改善。

尽管目前没有关于容积增量剂效力的明确证据，但其无疑能在一线治疗中有效治疗一些被动性大便失禁的患者；药物或保守治疗失败后，其为微创的替代疗法。应告知患者，想要达到大多数患者所得到的改善将需要进一步治疗（表 33.2）。

并发症

一般情况下，这些疗法的并发症在大多数研究中很少报告。并发症的严重性和持续时间都很少报道，在一些研究中，并没有提及是否有并发症。在大多数情况下，并发症轻微，包括不适、疼痛、出血和注射材料渗漏（图 33.7）。包含用不同试剂处理的 420 例患者的系统回顾中，Luo 等[76]报道 52 例不利事件，最常见的是未成年人，包括注射期间肛门瘙痒（$n=16$）和轻度疼痛（$n=13$）。其他常见的事件包括轻度肛门痛（$n=8$）、肛门炎症和肿胀（$n=6$）。更严重的事件包括肛门持续不适（$n=1$），需要引流的感染（$n=1$），排便期间疼痛（$n=1$）。一例患者在注射过程中疼痛显著，还报道了肛门出血（$n=2$）、肛门污染（$n=1$）、渗漏（$n=1$）、皮炎（$n=1$）。报道 14 例患者出现可注射填充剂的移动，2 例已注入矽胶颗粒悬浮液，其中 12 例已经接受了 PTQ 注射，没有出现与填充剂移动相关的严重后遗症，2 例患者有矽胶颗粒悬浮液与粪便的渗漏。

结　论

以本文的观点，关于使用容积增量剂治疗大便失禁，仍有许多未知的指标。虽然仍没有理想的试剂，且注射的容积、方法未知，然而，理想的候选人可能从这种疗法中受益。要回答其中一些重要的问题，必需选取精确数量的患者进行随机对照研究和长期随访。毫无疑问，未来局部治疗将联合再生医学，以恢复肌纤维或植入成纤维细胞，进行肛管的自发扩增。近来 Ratto 等[77]报道了新型试剂，在一小组植入过聚丙烯腈圆柱体（HYEXPAN；the Gatekeeper System；THD Corregio，意大利）的 14 例患者中，得到了中期的控便收益。这些圆柱体的容积迅速增加到其最大的 720%，始终够硬，以便他们不会分散，在超声引导下最完美地张开。90 天随访时，似乎会减少失禁发作，协助延迟排便功能。容积增量剂在括约肌间张开，可以减少侵蚀的风险，产品出现的内在退化和 / 或扩散少于其他植入体。热切期待对这些不同试剂进行临床比较。

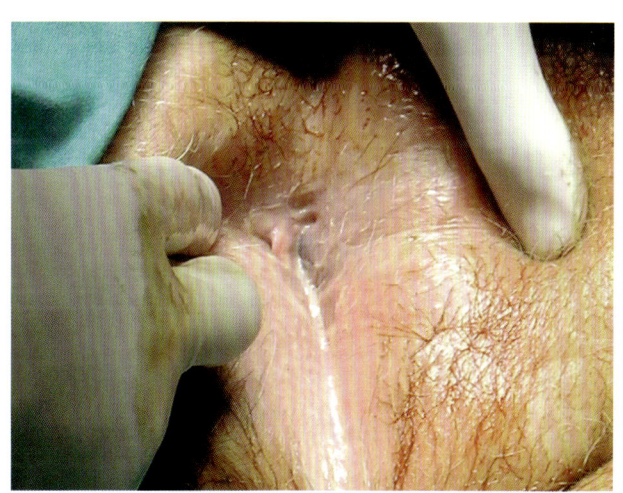

图 33.7　并发症。植入以后某天出现肛周脓肿

表 33.2　到目前为止，填充剂研究的概述

研究者	试　剂		n	改善（%）	随访（mo）
Shafik[18]	聚四氟乙烯/Polytef	黏膜下层	11	50	22
Shafik[23]	自体脂肪	黏膜下层	14	100	6
Bernardi[58]	自体脂肪	环周	1	10	12
Feretis[46]	微球	黏膜下层	6	100	8.6
Weiss[59]	矽胶颗粒悬浮液	括约肌间	10	60	3
Davis[38]	矽胶颗粒悬浮液	黏膜下层	18	83	12
Altomare[60]	矽胶颗粒悬浮液	黏膜下层	33	33	20.8
Aigner[61]	矽胶颗粒悬浮液	肛门周围	11	35	12
Tjandra[55]	矽胶颗粒悬浮液	黏膜下层	20	35	12
Aigner[62]	矽胶颗粒悬浮液	黏膜下层	11	–	24
Beggs[63]	矽胶颗粒悬浮液	括约肌间	23	71.3	12
Malouf[25]	PTQ 植入物	黏膜下层	10	60	6
Kenefick[26]	PTQ 植入物	黏膜下层	6	83	18
Jorge[64]	PTQ 植入物	–	12	75	4
Oliveira[65]	PTQ 植入物	–	6	83	4
Tjandra[57]	PTQ 植入物	括约肌间	82	55	6
Chan[66]	PTQ 植入物	括约肌间	7	100	14
Siproudhis[56]	PTQ 植入物	括约肌间	22	23	3
	含盐		22	27	
Van der Hagen[67]	PTQ 植入物	黏膜下层	24	45	12
Gaj[68]	PTQ 植入物	括约肌间	16	–	12
Maeda[69]	PTQ 植入物	黏膜下层	6	50	61
de la Portilla[70]	PTQ 植入物	黏膜下层	20	60	20
Soerensen[71]	PTQ 植入物	括约肌间	33	72	13
Tjandra[57]	PTQ 植入物	肛门周围	20	90	12
Bartlett[72]	PTQ 植入物	括约肌间	74	70	28
Smart[54]	Permacol	括约肌间	7	85	13
Maeda[45]	Bulkamid	黏膜下层	5	0	6
	Permacol		5		
Graf[73]	Zuidex	黏膜下层	34	56	12
Dehli[74]	Zuidex	黏膜下层	4	85	?
Danielson[41]	Solesta	黏膜下层	34	56	12
Kumar[34]	Contigen	黏膜下层	17	64	8
Stojkovic[75]	Contigen	黏膜下层	73	73	12
Ganio[40]	Coaptite	黏膜下层	10	80	12

参考文献

1. Nelson R, Norton N, Cautley E, Furner S. Community based prevalence of anal incontinence. JAMA. 1995;274:559–61.
2. Macmillan AK, Merrie AE, Marshall RJ, Parry BR. The prevalence of fecal incontinence in community-dwelling adults: a systematic review of the literature. Dis Colon Rectum. 2004;47:1341–9.
3. Gibbons CP, Trowbridge EA, Bannister JJ, Read NW. Role of anal cushions in maintaining continence. Lancet. 1986;1(8486):886–8.
4. Rao SS. Pathophysiology of adult fecal incontinence. Gastroenterology. 2004;126:14–22.
5. Vaizey CJ, Kamm MA, Bartram CI. Primary degeneration of the internal anal sphincter as a cause of passive fecal incontinence. Lancet. 1997;349:612–5.
6. Da Silva GM, Berho M, Wexner SD, Efron J, Weiss EG, Nogueras JJ, et al. Histologic analysis of the irradiated anal sphincter. Dis Colon Rectum. 2003;46:1492–7.
7. Altomare DF, Rinaldi M, Sallustio PL, Martino P, De Fazio M, Memeo V. Long-term effects of stapled hemorrhoidectomy on internal anal function and sensitivity. Br J Surg. 2001;88:1487–91.
8. Leroi AM, Kamm MA, Weber J, Denis P, Hawley PR. Internal anal sphincter repair. Int J Colorectal Dis. 1997;12:243–5.
9. Morgan R, Patel B, Beynon J, Carr ND. Surgical management of anorectal incontinence due to internal anal sphincter deficiency. Br J Surg. 1997;84:226–30.
10. Takahashi-Monroy T, Morales M, Garcia-Osogobio S, Valdovinos MA, Belmonte C, Barreto C, et al. SECCA procedure for the treatment of fecal incontinence: results of five-year follow-up. Dis Colon Rectum. 2008;51:355–9.
11. Edden Y, Wexner SD. Therapeutic devices for fecal incontinence: dynamic gracioplasty, artificial bowel sphincter and sacral nerve stimulation. Expert Rev Med Devices. 2009;6:307–12.
12. de la Portilla F, Rada R, Vega J, González CA, Cisneros N, Maldonado VH. Evaluation of the use of posterior tibial nerve stimulation for the treatment of fecal incontinence: preliminary results of a prospective study. Dis Colon Rectum. 2009;52:1427–33.
13. Keegan PE, Atiemo K, Cody J, McClinton S, Pickard R. Periurethral injection therapy for urinary incontinence in women. Cochrane Database Syst Rev. 2007;18:CD003881.
14. van Kerrebroeck P, ter Meulen F, Farrelly E, Larsson G, Edwall L, Fianu-Jonasson A. Treatment of stress urinary incontinence: recent developments in the role of urethral injection. Urol Res. 2003;30:356–62.
15. Pycha A, Klinger CH, Haitel A, Heinz-Peer G, Marberger M. Implantable microballoons: an attractive alternative in the management of intrinsic sphincter deficiency. Eur Urol. 1998;33:469–75.
16. Menard S, Porta GD. Incidence, growth and antigenicity of fibrosarcomas induced by Teflon disc in mice. Tumori. 1976;62:565–73.
17. Witherspoon P, Bryson G, Wright DM, Reid R, O'Dwyer PJ. Carcinogenic potential of commonly used hernia repair prostheses in an experimental model. Br J Surg. 2004;91:368–72.
18. Shafik A. Polytetrafluoroethylene injection for the treatment of partial fecal incontinence. Int Surg. 1993;78:159–61.
19. Politano VA. Periurethral polytetrafluoroethylene injection for urinary incontinence. J Urol. 1982;127:439–42.
20. Chaliha C, Williams G. Periurethral injection therapy for the treatment of urinary incontinence. Br J Urol. 1995;76:151–5.
21. Malizia AA, Reiman HM, Myers RP, Sande JR, Barham SS, Benson RC, et al. Migration and granulomatous reaction alter periurethral injection of polytef (Teflon). JAMA. 1984;251:3277–81.
22. Lightner DJ. Review of the available urethral bulking agents. Curr Opin Urol. 2002;12:333–8.
23. Shafik A. Perianal injection of autologous fat for treatment of sphincteric incontinence. Dis Colon Rectum. 1995;38:583–7.
24. Currie I, Drutz HP, Deck J, Oxorn D. Adipose tissue and lipid droplet embolism following periurethral injection of autologous fat: case report and review of the literature. Int Urogynecol J Pelvic Floor Dysfunct. 1997;8:377–80.
25. Malouf AJ, Vaizey CJ, Norton CS, Kamm MA. Internal anal sphincter augmentation for fecal incontinence using injectable silicone material. Dis Colon Rectum. 2001;44:595–600.
26. Kenefick NJ, Vaizey CJ, Malouf AJ, Norton CS, Marshall M, Kamm MA. Injectable silicone biomaterial for fecal incontinence due to internal anal sphincter dysfunction. Gut. 2002;51:225–8.
27. Uroplasty. Product-overview. Access online in http://www.uroplasty.com/Products.asp.
28. Smith DP, Kaplan WE, Oyasu R. Evaluation of polydimethylsiloxane as an alternative in the endoscopic treatment of vesicoureteral reflux. J Urol. 1994;152:1221–4.
29. Henly DR, Barrett DM, Weiland TL, O'Connor MK, Malizia AA, Wein AJ. Particulate silicone for use in periurethral injections: local tissue effects and search for migration. J Urol. 1995;153:2039–43.
30. Nijhuis PH, van den Bogaard TE, Daemen MJ, Baeten CG. Perianal injection of polydimethylsiloxane (bioplastique implants) paste in the treatment of soiling: pilot study in rats to determine migratory tendency and locoregional reaction. Dis Colon Rectum. 1998;41:624–9.
31. de la Portilla F, Vega J, Rada R, Segovia-Gonzáles MM, Cisneros N, Maldonado VH, et al. Evaluation by three-dimensional anal endosonography of injectable silicone biomaterial (PTQ) implants to treat fecal incontinence: long-term localization and relation with the deterioration of the continence. Tech Coloproctol. 2009;13:195–9.
32. Janowsky EC, Kupper LL, Hulka BS. Meta-analyses of the relation between silicone breast implants and the risk of connective-tissue diseases. N Engl J Med. 2000;342:781–90.
33. Bar-Meir E, Eherenfeld M, Shoenfeld Y. Silicone gel breast implants and connective tissue disease – a comprehensive review. Autoimmunity. 2003;36:193–7.
34. Kumar D, Benson MJ, Bland JE. Glutaraldehyde cross-linked collagen in the treatment of fecal incontinence. Br J Surg. 1998;85:978–9.
35. Stegman SJ, Chu S, Bensch K, Armstrong R. A light and electron microscope evaluation of Zyderm collagen and Zyplast implants in ageing human facial skin. A pilot study. Arch Dermatol. 1987;123:1644–9.
36. Leonard MP, Canning DA, Epstein JI, Gearhart JP, Jeffs RD. Local tissue reaction to the subureteral injection of glutaraldehyde cross-linked bovine collagen in humans. J Urol. 1990;143:1209–12.
37. Appell RA. New developments: injectables for urethral incompetence in women. Int Urogynecol J. 1990;1:117–9.
38. Davis K, Kumar D, Poloniecki J. Preliminary evaluation of an injectable anal sphincter bulking agent (Durasphere) in the management of fecal incontinence. Aliment Pharmacol Ther. 2003;18:237–43.
39. Pannek J, Brands FH, Senge T. Particle migration alter transurethral injection of carbon coated beads for stress urinary incontinence. J Urol. 2001;166:1350–3.
40. Ganio E, Marino F, Giani I, Luc AR, Clerico G, Novelli E, et al. Injectable synthetic calcium hydroxylapatite ceramic microspheres (Coaptite) for passive fecal incontinence. Tech Coloproctol. 2008;12:99–102.
41. Danielson J, Karlbom U, Sonesson AC, Wester T, Graf W. Submucosal injection of stabilized nonanimal hyaluronic acid with dextranomer: a new treatment option for fecal incontinence. Dis Colon Rectum. 2009;52:1101–6.
42. Dodi G, Jongen J, De la Portilla F, Raval M, Altomare DF, Lehur PA. An open-label, non comparative, multicenter study to evaluate efficacy safety of Nasha/Dx Gel as a bulking agent for the treatment of fecal incontinence, Castroenterol RES PRACT 2010; 2010: 467736.
43. Stenberg A, Larsson G, Johnson P, Heimer G, Ulmsten U. DiHA dextran copolymer, a new biocompatible material for endoscopic treatment of stress incontinent women. Short team results. Acta Obstet Gynecol Scand. 1999;78:436–42.
44. Stenberg AM, Sundin A, Larsson BS, Lackgren G, Stenberg A. Lack of distant migration after injection of a 125Iodine labeled dextranomer based implant into the Rabbit bladder. J Urol. 1997;158:1937–41.

45. Maeda Y, Vaizey CJ, Kamm MA. Pilot study of two new injectable bulking agents for the treatment of fecal incontinence. Colorectal Dis. 2008;10:268–72.
46. Feretis C, Benakis P, Dailianas A, Dimopoulos C, Mavrantonis C, Stamou KM, et al. Implantation of microballoons in the management of fecal incontinence. Dis Colon Rectum. 2001;44:1605–9.
47. Mitterberger M, Pinggera GM, Marksteiner R, Margreiter E, Plattner R, Klima G, et al. Functional and histological changes after myoblast injections in the porcine rhabdosphincter. Eur Urol. 2007;52:1736–43.
48. Kwon D, Kim Y, Pruchnic R, Jankowski R, Usiene I, de Miguel F, et al. Periurethral cellular injection: comparison of muscle-derived progenitor cells and fibroblasts with regard to efficacy and tissue contractility in an animal model of stress urinary incontinence. Urology. 2006;68:449–54.
49. Feki A, Faltin DL, Lei T, Dubuisson JB, Jacob S, Irion O. Sphincter incontinence: is regenerative medicine the best alternative to restore urinary or anal sphincter function? Int J Biochem Cell Biol. 2007;39:678–84.
50. Kang SB, Lee HN, Lee JY, Park JS, Lee HS, Lee JY. Sphincter contractility after muscle-derived stem cells autograft into the cryoinjured anal sphincters of rats. Dis Colon Rectum. 2008;51:1367–73.
51. Aghaee-Afshar M, Rezazadehkermani M, Asadi A, Malekpour-Afshar R, Shahesmaeili A, Nematollahi-mahani SN. Potential of human umbilical cord matrix and rabbit bone marrow-derived mesenchymal stem cells in repair of surgically incised rabbit external anal sphincter. Dis Colon Rectum. 2009;52:1753–61.
52. Miranda KYC, Tjandra JJ. Injectable silicone biomaterial (PTQ™) to treat fecal incontinence after hemorrhoidectomy. Dis Colon Rectum. 2006;49:433–9.
53. Maeda Y, Laurberg S, Norton C. Perianal injectable bulking agents as treatment for fecal incontinence in adults. Cochrane Database Syst Rev. 2010:CD007959.
54. Smart M, Merce-Jones M, Response to Maeda Y, Vaizey CJ, Kamm MA. Pilot study of two new injectable bulking agents for the treatment of fecal incontinence. Colorectal Dis. 2008;10:628.
55. Tjandra JJ, Chan MK, Yeh HC. Injectable silicone biomaterial (PTQ) is more effective than carbon-coated beads (Durasphere) in treating passive fecal incontinence-a randomized trial. Colorectal Dis. 2009;11:382–9.
56. Siproudhis L, Morcet J, Lainé F. Elastomer implants in fecal incontinence: a blind, randomized placebo-controlled study. Aliment Pharmacol Ther. 2007;25:1125–32.
57. Tjandra JJ, Lim JF, Hiscock R, Rajendra P. Injectable silicone biomaterial for fecal incontinence caused by internal anal sphincter dysfunction is effective. Dis Colon Rectum. 2004;47:2138–46.
58. Bernardi C, Favetta U, Pescatori M. Autologous fat injection for treatment of fecal incontinence: manometric and echographic assessment. Plast Reconstr Surg. 1998;102:1626–8.
59. Weiss EG, Efron JF, Nogueras JJ, Wexner SD. Submucosal injection of carbon coated beads is a successful and safe office-based treatment for fecal incontinence. Dis Colon Rectum. 2002;45:A46–7.
60. Altomare DF, La Torre F, Rinaldi M, Binda GA, Pescatori M. Carbon-coated microbeads anal injection in outpatient treatment of minor fecal incontinence. Dis Colon Rectum. 2008;51:432–5.
61. Aigner F, Conrad F, Margreiter R, Oberwalder M. Anal submucosal carbon bead injection for treatment of idiopathic fecal incontinence: a preliminary report. Dis Colon Rectum. 2009;52:293–8.
62. Aigner F. Injectables with special regard to Durasphere for the treatment of fecal incontinence. Colorectal Dis. 2007;9:13–60.
63. Beggs A, Irukulla S, Sultan AH, Ness W, Abulafi A. A pilot study of ultrasound guided Durasphere injection in the treatment of Fecal Incontinence. Colorectal Dis. 2010;12:935–40.
64. Jorge JM, Yusuf S, Alvarenga C, Habr-Gama A, Kiss DR, Gama-Rodrigues JJ. Transsphincteric injection of silicone biomaterial in the treatment of fecal incontinence due to internal anal sphincter defects. Dis Colon Rectum. 2004;47:565–660.
65. Oliveira LC, Neves Jorge JM, Yussuf S, Habr-Gama A, Kiss D, Cecconello I. Anal incontinence improvement after silicone injection may be related to restoration of sphincter asymmetry. Surg Innov. 2009;16:155–61.
66. Chan MK, Tjandra JJ. Injectable silicone biomaterial (PTQ) to treat fecal incontinence after hemorrhoidectomy. Dis Colon Rectum. 2006;49:433–9.
67. Van der Hagen SJ, van Gemert WG, Baeten CG. PTQ implants in the treatment of fecal soiling. Br J Surg. 2007;94:222–3.
68. Gaj F, Trecca A, Crispino P. Efficacia dell'agente PTQ nel trattamento dell'incontinenza fecale. Chir Ital. 2007;59:355–9.
69. Maeda Y, Vaizey CJ, Kamm MA. Long-term results of perianal silicone injection for fecal incontinence. Colorectal Dis. 2007;9:357–61.
70. de la Portilla F, Fernandez A, Leon E, Rada R, Cisneros N, Maldonado VH, et al. Evaluation of the use of PTQ™ implants for the treatment of incontinent patients due to internal sphincter dysfunction. Colorectal Dis. 2008;10:89–94.
71. Soerensen MM, Lundby L, Buntzen S, Laurberg S. Intersphincteric injected silicone biomaterial implants: a treatment for fecal incontinence. Colorectal Dis. 2009;11:73–6.
72. Bartlett L, Ho YH. PTQ anal implants for the treatment of fecal incontinence. Br J Surg. 2009;96:1468–75.
73. Graf W, Danielsson J, Sonesson AC. Results after submucous bulking therapy with NASHA/Dx for anal incontinence in relation to pretreatment clinical characteristics. Poster no. 280. In: 37th annual meeting of the International Continence Society, Rotterdam, 2007.
74. Dehli T, Lindsetmo RO, Mevik K, Vonen B. Anal incontinence assessment of a new treatment. Tidsskr Nor Laegeforen. 2007;127:2934–6.
75. Stojkovic SG, Lim M, Burke D, Finan PJ, Sagar PM. Intra-anal collagen injection for the treatment of fecal incontinence. Br J Surg. 2006;93:1514–8.
76. Luo C, Samaranayake CB, Plank LD, Bissett IP. Systematic review on the efficacy and safety of injectable bulking agents for passive fecal incontinence. Colorectal Dis. 2010;12:296–303.
77. Ratto C, Parello A, Donisi L, Litta F, De Simone V, Spazzafumo L, Giordano P. Novel bulking agent for faecal incontinence. Br J Surg. 2011;98:1644–53.

第34章　自体新建括约肌和排便控制的新技术

Ali A. Shafik

于向阳　译　王西墨　审校

摘　要

虽然具有统计学价值的数据寥寥无几，但是脂肪细胞移植和干细胞移植这两个最新的方法可能会为自体括约肌再造和新的排便控制技术提供保障。虽然本章介绍的是股薄肌成形术、臀大肌成形术以及其他新自体括约肌的重建技术，但是从技术角度来讲，细胞移植是可以实现的。但是，需要更多具备相应技术的专业人员准备注射用原料。随着时间的推移，我们可能会越来越熟悉这些各种各样的选择，而且其中的某些技术可能会成为大便失禁治疗方法的有益补充。

关键词

自体新建括约肌；排便控制；股薄肌成形术；臀肌成形术；闭孔内肌；半腱肌股二头肌长头；自体平滑肌；阔筋膜吊索替代物；耻骨直肠肌成形术；脂肪细胞移植；干细胞移植

引　言

人们曾在大便失禁患者身上试图以多种方式构造新肛门括约肌。这些内容在本书中第五部分的其他章节中已做了讨论，除了利用臀肌、股薄肌、闭孔内肌、股二头肌长头、半腱肌等进行肌肉转置术尚未描述。此外，很多平滑肌移位术（主要是作为动物体内实验的数据扩充）、各种再生和基因修饰的骨骼肌，还有干细胞都已经被认为是替代肛门括约肌的潜在技术。表34.1显示了各种可能的备选方案。

臀肌成形术

作为最古老的治疗大便失禁的外科方法之一，臀肌的外科转置正在悄然地重新引起学者们的兴趣。最初在1902年由Chetwood[1]报道以来，已经有各种各样的理由建议使用臀肌。首先，臀肌是由

表34.1　自体新建括约肌包括的肌肉、筋膜和细胞

肌肉皮瓣	
带蒂皮瓣	臀肌
	股薄肌
	闭孔内肌
	股二头肌长头
	半腱肌
	自体平滑肌
游离皮瓣	背阔肌
面部移植瓣	阔筋膜
	腹直肌
细胞移植	脂肪细胞移植
	干细胞移植

臀下动脉供血的血供丰富的肌肉；其次，臀肌较之股薄肌更大更强壮，能提供更多的组织块用于支持肛管；第三，当行走时，臀肌的收缩使得它能够成为外括约肌的重要补充；最后，臀肌的转移不会影响行走和骨盆的稳定。尽管很多技术已经被应用，但是研究最多的方法包括从骶骨上分离双侧臀肌，将一块肌肉劈开，皮下隧道式穿入，一条从前方，另一条从后方裹住直肠。首先将这些肌条缝合在一起，然后再与同侧的游离的肌肉缝合[2]。在一项对尸体的研究中，Pak-Art 等[3]建议对这一手术进行改良，他们发现使用近侧端蒂的臀肌瓣较之远侧端蒂者增加了肌肉长度，从而能减少肌肉张力。

股薄肌成形术

与臀肌类似，股薄肌是对于运动而言非必需的浅表内收肌，容易被获取，并在其近端有来自闭孔神经和股深动脉的固定的神经血管供应。股薄肌转置术已广泛用于大便失禁的治疗。这种技术最早是在 1952 年由 Pickrell 等[4]在治疗儿童神经源性失禁时提出的。由于股薄肌靠近肛管，容易获取，具有近端血和神经供应，股薄肌被认为是明智的选择。但是，由于股薄肌的快速易疲性使其对这些儿童的提高控制排便能力上的作用微乎其微。股薄肌无法持续收缩，因为它是易疲劳 II 型（快肌）肌肉。双股薄肌肛门直肠括约肌重建是一种用于肌肉远端坏死后重建的技术。这种技术似乎是利用残留股薄肌的潜在收缩能力的最佳方法，但目前尚缺乏无功能或缺血相关的纤维化的证据。

1981 年，Salmons 和 Henriksson[5]发现，电刺激在骨骼肌的形态学、生理学和生物化学特性上能引发深刻的变化。在他们的研究中，插入交流电刺激可使股薄肌转变为慢收缩（I 型）肌肉，使其发挥括约肌的功能。电刺激股薄肌成形术在 1991 年由 Baeten 等[6]首次发表。

待患者取截石体位后，在患者大腿内侧做一个长切口或 2~3 个短切口。肌肉经确认后被从胫骨粗隆的附着点上分离，小心保护近端的神经血管束。随后，肌肉通过两个横切口被转移至肛管周围，再缝合到对侧的胫骨粗隆。6~8 周后，电极通过皮下隧道被植入到肌肉组织，神经刺激器被植入腹壁。股薄肌的刺激需要对发生器进行的逐步增强活化。8 周后神经刺激器呈持续开启状态，患者可以用一块磁铁关闭神经刺激器来排便[7]。

在 Rongen 等[8]的一项长达 24 个月的研究中发现：对于没有进行造口的患者，16% 的患者完全可控制排便，43% 患者的失禁获得了高于基线 50% 以上程度的改善，11% 患者的失禁获得了高于基线 50% 以下程度的改善，7% 的患者转为造口，而 23% 的患者退出了研究。在股薄肌成形术之前已经造口的患者中，33% 的患者完全可控制排便，17% 的患者的失禁获得了高于基线 50% 以上程度的改善，22% 患者的失禁获得了高于基线 50% 以下程度的改善，6% 患者重新恢复造口，22% 的患者退出研究。对无造口患者的长期观察结果显示了包括固体和液体失禁的减少，以及 24 个月后护垫使用量的减少。然而，这些结果还不具有明显的统计学意义。

但是此项技术并非没有并发症。据 Matzel 等[9]的一份报告指出，在 121 例患者中有 211 项不良事件。89 例并发症被列为严重，需住院和甚至手术治疗。15% 的患者出现严重感染性并发症，需再次手术。9 例患者有麻木或明显的疼痛感。此外，也存在其他的一些并发症，包括轻微的感染、血栓栓塞性并发症、导线脱落、便秘及造瘘口闭塞相关并发症。虽然此手术并发症发生率高，但是大部分的并发症是可以成功治愈的，尽管手术后的排便控制并不完美，但患者确实可以明显改善他们的生活质量。

闭孔内肌

闭孔内肌同样也可发挥肛门新建括约肌的作用。肛门周围自体移植此肌肉的早期肌电图数据显示其被拉紧便产生收缩[10]。此肌肉可通过会阴部分离闭孔肌腱的途径可靠地获取。经过 Skácel 和 Laichman[11-15]一系列本主题的技术文献发表后，这项技术被学者们采纳，由于其产生肛门扩张的机制，这项技术也被采纳应用于治疗盆底失弛缓综合征的患者。在一项 20 例患者的小规模研究中，有半数患者取得了令人满意的结果[16]。

半腱肌和股二头肌长头

不常用的股薄肌的替代品包括半腱肌和股二头肌肌肉。Rab 等[17]所做的一项研究中，从人类尸体上切下 30 块半腱肌肌肉和 15 块股二头肌长头。股二头肌长头从第一和第二根穿支动脉获取其自主血供，从坐骨神经的运动分支获得神经供应。近端肌肉通常接收从臀下动脉与髂内动脉、髂外动脉、股动脉和股深动脉之间的吻合血管环路发出的分支[18]。虽然大多数情况下只有一条神经供应，且可用的肌肉长度占到大腿的一半长度，但是由于其肌肉长头内复杂的肌肉内吻合支，使得其用于多种用途[19]。半腱肌的肌肉显示血管供应的变异，从靠近坐骨结节的旋股内侧动脉接收自主血管蒂，也可从第二穿通支发出。神经供应包括两支坐骨神经的运动支。作为一个有潜力的新建括约肌，半腱肌因为它的血管供应和神经的走形而更有利，与此相同的方法已被用于犬缝匠肌的电刺激肛门置换试验[20]。

自体平滑肌在大便失禁治疗中的应用

一些动物模型使用自体平滑肌的袖口术来改善尿道和肛门括约肌的控制性[21-22]，并利用电刺激或非电刺激的游离的平滑肌移植瓣进行半可控的结肠造口术[23-24]。对于高度先天性肛门直肠发育异常的儿童，在拖出操作后立即完成平滑肌半桶状袖口成形已成为常规。除此之外，也适用于那些重复拖出手术、盆底筋膜成形术、术后直肠脱垂、巨结肠婴儿的后续治疗的一部分，或作为后矢状入路肛门直肠成形术的常规补充[25]。

阔筋膜吊带替代物和耻骨直肠肌成形术

单环或双环耻骨直肠肌成形术

此手术已经用于神经源性或创伤性大便失禁的治疗。操作时患者需摆成截石位，在肛管孔和尾骨之间做横向弧形切口。切口从肛尾缝深入，进入肛提肌上区域，从大腿取阔筋膜吊带移植瓣（20cm×2cm）沿其中间与肛管直肠交界上部背侧缝合4~6针。有关肛尾韧带最近的解剖学描述较之以前的描述更复杂——存在腹侧和背侧层[26]。腹侧层从骶前筋膜延续到肛管的联合丛肌层，而背侧层链接尾骨与外括约肌之间，在矢状位置达到最厚，肛提肌位于韧带背侧。

在耻骨下支靠近耻骨联合部位的皮肤和浅筋膜做一1cm长的切口，两个阔筋膜移植瓣的末端围住肛管形成"U"形吊带，在Hegar扩张器下呈大约90°的直肠角。然后两断端用2-3针不可吸收线与耻骨缝合固定。虽然支持此方法的数据很少，但是它遵循与泌尿外科文献所描述的大手术时使用尿道自体或合成吊带同样的原则[27]，专门作为耻骨直肠肌的加强而设计的。

利用其在肛管直肠结合部的吊带样作用，简单的耻骨直肠肌成形术改变直肠与肛管的角度使之更接近锐角。术前和术后的排粪造影发现肛管直肠角发生明显改变，由原来的广角变为接近直角。有可能产生一个高压区域，延迟大便下降，增加肛管有效存储长度。我们的研究团队在一项44例随机分成使用单环和双环吊带患者的研究中对双环耻骨直肠肌成形术进行了描述，显示双环组的排便控制力得到改善，对于某些表现为肛门开放的创伤性失禁或排便控制手术失败的神经源性失禁病例，我们提倡做这种手术[28]。

自体脂肪移植

由Shafik[29-31]在1995年首次报道的这项相对简单的技术被证明对不全性肛门失禁有效。它是将自体脂肪植入膀胱黏膜下层和/或尿道周围[32]。Shafic手术是从腹壁获取50~60ml脂肪黏膜下注射到肛管的3点钟和9点钟位置。一项随访18.6个月的14例患者的报道显示该手术能显著促进排便控制的改善，虽然半数的患者仍需要重复注射[29]。

自体干细胞移植

最近，该项技术已经由改善尿失禁的基础实验方法借鉴到到肛门失禁的临床治疗中，一系列细胞疗法已经用于加强尿道和肛门括约肌，包括干细胞[33]、体外诱导为成肌细胞的脂肪间充质干细胞[34]、骨髓间充质干细胞[35]，以及旨在局部产生血管内皮生长因子的附加基因处理的成肌细胞[36]等。后者能促进同时有肌源性干细胞不足和肌源性调节因子表达受损的先天性肛门直肠畸形和肌肉发育不良的新生儿的局部收缩力。肌源性调节因子包括：M-钙黏蛋白、肌细胞生成素、α-肌动蛋白和肌球蛋白H链。我们希望骨髓提取的肌源性干细胞能植入到后天肌肉中，能重新调整肌肉的生长、收缩力和神经营养素整合[37-38]。

结 论

即将来临的其他新兴的技术包括与主要阴部神经吻合术结合的各种肌成形术技术[39-41]。未来的研究方向可能集中在可注射的改良修饰过的自体可再生材料上，它们将更少引起过敏反应，并且不像合成材料一样容易移位。在这方面，注射的肌源性干细胞看来好像能够在肛门括约肌内存活，分化成肌原纤维，最终增强收缩力。肌源性干细胞在其注射的肛门括约肌内与肌肉结合，注射部位有新的肌肉生成，能够适应性转变为具有理想括约肌功能的慢肌纤维。

参考文献

1. Chetwood CH. Plastic operation of the sphincter ani with report of a case. Med Rec. 1902;61:529.
2. Devesa JM, Madrid JM, Gallego BR, Vicente E, Nuño J, Enríquez JM. Bilateral gluteoplasty for fecal incontinence. Dis Colon Rectum. 1997;40:883–8.
3. Pak-Art R, Silapunt P, Bunaprasert T, Tansatit T, Vajrabukka T. Prospective, randomized, controlled trial of proximally based vs. distally based gluteus maximus flap for anal incontinence in cadavers. Dis Colon Rectum. 2002;45:1100–3.
4. Pickrell KL, Broadbent TR, Masters FW, Metzger JT. Construction of a rectal sphincter and restoration of anal continence by transplanting the gracilis muscle; a report of four cases in children. Ann Surg. 1952;135:853–62.
5. Salmons S, Henriksson J. The adaptive response of skeletal muscle to increased use. Muscle Nerve. 1981;4:94–105.
6. Baeten CG, Konsten J, Spaans F, Visser R, Habets AM, Bourgeois IM, et al. Dynamic gracilloplasty for treatment of faecal incontinence. Lancet. 1991;338(8776):1163–5.
7. Baeten CG, Bailey HR, Bakka A, Belliveau P, Berg E, Buie WD, et al. Safety and efficacy of dynamic gracilloplasty for fecal incontinence: report of a prospective, multicenter trial. Dynamic Gracilloplasty Therapy Study Group. Dis Colon Rectum. 2000;43:743–51.
8. Rongen MJ, Uludag O, El Naggar K, Geerdes BP, Konsten J, Baeten CG. Long-term follow-up of dynamic gracilloplasty for fecal incontinence. Dis Colon Rectum. 2003;46:716–21.
9. Matzel KE, Madoff RD, LaFontaine LJ, Baeten CG, Buie WD, Christiansen J, et al.; Dynamic Gracilloplasty Therapy Study Group. Complications of dynamic gracilloplasty: incidence, management, and impact on outcome. Dis Colon Rectum. 2001;44:1427–35.
10. Farag A, Gadallah NA, el-Sherif EM. Obturator internus muscle autotransplantation: a new concept for the treatment of obstructive constipation. An anatomical, physiological and pathological study. Eur Surg Res. 1993;25:341–7.
11. Laichman S, Skácel V. The internal obturator muscles functioning as the neosphincter of the anus (I). An experimental study of the muscles used for replacing the sphincter of the anus. Acta Univ Palacki Olomuc Fac Med. 1986;113:271–9.
12. Laichman S, Skácel V. The internal obturator muscles functioning as the neosphincter of the anus (II). Accessibility of the internal obturator muscle from the point of view of topographical anatomy. Acta Univ Palacki Olomuc Fac Med. 1986;113:281–6.
13. Skácel V, Laichman S. The internal obturator muscles functioning as the neosphincter of the anus (III). Surgical technique of the reconstruction of the neosphincter of the anus. Acta Univ Palacki Olomuc Fac Med. 1986;113:287–310.
14. Skácel V, Laichman S. The internal obturator muscles functioning as the neosphincter of the anus (IV). Notes on the tactics and technique of muscle transposition. Acta Univ Palacki Olomuc Fac Med. 1986;113:311–6.
15. Skácel V, Laichman S. The internal obturator muscles functioning as the neosphincter of the anus (V). Neosphincter in short-term and long-term clinical evaluation. Acta Univ Palacki Olomuc Fac Med. 1986;113:317–24.
16. Farag A. Obturator internus muscle autotransfer: a new concept for the treatment of anismus. Clinical experience. Eur Surg Res. 1997;29:42–51.
17. Rab M, Mader N, Kamholz LP, Hausner T, Gruber H, Girsch W. Basic anatomical investigation of semitendinosus and the long head of biceps femoris muscle for their possible use in electrically stimulated neosphincter formation. Surg Radiol Anat. 1997;19:287–91.
18. Elbarrany WG, Al-Hayani A, Softa S. The blood and nerve supply of the longhead of the biceps femoris muscle; its possible use in dynamic neoanal sphincter. West Afr J Med. 2005;24:287–94.
19. Shanahan DA, George B, Williams NS, Sinnatamby CS, Riches DJ. The long head of the biceps femoris: anatomic basis for its possible use in the construction of an electrically stimulated neoanal sphincter. Plast Reconstr Surg. 1993;92:55–8.
20. Konsten J, Baeten CG, Havenith MG, Soeters PB. Canine model for treatment of faecal incontinence using transposed and electrically stimulated Sartorius muscle. Br J Surg. 1994;81:466–9.
21. Furness JB, Shafton AD, Hirst GD, O'Connell HE. Stimulated smooth muscle neosphincter in male intrinsic sphincter deficiency: proof of principle studies in a rabbit model. Neurourol Urodyn. 2010;29 Suppl 1:S24–8.
22. Holschneider AM, Amano S, Urban A, Donhauser G. Animal experimental studies on the free transplantation of smooth colon muscles as an artificial sphincter in the rat. Z Kinderchir. 1984;39:182–90.
23. Ruggiero R, Trere M, Ciliberti M, Iovino G. The smooth muscle autograft in continent colostomies. Experimental research on rabbits. Ann Ital Chir. 1991;62:75–80.
24. Schrag HJ, Karwath D, Grub C, Fragoza Padilla F, Noack T, Hopt UT. Electrodynamic smooth muscle sphincter: development and biomechanical evaluation of a novel porcine artificial smooth muscle sphincter in a new in vitro stoma simulator. Int J Colorectal Dis. 2005;20:321–7.
25. Hofmann-von-Kap-Herr S, Koltai IL, Tennant LJ. Anal sphincter substitute using autologous smooth muscle in a fold-over, half-cylinder, double plasty (SMFD-plasty): a new method of treatment of anorectal incontinence. J Pediatr Surg. 1985;20:134–7.
26. Shafik IA, Shafik A. Double-loop puborectoplasty: novel technique for the treatment of fecal incontinence. Surg Technol Int. 2009;18:103–8.
27. Kinugasa Y, Arakawa T, Abe SI, Ohtsuka A, Suzuki D, Murakami G, et al. Anatomical reevaluation of the anococcygeal ligament and its surgical relevance. Dis Colon Rectum. 2011;54:232–7.
28. Rehman H, Bezerra CC, Bruschini H, Cody JD. Traditional suburethral sling operations for urinary incontinence in women. Cochrane Database Syst Rev. 2005;20(3):CD001754.
29. Shafik A. Perianal injection of autologous fat for treatment of sphincteric incontinence. Dis Colon Rectum. 1995;38:583–7.
30. Bernardi C, Favetta U, Pescatori M. Autologous fat injection for treatment of fecal incontinence: manometric and echographic assessment. Plast Reconstr Surg. 1998;102:1626–8.
31. Ho KS, Ho YH. Diagnosing and managing faecal incontinence. Ann Acad Med Singapore. 1999;28:417–23.
32. Angioli R, Muzii L, Zullo MA, Battista C, Ruggiero A, Montera R, et al. Use of bulking agents in urinary incontinence. Minerva Ginecol. 2008;60:543–50.
33. Nikolavasky D, Stangel-Wójcikiewicz K, Stec M, Chancellor MB. Stem cell therapy: a future treatment of stress urinary incontinence. Semin Reprod Med. 2011;29:61–70.

34. Wu G, Zheng X, Jiang Z, Wang J, Song Y. Induced differentiation of adipose-derived stromal cells into myoblasts. J Huazhong Univ Sci Technolog Med Sci. 2010;30:285–90.
35. Aghaee-Afshar M, Rezazadehkermani M, Asadi A, Malekpour-Afshar R, Shaeshmaeili A, Nematollahi-mahani SN. Potential of human umbilical cord matrix and rabbit bone marrow-derived mesenchymal stem cells in repair of surgically incised rabbit external anal sphincter. Dis Colon Rectum. 2009;52:1753–61.
36. Delo DM, Eberli D, Williams JK, Andersson KE, Atala A, Soker S. Angiogenic gene modification of skeletal muscle cells to compensate for ageing-induced decline in bioengineered functional muscle tissue. BJU Int. 2008;102:878–94.
37. Deasy BM, Huard J. Gene therapy and tissue engineering based on muscle-derived stem cells. Curr Opin Mol Ther. 2002;4:382–9.
38. Aoi S, Shimotake T, Tsuda T, Deguchi E, Iwai N. Impaired expression of myogenic regulatory molecules in the pelvic floor muscels of murine embryos with anorectal malformations. J Pediatr Surg. 2005;40:805–9.
39. Pirro N, Konate I, Sielezneff I, Di Marino V, Sastre B. Anatomic bases of graciloplasty using end-to-side nerve pudendal anastomosis. Surg Radiol Anat. 2005;27:409–13.
40. Sato T, Konishi F, Endoh N, Uda H, Sugawara Y, Nagal H. Long-term outcomes of a ne-anus with a pudendal nerve anastomosis contemporaneously reconstructed with an abdominoperineal excision of the rectum. Surgery. 2005;137:8–15.
41. Schwabegger AH, Kronberger P, Obrist P, Brath E, Miko I. Functional sphincter ani externus reconstruction for treatment of fecal stress incontinence using free latissimus dorsi muscle transfer with coaptation to the pudendal nerve: preliminary experimental study in dogs. J Reconstr Microsurg. 2007;23:79–85.

第 35 章 尚有争议的骶神经调节

Klaus E. Matzel · Yasuko Maeda

石 洋 译 李国逊 审校

摘 要

骶神经调节在大便失禁患者的一线治疗和再次手术治疗中的作用越来越重要。本章介绍对这类患者永久性置入刺激电极后的疑难问题和微调。讨论当效果不佳甚至出现不良反应时，如何调节刺激直肠的技术。本章还介绍了再次修正手术治疗以及进行调整所需要的检测方法和技术。

关键词

骶神经调节；骶神经刺激；大便失禁；不理想效果；疗效；疼痛；感染；不良反应；调节；外科干预；电极移位；电极替换

引 言

骶神经刺激在过去 20 年已经发展成为治疗大便失禁的有效方法[1-2]。与传统的其他技术相比，它的侵入性更小，而且有一个 2~3 周的暂时调节期（经皮肤或经会阴的神经评估）。在永久性置入电极之前，提供了一个观察疗效的机会。

许多研究证明了骶神经刺激的作用，骶神经刺激也用于短期或者中期治疗肠功能障碍，包括便秘和肛门疼痛。然而有许多问题还没有解决，比如它的工作机制，如何对便秘和失禁同时调节，以及长期的疗效和耐受性[3]。而且随着我们经验的增加，发现效果不佳和治疗不良反应问题并不少见。一些患者需要不断调节刺激参数以提高疗效，一些患者因电极刺激导致疼痛和感染。这些往往需要外科手术进行干预和修正。目前置入的电极电池不能充电，如果电量耗尽，就需要再次置入新的电极。

本章介绍目前骶神经刺激相关的意外事件，其中一些需要手术去除已经放置的神经刺激装置。有关描述设备疗效不佳和不良反应的专业词汇，在表 35.1 中作出总结。

骶神经刺激相关问题

效果不佳

效果不佳分为两种情况。
- 无效：在经皮肤神经评估过程中所表现的效果不能再次显现，患者在植入电极后没有在临床治疗中获益。
- 失效：在经皮肤神经评估过程中所表现的效果再次显现，但逐渐或者突然消失。

无效或者失效是电极植入后最常见的问题之一。就可获得的资料而言，发生率高达 12%[4]。早期治疗失败的一个重要原因是永久性电极植入位置不理想（通常是分叉的四极有孔电极），通常是由于同步的 PNE 造成，在同步 PNE 过程中，把一个细的单极电极用于 PNE，永久性电极随之植入，这

第 35 章　尚有争议的骶神经调节

表 35.1　骶神经刺激术语

本章中使用词	定　义	文献中用词
可报道的事件	治疗效果欠佳和不良反应	并发症，治疗失败
1 治疗效果欠佳		
缺乏效果	治疗效果与预期不符或置入电极后效果减弱。在 PNE 过程中的改善未能再次表现。患者治疗效果很小或者没有满意的疗效	效果不佳，疗效不满意
失　效	在一段满意的疗效后效果减退，PNE 过程中表现的改善可以再现，但效果逐渐减弱或突然消失	效果减退，效果欠佳
2 不良反应	在骶神经刺激中新出现的症状或问题，影响导致患者不适，并被认为与骶神经刺激有关（机械相关或治疗相关）	包括术语：疼痛、感染、尿潴留、性功能改变、电击感、腹泻
刺激器名称		
刺激器	美敦力 3023，3058 台湾	IPG，起搏器，刺激器，刺激器Ⅱ
永久 / 分叉四象限电极	美敦力 3080，3093　螺旋分叉电极	电极，四象限电极
临时电极	美敦力 3057，041830 分叉螺旋 / 非螺旋 单极电极	临时导线 非螺旋导线　螺旋导线
临时刺激器	美敦力 3625	
设　备	置入刺激器和永久性电极	系统
移　除	将置入电极从置入部位部分或完全移除	移走，改变位置，迁移
断　裂	电极明显横断或弯曲	电极弯曲
外科介入		
替换永久电极	置入新的永久性电极	电极修改
永久电极重新定位	将新的电极或同一个电极置入在不同位置的骶孔	电极的再次定位
刺激器重新定位	在不同位置重新放置刺激器	电极再次定位
移　除	同时或单独移除电极及刺激器	IPG 或刺激器重新定位
其他临床方法		
调　整	改变刺激电极或参数（只改变振幅，频率和波宽保持不变）	调整
其他调整方法	改变刺激电极和参数（包括波宽和频率）	同时或单独增加或降低波宽及频率
终　止	结束刺激，不移除装置	结束治疗

PNE：经周围神经或经皮肤神经评估；IPG：置入脉冲发生器

可能导致电极并不在 PNE 过程中引起满意疗效的位置。如果想避免这个问题，可以通过分阶段手术进行。在进行 PNE 的时候，使用一个永久性电极，这个电极可以用来进行 PNE，如果治疗有临床效果，只需将刺激器和电极相连。后一种方法费用昂贵，一般都能固定在 PNE 测试中有效的电极位置。然而目前还没有研究对比这两种方法的疗效差别。

另一个造成治疗无效的原因是永久性电极术后的不稳定性和其周围组织纤维化。因此找到一种没有不适症状的刺激装置是很困难的。

造成最终无效的原因很多，是各因素共同作用的结果。目前还没有完全阐明。机械相关因素包括电极移位、内部纤维折断、连接不紧、周围组织纤维化导致传导受阻，这些被认为是导致无效的重要原因。刺激后期神经损伤和破坏是影响长期疗效的因素。但目前我们对于骶神经刺激有关的神经生理学和神经化学的了解还有限。此外，任何进行性的神经疾病都可能造成最初治疗有效，但经过一段时间后原先存在的疾病加重，导致骶神经刺激失效。

疼　痛

疼痛可能是由于植入的机械或电刺激引起，发生率估计在 13%[4-5]。通常报道在刺激器植入部位引起[3]。脉冲发生器本身可以引起皮肤腐蚀、血肿、蜂窝织炎、局部过敏、水肿或伤口裂开。如果患者体重下降明显或皮下组织萎缩严重，机器可能穿出。其他部位的疼痛，如会阴、腿、足也有报道，大多数病例看来与刺激的不良反应有关。

感　染

感染发生率报道为3.9%[6-7]。然而一个多中心研究（有关骶神经刺激治疗大便失禁）报道可达10.8%，大多数发生在植入机器3周之内[8]。最常见的致病菌是金黄色葡萄球菌[9]，可以在分叉的电极中发现。

刺激的不良反应

在应用骶神经刺激治疗大便失禁过程中，有此类报道，包括在排尿或排便时需要停止电刺激[10-11]、睡眠障碍或者在性行为时需要停止电刺激[12]。在一个个案的报道中，一例患者抱怨在经过电磁区域（例如防盗系统）时感到微小的电刺激。骶神经刺激应用于孕妇的效果也难以描述。一位孕妇应用骶神经刺激直至产前9周，最终早产1名患有唐氏综合征的婴儿[13]。

骶神经刺激治疗的效果欠佳及相关不良反应

骶神经刺激治疗肠功能障碍是在成功治疗尿失禁的基础上发展起来的，这已经通过长期随访得到验证。这些报道中，治疗效果欠佳和不良反应并不少见：53%~67%患者经历至少1种机械性或治疗相关的并发症[14-17]，30%~54%患者需要手术去除刺激装置。最常见的手术并发症是刺激设备周围的疼痛和感染。由于治疗失败或不良反应导致去除刺激装置据报道可达6%~50%[11]。

效果不佳和不良反应的处理方法：一种常用方法

首先要确定不良反应是由于治疗造成的，并确定可以纠正的因素。常用的排除方法见表35.1。第一步通过检查确定程序是否正常运转、电池是否还有电量，很重要的是要排除意外的关闭或开启，或者家属调整了系统。通过关闭机器一段时间，医生可以确定意外情况是由于刺激引起的而不是机器本身引起的。此外，这可以再次评价骶神经刺激治疗的效果。暂时的停止治疗还可以防止神经对于电刺激的适应。据我们的经验，在关闭骶神经刺激器一段较长的时间后（通常至少1个月），一些患者的神经对于刺激发生反应的数值有所下降。由于我们目前还不能确定关闭刺激器的具体时间，我们随机推荐2~4周，但这至少要确定不良反应是否是由于电刺激引起的。

在治疗过程中的疼痛分为机械性（设备植入后）和功能性（电流引起的），应该进行充分的体格检查确定疼痛是否是机械性的。如果排除后，需要关闭刺激器，确定疼痛是否由于电流引起。

如果发现伤口红肿，提示伤口感染，应该应用金黄色葡萄球菌敏感的抗生素（静脉应用或者口服）。无法治愈的感染或败血症，应该去除机械装置，但是还可以再次置入。

系统的评价和调试

测试系统

阻抗异常（<50或>4000Ω）可能与电路中断

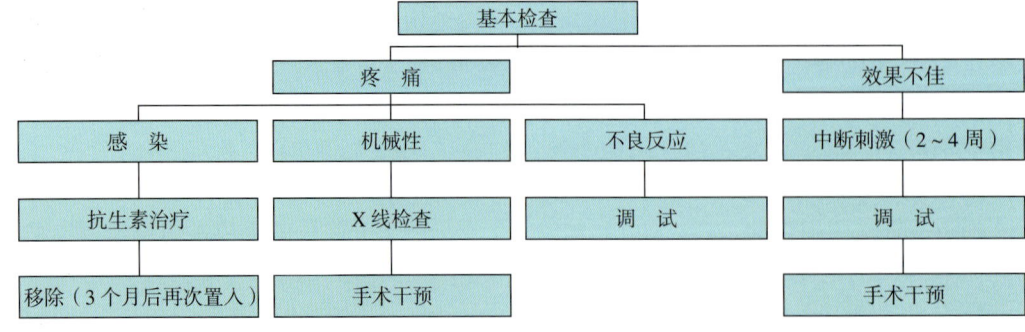

图35.1　骶神经刺激疑难问题处理流程

有关（电极断裂、短路、连接松弛或过紧）。高阻抗提示环路开放，如电极折断、断路或松弛；低阻抗提示短路，如连接过紧或体液混入到连接中。检测需要仔细进行单极检测。有时需要宽幅、高幅脉冲波或同时应用。因为这有时可以将阻抗正常化[8]。有时尽管存在阻抗异常，但是如果患者感觉或者运动反射可以得到改善，那么应该仔细考虑是否手术去除刺激装置。

调试

如果不存在机械故障导致疼痛或者骶神经刺激效果衰减，首先需要进行调试。目前常用的方法是改变电极的组合和波幅。目前还没有标准方法进行调试，但我们建议逐步进行调节。如对于刺激有异常感觉，应该首先进行单极调试（4连接），然后双极调节（12连接），以确定最高的组合连接方式，保证患者肛门周围在进行刺激时不会感觉到不适。如果没有理想的方式，可以尝试三极组合，对于功能性的疼痛，应该尝试调节电极以保证电极及其他位置没有疼痛。对于刺激器本身引起的疼痛，可以尝试将单极刺激器改为双极刺激器。因为在单极刺激器中，刺激器本身可以作为一个支点[18]引起疼痛。如果效果不佳，不能长时间进行调节。可以改变波幅和频率，但是目前还没有统一的调节规范。

手术干预

如果调节方法都已尝试或者确定是机械性因素引起的，那么需要通过手术停止对直肠的神经刺激。手术干预需要在特定的情况下应用。

电极移位

最新的电极上有分叉，可以使之难以移动。但仍有报道电极移位，大多数是向前方，也有向后方移位的[19]。骶骨侧位像可以确认疗效的急剧变化是由于电极脱落还是电极折断引起。如果移动幅度较小（<1cm），治疗效果可以通过调节电极组合或者刺激其他神经进行维持，这种情况下应该首选这种方法。

目前已有报道对于向前方移位的电极，可以将其向后方拉回。并通过网格或者扭锁固定于骶前筋膜上[20]。前提是患者应该不存在先天的组织薄弱或者萎缩导致新的电极再次发生移位。对于体质量指数较低者（<19kg/m^2），可以采用加强的方法。因为他们的肌肉组织较少，电极可以锚定在皮下组织内[21]。电极向后移位需要进行复位，可以同时给予加强固定。目前对于应用新的电极还是旧的电极还存在争议。还没有设备能够在术中检测电极是否破坏。因此我们建议置入新的电极。可以在身体同侧的不同位置的骶孔放置或者经过新一轮测试后在身体对侧置入新的电极。

对于失效或者无效患者再次置入电极

生产商建议如果患者有运动或者感觉方面的改善，就不应再次置入电极。因为疗效不佳可能是由于骶神经末梢对于电刺激反应减弱引起，而非电极位置引起。这种情况在尿潴留、尿失禁以及会阴疼痛患者中有报道。这些患者临床效果不佳，但神经肌肉反应性有所改善，进行再次电极置入后效果不佳。如果再次置入电极，应该考虑刺激不同位置的骶孔，可以对新的骶神经进行刺激[22]。

对于置入电极的修正手术

植入器械部位疼痛可能与发射器置入皮下位置有关，或者由于患者BMI显著降低导致皮下组织减少。如果没有感染的迹象，首选手术调整。可以将刺激器埋在对侧臀部皮下或者腹壁内。据报道，放置在臀部皮下与放置在腹壁下相比，再次手术几率更小[23]。较为少见的一些患者有意或者无意将刺激装置扭转，引起所谓的"旋弄者综合征"（在佩戴心脏起搏器患者中发生）[24]。因此必须在手术前仔细询问病史。

有关治疗的其他问题

这种治疗可以改善排尿功能和性功能。但对于孕妇效果还没有充分研究。任何与之有关的不良反应和意外事件都应停止治疗。已有报道骶神经刺激导致早产[4, 15]，因此育龄妇女在进行置入电极治疗之前，应该仔细进行交流询问。

结 论

由于相对简单的外科技术和较少的并发症，骶神经刺激被认为是治疗便失禁的微创、安全的方法。虽然手术方法简单，但效果满意[25]。一旦出现不理想的治疗效果或者意外事件（骶神经刺激相关）。首先要判断是意外还是治疗的不良反应。确定是机械性因素还是功能性因素是很重要的。保守治疗主要是调节，应该首先尝试。在调节无效后考虑手术治疗，手术干预适用于难治性的病例或者保守治疗难以纠正的机械性因素，手术方法主要包括纠正电极和刺激装置的位置。

参考文献

1. Matzel KE, Kamm MA, Stösser M, Baeten CGMI, Christiansen J, Madoff R, et al. Sacral nerve stimulation for fecal incontinence: a multicenter study. Lancet. 2004;363:1270–6.
2. Abrams P, Andersson KE, Birder L, Brubaker L, Cardozo L, Chapple C, et al. Fourth international consultation on incontinence recommendations of the international scientific committee: evaluation and treatment of urinary incontinence, pelvic organ prolapse, and fecal incontinence. Neurourol Urodyn. 2010;29:213–40.
3. Amend B, Matzel KE, Abrams P, de Groat WC, Sievert KD. How does neuromodulation work: ICI-RS 2010? Neurourol Urodyn. 2011; 30(5):762–5. Apr 1. doi: 10.1002/nau.21096 [Epub ahead of print].
4. Maeda Y, Matzel K, Lundby L, Buntzen S, Laurberg S. Postoperative issues of sacral nerve stimulation for fecal incontinence and constipation: a systematic literature review and treatment guideline. Dis Colon Rectum. 2011;54(11):1443–60.
5. White WM, Mobley 3rd JD, Doggweiler R, Dobmeyer-Dittrich C, Klein FA. Incidence and predictors of complications with sacral neuromodulation. Urology. 2009;73:731–5.
6. Washington BB, Hines BJ. Implant infection after two-stage sacral nerve stimulator placement. Int Urogynecol J Pelvic Floor Dysfunct. 2007;18:1477–80.
7. Wexner SD, Hull T, Edden Y, Coller JA, Devroede G, McCallum R, et al. Infection rates in a large investigational trial of sacral nerve stimulation for fecal incontinence. J Gastrointest Surg. 2010;14:1081–9.
8. Hijaz A, Vasavada SP, Daneshgari F, Frinjari H, Goldman H, Rackley R. Complications and troubleshooting of two-stage sacral neuromodulation therapy: a single-institution experience. Urology. 2006;68:533–7.
9. Huwyler M, Kiss G, Burkhard FC, Madersbacher H, Kessler TM. Microbiological tined-lead examination: does prolonged sacral neuromodulation testing induce infection? BJU Int. 2009;104:646–50.
10. Jarrett ME, Matzel KE, Christiansen J, Baeten CG, Rosen H, Bittorf B, et al. Sacral nerve stimulation for fecal incontinence in patients with previous partial spinal injury including disc prolapse. Br J Surg. 2005;92:734–9.
11. Matzel KE, Lux P, Heuer S, Besendorfer M, Zhang W. Sacral nerve stimulation for fecal incontinence: long-term outcome. Colorectal Dis. 2009;11:636–41.
12. Signorello D, Seitz CC, Berner L, Trenti E, Martini T, Galantini A, et al. Impact of sacral neuromodulation on female sexual function and his correlation with clinical outcome and quality of life indexes: a monocentric experience. J Sex Med. 2011;8:1147–55.
13. Wiseman OJ, v d Hombergh U, Koldewijn EL, Spinelli M, Siegel SW, Fowler CJ. Sacral neuromodulation and pregnancy. J Urol. 2002;167:165–8.
14. Siegel SW, Catanzaro F, Dijkema HE, Elhilali MM, Fowler CJ, Gajewski JB, et al. Long-term results of a multicenter study on sacral nerve stimulation for treatment of urinary urge incontinence, urgency-frequency, and retention. Urology. 2000;56:87–91.
15. Sutherland SE, Lavers A, Carlson A, Holtz C, Kesha J, Siegel SW. Sacral nerve stimulation for voiding dysfunction: one institution's 11-year experience. Neurourol Urodyn. 2007;26:19–28; discussion 36.
16. van Kerrebroeck PE, van Voskuilen AC, Heesakkers JP, Lycklama á Nijholt AA, Siegel S, Jonas U, et al. Results of sacral neuromodulation therapy for urinary voiding dysfunction: outcomes of a prospective, worldwide clinical study. J Urol. 2007;178:2029–34.
17. Siddiqui NY, Wu JM, Amundsen CL. Efficacy and adverse events of sacral nerve stimulation for overactive bladder: a systematic review. Neurourol Urodyn. 2010;29 Suppl 1:S18–23.
18. Hijaz A, Vasavada S. Complications and troubleshooting of sacral neuromodulation therapy. Urol Clin North Am. 2005;32:65–9.
19. Kessler TM, Madersbacher H, Kiss G. Bilateral migration of sacral neuromodulation tined leads in a thin patient. J Urol. 2005;173:153–4.
20. Deng DY, Gulati M, Rutman M, Raz S, Rodriguez LV. Failure of sacral nerve stimulation due to migration of tined lead. J Urol. 2006;175:2182–5.
21. Everaert K, De Ridder D, Baert L, Oosterlinck W, Wyndaele JJ. Patient satisfaction and complications following sacral nerve stimulation for urinary retention, urge incontinence and perineal pain: a multicenter evaluation. Int Urogynecol J Pelvic Floor Dysfunct. 2000;11:231–6.
22. Williams ER, Siegel SW. Procedural techniques in sacral nerve modulation. Int Urogynecol J Pelvic Floor Dysfunct. 2010;21 Suppl 2:S453–60.
23. Scheepens WA, Weil EH, van Koeveringe GA, Rohrmann D, Hedlund HE, Schurch B, et al. Buttock placement of the implantable pulse generator: a new implantation technique for sacral neuromodulation – a multicenter study. Eur Urol. 2001;40:434–8.
24. Zimmerman SA, Bright JM. Secure pacemaker fixation critical for prevention of Twiddler's syndrome. J Vet Cardiol. 2004;6:40–4.
25. Pettit P. Current opinion: complications and troubleshooting of sacral neuromodulation. Int Urogynecol J Pelvic Floor Dysfunct. 2010;21 Suppl 2:S491–6.

第六篇
肛门会阴重建手术的相关技术

引 言

Andrew P. Zbar

本篇包括了复发性和复杂性肛瘘的不同手术方法：儿童肛门前庭瘘的治疗方法，直肠阴道瘘的选择性手术入路，直肠尿道瘘和直肠前列腺瘘的治疗，术后持续性或复发性肛裂的治疗方法，治疗肛门狭窄以及广泛皮肤软组织切除后修复会阴的整形手术。近些年发展起来的一系列肛瘘的手术方法主要是为了应对瘘管切开/瘘管切除术用于复发性或顽固性复杂肛瘘时，治疗结果及远期功能较差等问题。虽然目前黏膜和皮肤前移肛门成形术的标准技术临床应用的结果相对较差，但这主要是因为操作的技巧和经验不足，而且似乎并没有被生物胶或肛瘘栓取代的趋势。结扎括约肌间瘘道似乎能解决所有这些问题，但仍需一段时间证明。显而易见的是，肛门内括约肌修复（因同时保证功能和减少复发而被众多研究者所认可）是这些技术中一个重要的组成部分，这也非常依赖于术者的技术。

先天性直肠畸形修复后的患者在肛肠科很少见，这方面的数据很有限。肛门位置过低或前庭肛门等肛门畸形的患者术后肛门狭窄再次手术成功的可能性很大；而显著性尿失禁患者术后功能恢复则相对较差。这些患者可能会从骶神经刺激或简单的肛周悬吊术中受益，改善尿失禁，但我们关于这部分患者的经验很少。

很多直肠阴道瘘的手术方式最终证明临床效果不佳。笔者认为，最简单的术式才是最好的，即使再手术失败也不会妨碍进一步的修复。马休球海绵肌移植对于许多低位的伴有会阴中心腱破坏的患者有较好的效果，如果患者没有伴随克罗恩病或周围损伤，这种简单的方法可能只有 20% 失败率。笔者在这些失败的病例中保留了股薄肌，这种保留并没有明确的治疗效果。在缺乏长期的成功率的统计的情况下，笔者倾向将植入生物补片作为最后的手段，而不是第一步，因为其手术失败、暴露或挤压会使得进一步的手术更加困难。

直肠前列腺（尿道）瘘发生率的上升与前列腺近距离放射治疗有关。在多数（但不是全部）病例中，如果在内镜下发现却不及时治疗，将会造成严重的后果。虽然有很多不同的手术方法，但是在经会阴修补术失败后，笔者仍然认为，Kraske 后路手术是一种可靠的选择，它是这种被忽视的术式的几个适应证之一。

对于顽固性慢性肛裂患者，特别是括约肌切开术存在较高的术后粪漏风险时，我们需要认真考虑保留括约肌功能的术式。必须广泛和充分地告知患者所有可选方案的预后。笔者认为影像学检查对于确定发生术后尿失禁高风险的患者是必需的，这些患者通常是由于肛门外括约肌受损或前肛管缩短。最简单的选择是肛裂切除术和改良肛门成形术，但是患者需要知道有一定的复发可能；但可能不会导致功能的恶化。当然，笔者并不完全相信目前关于肛裂切除术的有限的数据或以测压法为基础的局部、气囊扩张扩张术的安全性。我猜想小部分患者可因肉毒杆菌注射获益，但这可能发生严重的感染相关性并发症。

  幸运的是，只有一小部分痔切除术后的患者出现有症状的肛门狭窄并需要外科手术。同样，最简单的方法也是最好的。如果有周围皮肤狭窄可行传统的 S 成形术，如果有局部瘢痕可行局部的 house-style 修补。幸运的是，肛管很少出现明显的狭窄（结肠肛管吻合术发生缺血性狭窄）。单纯扩张术（有时在全身麻醉下进行）是一个合适的姑息治疗。我们不应该忽视局部皮肤移植在一些特殊情况下的临床价值，其在需要广泛的肛门重建术的特殊情况下，如在耳尼埃氏坏疽或严重会阴创伤后，治疗效果较好。后者也可以用于因布施克洛文斯顿肿瘤切除术、直肠癌局部切除术、复发或广泛湿疣病手术或侵袭性汗腺炎后遗留的较大肛裂。

第 36 章 复发性复杂肛瘘的再手术治疗

David D. E. Zimmerman · Litza Mitalas · W. Rudolph Schouten
石 洋 译 李国逊 审校

摘 要

本章讨论目前复发性肛瘘的手术治疗观点。对于这些患者的治疗已经成为一种专业，结直肠外科医师需要通过获得图像来取得成功的治疗。这最好能通过医生亲自进行超声检查来达到目的，并且对于脓毒症造成的破坏还要进行后续的重建手术。包括延期的括约肌修补、肛门成形术、直肠阴道瘘的治疗和会阴成形术。治疗这些患者需要处理这些破坏性的情况。

关键词

肛瘘；复发性复杂肛瘘；再手术；高位经括约肌肛瘘；经括约肌肛瘘；肛瘘切开术；大便失禁；克罗恩病；放射治疗；产伤；直肠阴道的；HIV；AIDS；胃肠道结核；继发性肛瘘；未引流感染；粪便转流；腺源性肛瘘；经直肠 / 直肠内皮瓣转移修补术；括约肌间瘘管结扎术（LIFT）；肛瘘切开同时括约肌修补；肛瘘栓；挂线术

引 言

许多医师因为治疗复杂性肛瘘损失了声誉。20 世纪早期 Lockhart-Mummery 爵士认识到了这一点[1]，他形象地描述了自己的失败："也许由于治疗肛瘘失败对于医生名声的破坏比切除直肠或胃失败更大。开腹手术的失败也许伴随着葬礼而消失，但失败的肛瘘手术会到处宣传着失败的疗效。"

30 多年前，Parks 和 Stitz[2] 的著名论著对肛瘘进行了解剖学分类，目前还在沿用，但当时并未包括复杂性肛瘘。过去的 20 多年中，复杂性肛瘘作为一种临床疾病出现。包括高位的经括约肌肛瘘（穿过外括约肌中上 1/3）和括约肌上方肛瘘。大多数医师认为如果不能通过不会造成大便失禁的肛瘘切除术治疗的肛瘘，应该称为复杂性肛瘘[3-4]。

很明显，由于克罗恩病、放射治疗、产伤引起的肛瘘应该属于复杂性肛瘘。由于肛管括约肌前方没有耻骨，直肠肌造成括约肌短且薄弱，Kodner[5] 将肛管前方的肛瘘也归为复杂性肛瘘，他们也将直肠阴道瘘归入其中。治疗复杂性肛瘘难度较大，治疗的目标不仅是去除肛瘘组织，同时（也许更为重要）需要防止发生大便失禁。

完善的术前准备和患者的选择

如果存在潜在的致病因素，那么治疗复发性肛瘘成功的机会要小一些。如果这些潜在的致病因素真的出现，那么手术后对控便功能的损伤可能会大于手术带来的效果。

相关因素：潜在病因

克罗恩病

据不同研究者报道，克罗恩病相关的肛瘘发生率在 10%～56%，与克罗恩病的部位及患者年龄相关。克罗恩病一旦出现，将是导致治疗失败的一个重要原因。因此，对于复发性肛瘘，有必要进行结肠镜检查、通过回肠插管或乙状结肠镜进行钡灌肠检查，以排除结直肠克罗恩病，也可以通过小肠系造影了解上消化道情况（参见第 22 章）。

即使是穿过外括约肌下 1/3 的肛瘘可以通过简单的肛瘘切除术治愈，仍有报道上述治疗失败的病例。许多医生建议性保守治疗，Keighley、Allan[6] 和 Buchmann 等[7] 观察有 35% 的肛瘘可以自愈。有报道表明一些患有克罗恩病、肛瘘穿过外括约肌下方的患者，手术治愈率相对较高，切开瘘管后愈合率可达 94%[8-9]。然而如果瘘管穿过上 2/3 括约肌或有不典型的瘘管，想达到预期效果就要多加注意。不同的手术技巧将在本章后面介绍。

人获得性免疫缺陷综合征

艾滋病患者有关肛瘘的报道资料十分有限[10]。由于抗蛋白酶疗法的应用，艾滋病患者肛瘘的发病率有所减少[11]。同性恋艾滋病患者中肛门直肠疾病发病率较高（6%～34%），静脉吸毒者发病率相对较低（仅为 3%）[12]。在这方面，Consten 等[12] 治疗 46 例艾滋病患者的肛周感染和肛瘘，手术成功率较低，愈合情况较差。这些作者建议充分引流脓肿和瘘管，避免引起转移性的坏死感染。

结核病

胃肠道结核占所有肛门会阴疾病比例 <1%，而且越来越少。在结核病流行地区传统数据已经不十分准确。一旦结核菌导致肛门会阴瘘形成，大部分是复杂性肛瘘。Sultan[13] 报道 6 例患者中 5 例是复杂性肛瘘。Kraemer 等报道 20 例此类疾病患者中 15 例有手术史，而且 18 例肛瘘中 17 例是复杂性肛瘘。复发病例只见于最初没有考虑结核菌感染而没有进行抗结核治疗的患者。治疗应包括抗结核治疗。一些结核性肛瘘患者可以通过单纯抗结核治疗而治愈。Stupart 等[15] 报道传统的组织病理学检查，包括 Ziehl-Neelsen 染色不足以对 1/3 患者明确诊断。他们建议在结核病高发地区应该在 Ziehl-Neelsen 染色组织病理学检查同时进行整个瘘管的活检。

相关因素：活动性感染和遗留的瘘管

许多医师认为马蹄状的瘘管是造成手术失败的原因。尽管还缺乏确切的证据，但这种瘘管如果不能充分引流，确实被证明有可能引起肛瘘的反复感染[2, 16, 17]。Barker 等[18] 研究证实了这种观点。他发现 9% 的患者术前 MRI 发现有瘘管而术中被遗漏造成肛瘘难以愈合。因此我们建议对于反复感染的患者应该在术前充分排查，排除继发的瘘管或不充分的引流。Buchana 也支持这种观点[19]，他对 71 例反复感染的患者进行了 MRI 检查，有 40 例手术所见与 MRI 相符，其中 5 例复发。31 例不相符的患者中有 16 例复发。他总结 MRI 检查可以减少瘘管复发率 75%，这种观点已被接受，并建议在术前进行详细的影像学检查[20]。

肛瘘的影像学检查的益处还在于能够确定肛瘘内口在括约肌的位置，估计手术需要切除的肌肉范围。尽管 H_2O_2 强化的直肠内超声与 MRI 的效果类似[21]，但这项检查是动态的，对操作者依赖性很大。大多数医生更倾向于 MRI 静态检查，而且在多数医院都能进行。

相关因素：粪便转流

复发性隐窝腺性肛瘘的粪便转流

一些复发性肛瘘的患者需要进行回肠或者结肠造瘘，还没有高级别证据支持这种做法。而临床工作中，粪便转流作为一种治疗肛瘘的方法，可以用于克罗恩病相关肛瘘或者反复发作的隐窝腺性肛瘘。研究表明，粪便转流对于经肛门的黏膜皮瓣转移手术有意义。有两项大型回顾研究[4, 22] 发现，是否造瘘对于皮瓣移植手术术后愈合率没有影响。而 Sonoda[22] 建议对于复杂病例可以进行造瘘，造瘘后将复杂肛瘘转变为相对简单的病例，以提高愈合率。

克罗恩病的粪便转流

特定患者行单纯粪便转流对于治疗肛瘘有效，但还纳造口的比例较低。还没有参数指标去确定哪些患者适宜造瘘[23]。曾有研究建议转流粪便对于提高严重克罗恩病患者生活质量有一定意义[24]。尽管已经获得了越来越多克罗恩病患者转流粪便和生活质量相关的数据，但是还没有高级别证据支持应用这种方法可以提高肛瘘的治愈率。

手术的选择

许多医师已经报道不同手术方法治疗复杂性肛瘘而失败。近年来，随着不同方法对肛瘘治愈率的提高，大便失禁的发生也有所增加。另一方面，也有看似能够保护肛门功能的方法，但疗效不佳。因此手术选择的关键在于权衡手术的风险和收益，因为存在一些临床因素对患者的满意度影响超过了功能对于患者满意度的影响[25]。如果能够取得满意疗效，对于控便功能一定限度的损伤也能够被患者接受。

单纯肛瘘切开术

手术技术

患者取折刀位，通过弧形的 Lockhart-Mummery 探针确定内口位置，完全明确瘘管走形，利用电刀或手术刀切开，充分引流。

技术相关观点

一些作者建议缝合伤口，可以加速愈合。在这方面，Ho 等[26]介绍了一种方法，缝合一半患者的伤口，另一半患者伤口开放。缝合伤口者愈合时间较开放伤口者少（6周 vs 10周），液体粪便失禁的比例较少（2%vs12%），对肛管最大收缩压损伤较小。

过去对于应该切开瘘管还是完全切除瘘管组织存在较多争议。现在，大多数医生使用瘘管切开术。完全切除瘘管组织，造成伤口较大，括约肌两侧断端缺损较大，因此愈合时间较长，大便失禁发生的可能性较大[27]。

评 价

单纯肛瘘切开较少用于复杂性肛瘘。切开肛管外括约肌的坚实部分可能会引起轻微的便失禁症状。如经括约肌肛瘘患者术后有 30%~50% 有污染衣物或气体、稀便失禁发生[28-29]。然而，如果操作正确，这种方法术后愈合率高达 95%[29]。理论上讲，这种手术失败的主要原因是医师未能找到正确的内口[29-30]。在 1996 年，Garcia-Aguilar 等已经证实了这一点[29]，他们对 299 例患者实行了肛瘘切开术，找到内口的患者，复发率为 7%，内口未能明确者，复发率为 56%。

关于复杂性肛瘘行单纯切开的数据较少。大多数作者报道的病例中，包含的复发性肛瘘患者较少。因此难以获得有意义的结论。我们认为再次行肛瘘切开术适用于上次手术未能明确内口或者合理的怀疑（详细造影）证实内口并不位于上次手术中所确定的位置。对于这类患者要特别注意，并且在术中仔细询问有无便失禁的症状。如前所述，这具有法律意义。在 Garcia 等[29]的研究中，复发性肛瘘患者的不满意率（61%）高于大便失禁患者的不满意率。有趣的是，由大便失禁引起的不满（84%）多于有肛瘘复发引起的不满（33%）。

经肛门（直肠内）的皮瓣移植修补术

手术技术[31]

患者取折刀位，暴露出肛瘘内口，切除内口周围的组织及上方的肛管皮肤。然后将瘘管组织从括约肌中切除。用可吸收缝线缝合内括约肌缺损，在齿线部位做一个包含黏膜、黏膜下层及部分肌肉纤维的皮瓣，并向近端拉近 4~6cm。皮瓣的长度一般是宽度的两倍。皮瓣移植后，用可吸收线缝合在新的齿线位置，见图 36.1 和图 36.2 a-e。

技术相关观点

有一些文献关注皮瓣的厚度和连续性。大多数作者[5,22,31-37]使用的皮瓣包括黏膜、黏膜下层和表浅的内括约肌组织。手术需要分离出一个相对的少血管区，使皮瓣有充分的弹性移动到内口位置。然而，也有研究者使用包含黏膜及黏膜下层的皮瓣[38]以及包含全层直肠壁的全层厚皮瓣[4,39-41]。有一些研究对比全层厚皮瓣和黏膜+黏膜下层皮瓣的疗效[40-42]。一项小的回顾性研究报道，使用全层皮瓣术后愈合较好，且没有控便功能的损害[40]。另一项 Khafagy 主持的近期小型、随机研究[41]也发现全层皮瓣患者术后效果较好，但是对控便功能影响较大。Roig 等[42]对 70 例行直肠内皮瓣移植的患者进行了一个精细的回顾性研究，发现全层皮瓣患者术后功能较差，但两者术后愈合率没有差别。尽管证据很少，但是在皮瓣下方谨慎地加上一些表浅的肌肉纤维组织可以加强皮瓣的覆盖功能。而且值得注意的是，目前大多数应用皮瓣技术发表的研究已经用部分厚的皮瓣配合表浅的肌肉组织。

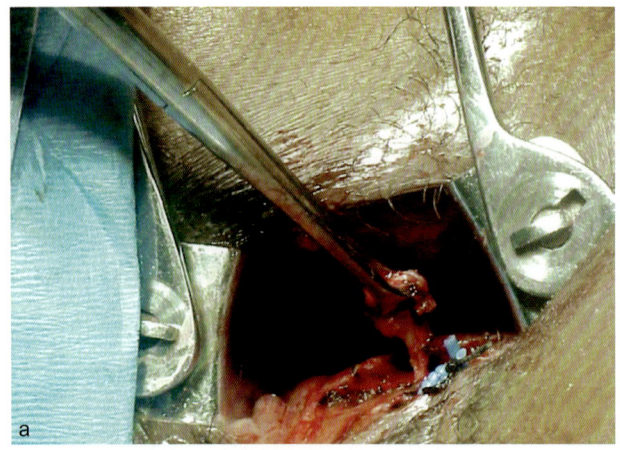
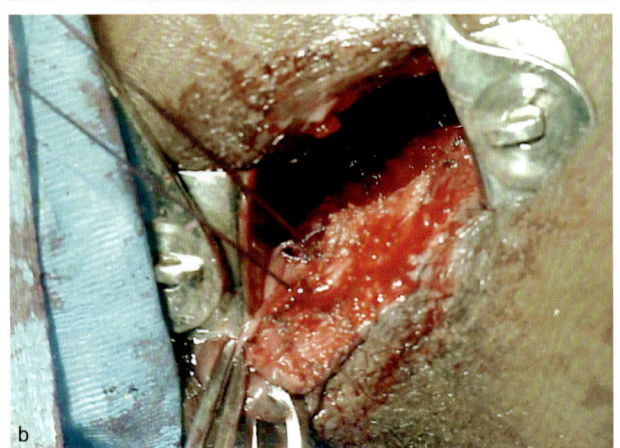
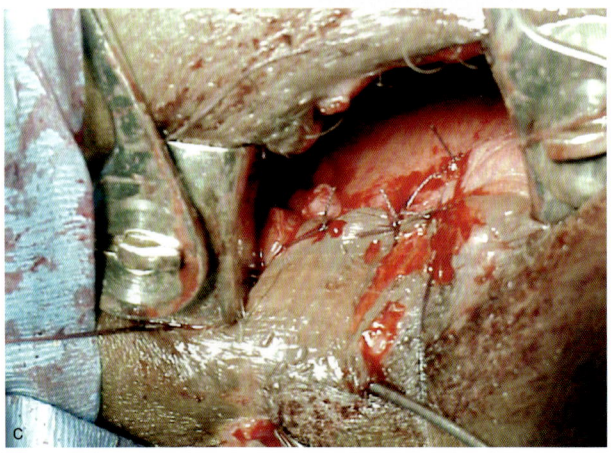

图 36.1 挂线术后延期黏膜移植肛门成形术同时的内外括约肌修补术。（a）切除内口部位肛瘘；（b）内括约肌修补；（c）黏膜移植缝合

影响因素：吸烟

据分析许多因素都可以影响经肛门皮瓣移植修补的疗效。一些研究者发现烟草有决定性的作用[43,46]，但其他研究者并不赞同[4,37]。在过去的一项观察吸烟者与非吸烟者皮瓣分离前后血运情况的研究中，Zimmerman 等发现在创造皮瓣后，直肠黏膜血运明显减少[32]。此外吸烟者在制作皮瓣前后，直肠壁的血流的明显低于非吸烟者，但并未发现血流与皮瓣手术成功率之间有关[45]。这个研究表明血流的减少并不是影响皮瓣手术的决定性因素。有多名研究者发现吸烟者术后愈合较慢，因此有必要向患者说明这点。对于准备行皮瓣手术的复发性肛瘘患者，应该有必要减少吸烟。Ellis 和 Clark[44] 发现吸烟对黏膜皮瓣有负面影响，而对肛管皮肤皮瓣没有影响。因此在这种病例中，应该考虑到修补方法的影响作用。

相关因素：术前挂线引流

一些研究者建议术前挂线引流。因为通过挂线使瘘管得到引流，减轻炎症反应，减少深部脓肿和继发瘘管的形成[2,46,47]，尽管一些研究者[2,22,46,47]发现术前切开引流可以促进皮瓣修复的愈合，但这种益处并未被其他研究者认可[43,48,49]。此外研究报道中的病理数目较少且病情多样，包括直肠阴道瘘和克罗恩病引起的肛瘘。总之，尽快挂线引流是一种分期治疗肛瘘的方法，但没有证据支持必须在皮瓣手术前进行挂线引流[50-51]，而在更复杂的病例中，挂线引流可以减轻术前的脓毒症，使复杂肛瘘术后的愈合率与一些直行的肛瘘相近。此外我们认为，在治疗复杂肛瘘前充分引流所有活动的肛周感染是很有必要的。因此挂线引流仍是治疗肛瘘的一种有用方法，是肛瘘术前治疗的一个重要组成部分。但我们不赞成用挂线进行切开，挂线切开可能会造成显著但不被认识的肛门控便功能障碍发生[52-53]。

经肛门皮瓣移植术治疗复发性肛瘘

Lindsey 等[49] 报道再次行皮瓣移植手术效果不佳。因为前次皮瓣移植失败形成的瘢痕会影响后次皮瓣手术的成功，但文献不支持这个结论。Kodner 等[5] 报道对 9 例皮瓣移植术后失败患者再次行皮瓣移植术，均获得成功。在另一项研究中，Mizrah[4] 对 12 例皮瓣移植术后失败者再次手术，8 例（67%）治愈。一些大规模研究[4,22,38,43,54] 已经建议用经肛门皮瓣移植治疗复发性肛瘘。研究[43,54] 发现，前次手术对术后愈合没有影响。我们相信对于应用这种技术治疗复发性肛瘘还存在很大争议。

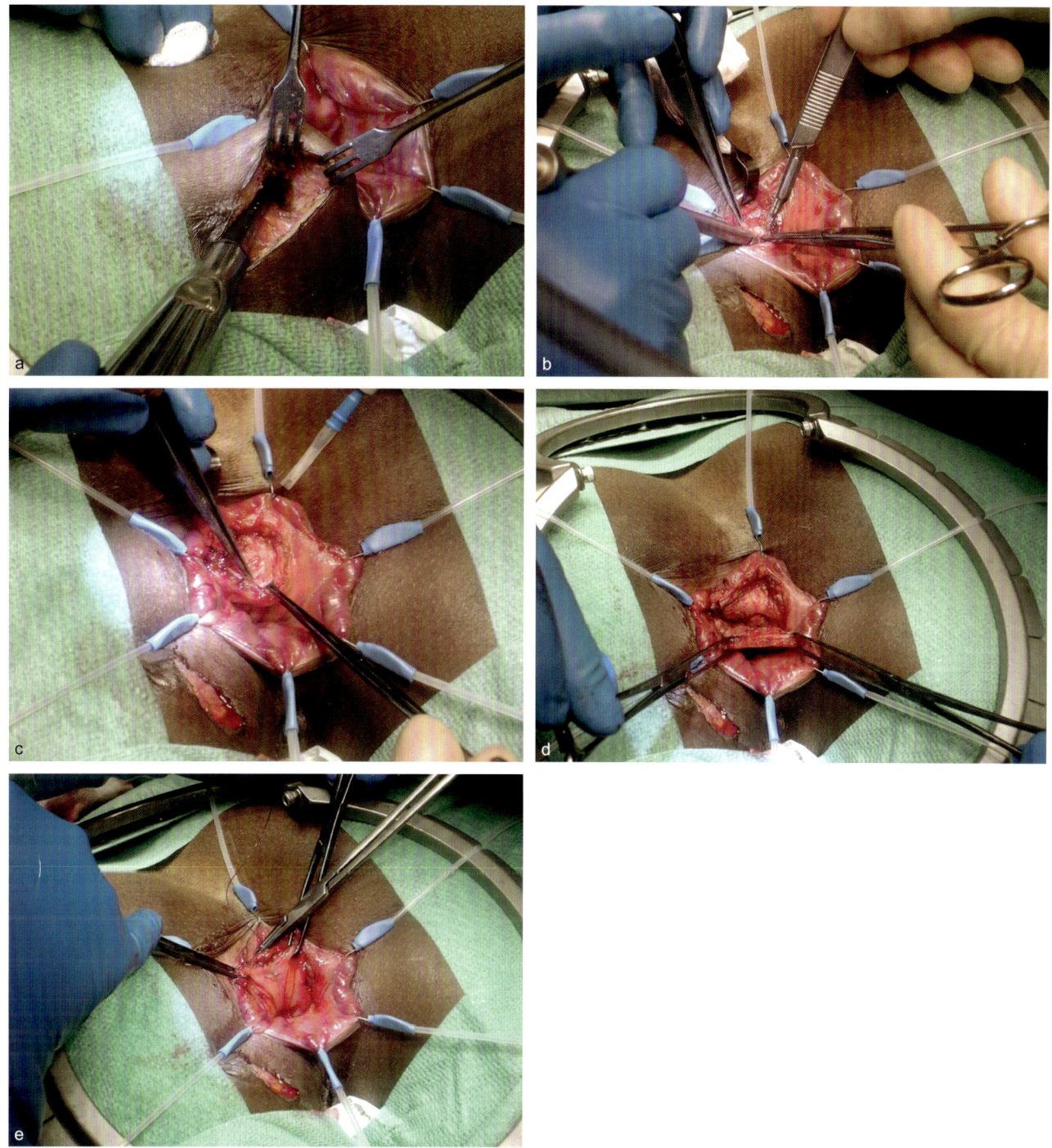

图36.2 经肛门皮瓣移植修补。（a）分离瘘管外部组织直到括约肌间隙；（b）切除内口，清理括约肌间隙。切除肛管表面皮肤。将含有黏膜、黏膜下层及表浅肌肉纤维的皮瓣拉起；（c）皮瓣自齿线拉起，向头侧移动4~6cm；（d）注意制作一个宽基底的皮瓣，保证血运；（e）皮瓣移植完成，用可吸收线缝合在新的齿线部位

功能相关问题

最近，几个大型研究[4,22,38,43,54]报道了移植皮瓣治疗复发性肛瘘，不幸的是，在这些研究中没有正确的评价控便功能。已有研究表明皮瓣移植会损害控便功能。据报道这种不良反应发生率为8%~30%[31,38]。这种影响一般是轻微的（液体或气体控制不良），一些研究表明是由于肛管内括约肌损伤引起。基于这种理论，二次皮瓣移植手术可能造成控便功能的进一步损害。最近Mitalas[54]等一

项 87 例患者的研究表明，二次手术与初次手术术后愈合率相当，且没有术后排便功能损害。

直肠内皮瓣移植用于克罗恩病患者

已有研究者研究移植皮瓣治疗克罗恩病患者的肛瘘。最初不推荐使用，因为据报道愈合率一般在 33%~83%[39,55]。而且报道病例数目都较少。Makowiec 等[56]报道相对较大的病例研究，对 32 例克罗恩病患者进行了 36 例皮瓣移植手术，虽然短期效果可以接受（只有 4 例失败），但有 17 例出现复发，导致肛瘘术后总的复发率达 66%。然而术后肛门功能较为满意。这些结果与 Mizrah[4] 和 Sonoda[22] 的结论极为类似。他们分别报道术后愈合率为 43% 和 50%，但这两项研究都没有详细描述术后肛门功能情况，值得注意的是，这些研究都发现克罗恩病是影响手术成功的一个不利因素。

近期 Soltani 和 Kaiser[57]的一项系统性回顾性研究统计采用黏膜皮瓣移植术治疗克罗恩病患者肛瘘，平均愈合率为 64%，但他们计算愈合率是基于术后短期愈合，其中包括两项相对较大的研究，分别报道治愈率为 75% 和 71%，这些研究也报道了远期疗效，使最终愈合率分别下降至 44% 和 55%。此外，在这项研究中，小规模的研究（<10 例）所占比例较大。

总之，采用黏膜皮瓣治疗克罗恩病患者肛瘘，术后愈合率较低，但仍有可能治愈，而且术后功能较好，尽管详细数据较少。因此对于能够接受这种手术率较低的手术的患者，可以考虑这种手术。

肛瘘切除术同时行括约肌修补

这种应用不多的技术，最初于 1993 年[58]出现在圣马可医院。而后被 Athanasiadis 等[60]改进。用这种技术已经取得了一些令人满意的效果，但是可能由于手术技巧较为困难，造成这种技术没有被广泛接受。

手术技术

完全切除内口和括约肌之间的瘘管组织，直至括约肌平面。刮除括约肌之间的瘘管，排出感染物质。然后以瘘管穿过外括约肌处为中心，在外口周围做一个宽椭圆形切口，将瘘管和周围皮肤脂肪组织整块切除。通过间断缝合关闭肛管内切除后残留的内口。第一行在内括约肌近端，然后逐行缝合，要包括部分肌肉纤维、黏膜和黏膜下层。肛门外括约肌的环形缺损可以通过肛周进行修补。

技术要点

很少有报道各方面均能取得良好的疗效[42,58,60,61]。肛门失禁问题已经得到充分的评估，而且手术方法已经描述得很清楚。最初有报道采用经括约肌手术途径，不被多数患者认可。后来这种技术发展成为 LIFT 并取得了令人鼓舞的效果[62]。最初看上去，在肛瘘可以经过肛门或肛周切除的前提下，在括约肌之间增加一个切口似乎不合逻辑。但随着发展，这种观点受到质疑。括约肌间的手术途径使内外括约肌之间的脓肿得到引流。现在关于肛瘘切除术后同时行括约肌修补的报道较少，但最初的报道和其他报道相比，愈合率要低很多。

Maos[58] 和 Perze[61]都缝合了外部伤口。在后一项研究中，伤口并发症发生率高达 71%。虽然 Matos 等没有报道术后伤口并发症，但很可能是这些并发症造成他们的手术成功率低于其他研究者。但外部伤口保持开放，术后伤口并发症发生率仍较高：一项研究报道为 15%[60]，另一项为 19%[42]。

一些研究者报道了应用肛管内皮瓣移植的方法[42,63]。没有研究发现术后并发症发生率有区别，但 Roig 等[42]报道肛管内皮瓣移植术后有控便功能的损害，尤其是全层皮瓣。有经验的研究者提出，经括约肌间肛瘘切除术并非适用于所有类型的肛瘘[60]。一些患者在内口周围或肛管内会形成瘢痕，对于这些病例，由于早期手术造成周围组织固定或缺乏弹性，不适于做直接的封闭。理想的患者是相对短且组织有弹性，并且肛瘘开口在肛管的背面。另一种方法是 Zbar 等[64]介绍的分期手术方法，在挂线引流术后，按照 Athanasiadis[60] 介绍的方法修补括约肌。但为了再次手术，挂线一般保留在内外括约肌之间。Zbar 等介绍的方法在复发率方面好于 Athanasiadis 等介绍的一项小型随机回顾性研究结果。而且，测压的结果也优于同时行内外括约肌修补的病例，但没有统计学意义。

克罗恩病患者行肛瘘切除同时括约肌修补

克罗恩病患者行肛瘘切除同时括约肌修补的资料有限。大多数研究都排除了克罗恩病患者。Matos 等描述了 5 例炎症肠病的患者。所有病例手术均失败，从这些有限的数据中没有得到有意义的结论。

通常的观点

据报道，这种技术术后成功率相当高（69%～93%），而且不同研究者报道愈合率之间差别不大。尽管只有少数报道了大便失禁的发生，但所有患者都评价了控便功能。术后大便失禁的发生率可以接受，为 6%～33%。因此在这种手术后应考虑到术后括约肌断裂和大便失禁的风险。只有 Perez 等[65]建议在术后行括约肌折叠缝合术。尽管他们报道术后愈合率较高（93%），但比不做括约肌折叠修补没有明显的优势。值得注意的是，正如几个研究观察的那样[42,65]，同时行括约肌修补并没有减低肛管压力。对于复发性肛瘘患者行肛瘘切除同时括约肌修补的资料有限，很少有研究者在研究中描述前次手术的情况。Athanasiadis 等的研究病例较多，包括 51 例患者有先前手术病史。有趣的是，他们发现术后愈合率没有差别，和 Roig 等的研究结果类似[42]。他们建议复发性肛瘘是这种手术的主要适应证。

肛门皮肤皮瓣移植术

Pino 等[66]介绍了对复发性肛瘘者采用肛管皮瓣移植术进行治疗的效果。他们报道病例数目较少，且达到理想效果。据研究者观点，这种手术不会造成肛管解剖结构的改变，后续还能进行其他手术治疗。其他研究者报道结果相近，但这种技术还没有被广泛接受。

手术技巧

首先切开肛瘘内口，清除周围的内容物，同时切除表面覆盖的肛管皮肤，然后切除外口至外括约肌之间的瘘管组织。瘘管穿过括约肌部分要切除或者刮除干净，用可吸收线缝合内括约肌缺损部分。制作一个倒 U 形的皮瓣，包括肛周皮肤和脂肪，注意防止局部缺血。皮瓣底宽度约为轴长的 2 倍。将皮瓣上提与黏膜和括约肌作单层缝合，用可吸收线间断缝合封闭内口，外部伤口保持开放。

技术相关问题

不同研究者采用的手术方式大不相同。最初报道使用梨形皮瓣，外部伤口保持开放[66-67]，另外一些研究者建议用钻石形皮瓣，外部伤口可以缝合[68]。其他可以封闭外部伤口的方法，包括 V-Y 肛管成形术[69-70]和应用 Burrow 三角形皮瓣[71]。我们使用过倒 U 形皮瓣[72-73]。为了预防感染，将外部伤口开放。Amin 和同事[69]使用 V-Y 皮瓣重建术，改良后保持伤口开放以防止感染，因为伤口感染并不被特别关注，因此这种方法很难得出有意义的结论。但看起来，将供体部位伤口缝合[68-71]会比保持供体部位开放[66,67,73]发生更多的伤口相关并发症。

一些研究者报道了皮瓣移植术后失败者再次行皮瓣移植术[67,69]。Nelson 等[67]对 13 例患者再次行皮瓣移植术，有 9 例获得成功（69%），因此研究者总结肛管皮瓣移植术的优点在于再次手术的成功率较高。Amin 等[69]的结论相同，虽然他们只对 2 例患者进行再次的皮瓣移植手术。

应用肛管皮瓣移植术治疗克罗恩病患者

应用肛管皮瓣移植术治疗克罗恩病患者肛瘘的资料有限。Nelson 等[67]用这种方法治疗 17 例克罗恩病肛瘘患者，只有 2 例复发。因为这是仅有的有关这种技术治疗克罗恩病患者的报道，因此不可能得到有意义的结论。

通常的观点

已有研究者报道应用这种技术治疗其他手术方法治疗失败的患者[67,70,71,73]，在小规模研究中[73]，发现之前没有手术和手术过 1 次的患者与术前有过 2 次或更多次手术患者相比，术后愈合率存在差异，这种差异别的研究者也注意到了，但没有统计学意义[67,70]。

结 论

肛管皮瓣移植手术相对简单,对于初次手术者效果满意,一些研究者对初次手术、没有克罗恩病的患者采用这种方法治疗,效果良好。对于复发性肛瘘,这种方法不太适合。如果用这种方法,建议保持外部伤口开放。

肛瘘栓

近年来,外科肛瘘栓(Cook 公司 Bloomington 市)已发展为传统手术的替代品。这种栓由猪小肠上皮提取的细胞外基质组成。这种基质使宿主组织重建,封闭瘘管,移植后不会被压缩。一些研究者认为这种微创技术为治疗肛瘘提供了一种简单、安全的方法。最初报道,有效率高达 87%[74-75],但近期也有疗效不理想的报道,愈合率降至 41%[76] 和 24%[77],对于复杂肛瘘达到 14%[78]。

手术技巧

在用 H_2O_2 冲洗瘘管后将圆锥体的栓通过瘘管拉入,将其剪至适合长度。用 8 字缝合的方法将其固定在内口部位,并且用黏膜覆盖内口部位。

要 点

Ellis 和 Clark[44] 最初比较了肛瘘栓和皮瓣移植术的效果。在他们的回顾性分析中,皮瓣移植术患者术后复发率为 33%,肛瘘栓为 12%,但没有统计学差异。Chung 等也有类似发现[79]。最近 2 项回顾性研究表明皮瓣移植术后愈合率明显高于应用肛瘘栓术后的愈合率[80-81]。这种结论也得到了另一个随机对照研究的支持[82]。

结 论

基于这些数据,皮瓣移植的效果看似好于肛瘘栓。但肛瘘栓的方法为简单低位的经括约肌肛瘘患者提供了一种新的治疗方法。但较高的费用是肛瘘栓的另一个缺点。目前而言,肛瘘栓并不是治疗复杂性肛瘘的理想方法。

LIFT 手术

最近,Rojanasakul 等[62] 介绍 LIFT 手术是一种比较新颖的手术图 36.3a-e,虽然以前也有关于这种手术的一些介绍[60, 64],只是相关数据较少,但效果看上去令人满意。

手术方法

将探针穿过瘘管,固定探针后标记内外括约肌间沟。在括约肌间沟做一弧形切口,保持探针的位置,并确认瘘管组织。注意不要分开任何括约肌。一旦将瘘管完全游离,瘘管会蜷缩,这时可以去除探针。下一步将瘘管两端缝合结扎,将外口保持开放,刮除瘘管内的坏死组织。也可以通过内口进行轻柔的刮除,然后封闭内口。最后用可吸收线间断缝合关闭皮肤切口。

技术相关问题

对于如何结扎瘘管存在一些不同方法,Bleier 等[83] 分离瘘管后去结扎瘘管两侧,而最初报道为切除外部瘘管[62]。Shaowani 等[84] 也去除外部瘘管。

观 点

肛瘘复发的原因被认为是粪便进入内口(由于肛管与肛周压力差造成)。LIFT 手术防止粪便进入瘘管,组织括约肌间形成脓肿,使肛瘘愈合。这种技术的优点包括保留了肛门括约肌、组织损伤小、缩短愈合时间,而且手术操作相对简单,可以用于其他任何手术治疗失败后的患者。这种技术术后愈合率也较高,据报道可达 57%~99%。Bleier 等用这种方法治疗患者中大部分曾接受过手术治疗[83],这可能是造成术后愈合率较低的原因。他们报道没有控便功能的损伤,也没有采用详细的问卷和其他

第36章 复发性复杂肛瘘的再手术治疗

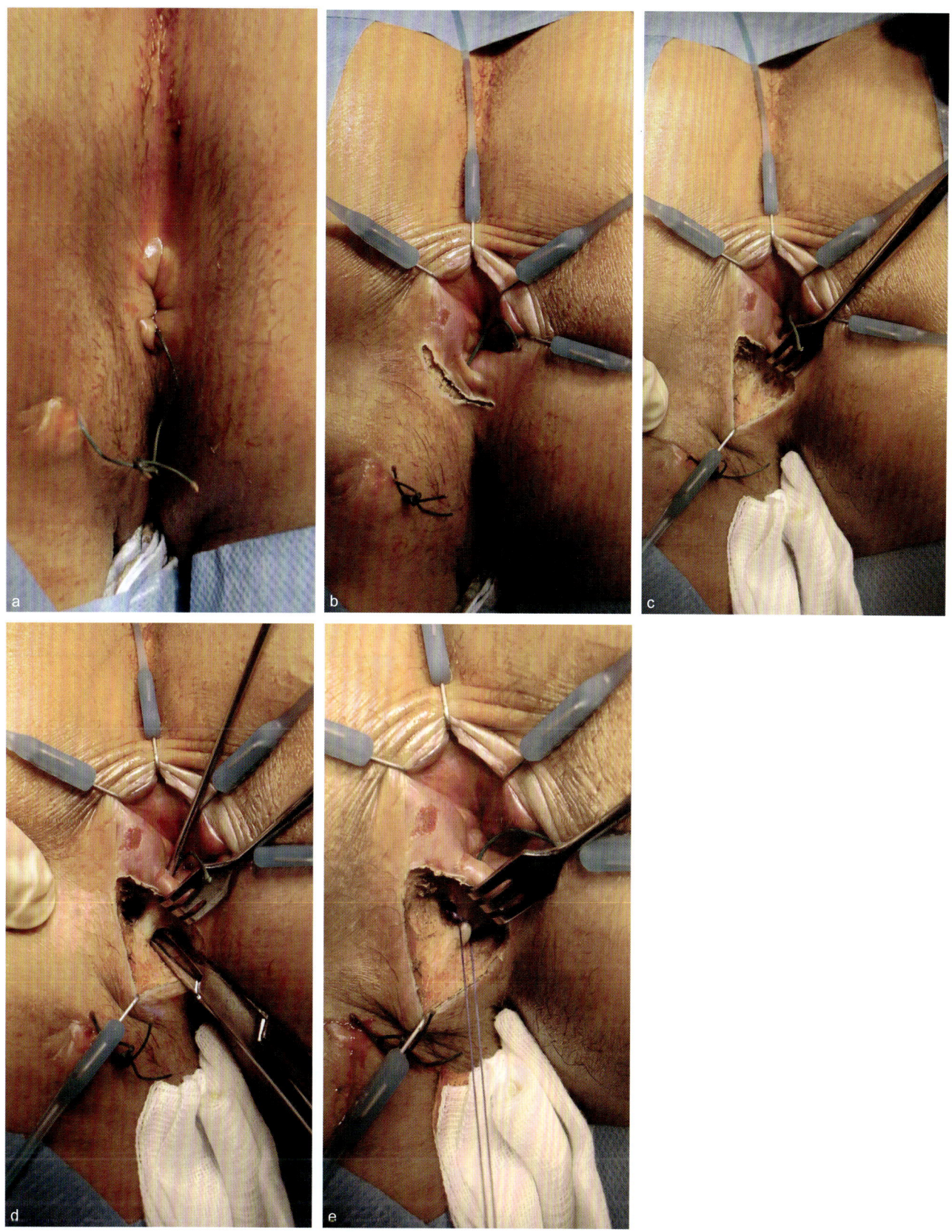

图 36.3 括约肌间瘘管结扎手术。(a) 将挂线穿过瘘管引起纤维化;(b) 在括约肌间沟做小切口;(c) 括约肌间隙分离完成;(d) 确认括约肌间瘘管组织;(e) 结扎括约肌间瘘管然后分离

有效工具进行评价。

LIFT 治疗克罗恩病患者的肛瘘

尽管在理论上，用这种方法治疗克罗恩病患者肛瘘有优势，但目前还没有可以获得的数据。

结　论

这种治疗肛瘘的新技术，着眼于保留括约肌。与其他保留括约肌的手术相比，已显示了良好的早期效果。通过随机对照试验来确定这种方法在肛瘘治疗中的作用和地位是值得的也是有必要的。

挂线术的应用

挂线术治疗肛瘘可以粗略分为3种类型，通过挂线对急性脓肿进行引流，已在前面进行了讨论。挂线作为最终治疗方法，有两种情况：挂线可以作为切开用途，或者作为长期引流的用途。后一种类型也称为长期引流挂线（LTIS）。这种技术多用于肛周克罗恩病引起的慢性感染，也有一些研究者应用这种技术治疗肛腺引起的高位经括约肌肛瘘[48,85,86]。

手术技术

切开挂线

用不可吸收缝线穿过瘘管，最初阶段保持松弛状态，每间隔2~4周收紧挂线。逐渐的压力及硬化形成导致挂线内所含内括约肌被缓慢、有计划地切开。当肌肉被切断以后，断端硬化并与括约肌粘连，这样可以确保防止肛门外括约肌的断端分开距离过大[87-88]。

长期挂线

这种技术是用不可吸收缝线或者硅胶环，穿过肛管及肛瘘。这种技术的原理是持续的引流可以防止脓肿的形成。此外，由于对于人体而言，挂线是一种异物，可以逐渐由括约肌向外迁移，可能为后期行简单的肛瘘切除术创造条件[85]。

要　点

切开挂线

Corman[89]认为这种方法是用绳子缓慢切开冰块。绳子通过后冰块还保持完整。尽管有理论上的优势，但用挂线切开后造成的缺损是否小于单纯的肛瘘切开术还不明确。用挂线切开后控便功能损伤的报道也有很大差异。一些研究者认为没有控便功能的损伤[90]。而大多数研究者报道控便功能损伤发生率相当高，在15%~67%之间[52,91-97]。这种技术的另一个缺点就是疼痛，且完全愈合需要相对较长的时间。

长期挂线引流

Lentner 和 Wienert[85] 报道他们应用LTIS治疗低位经括约肌和括约肌间肛瘘，有17.6%患者肛瘘被挂线切开，平均用时13.7个月，因此必须进行进一步手术治疗。有4%患者肛瘘复发。Buchanan 等[86] 对20例复杂肛瘘患者采用松弛挂线的方法治疗了平均13周（3~28周），据短期随访13例肛瘘愈合，但长期随访后发现由于脓肿复发，后来下降为4例。这可能是过早去除了挂线的原因[98]。很难理解，当内外括约肌之间伤口保持开放，挂线保留在原位时，伤口能够愈合。Neijenhuis 等[99] 对60例经括约肌肛瘘患者用长期挂线的方法进行治疗，其中13例患者在肛管上1/3部分有内口，有7例患者挂线后向外迁移，并行肛瘘切开术。在这方面，Eitan 等[91] 报道对41例高位穿括约肌肛瘘患者用这种方法进行治疗，并取得满意疗效。随访5个月，只有20%存在肛瘘组织残留，对这些患者再次用挂线方法进行治疗，也取得了成功。

挂线向远端移位只发生在少数患者中，LTIS多被用做瘘管引流，阻止脓肿形成。然而尚缺乏证据。总之，有一部分特定患者可以从中受益。理论上讲，虽然还缺乏临床研究证明这种方法的优势，但它特别适用于复发性复杂肛瘘的治疗。

肛瘘治疗流程

对于复发性复杂肛瘘治疗流程见图36.4和图36.5。

第36章 复发性复杂肛瘘的再手术治疗

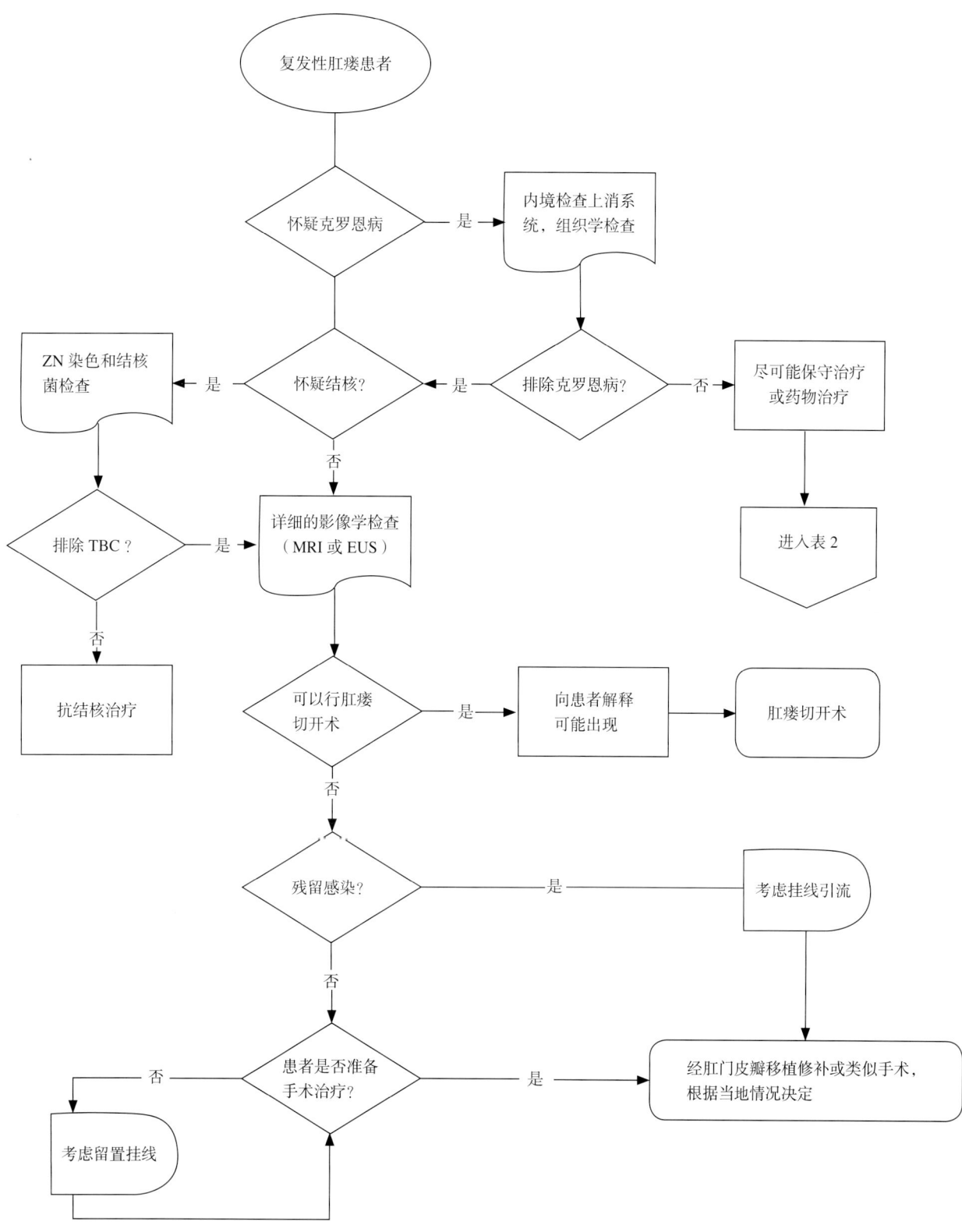

图 36.4 复发性肛瘘治疗流程

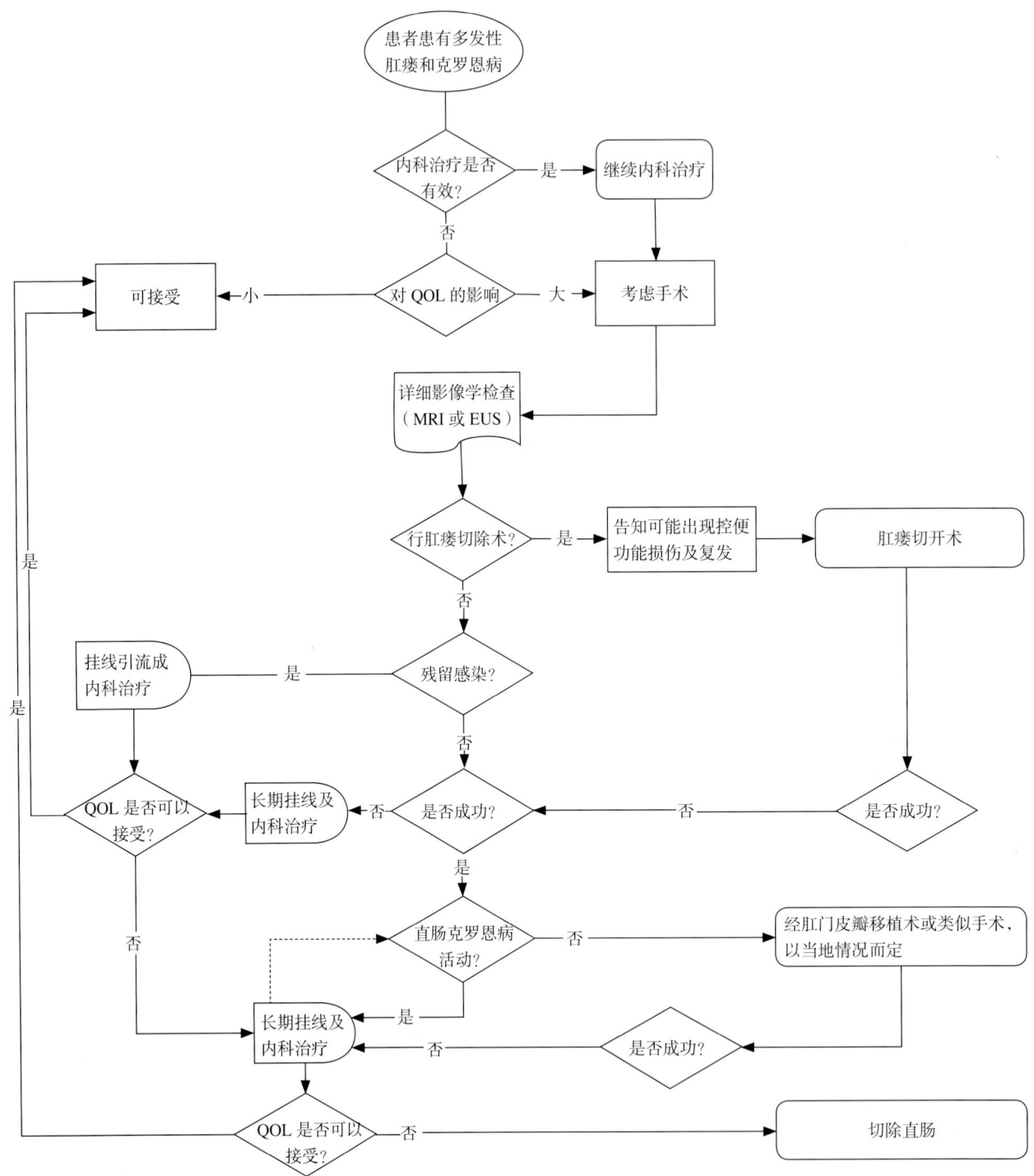

图 36.5 克罗恩病患者复发性肛瘘治疗流程

参考文献

1. Lockhart-Mummery HJ. Discussion on fistula-in-ano. Proc R Soc Med. 1929;22:1331–58.
2. Parks AG, Stitz RW. The treatment of high fistula-in-ano. Dis Colon Rectum. 1976;19:487–99.
3. Joy HA, Williams JG. The outcome of surgery for complex anal fistula. Colorectal Dis. 2002;4(4):254–61.
4. Mizrahi N, Wexner SD, Zmora O, Da Silva G, Efron J, Weiss EG, et al. Endorectal advancement flap: are there predictors of failure? Dis Colon Rectum. 2002;45:1616–21.
5. Kodner IJ, Mazor A, Shemesh EI, Fry RD, Fleshman JW, Birnbaum EH. Endorectal advancement flap repair of rectovaginal and other complicated anorectal fistulae. Surgery. 1993;114:682–90.
6. Keighley MR, Allan RN. Current status and influence of operation on perianal Crohn's disease. Int J Colorectal Dis. 1986;1:104–7.
7. Buchmann P, Keighley MR, Allan RN, Thompson H, Alexander-Williams J. Natural history of perianal Crohn's disease. Ten year follow-up: a plea for conservatism. Am J Surg. 1980;140:642–4.
8. Platell C, Mackay J, Collopy B, Fink R, Ryan P, Woods R. Anal pathology in patients with Crohn's disease. Aust N Z J Surg. 1996;66:5–9.
9. Levien DH, Surrell J, Mazier W. Surgical treatment of anorectal fistula in patients with Crohn's disease. Surg Gynecol Obstet. 1989;169:133–6.
10. Nadal SR, Manzione CR, Galvão VM, Salim VR, Speranzini MB. Perianal diseases in HIV-positive patients compared with a seronegative population. Dis Colon Rectum. 1999;42:649–54.
11. Hamadani A, Haigh PI, Liu IL, Abbas MA. Who is at risk for developing chronic anal fistula or recurrent anal sepsis after initial perianal abscess? Dis Colon Rectum. 2009;52:217–21.
12. Consten EC, Slors FJ, Noten HJ, Oosting H, Danner SA, van Lanschot JJ. Anorectal surgery in human immunodeficiency virus-infected patients. Clinical outcome in relation to immune status. Dis Colon Rectum. 1995;38:1169–75.
13. Sultan S, Azria F, Bauer P, Abdelnour M, Atienza P. Anoperineal tuberculosis: diagnostic and management considerations in seven cases. Dis Colon Rectum. 2002;45:407–10.
14. Kraemer M, Gill SS, Seow-Choen F. Tuberculous anal sepsis: report of clinical features in 20 cases. Dis Colon Rectum. 2000;43:1589–91.
15. Stupart D, Goldberg P, Levy A, Govender D. Tuberculous anal fistulae – prevalence and clinical features in an endemic area. S Afr J Surg. 2009;47:116–8.
16. Stoker J, Hussain SM, Lameris JS. Endoanal magnetic resonance imaging versus endosonography. Radiol Med. 1996;92:738–41.
17. Poen AC, Felt-Bersma RJ, Eijsbouts QA, Cuesta MA, Meuwissen SG. Hydrogen peroxide-enhanced transanal ultrasound in the assessment of fistula-in-ano. Dis Colon Rectum. 1998;41:1147–52.
18. Barker PG, Lunniss PJ, Armstrong P, Reznek RH, Cottam K, Phillips RK. Magnetic resonance imaging of fistula-in-ano: technique, interpretation and accuracy. Clin Radiol. 1994;49:7–13.
19. Buchanan G, Halligan S, Williams A, Cohen CR, Tarroni D, Phillips RK, et al. Effect of MRI on clinical outcome of recurrent fistula-in-ano. Lancet. 2002;360(9346):1661–2.
20. Zbar AP, Armitage NC. Complex perirectal sepsis: clinical classification and imaging. Tech Coloproctol. 2006;10:83–93.
21. West RL, Zimmerman DD, Dwarkasing S, Hussain SM, Hop WC, Schouten WR, et al. Prospective comparison of hydrogen peroxide-enhanced three-dimensional endoanal ultrasonography and endoanal magnetic resonance imaging of perianal fistulae. Dis Colon Rectum. 2003;46:1407–15.
22. Sonoda T, Hull T, Piedmonte MR, Fazio VW. Outcomes of primary repair of anorectal and rectovaginal fistulae using the endorectal advancement flap. Dis Colon Rectum. 2002;45:1622–8.
23. Yamamoto T, Allan RN, Keighley MR. Effect of fecal diversion alone on perianal Crohn's disease. World J Surg. 2000;24:1258–63.
24. Kasparek MS, Glatzle J, Temeltcheva T, Mueller MH, Koenigsrainer A, Kreis ME. Long-term quality of life in patients with Crohn's disease and perianal fistulae: influence of fecal diversion. Dis Colon Rectum. 2007;50:2067–74.
25. Garcia-Aguilar J, Davey CS, Le CT, Lowry AC, Rothenberger DA. Patient satisfaction after surgical treatment for fistula-in-ano. Dis Colon Rectum. 2000;43:1206–12.
26. Ho YH, Tan M, Chui CH, Leong A, Eu KW, Seow-Choen F. Randomized controlled trial of primary fistulotomy with drainage alone for perianal abscesses. Dis Colon Rectum. 1997;40:1435–8.
27. Kronborg O. To lay open or excise a fistula-in-ano: a randomized trial. Br J Surg. 1985;72:970.
28. van Tets WF, Kuijpers HC. Continence disorders after anal fistulotomy. Dis Colon Rectum. 1994;37:1194–7.
29. Garcia-Aguilar J, Belmonte C, Wong WD, Goldberg SM, Madoff RD. Anal fistula surgery. Factors associated with recurrence and incontinence. Dis Colon Rectum. 1996;39:723–9.
30. Jordán J, Roig JV, García-Armengol J, García-Granero E, Solana A, Lledó S. Risk factors for recurrence and incontinence after anal fistula surgery. Colorectal Dis. 2010;12:254–60.
31. Schouten WR, Zimmerman DD, Briel JW. Transanal advancement flap repair of transsphincteric fistulae. Dis Colon Rectum. 1999;42:1419–23.
32. Zimmerman DD, Gosselink MP, Mitalas LE, Delemarre JB, Hop WJ, Briel JW, et al. Smoking impairs rectal mucosal bloodflow – a pilot study: possible implications for transanal advancement flap repair. Dis Colon Rectum. 2005;48:1228–32.
33. Mitalas LE, Gosselink MP, Oom DM, Zimmerman DD, Ruud Schouten W. Required length of follow-up after transanal advancement flap repair of high transsphincteric fistulae. Colorectal Dis. 2009;11(7):726–8.
34. Aguilar PS, Plasencia G, Hardy Jr TG, Hartmann RF, Stewart WR. Mucosal advancement in the treatment of anal fistula. Dis Colon Rectum. 1985;28:496–8.
35. Ortiz H, Marzo J. Endorectal flap advancement repair and fistulectomy for high trans-sphincteric and suprasphincteric fistulae. Br J Surg. 2000;87:1680–3.
36. Willis S, Rau M, Schumpelick V. Surgical treatment of high anorectal and rectovaginal fistulae with the use of transanal endorectal advancement flaps. Chirurg. 2000;71:836–40.
37. van Koperen PJ, Wind J, Bemelman WA, Bakx R, Reitsma JB, Slors JF. Long-term functional outcome and risk factors for recurrence after surgical treatment for low and high perianal fistulae of cryptoglandular origin. Dis Colon Rectum. 2008;51:1475–81.
38. Golub RW, Wise Jr WE, Kerner BA, Khanduja KS, Aguilar PS. Endorectal mucosal advancement flap: the preferred method for complex cryptoglandular fistula-in-ano. J Gastrointest Surg. 1997;1:487–91.
39. Lewis P, Bartolo DC. Treatment of trans-sphincteric fistulae by full thickness anorectal advancement flaps. Br J Surg. 1990;77:1187–9.
40. Dubsky PC, Stift A, Friedl J, Teleky B, Herbst F. Endorectal advancement flaps in the treatment of high anal fistula of cryptoglandular origin: full-thickness vs. mucosal-rectum flaps. Dis Colon Rectum. 2008;51:852–7.
41. Khafagy W, Omar W, El Nakeeb A, Fouda E, Yousef M, Farid M. Treatment of anal fistulae by partial rectal wall advancement flap or mucosal advancement flap: a prospective randomized study. Int J Surg. 2010;8:321–5.
42. Roig JV, García-Armengol J, Jordán JC, Moro D, García-Granero E, Alós R. Fistulectomy and sphincteric reconstruction for complex cryptoglandular fistulae. Colorectal Dis. 2010;12:e145–52.
43. Zimmerman DD, Delemarre JB, Gosselink MP, Hop WC, Briel JW, Schouten WR. Smoking affects the outcome of transanal mucosal

advancement flap repair of trans-sphincteric fistulae. Br J Surg. 2003;90:351–4.
44. Ellis CN, Clark S. Effect of tobacco smoking on advancement flap repair of complex anal fistulae. Dis Colon Rectum. 2007;50:459–63.
45. Mitalas LE, Schouten SB, Gosselink MP, Oom DM, Zimmerman DD, Schouten WR. Does rectal mucosal blood flow affect the outcome of transanal advancement flap repair? Dis Colon Rectum. 2009;52:1395–9.
46. Williams JG, Rands PA, Williams AB, Taylor BA, Lunniss PJ, Sagar PM, et al. The treatment of anal fistula: ACPGBI position statement. Colorectal Dis. 2007;9 Suppl 4:18–50.
47. van der Hagen SJ, Baeten CG, Soeters PB, Beets-Tan RG, Russel MG, van Gemert WG. Staged mucosal advancement flap for the treatment of complex anal fistulae: pretreatment with noncutting Setons and in case of recurrent multiple abscesses a diverting stoma. Colorectal Dis. 2005;7:513–8.
48. Mitalas LE, van Wijk JJ, Gosselink MP, Doornebosch P, Zimmerman DD, Schouten WR. Seton drainage prior to transanal advancement flap repair: useful or not? Int J Colorectal Dis. 2010;25:1499–502.
49. Lindsey I, Smilgin-Humphreys MM, Cunningham C, Mortensen NJ, George BD. A randomized, controlled trial of fibrin glue vs. conventional treatment for anal fistula. Dis Colon Rectum. 2002;45:1608–15.
50. van der Hagen SJ, Baeten CG, Soeters PB, van Gemert WG. Long-term outcome following mucosal advancement flap for high perianal fistulae and fistulotomy for low perianal fistulae: recurrent perianal fistulae: failure of treatment or recurrent patient disease? Int J Colorectal Dis. 2006;21:784–90.
51. Zbar AP. Experience with staged mucosal advancement anoplasty for high trans-sphincteric fistula-in-ano. West Indian Med J. 2007;56:446–50.
52. Ritchie RD, Sackier JM, Hodde JP. Incontinence rates after cutting seton treatment for anal fistula. Colorectal Dis. 2009;11:564–71.
53. Vial M, Parés D, Pera M, Grande L. Fecal incontinence after seton treatment for anal fistulae with and without surgical division of internal anal sphincter: a systematic review. Colorectal Dis. 2010;12:172–8.
54. Mitalas LE, Gosselink MP, Zimmerman DD, Schouten WR. Repeat transanal advancement flap repair: impact on the overall healing rate of high transsphincteric fistulae and on fecal continence. Dis Colon Rectum. 2007;50:1508–11.
55. Jones IT, Fazio VW, Jagelman DG. The use of transanal rectal advancement flaps in the management of fistulae involving the anorectum. Dis Colon Rectum. 1987;30:919–23.
56. Makowiec F, Jehle EC, Becker HD, Starlinger M. Clinical course after transanal advancement flap repair of perianal fistula in patients with Crohn's disease. Br J Surg. 1995;82:603–6.
57. Soltani A, Kaiser AM. Endorectal advancement flap for cryptoglandular or Crohn's fistula-in-ano. Dis Colon Rectum. 2010;53:486–95.
58. Matos D, Lunniss PJ, Phillips RK. Total sphincter conservation in high fistula in ano: results of a new approach. Br J Surg. 1993;80:802–4.
59. Hyman N. Endoanal advancement flap repair for complex anorectal fistulae. Am J Surg. 1999;178:337–40.
60. Athanasiadis S, Helmes C, Yazigi R, Köhler A. The direct closure of the internal fistula opening without advancement flap for transsphincteric fistulae-in-ano. Dis Colon Rectum. 2004;47:1174–80.
61. Perez F, Arroyo A, Serrano P, Candela F, Sanchez A, Calpena R. Fistulotomy with primary sphincter reconstruction in the management of complex fistula-in-ano: prospective study of clinical and manometric results. J Am Coll Surg. 2005;200:897–903.
62. Rojanasakul A, Pattanaarun J, Sahakitrungruang C, Tantiphlachiva K. Total anal sphincter saving technique for fistula-in-ano; the ligation of intersphincteric fistula tract. J Med Assoc Thai. 2007;90:581–6.
63. Perez F, Arroyo A, Serrano P, Sánchez A, Candela F, Perez MT, et al. Randomized clinical and manometric study of advancement flap versus fistulotomy with sphincter reconstruction in the management of complex fistula-in-ano. Am J Surg. 2006;192:34–40.
64. Zbar AP, Ramesh J, Beer-Gabel M, Salazar R, Pescatori M. Conventional cutting vs. internal anal sphincter-preserving seton for high trans-sphincteric fistula: a prospective randomized manometric and clinical trial. Tech Coloproctol. 2003;7:89–94.
65. Perez F, Arroyo A, Serrano P, Candela F, Perez MT, Calpena R. Prospective clinical and manometric study of fistulotomy with primary sphincter reconstruction in the management of recurrent complex fistula-in-ano. Int J Colorectal Dis. 2006;21:522–6.
66. Del Pino A, Nelson RL, Pearl RK, Abcarian H. Island flap anoplasty for treatment of transsphincteric fistula-in-ano. Dis Colon Rectum. 1996;39:224–6.
67. Nelson RL, Cintron J, Abcarian H. Dermal island-flap anoplasty for transsphincteric fistula-in-ano: assessment of treatment failures. Dis Colon Rectum. 2000;43:681–4.
68. Robertson WG, Mangione JS. Cutaneous advancement flap closure: alternative method for treatment of complicated anal fistulae. Dis Colon Rectum. 1998;41:884–7.
69. Amin SN, Tierney GM, Lund JN, Armitage NC. V-Y advancement flap for treatment of fistula-in-ano. Dis Colon Rectum. 2003;46:540–3.
70. Sungurtekin U, Sungurtekin H, Kabay B, Tekin K, Aytekin F, Erdem E, et al. Anocutaneous V-Y advancement flap for the treatment of complex perianal fistula. Dis Colon Rectum. 2004;47:2178–83.
71. Jun SH, Choi GS. Anocutaneous advancement flap closure of high anal fistulae. Br J Surg. 1999;86:490–2.
72. Nahas SC, Sobrado Júnior CW, Marques CF, Imperiale AR, Habr-Gama A, Rocha JP, et al. Orifice Diseases Project – experience of the "Hospital das Clinicas" University of Sao Paulo Medical Center in day-hospital of anorectal disease. Rev Hosp Clin Fac Med Sao Paulo. 1999;54:75–80.
73. Zimmerman DD, Briel JW, Gosselink MP, Schouten WR. Anocutaneous advancement flap repair of transsphincteric fistulae. Dis Colon Rectum. 2001;44:1474–80.
74. Champagne BJ, O'Connor LM, Ferguson M, Orangio GR, Schertzer ME, Armstrong DN. Efficacy of anal fistula plug in closure of cryptoglandular fistulae: long-term follow-up. Dis Colon Rectum. 2006;49:1817–21.
75. Johnson EK, Gaw JU, Armstrong DN. Efficacy of anal fistula plug vs. fibrin glue in closure of anorectal fistulae. Dis Colon Rectum. 2006;49:371–6.
76. van Koperen PJ, D'Hoore A, Wolthuis AM, Bemelman WA, Slors JF. Anal fistula plug for closure of difficult anorectal fistula: a prospective study. Dis Colon Rectum. 2007;50:2168–72.
77. Lawes DA, Efron JE, Abbas M, Heppell J, Young-Fadok TM. Early experience with the bioabsorbable anal fistula plug. World J Surg. 2008;32:1157–9.
78. Cellini C, Safar B, Fleshman J. Surgical management of pyogenic complications of Crohn's disease. Inflamm Bowel Dis. 2010;16:512–7.
79. Chung W, Kazemi P, Ko D, Sun C, Brown CJ, Raval M, et al. Anal fistula plug and fibrin glue versus conventional treatment in repair of complex anal fistulae. Am J Surg. 2009;197:604–8.
80. Christoforidis D, Pieh MC, Madoff RD, Mellgren AF. Treatment of transsphincteric anal fistulae by endorectal advancement flap or collagen fistula plug: a comparative study. Dis Colon Rectum. 2009;52:18–22.
81. Wang JY, Garcia-Aguilar J, Sternberg JA, Abel ME, Varma MG. Treatment of transsphincteric anal fistulae: are fistula plugs an acceptable alternative? Dis Colon Rectum. 2009;52:692–7.

82. Ortiz H, Marzo J, Ciga MA, Oteiza F, Armendáriz P, de Miguel M. Randomized clinical trial of anal fistula plug versus endorectal advancement flap for the treatment of high cryptoglandular fistula in ano. Br J Surg. 2009;96:608–12.
83. Bleier JI, Moloo H, Goldberg SM. Ligation of the intersphincteric fistula tract: an effective new technique for complex fistulae. Dis Colon Rectum. 2010;53:43–6.
84. Shanwani A, Nor AM, Amri N. Ligation of the intersphincteric fistula tract (LIFT): a sphincter-saving technique for fistula-in-ano. Dis Colon Rectum. 2010;53:39–42.
85. Lentner A, Wienert V. Long-term, indwelling setons for low transsphincteric and intersphincteric anal fistulae. Experience with 108 cases. Dis Colon Rectum. 1996;39:1097–101.
86. Buchanan GN, Owen HA, Torkington J, Lunniss PJ, Nicholls RJ, Cohen CR. Long-term outcome following loose-seton technique for external sphincter preservation in complex anal fistula. Br J Surg. 2004;91:476–80.
87. Seow-Choen F, Nicholls RJ. Anal fistula. Br J Surg. 1992;79:197–205.
88. McCourtney JS, Finlay IG. Setons in the surgical management of fistula in ano. Br J Surg. 1995;82:448–52.
89. Corman M. Colon and rectal surgery. 2nd ed. Philadelphia: Lippincott; 2004. p. 146.
90. Walfisch S, Menachem Y, Koretz M. Double seton – a new modified approach to high transsphincteric anal fistula. Dis Colon Rectum. 1997;40:731–2.
91. Christensen A, Nilas L, Christiansen J. Treatment of transsphincteric anal fistulae by the seton technique. Dis Colon Rectum. 1986;29:454–5.
92. Eitan A, Duek DS, Barzilai A. The seton in the treatment of transsphincteric anal fistulae. Harefuah. 1990;119:134–6.
93. Williams JG, MacLeod CA, Rotghenberger DA, Goldberg SM. Seton treatment of high anal fistulae. Br J Surg. 1991;78:1159–61.
94. Graf W, Pahlman L, Ejerblad S. Functional results after seton treatment of high transsphincteric anal fistulae. Eur J Surg. 1995;161:289–91.
95. Hamalainen KP, Sainio A. Cutting seton for anal fistulae: high risk of minor control defects. Dis Colon Rectum. 1997;40:1443–7.
96. McCourtney JS, Finlay IG. Cutting seton without preliminary internal sphincterotomy in management of complex high fistula-in-ano. Dis Colon Rectum. 1996;39:55–8.
97. Garcia-Aguilar J, Belmonte C, Wong DW, Goldberg SM, Madoff RD. Cutting seton versus two-stage seton fistulotomy in the surgical management of high anal fistula. Br J Surg. 1998;85:243–5.
98. Schouten WR, Gosselink MP. Long term outcome following loose-seton technique for external sphincter preservation in complex anal fistula. Tech Coloproctol. 2005;9:79.
99. Neijenhuis P, van Tets W, Steur WD, Nellensteijn J. Dwelling seton treatment for perianal fistulae. Patience is a must. Dis Colon Rectum. 2008;51:695.

第 37 章 成人肛管前移畸形与肛管前庭瘘的治疗

F. Sergio P. Regadas · Rosilma Gorete Lima Barreto · Sthela Maria Murad-Regadas

陈　硕 译　李国逊 审校

摘　要

本章主要就复杂肛瘘的治疗介绍了一些特殊的方法，特别是对于肛门前庭瘘的治疗。没有任何一种单一的治疗方法可以治疗所有类型的肛门直肠瘘。治疗方法的选择主要依赖于外科医生的临床经验和判断。每一种治疗方法，包括直肠内皮瓣转移法，伴或不伴肛门成形术的内口关闭法、挂线疗法、内括约肌瘘管结扎法、生物蛋白胶和肛瘘塞填塞法，都应该是专家治疗方案中的备选方法之一。

关键词

肛门前移；肛门前庭瘘；复杂肛瘘的治疗；克罗恩病；前位瘘；术后失禁；肛周的；肛管直肠瘘；肛管直肠脓毒症；直肠内皮瓣转移；内口的闭合；挂线；生物蛋白胶；肛瘘栓；内括约肌瘘管结扎

引　言

这一章应该与复杂肛瘘的治疗和肛周克罗恩病的手术治疗案例两章相互参考阅读（详见第 22 章和第 36 章）。这章不但着重介绍了前庭瘘是造成术后尿失禁的高危因素之一，而且介绍了最新的肛瘘治疗方法。同时，在也讨论了肛门前庭瘘，并且在第 38 章直肠阴道瘘的治疗一章中还可能涉及。大部分肛周脓肿都是由肛门腺管的闭塞导致细菌过度繁殖进而形成脓肿而引起的[1]。一个脓肿一旦确诊应该尽早行切开引流术治疗，而不应该因没有波动感被延误，以免形成肛门周围败血症或是复杂肛门直肠瘘。治疗过程可以相对简单些，如做一个适当的切口或是切除表皮覆盖的皮肤，或是放置一个引流管或是挂线[2-3]。

肛瘘就是指慢性肛门直肠菌血症的慢性阶段，主要特征是长期的瘘口排脓或伴有复发脓肿的再积累，随后间断自发溃破减压的周期性疼痛。主要致病原因是皮瓣转移术后感染、创伤、克罗恩病、放射、恶性肿瘤和其他由细菌引起的非典型感染。瘘管的类型有很多种，其分类主要依据于瘘管相对于肛门括约肌的位置，先前帕克斯等曾报道过其分类类型主要包括括约肌间型、经括约肌型、括约肌上型、括约肌外型[4]。复杂肛瘘就是指那些穿过冠状位外括约肌的长度多于 30%~50% 或是位于前位的肛瘘，特别是对于有多个瘘道的临产孕妇，或是有尿失禁病史、局部照射病史、克罗恩病史的患者。这些特殊的瘘管都应通过仔细体格检查、三维成像、肛门直肠腔内超声，甚至通过核磁检查等进行术前评估。

没有任何一种单一的技术方法可以治疗所有类型的肛瘘。治疗的方法主要由外科医生的经验和判断决定，同时主要取决于瘘道的复杂性来选择具体的治疗方法，这些方法已经被全世界所认可。这些治疗方法主要包括直肠内旁路途径进展性激活法、内口的关闭法、挂线疗法、生物蛋白胶填塞法和肛瘘栓法。

在手术室就可以定义和分类前瘘管，然而Regadas等研究证实括约肌的分布规律是不对称的，女性的（2.2cm）前外括约肌长度要比男性（3.4cm）显著的短。基于这一发现，建议使用核磁共振成像或是使用注射过氧化氢溶液增强后的3D肛管直肠腔内超声来评估肛瘘的复杂性和制定最佳的外科手术方法[6-9]。Murad-Regadas等已经通过研究证实使用3D直肠腔内超声技术，通过测量被切断肌肉的长度来对经前括约肌间瘘进行术前评估是有用的（图37.1），有助于选择一种安全的治疗方法和降低术后自制障碍的比率。根据影像发现，瘘道可以分为简单的和复杂的两种。

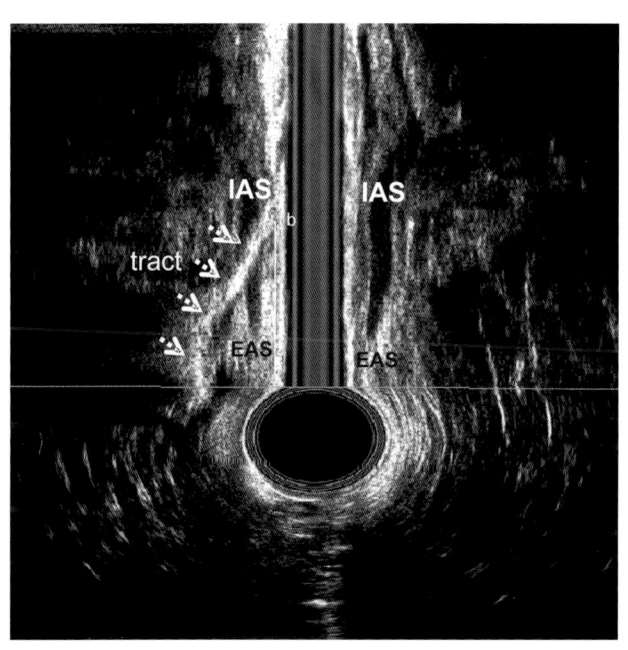

图37.1 管状的隧道显示连带肌肉贯穿它们的长度。IAS：肛门内括约肌；EAS：肛门外括约肌

简单前庭瘘

简单前庭瘘的定义是指瘘道仅位于皮下或内括约肌表浅部，或是瘘管穿过少于30%的前庭外括约肌的肛瘘。通过体格检查结合3D直肠腔内超声可以鉴别整个瘘道从内到外的走向。采用主要瘘管切除术来治疗简单前庭瘘是安全的，并且比单纯瘘管切除术要更好，这是因为前者包括两个开口和被腐蚀的瘘道的全部切除，而后者并没有切除这些。

复杂前庭瘘

复杂前庭瘘的治疗必需使用不同的治疗方法，例如挂线法、生物蛋白胶注射法、肛瘘栓法、直肠内皮瓣转移法、内括约瘘口结扎法（LIFT）。

挂线疗法

挂线疗法对穿过前庭外括约肌少于50%的复杂前庭肛瘘的治疗是一种有用的方法，特别是对于女性患者。穿过瘘道的挂线可以保证充分的引流。它通过逐渐拉紧肌肉来使伤口愈合。比较术前术后的价值，肛门有微小的括约肌损伤，但是不会导致严重的大便失禁，最终结果是令人满意的[11]，尽管在术后控制限制压和临床数据上是有一些争论，但是就切开挂线法而言是有益的[12]。

生物蛋白胶和肛瘘栓

这两种治疗方法都是很有发展前景的治疗方法，他们可以使大便失禁的风险最小化。最初，一些学者报道这两种方法的成功率只有60%~64%[13-14]，但是Buchanan等[15]通过一项前瞻性研究发现术后随访16个月仅有14%的治愈率。其他的一些研究也证实长期结果让人失望[16-17]，成功率低于16%[18-19]。就肛瘘栓而言，开始的结果很有前景，成功率为87%[20]，但是长期随访结果显示成功率为29%~48%[17]。

直肠腔内皮瓣转移法

直肠腔内皮瓣转移疗法对于治疗复杂前庭瘘是很有优势的，特别是对于女性患者，因为这种方法可以避免前庭外括约肌的严重损伤，因而可以防止大便失禁的发生。这种方法显示出关闭内口的优点同时不用切除括约肌，而且如果需要的话，这种方法还可以重建折叠联合括约肌。这种方法至少要游离到黏膜及黏膜下层，甚至包括肛门内括约肌和直肠壁。必须保证皮瓣有充足的血供，这要求游离的皮瓣基底部至少是顶部宽度的2倍。皮瓣必须保证向下没有张力，并且通过缝合消除残存的空隙，向外是开放的，以保证通畅引流。据报道，这一方法的成功率在 55%~98% 间[21-28]。Kodner 等[23]研究报道了通过这一方法治疗的 107 例患者，主要为低位直肠阴道瘘、前段肛门会阴瘘，还有较后位的肛门会阴瘘，成功率为 93%。然而 Mizrahi 等[27]报道了一组成功率为 59.6% 的病例，在 94 例患者，其中成功率偏低（57.1%）与克罗恩病的存在有关，而显著的复发率与推移皮瓣术后所致的肛瘘有关（33.3%）。此外，癌症、放射和直肠阴道瘘的瘘口直径大于 2.5cm 都是预后较差的原因[25,29]。因此尽管括约肌没有被切除，也导致了 31% 轻度失禁和 12% 的重度失禁[21,23,25,30,31]。

内括约肌瘘管结扎术（LIFT）

这一方法最早是由 Rojanasakul 等[32]报道的，主要过程包括使用探针沿瘘管探查并穿过内括约肌间隙于皮肤处标记。一个切口开在内括约肌槽处，同时在这里用探针探查瘘管。一旦瘘管被游离，探针就可以撤走。接下来，分离瘘道并结扎。外口敞开，切除瘘管。内口用刮匙刮出并关闭。皮肤切口用可吸收丝线缝合。Rojanasakul 等报道了 17 例患者，其中 94% 的成功率。然而，后来的研究报告指出成功治愈率在 57%~89% 之间[33-37]。最近，Ellis[37]报道了采用内括约肌结扎，瘘管采用生物补片加强的方法，在 31 例复杂肛瘘患者中成功率为 94%。

克罗恩病所致的肛瘘

无症状的克罗恩病所致肛瘘一般不需要任何干预，反之若是简单的低位前庭瘘采用传统的瘘管切除术就可以治疗，并且术后失禁率低于 12%[38-39]，但是需要 3~6 个月的长时间愈合[39]。

克罗恩病所致的复杂肛瘘患者治疗可以采用其正常的直肠黏膜行直肠腔内或是前移的黏膜皮瓣移植来治疗，但是有直肠炎的患者是禁忌的。可以替代直肠腔内皮瓣转移法的一种方法是姑息性的长期挂线引流术。挂线环绕瘘管 1 周，目的是通过持续的引流排脓和防止外口过早闭合来减少瘘道所致的后继脓毒症的发生。这种方法已经在 48%~100% 的患者中应用，且脓肿的复发率较低[38,40,41]。然而，即使应用所有的治疗手段，克罗恩病所致肛瘘的愈后仍然是不可预知的。由于此类疾病具有周期性，所谓永久的缓解是不可能的，12%~39% 的此类患者在随访中发现存在肠内疾病的进展而在最终需要行结肠造口术或是直肠切除术[42-44]。

进一步讨论克罗恩病所致的肛瘘，可以参阅第 22 章。

肛门前庭瘘

在肛门直肠畸形的类型中，直肠前庭瘘是女性中最常见的一种。拥有正常肛门的肛门前庭瘘是一种罕见的疾病，在西方国家只有 3.2% 的肛门直肠畸形患者肛门是正常的[45]。然而有报道称在亚洲国家发病率要高很多[46-47]。这种畸形被分为很多种类型，如 N 型瘘、H 型肛瘘、常见的会阴瘘和有两条瘘道的肛瘘[45-48]。在女性患者中比较少见相关的其他疾病，但是在男性患者常会合并严重的肾病、食道癌和脊柱畸形。在 10%~30% 的大型系列报道中，前庭瘘是女孩最常见的肛门直肠畸形类型[45]。直肠开口于阴道和阴唇系带之间。之前大多数报道都把这种前庭瘘划分为低位的前庭瘘，但是 Heinen[49]认为这种畸形是一类中间处的前庭瘘。这种畸形是有别于直肠前庭瘘和肛门前庭瘘的；前者是中间处的畸形（根据翼幅分类）因为直肠的末端在横纹肌的顶端适合前庭瘘长瘘管的产生。肛门前庭瘘是一种低位的畸形，在这里直肠穿透横纹肌的方式是很复杂的[50-51]。更重要的是，外科修复手术的重要性被普遍低估了；此外术后便秘发生率相比其他肛门直肠畸形手术要高，也使得肛门前庭瘘成为一种特殊类型的肛门畸形。这类疾病相比于男性患者或是其他类型的复杂肛瘘患者，女性的发病率要更高些，并且相对于它的严重性，其所受到的关注度要更少一些。诊断主要依靠临床体格检查或是使用子宫颈扩张器插入瘘管来确诊。在所有患者中行骶骨检查，如果发现任何异常，都应该行脊柱 X 线检查。腹部超声和心脏超声有助于排除腹腔和心脏的异常。在新生儿期，如果发现肛门前庭瘘，建议采用一个中止干预程序。之后，可以使用很多方法来给予矫正治疗。这些方法包括 Y-V 成形术[45]、肛门会阴重建术[46]、X 型成形术[47]、Z 型成形术[48]。暴露不充分，不完全的直肠阴道分离使得新建肛门向前移位，括约肌复合体处的直肠肛门的盲点是这个技术的主要缺点，因此导致其很少应用。较好的暴露和肛管直肠外括约肌复合体的精确定位使得前后矢状面更接近，这种新方法更受欢迎，并且对肛门前庭瘘进行了重建[46]。对于是否需要进行肛门重建和完成重建后的成人患者的控便能力的远期报道数据很有限[52-54]。

尽管对前庭瘘患者而言行预防性结肠造瘘非常安全，但是目前这种做法仍然存在争议[55-56]。一些外科医生认为行保护性结肠造口术对于瘘修补术患者而言可以降低伤口破损的风险[46,48]。但是即使做了保护性预防结肠造口术，复发的情况仍不少见[46,48,56]。Banu[57]等推荐最初的手术不用行保护性预防造口术，报道中指出伤口裂口主要多见于术前有会阴部脓肿的患者。另一种观点认为对于这类患者应该先治疗脓肿，然后第二阶段再完成瘘的治疗。

前庭成形术

在印度、亚洲以及美国、南美、欧洲，一些医学中心报道把前庭成形术作为治疗的初级[58-61]和第二阶段的内容[62]。初期的表皮上的肌电图评估对于准确定位新建肛门的位置很有帮助[63]。在新建肛门周围做一个球拍形状的切口，然后向阴道和瘘管方向扩展（图37.2a）。采用钝性和锐性相结合的方法游离直肠阴道间隙，注意要保护直肠壁的完整性（图37.2b）。通常，在瘘管处直肠和阴道间粘连很严重，一旦越过这里，那么对于分离异常的肛门前庭和直肠前庭就变得比较容易了（图

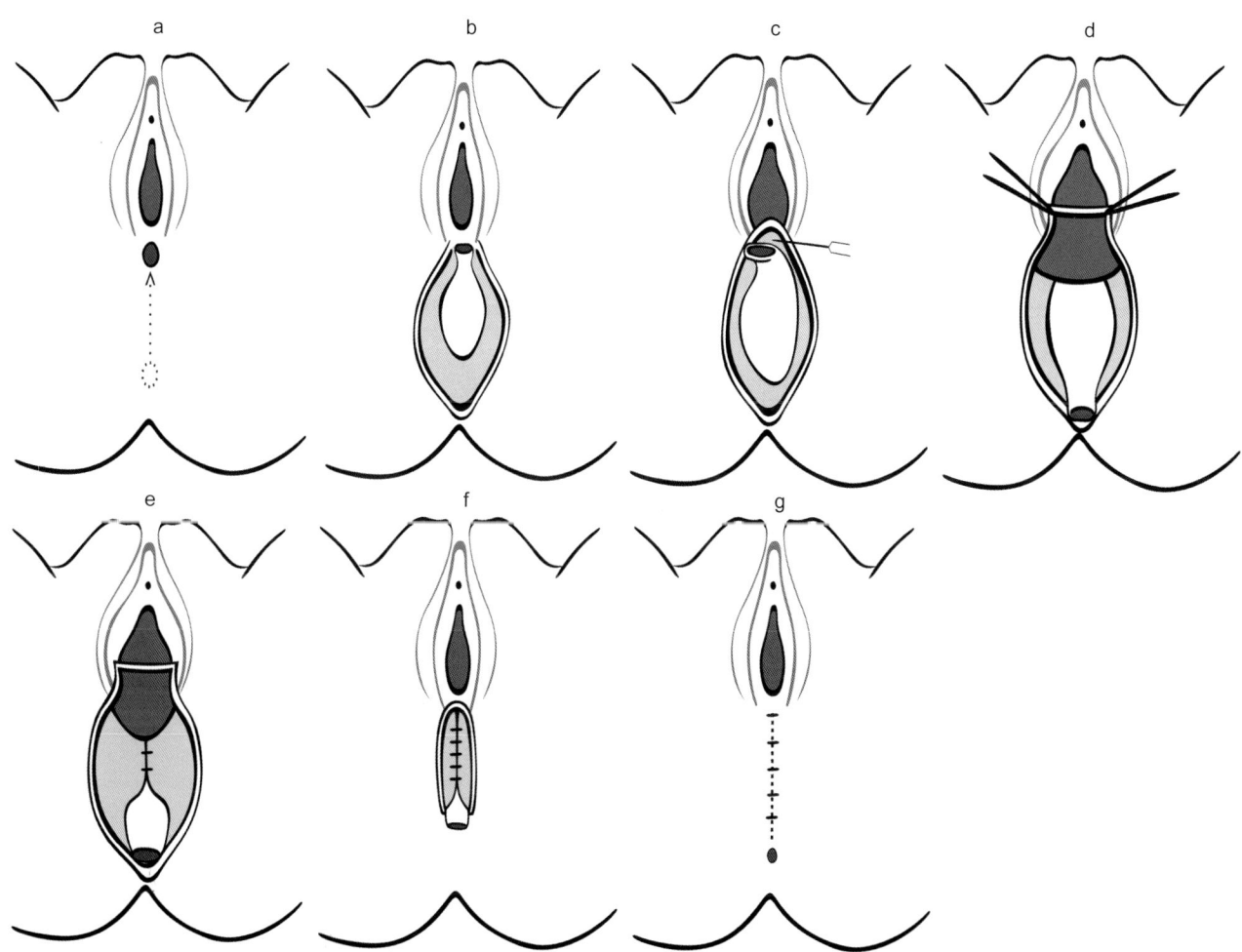

图37.2 （a）一个正中切口从瘘口到新建肛门的中心。切口深度通过会阴部肌肉和肛门外括约肌复合体的前庭纤维来划分；（b）直肠后壁被暴露，有一个很好的间隙，在这里可以进行锐性分离；（c）在阴道后壁和直肠之间的层面需要采用锐性分离；（d）直肠转移完成，开始进行更深层次的前方游离，同时进行后面和横向的游离。在游离后方时，前面的肛门的肛提肌不需切除；（e）会阴重建开始。肛门直肠转移于外括约肌复合体的范围内，先对最深处的软组织进行缝合；（f）会阴部重建完成，间断缝合后方和外侧的直肠周围肌肉；（g）缝皮后手术结束

37.2c）。有时，在分离的过程中很容易损伤阴道壁，但是当直肠分离完全时这种损伤是很容易缝合的。最终的解剖结果表明当直肠覆盖超过会阴皮肤 5mm 时是没有张力的（图 37.2d）。我们可以通过电刺激来界定横纹肌复合体的位置，同时利用直肠来固定这一区域的括约肌。通过缝合直肠和阴道之间的组织来重塑会阴体（图 37.2e, f）。最后重建阴唇系带，关闭切口，肛门成形术就完成了。

从前庭成形术在临床的全面开展到今天，前庭瘘的治疗方法没有再发生过改变；然而，整体并发症的发生率却下降了 7%[60]。影响结果改进的原因包括：增加更好的手术技术和解剖经验，较少的组织损伤，充分的直肠游离和不出血所致的血肿发生[60-61]。术后服用乳果糖来软化大便也是改善结果的一个好方法。在分娩时选择剖宫产的方法可以防止会阴体的损伤，这些患者的这一选择是很明智的[59]。

参考文献

1. Parks A. Pathogenesis and treatment of fistula-in-ano. BMJ. 1961;1:463–9.
2. Isbister WH. A simple method for the management of anorectal abscess. ANZ J Surg. 1987;57:771–4.
3. Read DR, Abcarian H. A prospective survey of 474 patients with anorectal abscess. Dis Colon Rectum. 1979;22:566–8.
4. Parks AG, Gordon PH, Hardcastle JD. A classification of fistula-in-ano. Br J Surg. 1976;63:1–12.
5. Regadas FS, Murad-Regadas SM, Lima DM, Silva FR, Barreto RG, Souza MH, et al. Anal canal anatomy showed by three-dimensional anorectal ultrasonography. Surg Endosc. 2007;21:2207–11.
6. West RL, Dwarkasing S, Felt-Bersma RJ, Schouten WR, Hop WC, Hussain SM, et al. Hydrogen peroxide-enhanced three-dimensional endoanal ultrasonography and endoanal magnetic resonance imaging in evaluating perianal fistulas: agreement and patient preference. Eur J Gastroenterol Hepatol. 2004;16:1319–24.
7. Ratto C, Grillo E, Parello A, Costamagna G, Doglietto GB. Endoanal ultrasound-guided surgery for anal fistula. Endoscopy. 2005;37:722–8.
8. Buchanan GN, Bartram CI, Williams AB, Halligan S, Cohen CR. Value of hydrogen peroxide enhancement of three-dimensional endoanal ultrasound in fistula-in-ano. Dis Colon Rectum. 2005;48:141–7.
9. Santoro GA, Fortling B. The advantages of volume rendering in three-dimensional endosonography of the anorectum. Dis Colon Rectum. 2007;50:359–68.
10. Murad-Regadas SM, Regadas FSP, Rodrigues LV, Holanda Ede C, Barreto RG, Oliveira L. The role of 3-dimensional anorectal ultrasonography in the assessment of anterior transsphincteric fistula. Dis Colon Rectum. 2010;53:1035–40.
11. Pinedo MG, Caselli MG, Urrejola SG, Niklitscheck LS, Molina PME, Bellolio RF, Zuñiga DA. Modified loose-seton technique for the treatment of complex anal fistulas. Colorectal Dis. 2012;12:31–313.
12. Vial M, Parés D, Pera M, Grande L. Faecal incontinence after seton treatment for anal fistulae with and without surgical division of internal anal sphincter: a systematic review. Colorectal Dis. 2010;12:172–8.
13. Sentovich SM. Fibrin glue for anal fistulas: long-term results. Dis Colon Rectum. 2003;46:498–502.
14. Cintron JR, Park JJ, Orsay CP, Pearl RK, Nelson RL, Sone JH, et al. Repair of fistulas-in-ano using fibrin adhesive: long-term follow-up. Dis Colon Rectum. 2000;43:944–9.
15. Buchanan GN, Bartram CI, Philips RK, Gould SW, Halligan S, Rockall TA, et al. Efficacy of fibrin sealant in the management of complex anal fistula: a prospective trial. Dis Colon Rectum. 2003;46:1167–74.
16. Loungnarath R, Dietz DW, Mutch MG, Birnbaum EH, Kodner IJ, Fleshman JW. Fibrin glue treatment of complex anal fistulas has low success rate. Dis Colon Rectum. 2004;47:432–6.
17. Christoforidis D, Etzioni DA, Goldberg SM, Madoff RD, Mellgren A. Treatment of complex anal fistulas with collagen fistula plug. Dis Colon Rectum. 2008;51:1482–7.
18. Ellis CN, Clark S. Fibrin glue as an adjunct to flap repair of anal fistulas: a randomized, controlled study. Dis Colon Rectum. 2006;49:1736–40.
19. Williams JG, Farrands PA, Williams AB, Taylor BA, Lunniss PJ, Sagar PM, et al. The treatment of anal fistula: ACPGBI position statement. Colorectal Dis. 2007;9:18–50.
20. Johnson EK, Gaw JU, Armstrong DN. Efficacy of anal fistula plug vs. fibrin glue in closure of anorectal fistulas. Dis Colon Rectum. 2006;49:371–6.
21. Aguilar PS, Plasencia G, Hardy TG, Hartmann RF, Stewart WR. Mucosal advancement in the treatment of anal fistula. Dis Colon Rectum. 1985;28:496–8.
22. Lowry AC, Thorson AG, Rothenberger DA, Goldberg SM. Repair of simple rectovaginal fistulas. Influence of previous repairs. Dis Colon Rectum. 1988;31:676–8.
23. Kodner IJ, Mazor A, Shemesh EI, Fry RD, Fleshman JW, Birnbaum EH. Endorectal advancement flap repair of rectovaginal and other complicated anorectal fistulas. Surgery. 1993;114:682–90.
24. Ozumer G, Hull TL, Cartmill J, Fazio VW. Long-term analysis of the use of transanal rectal advancement flaps for complicated anorectal vaginal fistulas. Dis Colon Rectum. 1996;39:10–4.
25. Schouten WR, Zimmerman DD, Briel JW. Transanal advancement flap repair of transsphincteric fistulas. Dis Colon Rectum. 1999;42:1419–23.
26. Ortiz H, Marzo J. Endorectal flap advancement repair and fistulectomy for high trans-sphincteric and suprasphincteric fistulas. Br J Surg. 2000;87:1680–3.
27. Mizrahi N, Wexner SD, Zmora O, Da Silva G, Efron J, Weiss EG, et al. Endorectal advancement flap: are there predictors of failure? Dis Colon Rectum. 2002;45:1616–21.
28. Sonoda T, Hull T, Piedmonte MR, Fazio VW. Outcomes of primary repair of anorectal and rectovaginal fistulas using the endorectal advancement flap. Dis Colon Rectum. 2002;45:1622–8.
29. Garcia-Aguilar J, Davey CS, Le CT, Lowry AC, Rothenberger DA. Patient satisfaction after surgical treatment for fistula-in-ano. Dis Colon Rectum. 2000;43:1206–12.
30. Kreis ME, Jehle EC, Ohlemann M, Becker HD, Starlinger MJ. Functional results after transanal rectal advancement flap repair of trans-sphincteric fistula. Br J Surg. 1998;85:240–2.
31. Gustafsson UM, Graf W. Excision of anal fistula with closure of the internal opening: functional and manometric results. Dis Colon Rectum. 2002;45:1672–8.
32. Rojanasakul A, Pattanaarun J, Sahakitrungruang C, Tantiphlachiva K. Total anal sphincter saving technique for fistula-in-ano: the ligation of intersphincteric fistula tract. J Med Assoc Thai. 2007;90:581–6.
33. Rojanasakul A. Intermediate outcome of total anal sphinctersaving technique for fistula-in-ano: the ligation of intersphincteric fistula tract (LIFT) [abstract]. Dis Colon Rectum. 2008;51:694–5.
34. Alfred KW, Roslani AC, Chittawatanarat K, et al. Short-term outcomes of the ligation of intersphincteric fistula tract (LIFT) procedure for treatment of fistula-in-ano: a single institution experience in Singapore [abstract]. Dis Colon Rectum. 2008;51:696.

35. Bleier JI, Moloo H, Goldberg SM. Ligation of the intersphincteric fistula tract: an effective new technique for complex fistulas. Dis Colon Rectum. 2010;53:43–6.
36. Shanwani A, Nor AM, Amri N. Ligation of intersphincteric fistula tract (LIFT): sphincter saving technique for fistula-in-ano. Dis Colon Rectum. 2010;53:39–42.
37. Ellis CN. Outcomes with the use of bioprosthetic grafts to reinforce the ligation of the intersphincteric fistula tract (BioLift procedure) for the management of complex anal fistulas. Dis Colon Rectum. 2010;53:1361–4.
38. Scott HJ, Northover JM. Evaluation of surgery for perianal Crohn's fistulas. Dis Colon Rectum. 1996;39:1039–43.
39. Michelassi F, Melis M, Rubin M, Hurst BD. Surgical treatment of anorectal complications in Crohn's disease. Surgery. 2000;128:597–603.
40. Pearl PK, Andrews JR, Orsay CP, Weisman RI, Prasad ML, Nelson RL, et al. Role of the seton in the management of anorectal fistulas. Dis Colon Rectum. 1993;36:573–9.
41. Takesue Y, Ohge H, Yokoyama T, Murakami Y, Imamura Y, Sueda T. Long-term results of seton drainage on complex anal fistulae in patients with Crohn's disease. J Gastroenterol. 2002;37:912–5.
42. Faucheron JL, Saint-Marc O, Guibert L, Parc R. Longterm seton drainage for high anal fistulas in Crohn's disease-a sphincter-saving operation? Dis Colon Rectum. 1996;39:208–11.
43. Sangwan YP, Schoetz Jr DJ, Murray JJ, Roberts PL, Coller JA. Perianal Crohn's disease: results of local surgical treatment. Dis Colon Rectum. 1996;39:529–35.
44. Hong MK, Craig Lynch A, Bell S, Woods RJ, Keck JO, Johnston MJ, et al. Faecal diversion in the management of perianal Crohn's disease. Colorectal Dis. 2011;13:171–6.
45. Rintala RJ, Mildh L, Lindhal H. H-type anorectal malformations: incidence and clinical characteristics. J Pediatr Surg. 1996;31:559–62.
46. Chatterjee SK. Double termination of the alimentary tract. A second look. J Pediatr Surg. 1980;15:623–7.
47. Tsuchida Y, Saito S, Honna T, Makino S, Kaneko M, Hazama H. Double termination of the alimentary tract in females: a report of 12 cases and a literature review. J Pediatr Surg. 1984;19:292–6.
48. White JJ, Haller JA, Scott JR, Dorst JP, Kramer SS. N-type anorectal malformations. J Pediatr Surg. 1978;13:631–7.
49. Heinen FL. The surgical treatment of low anal defects and vestibular fistulas. Semin Pediatr Surg. 1997;6:204–6.
50. Murphy F, Puri P, Hutson JM, et al. Incidence and frequency of different types and classification of anorectal malformations. In: Holschneider AM, Hutson JM, editors. Anorectal malformations in children. Berlin: Springer; 1996. p. 163–84.
51. Holschneider AM, Jesch NK, Stragholz E, Pfrommer W. Surgical methods for anorectal malformations from Rehbein to Peña–critical assessment of score systems and proposal for a new classification. Eur J Pediatr Surg. 2002;12:73–82.
52. Shaaban A, Heise C. Multimedia article. Posterior sagittal anorectoplasty for congenital rectovaginal malformations in the adult. Dis Colon Rectum. 2008;51:1569.
53. Ardelean MA, Bauer J, Schimke C, Ludwikowski B, Schimpl G. Improvement of continence with reoperation in selected patients after surgery for anorectal malformation. Dis Colon Rectum. 2009;52:112–8.
54. Senel E, Akbiyik F, Atayurt H, Tiryaki HT. Urological problems or fecal continence during long-term follow-up of patients with anorectal malformation. Pediatr Surg Int. 2010;26:683–9.
55. Brem H, Guttman FM, Laberge JM, Doody D. Congenital anal fistula with normal anus. J Pediatr Surg. 1989;24:183–5.
56. Bianchini MA, Fava G, Cortese MG, Vinardi S, Costantino S, Canavese F. A rare anorectal malformation: a very large H-type fistula. Pediatr Surg Int. 2001;17:649–51.
57. Banu T, Hannan MJ, Hoque M, Aziz MA, Lakhoo K. Anovestibular fistula with normal anus. J Pediatr Surg. 2008;43:526–9.
58. Okada A, Kamata S, Imura K, Fukuzawa M, Kubota A, Yagi M, et al. Anterior sagittal anorectoplasty for vestibular and anovestibular fistula. J Pediatr Surg. 1993;28:279–84.
59. Kumar V, Chattopdhay A, Vepakomma D, Shenoy D, Bhat P. Anovestibular fistula in adults: a rare presentation. Int Surg. 2005;90:27–9.
60. Jiwane A, Kumar T, Kutumbale R, Bhusare D, Kothari P, Kulkarni B. Perineal canal: an uncommon entity with good prognosis. Indian J Pediatr. 2003;70:667–9.
61. Terzi A, Coskun A, Yildiz F, Coban S, Akinci OF. Anovestibular fistula with imperforate anus in two adults. Ann Saudi Med. 2008;28:472–4.
62. Holschneider AM. Secondary sagittal posterior anorectoplasty. Prog Pediatr Surg. 1990;25:103–17.
63. Brain AJ, Kiely EM. Posterior sagittal anorectoplasty for reoperation in children with anorectal malformations. Br J Surg. 1989;76:57–9.

第 38 章 直肠阴道瘘的重复手术治疗

Oded Zmora · Nir Wasserberg

范朝刚 译 李 宁 审校

摘 要

本章列出了直肠阴道瘘的临床诊断方法，以及经阴道、直肠内、会阴或经腹途径的修补方法，具体修补方法取决于瘘位置的高低和病因学。也讨论近段肠管转流的作用及其危险因素。直肠阴道瘘的发生可能与一些原因有关，从简单的隐窝腺疾病到医源性损伤、会阴部创伤、克罗恩病、恶性疾病和放射治疗，潜在的病因是影响成功的外科修补机会的唯一的、最重要的因素。几乎所有类型的直肠阴道瘘的外科修补都可能被看作是初期修补失败病例的二线方案。

关键词

直肠阴道瘘；重复手术外科；隐窝腺疾病；产科损伤；医源性损伤；会阴部创伤；克罗恩病；恶性肿瘤；放射治疗

引 言

直肠阴道瘘定义为在肛管或低位直肠与阴道间不正常的交通，常常导致脓或粪便从阴道排出和不能控制的气体排出。在大多数病例中，这些症状显著损害患者的生活质量，影响患者的生理、心理、社会和妇女的性功能。在有克罗恩病或者恶性肿瘤的直肠阴道瘘的患者中，这些症状可能显著加重已经受损的生活质量。因此，大多数直肠阴道瘘的患者希望得到治疗，在大多数病例中需要外科手术修补。这些修补方法的成功率因各种不同的外科技术而呈现不同，主要依赖于瘘的病因和局部条件。因为没有外科技术能取得完美的疗效，有失败修补史、需要重新手术的直肠阴道瘘的患者在治疗中常见。

直肠阴道瘘有几个分类评分系统，但是均没有得到广泛接受。一些研究者试图根据解剖学标志如齿状线、肛管括约肌结构、子宫颈等相关的部位进行分类[1-2]。然而，不像其他类型的肛周瘘管，如没有涉及肛门括约肌结构大部分的低位瘘，常常能够用简单的瘘管切开术进行安全的处理，直肠阴道瘘几乎永远不能够用这些技术处理。差不多所有的直肠阴道瘘都环绕或位于会阴体之上，这是肛门括约肌前部的主要部分。妇女肛门括约肌结构的前部短而弱，并且相对缺乏耻骨直肠肌，任何在这个局部括约肌结构的切开均可能导致明显的损伤性失禁。大多数患者有独特的病史可以影响失禁，切开直肠和阴道间括约肌结构的任何部分都不很合适。因此，解剖分类可能并不能在直肠阴道瘘的外科治疗方面有所助益，除非最高位接近子宫颈的瘘，常常需要剖腹修补。因此，对于直肠阴道瘘的初次修补和再修补而言，按病因分类可能是临床上为外科医生使用的最有意义的分类[3]。

一些病因可以导致直肠阴道瘘的发生，从简单的隐窝腺疾病到医源性损伤、会阴部创伤、克罗恩病、恶性肿瘤和放射治疗。潜在的病因可能是影响成功外科修补唯一最重要的因素；由产科损伤或隐窝腺感染而导致的瘘与继发于克罗恩病或放射治疗的瘘相比，同样解剖位置的瘘，可能成功率更高。

大量的外科手术操作用于治疗直肠阴道瘘，从最小的操作如纤维蛋白胶注入或直肠阴道胶原蛋白塞塞入，到广泛的阴道、经肛门和经会阴修补，以及主要经腹腔的操作，尽管没有哪一种能够被广泛接受。总的成功率和与操作相关的并发症也与病因、修补类型、外科技术、外科医生的经验相关。治疗方法的多样性和中等成功率成为这种难治疾病的复杂性的佐证。差不多所有类型的直肠阴道瘘的外科修补方法都可能也被看作是初期修补失败的二线方案。

本章简要回顾了直肠阴道瘘的病因，讨论了患者流程，以及主要的、可靠的针对直肠阴道瘘再次手术的外科治疗意见，尤其强调了现代的方法。

病因学

几个疾病过程具有不同的特性，可能导致直肠阴道瘘的发生。确定准确的病因很重要，因为直接影响到手术方式的确定，并且必须仔细权衡再次手术的潜在风险和益处。直肠阴道瘘的病因可以归类于隐窝腺来源，创伤性会阴损伤相关的瘘、克罗恩病、恶性肿瘤或放射治疗相关的瘘。

隐窝腺直肠阴道瘘

肛周隐窝腺瘘通常起源于齿状线环周局部的肛腺感染。这样的腺体的引流不畅可能导致肛周脓肿，可能穿透肛周皮肤。前部脓肿可能穿入阴道，导致直肠阴道瘘。这种瘘的内部开口常常发生于齿状线，一般外科诊断不能明确区分那些在其他肛周局部的隐窝腺瘘。然而，因为会阴体肛门括约肌结构的解剖，这些瘘几乎总是包含明确的部分括约肌结构，并不能用单纯瘘管切除来治疗。

如果瘘引流较好，成功率非常高。Sonoda 等[4]报道在 48 例隐窝腺疾病患者用直肠内推进瓣治疗，成功率 77%。El-Gazzaz 等[5]从相同的机构报道一组用不同外科方法治疗的 40 例患者，成功率是 67%。

创伤性直肠阴道瘘

会阴局部创伤导致肛门直肠和阴道间瘘，可能由不同的损伤机制所导致，包括产科创伤、手术创伤或术后并发症，以及不同原因直接导致局部创伤的损伤。

产科损伤

产科损伤是直肠阴道瘘最常见的原因之一，常常与高级别的产科会阴体撕裂相关。4 级会阴体撕裂包括肛门括约肌结构前部的破裂，并伴有直肠黏膜的撕裂。高级别的产科会阴体损伤的风险在超重婴儿出生时可能增加，包括工具的应用如产钳和真空吸引，以及后正中线会阴切开术的应用[6]。没有识别出高级别的产科损伤、不适当的修补或术后感染可能导致直肠阴道瘘形成。在发展中国家，分娩后直肠阴道瘘的发病率似乎显著高于发达国家[7-8]，据推测是由于不能得到先进的医疗服务和高比例的产程过长导致对会阴的持续的压力。

手术创伤

正常会阴体上的直肠阴道隔很薄，可能被几乎所有涉及这一区域的外科手术所损伤。包括经阴道的手术，尤其是涉及阴道后壁的手术[9]；经肛门的手术，如对痔疮脱垂或经肛门直肠切除等用吻合器的手术[10]。然而，当由经验丰富的经过良好训练的外科医生实施手术时，这种医源性的直肠阴道瘘的发生率就低[11]。

经腹直肠切除术低位直肠吻合或肛管吻合需要切开直肠阴道隔，可能导致医源性损伤。低位结直肠吻合现在已经变成上 1/3 直肠癌的标准术式，结肠-肛管吻合常规用于全系膜切除后的中低位直肠癌。肛管吻合被常规实施在溃疡性结肠炎或家族性腺瘤型息肉病的回肠贮袋肛管吻合术中。这些病例中，在紧邻阴道后壁的区域需要用圆形吻合器进行肠吻合。将吻合钉置入阴道壁中将导致直肠阴道瘘的发生。另外，低位结直肠、结肠肛管、回肠-肛管吻合常伴高发生率的吻合口渗漏和感染并发症，这些可能影响到阴道而导致直肠阴道瘘，甚至当吻合口完成得很好的时候也会出现这种情况[12-13]。

其他形式的创伤

与产科创伤或手术无关的直肠阴道瘘已经很少作为一个病因被报道。这可能包括多器官钝性伤、贯穿创伤和继发于异物和性对象的局部创伤[14-15]。

通常，创伤性损伤后，因组织血供丰富，手术修补的成功率相当高。来自克利夫兰佛罗里达诊所的 Pinto 等[16]发现了36例产科创伤相关的直肠阴道瘘患者修补成功率为67%，20例其他各种会阴部创伤患者中成功率为70%。

克罗恩病

克罗恩病是一种慢性复发性炎性肠病。会阴区常常被会阴部克罗恩病所累及，通常大多数表现为会阴部脓肿和瘘，包括直肠（肛管）阴道瘘。直肠阴道瘘可能发生于3%~10%的克罗恩病女性中[17]，常常来源于穿透入阴道深部的肛管直肠前壁溃疡。可能是低位的，也可能是高位的，但常发生在直肠阴道隔的中部。慢性炎性组织和免疫抑制治疗，影响了外科手术修补的成功。Pinto 等[16]报道在77例克罗恩病直肠阴道瘘患者中成功率为44%。

肛门直肠和盆腔恶性肿瘤

肛门直肠和盆腔的恶性肿瘤可能通过肿瘤直接浸润相邻管腔结构引起直肠阴道瘘。另外，目前针对这些肿瘤的治疗，包括外科手术、放射治疗或两者都有，都可能导致直肠阴道瘘的发生。因为这个原因，在每个有局部恶性肿瘤病史的直肠阴道瘘的病例，必须排除肿瘤复发。

放射治疗

放射治疗是对不同类型的盆腔恶性肿瘤常用的治疗手段，或者作为治疗的主要模式，或者作为外科手术的辅助（或新辅助）。外粒子束放射治疗常用于肛管癌的治疗，也经常是进展期直肠癌、高危宫颈癌和高级别子宫内膜癌的联合治疗的一部分。放射治疗产生慢性炎症和缺血，均可能促使直肠阴道瘘的形成[18]。局部放射治疗，如短距离放射治疗，局部剂量较高，也可能导致直肠阴道瘘的形成[19]。

因为放射治疗导致组织的微血管化和灌注的不可逆效应，放射线引起的瘘的修补成功率通常有限。在这些病例中，应该考虑用血供丰富的组织如股薄肌或球海绵体肌移植[20-21]。

症　状

直肠阴道瘘的患者常常主诉脓或粪便从阴道流出，并不能控制地排气。然而，从阴道通过的内容物的数量可能不一样，依赖于瘘的大小、部位和粪便的稀稠度。在一些病例中，阴道流粪很明显，易于诊断。在其他病例中，阴道排粪极少，可能与肛门控制减弱混淆。在许多病例中，这些患者有肛门直肠疾病史或治疗史，可能被错误地解释这些症状。在有克罗恩病史、外科手术创伤或放射治疗的患者中，肛门直肠疼痛、活动性直肠炎和肛门直肠狭窄可能伴随存在，加剧了临床表现的复杂性。

评价和成像方法

复发性直肠阴道瘘的评价常常包括与检查原发瘘同样的方法。尽管瘘诊断的确立可能在复发时比较简单，重要的是排除失败的原因，如恶性肿瘤、放射损伤和炎性肠病。

应该从详细的病史和体格检查中直接调查瘘和失禁相关的症状，就像病因学调查一样。应该对以前的病情检查和手术进行仔细记录。在进一步调查之前，应该排除或治疗脓毒症。体格检查包括直肠和阴道的评价，瘘道用肛门镜或直肠镜检查，阴道开张器检查可能是看得见的。当证实了瘘道时，评估周围的组织有无炎症、裂伤和多发瘘很重要。如果有指征，应该实施活检，并评价肛门括约肌的健康状况和完整性。如果怀疑新的病因，应该进行一些特殊的检查，包括结肠镜排除克罗恩病或恶性肿瘤的转移。放射摄影的研究可能用于难以发现的瘘管的定位和指导外科手术路径。对比阴道 X 线摄影术可能证实瘘道的存在，敏感性为79%，但是对于低位直肠阴道瘘少有效果[22]。

CT 对于周围组织和邻近器官的影像可能很重要。Yee 等[23]和 Baig 等[24]报道，28%~73%怀疑有直肠阴道瘘的患者可以通过肛管内超声得到证实。肛管内超声的准确性可以用注射过氧化氢到瘘道的方法得到增强[25]。另外，肛管内超声在肛门括约肌的解剖评价中也很重要。Baig等在15例直肠阴道瘘的患者中发现9例有伴随的括约肌损伤。

MRI，包括肛门内MRI，在诊断直肠阴道瘘方面可能更准确些，准确性能达到100%[26]。而且，MRI是一种检查肛门括约肌损伤[27]和其他肛门周围异常[28-29]的敏感而特异的工具。CT可能对显示周围组织和邻近器官的影像是重要的，尽管由于容量平均效应，它较少提供关于在坐骨直肠窝的直肠周围脓毒症或有关同时发生的括约肌损害的准确信息。少数情况下，在麻醉下探查瘘道和邻近组织时是必要的。在瘘道不容易看到的病例中，亚甲蓝试验可以使用，在阴道中插入卫生棉塞，用亚甲蓝灌肠。作为选择，鼓泡试验可以证实瘘的存在，在阴道中灌满生理盐水，从肛门吹入空气。

内科治疗

直肠和阴道间的瘘管很少自愈，其修补大多数通过外科手术。如果外科手术失败，瘘管的修补常常需要重复尝试外科手术。不过，饮食增量剂、抗腹泻药物、温水坐浴和皮肤保护霜局部护理等保守治疗可能帮助患病女性减轻症状。在肛周克罗恩病和直肠阴道瘘的患者中，抗炎药物治疗活动性克罗恩病在减轻症状方面可能有效，偶尔也有瘘管完全闭合。抗TNF-α药物已经证实能够显著改善肛周克罗恩病，瘘管的完全闭合率为20%~50%[30-33]。不过，克罗恩病相关的直肠阴道瘘的完全闭合，比肛周区域其他位置相比，可能概率较低。Ricart等[30]报道用英夫利昔单抗治疗直肠阴道瘘治愈率33%，而其他肛周部位治愈率为49%，Parsi等[34]报道用英夫利昔单抗4~6周治疗直肠阴道瘘的闭合率为14%，而在所有克罗恩病性的外瘘中闭合率为78%。积极的内科治疗显著改善了大多数肛周克罗恩病患者的生活质量，包括直肠阴道瘘；并可能导致这些患者中的一部分瘘完全闭合，这让人有些难以理解。考虑到肛周克罗恩病活跃期的复杂性和增加重复外科手术修补的风险，内科治疗可能足以减轻一些患者的痛苦，在许多病例中值得做初始治疗。不过，有明显症状、希望手术修补的病例，应该考虑这样的干预。几个研究者建议，抗TNF-α单抗的治疗也可能作为外科手术的准备，使局部条件变好，提高成功的机会，但是这种方法的好处还没有得到充分的证明[35-36]。

外科处理

复发性直肠阴道瘘的手术修补是结直肠外科实践中最具挑战的任务之一。这种修补的复杂性由几个因素造成。在解剖学上，低位直肠和肛管靠近阴道，肛管直肠和阴道间的瘘管常常很短，并且两者间的组织量很少。外科手术创伤、放射损伤或克罗恩病引起的瘘可能起源于齿状线上的低位直肠，使得经肛门修补的技术操作比较困难。在许多病例，直肠阴道瘘和贮袋-阴道瘘与影响局部伤口愈合能力的条件相关，包括之前的放射治疗和克罗恩病。另外，之前失败的外科修补经常扰乱手术平面，引起局部瘢痕组织和纤维化，使得后续的修补更加复杂。心理上，之前修补失败的患者经常比较沮丧，并且可能对后续的外科治疗的尝试失去信心。由于修补尝试的失败和与不满意患者的交流，外科医生偶尔可能也会感到沮丧。鼓励他们对后续外科手术和结合各种外科修补选择的全面了解和现实预期（双方）的新治疗方法的态度，在处理这些患者时是必要的。这包括对负面结果预期因素的全面理解；克罗恩病可能需要平均1.8次手术才能最后成功[5, 16]，贮袋阴道瘘可能需要1.6次手术，产科相关的瘘可能仅需要1.3次手术。在这种情况下，年龄、体质量指数、糖尿病病史、激素或免疫抑制剂的使用、复发病例最初的和其后的修补的时间或近端转流术的应用，并不是其后复发的显著预后因素[16]。特别是克罗恩病、吸烟、免疫调节剂治疗和激素使用与复发和初期手术失败相关，尽管性交困难在失败病例中更常见，总体性功能和生活质量在愈合组和非愈合组间并没有显著不同[5]。

很多外科手术已经用来进行直肠阴道瘘的修补。这些手术可以被分为4个主要类别：经肛门修补、通过阴道修补、通过会阴路径修补和经腹修补。

经肛门修补

传统上，经肛门修补涉及肛门括约肌功能和保留下的直肠侧的内口的关闭。通常应用直肠内推进瓣技术，因其在局部高压侧瘘管的修补有理论上的益处。在这种技术中，患者取折刀位，以便对直肠前壁有足够的视野，肛管和瘘道用肛门镜进行探查。用电刀在低位直肠做一个宽基的U形切口，形成一个低位直肠瓣,包括被掀起的黏膜、黏膜下层和浅肌层。一些外科医生注射添加或没有添加肾上腺素的生理盐水或局部麻醉剂,以利于局部解剖和止血。瓣基部约3cm,向头侧开口,为到顶部的两倍宽,以确保足够的血供。随后移动,瘘道被清除,瓣下的内口用可吸收线关闭;瓣的顶部包括黏膜缺损处,被切除。瓣下拉覆盖内口,并用可吸收线在适当的位置间断缝合。瘘管的阴道部分保持开放以利引流(图38.1)。

使用这种技术,Rothenberger 等[37] 早在1982年报道用直肠内推进瓣修补成功率为86%。同组病例的成功率和之前修补的相关性分析发现在重复修补的病例中成功率降低。首次尝试修补病例中有88%成功修补,85%有1次先前修补史,55%有两次以前的尝试史[38]。Kodner 等[39] 在1993年报道71例直肠阴道瘘的患者经过经直肠内推进瓣修补的治疗,效果良好。所有经过初始手术失败的病例,再经过直肠内推进瓣手术,瘘口全部愈合。Hull 和 Fazio[40] 报道了35例克罗恩病病例,均经过直肠推进瓣治疗直肠阴道瘘,初始手术成功率为54%,5例患者手术失败,重复进行直肠内推进瓣手术获得成功。Mizrahi 等[41] 报道了106例经过直肠内推进瓣手术治疗的肛门周围复杂瘘,其中32例为直肠阴道瘘,5例贮袋阴道瘘。直肠阴道瘘的长期成功达到了66%,而在整个系列中为60%。在这个研究中,近半数病例有同样的之前修补的尝试,其中10例经过一次直肠内推进瓣手术。之前修补过的患者成功率为74%,特别是10例患者中8例经过重复推进瓣手术获得成功。这些结果,然而,所有类型的肛门直肠瘘和相关的直肠阴道瘘亚组并没有特别检查。近期,de Parades 等[42] 建议,在用瓣覆盖修补内口前,增加肌层的皱褶。在这些病例中,23例患者中9例之前尝试失败,65%的患者完全愈合。

近期,使用生物材料置入瘘道的修补技术已经有很大发展。在这些技术中,不需要切除组织,并发症发生的风险极小。生物材料是无细胞基质,促进炎性细胞向基质中迁移,引导伤口愈合,导致瘘道永久闭合。最初曾尝试使用纤维蛋白胶。纤维蛋白胶是一种用凝血酶活化物形成纤维蛋白凝块的血制品,可机械性地封闭瘘道,凝块促进组织愈合并逐步被纤维溶解吸收。不过,这种技术更容易在长而细的瘘道中获得成功,如在肛管和阴道开口间横穿会阴体的瘘道;并不适合用在直肠阴道隔那样的短瘘道。直肠阴道瘘用纤维蛋白胶的报道很少。Loungnarath 等[43] 尝试在3例患者中应用该技术,仅有1例成功。新的生物材料包括胶原蛋白塞,这种胶原蛋白无细胞基质,形成一种半刚性圆柱形塞子置入瘘道。为了防止塞子移位,尤其在短瘘道,

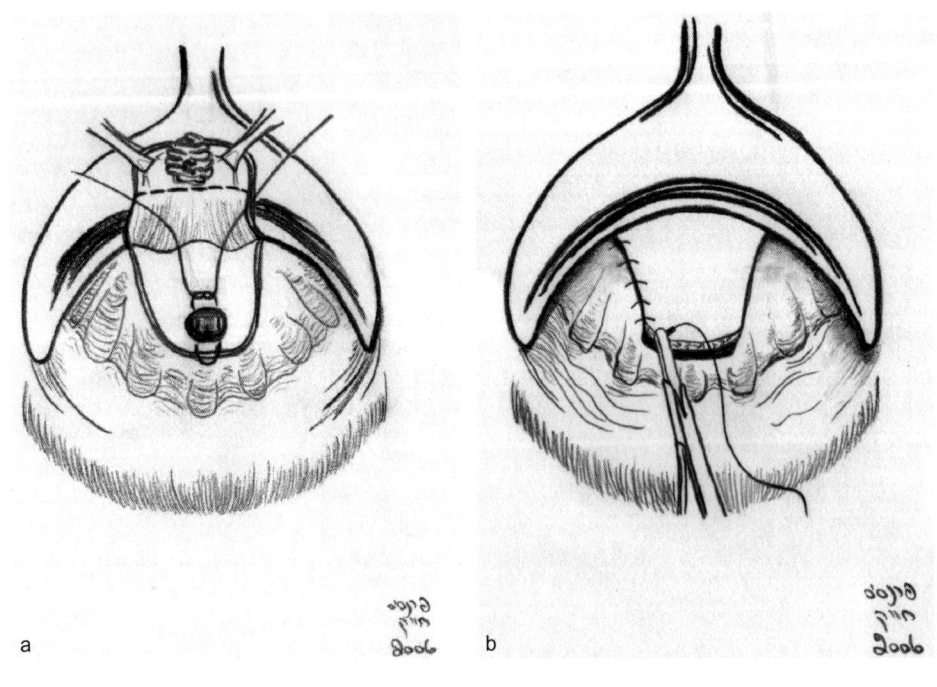

图 38.1 (a)制作一个直肠内推进皮瓣覆并关闭直肠的开口;(b)通过皮瓣覆盖瘘管的内口

塞子贴在固定扣上效果较好。这种塞子有几种针对不同瘘道宽度的尺寸，先彻底探查瘘道长度，再用商用的烟斗通条刷清理干净。然后将胶原蛋白塞经肛门内直肠开口和阴道插入瘘道，直到固定扣到达直肠壁。然后用可吸收线将固定扣固定在直肠壁。超过长度的塞子可以在阴道侧修剪，在阴道侧可以用另外的可吸收线松散缝合固定（图38.2）。塞子由于炎症过程逐渐被吸收，而代之以瘢痕组织，一旦固定固定扣的缝线被吸收，固定扣会脱落并随着肠蠕动排出。

Thekkinkattil 等[44]报道10例直肠阴道瘘或贮袋-阴道瘘的病例用没有固定扣的胶原蛋白塞子治疗。仅2例患者瘘道愈合，而不涉及到阴道的肛瘘成功率为50%。Ellis[45]用没有固定扣的胶原蛋白塞治疗了7例直肠阴道瘘的患者，5例是克罗恩患者。在所有病例中，这是修补的首次尝试。6例患者瘘道愈合，只有1例复发。Gonsalves 等[46]在12例女性患者中用有固定扣的塞子实施了20例瘘修补，7例是贮袋-阴道瘘。这12例患者，5例之前修补过，包括3例用没有固定扣的塞子。7例（58%）患者成功修补，所有用塞子的成功率35%。有趣的是，6例患者中只有1例两次用塞子后成功愈合，两例患者尝试3次没有获得成功，表明在第1次插入失败之后，重复插入的机会很少。Lupinacci 等[47]最近进行的15例研究的结果比较糟糕，其中7例经过之前的修补，在这些病例中肛瘘塞子的脱出率处于中等水平。

阴道修补

用阴道途径修补直肠阴道瘘易于进入，阴道瘘口有较好的视野。这个路径常常比经肛门手术容易进入，尽管存在潜在的从低压侧修补瘘管的不利因素。结直肠外科医生似乎很少应用这个路径。几种经阴道修补的外科技术已经被报道。最常用的手术操作是首先制造一个阴道壁瓣，在瓣下切开直肠阴道隔以分离瘘道，修补两侧瘘，将阴道壁瓣缝合，修补瘘道。这个技术的辅助措施是用可吸收的或生物补片，在关闭瓣之前可以插在直肠和阴道之间，增强瘢痕组织的形成，从而加固直肠阴道隔，支撑有缺陷的会阴体（图38.3a、b）。

Bauer 等[48]应用阴道径路治疗13例低位或中位直肠阴道瘘的克罗恩病患者，12例成功治愈。重要的是，这组病例的所有患者在修补前或同时都做了临时性粪便转流。Casadesus 等[49]应用同样的径路治疗了12例不同病因导致的瘘，9例成功治愈。其中1例患者用阴道径路进行重复修补，再次失败。Ruffolo 等[50]报道一个系统回顾，比较了经阴道修补和经肛门推进瓣修补治疗克罗恩病患者的成功率。经肛门修补的患者54%愈合，经阴道修补的患者69%愈合，但是两者并没有统计学差异。

会阴径路

会阴路径修补直肠阴道瘘时首先做会阴部皮肤切口，向头侧分开直肠阴道隔以分开瘘道，修补两侧瘘道，然后在直肠和阴道间插入组织。传统上，这样的插入物应该是血供良好、新鲜、非炎性、未经照射的组织，可能包括阴唇脂肪组织，一种蒂状肌瓣移植物；最近，有专家推荐生物补片。

Martius 移植物由阴唇脂肪组织构成，旋转进入直肠与阴道间形成的空间。在这个手术中，在大阴唇上做一个椭圆切口，随后瓣移动并与邻近的结构分离，保留后外侧蒂。然后通过隧道在阴道黏膜和小阴唇下面盖住直肠和阴道的闭合处。这样的操作可能更适合于直肠阴道隔下面部分的瘘的治疗，瓣

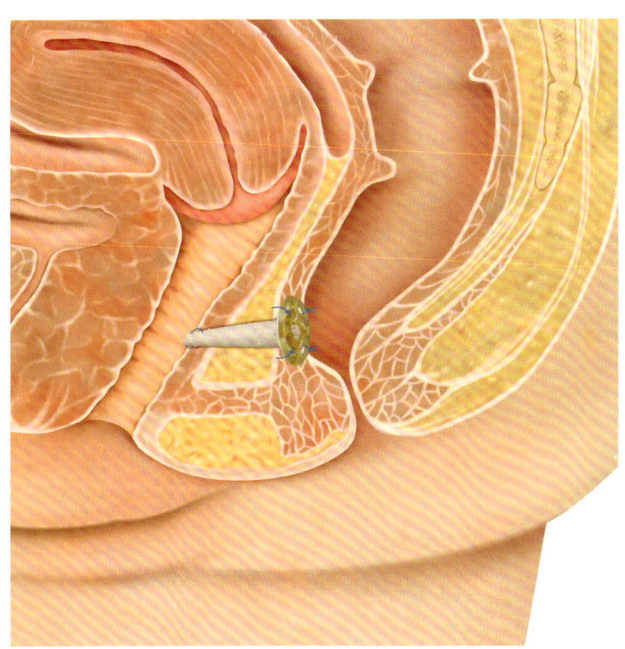

图38.2 带有固定扣的直肠阴道胶原蛋白塞（Permission for use granted by Cook Medical Incorporated, Bloomington Indiana）

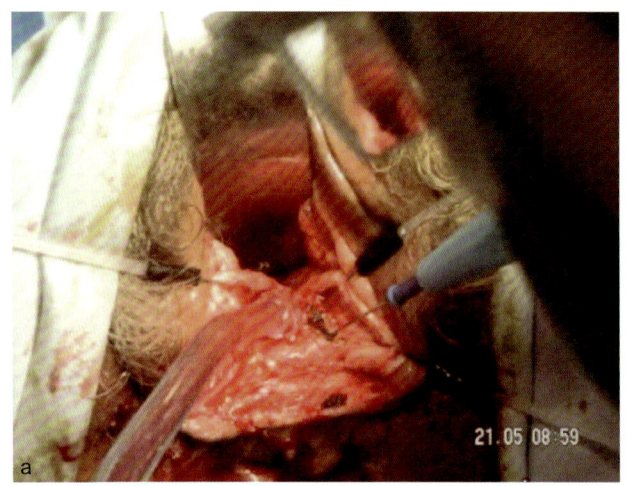 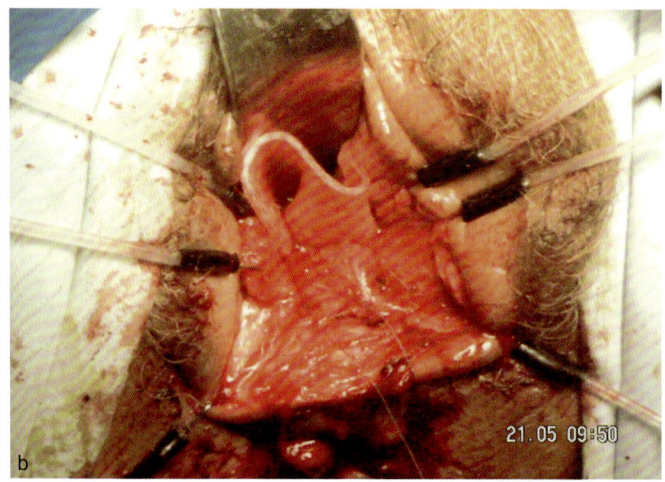

图 38.3 使用生物补片经阴道修复;(a)通过阴道途径制作阴道壁瓣。(b)放置生物补片

能够容易的无张力的插入。用 Martius 移植物修补一个病因不明的瘘的例子见图 38.4a-c。

McNevin 等[51]回顾了他们应用 Martius 瓣修补 16 例直肠阴道瘘患者的经验。这些患者中大多数瘘是由产科损伤导致。几例患者已经经过之前的用直肠黏膜推进瓣、局部经阴道修补和分层开放修补。在这项研究中,6 例患者在进行 Martius 瓣修补时做了转流。大多数患者的瘘成功愈合,除了一例患者,尽管有 5 例患者抱怨术后性交困难。Songne 等[52]报告用 Martius 瓣治疗直肠阴道瘘的经验,半数有克罗恩病,4 例是贮袋 - 阴道瘘。所有 14 例患者的瘘经 3 个月随访均完全愈合。然而 2 例患者复发,因肛周克罗恩病进展需要随后进行直肠切除术。

一些肌肉移植瓣已经用于修补直肠阴道瘘,其中股薄肌可能最常用。股薄肌的裁取可能需要做包括沿大腿内侧股薄肌上做 2~3 个 3~5cm 切口。在切口间皮下组织和肌肉间做隧道,切取足够通过隧道的肌肉(图 38.5a-e)。最接近的切口大约位于腹股沟韧带下方一手宽,以允许足够的神经血管束的显露。股薄肌从靠近胫骨平台的附着处被断开,然后游离并通过最近的切口传送。应该确认并保护神经血管束。从大腿近端至会阴部的嘴样切口形成皮下隧道,肌瓣置入最接近上部切口的凹处。

然后切开会阴。这样的径路可能用在截石位或俯卧折刀位。根据我们的经验,俯卧折刀位能够提供极好的直肠前壁的视野、优良的直肠和阴道间的会阴切开平面,容易对瘘口进行适当的修补,也易于插入肌瓣的固定。在肛门前的会阴作一个切口,大约在肛门和阴道口后缘间的中间。然后将直肠阴道隔切开,分离瘘道并到达头侧非炎症组织。在复发的直肠阴道瘘病例中,或者有影响直肠阴道隔的手术史时(如结肠肛门或回肠 - 肛门吻合),重新切开直肠阴道隔可能很困难,因为手术平面已经纤维化,并且没有间隙,不柔软。应该非常小心,证实在正确的平面解剖,避免切开时造成直肠和阴道的重复损伤。从两侧切开侧面的脂肪组织有时可能有助于确认解剖平面。然后直接关闭直肠缺损或用推进瓣修补。在会阴和大腿间的皮下隧道从会阴部切口可以接近,直到股薄肌被放置的口袋处。股薄肌被旋转并从会阴部切口轻轻引出。小心避免神经肌肉束的张力过高,避免任何血供问题。然后牵引股薄肌至之前切开的会阴部空间,置放在直肠阴道间。用 4-6 针缝合肌肉和切口的顶点,以保持肌瓣不移位。

Rius 等[53]报道 17 例直肠阴道瘘患者,3 例发生在回肠 - 直肠或结肠 - 直肠吻合术后。9 例患者是与克罗恩病相关的瘘。76% 的贮袋 - 阴道瘘患者在修补前经历过平均 2 次的失败尝试。75% 的非克罗恩病的直肠阴道瘘恢复正常,而克罗恩病的瘘仅有 33%。值得注意的是,2 例患者需要二次股薄肌移位。Ulrich 等[54]报道 9 例直肠阴道瘘患者(3 例有克罗恩病)经过股薄肌移位治疗。有克罗恩病的患者中 2 例瘘复发,而所有没有克罗恩病的患者完全恢复正常。Fürst 等[55]报道 12 例继发于克罗肌移位，均未成功。这个方法近来已被报道在盆腔恶性肿瘤的盆腔手术后的直肠阴道瘘病例中应用非常成功[57]。

最近，有学者推荐用生物补片植入直肠和阴道间。在切开足够的直肠阴道隔并修补两侧瘘口后，将补片放置在直肠阴道之间的空间中。尽管不是一个血管化的移植物，这些补片是用无细胞的胶原蛋白基质做成，能促进炎性细胞向内迁移并形成瘢痕组织和纤维化，之后补片被逐渐吸收。这些新近提出的补片植入的方法可以避免制作肌肉瓣或脂肪垫瓣，而它们可能导致明显的局部并发症。在这方面，Ellis[45]在27例患者中应用胶原蛋白补片，14例（52%）之前做过修补的尝试，只有2例患有克罗恩病，报告的成功率为81%。Shelton和Welton[58]对2例患者应用真皮胶原补片（AlloDerm），均获得成功。

腹部修补

直肠阴道瘘修补的腹部径路包含剖腹、深部盆腔前部解剖以分离瘘道。低位瘘需要更深的盆腔解剖。在一些病例，修补瘘道两侧组织并用大网膜瓣填入其中可能是合理的。然而，在个别病例，尤其是当瘘来源于低位吻合或与放射治疗相关，受影响的直肠或新的直肠肠段需要切除，重新做一个低位吻合。这个手术明显的缺点是手术创伤大以及相关的风险。另外，这个方法对于以前做过腹部手术的患者可能是一个挑战，这样的患者的大网膜可能不能用作植入瓣。

Nowacki[59]应用腹部路径对24例放射治疗后直肠阴道瘘的患者作结直肠袖状吻合。1例术后死亡，其余23例中18例修补成功。Cooke和Wellsted[60]报道在55例接受放射治疗并经过切除和结肠肛管吻合的患者中的成功率为93%。这个技术最近也由荷兰的Schouten和Oom[61]报告在8例患者中应用，5例获得成功，均通过后位Kraske或腹部-Kraske径路（Localio）应用直肠袖状前推技术。

手术考虑和选择

直肠阴道瘘的修补是有挑战性的外科工作，而无论何种手术方法，均有较高的失败率。因为这个原因，临床经常会碰见经过1次或多次修补尝试失

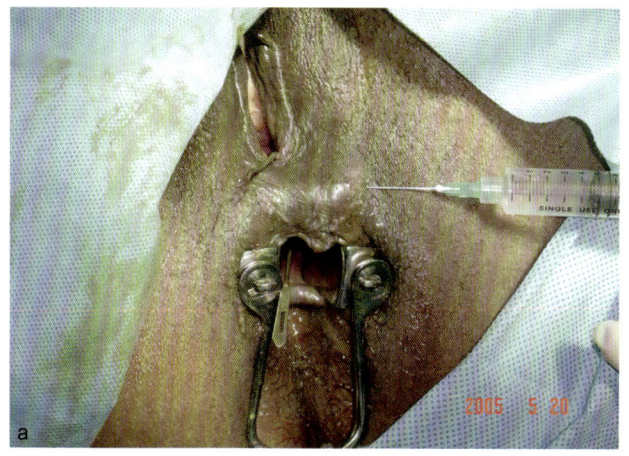
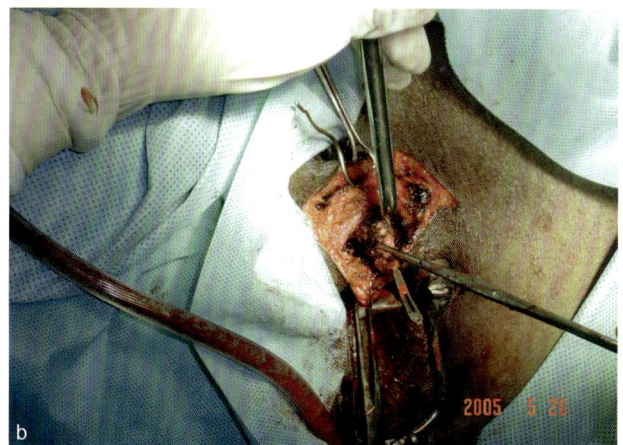
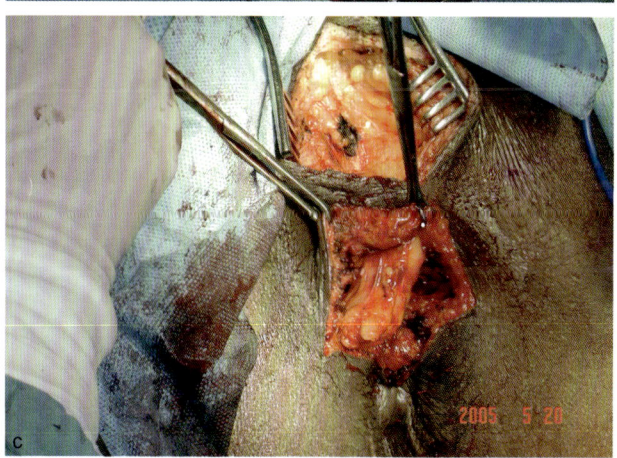

图38.4 在治疗隐发型直肠阴道瘘中使用Martius球海绵体肌移植物（a）将Lockhart-Mummery探针置入直肠阴道瘘；（b）阴道修复后将探针穿过会阴并改道；（c）将球海绵体肌（Martius）移植物进行塑形用来修补直肠阴道瘘

恩病的直肠阴道瘘，仅有1例失败。1例贮袋–阴道瘘的患者需要二次股薄肌移位术方愈合。最近，Lefèvre等[56]报道8例直肠阴道瘘患者，其中6例用股薄肌移位治愈。2例失败的病例经过二次股薄

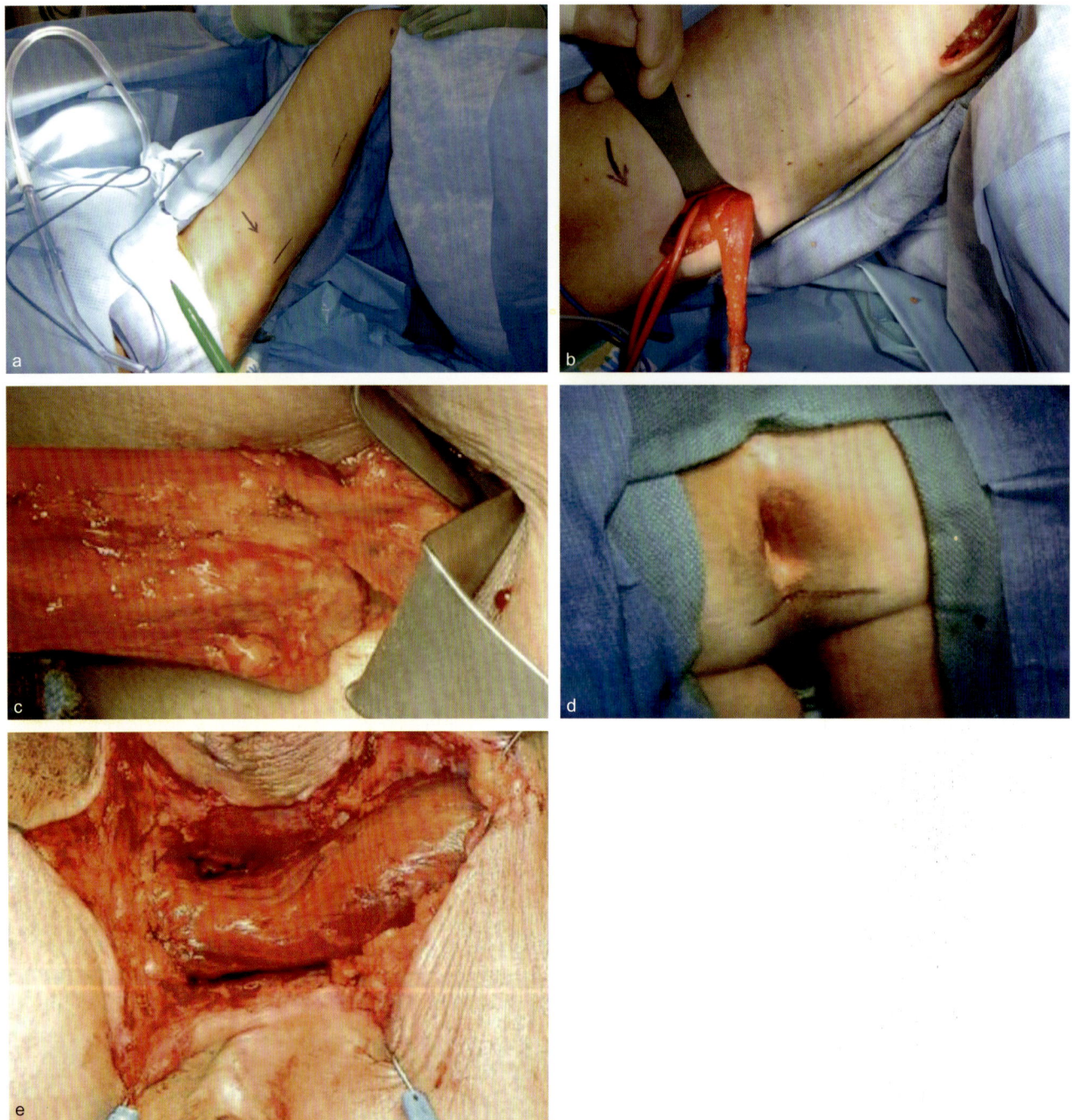

图 38.5 股薄肌移植。(a) 大腿皮肤切定位；(b) 切开肌肉；(c) 神经血管束；(d) 会阴皮肤切口定位；(e) 将肌肉插入直肠与尿道/阴道之间

败的直肠阴道瘘患者。除了由瘘的病因导致的复杂性，如克罗恩病或放射治疗，先前的手术修补所致的解剖层次不清晰和大范围的瘢痕组织可能使以后的尝试更加复杂。尽管如此，重复修补常常具有可能性，并经常成功。Halverson 等[62]报道 35 例患者 57 次用各种方法修补复发性直肠阴道瘘。79% 在经过平均 2 次手术后最终愈合。MacRae 等[63]回顾了 28 例经过复发性直肠阴道瘘修补的患者，61% 成功率。简单瘘的患者有 72% 成功愈合；相比之下，复杂瘘的患者仅有 40% 成功。

对于手术方式的选择，所有上面提及的修补直肠阴道瘘的外科技术也能应用于复发病例的修补，并没有绝对的指南决定哪种手术在其后的尝试中最好。总之，有 3 种主要选择：重复前面已经尝试过的手术，扩大到更大范围的手术，或者缩至小范围的手术。关于直肠阴道瘘再次手术的手术方式的选择方面的文献很有限，在大多数病例组中手术失败的复发性瘘的数量也是如此。几个应用如直肠内推进瓣[41]和股薄肌转移[53]的手术方法的病例群表明，用同样手术方式的二次尝试能与第一次尝试获得相似的成功率；然而，应用生物材料修补的患者群中重复修补的病例比第一次修补的成功率要低[46]。另外，还有一些偶尔报道的技术，包括氰基丙烯酸盐粘合剂[64]，作为确定性修补的一部分的外阴肛门切开术[65]、腹腔镜径路[66]，或者用作处理儿童先天性情况的新的血管化瓣[67-68]，但这些技术还不够成熟，无需讨论。在特殊的病例中，之前盆腔的手术已经应用了加强的补片，之前的证据表明，植入的修复材料需要取出并同时植入大网膜[69]。

许多外科医生和患者相信，如果一种手术失败了，自然的行为将是下一次采用范围更广的手术方式。例如，如果首次的手术使用经肛门或经阴道径路，下一次选择可能包括会阴部切开；如果会阴径路失败了，可能考虑经腹部手术。这样一种思路的根据是更广泛范围的手术大概成功率会高一些，让患者感觉更有希望，即使有更高的并发症发生率。反之，之前的失败的修补有可能在未来的尝试中增加外科手术的风险，外科医生和患者有时可能选择低估风险，选择低风险的手术，尽管只有中等成功率，尤其是如果这些选择在以前没有被尝试过。与患者全面讨论应该包括期望的成功率、可能的好处，以及每种手术的主要风险；下一次手术的选择应该考虑在适当的病例中，讨论对术后性功能可能的影响[5]。尽管外科医生的经验和偏好会掺进考虑之中，这些难治的病例应该由经过训练、已经掌握各种治疗方法，能够为不同患者选择合适手术方式的结直肠病学专家治疗。

另外需要考虑的是转流性造口以改善直肠阴道瘘修补结果的需要。如果患者有无法容忍的症状，而造口的目的是减轻这一症状，因而患者希望为此而造口，那么关于转流的决定相对较易作出。然而，在许多长期直肠阴道瘘的病例中，患者已经应付这种症状很长时间，并不希望仅仅因此而进行转流，尽管这些症状对生活质量有影响。理论上，可能粪便转流后，外科手术修补会更好地愈合，因此而改善修补的成功率。尽管存在理论上的好处，但没有研究比较用或不用转流性造口对各种不同手术方式的影响，仅有少量证据支持保护性造口。可能被广泛接受的转流指证仅仅是低位结肠肛门吻合后经腹修补。

重复修补的最佳时机也没有确定。足够的引流和脓毒症的解决在所有重复修补前都是必需的，并且以前的瘢痕要完全愈合。我们相信从解决脓毒症和伤口愈合最少延迟3个月才足以使组织瘢痕化。

结 论

直肠阴道瘘通常是一种生活质量问题，但也是法医学的问题（在54章讨论的问题）。患有这种令人难受的疾病的患者往往受到明显的心理或社会影响，并且损害到他们的生活质量。然而，身体的痛苦常常（并且幸运的）是中等程度的，并且这种状况很少危及生命。因此，修补手术的主要指证是改善生活质量。只有患者才能够确定这种状况如何糟糕地影响他/她的生活，愿意去做何种手术，在修补瘘的时候将面临哪些风险。通常，已经经过失败修补的患者会对疾病相关的处境更加沮丧，外科医生必须仔细地回顾患者的症状以及对生活质量的影响，因为这是重复手术的主要指证，需要治疗方案、主要风险、期望的益处和手术类型的成功率、瘘的病因和患者的内科外科治疗历史的全面讨论。在这种状况下，需要患者的期望和外科医生实际能够实现的结果密切结合。在这个方面，外科医生偶尔也可能因为失败的修补尝试感到沮丧，并且既不愿提供更进一步的外科干预，也没有动力去控制瘘，并说服患者不惜代价进行重复手术。重要的是记住主要手术指征是瘘对于患者生活质量的影响；因此，只有认识到影响成功（和失败）所有因素的患者，才能决定他/她是否希望实施更进一步修补手术的尝试。

参考文献

1. Champagne BJ, McGee MF. Rectovaginal fistula. Surg Clin North Am. 2010;90:69–82.
2. Lowry AC, Hoexter B. Rectovaginal fistulas. In: Wolff CB, Fleshman JW, Beck DE, Pemberton JH, Wexner SD, editors. The ASCRS textbook of colon and rectal surgery. New York: Springer; 2007. p. 215–27.
3. Saclarides TJ. Rectovaginal fistula. Surg Clin North Am. 2002;82: 1261–72.
4. Sonoda T, Hull T, Piedmonte MR, Fazio VW. Outcomes of primary repair of anorectal and rectovaginal fistulas using the endorectal advancement flap. Dis Colon Rectum. 2002;45:1622–8.
5. El-Gazzaz G, Hull TL, Mignanelli E, Hammel J, Gurland B, Zutshi M. Obstetric and cryptoglandular rectovaginal fistulas: long-term surgical outcome; quality of life and sexual function. J Gastrointest Surg. 2010;14:758–63.
6. Lowder JL, Burrows LJ, Krohn MA, Weber AM. Risk factors for primary and subsequent anal sphincter lacerations: a comparison of cohorts by parity and prior mode of delivery. Am J Obstet Gynecol. 2007;196:344.e1–5.
7. Raassen TJ, Verdaasdonk EG, Vierhout ME. Prospective results after first-time surgery for obstetric fistulas in East African women. Int Urogynecol J Pelvic Floor Dysfunct. 2008;19:73–9.
8. Narcisi L, Tieniber A, Andriani L, McKinney T. The fistula crisis in sub-Saharan Africa: an ongoing struggle in education and awareness. Urol Nurs. 2010;30:341–6.
9. Hilger WS, Cornella JL. Rectovaginal fistula after posterior intravaginal slingplasty and polypropylene mesh augmented rectocele repair. Int Urogynecol J Pelvic Floor Dysfunct. 2006;17:89–92.
10. Pescatori M, Gagliardi G. Postoperative complications after procedure for prolapsed hemorrhoids (PPH) and stapled transanal rectal resection (STARR) procedures. Tech Coloproctol. 2008;12:7–19.
11. Pescatori M, Dodi G, Salafia C, Zbar AP. Rectovaginal fistula after double-stapled transanal rectotomy (STARR) for obstructed defaecation. Int J Colorectal Dis. 2005;20:83–5.
12. Belliveau P, Trudel J, Vasilevsky CA, Stein B, Gordon PH. Ileoanal anastomosis with reservoirs: complications and long-term results. Can J Surg. 1999;42:345–52.
13. Kim NK, Lim DJ, Yun SH, Sohn SK, Min JS. Ultralow anterior resection and coloanal anastomosis for distal rectal cancer: functional and oncological results. Int J Colorectal Dis. 2001;16: 234–7.
14. Singhal SR, Nanda S, Singhal SK. Sexual intercourse: an unusual cause of rectovaginal fistula. Eur J Obstet Gynecol Reprod Biol. 2007;131:243–4.
15. Arias BE, Ridgeway B, Barber MD. Complications of neglected vaginal pessaries: case presentation and literature review. Int Urogynecol J Pelvic Floor Dysfunct. 2008;19:1173–8.
16. Pinto RA, Peterson TV, Shawki S, Davila GW, Wexner SD. Are there predictors of outcome following rectovaginal fistula repair? Dis Colon Rectum. 2010;53:1240–7.
17. Hull T, Fazio VW. Rectovaginal fistula in Crohn's disease. In: Phillips RK, Lunniss PJ, editors. Anal fistula: surgical evaluation and management. London: Chapman and Hall; 1996. p. 143.
18. Kim CW, Kim JH, Yu CS, Shin US, Park JS, Jung KY, et al. Complications after sphincter-saving resection in rectal cancer patients according to whether chemoradiotherapy is performed before or after surgery. Int J Radiat Oncol Biol Phys. 2010;78:156–63.
19. Houtmeyers P, Breusegem C, Ceelen W, Gillardin JM, Van De Putte D, Boterberg T, et al. Intraoperative high-dose-rate brachytherapy (IBT) for locally unresectable intraabdominal malignancy. Acta Chir Belg. 2007;107:523–8.
20. Zmora O, Tulchinsky H, Gur E, Goldman G, Klausner JM, Rabau M. Gracilis muscle transposition for fistulas between the rectum and urethra or vagina. Dis Colon Rectum. 2006;49:1316–21.
21. Cui L, Chen D, Chen W, Jiang H. Interposition of vital bulbocavernosus graft in the treatment of both simple and recurrent rectovaginal fistulas. Int J Colorectal Dis. 2009;24:1255–9.
22. Giordano P, Drew PJ, Taylor D, Duthie G, Lee PW, Monson JR. Vaginography–investigation of choice for clinically suspected vaginal fistulas. Dis Colon Rectum. 1996;39:568–72.
23. Yee LF, Birnbaum EH, Read TE, Kodner IJ, Fleshman JW. Use of endoanal ultrasound in patients with rectovaginal fistulas. Dis Colon Rectum. 1999;42:1057–64.
24. Baig MK, Zhao RH, Yuen CH, Nogueras JJ, Singh JJ, Weiss EG, et al. Simple rectovaginal fistulas. Int J Colorectal Dis. 2000;15: 323–7.
25. Poen AC, Felt-Bersma RJ, Eijsbouts QA, Cuesta MA, Meuwissen SG. Hydrogen peroxide-enhanced transanal ultrasound in the assessment of fistula-in-ano. Dis Colon Rectum. 1998;41: 1147–52.
26. Dwarkasing S, Hussain SM, Hop WC, Krestin GP. Anovaginal fistulas: evaluation with endoanal MR imaging. Radiology. 2004; 231:123–8.
27. Tan E, Anstee A, Koh DM, Gedroyc W, Tekkis PP. Diagnostic precision of endoanal MRI in the detection of anal sphincter pathology: a meta-analysis. Int J Colorectal Dis. 2008;23: 641–51.
28. Ziech M, Felt-Bersma R, Stoker J. Imaging of perianal fistulas. Clin Gastroenterol Hepatol. 2009;7:1037–45.
29. de Souza NM. Prospective comparison of endosonography, magnetic resonance imaging and surgical findings in anorectal fistula and abscess complicating Crohn's disease. Br J Surg. 1999;86(8): 1093–4.
30. Ricart E, Panaccione R, Loftus EV, Tremaine WJ, Sandborn WJ. Infliximab for Crohn's disease in clinical practice at the Mayo Clinic: the first 100 patients. Am J Gastroenterol. 2001;96: 722–9.
31. Ng SC, Plamondon S, Gupta A, Burling D, Swatton A, Vaizey CJ, et al. Prospective evaluation of anti-tumor necrosis factor therapy guided by magnetic resonance imaging for Crohn's perineal fistulas. Am J Gastroenterol. 2009;104:2973–86.
32. Colombel JF, Schwartz DA, Sandborn WJ, Kamm MA, D'Haens G, Rutgeerts P, et al. Adalimumab for the treatment of fistulas in patients with Crohn's disease. Gut. 2009;58:940–8.
33. Hagiu C, Badea R, Serban A, Petrar S, Andreica V. Rapid recovery of a rectovginl fistula with infliximab in a patient with Crohn's disease. J Gastrointestin Liver Dis. 2010;19:329–32.
34. Parsi MA, Lashner BA, Achkar JP, Connor JT, Brzezinski A. Type of fistula determines response to infliximab in patients with fistulous Crohn's disease. Am J Gastroenterol. 2004;99: 445–9.
35. Topstad DR, Panaccione R, Heine JA, Johnson DR, MacLean AR, Buie WD. Combined seton placement, infliximab infusion, and maintenance immunosuppressives improve healing rate in fistulizing anorectal Crohn's disease: a single center experience. Dis Colon Rectum. 2003;46:577–83.
36. Gaertner WB, Madoff RD, Spencer MP, Mellgren A, Goldberg SM, Lowry AC. Results of combined medical and surgical treatment of rectovaginal fistula in Crohn's disease. Colorectal Dis. 2011;13(6): 678–83.
37. Rothenberger DA, Christenson CE, Balcos EG, Schottler JL, Nemer FD, Nivatvongs S, et al. Endorectal advancement flap for treatment of simple rectovaginal fistula. Dis Colon Rectum. 1982;25: 297–300.
38. Lowry AC, Thorson AG, Rothenberger DA, Goldberg SM. Repair of simple rectovaginal fistulas. Influence of previous repairs. Dis Colon Rectum. 1988;31:676–8.
39. Kodner IJ, Mazor A, Shemesh EI, Fry RD, Fleshman JW, Birnbaum EH. Endorectal advancement flap repair of rectovaginal and other complicated anorectal fistulas. Surgery. 1993;114:682–9.
40. Hull TL, Fazio VW. Surgical approaches to low anovaginal fistula in Crohn's disease. Am J Surg. 1997;173:95.
41. Mizrahi N, Wexner SD, Zmora O, Da Silva G, Efron J, Weiss EG, et al. Endorectal advancement flap: are there predictors of failure? Dis Colon Rectum. 2002;45:1616–21.
42. de Parades V, Dahmani Z, Blanchard P, Zeitoun JD, Sultan S,

Atienza P. Endorectal advancement flap with muscular placation: a modified technique for rectovaginal fistula repair. Colorectal Dis. 2011;13(8):921–5. Epub 2010 May 28.
43. Loungnarath R, Dietz DW, Mutch MG, Birnbaum EH, Kodner IJ, Fleshman JW. Fibrin glue treatment of complex anal fistulas has low success rate. Dis Colon Rectum. 2004;47:432–6.
44. Thekkinkattil DK, Botterill I, Ambrose NS, Lundby L, Sagar PM, Buntzen S, et al. Efficacy of the anal fistula plug in complex anorectal fistulae. Colorectal Dis. 2009;11:584–7.
45. Ellis CN. Outcomes after repair of rectovaginal fistulas using bioprosthetics. Dis Colon Rectum. 2008;51:1084–8.
46. Gonsalves S, Sagar P, Lengyel J, Morrison C, Dunham R. Assessment of the efficacy of the rectovaginal button fistula plug for the treatment of ileal pouch-vaginal and rectovaginal fistulas. Dis Colon Rectum. 2009;52:1877–81.
47. Lupinacci RM, Vallet C, Parc Y, Chafai N, Tiret E. Treatment of fistula-in-ano with the Surgisys (®) AFP ™ anal fistula plug. Gastroenterol Clin Biol. 2010;34:549–53.
48. Bauer JJ, Sher ME, Jaffin H, Present D, Gelerent I. Transvaginal approach for repair of rectovaginal fistulae complicating Crohn's disease. Ann Surg. 1991;213:151–8.
49. Casadesus D, Villasana L, Sanchez IM, Diaz H, Chavez M, Diaz A. Treatment of rectovaginal fistula: a 5-year review. Aust N Z J Obstet Gynaecol. 2006;46:49–51.
50. Ruffolo C, Scarpa M, Bassi N, Angriman I. A systematic review on advancement flaps for rectovaginal fistula in Crohn's disease: transrectal versus transvaginal approach. Colorectal Dis. 2010;12:1183–91.
51. McNevin MS, Lee PY, Bax TW. Martius flap: an adjunct for repair of complex, low rectovaginal fistula. Am J Surg. 2007;193:597–9.
52. Songne K, Scotté M, Lubrano J, Huet E, Lefébure B, Surlemont Y, et al. Treatment of anovaginal or rectovaginal fistulas with modified Martius graft. Colorectal Dis. 2007;9:653–6.
53. Rius J, Nessim A, Nogueras JJ, Wexner SD. Gracilis transposition in complicated perianal fistula and unhealed perineal wounds in Crohn's disease. Eur J Surg. 2000;166:218–22.
54. Ulrich D, Roos J, Jakse G, Pallua N. Gracilis muscle interposition for the treatment of recto-urethral and rectovaginal fistulas: a retrospective analysis of 35 cases. J Plast Reconstr Aesthet Surg. 2009;62:352–6.
55. Fürst A, Schmidbauer C, Swol-Ben J, Iesalnieks I, Schwandner O, Agha A. Gracilis transposition for repair of recurrent anovaginal and rectovaginal fistulas in Crohn's disease. Int J Colorectal Dis. 2008;23:349–53.
56. Lefèvre JH, Bretagnol F, Maggiori L, Alves A, Ferron M, Panis Y. Operative results and quality of life after gracilis muscle transposition for recurrent rectovaginal fistula. Dis Colon Rectum. 2009;52:1290–5.
57. Nassar OA. Primary repair of rectovaginal fistulas complicating pelvic surgery by gracilis myocutaneous flap. Gynecol Oncol. 2011;121(3):610–4.
58. Shelton AA, Welton ML. Transperineal repair of persistent rectovaginal fistulas using an acellular cadaveric dermal graft (AlloDerm). Dis Colon Rectum. 2006;49:1454–7.
59. Nowacki MP. Ten years of experience with Parks' coloanal sleeve anastomosis for the treatment of post-irradiation rectovaginal fistula. Eur J Surg Oncol. 1991;17:563–6.
60. Cooke SA, Wellsted MD. The radiation-damaged rectum: resection with coloanal anastomosis using the endoanal technique. World J Surg. 1986;10:220–7.
61. Schouten WR, Oom DM. Rectal sleeve advancement for the treatment of persistent rectovaginal fistulas. Tech Coloproctol. 2009;13:289–94.
62. Halverson AL, Hull TL, Fazio VW, Church J, Hammel J, Floruta C. Repair of recurrent rectovaginal fistulas. Surgery. 2001;130:753–7.
63. MacRae HM, McLeod RS, Cohen Z, Stern H, Reznick R. Treatment of rectovaginal fistulas that has failed previous repair attempts. Dis Colon Rectum. 1995;38:921–5.
64. Ortiz-Moyano C, Guerrero-Jiménez P, Romero-Gómez M. Endoscopic closure of a rectovaginal fistula combining N-2-butyl-cyanoacrylate (Histoacryl) and resolution clips. Endoscopy. 2011;43 Suppl 2:E133–4.
65. Hull TL, El-Gazzar G, Gurland B, Church J, Zushi M. Surgeons should not hesitate to perform episioproctotomy for rectovaginal fistula secondary to cryptoglandular or obstetrical origin. Dis Colon Rectum. 2011;54:54–9.
66. Bailez MM, Cuenca ES, Di Benedetto V, Solana J. Laparoscopic treatment of rectovaginal fistulas. Feasibility, technical details and functional results of a rare anorectal malformation. J Pediatr Surg. 2010;45:1837–42.
67. Lee DT, Lee GK. Transverse Singapore flap for reconstruction of a congenital rectovaginal fistula in an 18-month-old infant. Ann Plast Surg. 2009;63:650–3.
68. Yun IS, Lee JH, Rah DK, Lee WJ. Perineal reconstruction using a bilobed pudendal artery perforator flap. Gynecol Oncol. 2010;118:313–6.
69. Ouaïssi M, Cresti S, Giger U, Sielezneff I, Pirrò N, Berthet B, et al. Management of recto-vaginal fistulas after prosthetic reinforcement treatment for pelvic organ prolapsed. World J Gastroenterol. 2010;28:3011–5.

第 39 章 直肠尿道瘘的处理

Mandeep S. Saund · Ronald Bleday
李 超 译　李国逊 审校

摘 要

本章将要讨论少见、但非常重要的直肠尿道瘘的诊断和处理方法。这种瘘常常是医源性因素造成的，如前列腺手术及前列腺近距离放射治疗都会造成直肠尿道瘘。这种瘘的手术入路需要依据患者个人情况而定，包括经腹入路、经肛周/肛管直肠内入路、经会阴入路、经括约肌间入路（York-Mason）、后入路（Kraske 术式）和直肠旁手术。这些术式的效果以及针对一些特殊情况下用生物胶填补的效果都将在本章中一一讨论。

关键词

直肠尿道瘘（rectourethral fistula, RUF）；泄殖腔；肛门直肠畸形；体外波放疗（external beam radiation therapy, EBRT）；近距离放疗；射频消融；冷冻疗法；克罗恩病；尿道周围脓肿；复发性会阴脓肿；前列腺癌；直肠癌；创伤；尿道感染；气尿；粪尿

引 言

由于女性盆底解剖与男性的差别，直肠尿道瘘（RUF）都发生在男性。尽管有多种原因可以导致 RUF，但 RUF 最常见的病因还是医源性损伤，这种医源性损伤通常都来源于良性前列腺疾病或前列腺癌的手术或治疗。前列腺癌患者接受近距离放疗后常发生 RUF，这一点已经得到确认，RUF 常在进行该治疗后的 2 年内出现[1]。

RUF 的病因包括以下几个方面：

- 先天性的病因——泄殖腔畸形、低位或高位的肛门直肠畸形
- 医源性的病因——前列腺手术或用以下手段对前列腺进行治疗，如体外波放疗（EBRT）、近距离放疗、射频消融和冷冻治疗
- 炎症——克罗恩病、尿道周围脓肿和复发性会阴脓肿
- 肿瘤——前列腺癌或直肠癌
- 创伤

解 剖

前列腺与直肠

前列腺呈卵圆形，其下端尖细，上端宽大，重约 18g。前列腺尖端位于尿生殖膈上。前列腺分 3 个面：前面、后面与侧面。耻骨前列腺韧带连接前列腺囊的前外侧，固定前列腺。前列腺由筋膜包裹，其后面厚约 0.5mm，称为前列腺囊。前列腺囊后面与 Denonvilliers 筋膜相贴，侧面与位于肛提肌之上

的内骨盆筋膜相融合。前列腺与直肠前壁之间由疏松结缔组织与和 Denonvilliers 筋膜分隔。

尿道于前列腺部向前弯曲成 35°，此角度可在 0°~90°之间变化。尿道分为近端尿道（前列腺前部）和远端尿道（前列腺部）。近端尿道由环形括约肌环绕，此肌肉不受意识控制。远端尿道通向前列腺尖端，称为膜部，长约 2~2.5cm（范围 0.5~5cm），周围被尿道膜部括约肌环绕，此肌延长了膜部的长度，远端插入到会阴体，并受自主意识控制。

直肠始于盆腔入口，此处结肠带消失，由完整的环形肌环绕而成。直肠是腹膜间位器官，其中段走形于精囊和前列腺的后方。腹膜在精囊前方和中段直肠后方反折形成隐窝。前列腺上端与直肠之间由 Denonvilliers 筋膜[2]（被认为是直肠与前列腺之间反折的两层腹膜形成）分隔。在 Denonvilliers 筋膜下方，前列腺下端与直肠之间有前列腺囊和系膜脂肪分隔。在前列腺下方，尿道膜部在延续为海绵体部之前，其紧贴下段直肠与上段肛管。

肛门三角

在前列腺尖端，直肠向后下方延伸为肛管。肛管长约 4cm，于肛门三角中心的会阴部通过。肛管由肛门内括约肌和肛门外括约肌包绕，前者不受意志控制，后者受意志控制。肛门外括约肌可分为 3 部：皮下部、浅部和深部[3]。

男性尿生殖三角

尿生殖膈位于肛提肌的下方，占据男性和女性会阴前方的尿生殖三角。在男性，位于皮肤及皮下脂肪下方的坐骨海绵体肌包绕阴茎海绵体，起自两侧的坐骨结节，止于尿生殖膈下筋膜。球海绵体肌包绕尿道海绵体并形成中线，其后方与会阴中心腱相融合。会阴浅、深横肌组成尿生殖膈后缘，也与会阴中心腱相融合[4]。

直肠尿道瘘的表现

直肠尿道瘘患者临床表现为以下几个方面：经直肠漏尿、反复尿生殖道感染、气尿与粪尿。此病常常与前列腺手术、前列腺放射治疗、直肠前入路手术等病史相关。此外，有些患者表现为尿酸在直肠的过度再吸收所导致的代谢性酸中毒[5]，也可表现为不育症[6]。

因前列腺癌行放射治疗（粒子植入内照射或体外照射）的患者，在瘘管形成之前，可先出现会阴部或直肠的疼痛。而且，这些患者在放射治疗多年之后，有可能造成直肠前壁溃疡和便血，进而发展并形成瘘管。由医源性损伤到直肠尿道瘘的发生所经历的时间不等，大致可以分为两类：早发型和迟发型。术后 30 天发生的直肠尿道瘘称为早发型。大部分在前列腺手术中造成医源性损伤的患者都能够被早期发现并修补。如果修补失败，则在术后约 7~10 天可发展为直肠尿道瘘。前列腺切除术中如发生未发现的直肠损伤，则患者表现为术后或 Foley 尿管拔除后 1~3 天出现经直肠漏尿。接受短距离放疗或外放射治疗的前列腺癌患者则表现为迟发型直肠尿道瘘。直肠尿道瘘的发病时间可以从 9 个月到 5 年不等。

历　史

Wagernus 在 1685 年首次描述了直肠尿道瘘。Astley Cooper 在 1823 年首次尝试利用外科手术行单纯会阴引流治疗直肠尿道瘘。1831 年，Bushe 尝试对直肠尿道瘘进行了手术分型。Weyrauch[7] 则最早对直肠尿道瘘进行了详尽的描述，并报道了直肠尿道瘘的修补原则。

发病率

多个研究中心所报道了前列腺手术致直肠尿道瘘的发生率。Eastham 和 Scardino[8] 在 3834 例行耻骨后根治性前列腺切除术（RRP）病例的研究中报道直肠尿道瘘的发病率为 0.2%~2.9%（平均 0.7%）。Thomas 等[9] 在 2447 例行前列腺根治性切除术患者的研究中报道其发病率为 0.53%。并非所有未被发现的直肠损伤或前列腺术后直肠修补都能造成直肠尿道瘘。Smith 和 Veenema[10] 报道，160 例耻骨后根治性前列腺切除术后 20 年的患者中，15 例发生直肠损伤，而在这 15 例患者中，只有 4 例罹患直肠尿道瘘。在另一项研究中，589 例接受耻骨后根治性前列腺切除术或者膀胱前列腺切除术的患者中有 23 例发生了直肠损伤，而在这 23 例患者中，12 例发生了直肠尿道瘘[11]。Castillo 等[12] 报道 110 例腹膜后腹腔镜前列腺切除术患者中9例发生直肠损伤，其中7例损伤术中及时被发现并行1期修补，其中1例修补失败。最终3例患者罹患直肠尿道瘘（1例行修补术，2例发生未被发现的直肠损伤）。

消融技术包括前列腺冷冻疗法、射频消融、短距离放射治疗和前列腺热疗，都可以导致直肠误伤，这种误伤常常是迟发性的。前列腺冷冻术、前列腺穿刺与短距离放射疗法致RUF率分别为2%~5%、2.5%、3.2%[13-15]。Theodorescu等[16]报道754例因前列腺癌接受短距离放射治疗的患者，其RUF的发病率为1%。对于单独行短距离放射治疗的患者，RUF发病率上下波动0.2%，对于行短距离放疗联合补救性前列腺切除术的患者，其发病率为8.8%。

直肠损伤也可发生在新型的前列腺手术当中。接受经耻骨后机器人或腹腔镜前列腺切除术后10年的11 452例患者中，18例发生了直肠损伤。其中12例为机器人手术（发病率0.12%），6例为腹腔镜手术（发病率0.47%）[17]。16例确认发生直肠损伤，并利用网膜植入分隔直肠与尿道缝合线的方法行1期修补。共4例发生RUF（其中2例发生直肠损伤被发现并做修补，另2例直肠损伤未被发现）。克罗恩病相关RUF发病率比较低，目前报道的只有13例，其中最近的1例报道于1995年[18]。

分　型

RUF有两种分型系统，一种与瘘管位置相关，另一种与患者功能相关。

解剖分型

高位：直肠膀胱型（直肠至膀胱或膀胱三角区）

中位：直肠前列腺型（直肠至尿道前列腺部或膜部）

低位：直肠尿道球型（直肠至尿道球）

功能分型[19]及建议的手术治疗方法

- Ⅰ级
  - 低位，距肛外缘<4cm，未经放射治疗
  - 经肛门修补
- Ⅱ级
  - 高位，距肛外缘>4cm，未经放射治疗
  - 经直肠/括约肌前直肠瓣修补
- Ⅲ级
  - 较小瘘管，<2cm，接受放射治疗
  - 经直肠/括约肌前直肠瓣修补
- Ⅳ级
  - 较大瘘管，>2cm，接受放射治疗
  - 股薄肌肌皮瓣行会阴修补
- Ⅴ级
  - 巨大坐骨褥疮瘘
  - 股薄肌肌皮瓣行会阴修补

调　查

大部分的RUF病例能够在体检时发现。肛门指诊通常能检测到直肠前壁的损伤并能够确定其大小、数量及瘘管开口的位置。在这方面，前列腺手术后94%的RUF病例能够通过单纯体格检查被确诊[20]。因此，我们需要更深入研究以确定瘘管的解剖，而非明确诊断。

可屈性乙状结肠镜检查是体格检查后另一种最好的检测方法。乙状结肠镜能够确定肛诊的检查结果并能够排除其他相关的病理，如直肠癌、复发的前列腺癌、克罗恩病和放射性直肠炎。瘘管开口边缘的组织活检将排除能妨碍单纯修补愈合的特殊病因（包括恶性肿瘤或克罗恩病）。当患者有前列腺或直肠恶性肿瘤病史时，应行组织活检以排除肿瘤复发，或者怀疑有特殊病因时，也应行组织活检。然而，如患者曾接受短距离放射治疗，在真性RUF形成之前如果对直肠前壁溃疡行组织活检有可能造成瘘，对于这些患者，除非恶性肿瘤，组织活检必须要精心操作。

由于在修补瘘管时尿失禁常常被忽略，因此在进行深入诊疗之前，必须对患者进行控尿评估。所有拟行瘘修补术的患者，建议做膀胱镜检查以确定瘘管尿道端开口的大小和位置。尿道损伤与输尿管口的位置关系对于在修补过程中防止对输尿管的损伤也非常关键。确定这些解剖关系对于高位直肠尿道瘘尤为重要。此外，膀胱镜检查还能排除重大RUF相关性尿道狭窄，如果存在狭窄，在RUF修补过程中应对其进行处理。

尿道动力学研究显示，在尿失禁或者尿道狭窄的患者中，尤其是接受骨盆照射之后发生尿失禁或尿道狭窄的患者，因为膀胱顺应性的改变有时会随

之出现尿动力学的改变[21]。排泄性膀胱尿道造影/逆行尿道膀胱造影也有助于确定瘘管的走形。本研究将对以往研究进行额外补充，尤其增加了由克罗恩病引发的复杂性瘘管的病例。泛影葡胺灌肠也可有助于确定瘘管的位置。尿动力学检查和泛影葡胺灌肠都最有助于评估修补的效果。会阴部核磁检查一直被用来确定瘘管走形，并能够关注到肛门括约肌和肛提肌的情况，此区域异常往往与先天性肛门直肠畸形有关[22]。

修补原则

RUF修补包括两层上皮表面的分离：尿道上皮和直肠黏膜。1958年Goodwin等[23]建议用不重叠缝合线进行修补，修补之前行尿流与粪流的改道，尿道上皮与直肠黏膜之间采用血管化组织填充。随着肠道准备、长期抗生素使用、长期Foley尿管留置的出现，无改道的RUF修补也已有报道[7, 23]。Kasraeian等[24]提出不进行改道行一期修补，得到了很好的效果。Kasraeian等只是在有腹膜炎、不可控制的败血症或有明显症状的脓肿的患者实施尿流与粪流的改道。在这方面，Nyam和Pemberton[20]提出作为单一治疗模式，仅仅行结肠造口术改道对于败血症患者或因瘘管巨大或经放射治疗的患者没有意义。

有些瘘管，尤其是无明显缺血组织的小直径或长的瘘管（尤体外放射治疗、短距离放射治疗、冷冻疗法或温热治疗），单独改道治疗可以治愈[20]。Wilhelm[25]介绍了13例接受单独改道治疗的病例（全部行结肠造口术），有9例全部治愈。同样，Goodwin等[23]介绍了22例不同瘘管长度的RUF患者单独行导尿管引流而未行手术治疗，其中9例治愈并且没有复发。

全身和局部因素影响创面愈合和任何位置瘘管的闭合。影响RUF愈合的因素包括瘘管本身长度偏短、上皮因修复而交错重叠、显著纤维化、照射治疗后血管减少，修补术有时还会造成尿道末端狭窄。首次修补无疑是最佳的时机，所以上文介绍的主要原则和最佳的修补方法必须在第一步实施。1964年Culp和Calhoon[26]强调外科医生要始终选择他们最舒服的手术方式。这一点直到今天仍然十分适用，就像早期Weyrauch[7]的观点一样，他曾于1951年这样写道："为了使一般泌尿科医师都能够轻易实施，手术技术必须简洁。像所有的手术一样，手术效果与其操作的简单性直接相关。一次手术必须保证快速愈合，对控制排尿排便的功能方面的恢复非常关键。"

现今，由于短距离放射治疗、EBRT或其他消融技术在前列腺癌治疗中的使用，RUF的发病率有所升高。在前列腺切除术中发生直肠损伤导致RUF的发生率相对稳定在2%以下。由于放射治疗导致的血管减少，广泛组织纤维化以及大瘘管，使得放射致RUF的修补术面临很大的挑战。随着新类型放射致瘘管的出现，使用血管化的皮瓣来填充大的缺损，并使瘘管愈合显得尤为重要。

前列腺切除术中直肠损伤的修补

在前列腺切除术和其他泌尿系统的手术中，直肠损伤是相对比较少见的。膀胱镜检查过程中造成的直肠损伤可以通过放置几个星期的导尿管使尿道和直肠损伤治愈。当在前列腺手术中出现损伤，尤其是热损伤时，外科医生要清创直肠壁，然后通过使用可吸收的缝合线缝合健康组织进行1期修复。如果可能的话，要用大网膜瓣来分隔尿道膀胱吻合口与修补的直肠。进行结肠造口术不是必须的[27-28]，但是在某些情况下这可以作为保守治疗的补充。另一种方法是在直肠修补后，即让患者低纤维饮食或者肠外营养，并结合使用广谱抗生素。是否进行分流造口术要取决于损伤时肠道准备程度，损伤的程度，以及是否即时或延迟发生脓毒血症或脓肿。

直肠尿道瘘修补技术

对于直肠尿道瘘，Munoz[29]等已经介绍了40种不同的手术方式，而Mayo门诊的Nyam和Pemberton[20]则描述了8种不同的方法，并修复了16例RUF患者。我们将仅就我们认为当前最佳的手术方式做如下探讨，而小儿先天肛门直肠畸形相关性RUF则不做讨论。

手术方式选择

- 经腹入路：
  — 瘘管的修补和结肠肛管的拉脱
  — 切除术（膀胱及直肠切除术）
- 前入路：

- 经会阴路径
- 经肛门入路：
  - Parks 与 Motson 入路
  - 经肛门内窥镜手术
  - 单孔腹腔镜手术（SILS port）入路
- 后入路手术：
  - 经括约肌 (York-Mason) 入路
  - Kraske/ 经尾骨入路
  - Laterosacral 入路

经腹入路

由于再次行开腹手术，经腹入路行 RUF 修补有发生相关的并发症或导致患者死亡的风险。此外，这还需要分离 Denonvilliers 筋膜，而 Denonvilliers 筋膜通常由于以前的手术或者放射治疗而纤维化，使分离变得非常困难。尽管此入路可以修补直肠，但直肠前方暴露受限，为尿道修补带来困难。经腹入路可以获取大网膜瓣来分隔两个上皮层，这在需要行膀胱或直肠切除术中是必需的。通常情况下，这些切除只有在其他修复 RUF 的尝试都失败后才实施。经腹入路修补术结果如表 39.1 所示。

经会阴路径

此术式患者可以选择膀胱结石位或者俯卧折刀位，沿会阴中线纵切口或横切口，到达介于尿道和肛门外括约肌之间的直肠 / 尿道层面。这种方法可能需要分离横向会阴部肌肉。采用此种术式时，Foley 导尿管对于尿道的确认非常重要。有时 Foley 导尿管需要通过膀胱镜的引导或者通过膀胱逆行的方式来放置。当确定瘘管后，如果可行的话，需继续在瘘管周围解剖其外侧和近端。或者分离 RUF 远端，通过界定周边外侧和近端正常组织边缘以区分尿道上皮与直肠黏膜。我们尝试分别修复直肠和尿道，然后将皮瓣或其他填充物放置在缝合线之间。

股薄肌瓣，带血管白膜和阴囊肉膜瓣都被使用过。此外，肛提肌也曾被作为填充物填在修复缝合线之间。作为另外一种选择，Young 和 Stone[32] 曾报道先将近端直肠与肛门会阴侧缝合，然后将瘘管的直肠段拉至肛门外切除。此外，他们修补尿道上皮并切除瘘管。

经会阴入路结果

表 39.2 列出了经会阴入路的结果。1947 年，Lewis[41] 报道使用经会阴入路修补了 13 例 RUF 患者，其中 11 例获得成功。1 例患者没有治愈，另 1 例患者的治疗效果不确定。然而，他们的这种方法涉及到 RUF 的识别和分离。尿道与直肠采用铬肠线双层缝合。游离直肠以补偿尿道修补远端的直肠修补部位。Goodwin 等[23] 随后提出了在上述手术中还需游离肛提肌至尿道与直肠修补处之间并缝合。

Culp 与 Calhoon[26] 报道了 20 例诊断为 RUF 的病例。他们在会阴部采用了倒 U 形切口，于会阴横肌后方仔细分离直肠与尿道。然后确认瘘管并分离，单层缝合修补尿道，双层缝合修补直肠。他们用丝线缝合修补直肠肌层与浆膜层，丝线的使用与会阴部长时间引流能确保瘘管的愈合。15 例行此方法单纯修补的患者中 9 例获得了治愈，而其余 6 例复发并进行了 1～4 次会阴修补。其中两例 RUF 患者具有潜在复发性癌风险，他们认为尝试对其行修补术不妥。

Zmora 等[33] 在 2003 年报告了 11 例 RUF 患者利用股薄肌植入进行直肠尿道瘘会阴修补术。其中 6 例有放射治疗史，5 例之前行修补术失败。1 例修补失败，需要进行股薄肌植入的重新修补。1 位患者瘘管通过会阴部皮肤破溃，利用纤维蛋白凝胶剂滴注被成功治愈。这 11 例患者中没有人出现大小便失禁现象。1 例迁延不愈的患者在经过额外 5 个月的排泄物改道后被治愈。Wexner 等[39] 更新了这个数据，据报道称他们成功治愈了 36 例男性直

表 39.1 经腹入路 RUF 修补术结果

研究者（年份）	病例数	放射疗法 / 冷冻疗法	移植物	控便	控尿	复发	总成功率(%)
Nyam 和 Pemberton（1999）[20]	3	0/0	无	未说明	未说明	1	66
Lane 等（2006）[30]	9	9/0	面颊	5	5	0	100
Sotelo 等（2007）[31]	3	0/0	无	未说明	未说明	0	100

表 39.2 经会阴入路 RUF 修补术结果

研究者（年份）	病例数	放射疗法/冷冻疗法	移植物	控便	控尿	复发	总成功率（%）
Wilhelm（1945）[25]	4	0/0	无	不详	不详	0	100
Culp and Calhoon（1964）[26]	15	1/0	无	15	12	6-2P	60~86.6 重复修补术后
Nyam and Pemberton（1999）[20]	3	0/0	未说明	未说明	未说明	1	66
Zmora 等（2003）[33]	11/5 曾接受过修补	6/0	股薄肌	11	6[a]	2	81~100 重复修补术后
Rabau 等（2006）[34]	4/4 曾接受过修补	0/0	股薄肌	未说明	未说明	0	100
Elliot 等（2006）[35]	7	1/1	阴囊肉膜（2）	未说明	未说明	1	85.7
Varma 等（2007）[36]	8	0/0	阴囊肉膜	未说明	未说明	2	75
Gupta 等（2008）[37]	15/3 曾接受过修补	0/0	股薄肌	14	15	1（肌瓣脱出）	100
Ghoniem 等（2008）[38]	25	17/2	股薄肌	19	13+5[b]	2（肌瓣失活）	100
Wexner 等（2008）[39]	36/13 曾接受过修补	17/4	股薄肌	29[c]		8-1P 顽固性瘘管	78~97 重复修补术后
Nerli 等（2009）[40]	3	0/0	睾丸鞘膜	未说明	未说明	0	100

a：5 例患者 RUF 修补之前尿失禁
b：5 例患者因植入人工尿道括约肌恢复了控尿能力，修补前控尿能力未知
c：6 例患者造口仍未还纳，30 例造口还纳后的患者中 29 例恢复控便能力

肠尿道瘘，其中有 13 例曾经接受过失败的修补术。在这些患者中有 8 例首次行股薄肌植入修补术失败，其中的 5 例患者再次接受了修补术，其中有 4 例成功治愈。在这些患者中有 1 例在还实施了直肠内推进瓣修补术。

功 能

除治愈瘘管外，一些研究还探讨了修补术后尿道和肛门功能。前列腺癌根治术后经过放射治疗和（或）冷冻治疗后出现较大瘘管（直径大于 2cm）的患者，几乎观察不到尿粪排泄物[38]。

经肛门入路

经肛门入路包含经会阴联合肛门外括约肌前部的分离并直肠前壁推移瓣覆盖瘘口，行瘘管切除及直肠、括约肌与尿道的修补[42]。对于经肛门入路，患者常常取俯卧折刀位。游离瘘管周围直肠黏膜并切除瘘管。尿道与直肠的游离是有限的，而暴露不充分可能给尿道上皮修补和重叠缝合带来困难。

1949 年，Vose[43] 报道了 3 个前列腺切除术后直肠尿道瘘经肛门入路修补成功的病例。从尿道游离直肠壁和黏膜，直肠用铬缝合线行双层缝合。术后 10d 拔除尿管后，2 例患者可见残破细小开口并行硝酸银烧灼。Latzko[44] 建议用可吸收缝合线分别独自缝合尿道上皮、Denonvilliers 筋膜和直肠 3 层，安置 Foley 导尿管 3 周。Parks 和 Motson[45] 报道了一种改良的经肛门入路修补术，在瘘管的直肠末端切除 2cm 的直肠黏膜后，生成一个全层的直肠内瓣并将其置于暴露的瘘管末端黏膜的边缘。这样直肠修补后的缝合线处于尿道缺损或者尿道缝合线的远端，从而避免了重叠缝合。全层瓣是通过在瘘口上缘做侧切口，然后在尿道和直肠之间靠近瘘 2cm 处做水平切口来建立的。表 39.3 示已报道的经肛门入路修补的结果。

经肛门内窥镜手术

两个团队利用经肛门内窥镜手术行 RUF 修补。在 2 例 RUF 患者中，Bochove-Overgaauw 等[51] 通

过切除 RUF 处 1cm 直肠组织然后修补尿道与直肠壁成功治愈了其中 1 例患者。其中失败的 1 例被认为既往行股薄肌成形术失败后出现了广泛纤维化。Andrews[52] 等报道利用经肛门内窥镜手术成功修复 1 例前列腺癌行高频聚焦超声治疗后 RUF 患者。他们切除瘘管、修补尿道并建立了全层直肠内瓣。

经括约肌后入路 (York-Mason)

表 39.4 列出了经括约肌后入路修补术的结果。Kilkpatrick 与 Mason[53] 在 1969 年提出了这种处理 RUF 的入路方式，但是直到那时，这种方法只是被用于直肠中 1/3 的绒毛状腺瘤和腺癌患者[60-62]。此

表 39.3 经肛门入路 RUF 修补术结果

研究者（年份）	病例数	放射疗法/冷冻疗法	移植物	控便	控尿	复发	总成功率（%）
Vose（1949）[43]	3	0/0	无	未说明	未说明	0	100
Park and Motson（1983）[45]	5	0/0	全层直肠推进瓣	3ª	3ª	0	100
Al-Ali 等（1997）[46]	6	0/0	全层直肠推进瓣	未说明	未说明	3	50
Nyam and Pemberton（1999）[20]	2	0/0	无	未说明	未说明	1	50
Dreznik 等（2003）[47]	2	0/0	部分厚度直肠推进瓣	2	2	0	100
Garofalo 等（2003）[48]	12	0/0	全层直肠推进瓣	12	12	4	66～83.3 重复修补术后
Rivera 等（2006）[19]	3	0/0	全层直肠推进瓣	3	未说明	0	100
Razi 等（2008）[49]	5	0/0	Latzko 技术	未说明	未说明	0	100
Joshi 等（2011）[50]	5	1/0	全层直肠推进瓣	未说明	未说明	1	80～100 重复修补术后

a: 控便与控尿能力无法评估。2 例患者造瘘还纳前死于非相关因素

表 39.4 经括约肌入路 RUF 修补术结果

研究者（年份）	病例数	放射疗法/冷冻疗法	移植物	控便	控尿	复发	总成功率（%）
Kikpatrick and Mason（1969）[53]	4	0/0	无	4	4	0	100
Wood and Middleton（1990）[54]	2	0/0	直肠推进瓣	2	2	0	100
Bukowski 等（1995）[55]	3	0/0	无	3	3	0	100
Stephenson and Middleton（1996）[27]	15	0/0	直肠推进瓣	15	11/4ª	1	93.3/100 重复修补术后
Al-Ali 等（1997）[46]	10	0/0	直肠推进瓣	未说明	未说明	0	100
Boushey 等（1998）[56]	2	0/0	直肠推进瓣	未说明	未说明	0	100
Renschlerand and Middleton（2003）[57]	24	0/0	直肠推进瓣	未说明	未说明	2/1 顽固性瘘管	91.6/96 重复修补术后
Barisic and Krivokapic（2006）[58]	6/3 曾接受过修补	0/0	直肠推进瓣	未说明	未说明	0	100
Rivera 等（2007）[19]	7	4/0	直肠推进瓣	4ᵇ	未说明	0	100
Pera 等（2008）[59]	5	0/0		未说明	未说明	0	100
Kasraeian 等（2009）[24]	12	0/0	无	12	未说明	3+1	75/92 重复修补术后/100 重复修补术后

a: 4 例患者修补术前尿失禁，植入人工括约肌后恢复控尿能力
b: 3 例 RUF 患者同时合并脊髓损伤，修补术前大便失禁

方法中，患者取俯卧折刀位，做从肛门边缘至尾骨顶部的后正中切口，分离肛门内、外括约肌，切除或不切除尾骨。这种方法充分暴露了直肠前壁，但是无法在尿道和直肠之间填充肌瓣。此外，它还要求标记括约肌束以便进行括约肌重建，在原则上这不会导致尿失禁。然而，从已报道的尿失禁的结果来看，这一方法的效果不一并且常常效果很差[57]。

在 1973 年又后续报道了 9 例成功修复直肠尿道瘘的患者，其中 1 例既往接受过肛门闭锁成形术的患者出现了大便失禁的现象[63]。1990 年 Wood 与 Middleton[54] 使用改良的 York-Mason 术式成功对 7 例医源性 RUF 患者进行了 1 期修复，且没有出现大小便失禁的现象。这些患者在手术前都预防应用了抗生素并进行了机械性肠道准备。1996 年 Stephenson 与 Middleton[27] 使用改良的 York-Mason 技术成功修复了 15 例直肠尿道瘘（14 例医源性，1 例创伤性），没有出现大便失禁，肛门狭窄或控尿能力变化的现象。其中 6 例患者没有进行粪便改道。Renschler 和 Middleton[57] 报道的 24 例患者中有 22 例一次成功修复而没有进行结肠造口术。1 例患者接受了二次改良的 York-Mason 修补术并成功治愈。这些患者无一出现大便失禁。在 2007 年 Rivera[19] 等报告了 13 例直肠尿道瘘患者，其中 7 例使用了这种修补技术并没有出现大小便失禁，实现了 100% 治愈。Kasraeian 等[20] 描述了 12 例使用改良的 York-Mason 技术治疗直肠尿道瘘的患者。一次、二次、三次手术修补成功率分别为 75%，92% 与 100%。尽管重复手术，却无一出现大小便失禁。

Kraske/ 经尾骨入路

1885 年，Kraske 提出了经括约肌复合体上方，骶骨侧方行后外侧切口以切除低位直肠病变的术式。这种方法避免了对括约肌进行分离并且为尿道与直肠的 1 期修补提供了到达直肠前壁的入路。在不联合经会阴入路的情况下，此方法也无法填充肌瓣。术中将尾骨和下段骶骨（S_3，S_4 和 S_5）切除可以使暴露更充分，但这在 RUF 的修补中往往是不需要的。Kilpatrick 和 Thompson[64] 通过改进 Kraske 的方法，环形切除临近瘘管的直肠边缘以便分离瘘管，然后沿切除的直肠壁修补尿道并修补直肠。被修复的直肠呈旋转位以免与缝合线重叠。肛提肌的后方在入路时被分离，在缝合皮肤前将其修补。通过使用这种方法，13 例患者中有 12 例得到成功修补，1 例患者在修补 1 年后复发。有 2 例患者在修补之前有大小便失禁的情况，修补后无一复发尿失禁或大便失禁。从过去 20 年已公布的数据来看，我们没有发现有使用 Kraske 方法来进行 RUF 治疗的例子，但是我们在 1990 年—2010 年期间，亲自试用这种技术修补 RUF，在某些患者取得了很好的效果。表 39.5 展示了使用 Kraske 方法行 RUF 修补的部分结果。

后矢状直肠旁入路

做后正中切口，起自尾骨上方臀沟，经过肛周左侧向下延伸至会阴，止于近阴囊处。切除尾骨逐层分离肛门后肌群；对匹配慕丝缝合线牵引标记各层肛门括约肌以便准确重建。暴露直肠并切开其左侧，直肠缩至右侧。前侧向直肠切口暴露 Denonvilliers 筋膜，确认 RUF 并切除。修补尿道与直肠并充填臀大肌皮瓣分隔两侧缝合线。逐层关闭各层并引流。只有 Abdalla[65] 的 1 个病例曾经使用这种方法修复 RUF 并且取得了非常好的效果（表 39.6）。

生物制剂的作用

纤维蛋白胶

纤维蛋白胶或类似的生物止血制剂偶尔已单独使用或结合皮瓣来修补 RUF。Dolay 等[66] 使用内窥镜将纤维蛋白胶滴入直肠尿道瘘管里来阻断瘘口。Bhandari 等[67] 也向瘘管内滴入纤维蛋白胶修补 1 例 RUF。Verriello[68] 等使用纤维蛋白胶制剂 Quixil（OMRIX 生物制药有限公司，Kiryat Ono，以色列）联合直肠直肠黏膜瓣修补了 1 例 RUF。此例 RUF

表 39.5 Kraske 入路 RUF 修补术结果

研究者（年份）	病例数	放射疗法/冷冻疗法	移植物	控便	控尿	复发	总成功率(%)
Kilpatrick and Thompson(1962)[64]	13	0/0	无	13	11[a]	1	92.3

a：2 例患者修补术前存在尿失禁

表 39.6 后矢状直肠旁入路 RUF 修补术结果

研究者（年份）	病例数	放射疗法/冷冻疗法	移植物	控便	控尿	复发	总成功率(%)
Abdalla（2009）[65]	8	0/0	臀大肌	未说明	未说明	0	100

被成功修补，并在 1 年后的随访中没有复发。这些患者都是前列腺手术后形成的 RUF，3 例患者中无一在前列腺切除术前接受过放射治疗。

人造真皮

Lesser 等[69]经肛门入路利用人造真皮 Alloderm（Life Cell 公司，布兰斯堡，新泽西）联合直肠内肌瓣分离尿道与直肠黏膜并填充，修补了 1 例因前列腺癌行放疗与冷冻消融治疗而形成 RUF 的患者。

建议/结论

面对这么多的可供选择的修复方案，很难决定哪种方法最适合某一个特定患者。我们通常把患者分为 5 类，并为每类患者推荐不同的治疗方式。

1. 观察：有些患者可能只有气尿且很少发生尿路感染。对于这样的患者，最佳选择是长期抗生素抗感染治疗，不需修复。

2. 单纯改道：大小便失禁情况非常严重的患者适合进行单纯粪便或尿流改道。结肠造口术并长期尿管导尿或耻骨上导尿最适合老年患者、具有严重大小便失禁的患者以及出现严重合并症的患者。

3. 经肛门修补：对于那些行前列腺手术且术后未行放射治疗而导致的 RUF 患者最好尝试进行经肛门入路修补术，亦可联合临时粪流改道。我们通常行粪流改道，但也可尝试不进行临时性结肠造口术。

4. 经会阴入路联合股薄肌填充（图 39.1a, b）：接受任何放射治疗的 RUF 患者都是最难处理的。根据我们的经验，只有 67% 的患者有希望成功闭合瘘管并还纳临时改道。这种瘘的治疗需要经过三个阶段：改道；经会阴修补并带肌瓣填充，以提供丰富的血供；改道还纳。重复修补或修补失败很常见。

5. 经腹入路修补并切除：对于那些经会阴或经后入路修补失败患者，可以考虑经腹入路修补。一种方法是直肠切除术，亦可联合结肠肛管吻合术；另一种方法是膀胱切除术。此外，除非高位瘘管，我们一般最后考虑经腹入路修补。

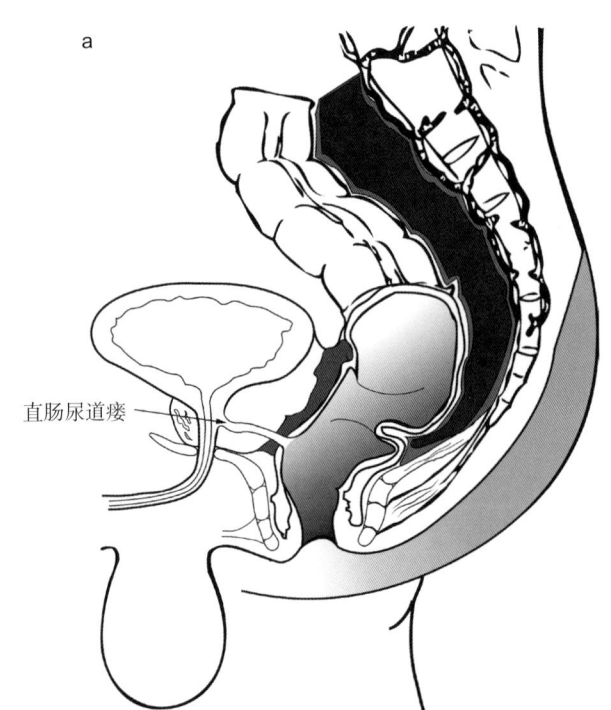

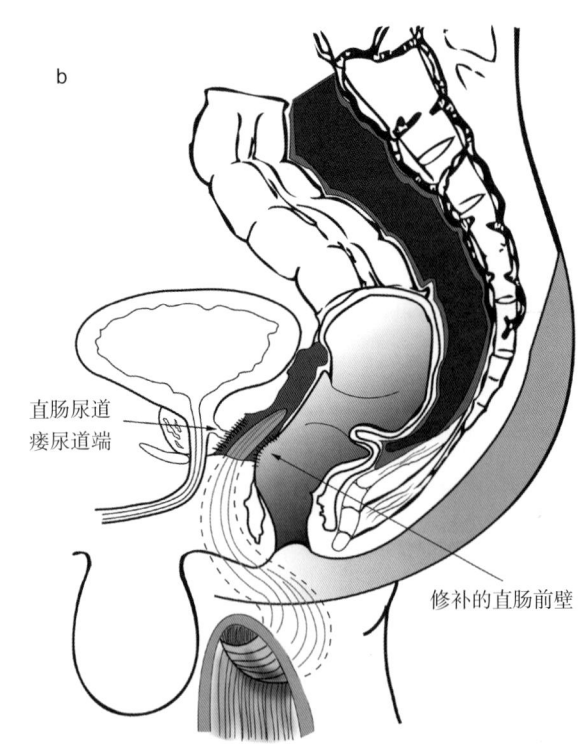

图 39.1 （a）直肠尿道瘘矢状位观；（b）直肠尿道瘘股薄肌瓣修补矢状位观

参考文献

1. Shakespeare D, Mitchell DM, Carey BM, Finan P, Henry AM, Ash D, et al. Recto-urethral fistula following brachytherapy for localized prostate cancer. Colorectal Dis. 2007;9:328–31.
2. Benoit G, Delmas V, Quillard J, Gillot C. Surgical significance of Denonvillier's aponeurosis. Ann Urol (Paris). 1984;18:284–7.
3. Al-Ali S, Blyth P, Beatty S, Duang A, Parry B, Bissett IP. Correlation between gross anatomical topography, sectional sheet plastination, microscopic anatomy and endoanal sonography of the anal sphincter complex in human males. J Anat. 2009;215:212–20.
4. Zhai LD, Liu J, Li YS, Ma QT, Yin P. The male rectourethralis and deep transverse perineal muscles and their relationship to adjacent structures examined with successive slices of celloidin-embedded pelvic viscera. Eur Urol. 2011;59:415–21.
5. Iwai N, Ogita S, Shirasaka S, Yamamoto M, Majima S. Hyperchloremic acidosis in an infant with imperforate anus and rectourethral fistula. J Pediatr Surg. 1978;13:437–8.
6. Hershman M, Kallmeyer V, Wood CB, Williams G. Rectourethral fistula: a rare cause of infertility. Urology. 1986;28:399–400.
7. Weyrauch HM. A critical study of surgical principles used in repair of urethrorectal fistula. Presentation of a modern technique. Stanford Med Bull. 1951;9:2.
8. Eastham JA, Scardino PT. Radical prostatectomy. In: Walsh PC, Retik AB, Vaughan ED, Wein AJ, editors. Campbell's urology. 7th ed. Philadelphia: WB Saunders; 1997. p. 2554.
9. Thomas C, Jones J, Jäger W, Hampel C, Thüroff JW, Gillitzer R. Incidence, clinical symptoms and management of rectourethral fistulas after radical prostatectomy. J Urol. 2010;183:608–12.
10. Smith AM, Veenema RJ. management of rectal injury and rectourethral fistulas following RRP. J Urol. 1972;108:778.
11. Noldus J, Graefen M, Huland H. An "old technique" for a new approach for repair of rectourinary fistulas. J Urol. 1997;157:1547.
12. Castillo OA, Bodden EM, Vitagliano GJ, Gomez R. Anterior transanal, transsphincteric sagittal approach for fistula repair secondary to laparoscopic radical prostatectomy: a simple and effective technique. Urology. 2006;68:198–201.
13. Kleinberg L, Wallner K, Roy J, Zelefsky M, Arterbery VE, Fuks Z, et al. Treatment-related symptoms during the first year following transperineal 125I prostate implantation. Int J Radiat Oncol Biol Phys. 1994;28:985–90.
14. Zippe CD. Cryosurgery of the prostate: techniques and pitfalls. Urol Clin North Am. 1996;23:147–63.
15. Porter CR, Gamito EJ, Crawford ED, Bartsch G, Presti Jr JC, Tewari A, et al. Model to predict prostate biopsy outcome in large screening population with independent validation in referral setting. Urology. 2005;65:937–41.
16. Theodorescu D, Gillenwater JY, Koutrouvelis PG. Prostatourethral-rectal fistula after prostate brachytherapy. Cancer. 2000;89:2085–91.
17. Roberts WB, Tseng K, Walsh PC, Han M. Critical appraisal of management of rectal injury during radical prostatectomy. Urology. 2010;76:1088–91.
18. Santoro GA, Bucci L, Frizelle FA. Management of rectourethral fistulas in Crohn's disease. Int J Colorectal Dis. 1995;10:183–8.
19. Rivera R, Barboglio P, Helinger M, Gousse A. Staging of rectourinary fistulas to guide surgical treatment. J Urol. 2006;68(suppl 5A).
20. Nyam DCNK, Pemberton JH. Management of iatrogenic rectourethral fistula. Dis Colon Rectum. 1999;42:994–9.
21. Shin PR, Foley E, Steers WD. Surgical management of rectourinary fistulae. J Am Coll Surg. 2000;191:547–53.
22. Kim SM, Chang HK, Lee MJ, Shim KW, Oh JT, Kim DS, et al. Spinal dysraphism with anorectal malformation: lumbosacral magnetic resonance imaging evaluation of 120 patients. J Pediatr Surg. 2010;45:769–76.
23. Goodwin WE, Turner RD, Winter CC. Rectourinary fistula: principles of management and a technique of surgical closure. J Urol. 1958;80:246–54.
24. Kasraeian A, Rozet F, Cathelineau X, Barret E, Galiano M, Vallancien G. Modified York-Mason technique for repair of iatrogenic rectourinary fistula: the Montsouris experience. J Urol. 2009;181:1178–83.
25. Wilhelm SF. Treatment of recto-urethral and recto-vesical fistula. J Urol. 1945;53:719–22.
26. Culp OS, Calhoon HW. A variety of rectourethral fistulas: experience with 20 cases. J Urol. 1964;91:560.
27. Stephenson RA, Middleton RG. Repair of rectourinary fistulas using posterior sagittal transanal transrectal (modified York-Mason) approach: an update. J Urol. 1996;155:198.
28. Crippa A, Dalloglio MF, Nesrallah LJ, Hasegawa E, Antunes AA, Strougi M. The York-Mason technique for recto-urethral fistulas. Clinics (Sao Paulo). 2007;62:699–704.
29. Munoz M, Nelson H, Harrington J. Management of acquired rectourinary fistulas: outcome according to cause. Dis Colon Rectum. 1998;41:1230–8.
30. Lane BR, Stein DE, Remzi FH, Strong SA, Fazio VW, Angermeier KW. Management of radiotherapy induced rectourethral fistula. J Urol. 2006;175:1382–7.
31. Sotelo R, Mirandolino M, Trujillo G, Garcia A, de Andrade R, Carmona O, et al. Laparoscopic repair of rectourethral fistulas after prostate surgery. Urology. 2007;70:515–8.
32. Young HH, Stone HB. The operative treatment of recto-urethral fistula. Presentation of a method of radical cure. J Urol. 1917;1:289.
33. Zmora O, Potenti FM, Wexner SD, Pikarsky AJ, Efron JE, Nogueras JJ, et al. Gracilis muscle transposition for iatrogenic rectourethral fistula. Ann Surg. 2003;237:483–7.
34. Rabau M, Zmora O, Tulchinsky H, Gur E, Goldman G. Rectovaginal/urethral fistula: repair with gracilis muscle transposition. Acta Chir Iugosl. 2006;53:81–4.
35. Elliot SP, McAninch JW, Chi T, Doyle SM, Master VA. Management of severe urethral complications of prostate cancer therapy. J Urol. 2006;176:2508–13.
36. Varma MG, Wang JY, Garcia-Aguilar J, Shelton AA, McAninch JW, Goldberg SM. Dartos muscle interposition flap for the treatment of rectourethral fistulas. Dis Colon Rectum. 2007;50:1849–55.
37. Gupta G, Kumar S, Kekre NS, Gopalakrishnan G. Surgical management of rectourethral fistula. Urology. 2008;71:267–71.
38. Ghoniem G, Elmissiry M, Weiss E, Langford C, Abdelwahab H, Wexner S. Transperineal repair of complex rectourethral fistula using gracilis muscle flap interposition – can urinary and bowel functions be preserved. J Urol. 2008;179:1882–6.
39. Wexner SD, Ruiz DE, Genua J, Nogueras JJ, Weiss EG, Zmora O. Gracilis muscle interposition for the treatment of rectourethral, rectovaginal, and pouch-vaginal fistulas: results in 53 patients. Ann Surg. 2008;248:39–43.
40. Nerli R, Amarkhed SS, Hiremath MB. Vascularized tunica vaginalis interposition flap for the treatment of recto-urethral fistulas. Indian J Urol. 2009;25:467–9.
41. Lewis LG. Repair of recto-urethral fistulas. J Urol. 1947;57:1173–83.
42. Gecelter L. Transanorectal approach to the posterior urethra and bladder neck. J Urol. 1973;109:1011–6.
43. Vose SN. A technique for the repair of recto-urethral fistula. J Urol. 1949;61:790.
44. Latzko W. Postoperative vesicovaginal fistulas. Am J Surg. 1942;58:211.
45. Parks AG, Motson RW. Peranal repair of rectoprostatic fistula. Br J Surg. 1983;70:725.
46. Al-Ali M, Kashmoula D, Saoud IJ. Experience with 30 post traumatic rectourethral fistulas: presentation of posterior transsphincteric anterior rectal wall advancement. J Urol. 1997;158:421–4.
47. Dreznik Z, Alper D, Vishne TH, Ramadan E. Rectal flap advancement – a simple and effective approach for the treatment of rectourethral fistula. Colorectal Dis. 2003;5:53–5.
48. Garofalo TE, Delaney CP, Jones SM, Remzi FH, Fazio VW. Rectal advancement flap repair of rectourethral fistula: a 20-year experience. Dis Colon Rectum. 2003;46:762–9.
49. Razi A, Yahyazadeh SR, Gilani MA, Kazemeyni SM. Transanal repair of rectourethral and rectovaginal fistulas. Urol J. 2008;5(2):111–4.

50. Joshi HM, Vimalachandran D, Heath RM, Rooney PS. Management of iatrogenic recto-urethral fistula by transanal rectal flap advancement. Colorectal Dis. 2011;13(8):918–20.
51. Bochove-Overgaauw DM, Beerlage HP, Bosscha K, Gelderman WAH. Transanal endoscopic microsurgery for correction of rectourethral fistulae. J Endourol. 2006;20(12):1087–90.
52. Andrews EJ, Royce P, Farmer KC. Transanal endoscopic microsurgery (TEM) repair of rectourethral fistula after high intensity focused ultrasound (HIFU) ablation of prostate cancer. Colorectal Dis. 2011;13:342–3.
53. Kilkpatrick FR, Mason AY. Post-operative recto-prostatic fistula. Br J Urol. 1969;41:649–54.
54. Wood TW, Middleton RG. Single-stage transrectal transphincteric (modified York-Mason) repair of rectourinary fistulas. Urology. 1990;35:27–30.
55. Bukowski TP, Chakrabarty A, Powell IJ, Frontera R, Perlmutter AD, Montie JE. Acquired rectourethral fistula: methods of repair. J Urol. 1995;153:730–3.
56. Boushey RP, McLeod RS, Cohen Z. Surgical management of acquired rectourethral fistula, emphasizing the posterior approach. Can J Surg. 1998;41:241–4.
57. Renschler TD, Middleton RG. 30 years of experience with York-Mason repair of recto-urinary fistulas. J Urol. 2003;170:1222–5.
58. Barisic GI, Krivokapic ZV. Long term results of surgically treated traumatic rectourethral fistulas. Colorectal Dis. 2006;8:762–5.
59. Pera M, Alonso S, Pares D, Lorente JA, Bielsa O, Pascual M, et al. Treatment of rectourethral fistula after radical prostatectomy by York Mason posterior trans-sphincter exposure. Cir Esp. 2008;84:323–7.
60. Mason AY. Surgical access to the rectum – a trans-sphincteric exposure. Proc R Soc Med Suppl. 1970;63:91.
61. Mason AY. The place of local resection in the treatment of rectal carcinoma. Proc R Soc Med. 1970;63:1259.
62. Oh C, Kark AE. The trans-sphincteric approach to mid and low rectal villous adenoma: anatomic basis of surgical treatment. Ann Surg. 1972;176:605–12.
63. Mason AY, Kilpatrick FR. Rectoprostatic and rectourethral fistulae. Proc R Soc Med. 1973;66:245–6.
64. Kilpatrick FR, Thompson HR. Post-operative rectoprostatic fistula and closure by Kraske's approach. Br J Urol. 1962;34:470–4.
65. Abdalla MA. Posterior sagittal pararectal approach with rectal mobilization for repair of rectourethral fistula: an alternative approach. Urology. 2009;73:1110–4.
66. Dolay K, Aras B, Tugcu V, Ozbay B, Aygun E, Tasci AI. Combined treatment of iatrogenic RUF with endoscopic fibrin glue application and clipping. J Endourol. 2007;21:433–6.
67. Bhandari Y, Khandkar A, Chaudhary A, Srimali P, Desai D, Srinivas V. Post-radical prostatectomy rectourethral fistula: endoscopic management. Urol Int. 2008;81:474–6.
68. Verriello V, Altomare M, Masielo G, Curatolo C, Balacco G, Altomare DF. Treatment of post-prostatectomy rectourethral fistula with fibrin sealant(Quixil) injection: a novel application. Tech Coloproctol. 2010;14:341–3.
69. Lesser T, Aboseif S, Abbas MA. Combined endorectal advancement flap with Alloderm graft repair of radiation and cryoablation-induced rectourethral fistula. Am Surg. 2008;74:341–5.

第 40 章　复发性肛裂的个体化治疗

Jonathan N. Lund

李　鹏 译　李国逊 审校

摘　要

判断患者是否需要手术，应关注侧方肛门内括约肌切断术的控便效果。在确定需要手术后，有持续性症状肛裂患者的风险控制尤为重要。本章概述了当常规手术失败时，保留肛门括约肌的各种外科治疗方法。

关键词

复发性肛裂；非手术治疗；括约肌切断术；指南；硝酸盐；钙通道阻滞剂；高纤维；硝酸甘油（GTN）；侧方内括约肌切断术（LIS）；肉毒杆菌毒素

引　言

肛裂是远端肛管皮肤层的裂伤，是一种常见病，欧洲约有一百万例患者，在青壮年中更常见。肛裂常发生于分娩后，也可能由复杂性克罗恩病及其他情况引起。肛裂在排便时会引起剧痛，经常被描述为"像是在排泄碎玻璃"，便后肛门处往往有 2～3h 的烧灼感。此外，排便时可能会有少量的鲜血流出。肛裂对生活质量的负面影响显而易见 [1]。

治疗的目的是缓解症状并治愈肛裂。绝大多数治疗方法是依靠降低肛门内括约肌（IAS）的压力，此时溃疡面的血供也随之增加 [2-3]。通过调整饮食来软化大便可以辅助缓解症状；治愈后，高纤维饮食能减少复发概率 [4]。

所有的治疗都不可能做到完全不复发，当准备治疗复发性肛裂时，最应该注意的是肛裂的类型、以前的治疗方法以及患者个体差异，而不仅仅是性别和生育史 [5]。

急性复发性肛裂

急性肛裂持续几天，症状在摄入纤维性食物后迅速缓解 [4]。然而，症状可能重新出现，一些患者会经历周期性过程，这时的治疗是建议维持足够的高纤维饮食，并外用药膏来松弛肛门括约肌以减轻疼痛 [5]。在欧洲和许多其他国家，硝酸甘油被用于减轻肛裂引起的疼痛，但是它会使少数患者产生头痛 [6-7]。钙通道阻滞剂能有效减轻疼痛并且不良反应很少，但目前没有得到使用许可 [8-11]。应考虑能引起急性肛裂的潜在疾病；便秘或腹泻会导致急性肛裂，一些引起溃疡和表皮脱落的情况也会导致急性肛裂。痔疮切除术后遗留的裂隙状创面可以被局部平滑肌松弛剂成功治愈。

慢性复发性肛裂

慢性肛裂没有明确的定义，但大多数学者认为超过6周的肛裂，伴或不伴有其慢性特征（可见的内括约肌纤维、前哨痔及肛乳头肥大），均为慢性肛裂[7,12,13]。如果病程持续很长时间的话，患者很可能会提供不可靠的病史，这导致了一些早期肛裂治疗随机实验的错误。在这些实验中，安慰剂的有效率一直很高[11]。慢性肛裂的治疗可以参考多种指南[5,14-16]，但普遍应用的是先采用局部用药的方法，无效再采用更具侵入性的方法。

局部治疗后未愈或复发的肛裂

经过几天至数周局部应用平滑肌松弛剂后，如硝酸盐、钙通道阻滞剂等，会使症状得到明显改善[6]，成功再上皮化的患者只有1/2~2/3[17]。有研究表明，患者外用硝酸甘油软膏3个月后能痊愈，这时肛管静息压力可达到预设值[18]。经过局部用药治疗治愈后有12%~57%的复发率[11,19,20]。

也许诊断和最初的治疗是在初级保健机构和其他类似的机构中，而那里没有专业的结直肠医生。需要从复发或未愈的患者身上采集病史，显著症状，疾病史（特别是能引起肛裂的其他疾病，如克罗恩病、结核、结节病、人类免疫缺陷病毒），用药史（众所周知，尼可地尔可以引起皮肤黏膜溃疡），其他原因引起的皮肤疾病（如坏疽性脓皮病），并且应该询问女性的生育史。检查时应该轻柔，轻轻分开臀部，在进行直肠指检或引起疼痛时应该安抚患者，将肛门分开，会发现在肛裂的下端是皮肤的裂伤。通过一些皮肤标志，可以判断为慢性肛裂，如肛裂边缘的硬结及可见的括约肌纤维的基底部。侧方肛裂不常见，若有应考虑其他潜在的疾病[7,13]。如果患者的病史或者肛裂的表现不常见，那么应在麻醉下进行检查，以便能充分查看，检查直肠黏膜，必要时取活检来排除直肠或肛管的肿瘤，这一步对于肛裂持续存在的老年患者尤为重要[5]。一旦判断没有引起肛裂的其他潜在性疾病，就应该和患者进行探讨，以进一步证实。

在肛裂复发的最初一段时间内没有症状，前期的治疗方案就有可能治愈[20]。许多患者，尤其是应用硝酸甘油软膏后出现头痛的患者，不能严格进行局部治疗。除了头痛，很多患者不能很好遵守一日两次用药的医嘱或者症状一减轻就停止治疗，导致了早期复发。所以，在局部治疗之前，应该告知患者药物潜在的不良反应，这样会提高他们忍受的程度，而向患者强调治疗过程要6~8周也是至关重要的。在这方面，Gagliardi等[21]最近的研究评估局部应用高剂量硝酸甘油软膏治疗慢性肛裂的短期和长期疗效，结果表明如果刚开始疗效欠佳，预示以后创面也不会很好愈合，应该放弃传统的治疗理念，尽早手术治疗。

应提供二线治疗方案供患者选择，如果头痛的不良反应一直存在，那么硝酸盐制剂应改为钙通道阻滞剂[9,17]；如果患者遵医嘱外用硝酸甘油软膏6~8周后仍然有症状，此时改用钙通道阻滞剂可能会有改善，仅有1/10的患者会因此痊愈。其他的二线治疗方案，包括肉毒杆菌毒素、肉毒杆菌毒素联合肛裂切除术、侧方内括约肌切断术（LIS），而皮瓣移植需要考虑患者的个体情况和意愿。

侧方内括约肌切断术（LIS）后的失禁情况

内括约肌切断术是通过对内括约肌造成永久性损伤使肛门静息压力降低，正是这一关键作用能有效治疗慢性肛裂，疼痛常在2周内消失，治愈率约为95%左右，复发率为1/20[13]。术后尿失禁的发生率经常被高估和低估，幸运的是术后很少见到大便失禁，但是LIS后失禁病例经常被报道。有些外科医生声明从没有患者在LIS后说有过失禁，这很可能是由于医生没有以正确的方式向患者提出正确的问题，一份来自美国俄亥俄州克利夫兰诊所的报告很好地说明了这一点[22]。一项评估LIS后患者显著症状的回顾性分析表明，不能控制排气的仅有4.4%，大便失禁的占2.8%。而来自同一批患者的匿名问卷调查结果则截然不同，术后不能控制排气的占31.5%，大便失禁的患者则高达28.7%；术后3个月这两项分别为30%和8%。患者诉说这些症状时有些尴尬，而且他们普遍希望取悦他们的外科医生。失禁必然导致生活质量的下降[23-24]。

妇女LIS术后尿失禁的风险高于男性[22]，因为分娩是导致内括约肌损伤的重要机制。分娩后的妇女出现尿失禁的比例很高，35%~40%有内括约肌损伤的证据[25]。较长的第二产程、产钳助产、撕裂或侧切都会增加括约肌损伤的风险。此外，妇女的肛门内括约肌比男子短，而不恰当选用 LIS 造成括约肌的损伤所占比例更高[12, 26]。在决定对一位女性患者施行 LIS 之前一定要仔细分析，并且应该让患者充分了解尿失禁的影响以及替代疗法，这样她们就能比较这些方法与 LIS 的优劣。这个问题有法医学的意义，并且在本书的其他部分也有提及。如果有产科创伤的病史或者存在失禁症状，那么评估括约肌的形态和功能，并测量肛管静息压力能提供有用信息。相同的原则也适用于直肠肛管前壁的肛裂手术，产妇很可能有固有的隐匿性肛门外疾病[27]。我们应该意识到，慢性肛裂术后轻度尿失禁的发生率达到了 28%[28]，出于类似的原因，伴有腹泻型肠易激综合征及其他疾病的患者应仔细考虑 LIS 的利与弊。

尽管有以上原则，但对慢性肛裂（顽固性或局部用药后复发）来说 LIS 仍然是简单有效的治疗方案。由于 LIS 后有发生轻度尿失禁的风险，必须有备选方案并提供给患者参考[29]。

肉毒杆菌毒素

肉毒杆菌毒素是人类已知的毒性最强的物质，它是一种神经毒素，与突触前胆碱能受体结合，造成神经末梢受损而阻断传导，直至大约 3 个月后神经末梢重新生长才能恢复[13, 30]。自 20 世纪 90 年代初以来，已被用来作为一个长效的、"可逆的"内括约肌切断术，让肛门压力降低，血液供应增加，有效期达 3 个月[31-33]，并发症罕见，报道过的有血肿、肛周感染以及极少见的长期大小便失禁[34]。

如果局部治疗失败或局部治疗后复发，可以考虑用肉毒杆菌毒素，特别对女性患者更有效。常用剂量是 50IU，虽然不清楚最佳注射部位（肛门内括约肌或肛门外括约肌），不过括约肌内的注射点应该没有什么差别，因为它的作用是松解肌环。尽管肉毒杆菌毒素效果明显，然而有荟萃分析显示，对于慢性肛裂，肉毒杆菌毒素与安慰剂没有任何差别[35]。肉毒杆菌毒素能加强括约肌切除术的效果（使肛裂有新鲜的边缘和易于刮除的基底部），有很高的初始治愈率，但是复发率也很高，在第一年甚至高达 50%[36-38]。当考虑括约肌切断术很可能会导致排便失禁时，就应该考虑选用这种方法。

侧方内括约肌切断术（LIS）后未愈或复发

侧方内括约肌切断术（LIS）后未愈或复发很少见，二者的发生率最多为 5%。导致侧方内括约肌切断术后肛裂未愈的最常见原因是手术时切除不完全。Farouk 等[39] 应用腔内超声检查 LIS 后未愈的患者，发现绝大多数患者的内括约肌仍然完好无损，没有被切断，显然手术中被认为已经切断了，因此 LIS 应该由经验丰富的外科医师来操作。由于 LIS 后大便失禁的关注度不断增加，外科医生对分离括约肌的长度越来越保守。有时切除少量括约肌也能降低肛门静息压，但肛裂不会愈合。应该记住的是，个体化 LIS 中切除内括约肌的数量基本上等于肛裂的长度。在这方面，个体化治疗方法（即括约肌切断术止于肛裂的顶点，而非齿状线）虽然能降低便失禁的发生率，但是复发或未愈率却很高[40-41]。这些研究使我们对括约肌切断术的不精确性产生了一些质疑，而且目前仍不清楚术前肛门测压为静息压力减低或者正常时[42]，能否作为精确括约肌切断术的适应证[43-44]。

如果腔内超声和肛门测压提示括约肌切断充分，那么就应该考虑是否有其他的潜在疾病[5]，应该再一次详问病史，找出与肛裂情况不同的特征；值得注意的是，药物也可以引起如同肛裂的损伤。应进行适当的检查以排除其他诊断，如麻醉下检查并取活检。如果损伤是由尼可地尔或坏疽性脓皮病引起的话，这样的检查会加重损伤[13]。如果发现这些潜在的原因，那么针对病因的治疗会使肛裂得到明显改善。低位直肠癌或肛管癌偶尔会引起类似肛裂的症状，但是麻醉下检查取活检能排除这些诊断。

如果没有发现潜在疾病，而且患者症状明显，那么应该根据肛门测压结果制定进一步的治疗方案；如果肛门静息压力很高，再次衡量症状缓解和便失禁并发症孰轻孰重，并告知患者，在征得患者同意后施行 LIS。如果静息压力低于正常，而且没有潜在疾病，肛周皮肤皮瓣移植就应列入治疗方案中。

皮瓣移植

低压肛管的复发性肛裂如果没有潜在性疾病，肛周皮肤的皮瓣移植是一种治疗方案[45-46]。V-Y 成形皮瓣移植技术很简单，但是由于距离肛门太近，偶尔也会失败。

结 论

肛裂复发后应注意以下关键点：

1. 排除其他潜在肿瘤疾病；
2. 达到症状缓解；
3. 避免失禁并发症，并根据个体情况来治疗慢性肛裂[47]。

由于大便失禁被高度关注，因此只有在局部治疗失败的情况下才考虑 LIS；即使施行手术，也呈现出保留括约肌的趋势[48]。在这种情况下存在一定的不确定性，传统 LIS 后功能可能会更差，仅有少量有用的数据帮助结直肠学家决定是否施行括约肌切除术及肛门成形术，这两种手术都有很低的失禁发生率，但是复发率较高。近来，有报道称简单肛裂切除术能成功解决问题，很少造成失禁的发生，但仍需要进一步的研究[49]。鉴于此情况下，局部治疗已经取得了一些成功，那么可控、随机、前瞻性研究的进行就有可能为是否手术治疗提供依据。在特殊的亚组中，局部治疗能否消除影响生活质量的症状才是评估是否要转为手术治疗的关键。这可能很容易理解，有早期肛裂的产妇患者、肛裂不是位于后正中位的患者、合并失禁的患者以及仍未手术的慢性肛裂患者都能从上述治疗方案中获益，即不用切断括约肌或者将括约肌损伤降至最小。

参考文献

1. Griffin N, Acheson AG, Tung P, Sheard C, Glazebrook C, Scholefield JH. Quality of life in patients with chronic anal fissure. Colorectal Dis. 2004;6:39–44.
2. Schouten WR, Briel JW, Auwerda JJ, Boerma MO. Anal fissure: new concepts in pathogenesis and treatment. Scand J Gastroenterol Suppl. 1996;218:78–81.
3. Schouten WR, Briel JW, Auwerda JJ, De Graaf EJ. Ischaemic nature of anal fissure. Br J Surg. 1996;83:63–5.
4. Jensen SL. Maintenance therapy with unprocessed bran in the prevention of acute anal fissure recurrence. J R Soc Med. 1987;80:296–8.
5. Lund JN, Nyström PO, Coremans G, Herold A, Karaitianos I, Spyrou M, et al. An evidence-based treatment algorithm for anal fissure. Tech Coloproctol. 2006;10:177–80.
6. Lund JN, Scholefield JH. A randomised, prospective, double-blind, placebo-controlled trial of glyceryl trinitrate ointment in treatment of anal fissure. Lancet. 1997;349(9044):11–4.
7. Lindsey I, Jones OM, Cunningham C, Mortensen NJ. Chronic anal fissure. Br J Surg. 2004;91:270–9.
8. Cook TA, Humphreys MM, McC Mortensen NJ. Oral nifedipine reduces resting anal pressure and heals chronic anal fissure. Br J Surg. 1999;86:1269–73.
9. Ezri T, Susmallian S. Topical nifedipine vs. topical glyceryl trinitrate for treatment of chronic anal fissure. Dis Colon Rectum. 2003;46:805–8.
10. Madoff RD, Fleshman JW. AGA technical review on the diagnosis and care of patients with anal fissure. Gastroenterology. 2003;124:235–45.
11. Nelson R. Non surgical therapy for anal fissure. Cochrane Database Syst Rev. 2006;(4):CD003431
12. Lund JN, Scholefield JH. Aetiology and treatment of anal fissure. Br J Surg. 1996;83:1335–44.
13. Collins EE, Lund JN. A review of chronic anal fissure management. Tech Coloproctol. 2007;11:209–23.
14. American Gastroenterological Association medical position statement. Diagnosis and care of patients with anal fissure. Gastroenterology. 2003;124:233–4.
15. Cross KL, Massey EJ, Fowler AL, Monson JR. The management of anal fissure: ACPGBI position statement. Colorectal Dis. 2008;10 Suppl 3:1–7.
16. Perry WBD, Sharon L, Buie DW, Rafferty JF. On behalf of the Standards Practice Task Force of the American Society of Colon and Rectal Surgeons. Practice Parameters for the Management of Anal Fissures (3rd Revision). Dis Colon Rectum. 2010;53:1110–5.
17. Nelson R. Anal fissure (chronic). Clin Evid (Online). 2007;pii:0407.
18. Lund JN, Scholefield JH. Internal sphincter spasm in anal fissure. Br J Surg. 1997;84:1723–4.
19. AbdElhady HM, Othman IH, Hablus MA, Ismail TA, Aboryia MH, Selim MF. Long-term prospective randomised clinical and manometric comparison between surgical and chemical sphincterotomy for treatment of chronic anal fissure. S Afr J Surg. 2009;47:112–4.
20. Lund JN, Scholefield JH. Follow-up of patients with chronic anal fissure treated with topical glyceryl trinitrate. Lancet. 1998;352(9141):1681.
21. Gagliardi G, Pascariello A, Altomare DF, Arcanà F, Cafaro D, La Torre F, et al. Optimal treatment of glyceryl trinitrate (GTN) for chronic anal fissure (CAF): results of a prospective randomized trial. Tech Coloproctol. 2010;14:241–8.
22. Casillas S, Hull TL, Zutshi M, Trzcinski R, Bast JF, Xu M. Incontinence after a lateral internal sphincterotomy: are we underestimating it? Dis Colon Rectum. 2005;48:1193–9.
23. Hyman N. Incontinence after lateral internal sphincterotomy: a prospective study and quality of life assessment. Dis Colon Rectum. 2004;47:35–8.
24. Menteş BB, Tezcaner T, Yilmaz U, Leventoğlu S, Oguz M. Results of lateral internal sphincterotomy for chronic anal fissure with particular reference to quality of life. Dis Colon Rectum. 2006;49:1045–51.
25. Sultan AH, Kamm MA, Hudson CN, Thomas JM, Bartram CI. Anal-sphincter disruption during vaginal delivery. N Engl J Med. 1993;329:1905–11.
26. Sultan AH, Kamm MA, Nicholls RJ, Bartram CI. Prospective study of the extent of internal anal sphincter division during lateral sphincterotomy. Dis Colon Rectum. 1994;37:1031–3.
27. Zbar AP, Aslam M, Allgar V. Faecal incontinence after internal sphincterotomy for anal fissure. Techn Coloproctol. 2000;4:25–8.
28. Ammari FF, Bani-Hani KE. Faecal incontinence in patients with anal fissure: a consequence of internal sphincterotomy or a feature of the condition? Surgeon. 2004;2:225–9.
29. Zbar A, Beer-Gabel M, Chiappa AC, Aslam M. Fecal incontinence after minor anorectal surgery. Dis Colon Rectum. 2001;44:1610–23.
30. Jost WH, Aoki KR. Botulinum toxin A in anal fissure: why does it work? Dis Colon Rectum. 2004;47:257–8.
31. Jost WH, Schimrigk K. Use of botulinum toxin in anal fissure. Dis Colon Rectum. 1993;36:974.
32. Jost WH. Ten years' experience with botulin toxin in anal fissure. Int J Colorectal Dis. 2002;17:298–302.
33. Brisinda G, Cadeddu F, Brandara F, Marniga G, Maria G. Randomized clinical trial comparing botulinum toxin injections

34. Brown SR, Matabudul Y, Shorthouse AJ. A second case of long-term incontinence following botulinum injection for anal fissure. Colorectal Dis. 2006;8:452–3.
35. Nelson R. Anal fissure (chronic). Clin Evid (Online). 2010;pii:0407.
36. Baraza W, Boereboom C, Shorthouse A, Brown S. The long-term efficacy of fissurectomy and botulinum toxin injection for chronic anal fissure in females. Dis Colon Rectum. 2008;51:239–43.
37. Mousavi SR, Sharifi M, Mehdikhah Z. A comparison between the results of fissurectomy and lateral internal sphincterotomy in the surgical management of chronic anal fissure. J Gastrointest Surg. 2009;13:1279–82.
38. Witte ME, Klaase JM, Koop R. Fissurectomy combined with botulinum toxin A injection for medically resistant chronic anal fissures. Colorectal Dis. 2010;12:e163–9.
39. Farouk R, Monson JRT, Duthie GS. Technical failure of lateral sphincterotomy for the treatment of chronic anal fissure: a study using endoanal ultrasonography. Br J Surg. 2005;84:84–5.
40. Littlejohn DR, Newstead GL. Tailored lateral sphincterotomy for anal fissure. Dis Colon Rectum. 1997;40:1439–42.
41. Menteş BB, Ege B, Leventoglu S, Oguz M, Karadag A. Extent of lateral internal sphincterotomy: up to the dentate line or up to the fissure apex? Dis Colon Rectum. 2005;48:365–70.
42. Bove A, Balzano A, Perrotti P, Antropoli C, Lombardi G, Pucciani F. Different anal pressure profiles in patients with anal fissure. Techn Coloproctol. 2004;8:151–7.
43. Mentes BB, Güner MK, Leventoglu S, Akyürek N. Fine-tuning of the extent of lateral internal sphincterotomy: spasm-controlled vs. up to the fissure apex. Dis Colon Rectum. 2008;51:128–33.
44. Rosa G, Lolli P, Piccinelli D, Mazzola F, Zugni C, Ballarin A, et al. Calibrated lateral internal sphincterotomy for fissure. Techn Coloproctol. 2005;9:127–32.
45. Giordano P, Gravante G, Grondona P, Ruggiero B, Porrett T, Lunniss PJ. Simple cutaneous advancement flap anoplasty for resistant chronic anal fissure: a prospective study. World J Surg. 2009;33:1058–63.
46. Patti R, Fama F, Tornambe A, Restivo M, Di Vita G. Early results of fissurectomy and advancement flap for resistant chronic anal fissure without hypertonia of the internal anal sphincter. Am Surg. 2010;76:206–10.
47. Pascual M, Pares D, Pera M, Courtier R, Gil MJ, Puig S, et al. Variation in clinical, manometric and endosonographic findings in anterior chronic anal fissure: a prospective study. Dig Dis Sci. 2008;53:21–6.
48. Zbar AP. Sphincter-sparing surgical alternatives for chronic anal fissure: the place of fissurotomy. Dis Colon Rectum. 2008;51:1299.
49. Pelta AE, Davis KG, Armstrong DN. Subcutaneous fissurotomy: a novel procedure for chronic fissure-in-ano. A review of 109 cases. Dis Colon Rectum. 2007;50:1662–7.

第 41 章 肛管狭窄的肛管皮肤填补术

Jennifer Blumetti · Herand Abcarian
李淑媛 译　王西墨 审校

摘　要

肛管狭窄虽不常见，但令人苦恼。本章主要介绍肛管狭窄的手术方法。肛管狭窄病因为肛门上皮切除过多，最常见于痔切除术后，也可发生于肛门尖锐湿疣或 Buschke-Loewenstein 癌的切除术后。在过去几年里，针对严重或高位的肛管狭窄，外科手术从简单的括约肌切开发展为复杂的皮瓣成形术。

关键词

肛管狭窄；肛管；肛门上皮；瘢痕；痔切除术；狭窄缓解；括约肌切开术；黏膜皮瓣推移；Y-V 肛门成形术；菱形皮瓣；U 形皮瓣；房式皮瓣；S 成形

引　言

肛管狭窄非常少见[1-2]，定义为肛管上皮被瘢痕或结缔组织替代并导致其收缩，从而导致肛管异常的狭窄[3]。肛管上皮的缺失是瘢痕和狭窄形成的主要原因[2,4]。肛管上皮瘢痕形成的任何原因均可导致肛管狭窄[1]，最常见于肛门直肠术后，尤其是痔除术[1,5-10]，发病率在 5%～10%[11]。一项研究表明，痔切除术后肛管狭窄的发病率高达 87%[12]。肛管狭窄也可发生在其他需广泛切除肛管上皮的肛门直肠手术（表 41.1）[1,2,4-6,13-16]。

肛管狭窄的症状在表 41.2 中列出[1,4,12-14,17,18]。肛管狭窄通过体格检查即可确诊。指肛检查时，排除不适和疼痛导致的肛管收缩，手指不能通过肛管即可确诊[3-4]。患者不适可导致检查不充分，因此，为了诊断肛管狭窄常需在麻醉状态下，并且麻醉状态下检查能够区分功能性狭窄和真性狭窄。功能性狭窄在麻醉状态下可缓解，但是由瘢痕组织导致的真性狭窄在麻醉状态下仍不能缓解[1]。

表 41.1　导致肛管狭窄的原因

肛肠手术
痔切除术 /whitehead 痔切除术
肛管或回肠肛管吻合口狭窄
低位直肠肿瘤切除术
尖锐湿疣广泛的清创术或电灼术
Paget 病或 Bowen 病的广泛切除术
创伤
炎症性肠病
辐射
感染
性传播疾病
肺结核
慢性泻药滥用
肿瘤
先天性畸形

需根据狭窄的严重程度和部位对肛管狭窄进行治疗。Milson 和 Mazier[12] 对肛管狭窄进行了分类（表 41.3）。对于轻度的和低位的肛管狭窄，可采用球囊

或手指或扩肛器等扩肛[1,4,15]。但是很少有研究证实肛管扩张对肛管狭窄治疗的有效性[1]。对于严重的和高位的肛管狭窄，需外科手术干预。过去的几年里，手术方法已经从简单的括约肌切开术发展为复杂的皮瓣成形术。本章主要介绍各种手术方法和其适应证。

表 41.2　肛管狭窄的症状

便秘
大便变细
排便困难
排便不尽
里急后重
腹泻
出血
肛门渗液和潮湿（伴随黏膜外翻时）

表 41.3　肛管狭窄的分级

根据严重程度分级：	根据位置分级：
轻度：手指或 Hill Ferguson 扩张器可以完成肛门检查	低位：狭窄边缘距离齿状线至少 0.5 cm
中度：需要扩张后才能用手指或者 Hill Ferguson 扩张器完成肛门检查	中位：狭窄边缘在齿状线上下 0.5 cm 范围内
重度：除非大力扩张，否则不能用手指或者 Hill Ferguson 扩张器完成肛门检查	高位：狭窄边缘高十齿状线 0.5 cm

术前准备和术后护理

对于大多数患者来说，很多患者不能耐受在门诊进行检查，因此需行最简单的术前检查。在大部分患者，肛管狭窄与前次手术相关，并且行肛管皮肤修复术后会发生肛门失禁。因此许多医师术前行肛管测压和经直肠超声检查。Gonzalez 等[17]对 17 例患者中的 14 例患者进行了肛管测压，79% 的患者肛管静息压和收缩压正常。剩余的 3 例患者因疼痛而无法耐受肛管测压。同样因为疼痛，只有 9 例患者进行了直肠超声检查，78% 的患者超声检查正常。尽管只有一半患者进行了术前检查，但研究者认为大部分患者术前不需行肛管测压和直肠超声检查，而术前伴随有括约肌缺陷或神经损伤的患者需行检查。

麻醉状态下检查非常重要，并且对术前评估很有意义[1,13,17]。麻醉状态下，检查者可充分评估肛管狭窄的严重程度和范围，并能对狭窄部位取活检。大多数肛管狭窄的患者不需取活检，但是有尖锐湿疣、Pgaet 病或 Bowen 病、肿瘤或 Crohn 病行直肠肛管手术史的患者，必须取活检获得病理以明确肛管狭窄的病因。麻醉状态下检查还可以鉴别因瘢痕形成造成的功能性狭窄[1]。

一旦诊断为重度狭窄，非手术治疗对改善患者症状无效，需手术治疗。术前准备相同。如果患者可以耐受，最好行全肠道准备或术前 1 天灌肠。对不能耐受的患者，术中需行直肠灌洗。

术后期间，所有接受肛管狭窄手术的患者均需预防便秘以促进伤口愈合[4-6,9,11,18]。术后 2~5 天，患者需流质饮食。近来的许多研究认为，术后并不需要流质饮食[1,2,13,19,20]，患者可采用高纤维饮食联合服用大便软化剂或溶剂性泻药即可。术后 2 天，根据患者的手术范围和对疼痛的控制力，患者可出院。

手术方案

肛管狭窄的手术治疗方案有很多种，由于缺乏相互间的比较，没有一种手术治疗方案被认为是理想的。根据 Angelchik 等[21]，理想的手术方案为："最小的并发症发生率，良好的患者耐受，技术操作简单和理想的远期效果。"

下面讲述的手术方案均是在折刀卧位下进行的，需用臀垫进行更好的暴露并留出足够的皮肤行皮瓣游离。围术期需放置 Foley 导尿管并应用抗生素。尽管全麻可以维持更长的手术时间，但大部分患者仍采用局麻。局麻药物里含稀释的肾上腺素，可以减少出血。需用无菌记号笔仔细的标记切口线并保证足够的皮瓣游离。

皮瓣前移术

黏膜皮瓣前移术与 1944 年首次报道的 Martin 手术相似或经过改良，已在肛管狭窄的治疗中应用[3,14,18,22,23]。手术包括切除瘢痕组织、内括约肌切开术以及远端直肠黏膜前移，并将其缝至齿状线。

最初，采用 Khubchandani 技术（采用侧向皮瓣前移）[3]，皮瓣均取自后 1/4 象限[22-23]。一般从侧面与齿状线垂直切开瘢痕，一直到肛外缘。切除瘢痕后，行远端的内括约肌切开术。横行切口游离2~5cm长黏膜皮瓣。将皮瓣横向缝合至括约肌间沟，应该避免黏膜外翻。肛周皮肤遗留的小切口可通过二次手术愈合。Khubchandani 报道[3]，采用这种手术方案，有82%的患者取得了良好的效果。其他研究报道，90%的患者取得的良好效果，仅10%的患者需再次手术[15]。黏膜皮瓣前移术的优点是，并发症率低（研究报道仅3%[15]），与皮肤皮瓣相比，肛周伤口小。采用侧向皮瓣可以避免锁孔畸形。对于重度肛管狭窄，可采用双向皮瓣，单侧皮瓣手术失败的患者可采用对侧皮瓣[17]。大部分患者在术后当天可出院[17]。

这一手术方案的缺点是，技术要求比较高，并可导致黏膜外翻[24]。这一手术方案不适用于重度远端狭窄患者，其复发率可达20%[15]。对于远端重度肛管狭窄，可以采用黏膜前移肛门成形术辅助皮肤皮瓣前移术[16]。

Y-V 肛门成形术

Y-V 皮瓣成形采用的是带蒂皮瓣，是1944年由Penn 首先报道的。Gingold 和 Arvanitis 等[25]的手术技术为 Y 形切开，V 形缝合。Y 的底部是指中部切开，Y 的分叉是指侧面切开（图41.1）。这一技术必须仔细测量切口，因为皮瓣的基底部需长于皮瓣长度，以确保皮瓣足够的活动性及良好的血供。

必须小心的游离全层皮瓣避免皮瓣缺血。切口可做成放射状与狭窄垂直（图41.1b），然后行内括约肌切开术[11]。全层皮瓣分别按 Y 形缝合切口并不留创面（图41.1c）。根据肛管狭窄的严重程度，这一方案可选用单边或双边皮瓣成形。

Y-V 成形术的成功率为90%~100%[11, 25]。在一项对29例肛管狭窄患者行 Y-V 成形术的研究中报道，3例患者早期出现了皮瓣并发症，并导致了长时间的不良后果[11]。与其他手术相比，Y-V 成形术的优点是操作简单，并没有导致开放性伤口。其显著的缺点是，由于皮瓣固定于侧面，可使中间部皮瓣张力增高，进而导致皮瓣缺血坏死甚至回缩；此外，整个皮瓣的血供也不一致，可导致肛管顶部皮瓣的缺血和坏死[26]。这些并发症可导致再狭窄。Maria 研究报道[11]，远期效果不理想的患者，或者存在早期缝合裂开，或者存在皮瓣的缺血性挛缩。Angelchik 等发现[21]，与其他手术相比，由于挛缩、感染或顶端皮瓣坏死等并发症，Y-V 成形术只适用于中度的肛管狭窄。最适用于齿状线以下的低位肛管狭窄[1, 20]。

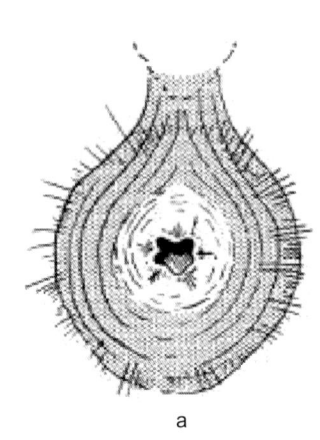
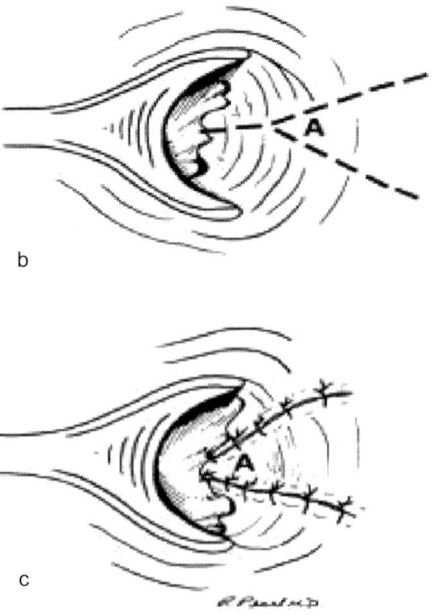

图41.1 Y-V 肛门成形术。(a) 肛管狭窄；(b) Y-V 肛门成形术时要注意从上至下切开的长度应大于或等于 Y 的两臂之间的长度；(c) 完成 Y-V 肛门成形术并缝合所有切口

菱形皮瓣成形术

菱形皮瓣成形术由 Caplin 和 Kodner 在 1986 年首先报道[5]。与前述的 Y-V 成形术不同，菱形皮瓣是在切口周围环形游离。因不受邻近皮肤限制，可使皮瓣前移到肛管治疗更高位的狭窄。这一技术以及其他类似技术均由于上述原因被称作岛状皮瓣[4]。首先瘢痕松解通过侧面的放射状切开进行。如果存在括约肌狭窄，切口必须深达括约肌，类似于括约肌切开术。这样造成的缺陷形状类似于菱形。此时，记号笔标记出菱形皮瓣，紧邻肛门的皮瓣应该与切口大小相同（图41.2a）。为避免皮瓣缺血，分离全层皮瓣时需仔细保护皮下血管蒂。皮瓣完全游离后，应确保足够的游离度保证与菱形切口的无张力吻合。菱形的后缘和取皮处也需缝合，不留伤口（图41.2b，c）。同其他手术方案一样，当单边皮瓣不能完全解除狭窄时可采用双边皮瓣。

Caplin 和 Kodner 为 7 例肛管狭窄患者成功实施了菱形皮瓣成形术[5]。Anderson 等对 8 名 1～5 岁肛管狭窄儿童的治疗取得了成功[26]，只有 1 例儿童出现皮瓣部分坏死，且不需再次手术治疗。儿童可采用扩张术治疗肛管狭窄并能取得不错的远期效果[26]。Maria 等[11] 对 13 例肛管狭窄患者实施了手术治疗。菱形皮瓣成形术没有出现伤口并发症，而 Y-V 成形术伤口并发症发生率为 10%。所有接受菱形皮瓣成形术的患者，术后 2 年内肛管狭窄症状完全缓解。因此，Maria 等认为菱形皮瓣成形术比 Y-V 成形术更适合于肛管狭窄患者。Pearl 等也成功应用了菱形皮瓣成形术，并且没有皮瓣缺血或感染[4]。

菱形皮瓣成形术的优点为，操作简单并且没有遗留开放伤口。由于皮瓣血供来自于深部皮下组织，皮瓣的缺血坏死较少发生[2, 20, 26]。在 Y-V 成形术失败后仍可采用这一技术[26]。菱形皮瓣的完全游离保证了无张力吻合[11, 20]，适用于低位或高位肛管狭窄。

U 形皮瓣

U 形皮瓣由 Pearl 等报道，最初用于治疗肛门狭窄和黏膜外翻[4]（图41.3）。U 形皮瓣也被认为是岛状皮瓣。这一手术包括切除括约肌的瘢痕。U 形

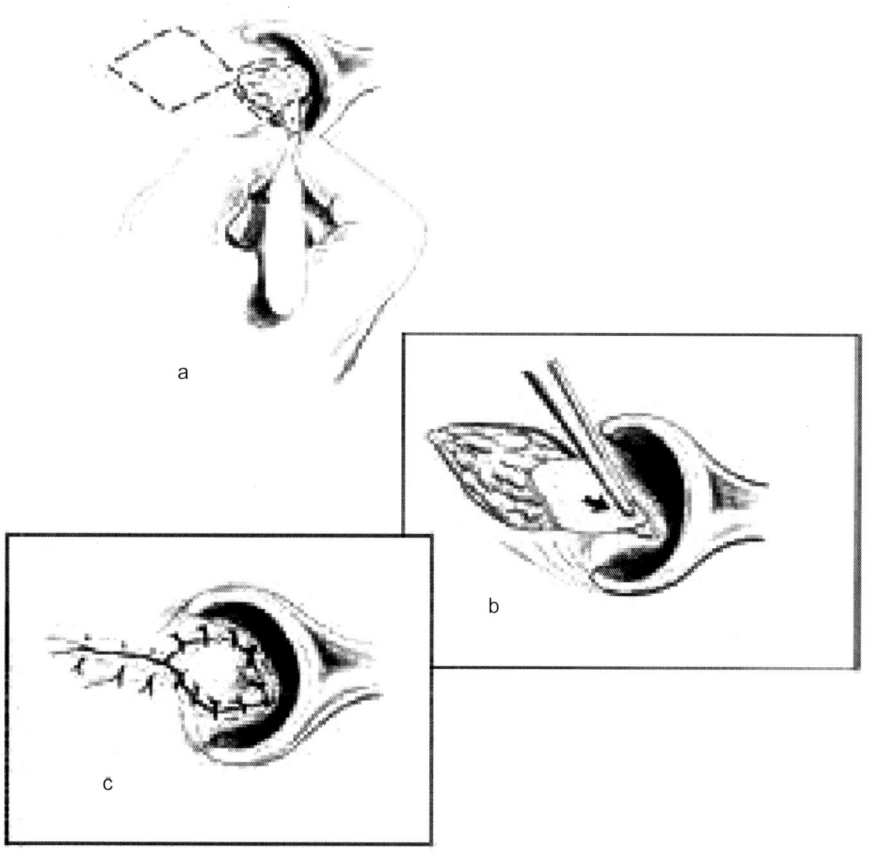

图 41.2 菱形皮瓣成形术。(a) 菱形皮瓣成形术的切开线，皮瓣前缘应于肛管缺损的大小相一致；(b) 将切开的皮瓣充分松解然后填入肛管的缺损处；(c) 完成菱形皮瓣成形术

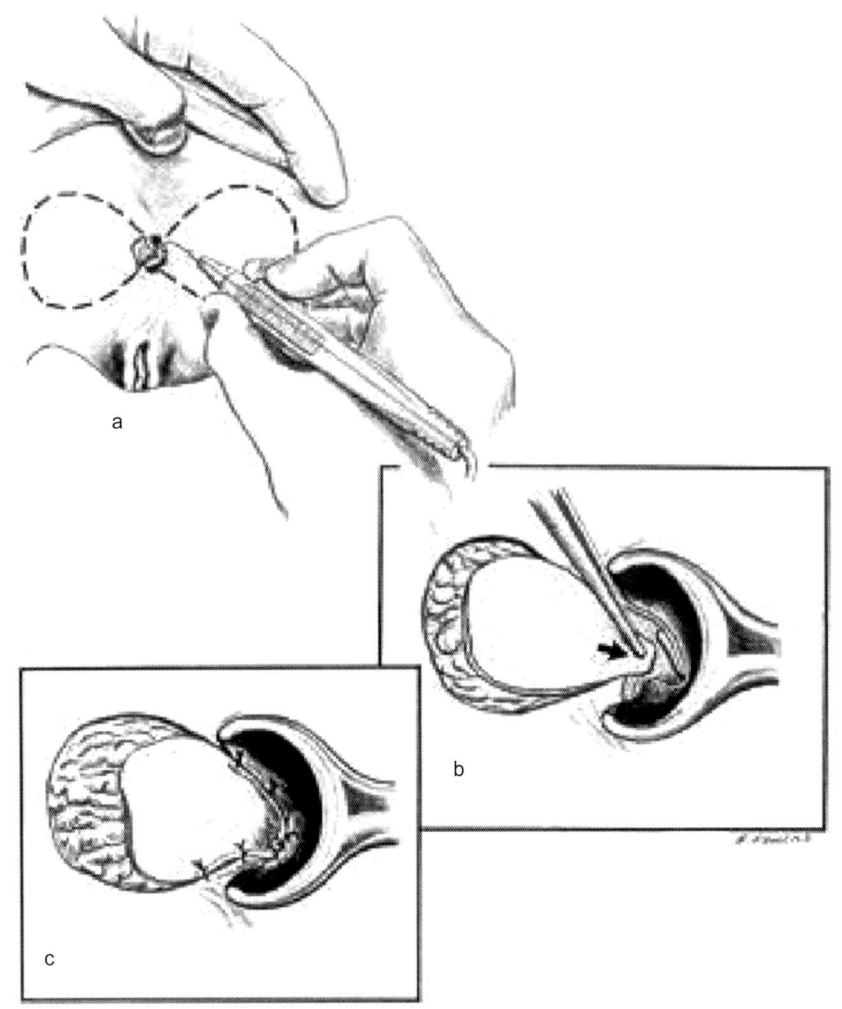

图 41.3　U 形皮瓣成形术。（a）设计双边 U 形皮瓣成形术的切口；（b）充分松解皮瓣使其能够覆盖缺损处；（c）将皮瓣妥善缝合固定。注意侧部供皮处的开放创口愈合需行二期手术

切开肛周皮肤和皮下组织，建立全层皮瓣，然后将皮瓣移入肛管并缝合（图 41.3a，b）。皮瓣处的愈合需行二次手术（图 41.3c）。Pearl 等报道 U 形皮瓣均没有缺血或感染，只有 2 例患者手术失败。一例因为回肠储袋吻合裂开导致的较长的肛管狭窄，U 形皮瓣不能达到储袋的黏膜处；另一例可能因为炎症性肠病继发的皮瓣边缘顽固性溃疡[4]。其他患者均恢复完好。

U 形皮瓣的优点是操作简单并且适合任何重度的肛管狭窄。U 形皮瓣成形术可用于 50% 环形狭窄的肛管狭窄并且能治疗重度和高位狭窄的黏膜外翻[1,4]。它也可使用双边皮瓣治疗环形狭窄（图 41.3a）。U 形皮瓣主要依靠皮下组织供血，因此能降低缺血的风险[16]。U 形皮瓣最大的缺陷是，与一期缝合的皮瓣相比，取皮瓣处的伤口，需要长时间的愈合。

房式皮瓣

为了避免其他手术的缺陷，Christensen 等发明了房式皮瓣[20]。房式皮瓣是矩形皮瓣（由 Sarner 在 1969 年发明[27]）和前述 Y-V 皮瓣的综合。当狭窄扩展到齿状线以上时可采用房式皮瓣。需从齿状线一直切开到狭窄远端。切开长度相当于皮瓣长度（图 41.4）。皮瓣需以切口为中心，距离并不能超过肛管狭窄周径的 25%。房式皮瓣的"屋顶"需与个壁大约相等。根据情况决定是否行内括约肌切开术。皮瓣可以完全游离并可轻松移入肛管内，然后缝合皮瓣及供皮瓣区。

房式皮瓣成功率在 89% ~ 100%[2,17,24,28]。一项研究发现，尽管 100% 患者术后能改善症状，但所有患者解剖缺陷的修整只有 50%[18]。Alver 等报道

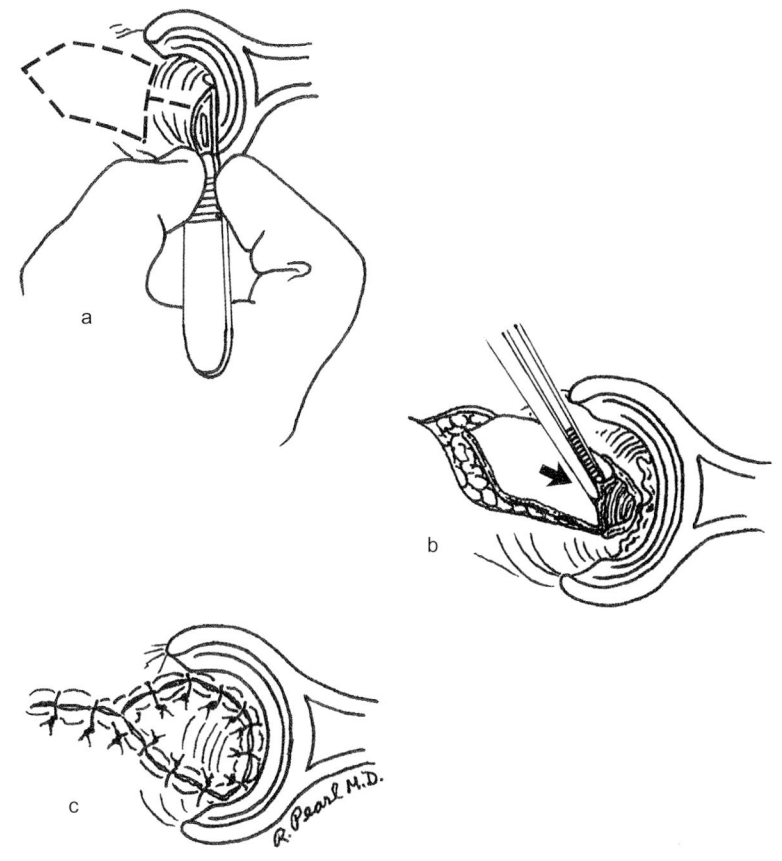

图 41.4 房式皮瓣成形术。（a）设计房式皮瓣成形术的切口；（b）充分松解房式皮瓣使其移入肛管；（c）妥善缝合固定皮瓣

28 例患者（包括各种直肠肛管疾病、瘘）成功进行了房式皮瓣成形术[24]。除 1 例患者发生直肠阴道瘘需 Martius 修复外，其他所有患者完全治愈。8 例肛管狭窄患者，治疗效果良好，但有 2 例伤口裂开需局部治疗[24]。

在少数的前瞻性研究中，Farid 等对 60 例患者进行了房式、菱形和 Y-V 皮瓣成形术的随机研究[2]。研究发现，房式皮瓣成形组达到了 90% 临床改善率，比菱形或 Y-V 皮瓣成形术高出很多（分别为 60% 和 30%）。患者的满意度和生活质量与临床改善相关。Farid 等认为，房式皮瓣整形术是首选的手术方式，唯一的缺陷是比其他手术方式手术时间长。

Christensen 等报道[20] 房式皮瓣的优点在于提供了一个广基的皮瓣，能够覆盖整个肛管，并可以一期愈合。作为一个岛状皮瓣，它的血供良好，并不依赖于皮瓣自身皮肤或黏膜桥的血管，因此很少发生缺血性并发症[1, 2, 13, 24]。还避免了过度游离组织并且操作简便[2, 24]。因为皮瓣足够长，它可用来治疗高位或长的齿状线以上的狭窄[1, 24, 28]。房式皮瓣的缺点是，手术时间较长，平均手术时间为 62min，而 Y-V 成形术手术时间为 35min[2]。单一的房式皮瓣只能覆盖 25% 肛管周径，尽管可采用双边皮瓣，但也只能覆盖 50% 肛管周径，因此对于严重的肛管狭窄，房式皮瓣成形术较少。

S-成形术

S-成形术是 Ferguson 于 1965 年报道的一种旋转皮瓣[5]。1973 年 Faulconer 和 Ferguson 再次报道并第一次应用于怀特海德法痔切除术后的肛管狭窄和黏膜外翻[7]。S-成形术是目前最复杂的手术方式（图 41.5）。手术以环形切除瘢痕开始，需将瘢痕从括约肌上分离（图 41.5a）。然后以环形切口为中心，仔细标记 S 形状的皮瓣。皮瓣需与切口等长或比切口更长（图 41.5b）。然后游离全层皮瓣并旋转向肛门，以便于上面的皮瓣与下面的切口缝合（图 41.5c, d）。Ferguson 最初报道的 S-成形术，为避免伤口的张力过大，皮瓣处皮肤缺损是敞开的。

在 Ferguson 最初的文章中，有 4 例患者成功实施了 S-成形术，仅在 1 例患者中出现了较小的皮瓣

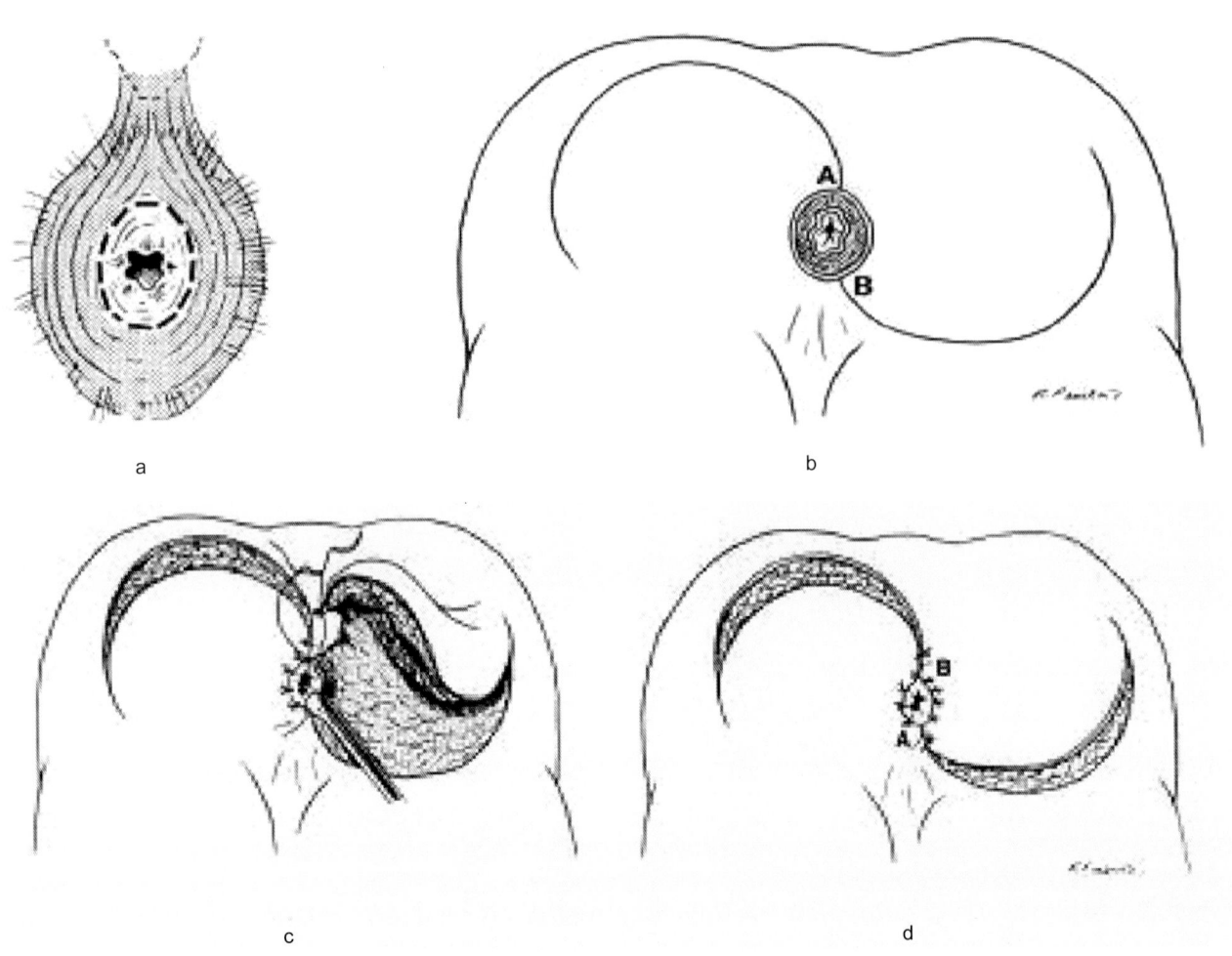

图 41.5 S- 成形术。(a) 设计狭窄或外翻部位的切除线（虚线所示）；(b) 设计 S- 成形术的切口。A 点至左侧边缘的距离是基于上面皮瓣的长度。注意这一距离应该长于上下两个皮瓣的高度；(c) 如图所示，松解游离下方的皮瓣，上方的皮瓣已完成；(d) 最终完成后的外观。注意上方皮瓣的尖端（A 点）被旋转缝合于创口的下部皮瓣侧，而下方皮瓣的尖端（B 点）则位于上方皮瓣侧。供皮处的缺损是敞开的，但是可以一期关闭

坏死，在没有任何干预措施下自行愈合。Faulconer 和 Ferguson 报道[7]，13 例患者中 12 例行 S- 成形术取得成功 (92%)，1 例患者因脓肿而需再次行 S- 成形术。其他发生皮瓣坏死的患者采用了保守治疗。据另一报道，6 例患者经 S- 成形术后获得了完全改善，而经房式成形术后的改善率仅 50%[18]。

S- 成形术最大的优势为，能够切除并覆盖大的缺损，如肛管狭窄合并整个肛管的外翻[1, 9, 16, 18]。S- 成形术主要的缺点是操作复杂，作为旋转皮瓣，其血供来源于附近组织，这可导致皮瓣收紧，导致缺血、坏死和裂开[18, 26]。因此，S- 成形术仅适用于最严重的高位狭窄或其他手术方式失败时[2]。

如何选择手术方式？

很少有前瞻性研究比较肛管狭窄的不同手术方式，并且没有任何一种手术方式能解决这一复杂问题。本章中所讲述的成功治疗肛管狭窄的手术方式既有明显优点，也有缺点。如前所述，理想的手术方式应该包括操作简单、良好的患者满意度和最小的并发症发生率[21]。每一患者均需选择特定的手术方式。这可根据 Milsm 和 Mazier[12] 的分类进行选

择（表 41.3）。一旦肛管狭窄分类完成，外科医生需选择手术方式。尽管有原则可做参考（表 41.4），但手术医师应根据自身熟悉的不同术式做出最终决定。

在笔者研究所，对于肛管狭窄，我们习惯首选 Pearl 等报道的 U 形皮瓣成形术[4]。U 形皮瓣成形术操作简单，可用于低位或高位狭窄，必要时还可以采用双边皮瓣。尽管皮瓣处伤口需二次干预才能愈合，但是患者的并发症率较低，且无张力皮瓣可促进较高的成功率。此外，U 形皮瓣成形术还可成功用于其他肛门直肠疾病，如肛瘘[29]。

结　论

肛管狭窄是一个复杂的疾病过程，常常发生于肛门直肠术后。很多患者可采取球囊扩张等保守治疗，但是严重的肛管狭窄患者需通过手术干预缓解症状。肛管狭窄的手术方式很多，每一种手术方式均有优点和缺点。尽管肛管狭窄最佳治疗为最小化的减轻肛门直肠手术时相关的肛门上皮损伤，但外科医生必须熟悉该病的各种治疗方案，并为患者选择合适的方案。

表 41.4　肛管狭窄的治疗选择

	低位	中位	高位
中度狭窄	V-Y 肛门成形术	黏膜皮瓣前移术	黏膜皮瓣前移术
		U 形皮瓣成形术	U 形皮瓣成形术
		房式皮瓣成形术	房式皮瓣成形术
		菱形皮瓣成形术	
重度狭窄	U 形皮瓣成形术	U 形皮瓣成形术	S- 成形术
	房式皮瓣成形术	房式皮瓣成形术	U 形皮瓣成形术
	菱形皮瓣成形术	菱形皮瓣成形术	房式皮瓣成形术

参考文献

1. Liberman H, Thorson AG. Anal stenosis. Am J Surg. 2000; 179:325–9.
2. Farid M, Youssef M, El Nakeeb A, Fikry A, El Awady S, Morshed M. Comparative study of the house advancement flap, rhomboid flap and y-v anoplasty in treatment of anal stenosis: a prospective randomized study. Dis Colon Rectum. 2010;53:790–7.
3. Khubchandani IT. Mucosal advancement anoplasty. Dis Colon Rectum. 1985;28:194–6.
4. Pearl RK, Hooks VH, Abcarian H, Orsay CP, Nelson RL. Island flap anoplasty for the treatment of anal stricture and mucosal ectropion. Dis Colon Rectum. 1990;33:581–3.
5. Caplin DA, Kodner IJ. Repair of anal stricture and mucosal ectropion by simple flap procedures. Dis Colon Rectum. 1986;29:92–4.
6. Rosen L. V-Y advancement for anal ectropion. Dis Colon Rectum. 1986;29:596–8.
7. Ferguson JA. Repair of "whitehead deformity" of the anus. Surg Gynecol Obstet. 1959;108:115–6.
8. Hudson AT. S-plasty repair of whitehead deformity of the anus. Dis Colon Rectum. 1967;10:57–60.
9. Faulconer HT, Ferguson JA. Anal S-plasty for whitehead deformity. Dis Colon Rectum. 1973;16:388–91.
10. Oh C, Zinberg J. Anoplasty for anal stricture. Dis Colon Rectum. 1982;25:809–10.
11. Maria G, Brisinda G, Civello IM. Anoplasty for the treatment of anal stenosis. Am J Surg. 1998;175:158–60.
12. Milsom JW, Mazier WP. Classification and management of postsurgical anal stenosis. Surg Gynecol Obstet. 1986;163:60–4.
13. Katdare MV, Ricciardi R. Anal stenosis. Surg Clin North Am. 2010; 90:137–45.
14. Rakhmanine M, Rosen L, Khubchandani I, Stasik J, Riether RD. Lateral mucosal advancement anoplasty for anal stricture. Br J Surg. 2002;89:1423–4.
15. Saldana E, Paletta C, Gupta N, Vernava AM, Longo WE. Internal pudendal flap anoplasty for severe anal stenosis. Dis Colon Rectum. 1996;39:350–2.
16. Gambiez LP, Finzi LS, Brami FC, Karoui MG, Denimal FA, Quandalle PA. Posterior transsacral approach: an alternative for the resection and reconstruction of severe ileoanal anastomotic strictures. J Am Coll Surg. 2000;190:379–84.
17. Gonzalez AR, De Oliveira O, Verzaro R, Nogueras J, Wexner SD. Anoplasty for stenosis and other anorectal defects. Am Surg. 1995;61:526–9.
18. Khubchandani IT. Anal stenosis. Surg Clin North Am. 1994; 74:1353–60.
19. Lopez-Rios FL. Rhomboid flap in proctologic reconstruction. Dis Colon Rectum. 1990;33:73–7.
20. Christensen MA, Pitsch RM, Cali RL, Blatchford GJ, Thorson AG. "House" advancement pedicle flap for anal stenosis. Dis Colon Rectum. 1992;35:201–3.
21. Angelchik PD, Harms BA, Starling JR. Repair of anal stricture and mucosal ectropion with Y-V or pedicle flap anoplasty. Am J Surg. 1993;166:55–9.
22. Shropshear G. Posterior and anterior anal proctotomy: a simplified technic for postoperative anal stenosis. Dis Colon Rectum. 1971;14:62–6.
23. Malgieri JA. Anoplasty to correct anal stenosis. Dis Colon Rectum. 1961;4:289–91.
24. Alver O, Ersoy YE, Aydemir I, Erguney S, Teksoz S, Apaydin B, et al. Use of "house" flap in anorectal diseases. World J Surg. 2008;32:2281–6.

25. Gingold BS, Arvanitis M. Y-V anoplasty for treatment of anal stricture. Surg Gynecol Obstet. 1986;162:241–2.
26. Anderson KD, Newman KD, Bond SJ, Sherman NJ. Diamond flap anoplasty in infants and children with an intractable anal stricture. J Pediatr Surg. 1994;29:1253–7.
27. Sarner JB. Plastic relief of anal stenosis. Dis Colon Rectum. 1969;12:277–80.
28. Sentovich SM, Falk PM, Christensen MA, Thorson AG, Blatchford GJ, Pitsch RM. Operative results of house advancement anoplasty. Br J Surg. 1996;38:912–5.
29. Del Pino A, Nelson RL, Pearl RK, Abcarian H. Island flap anoplasty for the treatment of transsphincteric fistula in ano. Dis Colon Rectum. 1996;39:224–6.

第 42 章　会阴皮肤填补与重建

William Samson · Mitchell Bernstein · Jamie Schwartz
于向阳 译　王西墨 审校

摘　要

很多累及会阴部的良、恶性疾病在治疗原发病后所留下的会阴伤口，在处理时是具有挑战性的。本章概述复杂伤口的手术方法。成功的治疗取决于基础条件并且受诸如软组织缺损的大小、盆腔死腔的存在、之前放射治疗所致的缺血、继发于慢性炎症或脓毒症的组织硬化，以及炎性肠病或相关感染过程所致的瘘管形成等局部因素的影响。会阴软组织闭合失败的结局是毁灭性的，这往往造成辅助治疗的延误。此外，本章还讨论了一系列特殊的复杂肛门直肠疾病的会阴皮肤再造问题。

关键词

会阴；会阴表皮再造；会阴重建；肛门生殖器疣；人乳头瘤病毒；尖锐湿疣；布－洛二氏瘤；刃厚皮肤移植；会阴化脓性汗腺炎；福耳尼埃坏疽；辅助放疗；纵向腹直肌肌皮（VRAM）瓣；股薄肌肌皮瓣

引　言

很多累及会阴部的良、恶性疾病在其原发病治疗后所留下的会阴伤口的处理具有挑战性。那些能够一期缝合的简单会阴伤口也会因为细菌污染和特殊的解剖位置所致的剪切力和压迫点而存在伤口并发症的风险，复杂伤口的缝合则提出更大的挑战[1-2]。复杂伤口可能会受诸如软组织缺损大小、盆腔死腔、之前放射治疗所致的缺血、继发于慢性炎症和脓毒症的组织硬化，以及炎性肠病或相关感染过程所致的瘘管形成等局部因素的影响。此类伤口的复杂性可能由于患者的某些特殊状况而恶化，包括营养不良、糖尿病、免疫抑制和围术期放疗等。会阴软组织关闭失败的结局是毁灭性的，常造成必要的辅助治疗的延误。长期的伤口护理要求持久的医疗关注，并可能需要再次手术，所以花费昂贵。另外，来自慢性会阴伤口的恶臭会造成社交的尴尬，会阴伤口迟迟不能牢固闭合势必对患者整个生活质量带来不利影响[3]。

人乳头瘤病毒引起的肛门生殖器疣（图42.1）伴随的会阴部伤口的处理所面临的挑战就属于此种情况。肛门疣常被患者忽视，一旦治疗延误，结局就是需要覆盖的巨大组织缺损。当遇到巨大尖锐湿疣（布－洛二氏瘤）（图42.2和图42.3）的处理时，疣切除后刃厚皮肤移植的应用可能带来高成功率[4]。

对于会阴化脓性汗腺炎（图42.4）或福耳尼埃坏疽（图42.5）治疗过程中产生的会阴伤口单靠刃厚皮肤移植恐怕还不够。这两种疾病的治疗结局常常是以大的组织缺损及局部组织硬结和感染为特征的会阴部伤口。对全部坏死和感染组织的清创之后，

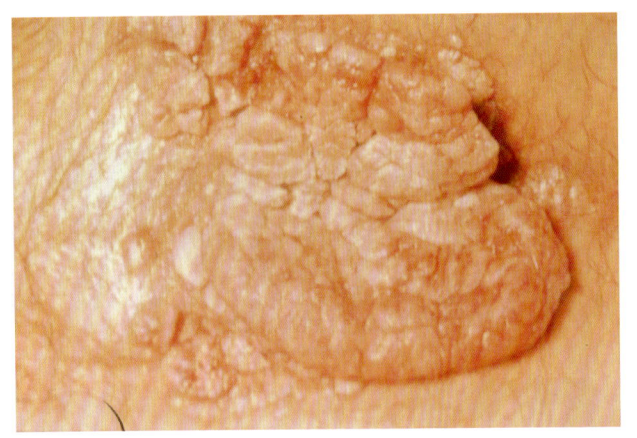

图 42.1 肛门生殖器疣（尖锐湿疣）

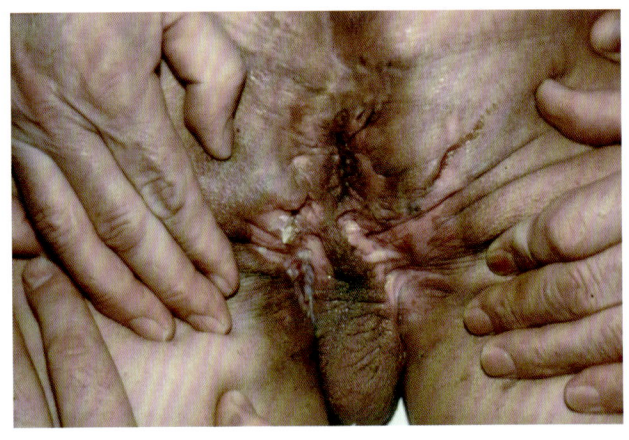

图 42.4 化脓性汗腺炎

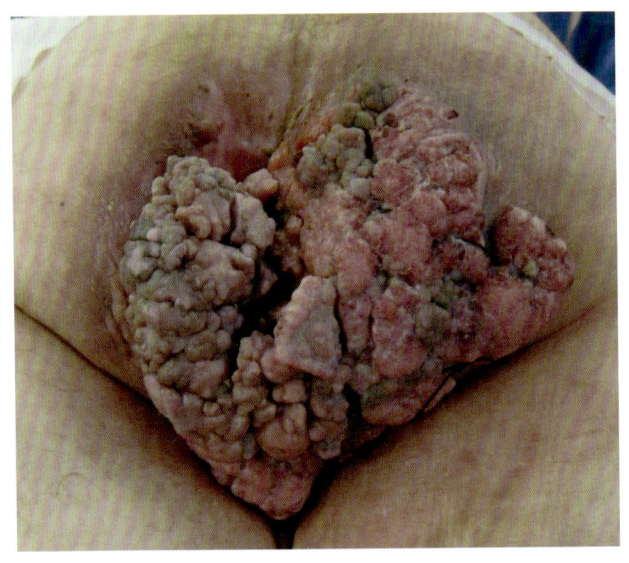

图 42.2 巨大尖锐湿疣（布-洛二氏瘤）

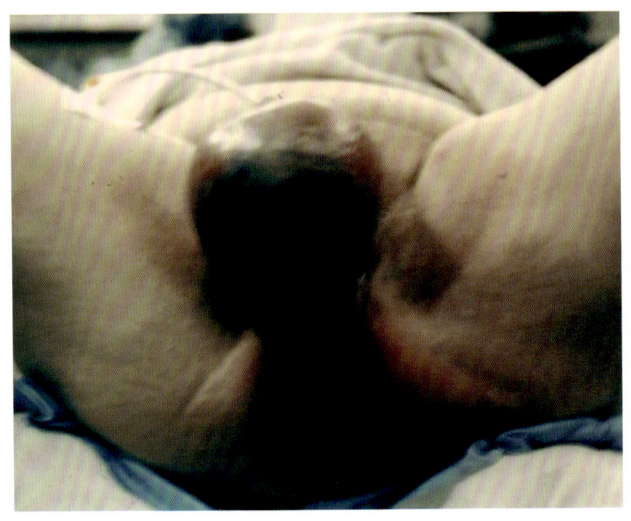

图 42.5 福耳尼埃坏疽

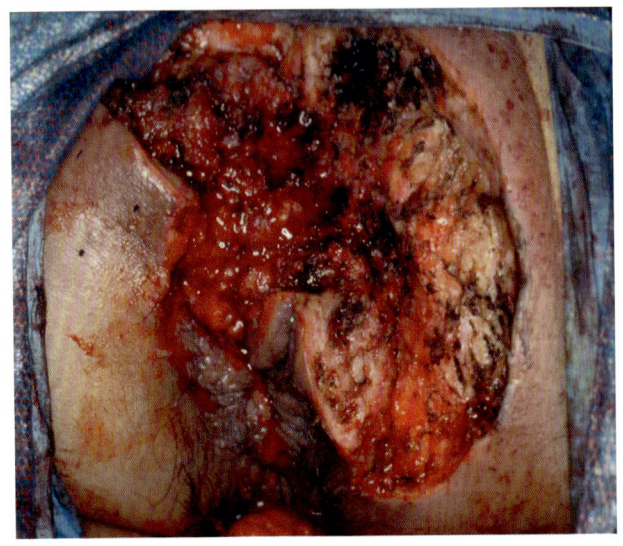

图 42.3 巨大尖锐湿疣（布-洛二氏瘤）广泛切除后的组织缺损

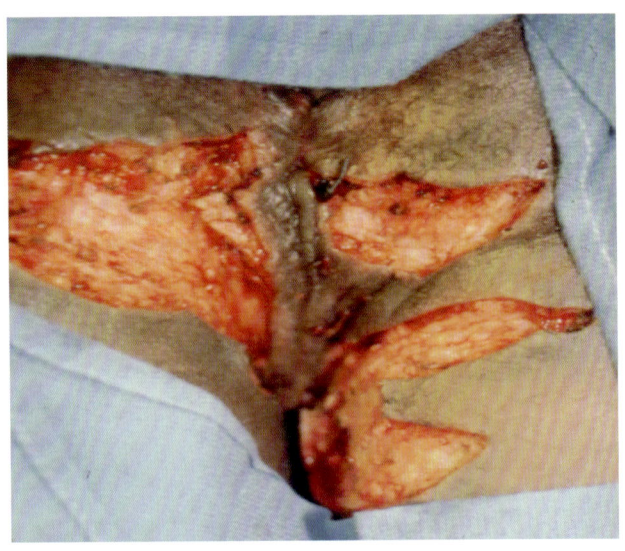

图 42.6 化脓性汗腺炎切除和清创后的组织缺损

也许就决定了单纯二期愈合或刃厚皮肤移植的覆盖都是不足的。在这些病例中，皮瓣覆盖可能是必须的。

如果说皮瓣覆盖对此类复杂会阴伤口重建是必需的，那么成功的重建取决于能够因地制宜（图42.7a-h）地裁取局部区域血供丰富组织[7-9]行简单随机方式的重建。大量的更复杂的皮瓣选择可以根据伤口的特点和重建需求而被采用。结直肠外科医生所遇到的大多数情况是由低位直肠肛门恶性肿瘤根治术带来的（图42.8和图42.9）。复杂的重建技术对那些有需求或者曾接受辅助放疗的患者尤其必要。大多数这种缺损是用纵向腹直肌肌皮瓣（VRAM）（图42.10）以及单侧或双侧股薄肌肌皮瓣来填补的。这些局部区域皮瓣能够可靠地从其正常解剖位置旋转到复杂会阴缺损处进行重建，并能依靠其自主血供来维持循环。肌皮瓣的皮肤部分正好可以用来对大量软组织缺损行表皮修复，而皮瓣本身提供的大块组织则用来消灭死腔。这些相对远隔的组织自然是位于放疗区域之外，将该皮瓣旋转到先前的辐照区域，正好可以为相对缺血的伤口床提供血供丰富的组织，从而促进愈合[10-11]。此外，肌皮瓣对会阴伤口常见的细菌污染相对更具有抵抗力[10-13]。

整形外科重建的一般原则包括恢复外形和功能的同时将皮瓣供区的并发症最小化。患者整体的安全性也是至关重要的。股薄肌和腹直肌肌皮瓣都具有相对较低的皮瓣供区的并发症发生率。根据患者的个体差异，皮瓣的特点也有所变化。手术技巧方面的文献描述详尽，其应用于会阴重建的理由非常充分[14-18]。

蒂在下的纵向腹直肌肌皮瓣保留着深部的腹壁下动静脉。腹直肌的肌肉起止于耻骨和肋缘下。穿通支血管发于血管主干，从肌肉后面穿入，供应上面的皮肤和皮下脂肪[19]。在进行皮瓣设计的时候了解皮肤替换的需求是重要的。因为皮瓣需要隧道式穿过腹盆腔来覆盖会阴部，所以皮岛通常在远离腹壁下血管蒂靠近肋下缘的地方选取。如果需要超大块组织，则皮瓣设计时应选取更大的皮肤区域，且更多的远侧皮肤被去表皮化，余下的脂肪增加了皮瓣容积从而能消灭更大的死腔。除修复会阴的表皮之外，皮岛还可用于重建部分或完全阴道切除术后的缺损。除了其多种多样的皮岛设计方案提供组织块满足消除死腔的需求外，纵向腹直肌肌皮瓣还有利于腹、盆腔的分隔，防止内脏下垂，从而能够避免放射性肠炎和肠外瘘等并发症。我们习惯于首先将纵向腹直肌肌皮瓣游离提起，然后就在供区靠近中线附近的腹直肌后鞘切开进入腹腔。因为血管的解剖和皮瓣的可靠性都是早有预见的，所以皮瓣能够迅速地被游离。然后安置牵开器拉开进腹切口以使皮瓣获得适当的保护。当皮瓣需求不确定时，比较明智的做法是暂时推迟游离皮瓣，直至弄清楚重建需求。

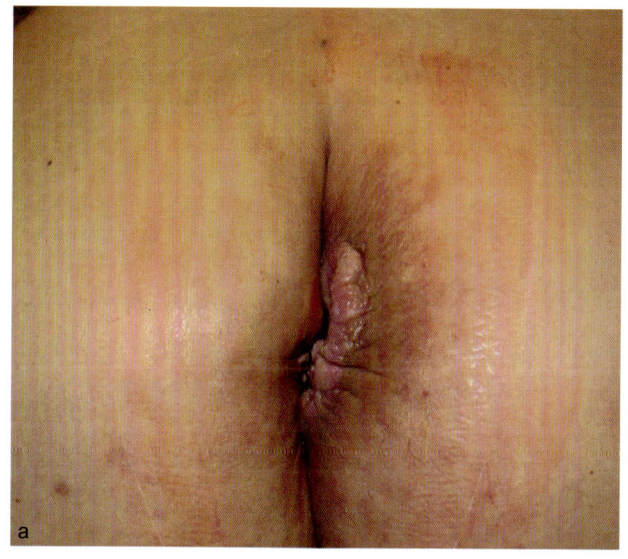 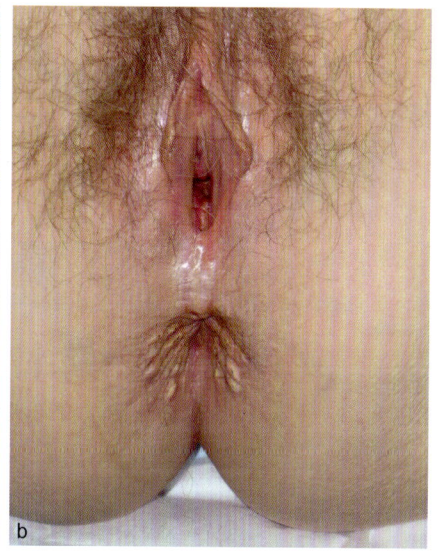

图42.7 （a）直肠癌腹会阴联合切除术后会阴切口瘢痕的肿瘤复发；（b-h）肛周Paget病切除后专门的前徙瓣覆盖（Courtesy of A.P.Zbar）

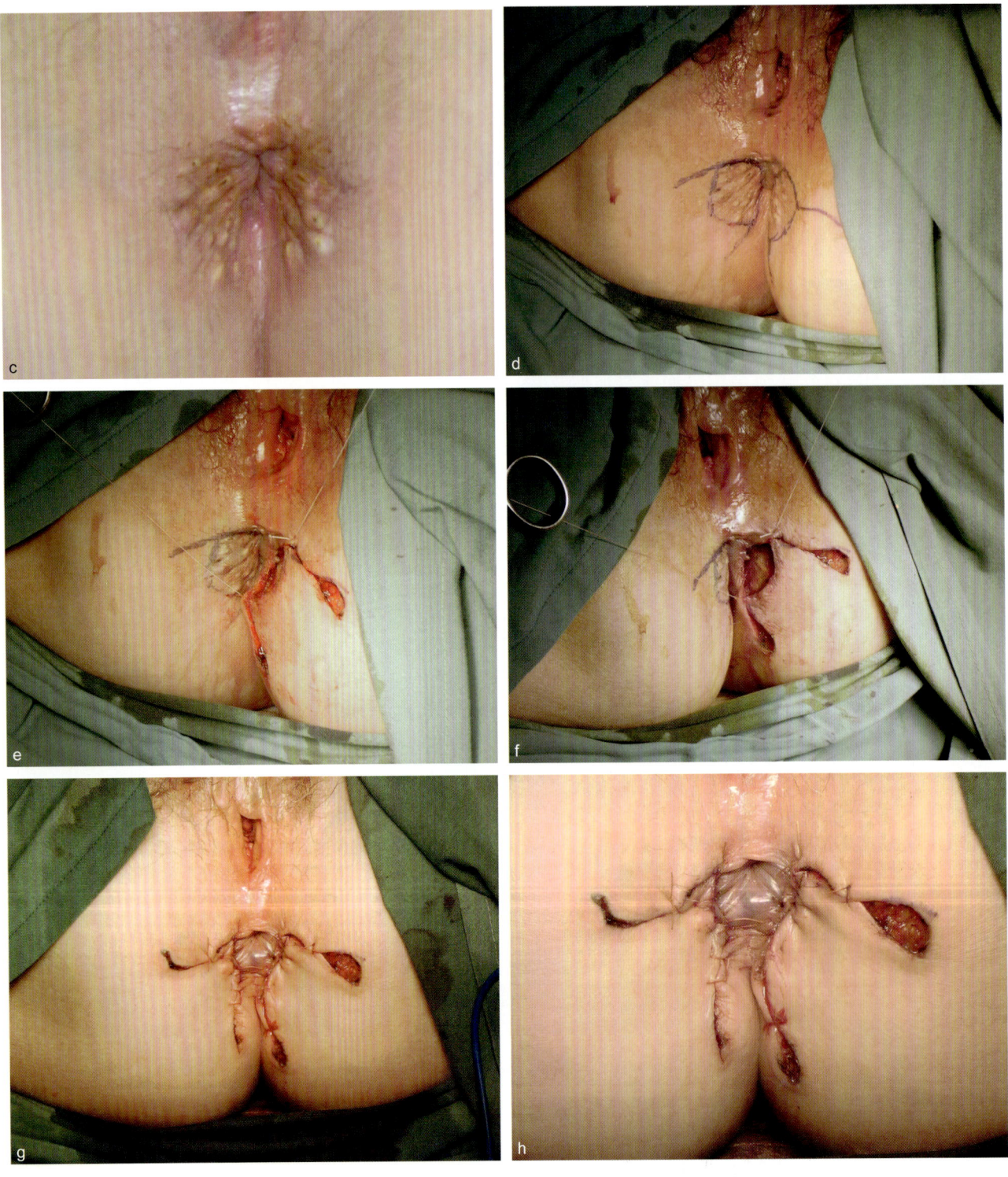

图 42.7 续

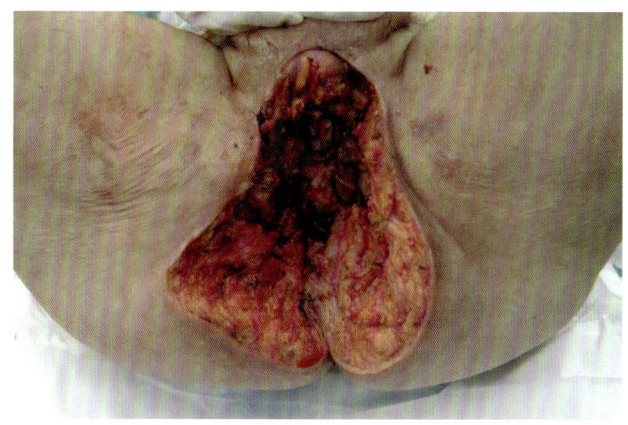

图 42.8　复发癌根治术后的组织缺损

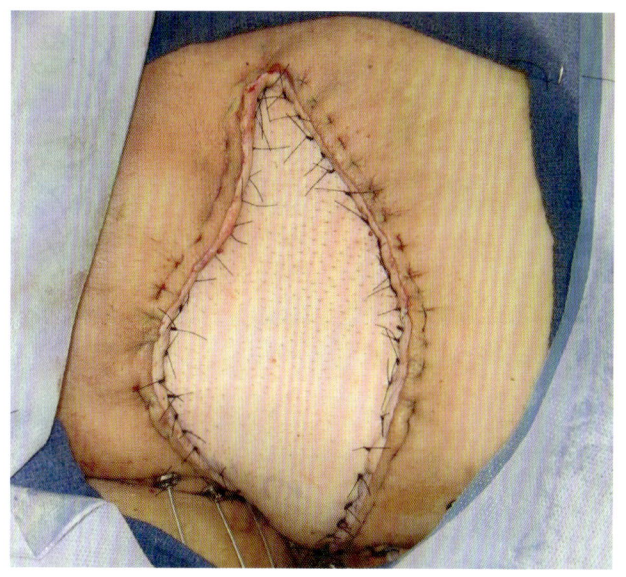

图 42.10　纵向腹直肌肌皮瓣填补的组织缺损

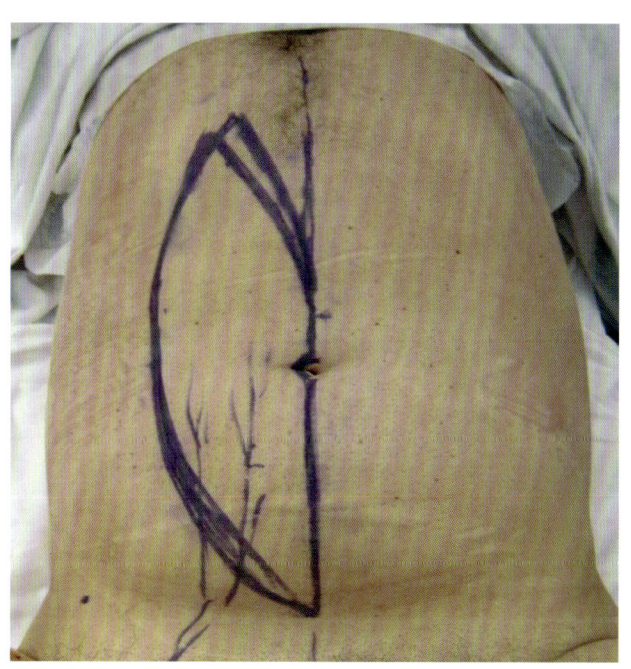

图 42.9　计划的纵向腹直肌肌皮瓣

一般来说，要保持耻骨上肌肉起始处的完整，以使皮瓣穿过腹腔的时候避免腹壁下血管蒂的张力。虽然源于获取纵向腹直肌肌皮瓣的不良问题发生率较低，但仍然有造成腹壁薄弱从而形成疝的风险，所以必须仔细地缝合腹壁筋膜。另外纵向腹直肌肌皮瓣的应用也对腹壁造瘘位置的选择造成了限制。当经腹入路不是十分必要的时候，纵向腹直肌肌皮瓣并不总是最理想的重建方案。

股薄肌肌皮瓣由内侧旋股动脉升支及其伴行静脉供血，肌肉位于股内侧，发于耻骨联合并延伸至胫骨内髁。虽然股薄肌是大腿的内收肌，但更多强有力的长收肌和大收肌的存在使股薄肌成为可牺牲的肌肉。除了股薄肌和上面覆盖的皮肤之间的血管交通之外，还有发自于肌肉周围主干的筋膜血管供应皮肤和皮下组织。这些血管在皮瓣游离的时候予以保留很重要。另外，覆盖股薄肌远端 1/3 的皮肤的血运通常不太可靠，所以皮瓣设计时不应该将其包括在内[20]。当患者摆成截石位的时候，皮肤会跟随肌肉下垂而相应向后移位，这一点应引起特殊重视。因此，建议术前患者直立情况下在皮岛上做标记。一旦肌皮瓣被游离至内侧旋股血管蒂水平，它就能很容易地被旋转到会阴缺损处。当皮肤缺损较大时，皮瓣可以直接转置，而当会阴皮肤缺损较小时，可经皮下隧道转置。股薄肌皮瓣的皮肤区域要小于纵向腹直肌肌皮瓣，另外，整个皮瓣的组织块往往也更小。从特殊皮瓣需求角度来说，这可能是优点也可能是缺点。当同时需要做较大面积的表皮覆盖和大的死腔填补的时候，就必须做双侧股薄肌皮瓣。如纵向腹直肌肌皮瓣，肌皮瓣上的皮岛可以用来修复部分阴道切除术后的阴道壁缺损，而全阴道切除就要用双侧皮瓣来修补[21]。因为主血管蒂位于耻骨结节下大约 10cm，所以重力可能阻碍肌皮瓣的填入。于是要求进行仔细地缝合悬吊，以防止皮瓣下垂。

当计划经腹入路并且对皮瓣的要求能在术前准确预测时，股薄肌皮瓣可以同时进行游离。然而，如果是计划会阴入路或皮瓣需求不确定时，那么同时游离皮瓣就可能考虑欠周。此类病例的皮瓣游离应在缺损完全清创之后进行。相比纵向腹直肌肌皮瓣而言，股薄肌肌皮瓣的供区并发症略少一些，因为它没有造成腹壁主要核心肌肉组织结构的附加损伤。正因如此，术后呼吸受限的机会才更少。并且应用股薄肌皮瓣也不会影响腹部造口位置的选择。股薄肌仅为次要的内收肌，所以一般不会对患者术后行走和活动方面产生不利影响。当不必要经腹入路的时候（如会阴伤口一期缝合愈合失败的二次重建或低位瘘形成等其他并发症的治疗），使用股薄肌肌皮瓣的确有利。

结　论

一系列累及会阴的良性和恶性疾病都可能出现难以处理的会阴伤口。伤口处理的选择包括二期愈合、刃厚皮肤移植和皮瓣覆盖。然而在复杂会阴缺损的众多皮瓣选择中，最常用的方法仍无非是前面描述的股薄肌和腹直肌肌皮瓣的应用。对预计出现的缺损准确预估，个体化考虑患者情况有利于做出恰当的皮瓣选择，并且皮瓣设计必须符合患者的实际需要。仔细地斟酌哪些患者能够从局部皮瓣重建获益，并适当地与整形外科团队进行会诊磋商，能够减少并发症并促进预后。

参考文献

1. Bullard K, Trudel J, Baxter N, Rothenberger D. Primary perineal wound closure after preoperative radiotherapy and abdominoperineal resection has a high incidence of wound failure. Dis Colon Rectum. 2005;48:438–43.
2. Wiatrek RL, Thomas S, Papaconstantinou HT. Perineal wound complications after abdominoperineal resection. Clin Colon Rectal Surg. 2008;21:76–85.
3. Loessin SJ, Meland NB, Devine RM, Wolff BG, Nelson H, Zincke H. Management of sacral and perineal defects following abdominoperineal resection and radiation with transpelvic muscle flaps. Dis Colon Rectum. 1995;38:940–5.
4. Balik E, Eren T, Bugra D. A surgical approach to anogenital Buschke Loewenstein Tumours (Giant Condyloma Acuminata). Acta Chir Belg. 2009;109:612–6.
5. Balik E, Eren T, Bulut T, Büyükuncu Y, Bugra D, Yamaner S. Surgical approach to extensive hidradenitis suppurativa in the perineal/perianal and gluteal regions. World J Surg. 2009;33:481–7.
6. Chen SY, Fu JP, Wang CH, Lee TP, Chen SG. Fournier gangrene: a review of 41 patients and strategies for reconstruction. Ann Plast Surg. 2010;64:765–9.
7. Butler CE, Gündeslioglu AO, Rodriguez-Bigas MA. Outcomes of immediate vertical rectus abdominis myocutaneous flap reconstruction for irradiated abdominoperineal resection defects. J Am Coll Surg. 2008;206:694–703.
8. Chessin DB, Hartley J, Cohen AM, Mazumdar M, Cordeiro P, Disa J, et al. Rectus flap reconstruction decreases perineal wound complications after pelvic chemoradiation and surgery: a cohort study. Ann Surg Oncol. 2005;12:104–10.
9. Khoo AKM, Skibber JM, Nabawi AS, Gurlek A, Youssef AA, Wang B, et al. Indications for immediate tissue transfer for soft tissue reconstruction in visceral pelvic surgery. Surgery. 2001;130:463–9.
10. Chang N, Mathes SJ. Comparison of the effect of bacterial inoculation and musculocutaneous and random pattern flaps. Plast Reconstr Surg. 1982;70:1–10.
11. Shibata D, Hyland W, Busse P, Kim HK, Sentovich SM, Steele Jr G, et al. Immediate reconstruction of the perineal wound with gracilis muscle flaps following abdominoperineal resection and intraoperative radiation therapy for recurrent carcinoma of the rectum. Ann Surg Oncol. 1999;6:33–7.
12. Rius J, Nessim A, Nogueras J, Wexner S. Gracilis transposition in complicated perianal fistula and unhealed perineal wounds in Crohn's disease. Eur J Surg. 2000;166:218–22.
13. Schaden D, Schauer G, Haas F, Berger A. Myocutaneous flaps and proctocolectomy in severe perianal Crohn's disease – a single stage procedure. Int J Colorectal Dis. 2007;22:1453–7.
14. Shukla HS, Hughes LE. The rectus abdominis flap for perineal wounds. Ann R Coll Surg Engl. 1984;66:337–9.
15. Vermaas M, Ferenschild FTJ, Hofer SOP, Verhoef C, Eggermont AMM, de Wilt JHW. Primary and secondary reconstruction after surgery of the irradiated pelvis using a gracilis muscle flap transposition. Eur J Surg Oncol. 2005;31:1000–5.
16. Bell SW, Dehni N, Chaouat M, Lifante JC, Parc R, Tiret E. Primary rectus abdominis myocutaneous flap for repair of perineal and vaginal defects after extended abdominoperineal resection. Br J Surg. 2005;92:482–6.
17. Tobin GR, Day TG. Vaginal and pelvic reconstruction with distally based rectus abdominis myocutaneous flap. Plast Reconstr Surg. 1988;81:62–73.
18. de Haas WG, Miller MJ, Temple WJ, Kroll SS, Schusterman MA, Reece GP, et al. Perineal wound closure with the rectus abdominis musculocutaneous flap after tumor ablation. Ann Surg Oncol. 1995;2:400–6.
19. Mathes SJ, Nahai F. Chapter 10: Abdomen – rectus abdominis flap. In: Mathes SJ, Nahai F, editors. Reconstructive surgery: principles, anatomy, and technique, vol. II. New York: Churchill Livingstone; 1997. p. 1043–83.
20. Mathes SJ, Nahai F. Chapter 12: Thigh – gracilis flap. In: Mathes SJ, Nahai F, editors. Reconstructive surgery: principles, anatomy, and technique, vol. II. New York: Churchill Livingstone; 1997. p. 1173–91.
21. McCraw J, Massey F, Shanklin K, Horton C. Vaginal reconstruction with gracilis myocutaneous flaps. Plast Reconstr Surg. 1976;58:176–83.

第七篇
改良式造瘘术

引 言

Robert D. Madoff

很多有经验的盆底外科医生认为在常规结直肠手术中，Hartmann 封闭的难度是最被低估的。Hartmann 手术通常在不利的条件下实施，如憩室炎穿孔或结肠癌、远端结肠梗阻、拟切除前需要放化疗的局部侵袭性直肠癌或尝试低位前切除术后的吻合口瘘。在以上情形中，腹部情况较差，往往存在技术难度。对于外科医生，有责任预料到这些困难，并采取相应措施，如留置导尿管，这样可以提高切除手术的安全性和效率。

结肠造瘘关闭术的另一方面是永久性造瘘的发明。尽管人们无论在理论还是实践中十分注重挽救肛门括约肌，但事实是许多患者仍需要永久性造瘘，包括难治性严重大便失禁的患者、因术前括约肌功能不良致不能采取可复性切除的患者、低位直肠癌或肛门癌需要经腹会阴联合切除以达根治的患者，以及直肠前切除术后控便能力相当不满意的患者。因此，所有的选择性造瘘术前都应做造口标记，并尽力使造瘘口血供丰富与舒适外翻。然而，即使最好的造瘘也存在并发症，如最常见的造口旁疝。小儿患者造瘘存在特殊的挑战。

第七篇将讨论造瘘术面临的特殊挑战，分别重点讨论 Hartmann 结肠造口闭合术、成人及小儿造瘘术后并发症的处理与临时改良式手术的必要性。

第43章 造口重造、移位和关闭

C. Neal Ellis · Jack W. Rostas III

尹注增 译　王西墨 审校

摘 要

造口手术可导致多种并发症，其总的并发症发生率为21%～71%。本章讲述造口缺血、回缩、狭窄、脱垂以及造口位置不当等并发症的处理及修复。此外，还将讨论造口关闭和重造的相关技术和并发症。

关键词

造口修复；造口重造；造口关闭；造口术；造口坏死；造口回缩；造口分离；造口狭窄；造口梗阻；造口脱垂

引 言

造口手术可导致多种并发症，总并发症发生率为21%～71%[1-2]。不幸的是，造口并发症常常发生在因疾病进展而必须行造口手术时，最常见的为炎性肠病及癌症[3-4]。高龄、肥胖和急性肠梗阻均可增加并发症的发生率[1,5,6]。造口术后出现严重并发症时，必需考虑重新行造口手术的可能。如果需要持续保留造口，首先应该尝试非手术方案。造口修复和重造通常限于经局部或系统性治疗仍未好转的患者。

造口术的一般原则

修复或重建有问题造口的原则是尽可能地减少并发症的复发。尽管大部分造口问题可以避免，但造口位置不当是常见原因。如果技术条件允许，造瘘口应该在"造口三角区"（髂前上棘、耻骨结节及脐）范围中间。典型的回肠造口位置是在右腹，结肠造口是在左腹，造口位置在"造口三角区"并略低于脐，并且无论患者在坐位或站立位时均能看见造口。如果有可能，造口术前需经有经验的造口师行造口评估并标记合适的造口位置，以尽可能地减少远期并发症[7-9]。造口应位于腹部皱褶线上方，远离患者腰线、皮肤裂隙、瘢痕以及骨性隆起5cm，造口应高于皮肤1～2cm，以便于放置造口袋，造口术不能影响患者日常行为[2-10]。造口术时可考虑应用可吸收的黏附隔膜保护造口周围皮肤，尤其是将来可还纳的造口[11-12]。

造口术后造口旁疝的发病率可达48%，很多技术可以减少造口旁疝的发病率[13]见第44章。在初次手术时，为避免造口旁疝的标准方法包括，经腹膜外造口，并与腹部筋膜固定。尽管在非随机试验中，上述措施仅有部分效果，但这些措施无不良反应，并被广泛采取[14-18]。造口术时放置合成补片是新技术，但它是预防造口旁疝的最有效措施。放置补片的安全性已被证实，但仍需大量前瞻性研究验证其适应证[19-20]。预防性放置补片，对永久性造口或长时间造口患者有重要意义。此外，对有潜在造口旁疝危险因素的患者也有意义，如袢式造口、高龄、慢性阻塞性肺病以及肥胖患者[17, 21-24]。

减少造口手术远期并发症的另外一个关键点是造口肠管的活性，需保证造口无张力并有足够的血运。如果术中发现造口肠管血运差，需高度警惕并触摸肠系膜血管搏动。术中处理造口肠管和腹壁造口通路时，有足够的时间发现造口肠管的局部缺血[10]。保证足够长度的造口肠管包括充分游离脾区、分离腹膜和腹外斜肌腱膜、结扎靠近肠系膜下动脉根部并保护左结肠动脉。通过游离小肠系膜和回结肠动脉根部结扎来增加回肠造口肠管长度的方法很少应用[25]。结肠或小肠的单腔造口，尤其是在肥胖患者，需保证足够的肠管长度和良好的血运[9, 25]。

特殊并发症和处理

造口并发症可分为非手术并发症和手术并发症，这两种分类有重叠部分（表43.1）。非手术并发症（内科并发症）是指需有经验的造口师协助处理，不需手术治疗[26]。手术并发症（外科并发症）是指与手术本身相关，并需手术干预处理。文献报道的手术并发症发病率在表43.2列出。造口旁疝的特殊处理，还有Hartmann手术造口的指南，以及儿科造口并发症在本书后续章节里有详细介绍。

造口坏死

肥胖患者行急症造口、结肠炎或Crohn病患者，造口坏死的发生非常普遍。局部创伤、张力过大以

表43.1 造口并发症的分类[1, 26, 27, 35, 37, 58]

非手术并发症（内科并发症）	手术并发症（外科并发症）
皮肤病	造口旁疝
造口漏	位置不佳
改道性结肠炎	造口分离
局部缺血	造口回缩
新陈代谢紊乱	梗阻
脱水	生活质量不佳
肾结石	造口坏死
胆石病	造口脱垂
	造口狭窄
	造口感染/脓肿
	复发
	肿瘤
	静脉曲张

表43.2 造口手术并发症[1, 2, 5, 10, 13, 27, 28, 35-37, 47, 50, 56, 58]

并发症	发生率（%）	平均（%）
造口皮肤病	10%~70%	40%
造口旁疝	4%~48%	26%
造口位置不佳	8%~44%	26%
结肠炎	0~50%	25%
造口分离	25%	25%
造口回缩	1%~40%	21%
梗阻	12%	12%
生活质量不佳	8%~11%	10%
造口坏死	1%~17%	9%
造口脱垂	2%~22%	8%
造口感染	1%~15%	8%
造口狭窄	0~15%	8%

及造口肠管缺血（包括动脉缺血和静脉淤血）均可导致造口肠管坏死[10, 27]。造口坏死常发生在24h内，可通过造口透光试验及结肠镜发现[25, 28]。带有微小坏死的造口肠管表面颜色差不会侵及全层的坏死，可观察处理，但可增加造口狭窄或回缩的风险，需长期观察。任何筋膜下的造口肠管坏死需进行完全修复，并特别注意和去除上述可产生造口坏死的各种病因。必要时需剖腹探查，切除病变肠管，并重新行无张力造口[25]。

造口回缩

造口回缩是指造口肠管的高度低于皮肤水平，常见原因为肠管张力、未处理的造口坏死、皮肤瘢痕以及肥胖患者的腹围增加和体重减轻后皮肤松弛[29-31]。严重的造口回缩主要表现为不能正常放置造口袋，导致周围皮肤刺激、渗液和异味。初步处理为非手术治疗，请有经验的造口师合理放置造口袋[32]。持续存在的造口回缩，需通过手术修复或再次造口解决，手术的关键点为游离足够的肠管并确保造口肠管高出皮肤至少1cm[10]。腹壁成形术可避免造口修复或重造手术，或作为手术的辅助手段。腹壁成形术包括局限性抽脂、切除造口周围脂肪组织、脂膜切除术或造口周围皮瓣迁移[29, 33]。造口创面皮肤良好的患者可采用局部治疗措施，否则应行腹壁成形术[34]。图43.1a-d显示了腹壁成形术治疗严重造口回缩。腹壁成形术包括：脂肪抽吸（图43.1a）、造口肠管周围脂肪清除（图43.1b）、脂膜切除术（图

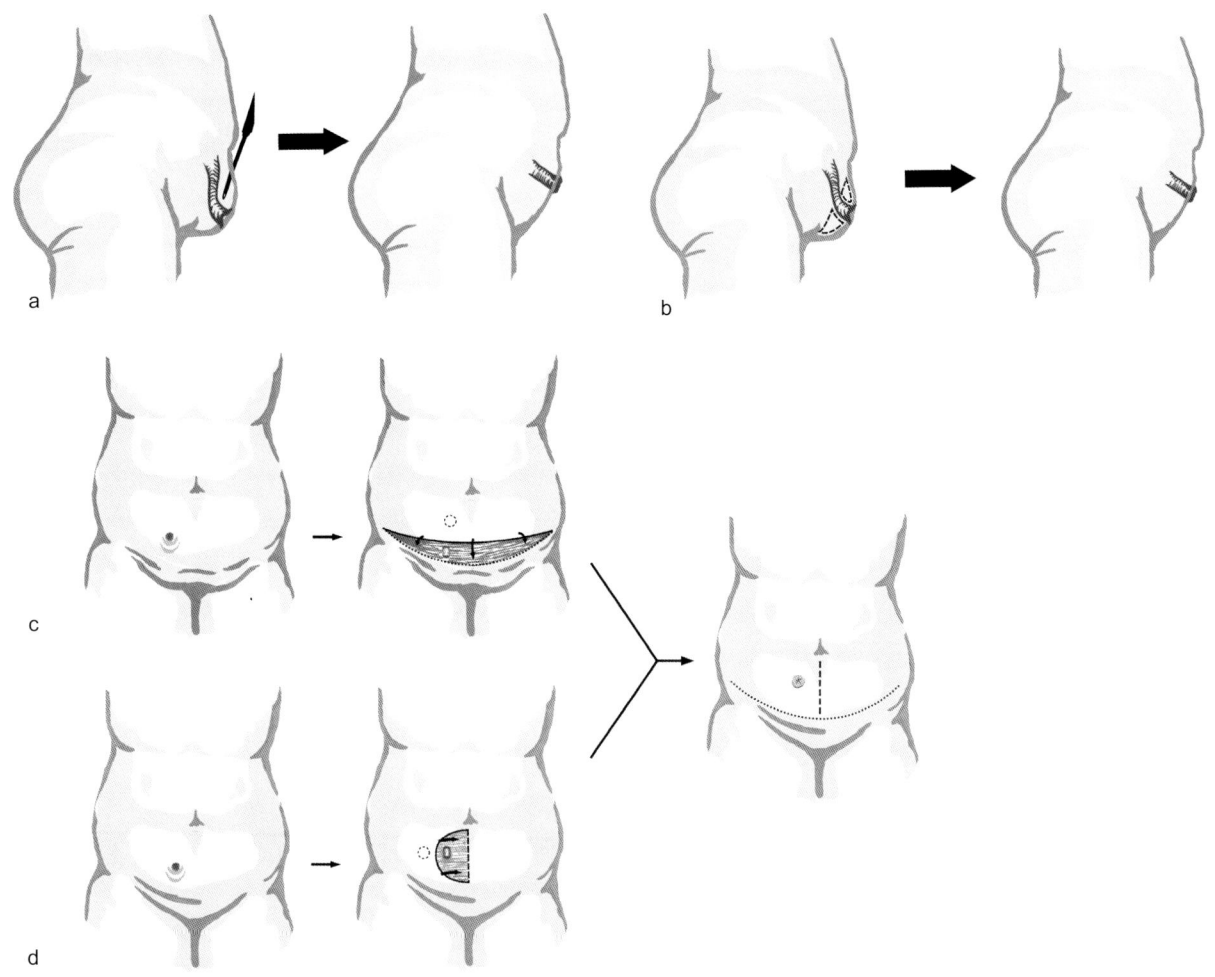

图 43.1 造口回缩的腹壁整形术。(a) 抽脂；(b) 造口周围脂肪修剪；(c) 脂膜切除术；(d) 造口周围皮瓣迁移，通过造口修复手术减少腹壁松弛和创建合适的造口高度，使放置造口袋更容易（Illustration by J.Jordan）

43.1c）以及造口肠管周围皮瓣迁移（图 43.1d）。

造口分离

造口分离类似于上述的造口回缩，原因为造口张力、坏死导致的部分或全部皮肤黏膜分离。任何围术期影响愈合的因素均可导致造口回缩，如糖尿病、应用激素、感染等。部分造口分离通常采用保守治疗，包括全身或局部治疗促进愈合[10]。造口狭窄是反复造口回缩的并发症[28]。完全造口分离非常少见，可导致腹膜炎，并需要急症重新造口术[10, 27]。

造口狭窄和梗阻

造口狭窄与造口缺血、造口回缩和皮肤瘢痕形成有关[35]。早期可采用避免进食不好消化的食物和排除潜在肠梗阻等非手术方法治疗。对于长期的造口狭窄，造口扩张术常常无效并可增加瘢痕形成加重狭窄。顽固的造口狭窄需行完全修复，尤其应注意腹筋膜层的开孔大小[32]。Z 成形术或 W 成形术可作为修复手术或扩大皮肤切口的辅助手段[33, 36]。完全造口梗阻可通过病因学分类，如粘连、嵌顿、造口旁疝、Crohn 病或癌症的复发等[28]。早期可通过非手术治疗，包括胃肠减压或灌肠等。非手术治疗无效或完全梗阻、甚至发生肠缺血坏死或穿孔时需剖腹手术[37]。

造口脱垂

造口脱垂是指造口脱出腹壁外（图 43.2）。双

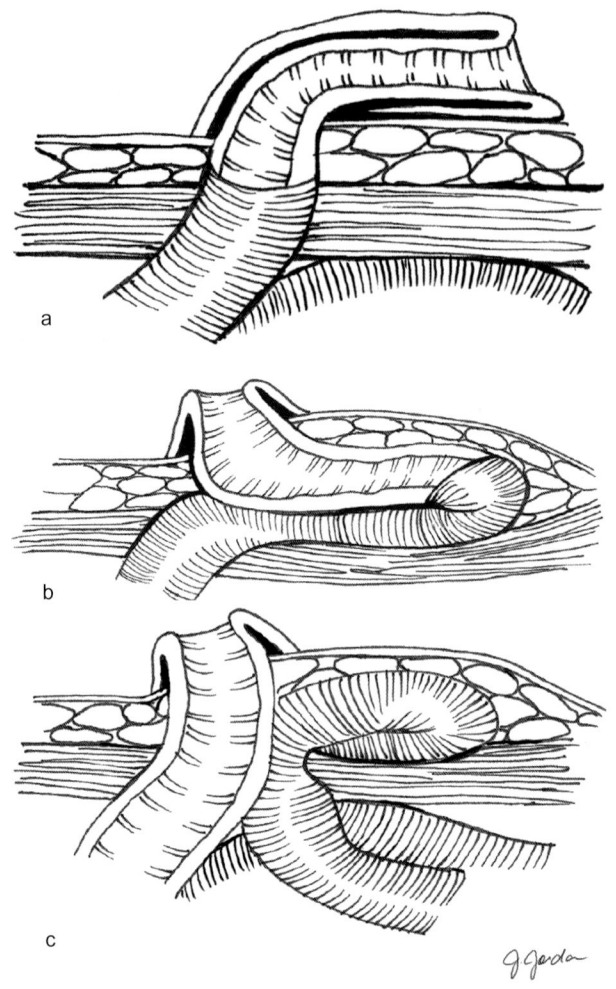

图 43.2 （a）造口脱垂；（b）皮下脱垂；（c）造口旁疝；筋膜缺损导致的脱垂和皮下脱垂的修复手术类似

腔造口比单腔造口脱垂常见，文献报道横结肠双腔造口脱垂发病率最高[28, 38-41]。造口脱垂的危险因素包括急症手术、高龄、筋膜结构薄弱或大面积缺损以及慢性阻塞性肺病[42]。造口脱垂发生嵌顿相当少见，急性脱垂时，轻柔还纳能避免或延迟手术，并能选择更好的治疗方案。通过冷敷、干燥，如糖等，使肠管消肿、收缩可便于还纳[43]。皮下脱垂是造口肠管脱出至皮下间隙（图 43.2b）。皮下脱垂类似于造口旁疝（图 43.2c），但症状比较局限，如放置造口袋困难、不舒适以及梗阻症状。皮下脱垂的诊断为指检时皮下间隙疏松、扩张；CT 可明确诊断[37]。皮下脱垂与完全脱垂的局部治疗方案不同，但手术方案相同。各种造口脱垂必须还纳脱垂肠管。如果不能还纳，可选择造口修复或重新造口，当需切除多余肠管时需重新造口

并保证腹筋膜足够的张力。如果能证实为远端梗阻时，将双腔造口改为单腔造口，可明显减少造口脱垂的复发率。或将复杂的结肠造口改为回肠造口。然而，所有治疗方案均有相当高的复发率[28]。局部切除脱垂的肠管是较新的治疗方案，它不需要全麻并可在腹膜外操作。但这一方案的远期效果仍需进一步研究[44-49]。

造口皮肤和肿瘤并发症

造口术后可导致皮肤并发症，如化学和机械因素导致皮肤损害、抗原刺激、局部及全身感染[50]。上述并发症与持续造口缺血、造口类型（常见于回肠造口）和肥胖有关[51]。尽管皮肤并发症令人苦恼、疼痛和难以护理，但一般不需要有经验的造口师处理。只有当患者局部皮肤并发症难以修复时，才考虑造口修复和重新造口。避免造口术后皮肤并发症，首先从造口技术来讲，高于皮肤的造口比皮肤水平造口有效。皮肤水平造口难以合理的放置造口袋，并可导致造口周围皮肤持续刺激和脱皮。任何手术干预措施必须特别注意，尽可能地保证造口肠管高于皮肤至少 1cm[10]。

造口坏疽性脓皮病非常少见，但治疗困难，主要是由于造口袋对周围皮肤刺激导致。确切的治疗包括造口翻转；其他治疗包括局部或系统性应用免疫调节剂。据报道，造口坏疽性脓皮病复发率为 40%~100%，因此应该避免造口修复或重造[32,52]。

造口感染的危险因素包括全身疾病（糖尿病）、全身健康状况差、免疫抑制（激素或化疗）[53]。葡萄球菌和白色念珠菌是分离出的最常见的细菌和真菌感染。治疗包括合理选择抗生素、营养支持和清除坏死组织。脓肿形成后需行引流术。免疫受损患者发生坏死性筋膜炎时，需切开引流和造口重造[28]。

造口周围瘘管最常见于回肠造口术，而横结肠袢式造口发病率最低。危险因素包括反复的创伤、Crohn 病、造口术时黏膜层的异位缝合[27, 42]。永久性的造口瘘管应行瘘管切除术[28]。部分结肠与皮肤交通的瘘管患者可采用自展式支架治疗避免再次剖腹手术[54]。Crohn 病侵犯皮肤时，首选治疗方案为免疫抑制剂；但是，永久性溃疡或复杂瘘管除内科强化治疗外，需造口修复或造口再造[32,55]。

造口皮肤黏膜种植（移位）是因造口手术时黏膜层缝合错误导致肠黏膜种植于黏膜与表皮连接部所致。这一问题可通过造口黏膜固有层的成熟预防。局部治疗措施，如硝酸银，常导致复发[56]。严重的造口肠黏膜移位患者，可考虑造口修复或重造，并避免黏膜的错误缝合。

造口肿瘤发病率极低，原因常为肿瘤的多基因和转移特性，如结肠癌的异时或同时转移；或者不相关的肿瘤，如鳞癌[57]。治疗包括肿瘤的充分评估、分期、广泛切除及造口重造[27]。

改道性结肠炎

改道性结肠炎是因粪便或肠液转流而出现的闭锁肠段的综合症，可表现为腹部或盆腔疼痛、下消化道出血以及直肠排恶臭黏液。最有效的治疗为造口还纳。非手术治疗只用于造口还纳前暂时出现的改道性肠炎症状，或者是造口不能还纳的患者。非手术治疗包括 5-乙酰水杨酸栓剂或应用含 5-氨基水杨酸溶液、激素或短链脂肪酸等行结肠灌洗。经内科治疗仍持续存在改道性肠炎症状或行永久性造口患者，可考虑切除远端残留肠管。局限性切除是指靠近病灶切除，但为了清除所有病变肠管需行系膜切除[28,58,59]。

造口静脉曲张

各种原因的重度门脉高压症可使造口黏膜皮肤连接处出现静脉曲张[60]。溃疡性结肠炎并发原发性硬化性胆管炎是造口静脉曲张的高危因素[61]。初始局部治疗包括凝胶填塞压迫、缝扎以及注射硬化剂，但复发率均较高。注射硬化剂还有一特殊风险，即黏膜溃疡或狭窄可能[60]。手术治疗更有效，如造口修复、门腔静脉分流、造口黏膜皮肤曲张血管断流术以及肝移植，但肝硬化时手术风险较大。肠系膜静脉栓塞对于造口静脉曲张有效，但存在肠坏死风险。经皮穿刺放置钢圈或凝胶直接栓塞曲张静脉是有效的[62-63]。气囊阻塞对曲张静脉出血时有效[64]。与上述方法相比，门腔分流术后再出血概率最低。因此，对于静脉曲张出血，单纯经颈静脉肝内门体分流术或联合栓塞术可有效控制出血。经颈静脉肝内门体静脉分流术的禁忌证为终末期肝病、肝性脑病或不能进行肝移植的患者。

人工肛门患者的生活质量

造口不能替代正常肛门的功能，因此，每一例需行造口的患者，其生活质量将受到不同程度的影响[65-66]。尽管造口手术可导致很多并发症，但患者的生活质量首先取决于对造口装置的应对能力[67]。因此，在择期行造口术前，必须个体化评估粪便转流后的潜在影响。尽管低位直肠吻合可导致严重的排便功能障碍，但患者避免了行永久性造口，其生活质量评分仍较高[68]。术前知情同意谈话需给患者及家属详细介绍造口的后果[69]。造口可导致患者身体和精神上的严重损失，实施肠造口术的干预非常困难。对于可能为永久性造口的患者，需适时的讨论和评估造口还纳的可能性，持续进行支持治疗，不间断咨询及随访[70-71]。

最近的一项前瞻性研究认为，对直肠癌行保留括约肌手术的患者，其临时造口对全身生活质量评分（包括生理和社会功能）影响较小。但是，造口可导致身体损害，如性欲减退、个人隐私等问题[72]。患者的负面影响因素包括急症手术、造口与脐的距离、老年患者、造口旁疝[6]。

造口位置不当

造口位置不当是不幸的，且是最可能避免的并发症。造口位置不当包括影响造口功能和妨碍放置造口袋，如靠近瘢痕或皮肤皱褶处。因造口位置不当，如靠近下垂的乳房或在患者腰线以下，尽管这些造口功能正常，但仍导致患者压抑或不满[31,73]。术前经有经验的造口师评估，可以显著降低因造口位置不当导致的并发症[9-10]。但是，有时难以请造口师会诊或需急症手术，因此外科医师必须熟知造口术的原则。正确的造口相当重要，因为近 1/3 的临时性造口可能变为永久性造口[74]。

在肥胖患者，由于腹壁肥厚，在常规位置造口非常困难，因此选择合适的造口位置比较有挑战性。靠近头侧位置造口可以更容易达到无张力，因为脐以上腹壁相对薄弱[25]。对于腹部膨隆的患者，很难触及传统位置的造口，靠近头侧位置造口更有利。相反，体重过轻的患者，由于皮肤的松弛，也存在造口位置不当导致的上述类似问题，有时需进行干预。这些问题和并发症主要表现为不能准确的放置造口袋。借助有经验的造口师完全可以解决上述问题。但是，对于顽固的造口位置问题需进行治疗，如可以考虑造口修复或重造。

造口再造原则

局部治疗不能解决的并发症需要通过造口再造达到确定性的治疗。重新造口可能面临二次剖腹手术的并发症。造口再造的一般原则为在上次造口的对侧腹壁行造口术。严格遵循造口术的原则可有效减少任何并发症的复发。腹壁筋膜层缝合后，腹壁伤口的处理将在"伤口处理"章中介绍。

造口关闭

患者的选择

对于充分的粪便转流和后期的造口还纳已经有了很多研究进展。尽管有些进展仍有争议，但研究一致认为回肠袢式造口最容易行造口还纳。回肠袢式造口还纳术后并发症发生率为17.3%，死亡率为0.4%，再次剖腹手术的并发症发生率为3.7%[75]。造口还纳手术的实施取决于患者的个体化因素，并且需没有感染疾病，如盆腔脓肿或吻合口瘘等症状。腹膜炎病史或严重的腹腔感染常预示还纳并发症。预防性应用生物可吸收补片可简化造口还纳[11-12]。年龄也是造口还纳的一个重要危险因素[76]。其他危险因素包括单腔造瘘、合并糖尿病、服用激素、放化疗以及低蛋白血症。与回肠造口还纳相比，结肠造口还纳可增加总体并发症发病率（见第45章）[77-78]。术前评估造口还纳的可能危险因素相当重要，如有可能，需在行造口术时考虑这些危险因素[75]。

还纳时机

传统上，最少间隔6周考虑行造口还纳，平均都在2~3个月后行造口还纳。但是如果条件允许，可在数周后考虑行回肠袢式造口还纳[27-28]。早期的文献报道造口术后发生了激烈的病理变化过程，因此需经过较长时间才能行还纳，如造口术后患者的恢复以及腹腔粘连的减少[79-80]。严重的术后并发症，尤其是吻合口瘘，将延迟造口还纳，并且必然使进一步的干预措施受阻。任何严重的延迟造口还纳都会导致患者维持长时间的造口生活。更不幸的是，在造口还纳前，患者因疾病进展为失代偿或死亡[81]。因上述原因导致临时造口不能被还纳的几率达15%~25%，甚至存在合适还纳时机[74,82]。辅助化学治疗或放射治疗都可以增加造口还纳的并发症，因此应该避免同时进行[3]。可行的方案为，造口还纳应该在治疗周期之间，既能减少辅助治疗的不良反应又能防止造口还纳的延迟[81]。

术前评估

造口还纳前，第一次手术时的任何吻合口均应进行评估。低位的盆腔吻合口可通过指肛检查或直肠镜检查证实吻合口的愈合。当临床怀疑存在并发症时，可用结肠镜来评估近端的吻合口[83]。当结肠镜不能发现异常时，钡剂灌肠作为替代结肠镜的辅助检查[84-87]。

造口还纳前推荐传统的肠道准备。如回肠造口还纳前简单的禁食或要素饮食，结肠造口还纳前用抗生素或机械法行肠道准备。但是，必须根据个体差异进行准备。近期的研究并没有证明机械或抗生素肠道准备对结直肠造口还纳更有意义[88-90]。

手术方法

造口还纳的手术方式主要取决于造口方式。对于大多数患者，袢式造口还纳仅需简单肠切除吻合或局部分离吻合[91]。造口还纳首先要环形切除造口周围皮肤。如果考虑到需通过二次或三次手术关闭造口，可行圆形切口；如果计划一次性闭合原伤口，需行椭圆行切口[92]。如果能确定一次性关闭造口，圆形切口可以扩展为椭圆形切口。最近发现，造口还纳可采用三角皮瓣推进技术，不仅能改善肠管的暴露，还能促进皮肤切口的愈合[93]。

仔细解剖分离所有造口周围的粘连，可实现造口的暴露。充分游离肠管与皮下组织、筋膜以及腹腔内容物后，可以行肠切除吻合或造口切除吻合。必须修整肠管周围的纤维组织，然后通过间断内翻缝合或吻合器吻合。回肠袢式造口还纳通常采用侧侧吻合完成肠吻合。尽管有争议，但仍有研究报道，吻合器可以缩短手术时间[94]。没有足够的证据表明，用吻合器行大口径的功能性端端吻合，能够减少肠梗阻的发病率[95-98]。吻合器能够减少术后肠梗阻的发病率，可能是因为能缩短手术及麻醉时间[98]。与吻合器相比，手工吻合不能保证足够的灵活度。

吻合完成后，肠管需还纳腹腔并关闭腹膜[91]。预防性放置腹腔引流应该避免[76, 99, 100]。目前有很多方案处理造口皮肤创伤，后面将进行讨论。尽管回肠袢式造口最常见，但在某些情况下，为了造口重建，提倡远端肠管埋入皮下的末端回肠造口[101]。尽管这一手术方式与减少造口并发症无关，但这种方法可减少造口周围皮肤和造口漏等问题。

袢式结肠造口还纳一般可通过局部手术完成，而不需要常规的开腹手术。与前述相同，吻合器亦可用于结肠袢式造口还纳，但是由于结肠的口径较大，手工吻合需行双层吻合。如果同时需要回肠吻合，通常需先行回肠吻合，这样可以减少吻合口瘘的发生率[102]。并不是所有的造口还纳均能通过局部手术完成，如果不能定位远端的肠管残端，需通过正中切口或其他入路。

末端造口还纳需腹腔内暴露远端肠管残端，并保证远端和近端肠管足够的游离度以确保吻合口无张力[63]。传统上，这需要常规的开腹手术，但是近来的研究表明，腹腔镜辅助手术是趋势。目前，结直肠吻合通常选择圆形吻合器行端端吻合。吻合完成后常常进行吻合口测试，夹闭近端肠管后，通过充分的盆腔灌洗浸没吻合口并通过硬式直肠镜行肠道充气，检查是否存在吻合口瘘。如果发现任何气泡则证明存在吻合口瘘，可在直视下缝合修补或拆除吻合口重新吻合[103]。末端造口还纳将在第 45 章进行详细讨论。

伤口处理

结肠造口还纳术后切口疝的发病率比回肠造口还纳术后的发病率高[48, 70, 102]，这可能与结肠造口术后大的筋膜切口有关[27, 39, 104-106]。疝也常发生在急症造口手术的还纳术后，患者易发生疝的危险因素包括吸烟、伤口并发症、高龄或男性患者[106-107]。需警惕腹直肌前鞘的关闭，当存在切口疝的危险因素，如有较大的缺损，可使用补片。局部使用补片修复是切口疝的治疗进展[27]。

造口还纳术后皮肤缺损的处理方法有很多，当需要行整形手术时，必须很好地预防手术部位的感染[93]。据报道，手术部位的感染有很多手术技术原因以及其他复合因素，如肠道准备和围术期应用抗生素等。关于手术部位感染有很多定义和主观定义。回肠还纳术手术部位的感染率可达 18%[27]，结肠造口还纳感染率更高[27, 105]，可达 41%[92, 108]。危险因素包括糖尿病和免疫抑制剂的应用。当临床怀疑局部有脓肿形成时需局部探查。

广义讲，伤口缝合包括一期缝合、部分一期缝合以及二期或延期缝合。传统上讲，如果怀疑伤口感染，可通过伤口冲洗、伤口敞开，采用二期或延迟缝合。近来研究报道，采用上述方法处理后伤口感染率为 5%~20%[108-110]。但这些方法仍然有争议，如与一期缝合相比，上述方法可增加伤口感染率，延长住院时间，加重伤口护理负担，发生切口疝的危险率更高，以及增加医疗费用[27, 111]。

一期缝合的伤口感染率文献报道在 0~40% 不等[112-113]。一期缝合优点包括减少大部分患者术后的护理、相对低的伤口感染发病率、切口疝的发病率最低[77, 108, 110]。部分一期缝合通过荷包缝合皮下组织缩小皮肤缺损（图43.3）。这一方法可降低伤口感染率并可减少瘢痕形成，但与一期缝合相比，仍能需要加强术后护理[92, 113]。皮下引流没有任何优势，应该避免[114]。总之，尽管二期或部分一期缝合对患者有利，但可增加伤口感染的风险，因此应该熟悉并慎重选用各种缝合技术[111]。希望通过标准化或预防伤口感染的措施，使上述缝合技术更容易应用，以改善造口还纳术的伤口感染率。

术后处理

理想的情况是在造口还纳术后让患者提前进食，并及时改为门诊随访[115-116]。患者相关的危险因素（如放疗、糖尿病、低蛋白血症、肥胖），或手术难度、手术时间的增加，均需术后密切观察[107]，并包括患者感受能力的评估以及出院时间的判断。

表 43.3 列出了造口还纳术后最常见并发症的发病率。造口还纳术后最常见的肠道并发症是小肠梗阻，这也是回肠造口还纳术后最常见的并发症[27, 39]。梗阻原因包括，腹腔粘连、腹壁与肠管粘连[115]。初始治疗为肠减压以及补液，当梗阻不缓解或患者状态进一步恶化时需剖腹手术。

近来的研究报道，造口还纳术后吻合口瘘的发病率为 0~3.8%[28, 75, 77, 117]。吻合口瘘形成脓肿的患者应行引流，如果出现腹膜炎时，应考虑早期腹腔探查[27]。形成瘘管的吻合口瘘比较少见，其治疗为肠道休息并肠外营养。顽固性的瘘管，或瘘管需肠非手术治疗有效[114]。

结 论

尽管行造口术时非常仔细，但偶尔仍能出现并发症。因此，造口术后必须随访、与造口师合作，周期性排除造口相关问题，这是临床医师和患者的惯例。结直肠科医师必须熟悉造口的管理及修复。当前，很多权威的造口护理并不是结直肠医师的正式培训内容[119, 120]。预防和处理造口并发症的新方法层出不穷，并不断更新，目前很多造口修复和重造的技术只是姑息性的，并且有很高的复发率。如重度肥胖患者的造口回缩通过脂膜切除进行修复[31-34, 121]和吻合器行造口修复[49, 122]都是比较新的技术。为了确切治疗，必须适时评估，当造口还纳手术以及新的造口修复手术将导致严重的、难治的并发症（如瘘管、严重回缩和复杂的造口旁疝）时，如果条件允许，需考虑选择有经验的结直肠外科医师手术。

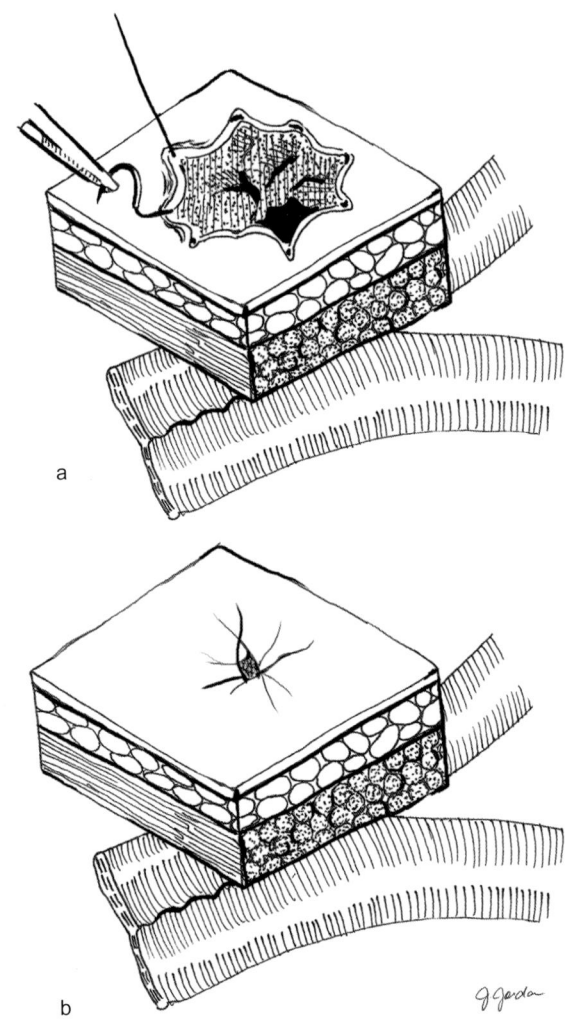

图 43.3 部分一期缝合。(a) 环形缝合皮下组织；(b) 皮肤缺损的部分靠拢

表 43.3 造口还纳术并发症

并发症	发生率（%）	平均（%）
创口感染	0~41%	21%
肠梗阻	0~10%	5%
切口疝	3.8%~5.5%	5%
吻合口漏	0~3.8%	2%

切除时，应剖腹探查行确定性手术治疗[106]。

残留肠道重建术后继发的肛门失禁非常多见，在初次手术术后时间越长越常见。大多数患者及外科医师选择非手术治疗，通过让患者逐步适应出现的症状，避免二次造瘘[118]。幸运的是，这些症状通常比较轻并能随时间而改善[81]。其他并发症，如出血、吻合口狭窄及梗阻比较少见，并且大多数对

参考文献

1. Parmar K, Zammit M, Smith A, Kenyon D, Lees N. A prospective audit of early stoma complications in colorectal cancer treatment throughout the Greater Manchester and Cheshire Colorectal Cancer Network. Colorectal Dis. 2011:13(8):935–8.
2. Shabbir J, Britton DC. Stoma complications: a literature overview. Colorectal Dis. 2010;12:958–64.
3. Thalheimer A, Bueter M, Kortuem M, Thiede A, Meyer D. Morbidity of temporary loop ileostomy in patients with colorectal cancer. Dis Colon Rectum. 2006;49:1011–7.
4. Takahashi K, Funayama Y, Fukushima K, Shibata C, Ogawa H, Kumagai E, et al. Stoma-related complications in inflammatory bowel disease. Dig Surg. 2008;25:16–20.
5. Cottam J, Richards K, Hasted A, Blackman A. Results of a nationwide prospective audit of stoma complications within 3 weeks of surgery. Colorectal Dis. 2007;9:834–8.
6. Scarpa M, Ruffolo C, Boetto R, Pozza A, Sadocchi L, Angriman I. Diverting loop ileostomy after restorative proctocolectomy: predictors of poor outcome and poor quality of life. Colorectal Dis. 2009;12:914–20.
7. Erwin-Toth P. Ostomy pearls, a concise guide to stoma siting, pouching systems, patient education, and more. Adv Skin Wound Care. 2003;16(3):146–52.
8. Brand M, Dujovny N. Preoperative considerations and creation of normal ostomies. Clin Colon Rectal Surg. 2008;21(1):005–16.
9. Millan M, Tegido M, Biondo S, García-Granero E. Preoperative stoma siting and education by stomatherapists in colorectal cancer patients: a descriptive study of 12 colorectal surgery units in Spain. Colorectal Dis. 2009;12:88–92.
10. Kann B. Early stomal complications. Clin Colon Rectal Surg. 2008;21:23–30.
11. Tang C-L, Seow-Choen F, Fook-Chong S, Eu K-W. Bioresorbable adhesion barrier facilitates early closure of the defunctioning ileostomy after rectal excision. Dis Colon Rectum. 2003;46:1200–7.
12. Schnüriger B, Barmparas G, Branco BC, Lustenberger T, Inaba K,

Demetriades D. Prevention of postoperative peritoneal adhesions: a review of the literature. Am J Surg. 2010;201:111–21.
13. Ellis C. Short-term outcomes with the use of bioprosthetics for the management of parastomal hernias. Dis Colon Rectum. 2010;53:279–83.
14. Carne PWG, Robertson GM, Frizelle FA. Parastomal hernia. Br J Surg. 2003;90:784–93.
15. Israelsson L. Parastomal hernias. Surg Clin North Am. 2008;88:113–25.
16. Lo Menzo E, Martinez JM, Spector SA, Iglesias A, DeGennaro V, Cappellani A. Use of biologic mesh for a complicated paracolostomy hernia. Am J Surg. 2008;196:715–9.
17. Szmulowicz UM, Hull TL. The role of biological implants in the repair and prevention of parastomal hernia. Semin Colon Rectal Surg. 2009;20:131–8.
18. Pilgrim CHC, McIntyre R, Bailey M. Prospective audit of parastomal hernia: prevalence and associated comorbidities. Dis Colon Rectum. 2010;53:71–6.
19. Jänes A, Cengiz Y, Israelsson LA. Preventing parastomal hernia with a prosthetic mesh, a randomized study. Arch Surg. 2004;139:1356–8.
20. Marimuthu K, Vijayasekar C, Ghosh D, Mathew G. Prevention of parastomal hernia using preperitoneal mesh: a prospective observational study. Colorectal Dis. 2006;8:672–5.
21. Gögenur I, Mortensen J, Harvald T, Rosenberg J, Fischer A. Prevention of parastomal hernia by placement of a polypropylene mesh at the primary operation. Dis Colon Rectum. 2006;49:1131–5.
22. Helgstrand F, Gögenur I, Rosenberg J. Prevention of parastomal hernia by the placement of a mesh at the primary operation. Hernia. 2008;12:577–82.
23. Tam K-W, Wei P-L, Kuo L-J, Wu C-H. Systematic review of the use of a mesh to prevent parastomal hernia. World J Surg. 2010;34:2723–9.
24. Jänes A, Cengiz Y, Israelsson LA. Experiences with a prophylactic mesh in 93 consecutive ostomies. World J Surg. 2010;34:1637–40.
25. Cataldo P. Technical tips for stoma creation in the challenging patient. Clin Colon Rectal Surg. 2008;21:17–22.
26. Hyman N, Nelson R. Stoma complications. In: Wolff B, editor. The ASCRS textbook of colon and rectal surgery. New York: Springer; 2007. p. 643–52.
27. Delrio P, Conzo G. Complications of ileostomy. Semin Colon Rectal Surg. 2008;19:140–5.
28. Mirnezami A, Moran B. Complications of colostomy. Semin Colon Rectal Surg. 2008;19:160–6.
29. Shellito PC. Complications of abdominal stoma surgery. Dis Colon Rectum. 1998;41:1562–72.
30. Beck DE. Stomal revision using abdominal wall contouring. Ochsner J. 2007;7:35–6.
31. Wright J. Managing retracted stomas. Br J Community Nurs. 2008;22:16–21.
32. Yeo H, Abir F, Longo WE. Management of parastomal ulcers. World J Gastroenterol. 2006;12:3133–7.
33. Beck D. Abdominal wall modification for the difficult ostomy. Clin Colon Rectal Surg. 2008;21:71–5.
34. Bisaccia E, Saap L, Scarborough D. Reduction of excess abdominal skin via liposuction and surgical excision. In: Alam M, Pongprutthipan M, editors. Body rejuvenation. 1st ed. New York: Springer; 2010. p. 250.
35. Duchesne JC, Wang Y, Weintraub S, Boyle M, Hunt J. Stoma complications, a multivariate analysis. Am Surg. 2002;68:961–6.
36. Beraldo S, Titley G, Allan A. Use of W-plasty in stenotic stoma: a new solution for an old problem. Colorectal Dis. 2006;8:715–6.
37. Husain S, Cataldo T. Late stomal complications. Clin Colon Rectal Surg. 2008;21:31–40.
38. Gastinger I, Marusch F, Steinert R, Wolff S, Koeckerling F, Lippert H. Protective defunctioning stoma in low anterior resection for rectal carcinoma. Br J Surg. 2005;92:1137–42.
39. Guenaga FK, Lustosa SAS, Saad SS, Saconato H, Matos D. Ileostomy or colostomy for temporary decompression of colorectal anastomosis. Cochrane Database Syst Rev. 2007;(1):CD004647.
40. Güenaga KF, Lustosa SA, Saad SS, Saconato H, Matos D. Ileostomy or colostomy for temporary decompression of colorectal anastomosis. Systematic review and meta-analysis. Acta Cir Bras. 2008;23:294–303.
41. Rondelli F, Reboldi P, Rulli A, Barberini F, Guerrisi A, Izzo L, et al. Loop ileostomy versus loop colostomy for fecal diversion after colorectal or coloanal anastomosis: a meta-analysis. Int J Colorectal Dis. 2009;24:479–88.
42. Butler DL. Early postoperative complications following ostomy surgery, a review. J Wound Ostomy Continence Nurs. 2009;36:513–9.
43. Shapiro R, Chin EH, Steinhagen RM. Reduction of an incarcerated, prolapsed ileostomy with the assistance of sugar as a desiccant. Tech Coloproctol. 2009;14:269–71.
44. Maeda K, Maruta M, Utsumi T, Sato H, Aoyama H, Katsuno H, et al. Local correction of a transverse loop colostomy prolapse by means of a stapler device. Tech Coloproctol. 2004;8:45–6.
45. Tepetes K, Spyridakis M, Hatzitheofilou C. Local treatment of a loop colostomy prolapse with a linear stapler. Tech Coloproctol. 2005;9:156–8.
46. Hata F, Kitagawa S, Nishimori H, Furuhata T, Tsuruma T, Ezoe E, et al. A novel, easy, and safe technique to repair a stoma prolapse using a surgical stapling device. Dig Surg. 2005;22:306–10.
47. Seamon L, Richardson D, Pierce M, Omalley D, Griffin S, Cohn D. Local correction of extreme stomal prolapse following transverse loop colostomy. Gynecol Oncol. 2008;111:549–51.
48. Chang S-C, Shen M-H, Lee HH-C. Local repair for a loop colostomy prolapse using a linear stapling device. J Soc Colon Rectal Surgeon. 2008;19:22–6.
49. Ferguson HJM, Bhalerao S. Correction of end colostomy prolapse using a curved surgical stapler, performed under sedation. Tech Coloproctol. 2010;14:165–7.
50. Alvey B, Beck D. Peristomal dermatology. Clin Colon Rectal Surg. 2008;21:41–4.
51. Nybæk H, Knudsen DB, Laursen TN, Karlsmark T, Jemec GBE. Skin problems in ostomy patients: a case–control study of risk factors. Acta Derm Venereol. 2009;89:64–7.
52. Poritz L, Lebo M, Bobb A, Ardell C, Koltun W. Management of peristomal pyoderma gangrenosum. J Am Coll Surg. 2008;206:311–5.
53. Meisner S, Balleby L. Peristomal skin complications. Semin Colon Rectal Surg. 2008;19:146–50.
54. Nikfarjam M, Champagne B, Reynolds HL, Poulouse BK, Pnsky JL, Marks JM. Acute management of stoma-related colocutaneous fistula by temporary placement of a self-expanding plastic stent. Surg Innov. 2009;16:270–3.
55. Lyon CC, Smith AJ, Griffiths CEM, Beck MH. The spectrum of skin disorders in abdominal stoma patients. Br J Dermatol. 2000;143:1248–60.
56. Erwin-Toth P. Wound wise, peristomal skin complications. Am J Nurs. 2010;110:43–8.
57. Carne PWG, Farmer KCR. Squamous-cell carcinoma developing in an ileostomy stoma. Dis Colon Rectum. 2001;44:594.
58. Eggenberger JC, Farid A. USA diversion colitis. Curr Treat Options Gastroenterol. 2001;4:255–9.
59. Haugen V, Rothenberger DA, Powell J. Antegrade irrigations of a surgically reconstructed Hartmann's pouch to treat intractable diversion colitis. J Wound Ostomy Continence Nurs. 2008;35:231–2.
60. Ryu RK, Nemcek AA, Chrisman HB, Saker MB, Blei A, Omary RA, et al. Treatment of stomal variceal hemorrhage with TIPS: case report and review of the literature. Cardiovasc Intervent Radiol. 2000;23:301–3.
61. Alkari B, Shaath NM, El-Dhuwaib Y, Aboutwerat A, Warnes TW, Chalmers N, et al. Transjugular intrahepatic porto-systemic shunt and variceal embolisation in the management of bleeding stomal varices. Int J Colorectal Dis. 2005;20:457–62.
62. Minami S, Okada K, Matsuo M, Kamohara Y, Sakamoto I, Kanematsu T. Treatment of bleeding stomal varices by balloon-

63. Naidu SG, Castle EP, Kriegshauser JS, Huettl EA. Direct percutaneous embolization of bleeding stomal varices. Cardiovasc Intervent Radiol. 2009;33:201–4.
64. Arulraj R, Mangat KS, Tripathi D. Embolization of bleeding stomal varices by direct percutaneous approach. Cardiovasc Intervent Radiol. 2011;34 Suppl 2:S210–3.
65. Sharma A, Sharp DM, Walker LG, Monson JRT. Predictors of early postoperative quality of life after elective resection for colorectal cancer. Ann Surg Oncol. 2007;14:3435–42.
66. Wilson TR, Alexander DJ. Clinical and non-clinical factors influencing postoperative health-related quality of life in patients with colorectal cancer. Br J Surg. 2008;95:1408–15.
67. Siassi M, Weiss M, Hohenberger W, Lösel F, Matzel K. Personality rather than clinical variables determines quality of life after major colorectal surgery. Dis Colon Rectum. 2009;52:662–8.
68. Fucini C, Gattai R, Urena C, Bandettini L, Elbetti C. Quality of life among five-year survivors after treatment for very Low rectal cancer with or without a permanent abdominal stoma. Ann Surg Oncol. 2008;15:1099–106.
69. Çakmak A, Aylaz G, Kuzu MA. Permanent stoma not only affects Patients' quality of life but also that of their spouses. World J Surg. 2010;34(12):2872–6.
70. Nugent KP, Daniels P, Stewart B, Patankar R, Johnson CD. Quality of life in stoma patients. Dis Colon Rectum. 1999;42:1569–74.
71. Tsunoda A, Tsunoda Y, Narita K, Watanabe M, Nakao K, Kusano M. Quality of life after low anterior resection and temporary loop ileostomy. Dis Colon Rectum. 2008;51:218–22.
72. Neuman HB, Patil S, Fuzesi S, Wong WD, Weiser MR, Guillem JG, et al. Impact of a temporary stoma on the quality of life of rectal cancer patients undergoing treatment. Ann Surg Oncol. 2011;18(5):1397–403. Epub 2010 Dec 3.
73. Mahjoubi B, Kiani Goodarzi K, Mohammad-Sadeghi H. Quality of life in stoma patients: appropriate and inappropriate stoma sites. World J Surg. 2009;34:147–52.
74. David GG, Slavin JP, Willmott S, Corless DJ, Khan AU, Selvasekar CR. Loop ileostomy following anterior resection: is it really temporary? Colorectal Dis. 2010;12:428–32.
75. Chow A, Tilney HS, Paraskeva P, Jeyarajah S, Zacharakis E, Purkayastha S. The morbidity surrounding reversal of defunctioning ileostomies: a systematic review of 48 studies including 6,107 cases. Int J Colorectal Dis. 2009;24:711–23.
76. Pokorny H, Herkner H, Jakesz R, Herbst F. Mortality and complications after stoma closure. Arch Surg. 2005;140:956–60.
77. Kaiser AM, Israelit S, Klaristenfeld D, Selvindoss P, Vukasin P, Ault G, et al. Morbidity of ostomy takedown. J Gastrointest Surg. 2008;12:437–41.
78. Hindenburg T, Rosenberg J. Closing a temporary ileostomy within two weeks. Dan Med Bull. 2010;57:1–5.
79. Perez RO, Habr-Gama A, Seid VE, Proscurshim I, Sousa AH, Kiss DR, et al. Loop ileostomy morbidity: timing of closure matters. Dis Colon Rectum. 2006;49:1539–45.
80. Martínez JL, Luque-de-León E, Andrade P. Factors related to anastomotic dehiscence and mortality after terminal stomal closure in the management of patients with severe secondary peritonitis. J Gastrointest Surg. 2008;12:2110–8.
81. Chand M, Nash GF, Talbot RW. Timely closure of loop ileostomy following anterior resection for rectal cancer. Eur J Cancer Care. 2008;17(6):611–5.
82. Bailey CMH, Wheeler JMD, Birks M, Farouk R. The incidence and causes of permanent stoma after anterior resection. Colorectal Dis. 2003;5:331–4.
83. Bax T, McNevin M. The value of diverting loop ileostomy on the high-risk colon and rectal anastomosis. Am J Surg. 2007;193:585–8.
84. Silva GM, Wexner SD, Gurland B, Gervaz P, Moon SD, Efron J, et al. Is routine pouchogram prior to ileostomy closure in colonic J-pouch really necessary? Colorectal Dis. 2004;6:117–20.
85. Karsten BJ, King JB, Kumar RR. Role of water-soluble enema before takedown of diverting ileostomy for low pelvic anastomosis. Am Surg. 2007;75:941–4.
86. Khair G, Alhamarneh O, Avery J, Cast J, Gunn J, Monson JRT, et al. Routine use of gastrograffin enema prior to the reversal of a loop ileostomy. Dig Surg. 2007;24:338–41.
87. Kalady MF, Mantyh CR, Petrofski J, Ludwig KA. Routine contrast imaging of low pelvic anastomosis prior to closure of defunctioning ileostomy: is it necessary? J Gastrointest Surg. 2008;12:1227–31.
88. Slim K, Vicaut E, Launay-Savary M-V, Contant C, Chipponi J. Updated systematic review and meta-analysis of randomized clinical trials on the role of mechanical bowel preparation before colorectal surgery. Ann Surg. 2009;249:203–9.
89. Guenaga KKFG, Matos D, Wille-Jørgensen P. Mechanical bowel preparation for elective colorectal surgery. Cochrane Database of Systematic Reviews. 2009;(1):CD001544.
90. Ellis CN. Bowel preparation before elective colorectal surgery: what is the evidence. Semin Colon Rectal Surg. 2010;21:144–7.
91. Bell C, Asolati M, Hamilton E, Fleming J, Nwariaku F, Sarosi G, et al. A comparison of complications associated with colostomy reversal versus ileostomy reversal. Am J Surg. 2005;190:717–20.
92. Marquez TT, Christoforidis D, Abraham A, Madoff RD, Rothenberger DA. Wound infection following stoma takedown: primary skin closure versus subcuticular purse-string suture. World J Surg. 2010;34(12):2877–82.
93. Lim JT, Shedda SM, Hayes IP. "Gunsight" skin incision and closure technique for stoma reversal. Dis Colon Rectum. 2010;53:1569–75.
94. Hull TL. Comparison of handsewn and stapled loop ileostomy closures. Dis Colon Rectum. 1996;39:1086–9.
95. Kraemer M, Seow-Choen F, Ho YH, Eu KW. A comparison of sutured and stapled closure of diverting loop ileostomies. Tech Coloproctol. 2000;4:89–92.
96. Hasegawa H, Radley S, Morton DG, Keighley MRB. Stapled versus sutured closure of loop ileostomy. Ann Surg. 2000;231:202–4.
97. Leung TTW, MacLean AR, Buie WD, Dixon E. Comparison of stapled versus handsewn loop ileostomy closure: a meta-analysis. J Gastrointest Surg. 2007;12:939–44.
98. Shelygin YA, Chernyshov SV, Rybakov EG. Stapled ileostomy closure results in reduction of postoperative morbidity. Tech Coloproctol. 2009;14:19–23.
99. Pokorny H, Herkner H, Jakesz R, Herbst F. Predictors for complications after loop stoma closure in patients with rectal cancer. World J Surg. 2006;30(8):1488–93.
100. de Jesus E, Karliczek A, Matos D, Castro A, Atallah Á. Prophylactic anastomotic drainage for colorectal surgery. Cochrane Database Syst Rev. 2004;(4):CD002100.
101. Van der Sluis FF, Schouten N, de Graaf PW, Karsten TM, Stassen LP. Temporary end ileostomy with subcutaneously buried efferent limb: results and potential advantages. Dig Surg. 2010;27:403–8.
102. Choy PYG, Bissett IP, Docherty JG, Parry BR, Merrie A. Stapled versus handsewn methods for ileocolic anastomoses. Cochrane Database Syst Rev. 2007;(3):CD004320.
103. Ricciardi R, Roberts PL, Marcello PW, Hall JF, Read TE, Schoetz DJ. Anastomotic leak testing after colorectal resection. Arch Surg. 2009;144:407–11.
104. Edwards DP, Leppington-Clarke A, Sexton R, Heald RJ, Moran BJ. Stoma-related complications are more frequent after transverse colostomy than loop ileostomy: a prospective randomized controlled trial. Br J Surg. 2001;88:360–3.
105. Tilney HS, Sains PS, Lovegrove RE, Reese GE, Heriot AG, Tekkis PP. Comparison of outcomes following ileostomy versus colostomy for defunctioning colorectal anastomoses. World J Surg. 2007;31:1143–52.
106. Kaidar-Person O, Person B, Wexner S. Complications of construction and closure of temporary loop ileostomy. J Am Coll Surg. 2005;201:759–73.
107. Saha AK, Tapping CR, Foley GT, Baker RP, Sagar PM, Burke DA, et al. Morbidity and mortality after closure of loop ileostomy. Colorectal Dis. 2009;11:866–71.

108. Harold DM, Johnson EK, Rizzo JA, Steele SR. Primary closure of stoma site wounds after ostomy takedown. Am J Surg. 2010;199:621–4.
109. Lahat G, Tulchinsky H, Goldman G, Klauzner JM, Rabau M. Wound infection after ileostomy closure: a prospective randomized study comparing primary vs. delayed primary closure techniques. Tech Coloproctol. 2005;9:206–8.
110. Vermulst N, Vermeulen J, Hazebroek EJ, Coene PPLO, van der Harst E. Primary closure of the skin after stoma closure. Dig Surg. 2006;23:255–8.
111. Akiyoshi T, Fujimoto Y, Konishi T, Kuroyanagi H, Ueno M, Oya M, et al. Complications of loop ileostomy closure in patients with rectal tumor. World J Surg. 2010;34:1937–42.
112. Milanchi S, Nasseri Y, Kidner T, Fleshner P. Wound infection after ileostomy closure can be eliminated by circumferential subcuticular wound approximation. Dis Colon Rectum. 2009;52:469–74.
113. Reid K, Pockney P, Pollitt T, Draganic B, Smith SR. Randomized clinical trial of short-term outcomes following purse-string versus conventional closure of ileostomy wounds. Br J Surg. 2010;97:1511–7.
114. Williams LA, Sagar PM, Finan PJ, Burke D. The outcome of loop ileostomy closure: a prospective study. Colorectal Dis. 2008;10:460–4.
115. Ihedioha U, Muhtaseb S, Kalmar K, Donnelly L, Muir V, Macdonald A. Closure of loop ileostomies, Is early discharge safe and achievable. Scott Med J. 2010;55:27–9.
116. Baraza W, Wild J, Barber W, Brown S. Postoperative management after loop ileostomy closure: are we keeping patients in hospital too long? Ann R Coll Surg. 2010;92:51–5.
117. Wong K-S, Remzi FH, Gorgun E, Arrigain S, Church JM, Preen M, et al. Loop ileostomy closure after restorative proctocolectomy: outcome in 1,504 patients. Dis Colon Rectum. 2005;48:243–50.
118. Williams NS. Stoma reversal: limitations and pitfalls. Lancet Oncol. 2007;8:278–9.
119. Burch J. An update on stoma appliance flanges and base-plates. Br J Community Nurs. 2009;14(338):340–2.
120. Scheicher C, Senninger N, Vowinkel T, Anthoni C. Stoma prolapse and stoma retraction. Chirurg. 2010;81:978–81.
121. Kahoori D, Samavedi S, Kava B, Soloway MS, Manoharan M. Synchronous panniculectomy with stomal revision for obese patients with stomal stenosis and retraction. BJU Int. 2010;105:1586–9.
122. Skaerlund ML, Jacobsen L, Tottrup A. Ileostomy revision using a noncutting linear stapler. Colorectal Dis. 2008;10:833–6.

第 44 章 造口旁疝的治疗

Edward C · Borrazzo · Neil Hyman

张 帅 译 王荫龙 审校

摘 要

造口旁疝是肠造瘘手术的常见并发症。因诊断标准的不同（临床、影像），各处报道的发病率差异较大。大量确凿数据证明放置表层或深层的补片进行加强，可阻止延迟性造口旁疝的发生。通过比较，发现身体状况好的志愿者进行腹腔镜修补可获得较好的效果，应该通过 Sugarbarker 技术将补片固定于深层，而不是 slit 或者锁孔方式。身体状况较差的手术志愿者通过造口旁疝侧入路进行修补，有相对高的复发率。最佳的入路、最合适的技术及补片还待进一步确定。

关键词

造口旁疝；随访；外科学；腹腔镜；修补；危险因素；网片造口术；造瘘；结肠造口术；回肠造口术；复发率；生物补片

引 言

造口旁疝是肠造瘘术的常见并发症。其发生率极高，甚至有些言论指出造口旁疝并非造瘘术的"并发症"[1]。但造口旁疝的真实发病率的高低受定义影响较大。严格地讲，腹壁的缺损一般会伴随脏器疝出。大多数造口患者的造瘘处都会至少存在少许腹腔内器官（如网膜或肠脂垂）突出瘘口。在这个背景下，通过腹壁 CT 诊断造口旁疝发病率高达 78%[2]。然而，有时造口周围筋膜及皮下组织的广泛塌陷也会造成瘘口周围组织的隆起，但并不代表形成了真正的疝。

如此看来，造成造口旁疝发病率如此巨大波动的主要原因是，诊断的标准是临床还是影像，以及症状是否是诊断所必须。而真实的发病率只能靠长久的随访来获得。被报道的造口旁疝发病率中，结肠造口波动于 4%~48% 之间，而回肠造口波动于 1.8%~28% 之间[3]。生命量表分析表明造口旁疝的发病率随着随访时间的延长而不断升高，突出了长期随访在诊断此并发症中的重要性[4-6]。

表 44.1 造口旁疝发展的危险因子

造口旁疝危险因子
肥胖 / 腰围
伴随切口疝
腹腔内压力增加
慢性阻塞性肺疾病
术后脓肿
年龄
吸烟史
营养不良
急诊手术
结肠造口
高胆固醇血症

尽管大多数造口旁疝临床症状不明显，但少数会造成疼痛、梗阻及造口护理的困难。并且，一个大的疝囊会造成非常难看的隆起伴随着难以接受的整容术。

对于造口旁疝的患者，会经常采取仰卧或站立体位检查。瓦尔萨尔瓦动作（将口鼻闭住，作深呼气）一般可使疝囊突出。CT检查可明确筋膜孔洞及周围缺损。大多数患者体格检查就可以确诊，然而，CT检查对于隐秘疝的诊断更加有益（如病态肥胖），可评估需手术治疗患者的疝囊情况。造口疝根据疝囊位于皮下、腹壁、是否有疝内容物、位于造口内还是造口旁进行分类[7]。然而，此分类方法在临床上的应用有局限性。

进行造口旁疝修补的决定需十分小心。术前应仔细评估患者存在的与手术相关的疾病及耐受能力。大多数患者的病情可通过经验丰富的造口医师的治疗得到控制。束带装置或支撑装置可减轻患者的不适。患者及医生仔细考虑修补手术的时候，应该把重点放置在可能出现的不良后果上，此种情况已被多次报道过，特别是在一些长时间随访的患者中。

虽然经过仔细的考虑，对于症状不典型的患者是否需要手术，手术是否只解决了疝囊膨出及切口疝，很难考证。针对症状不典型患者的治疗，保险起见，患者常常需要就诊于造口医师。然而对于存在顽固性疼痛、梗阻及长期依赖固定装置的患者，若经验丰富的造口师也无能为力，那么将建议进行手术治疗。

预 防

目前，已经制定了一个存在多种变量的有关造口旁疝发展的危险因素量表[3, 7-9]，大多数促成因素都在外科医生的掌控之外（图44.1）。大多数介绍减少造口旁疝发生率的外科技术大多不被文献所支持。在这方面，使造口穿过直肠肌、严格的筋膜层固定及造口周围间隙的关闭等措施，并不能减低造口旁疝的发病率，制作一个无张力及血运丰富的瘘口才是精明的做法[10]。

近几年来，在行造口手术的同时放置补片于瘘口的表层[11]或内层[12]，加强腹壁可降低造口旁疝的发病率。在这方面，腰围成为造口旁疝形成的独立危险因素，而在此研究中是否决定使用补片、放

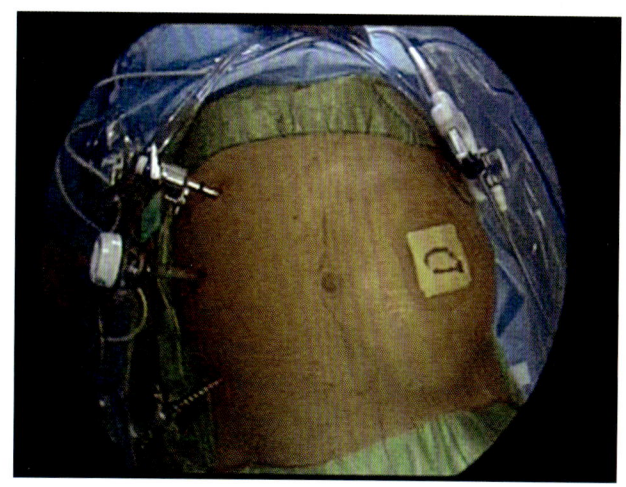

图 44.1 腔镜修补术中戳克放置在瘘口的对面

置补片的方法及手术方式影响发病率等证据并不很明显[9]。早期结果已经明确提示，非肥胖患者应用补片可大大降低造口旁疝的发病率，特别是将补片放置于下层组织后方，即腹直肌的后面后鞘之前。一项评估常规使用补片的优点及缺点的长期随访计划已经开展，有关预防性应用生物补片的试验也在进行。如果长期随访证明预防性使用补片的确安全有效，主要的问题就集中在使用哪种补片合适及放置位置的选择。

外科手术

手术应用于出现疼痛、梗阻及造口医师难以解决的造瘘袋问题的患者。可能最先考虑的问题是瘘口是否能还纳。的确，如果患者既往所经历的是Hartmann术，那么当出现造口旁疝的时候行瘘口还纳是理想的选择。任何造口旁疝的修补术都是通过保护或创造腹壁缺损使得肠管通过或瘘口还纳。

不幸的是，在很多患者中，瘘口还纳并不是解决问题的方法，这些患者的治疗结果提示该治疗效果极差，必须行正规的造口旁疝修补。常见方法包括局部组织修复、造口再造及补片修补术等。局部组织修复存在46%~100%的复发率。瘘口再造的手术效果也并不满意，但当现存的瘘口位置必须更改或不满意时仍是有效的。除了发生在新位置的复发疝，患者如果经历正规的剖腹术，原造口位置及中线伤口位置发生疝的概率相当高，一般要求瘘口再造。鲁宾及其团队[13]曾经报导局部修复复发率为76%，瘘口再造为36%。

显而易见，补片修补是最有效的治疗方法。然而，补片种类及放置位置尚未确定，补片或许可以放置于腹膜内、腹膜外筋膜下层或筋膜表面。如果补片放置于腹膜内，肠管可能会穿过补片（如锁眼技术）或者位于补片侧面，如Sugarbaker所描述的那样[14-15]。一般来说，将补片放置在下层更加合适，补片既可以被腹腔内压力固定，又可以远离一些外在的压力。在复发率方面，腹膜内补片比表层补片效果好[16]。

瘘口侧方修补比锁孔技术更具优势，因为随着时间延长，后者补片周围的缝隙会逐渐扩大[17]。在这方面，Hansson等发表过一例报道，即利用锁孔技术及聚四氟乙烯补片修补造口疝37%复发率的时间中位数是36个月。然而，Mancini等[19]利用同样的补片，利用侧方修补技术，4%复发率的时间中位数为19个月。Sugarbaker方法，或侧方修补技术，确保肠管与侧腹壁间不存在间隙或锁孔，被补片覆盖，呈现出一种"活瓣阀"的效果。理论上这种技术会出现肠道梗阻，而实际临床经验中并不多见。然而，由于补片感染的问题[20-21]，使得具有显著抗感染功能的生物补片[22]得到广泛应用，特别是在感染的病例中。理想的补片应具有足够的强度、轻微的组织反应性、组织内生性、合理的价格及简单易用的优点。

作者的方法

我们的目标是尽量避免对不必要手术患者行手术治疗。当手术不可避免且瘘口还纳并不适用时，我们一般推荐腔镜下于腹壁下层放置合成补片。健康且腹腔内排斥较小、可以耐受气腹的患者可以进行腹腔镜补片修补术。许多患者并存切口疝，可被同时修补。

为了保证造口侧面被补片覆盖，可以使用垫子或者摇床使同侧髋关节升高。在瘘口处做一荷包缝合，防止肠内容物对手术区域的污染。然后瘘口处覆盖纱布吸收黏液，并且用手术贴膜覆盖整个腹壁以隔离瘘口，会避免当补片接触腹壁时造成的污染（图44.1）。

在瘘口对侧腹壁进入腹腔。气腹针技术对于肥胖患者建立气腹非常有益。如果没有应用开放式气腹技术建立气腹，我们首先建立可视戳克作为腹腔的第一个入路。同侧放置3个戳克有利于进行分离。

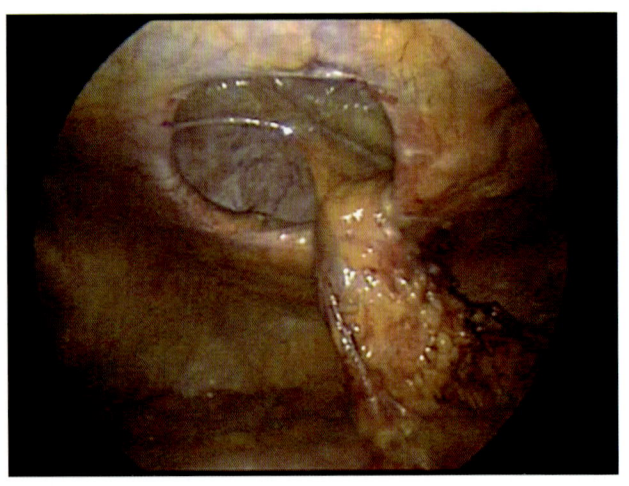

图44.2 造口旁疝合并筋膜缺损及瘘口肠管

利用俯视镜头（直径5mm，30°角镜头）将获得瘘口侧面腹壁及其余肠管的图像。为了探查同时存在的切口疝，需要松解腹壁的粘连。如果确诊，应用一个补片进行两处缺损的修补。

分解粘连的过程中应十分小心，避免造成肠管损伤。大多数位于缺损部位的肠管在粘连及牵拉的作用下缩窄。还应避免粘连分离过程中腔镜器械与周围组织接触造成的肠管或瘘口边缘的损伤。有时很难将瘘口肠管与周围肠管分辨开来。应保留瘘口肠管的系膜及其供应血管；否则，瘘口将存在缺血的风险（图44.2）。

有时，助手可以用手指确定瘘口肠管位置，并于肠管与瘘口肠管间分离出一个平面。当所有腹壁的粘连都被分离下来后，在腹壁上标记筋膜的缺损范围。裁剪聚四氟乙烯补片，边缘应超过瘘口缺损至少5cm。将一个尺子放置于腹腔内，用于精确地测量补片的大小（图44.3）。因为瘘口一般位于腹壁中线的一侧，为了方便进行适当的锚钉缝合，避免补片过度松弛，应认真选择穿刺缝合的位置。可穿透侧腹壁的细针可以准确定位补片边缘在腹壁上位置。在补片边缘进行牢固的锚钉缝合，间距约6cm（图44.4）。将瘘口及瘘口肠管的位置标记在补片上，确定瘘口肠管在补片表层通过。这样能确保补片边缘锚钉缝合准确，并且可以有效防止钉子损伤肠管，或距离太近。

筋膜固定装置将缝合锚钉刺入腹壁，就像Endoclose™（Covidien, Mansfield, MA）。首先，进行补片侧面的固定,将操作部位放于戳克的中间（图44.5）。应该避免缝合贯穿疝囊，这样会引起较长时

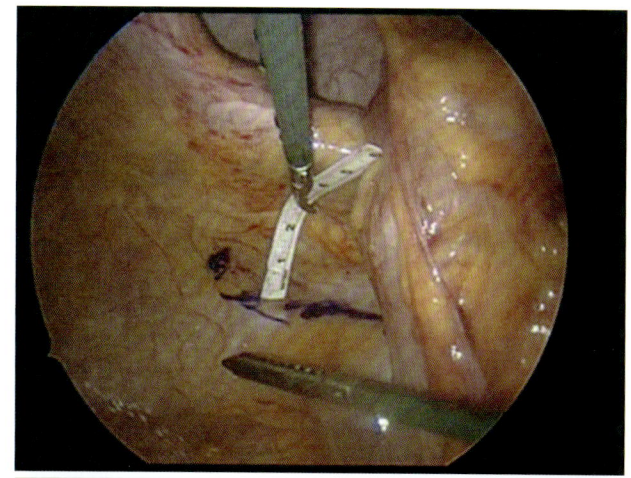

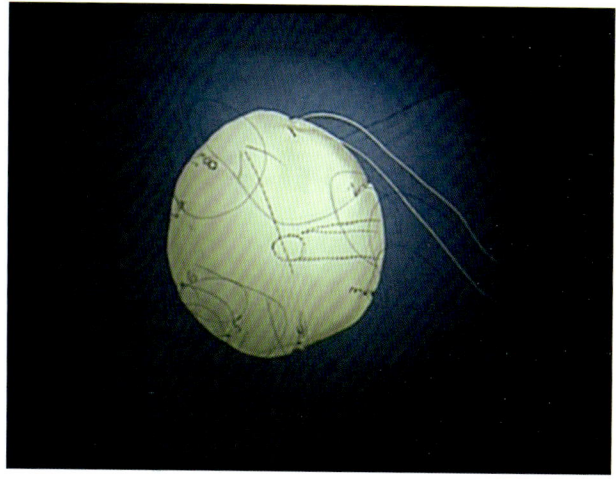

图 44.4　补片进行锚钉缝合，并标记瘘口肠管位置

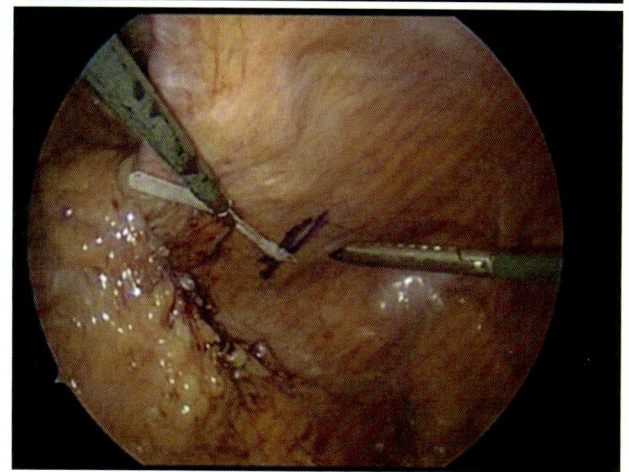

图 44.3　利用量尺精确测量补片

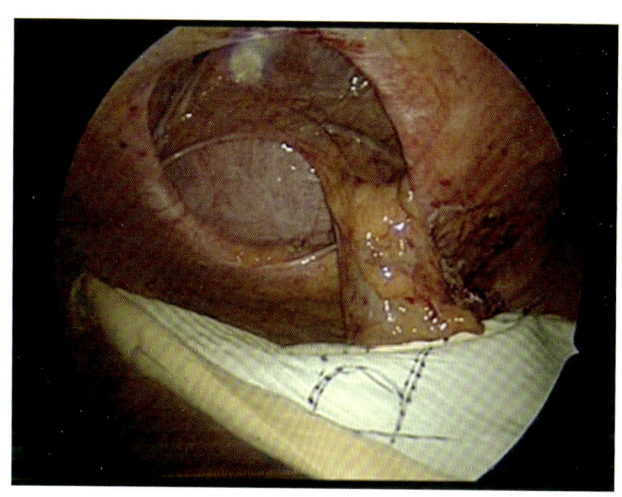

图 44.5　放置补片，首先进行侧方固定

间的血肿。补片边缘的固定相隔 1cm。这样不仅可以防止小肠自缝合线之间疝出，而且使得补片与腹壁紧密结合。推荐 Protack™ 系列装置（Covidien），该装置利用金属螺旋线进行牢靠的固定，也可选择可吸收固定装置，但长期使用后的复发率问题尚未确定。

瘘口肠管周围也需要固定。千万不要将钉子钉偏，这样可以防止瘘口肠管位于补片的后方。缝合过程中应为瘘口肠管预留空隙，如果此处有过大的张力，将会出现瘘口肠梗阻。降低腹腔内压力有助于指导造口边缘补片放置的强度（图 44.6）。最后，将大网膜放置在补片下方并固定，将内脏与补片隔开。

有些瘘口经常在短短几天内丧失功能。原因可能与术后肠梗阻有关，但是更直接的原因应该是瘘口肠管的梗阻。这些瘘口在修补术期间完成，在术后短期时间内出现水肿。而且，侧方修补术可造成瘘口肠管的直角折叠，术后几天当肠鸣音恢复后，通过手指扩张瘘口肠管，并测量瘘口张力。此种简

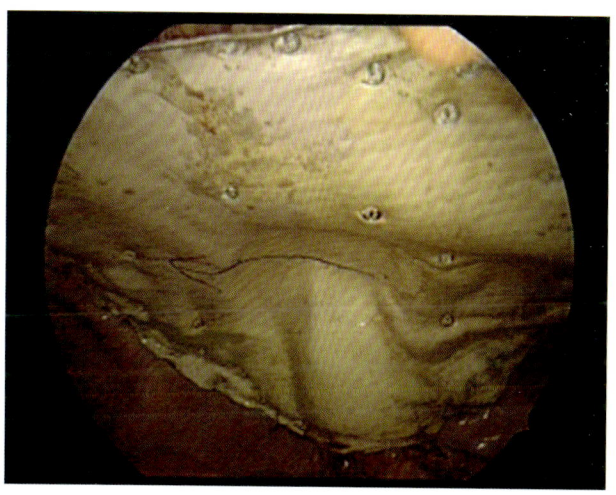

图 44.6　补片被锚钉固定。减低腹腔内压力来评估瘘口肠管周围的压力

单的方法对于敞开的肠管功能恢复非常有效，在此之后，肠内容物常常很快排出瘘口。

术后血肿是腹腔镜疝修补术的常见并发症。患者常出现腹壁肿块，和术前的造口旁疝形状很像。血肿最终会被吸收消失，但可能会持续几个月，应向患者告知相关并发症。

尽管认识到较高的复发率，我们仍坚信在筛选的部分患者中仍可使用表层入路放置补片。一些患者腹腔镜手术较难进行，开腹手术也存在较高风险，如患有严重疾病、腔镜禁忌证的患者及有腔镜潜在风险的患者。造口旁疝的患者术后即使出现复发，也可通过非手术治疗轻易得到控制，这点已经被经验所证实。

沿着造口旁疝的边缘切开皮肤。切口通过皮下组织，将肠管分离开来。反向推拉肠管，疝囊被确认，打开疝囊，在筋膜背面各个方向分离。围绕缺损360°范围内严格确定筋膜的边缘，分离筋膜下粘连，分离出足够的筋膜用于缝合。任何疝出的肠管及网膜应还纳回腹腔。行一组不规则的较粗糙的聚丙烯缝线缝合，并且利用止血钳标记，但不要打结。保留约1/2指头大小的缺损，使得小肠能够通过。然后，所有缝线打结，确保筋膜宽松的放置在肠管周围，不影响血运及遗留死腔。通过可吸收重叠5cm缝合使得可吸收补片更加牢靠。利用闭式引流减低术后血肿的形成。

结　论

造口旁疝是肠造瘘手术后极其常见的并发症。因传统外科手术修补的缺点，保守的治疗方法在大多数病例中被认同。非随机统计上来讲，腔镜造瘘术的术后并发症比开腹外科手术的低[23]。通过对需要进行修补的志愿者的手术随访，得出利用Sugarbaker技术将补片放置于下层位置比裂缝或锁孔法的复发率及并发症发生率低[24-25]。大多数患者最好通过腹腔镜完成手术，不能耐受腔镜手术的患者也可通过侧方修补完成，但复发率相对高些[26]。对于反复腔镜手术的复发患者中也可使用上述方法[27]。我们寄希望于长期的术后随访及对比来验证技术的提高，以及补片选择是否合适。然而，最终的手术方式、技术要点及最合适的补片材料仍有待确定[28]。

参考文献

1. Goligher J. Surgery of the anus, colon, and rectum. 5th ed. London: Ballière Tindall; 1984. p. 703–4.
2. Cingi A, Cakir T, Sever A, Aktan AO. Enterostomy site hernias: a clinical and computerized tomographic evaluation. Dis Colon Rectum. 2006;49:1559–63.
3. Carne PW, Robertson GM, Frizelle FA. Parastomal hernia. Br J Surg. 2003;90:784–93.
4. Leong AP, Londono-Schimmer EE, Phillips RK. Life-table analysis of stomal complications following ileostomy. Br J Surg. 1994;81:727–9.
5. Londono-Schimmer EE, Leong AP, Phillips RK. Life table analysis of stomal complications following colostomy. Dis Colon Rectum. 1994;37:916–20.
6. Mylonakis E, Scarpa M, Barollo M, Yarnoz C, Keighley MR. Life table analysis of hernia following end colostomy construction. Colorectal Dis. 2001;3:334–7.
7. Israelsson LA. Parastomal hernias. Surg Clin North Am. 2008;88:113–25.
8. Shellito PC. Complications of abdominal stoma surgery. Dis Colon Rectum. 1998;41:1562–72.
9. De Raet J, Delvaux G, Haentjens P, Van Nieuwenhove Y. Waist circumference is an independent risk factor for the development of parastomal hernia after permanent colostomy. Dis Colon Rectum. 2008;51:1806–9.
10. Pilgrim CH, McIntyre R, Bailey M. Prospective audit of parastomal hernia: prevalence and associated comorbidities. Dis Colon Rectum. 2010;53:71–6.
11. Gögenur I, Mortensen J, Harvald T, Rosenberg J, Fischer A. Prevention of parastomal hernia by placement of a polypropylene mesh at the primary operation. Dis Colon Rectum. 2006;49:1131–5.
12. Jänes A, Cengiz Y, Israelsson LA. Randomized clinical trial of the use of a prosthetic mesh to prevent parastomal hernia. Br J Surg. 2004;91:280–2.
13. Rubin MS, Schoetz Jr DJ, Matthews JB. Parastomal hernia: is stomal relocation superior to fascial repair? Arch Surg. 1994;129:413–9.
14. Sugarbaker PH. Prosthetic mesh repair of large hernias at the site of colonic stomas. Surg Gynecol Obstet. 1980;150:576–8.
15. Sugarbaker PH. Peritoneal approach to prosthetic mesh repair of paraostomy hernias. Ann Surg. 1985;201:344–6.
16. Pastor DM, Pauli EM, Koltun WA, Haluck RS, Shope TR, Poritz LS. Parastomal hernia repair: a single center experience. JSLS. 2009;13:170–5.
17. Moisidis E, Curiskis JI, Brooke-Cowden GL. Improving the reinforcement of parastomal tissues with Marlex mesh: laboratory study identifying solutions to stomal aperture distortion. Dis Colon Rectum. 2000;43:55–60.
18. Hansson BME, Bleichrodt RP, de Hingh IH. Laparoscopic parastomal hernia repair using a keyhole technique results in a high recurrence rate. Surg Endosc. 2009;23:1456–9.
19. Mancini GJ, McClusky 3rd DA, Khaitan L, Goldenberg EA, Heniford BT, Novitsky YW, et al. Laparoscopic parastomal hernia repair using a nonslit mesh technique. Surg Endosc. 2007;21:1487–91.
20. Geisler DJ, Reilly JC, Vaughan SG, Glennon EJ, Kondylis PD. Safety and outcome of use of nonabsorbable mesh for repair of fascial defects in the presence of open bowel. Dis Colon Rectum. 2003;46:1118–23.
21. Steele SR, Lee P, Martin MJ, Mullenix PS, Sullivan ES. Is parastomal hernia repair with polypropylene mesh safe? Am J Surg. 2003;185:436–40.
22. Ellis CN. Short-term outcomes with the use of bioprosthetics for the management of parastomal hernias. Dis Colon Rectum. 2010;53:279–83.
23. Liu J, Bruch HP, Farke S, Nolde J, Schwandner O. Stoma formation

for fecal diversion: a plea for the laparoscopic approach. Tech Coloproctol. 2005;9:9–14.
24. Muysoms EE, Hauters PJ, Van Nieuwenhove Y, Huten N, Claeys DA. Laparoscopic repair of parastomal hernias: a multi-centre retrospective review and shift in technique. Acta Chir Belg. 2008;108:400–4.
25. Wara P, Andersen LM. Long-term follow-up of laparoscopic repair of parastomal hernia using a bilayer mesh with a slit. Surg Endosc. 2011;25(2):526–30.
26. López-Cano M, Lozoya-Trujillo R, Espin-Basany E. Prosthetic mesh in parastomal hernia prevention. Laparoscopic approach. Dis Colon Rectum. 2009;52:1006–7.
27. Zacharakis E, Shalhoub J, Selvapatt N, Darzi A, Ziprin P. Revisional laparoscopic parastomal hernia repair. JSLS. 2008;12:403–6.
28. Lo Menzo E, Martinez JM, Spector SA, Iglesias A, Degennaro V, Cappellani A. Use of biologic mesh for a complicated paracolostomy hernia. Am J Surg. 2008;196:715–9.

第 45 章 哈特曼手术后重建的相关问题

Zoran Krivokapić · Goran I. Barišić

张明庆 译　王荫龙 审校

摘要

哈特曼手术后还纳通常充满挑战，并需要规划设计，而直肠残端的评估取决于非恢复性手术的最初适应证。哈特曼术后还纳的并发症率很高，发病率约 30%～40%，吻合口瘘的发生率高达 15%，而有报道死亡率达到 10%。大部分哈特曼术后重建的患者存在高龄和多种并存病，这往往进一步阻碍外科医生和患者选择重建；40% 哈特曼手术后的患者从未进行造口还纳。本章中将讨论哈特曼术后重建的技术现状，提供手术技术的提示，也会探讨腹腔镜辅助入路的选择性应用。

关键词

哈特曼手术；重建；切除术；憩室病；癌症；左半结肠缺血；穿孔；肠扭转；吻合口漏；乙状结肠切除术；结肠造口术

引言

哈特曼手术最早于 1921 年被法国外科医生 Henri Albert 描述[1]，用于左半结肠癌切除术。主要用于减少吻合口瘘引起的并发症发生率和死亡率，吻合口瘘很常见，这是高死亡率的主要原因。自从首次描述以来，该手术被广泛应用于主要由憩室病及恶性肿瘤引起的复杂左半结肠病变的手术治疗。近一个世纪后，该手术仍为急症状况下常用的方式。如今，其适应证包括治疗严重的左半结肠缺血、穿孔、肠扭转、吻合口瘘，以及其他乙状结肠切除术后需慎重避免创建吻合的情况。最近来自英国的全国数据显示，几乎 1/3 的哈特曼手术是择期进行的，同时择期状况下癌症的手术比例更高，而急症情况下急性憩室病的比例更高[2]。

最初，手术过程包括乙状结肠切除术，并随之封闭直肠残端，行端式结肠造口术。随着时间推移，术语"哈特曼手术"被提出，即定义为部分乙状结肠或直肠切除后，继而封闭残留的直肠，并行端式结肠造口术的手术过程。还不能确定哈特曼手术是否实际上能预料到结肠造口术还纳。现在，绝大多数外科医生认为应尽最大努力恢复肠道的连续性，主要为了提高患者的生存质量和自我形象，并减少结肠造口术相关的并发症。然而，尽管外科技术和设备有了巨大进步,但仍有很大比例 (30%～90%)[3-4] 的患者从未进行重建，在大多数病例组中总体还纳率接近 60%[5]。如此高比例的永久性结肠造口术有很多原因。首先哈特曼术后还纳是较大的、具有技术挑战性的手术，需要经验丰富的结直肠外科医生来完成。除此之外，重建中吻合器的常规应用，使得很容易决定首次手术选用哈特曼手术[4]。第二个原因是，哈特曼术后重建的并发症率很高，发生率约

30%~40%，吻合口瘘的发生率高达15%，而有报道死亡率达到10%[6-7]。哈特曼术后重建的患者大多存在高龄和多种并存病，这往往进一步阻碍外科医生和患者选择重建。美国麻醉医师协会评分系统能够提供一些预测术后并发症发生率和死亡率可能性的价值[8-9]。克利夫兰医院根据初次术后一年内未还纳病例的回顾性研究，创立了不能还纳的预测评分系统，确定ASA评分、肺部合并症、术前输血以及抗凝治疗的应用作为负的预测指标[10]。

由于恢复肠道连续性的目的是提高患者的生存质量和自我形象，对于患者一般健康状况几乎或根本没有影响，一些患者并不愿意承受可能危及生命的大的外科手术的风险，尤其是初次术后恢复过程复杂的患者[11-12]。另一方面，永久性结肠造口术会降低患者生活质量，以及影响常规的社交活动和性生活，而且易于出现并发症（造口旁疝、吻合口脱垂和皮肤并发症）。

此外，由于降低了劳动能力和造口并发症需要的额外花费造成的经济上的负面影响。因此，进行哈特曼术后重建的决定复杂而困难，术前许多重要的因素需要考虑。

患者的一般健康状况

一般健康状况是决定哈特曼术后还纳的首要因素。在绝大多数病例中，高龄和并存病可能是造口还纳率较低的主要原因[2,7]。这可能是初次手术进行患者选择的后果，因为在大多数情况下，进行哈特曼手术的患者通常高龄、高危，并且有复杂的左半结肠疾病，经常有严重的合并症而病情危重，以及其他不适合大手术的原因。选定的患者群通常排除了一期手术切除并原位吻合的可能。因而，这些患者中的大多数已经自我选择为"高危"，所以影响了恢复肠道连续性的决策。尽管如此，单独的合并症并不妨碍还纳。如上所述，一些学者报道ASA分值大于2分的患者并发症发生率较高[9,11,13-15]。然而关于ASA评分的文章有一些混乱。一些研究显示ASA评分和合并症的数量对于哈特曼术后还纳的预后并没有显著的影响[8,16]。一些研究显示血清白蛋白水平低是一个重要的术后并发症的预测指标[8]，而吸烟和高血压影响术后并发症的总体发生率[7]。一些研究者认识到高龄是并发症发生率和死亡率升高的危险因子[17]，然而其他研究者没有报道年龄的任何影响[8,9,18]。

在这方面，最近发表的一篇文献综述，汇总了35项研究共计6249例进行哈特曼术后还纳的患者，平均还纳率为44%（范围19%~71%），放弃还纳最常见的原因分别是ASA评分高、患者拒绝、高度恶性肿瘤或高龄[19]。这项研究中，哈特曼术后还纳的患者中，67%为ASA Ⅰ、Ⅱ级，31%为ASA Ⅲ级，只有2%的患者为ASA Ⅳ级。性别也被认为与还纳率相关；尽管男性骨盆狭窄往往技术难度更大，但众多研究显示男性总体还纳率较高[4,7,16]。

原发病（哈特曼手术的适应证）对哈特曼术后还纳的影响

哈特曼手术最初设计用于治疗肿瘤性梗阻，而现在的适应证也包括良性疾病，比如复杂的憩室炎、外伤性损害、左半结肠缺血、穿孔、乙状结肠扭转以及吻合口瘘等。最近发表的一篇文献综述显示，良性疾病是哈特曼手术最常见的适应证（83%），其次才是结肠恶性肿瘤（17%）[19]。哈特曼手术的最初适应证对于哈特曼术后还纳的决定具有重要的影响，同样也影响还纳的时机。在大多数病例组中，由于良性疾病行哈特曼手术的患者还纳的百分比更高。这与资料显示的一致，即晚期恶性肿瘤是放弃还纳的重要因素[5,12,16,20-22]。

此外，最初行哈特曼手术的适应证能直接影响还纳的时机，治疗良性疾病的哈特曼手术的中位还纳时间始终早于治疗恶性肿瘤的还纳时间[2]。良性疾病术后还纳的时间应当仔细评估，以提供足够的时间来使瘢痕组织和粘连成熟，以及改善的患者一般健康状况。通常，评估依赖于剖腹手术所见、患者术后的恢复、如Hinchey评分所定义的初始腹膜炎指数、术后并发症的发病率以及伤口愈合的初期问题。恶性疾病还纳时间通常延迟，因为大多数外科医生重建之前需要除外盆腔复发，同时由于完全辅助治疗花费的时间，可能延迟更多。由于哈特曼手术通常用于局部晚期的肿瘤（恶性梗阻、癌性穿孔），大多数患者需要辅助治疗，而且局部或远处复发的概率较高。

还纳的时机

哈特曼术后还纳的时机问题仍旧是许多争论的

关键。在大多数病例组中，患者一般在初次手术后7～8个月进行还纳[7, 13, 23, 24]。然而，一些研究者认为在不增加术后并发症危险或者术中技术难度的情况下，这一时间可以缩短。Roe 等[20] 对比了 4 个月前和 4 个月后行还纳手术的患者的并发症发生率和死亡率，没有发现明显差异，提示还纳前的时间不应超过 4 个月。其他研究者认为在不增加并发症风险的情况下，这一时期可以缩短至 1 个月，声称在此期间，手术技术更为容易，而且直肠残端的辨认和解剖更为简单[21]。另一方面，相当长的时间后再行还纳经常导致残余直肠的萎缩，使得还纳在技术上更加困难。在这一点上，Mortensen 等[25] 指出：在哈特曼术后还纳之前向直肠残端滴注短链脂肪酸能够增加肠黏膜的血流和肠黏膜隐窝的高度，建议还纳前直肠残端应进行局部处理。无论如何，绝大多数中心均没有哈特曼术后还纳前评估直肠残端的确切方案[26]。目前，X 线或内镜学对直肠残端的评估能否事实上影响最终的手术方案尚未明确，尤其是当初次手术治疗良性疾病时。由于文献中关于时机问题并没有一致意见，肛肠科专家考虑到患者的状况、适应证、初次手术所见，以及初次手术的并发症，最值得关注的是直肠残端的长度，再为每一个特定的病例做最后决定[27-29]。

术后并发症对于哈特曼术后还纳的影响

初次手术的术后并发症可能直接影响是否进行重建以及手术的时机。虽然它从技术上增加了重建中的难度及重建之后的并发症发生率，但这一重要问题在文献中被忽视，哈特曼手术最重要的并发症是直肠残端裂开及造口相关并发症。这两种并发症都将危及患者的生命，并对幸存患者有长期的影响。直肠残端裂开可能导致残端上方盆腔脓肿的形成，如处理不当，它将扩散为弥漫性腹膜炎。在大多数病例，脓肿可以通过肛门经残端开放引流来治疗。这一治疗要在作出诊断后尽快完成，因为任何的延误都可能导致严重的感染和盆腔脓毒症。结果，在试图恢复肠道连续性时可以预料到过度的残端纤维化。过度的纤维化使纤维变性，且易于撕裂，可能导致在进入盆腔或分辨及解剖直肠残端时出现很多困难。如果在初次手术时直肠系膜被游离，它可能附着在盆筋膜上，使得后壁解剖较为困难，因为其有导致骶前静脉丛严重出血的风险。小肠、直肠残端、膀胱及周围组织比如邻近输尿管的粘连可能使重建更为复杂。

难易程度也与直肠残端封闭的水平相符，有时这些困难可能是放弃还纳的原因。初次术后治愈的弥漫性腹膜炎可能会促进腹腔和盆腔僵硬致密粘连的进展，使重建手术充满挑战。伤口裂开以及术后疝的发展也常见于这类患者，构成了重建手术的一部分。

残余直肠长度对于哈特曼术后还纳的影响

在剩余直肠长度和哈特曼术后重建的难度水平之间存在负相关，即直肠残端越短，还纳难度越大。在此方面，哈特曼术后肠道连续性的恢复根据残余直肠的长度可以分为三组。这三组中的每一种均存在着特殊的问题、技术挑战以及并发症。

"高位"重建定义为在首次手术时保留大部分直肠，直肠残端封闭于或高于骨盆缘（即残余直肠的长度通过硬式直肠镜检查自肛缘超过 10cm）。

"中位"重建是指直肠系膜被横断，残余直肠在盆腔深部被封闭（即通过硬质直肠镜测量残余直肠长度自肛缘约 5～10cm）。

"低位"重建是指进行了全直肠系膜切除术，残余直肠在盆膈水平或稍靠上被封闭。为准确定义，在仅残存肛管的病例，剩余直肠（肛管）长度用硬式直肠镜测量距肛外缘最多 5cm。

高位重建

在大多数哈特曼术后还纳的病例采用高位重建。Banerjee 等发表的研究中[7]，81% 的修复手术是"高位直肠或远端乙状结肠"。这一现象有一定原因。首先，憩室病是哈特曼手术最常见的适应证。在这些病例中，直肠被保留，并在骶骨岬水平封闭。其次，高位重建技术要求较低，可由普通外科医生完成，此种重建占现有文献的绝大部分。手术的附加操作包括术中直肠镜检查以及子宫扩张器或扩张器大小的圆形吻合器的插入。再者，术中并不需要游离残余直肠，因为结直肠吻合可以通过在直肠前壁的端侧吻合安全实现，如图 45.1。

这种方式尤其适用于哈特曼手术治疗良性疾病的患者。在因癌症而进行的手术中，尤其是担心残

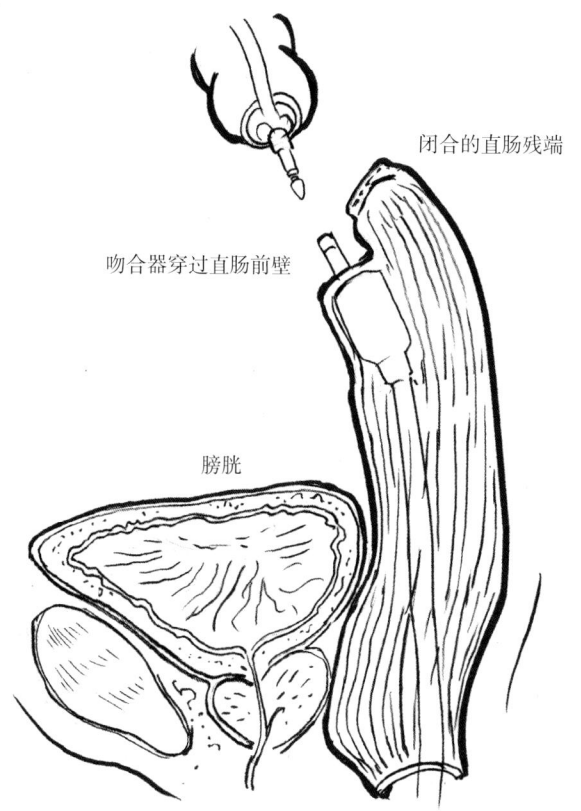

图 45.1 高位重建时通过直肠前壁插入吻合器。注意吻合器至少在直肠残端远端 3~4cm（依据其尺寸）插入

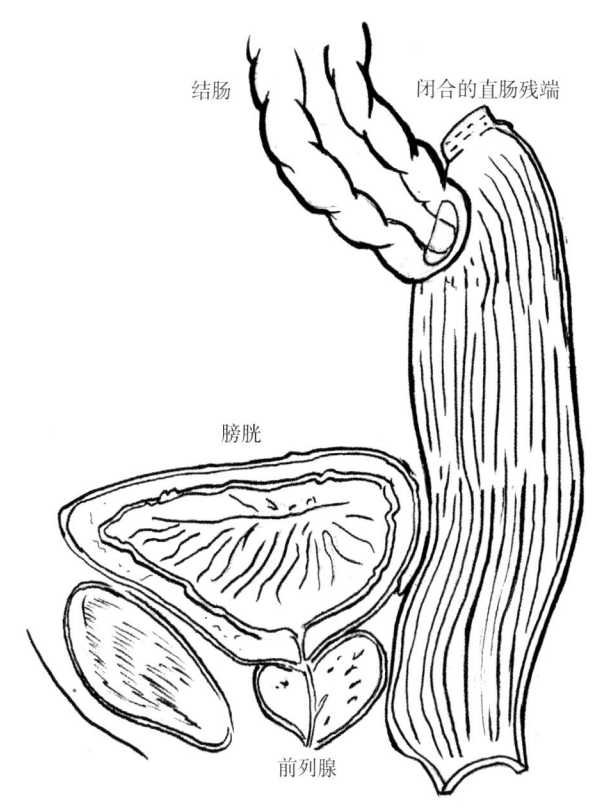

图 45.2 高位重建时在直肠前壁建立结直肠吻合术。注意吻合口需要远离膀胱及其他盆腔器官

余直肠局部复发的患者，可以适当游离直肠，将残余直肠部分切除，根据术中病理检查所见，最终确定是否再吻合。在这样的病例，端端吻合术是可取的。在直肠前壁进行端侧吻合的病例值得思考（不游离直肠残端），需要注意吻合口要距离先前直肠残端的封闭口至少约2cm，因为这一区域由于血供减少可能会增厚（图45.2）。

如果可能，外科医生需要知道初次手术中直肠残端封闭的技术。如果运用荷包缝合（通常双层缝扎），与闭合器相比，残端更厚，吻合口需要移至更远端。同样，在这一区域过度纤维化的患者（由于先前的缝线渗漏），吻合口需要建立在更远端没有增厚并且具有更好血液供应的区域。吻合可以手法缝合，或者更好的是利用圆形吻合器（单排或双排钉技术）。当尝试吻合器吻合时，在直肠前壁没有必要建立荷包缝合（或者不合适），因为单纯将圆形吻合器的钉砧通过直肠壁的小孔在可以让绝大多数病例满意。孔需要在直肠残端远端至少 3~4cm 的位置建立（取决于圆形吻合器的尺寸）。出于这一目的，我们选择弯曲、中等尺寸（28~29mm）圆形吻合器，因为他们更容易通过直肠插入。在直肠前壁建立吻合简化了步骤，缩短了手术时间，彻底消除了游离直肠残端带来的并发症。

应主要避免的并发症包括损伤输尿管（在这一部位曾行放射治疗或恶性肿瘤患者通常需要支架支撑）、生殖器血管、腹下神经，它们中的任何一个都可能粘连到直肠残端的纤维组织[30]。在预期放置输尿管支架的情况下进行初步的 CT 扫描可以提供包括输尿管位置（以及数目）和双侧排泄功能的信息，可能影响这一决定[31]。输尿管支架在重建手术中易被触及，或能被透视。如果直肠残端明显萎缩（尤其哈特曼术后还纳耽搁较久），在吻合器插入的过程中存在直肠壁撕裂的风险。直肠壁的全层撕裂是严重的并发症，但它在术中易被发现。可更为隐蔽的是直肠黏膜层的撕裂，也可导致严重的并发症。

这些黏膜层撕裂易被忽略，直到由于术后直肠出血、或脓毒性并发症，或二者并存而变得明显。我们认为，在哈特曼术后还纳前1月内对残余直肠进行重复的球囊扩张术，或利用硬性扩张器进行持续的扩张，对于预防此类特殊的术中并发症可能有效。在这些情况下可以应用28~29mm的圆形吻合器。强烈推荐在插入吻合器前用硬质U型扩张器测量直肠直径，来避免直肠壁的损伤。在经过上述处理之后插入吻合器仍不安全的病例，如果可能，应尽量尝试手法吻合。结肠近端应该在结肠造口上方切除几厘米以准备吻合。在结肠造口术近端残存不复杂憩室病的患者，如果该结肠肠段较短而且不需要结肠大部切除术，该肠段应被切除。如果该肠段较长并可能需要结肠大部切除术，应原位保留该肠段，并注意不要将憩室部分并入吻合口。大多数情况下，并不需要游离结肠脾曲以获得足够长度来完成无张力的可靠吻合。

中位重建

中位重建通常适用于因直肠癌而进行的哈特曼手术。在这些病例中，直肠系膜被横断，残余直肠在盆腔深部被封闭。此种重建技术要求高，需要由有经验的结直肠外科医生完成。这种情况下的手术技巧与高位重建完全不同。在大多数情况下，尤其男性，不可能在直肠前壁解剖出足够的长度来为可靠的吻合获得额外的游离空间。在女性，可能能从阴道上游离直肠壁，使得在直肠前壁建立吻合成为可能。在这些情况下，要注意避免将部分阴道后壁并入吻合口，这将导致阴道直肠瘘的形成。然而直肠残端的解剖，尤其是前部，充满挑战，男性或女性患者均易出现并发症；无论何时均应避免，这种情况下端-端吻合更为安全。此外，小肠和盆腔脏器（膀胱、子宫、卵巢、前列腺和精囊）在直肠切除术后易于填充盆腔空间，而使粘连松解术特别困难（图45.3）。

直肠残端在腹膜外封闭而没有完全关闭盆腔腹膜的患者尤其困难。我们认为用腹膜覆盖骨盆腔是哈特曼手术重要的一步，能使还纳简化并减少小肠损伤的风险。然而，在术中向前牵拉盆腔腹膜的过程中，如果在缝合之前没有特别注意去解剖双侧输尿管，他们可能被向中间牵拉。解剖要始终从直肠残端的中后方开始，并向侧面进行，这样更为安全而且要求不高。需要强调的是如果解剖并没有从这一位置开始，双侧输尿管由于前述的盆腔腹膜化可能向中间移位，损伤的风险较高。在合并直肠残端裂开以及已愈合或正在愈合的盆腔脓肿病例，直肠残端和周围器官的粘连可能致密且纤维化，使粘连松解术充满挑战。小肠和膀胱损伤的风险较高，尤其是男性，因为膀胱有向下进入盆腔并附着在直肠残端的趋势。由于骨盆狭窄，空间缺乏，男性患者的解剖更加困难，膀胱、精囊、前列腺和盆腔神经损伤的风险更高（图45.4）。

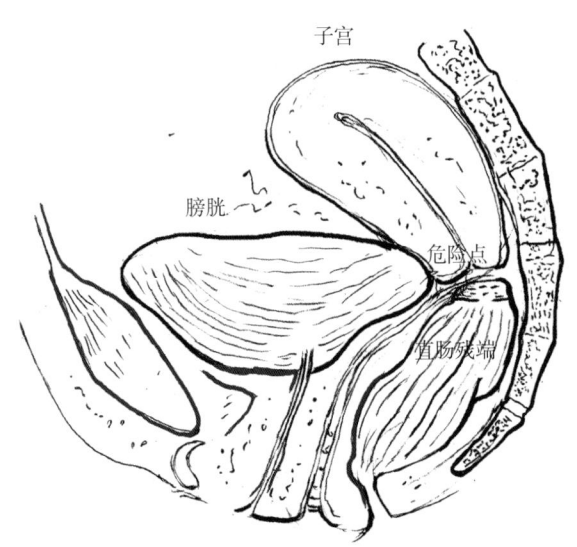

图45.3 女性盆腔器官（膀胱和子宫），在直肠切除术后倾向于填充盆腔空间，使得粘连松解术尤为困难

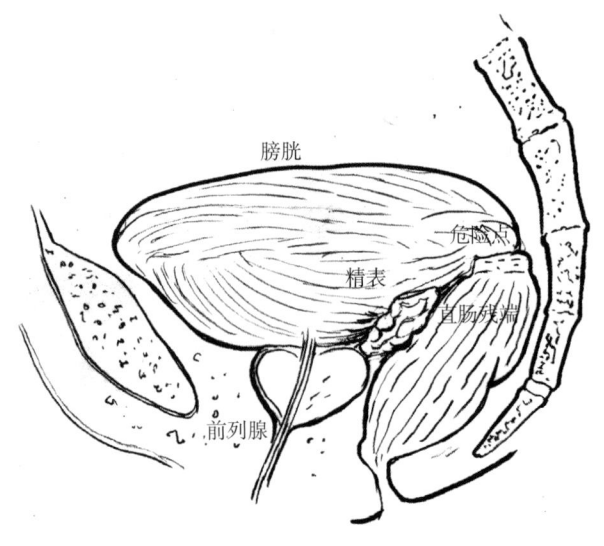

图45.4 男性患者，膀胱倾向于降入盆腔并附着在直肠残端。注意男性解剖由于骨盆狭窄空间狭小更为困难，相比有较高风险出现膀胱、精囊、前列腺和盆腔神经的损伤

有过子宫切除术的女性患者，损伤膀胱或阴道的风险以及大量骶前出血的风险都很高。进行过前骶骨阴道固定术的女性，远期并发症是其一个特征，骶前解剖是不明智的。如果其真要进行，后壁解剖应尽可能在肌肉周围层面（贴近直肠壁）进行。通过向直肠残端和阴道内插入金属扩张器或者手指来辨认二者，有助于困难盆腔的解剖。当经过最小的解剖能够肯定分辨直肠残端时，环形吻合器的钉砧通过一个小孔插入，该小孔需要朝向后壁建立，尤其是前壁分离困难的病例。需要注意不要将膀胱或阴道的一部分并入吻合。如果前壁解剖极为困难，伤及周围脏器的风险很高，手术医生应该集中于后壁的解剖并在直肠后壁建立吻合。如前所述，虽然直肠后壁的解剖较前壁解剖要求低，骶骨前解剖使得如此的后壁解剖尤为危险。

低位重建

低位重建通常用于对中位直肠癌采用哈特曼手术的患者。在大多数情况下进行了全直肠系膜切除术，直肠残端被封闭在盆腔深部肛提肌水平。此类重建手术只能由有经验的结直肠外科医生完成。在这些病例进行哈特曼术后还纳时，主要注意的是较短的直肠残端、盆腔粘连，以及不确定的术后功能结果。所有先前描述的中位重建中关于盆腔粘连松解术的问题，都将在低位重建中出现，而且更严重。从盆腔移除了小肠粘连之后，然后开始解剖直肠残端。周围脏器都要从直肠残端上小心的游离，尤其要注意避免损伤膀胱、男性的前列腺、精囊以及女性的子宫和阴道。将一根手指插入肛管或者阴道将使直肠残端的解剖更为容易。如果直肠残端游离出了足够长度进行可靠的吻合，可以运用圆形吻合器完成端端吻合术。在大多数情况下，直肠残端较厚，使得用吻合器进行吻合的安全性更差。

在这种情况下，在直肠残端做小的深达固有肌层的放射状切开可能解决这一问题；然而，在大多数情况下，在如此短小的直肠残端进行安全切开是不可能的，因此推荐黏膜切除术并经肛手法缝合结直肠吻合术。运用这种技术，就不必进行广泛而危险的直肠残端的游离。进行全直肠系膜切除术后直肠残端很容易分辨，其开始于齿状线上约1cm，而结束于直肠残端的尖端。黏膜切除术可以经肛和经腹手法辅助，可以通过黏膜下注射稀释肾上腺素来减少出血，增加可见度和在正确层面解剖，从而使其更容易。针对同样的技术最初描述为部分的回肠贮袋肛管吻合术，用于炎性肠病或家族性息肉病的治疗[32]，移行区一般需要保留以改善功能效果。在全黏膜切除术后，直肠残端应该经肛穿过瘢痕组织在直视下切开。切口应足够大以容纳经肛管带出的结肠，然后进行直肠肛管手法缝合吻合术，如 Parks 所述[33]。我们认为在手术结束时应进行辅助性回肠造口术。在大多数情况下，结肠脾曲需要通过高位结扎肠系膜下动静脉来充分游离，以获得足够长度的结肠来建立无张力吻合。结肠脾曲游离过程中的脾脏损伤是少见但严重的并发症。据报道，结肠切除术中脾脏损伤的发生率约 0.42%，而在需要游离脾曲的患者发生率升高至 3.1%[34, 35]。

先前的控便功能

先前的控便功能是一个重要的问题，尤其是在考虑低位重建的情况下。低位前切除术后的功能恢复和结肠肛管吻合可能不令人满意，主要是因为大便失禁和以便频和不成形便为表现的排便障碍（即所谓的低位前切除综合征）[36]。这些问题可能在哈特曼术后还纳之后出现，尤其是低位重建的病例，因此还纳前患者对功能恢复需要充分的认识。大多数患者还纳前并不需要常规的控便功能的评估，然而有轻症失禁病史及明显的肛门直肠手术的患者需要评估。由于直肠储袋的减少、骨盆神经病变以及经肛吻合的建立中对于肛门括约肌的牵拉造成的可能的括约肌损伤，低位重建与大便失禁的高风险有关。有一组多数为女性患者的病例，在哈特曼术前有控便功能受损但没有便失禁的症状。在大多数病例，她们都有不易察觉的产科括约肌损伤或阴部神经病变。

在低位重建之后，已经受损的控便机制在新的解剖结构中已不适用（直肠储存功能的丧失），而导致大便失禁。这一组患者难以区分。控便功能可疑的患者需要被选出，并利用调查问卷、肛门测压和直肠内超声进行评估。在预计严重失禁的病例，应当避免进行哈特曼术后还纳。

直肠残端的评估

剩余直肠残端的长度对于哈特曼术后还纳后的排便功能最为重要，因为直肠有较大容量，在粪便排出之前充当储存器。直肠切除的总量越大，直肠容积和顺应性丧失越多，导致排便急迫、频繁。此外，在初次手术和还纳间隔较长的患者，可能出现直肠残端的萎缩和改道性结肠炎，使得还纳后的功能效果更差。幸运的是，直肠残端萎缩和改道性结肠炎能够通过重建手术逆转，而不妨碍哈特曼术后还纳[37-39]。虽然缺乏证据支持[26]，但重建术前应常规反复对直肠残端进行内镜检查并对比。在此方面，Cherukuri 等[40]指出哈特曼术后还纳前无症状的患者 X 线的直肠残端异常的发生率较低，而大多异常的 X 线或内镜学发现似乎并不影响确定性治疗[26, 41]。我们中心术前常规进行直肠残端的 X 线和内镜学检查，除了文献中记录的具体价值外，还可以确定直肠残端的长度、意外瘘的存在、狭窄、感染、肿瘤复发以及直肠残端的萎缩。这种评估的方式在异地进行哈特曼手术的患者是必需的，可以协助手术设计，以及预期功能恢复的预测和咨询。在某些情况下，这样的信息可以为一些患者转诊至更有经验的肛肠科医生提供根据。

功能效果与生活质量

现有的关于哈特曼术后重建的文献，主要报道了手术的短期预后，包括死亡率和并发症发生率，而没有探讨生活质量和功能恢复。现代外科学认为在评估外科手术术后临床结果时，标准化的生活质量评估是重要因素。虽然很多患者组并没有严格的对比[44]，传统认为，与永久性结肠造口术相比，保留括约肌式的术后生活质量更好[42-43]。直观上大多数哈特曼术后患者愿意选择恢复肠道的连续性，原因是他们面对生理和心理的双重压力，大多都和造口相关[45]。在这方面，造口还纳能够使其整体生活质量以及生理和社交功能都有显著的提高[46]。最近研究显示哈特曼术后造口的存在是总体生活质量更差的独立因素，而且生活质量的恶化主要由于生理功能和身体形象的问题[47]。Vermeulen 等[12]最近一项评价憩室性腹膜炎术后数年生活质量的研究表明，与进行哈特曼手术的患者相比，一期手术患者生活质量更高；只有严重术后并发症的发生率超过 40% 时，将妨碍患者生活质量。然而，在大多数病例，哈特曼术后还纳的功能恢复和生活质量令人满意；Constantinides 等[48]指出哈特曼术后还纳患者的生活质量与一期手术患者及一般人群生活质量相仿。尤其是在进行高位重建（如所定义）患者的情况下，其直肠及控便机制均保持原状。低位重建的患者功能恢复不满意和生活质量下降的风险最高，因为他们的大部分直肠在初次手术中被切除，直肠顺应性和容积大大减小，同时还有肛门括约肌损伤的风险，这取决于所用的吻合技术。存在吻合口并发症的患者功能恢复和生活质量可能下降更多，需要经历不同程度的大便失禁和排便功能障碍。在一些极端情况下，对于某些患者，结肠造口再造是他们唯一的解决办法。虽然很难预测低位哈特曼术后还纳的最终预后，肛肠专家需要尽量去分辨较差功能恢复危险性高的患者，当需要时，在还纳前进行额外的检查（如前所述）。肛门直肠生理测试在再手术患者功能失调风险中的作用在本书第一篇有涉及。

腹腔镜哈特曼术后还纳：一个可行的选择

很多中心将哈特曼术后还纳的技术改为全腹腔镜或腹腔镜辅助的方式。毫无疑问这导致了一项要求更高的技术，依照开腹手术的步骤，可以进行粘连松解术、直肠残端的辨认和游离，如果需要的话可进行脾曲的游离，通过腹腔内定位经吻合口插入吻合器钉砧[48]。这一步骤与开腹手术相比，具有可接受的平均手术时间、几乎没有差别的术后并发症发生率，似乎选择性可行[49-52]。关于这两项还纳技术的前瞻性[52]和回顾性[50, 53]对比研究发现腹腔镜组中转开腹率约 9%~19%，缩短了住院时间，减少了输血量，肠道功能恢复更早，弥补了手术器械花费的增加。术中中转开腹的主要原因如所预料一样，在低位重建患者，粘连松解术或者寻找挛缩的直肠残端的困难。如同最近一项针对 8 组对照研究 450 例患者的荟萃分析，许多此类研究都是病例对照研究而不是随机试验。腹腔镜治疗组的晚期并发症率略低于开腹手术组，开腹手术组中 6 个月的并发症和再手术大多是与腹壁相关[53]。两组患者的再次住院率相似，但开腹组更多由于外科原因，而腹腔镜组则多由于内科原因。如我们所预想的，随机临床对照试验显示，在高位和中位直肠病例可能会有更多常规转变为腹腔镜还纳的尝试，尤其是那些通常由 ASA 评分评判为高危和妨碍开腹重建者。

参考文献

1. Hartmann H. Note sur un procéde nouveau d'extirpation des cancers de la partie du côlon. Bull Mem Soc Chir Paris. 1923;49:1474–7.
2. David GG, Al-Sarira AA, Wilmott S, Cade D, Corless DJ, Slavin JP. Use of Hartmann's procedure in England. Colorectal Dis. 2009;11:308–12.
3. Oomen JL, Cuesta MA, Engel AF. Reversal of Hartmann's procedure after surgery for complications of diverticular disease of the sigmoid colon is safe and possible in most patients. Dig Surg. 2005;22:419–25.
4. Wigmore SJ, Duthie GS, Young IE, Spalding EM, Rainey JB. Restoration of intestinal continuity following Hartmann's procedure: the Lothian experience 1987–1992. Br J Surg. 1995;82:27–30.
5. Leong QM, Koh DC, Ho CK. Emergency Hartmann's procedure: morbidity, mortality and reversal rates among Asians. Tech Coloproctol. 2008;12:21–5.
6. Pearce NW, Scott SD, Karran SJ. Timing and method of reversal of Hartmann's procedure. Br J Surg. 1992;79:839–41.
7. Banerjee S, Leather AJ, Rennie JA, Samano N, Gonzales JG, Papgrigoriadis S. Feasibility and morbidity of reversal of Hartmann's. Colorectal Dis. 2005;7:454–9.
8. Schmelzer TM, Mostafa G, Norton HJ, Newcomb WL, Hope WW, Lincourt AE, et al. Reversal of Hartmann's procedure: a high-risk operation. Surgery. 2007;142:598–607.
9. Albarran SA, Simoens C, Van De Winkel N, da Costa PM, Thil V. Restoration of digestive continuity after Hartmann's procedure: ASA score is a predictive factor for risk of postoperative complications. Acta Chir Belg. 2009;109:714–9.
10. Riansuwan W, Hull TL, Millan MM, Hammel J. Nonreversal of Hartmann's procedure for diverticulitis: derivation of a scoring system to predict nonreversal. Dis Colon Rectum. 2009;52:1400–8.
11. Aydin HN, Remzi FH, Tekkis PP, Fazio VW. Hartmann's reversal is associated with high postoperative adverse events. Dis Colon Rectum. 2005;48:2117–26.
12. Vermeulen J, Gosselink M, Busschbach JJ, Lange JF. Avoiding or reversing Hartmann's procedure provides improved quality of life after perforated diverticulitis. J Gastrointest Surg. 2010;14:651–7.
13. Paredes JP, Caínzos M, García J, Parada P, Fernández E, Paulos A, Potel J. Colostomy closure: is it an intervention without risk? Rev Esp Enferm Dig. 1994;86:733–7.
14. Ghorra SG, Rzeczycki TP, Natarajan R, Pricolo VE. Colostomy closure: impact of preoperative risk factors on morbidity. Am Surg. 1999;65:266–9.
15. Albarran SA, Simoens C, Takeh H, Mendes da Costa P. Restoration of digestive continuity after Hartmann's procedure. Hepatogastroenterology. 2004;51:1045–9.
16. Roque-Castellano C, Marchena-Gomez J, Hemmersbach-Miller M, Acosta-Merida A, Rodriguez-Mendez A, Fariña-Castro R, et al. Analysis of the factors related to the decision of restoring intestinal continuity after Hartmann's procedure. Int J Colorectal Dis. 2007;22:1091–6.
17. Pessaux P, Muscari F, Ouellet JF, Msika S, Hay JM, Millat B, et al. Risk factors for mortality and morbidity after elective sigmoid resection for diverticulitis: prospective multicenter multivariate analysis of 582 patients. World J Surg. 2004;28:92–6.
18. Longo WE, Virgo KS, Johnson FE, Oprian CA, Vernava AM, Wade TP, et al. Risk factors for morbidity and mortality after colectomy for colon cancer. Dis Colon Rectum. 2000;43:83–91.
19. van der Wall BJ, Draaisma WA, Schouten ES, Broeders I, Consten E. Conventional and laparoscopic reversal of the hartmann procedure: a review of literature. J Gastrointest Surg. 2010;14:743–52.
20. Roe AM, Prabhu S, Ali A, Brown C, Brodribb AJ. Reversal of Hartmann's procedure: timing and operative technique. Br J Surg. 1991;78:1167–70.
21. Geoghegan JG, Rosenberg IL. Experience with early anastomosis after the Hartmann procedure. Ann R Coll Surg Engl. 1991;73:80.
22. Khan AL, Ah-See AK, Crofts TJ, Heys SD, Eremin O. Reversal of Hartmann's colostomy. J R Coll Surg Edinb. 1994;39:239–42.
23. Bielecki K, Kami ski P. Hartmann procedure: place in surgery and what after? Int J Colorectal Dis. 1995;10:49–52.
24. Khosraviani K, Campbell WJ, Parks TG, Irwin ST. Hartmann procedure revisited. Eur J Surg. 2000;166:878–81.
25. Mortensen FV, Hessov I, Birke H, Korsgaard N, Nielsen H. Microcirculatory and trophic effects of short chain fatty acids in the human rectum after Hartmann's procedure. Br J Surg. 1991;78:1208–11.
26. Ballian N, Zarebczan B, Munoz A, Harms B, Heise C, Foley EF, et al. routine evaluation of the distal colon remnant before Hartmann's reversal is not necessary in asymptomatic patients. J Gastrointest Surg. 2009;13:2260–7.
27. Keck JO, Collopy BT, Ryan PJ, Fink R, Mackay JR, Woods RJ. Reversal of Hartmann's procedure: effect of timing and technique on ease and safety. Dis Colon Rectum. 1994;37:243–8.
28. Roque-Castellano C, Marchena-Gomez J, Hammersbach-Miller M, Acosta-Merida A, Rodriguez-Mendez A, Farina-Castro R, et al. Analysis of the factors related to the decision of restoring intestinal continuity after Hartmann's procedure. Int J Colorectal Dis. 2007;22:1091–6.
29. Tokode AM, Akingboye A, Coker O. Factors affecting reversal following Hartmann's procedure: experience from two district general hospitals in the UK. Surg Today. 2011;41:79–83.
30. Bothwell WN, Bleicher RJ, Dent TL. Prophylactic ureteral catheterization in colon surgery. Dis Colon Rectum. 1994;37:330–4.
31. Zbar AP, Rambarat C, Shenoy RK. Routine preoperative abdominal computed tomography in colonic cancer: a utility study. Tech Coloproctol. 2007;11:105–9.
32. Bülow S. Mucosectomy and stapled pouch-anal anastomosis in familial adenomatous polyposis. Colorectal Dis. 2012;14(1):68–70.
33. Parks A. Transanal technique in low rectal anastomosis. Proc R Soc Med. 1972;65:975–6.
34. Langevin JM, Rothenberger DA, Goldberg SM. Accidental splenic injury during surgical treatment of the colon and rectum. Surg Gynecol Obstet. 1984;159:139–44.
35. Holubar SD, Wang JK, Wolff BG, Nagorney DM, Dozois EJ, Cima RR, et al. Splenic salvage after intraoperative splenic injury during colectomy. Arch Surg. 2009;144:1040–5.
36. Matsuoka H, Masaki T, Kobayashi T, Sato K, Mori T, Sugiyama M, et al. Neurophysiologic investigation of anal function following double stapling anastomosis. Dig Surg. 2010;27:320–3.
37. Haas PA, Fox Jr TA. The fate of the forgotten rectal pouch after Hartmann's procedure without reconstruction. Am J Surg. 1990;159:106–10.
38. Deruyter L, Delvaux G, Willems G. Restoration of colorectal continuity reverses atrophy in human rectal mucosa. Dig Dis Sci. 1990;35:488–94.
39. Orsay CP, Kim DO, Pearl RK, Abcarian H. Diversion colitis in patients scheduled for colostomy closure. Dis Colon Rectum. 1993;36:366–7.
40. Cherukuri R, Levine M, Maki DD, Rubesin SE, Laufer I, Rosato EF. Hartmann's pouch: radiographic evaluation of postoperative findings. Am J Roentgenol. 1998;171:1577–82.
41. da Silva GM, Wexner SD, Gurland B, Gervaz P, Moon SD, Efron J, et al. Is routine pouchogram prior to ileostomy closure in colonic J-pouch really necessary? Colorectal Dis. 2004;6:117–20.
42. Williams NS, Johnston D. The quality of life after rectal excision for low rectal cancer. Br J Surg. 1983;70:460–2.
43. Hassan I, Larson DW, Cima RR, Gaw JU, Chua HK, Hahnloser D, et al. Long-term functional and quality of life outcomes after coloanal anastomosis for distal rectal cancer. Dis Colon Rectum. 2006;49:1266–74.

44. Grumann MM, Noack EM, Hoffmann IA, Schlag PM. Comparison of quality of life in patients undergoing abdominoperineal extirpation or anterior resection for rectal cancer. Ann Surg. 2001;233:149–56.
45. Nugent KP, Daniels P, Stewart B, Patankar R, Johnson CD. Quality of life in stoma patients. Dis Colon Rectum. 1999;42:1569–74.
46. Camilleri-Brennan J, Steele RJ. Prospective analysis of quality of life after reversal of a defunctioning loop ileostomy. Colorectal Dis. 2002;4:167–71.
47. Constantinides VA, Heriot A, Remzi F, Darzi A, Senapati A, Fazio VW, et al. Operative strategies for diverticular peritonitis: a decision analysis between primary resection and anastomosis versus Hartmann's procedures. Ann Surg. 2007;245:94–103.
48. Leroy J, Constantino F, Cahill RA, D'Agostino J, Wu WH, Mutter D, et al. Technical aspects and outcome of a standardized full laparoscopic approach to the reversal of Hartmann's procedure in a teaching centre. Colorectal Dis. 2011;13(9):1058–65.
49. Carus T, Bollman S, Lienhard H. Laparoscopic reversal of Hartmann's procedure: technique and results. Surg Laparosc Endosc Percutan Tech. 2008;18:24–8.
50. Mazeh H, Greenstein AJ, Swedish K, Nguyen SQ, Lipskar A, Weber KJ, et al. Laparoscopic and open reversal of Hartmann's procedure – a comparative retrospective analysis. Surg Endosc. 2009;23:496–502.
51. Chouillard E, Pierard T, Campbell R, Tabary N. Laparoscopically assisted Hartmann's reversal is an efficacious and efficient procedure: a case control study. Minerva Chir. 2009;64:1–8.
52. Siddiqui MR, Sajid MS, Baig MK. Open vs laparoscopic approach for reversal of Hartmann's procedure: a systematic review. Colorectal Dis. 2010;12:733–41.
53. Haughn C, Ju B, Uchal M, Arnaud JP, Reed JF, Bergamaschi R. Complication rates after Hartmann's reversal: open vs laparoscopic approach. Dis Colon Rectum. 2008;51:1232–6.

第 46 章 儿童肠造口并发症的再手术治疗

Andrea Bischoff · Marc A. Levitt · Alberto Peña

王树森 译　王西墨 审校

摘 要

结肠造口术在儿童中并不罕见，尤其常常被应用在肛门直肠畸形的病例。针对经常由于不易定位和下垂造成的并发症，专家们关于如何进行专门的手术途径进行了讨论。手术途径需要考虑到直肠和肛门的重塑及这群特殊患者中是否存在与尿道相关的瘘管。

关键词

小儿造口；结肠造口术；肛门直肠畸形；倒置造口；右上乙状结肠造口术；造口脱垂；右横结肠造口术；左横结肠造口术；降结肠造口术；器官狭窄；缩复

引 言

结肠造口术是一种常见的儿科手术，尤其被经常应用于肛门直肠畸形的病例。由于儿科结肠直肠手术本身的特殊性，患者因为先天肛门直肠畸形，往往在出生时已经在其他地方接受了结肠造口术，到医院是为了进行最后的结构重塑。因此，我们进行了大量的结肠造口术，也由此获得了关于不同类型造口术存在的优缺点、最常见的难点、各自的特殊性及如何解决和避免这些难点的丰富经验[1]。

结肠造口术的目的是改变排泄物流向。这种转向包括完全性（分离的造口）和部分性（环形造口术）。然而针对肛门直肠畸形的处理，结肠造口术的目的稍有不同，手术除了必须达到降低胃肠道的压力外，还需做到完全改变粪便的流向以避免泌尿生殖器的污染，因为超过85%的肛门直肠畸形的患者在远端处和泌尿系统相通。为了达到这些目的，我们建议在左下1/4部位进行结肠造口术（图46.1），即利用降结肠接触腹膜后腔的优点在降结肠远端可移动的结肠部位进行。这种构建有助于避免随后的脱垂。为了术后的康复，结肠造口术必须留出足够的远端肠管，再者近端必须位于由最后一个左侧肋骨、脐及髂嵴所形成的三角形的中心，从而使结肠瘘袋适应于腹部表面的平坦部分。近端造口必须与远端造口完全分离以保证造口附件不会覆盖黏膜瘘。因此这些手术目的与在成年患者机体进行的传统造口术目的相差甚远。另外，因为黏膜瘘只是用来灌注和冲洗造影剂以明确修复前畸形的解剖结构，所以黏膜瘘需要小而且平坦（图46.1和图46.2）。

应用生理盐水完全冲洗远端肠管的胎粪是结肠造口术中一个重要的步骤。因为在直肠上的瘘管时，远端部分胎粪可造成粪瘤和泌尿道的污染。

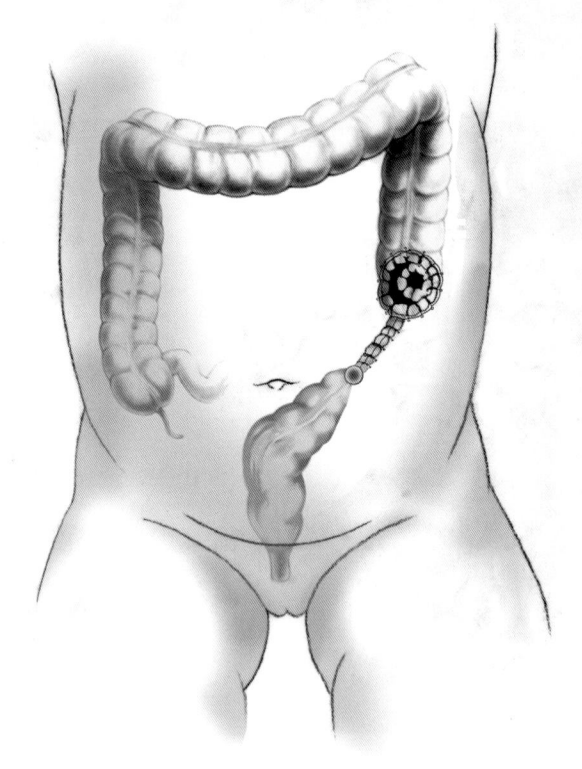

图 46.1 降结肠造口术

造口最常见的过失

造口定位错误

造口定位错误可由几种方式造成。

近端和远端造口之间距离太近

当近端和远端造口之间距离太近时，由于造口袋覆盖在两个造口上而使一段粪便从近端传至远端。因而造成一些患者反复尿道感染。可以通过两种方案解决这个问题：提前修复或加大两个造口的距离。

而这种两种方案的选择多少依赖于特定的临床情况。如果选择进行主要修复，经过重塑肠管的粪便将增加患者感染的危险性。鉴于这种情况可进行以下措施：

（1）术前清洗胃肠道，患者禁食大约一周，采取胃肠外营养供给；

（2）通过在远端造口制作一个密集的荷包缝合而暂时阻断肠管，以避免远端粪便经过。

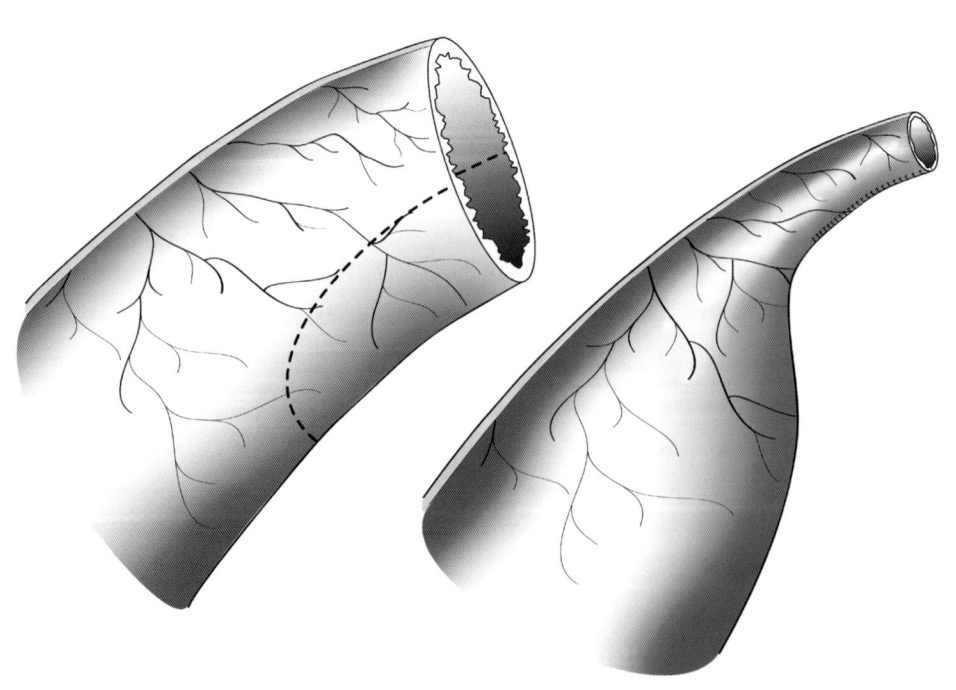

图 46.2 小而平坦的远端造口

结肠造口术在乙状结肠的过远侧进行，造成远端部分不够长以进行直肠拖出

在这种情况下，医生可有以下几种选择（图46.3）。第一种是通过下拉远端造口（黏膜瘘）并结扎成一个哈氏袋。有时这段肠管太短而使造口闭合术难度加大，因为这时吻合必须在膀胱后面的盆腔深部进行。第二种选择是在进行主要修复的时候实施造口关闭，然后下拉直肠，这种情况则使患者没有获得保护性的结肠造口术。在这种情况下，我们建议术前完全清洗胃肠道，患者禁食7～10天，胃肠外供给营养。第三种选择是关闭造口，下拉直肠，制作一个新的近端结肠造口术来转移粪便和保护会阴。

倒置造口

由于疏忽使近端造口位于不恰当位置，造口则很难适应造口袋（图46.4a，b）。另外一个问题是医生错误的缩窄肠管，臆断此肠管是黏膜瘘，结果引起阻塞发生，这种情况需要重新手术。关于倒置造口的另一问题是远端肠管存在张力，需要移动远端造口而留出足够长度的肠管进行随后的直肠拖出。

上腹部的乙状结肠造口术

在这种情况下外科医生计划进行横结肠造口术。因此，医生在上腹部做切口，找到一段结肠，认为它就是横结肠而取出进行结肠造口术。反而在上腹部进行的乙状结肠造口术则会干扰随后进行的拖出（图46.5）。在进行横结肠造口术时，医生必须记得患有肛门直肠畸形的新生儿具有一个非常膨胀的可以抵达膈的乙状结肠。当查明此情况后，在直肠拖出之前必须在下腹部重新进行结肠造口术。确定结肠造口术定位不适宜的最好诊断方法是远端结肠造影[3]，它是一种肛门结肠畸形主要修复术前的常规检测。

脱 垂

第二种最常见的并发症是结肠造口脱垂[3]。这是一种严重的并发症，往往由于缺血而造成肠缺失。我们认为在紧挨着结肠固定部位进行结肠造口可以避免大多数拖出并发症。如果结肠造口必须在肠管的移动部分进行，我们建议将距离造口大约6～7cm近端部位固定在前腹壁。在图46.6a-c可以识别出正常旋转结肠的可移动及固定部分，并且可以理解哪一部分易于脱垂而需要固定于腹前壁。

当一个患者患有严重脱垂时，我们会建议进行手术修复。首先将大量浸透聚烯吡酮碘的压缩棉嵌入脱垂肠管，稍稍缩短脱垂部分。然后通过触诊判断触摸到的团块正是朝向腹内侧的肠管内的压缩棉。在触诊到的团块上方做一个横切口，通常距离造口5cm。相继打开皮肤、皮下组织、肌肉、筋膜、腱膜和腹膜后，则很容易就识别出充填棉球的肠管。而后应用间断性vicry缝线缝合结扎腹膜和腱膜，每一个缝合内均包含一段肠管壁（没有带出压缩棉），将肠管牢固的固定在腹壁而防止脱垂发生。

狭 窄

因狭窄而患有阻塞症状的患者比我们预测的多。当打开造口，特别建议建造一个适当空间，有利于功能性肠管通过而不受筋膜压迫。这是为避免

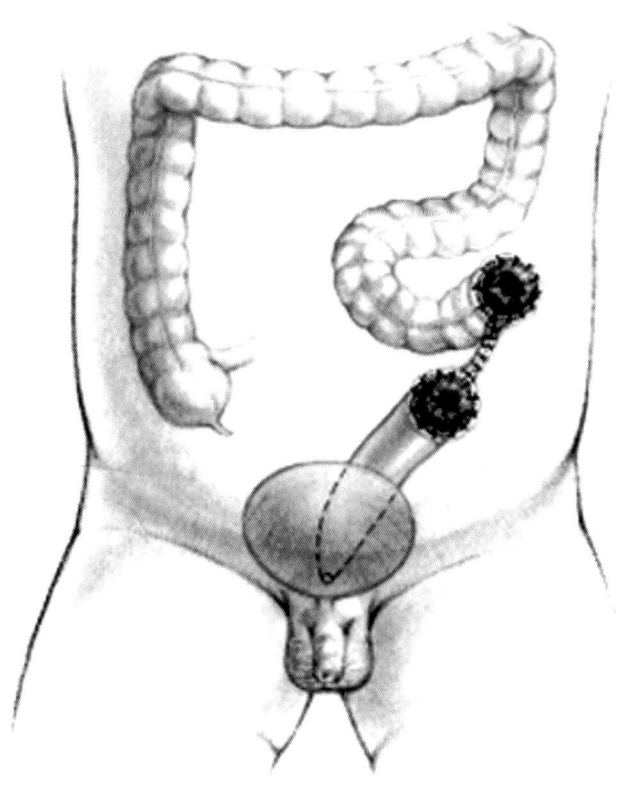

图46.3 太远端的结肠造口术致使远端肠管不够长来进行拉出操作[2]

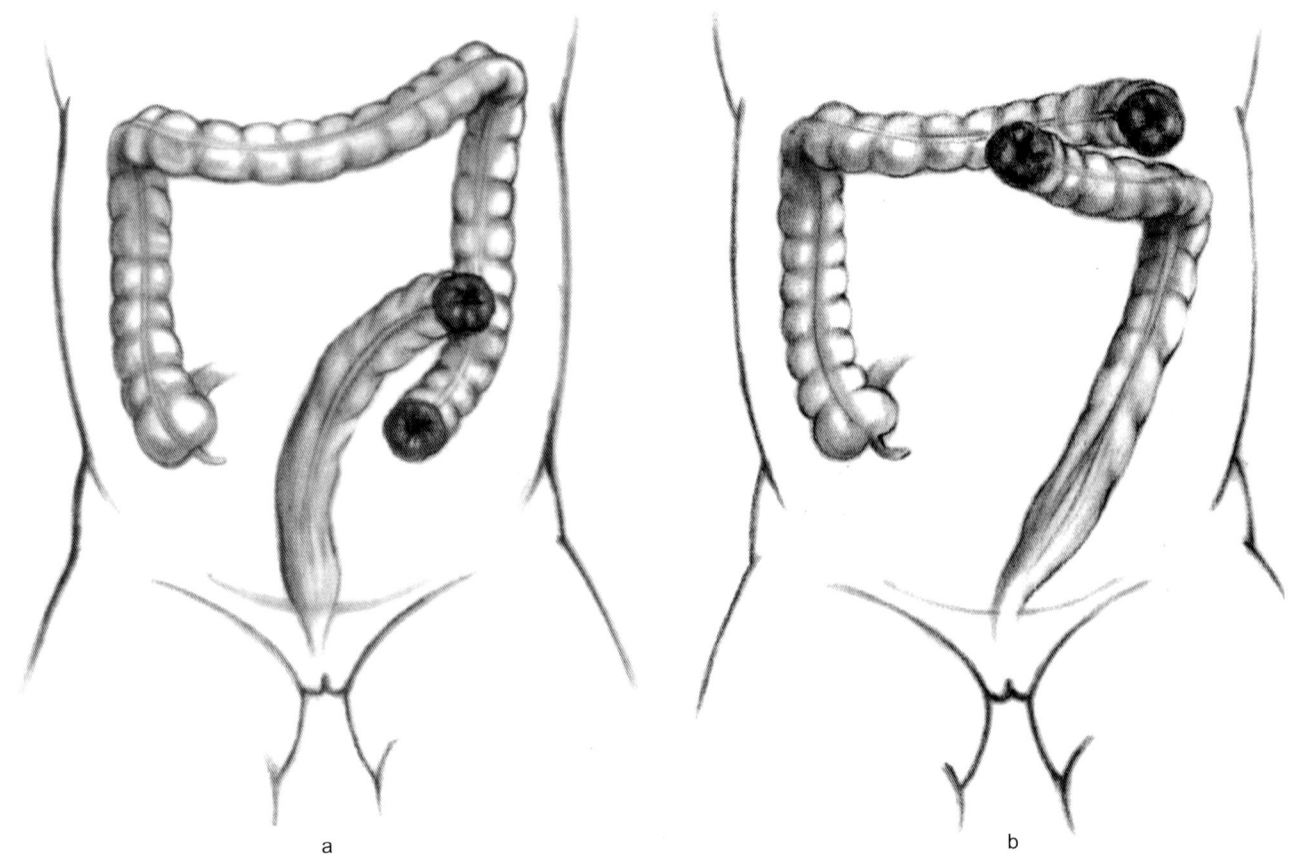

图46.4（a,b）倒置造口[1]

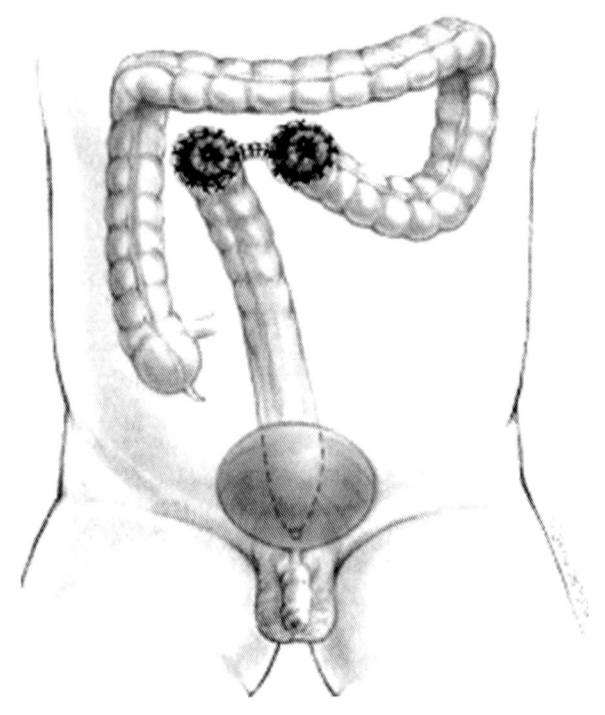

图46.5 右上乙状结肠造口术代替右横结肠造口术[2]

由简单的戳伤而制作造口所必须。在这种情况下，构建一个由皮肤、筋膜、肌肉和腹膜组成的环形区域，根据我们的经验，这是必须的，因为大多数造口狭窄不会因为简单或重复的膨胀引起。

回 缩

这种并发症是因为技术上的错误造成，因此是可以避免发生。急性早期的回缩是一种外科急症。晚期的回缩将使造口很难处理，因为它很难适应造口袋。将造口移动至皮肤表面更高的部位。

根据我们的经验，在制作造口时，需要特别考虑患有先天泄殖腔外翻的患者[4-5]。因为一个普遍存在的错误概念是这类患者具有短小因而相对无用的结肠。因此许多外科医生在患者出生时实施回肠造口术，而用结肠进行泌尿生殖道重塑（有时简单弃掉）。然而这段结肠对于患者是非常珍贵的，可

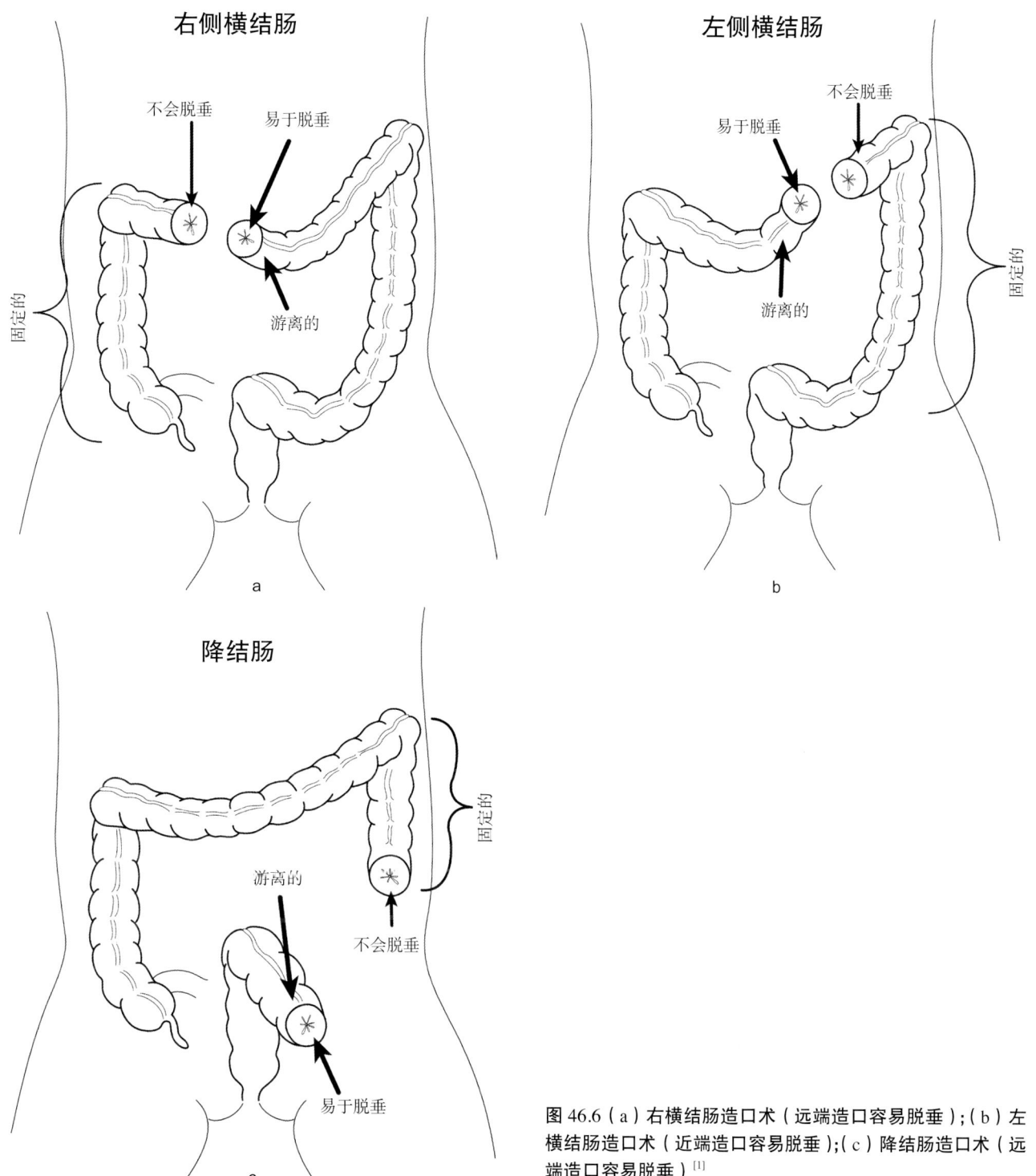

图 46.6 （a）右横结肠造口术（远端造口容易脱垂）；（b）左横结肠造口术（近端造口容易脱垂）；（c）降结肠造口术（远端造口容易脱垂）[1]

以应用它们来形成固体粪便而在以后的结肠回复术中成为备选肠管[6]。鉴于这种情况，使每一小段结肠都参与粪便流向是很重要的，尽管它很小，但是随着时间的延长，这些肠管会长相当大。结肠参与粪流的另外一个优点是这类患者比进行回肠造口术的患者容易修复。我们医院已经将一个在其他地方应用废弃结肠合并的患者重新完成此手术。

参考文献

1. Peña A, Migotto-Krieger M, Levitt MA. Colostomy in anorectal malformations: a procedure with serious but preventable complications. J Pediatr Surg. 2006;41:748–56.
2. Pena A. Atlas of surgical management of anorectal malformations. New York: Springer; 1989.
3. Gross GW, Woflson PJ, Peña A. Augmented-pressure colostogram in imperforate anus with fistula. Pediatr Radiol. 1991;21:560–2.
4. Soffer SZ, Rosen NG, Hong AR, Alexianu M, Peña A. Cloacal exstrophy: a unified management plan. J Pediatr Surg. 2000;35:932–7.
5. Levitt MA, Mak GA, Falcone RA, Peña A. Cloacal exstrophy – pull through or permanent stoma? A review of 53 patients. J Pediatr Surg. 2008;43:164–70.
6. Bischoff A, Levitt MA, Lawal TA, Peña A. Colostomy closure: how to avoid complications. Pediatr Surg Int. 2010;26:1087–92.

第八篇
肛肠再手术学的特殊论题

引 言

Andrew P. Zbar

本篇涵盖了结直肠再手术的一系列较常见但很重要的问题，包括再手术中的麻醉方式、急慢性憩室炎的再手术、吻合口瘘的注意事项、骶前肿瘤的手术入路、直肠脱垂的再手术方式、复发性藏毛窦的处理及结直肠子宫内膜异位再重建手术中的注意事项。最后将通过实例重点讨论关于再手术患者的医学法律问题。尤其对于择期结肠癌手术的老年患者，快速康复疗法比传统治疗更适合作为最佳治疗方案。这种方法的发展得益于微创技术的使用增加，且不受年龄限制；它大大减少了患者围术期的失血和住院时间，使患者更快地恢复经口进食和胃肠功能。

对于需要入院治疗的憩室病患者，我们几乎没有数据来告知他们再次入院的可能性。腹腔镜技术在某种程度上干扰了我们对选择性切除适应证的判断，特别是对于反复入院的年轻患者。腹腔镜技术对于适用于简单灌洗的病例是最简单的诊疗方法，并且得力于计算机断层扫描的常规使用，尤其在病程短且无腹膜后穿孔相关并发症的情况下。有严重肺部并发症，特别当患者高龄、ASA（American Society of Anesthesiologists）分期差、初期即需要输血或者长期进行抗凝治疗的患者，进行 Hartmann 造口还纳的可能性会降低。

无论何种吻合技术，其发生吻合口瘘的影响因素都已阐明。最近在处理低位直肠吻合口瘘方面，随着真空辅助仪器的引入，已经彻底排除了再次开腹手术的必要性。

骶前肿瘤相对比较少见，似乎需要一个更加实用的分类体系。绝大多数骶前肿瘤为良性，并且得益于精确的矢状位图像可准确确定骶骨受侵蚀的可能性。大多数情况下，如果已经通过病变的范围确定了手术方式，术前活组织检查是禁忌的；大多数情况下经骶入路（Kraske 入路）手术伴或不伴尾骨切除术是合适的。严重或复发性的病例可能需要经腹会阴入路（Localio 入路），并且在笔者看来，应尽量限制使用经肛或阴道旁技术，这些技术导致复发或边缘性切除可能性大。

对于棘手的复发性藏毛疾病，单纯环钻术似乎是最安全的选择，它可以在门诊局麻下实施，并且在大样本研究中发现其复发率在可接受范围，对于难治性复发病例与棘手的双侧病例，此术式可以保留更广泛的皮瓣。双侧藏毛疾病发病率高。

随着耐用的腹腔镜技术的出现，经会阴入路手术似乎越来越少地用于直肠脱垂治疗。腹腔镜技术可能适用于很多情况，而开腹手术迄今已不作为首选。对于复发病例仍然沿用以往的治疗方法。由于招募对象少及患者随机化中出现的偏倚，对于手术随机化的尝试，如英国 PROSPER 试验，大部分都以失败告终。经腹腔直肠固定术后发生全层复发需要再次评估，并且可能再次切除直肠固定，但幸运的是临床上很少发生。对于有二次残余和难治性大便失禁的会阴部复发患者，腹腔镜的治疗效果最好。在这些患者中，经会阴乙直肠切除术要慎重使用，可通过术前测压决定是否采用此术式。

人们越来越多地使用腹腔镜技术治疗结直肠子宫内膜异位症，虽然客观上此疾病也被定义为腹腔内疾病，但腹腔镜技术并非具有绝对优势，腹腔镜技术和开腹手术都需要应用，这也许会导致腹腔镜技术在肛肠学中发展成为一门单独的附属学科。

在三级肛肠转诊基地，直肠、肛门与会阴部重建手术的患者占大部分，而避免与其相关的医学法律诉讼是成功实践的关键。从这个意义上来说，与以往一样，在患者的期望值与外科医生达到患者期望值的能力之间必须建立一种明确的关系，这些患者所患疾病往往发病率高而以往手术治疗效果不佳。对于特殊的肛门直肠功能紊乱有很多已知和未知的方面，在面对已通过互联网部分了解这些疾病的患者的时候，循证基础所代表的概念已经改变。某种程度上，一系列肛肠手术的创新使得这个问题更复杂。经过试验论证并被批准的新技术并没有被严格应用，并且在某种程度上，在缺少随机化数据的情况下，市场力量主导了某些技术的特殊使用。

对于专注于治疗困难盆底紊乱的外科医生来说，如果矫正术后症状改善不明显，其必将处于危险的境地。对于多分隔疾病，可能已经进行了大体病理检查，而术前和术后症状评分系统相当主观。对于并发症的治疗，随着新型技术的出现，如纤维蛋白胶治疗、瘘插头、脱垂、痔疮治疗/痔切除吻合器、经肛吻合器直肠切除术（STARR）治疗脱肛、直肠脱垂及出口梗阻等，已使上述治疗方法的适应证变得模糊。在很多病例中，相对不理想的中期疗效与术后严重的难治性新综合征已使最初的兴奋大打折扣。

在专业领域，腹腔镜技术及最近出现的机器人手术被快速引进。虽然其在结直肠手术中的效果已被确认，如果非选择性地使用这些技术，其效果让人怀疑。人们支持将其用于复杂盆底功能紊乱的病例中，可以引导手术操作而带来便利，虽然其疗效还没有得到随访病例的证实，但在治疗多隔室综合征的病例中被誉为"圣杯"。患者需要注意的是，手术就是手术，没必要因为这种微创技术昂贵，但却有其令人兴奋的效果而使其合法化。

第47章 结直肠及肛门再次手术的麻醉相关问题——快速康复外科的作用

Timothy A. Rockall · Bruce F. Levy · M.J. P. Scott

王 刚 译 李 宁 审校

摘 要

本章讨论术后康复治疗对结直肠切除患者的意义,对于某些特定病例,术后快速康复具有较高的成本效益,且并发症发生率可以让人接受。文章主要对结直肠手术的麻醉相关问题进行讨论。

目标导向液体治疗,有效地镇痛以及早期进食是实现最佳预后的关键。实现每搏输出量最优化的目标导向液体治疗可以确保最佳的总体氧供,且在术后避免开放性输入大量含盐液体,可以减少术后肠麻痹的发生。手术期间应用区域阻滞可以帮助调节应激反应和减少肠麻痹的发生。这些新的方法在腹腔镜辅助手术中显示出更好的优势。

关键词

麻醉;快速康复外科;再次手术;结直肠手术;心肺评估;鼻胃管;术后恶心呕吐;抗生素预防;尿管引流;围术期低体温;液体治疗

引 言

除了导致发生并发症和死亡率的直接风险,大手术中发生的并发症还具有其他重要意义。2005年,Khuri等[1]对其研究进行了报道,该研究基于105951例手术患者的临床数据库,总结了8种常见的手术,8年随访观察显示术后30天内发生并发症是导致术后生存率降低的关键因素。因此,麻醉师必须在循证的基础上,利用可行的技术及相关的药物治疗来减少术后并发症的发生。

麻醉师的地位

过去10年中,结直肠手术后可能出现的预后发生了巨大变化。过去接受结肠切除的患者往往至少需住院14天。而现在,麻醉师对患者的临床转归发挥着不可或缺的作用。麻醉师的作用包括:

- 术前评估及优化治疗患者的合并症;
- 在循证的基础上利用可行的技术与药物治疗降低患者的围术期风险;
- 使用现代麻醉技术尽可能减少术后恶心、呕吐(PONV),以早期恢复胃肠功能;
- 使用局部麻醉技术与多模式镇痛有效为患者止痛,以实现早期进食与活动;
- 围术期目标导向液体治疗的个体化;
- 尽可能减少并发症的发生,如血栓栓塞性疾病、创伤和胸部感染。

预评估与患者优化治疗

择期大手术患者在到医院接受手术之前应在特定的术前评估门诊由麻醉师进行评估，期间可以就麻醉事项与快速康复（Enhanced Recovery，ER）计划（Enhanced Recovery Program，ERP）对患者进行说明，也可安排患者与 ER 以及造口护理的护士会面，并取得患者的知情同意。

临床检查与基本检查可以提供进一步的信息，如全血细胞计数、尿及电解质测定、肝功能检查、肺功能检查以及静息心电图。耐甲氧西林金黄色葡萄球菌的筛选可于此时进行。对每位患者均需完成以下几项内容：
- 功能状态评估
- 心血管风险指数测定
- 基础疾病的优化治疗
- 若有指证，可开始使用β-受体阻滞剂与他汀类药物

下面对以上内容做进一步详述。

功能状态

功能状态的评估是患者评估的重要开始。功能状态用代谢当量（MET）测定，1MET 等于静息时的基础代谢率。爬两层楼梯需要 4MET，剧烈活动如体育运动或游泳需要 10MET 以上。无法完成需 4MET 的活动提示功能状态较差，发生术后心脏事件的可能性较大。如果功能状态较好，即使患者存在稳定性缺血性心脏病或其他危险因素，预后仍较为乐观[1]。

非心脏手术中的心脏风险：Lee 指数

1999 年，Lee 等[2] 提出 Lee 指数，即对 Goldman 心脏风险指数的修正。Lee 指数包含围术期严重心脏事件的 6 项独立临床决定因素：
- 缺血性心脏病（IHD）病史
- 脑血管疾病病史
- 心力衰竭
- 胰岛素依赖型糖尿病
- 肾功能损害
- 高危手术

所有因素均为 1 分，指数即为总分。指数为 0、1、2、3 分的患者严重心脏并发症的发生率估计分别为 0.4%、0.9%、7% 和 11%。

使用心肺运动试验评估心肺状态

心肺运动试验（CPET）可以动态、无创、客观地评估患者的心肺系统对需氧量急剧上升的适应能力。极量运动试验通过踏车运动完成，随着运动量的增加，耗氧量最终将超过供氧量，有氧代谢不足以满足代谢的需求，因此无氧代谢增加，血乳糖上升。此时的耗氧量即无氧阈值（AT），单位为 $ml/(kg \cdot min)$。Older 等[3-4] 最初的研究表明，AT 值为 $11ml/(kg \cdot min)$ 以下的患者在进行腹部大手术时死亡率较高，若患者有缺血性心脏病则风险进一步增加。Snowden 等[5] 之后的一项研究则通过次极量心肺运动试验证实患者术后并发症的发生率及住院时间有所增长。该研究显示，与患者填写术前问卷相比，CPET 作为预测指标具有更高的灵敏度。该组患者中，$AT \geq 10.1\ ml/(kg \cdot min)$ 者发生术后并发症的风险较低[5]。CPET 达到的 VO_{2max} 也已证实为大手术预后判断的一项重要变量，尤其是胸外科手术。

基础疾病的优化治疗

有基础心肺疾病的患者应由全科医师或内科医师进行优化治疗。糖尿病患者应稳定血糖水平。同时，患者应做贫血筛查，如果存在贫血，在手术之前应予以纠正。手术前鼓励患者戒烟。

降低心血管风险

使用他汀类药物和β-受体阻断药降低围术期心肌缺血事件及心肌梗死已得到广泛关注。以下为美国心脏协会[6] 所提出的一级循证治疗建议：
- 对术前负荷试验显示有 IHD 或心肌缺血的患者建议使用β-受体阻断药；
- 对之前因 IHD、心律失常或高血压而接受过β-受体阻断药治疗的患者建议继续使用β-受体阻断药；
- 他汀类药物在围术期应连续使用；

- 对于高危患者，开始给予他汀类药物的最佳时间为术前30天到术前至少1周。

术前应确认患者是否有服用某些特定药物，因为这些药物在围术期需要特殊处理，如果处理不当，可能会增加围术期并发症的风险。这些药物包括：
- 阿司匹林——遵循当地医院的政策
- 冠状动脉支架植入后使用氯吡格雷——联系患者的心脏病医师
- 华法林——联系患者的血液科医师
- 血管紧张素转化酶抑制剂——考虑手术当天早上停止服药

术后快速康复

快速康复计划（ERP）由Kehlet等提出，意指加速手术后患者的康复。术后加速康复小组针对加速康复提出了关键治疗方案，并于近期发表了指南[7]。2009年，Levy等[8]将这些关键治疗相结合，并使用硬膜外麻醉联合全身麻醉首次使一批结直肠切除术患者的住院时间缩短至23h。

液体治疗和镇痛是ERP的关键，由麻醉师控制。另外几项主要的非手术因素可以通过ER实施，给予患者持续的护理，帮助患者早期达到术后目标。下面针对以上几点以及ERP的其他方面进行讨论。

手术当天

住 院

患者比较倾向于手术当天住院，因为睡自己的床可以使其在手术前一天有较佳的睡眠质量，并且这也可以改善医院的床位使用。术前不可给予镇静剂和抗焦虑药。手术前一天晚上至术前2h服用碳水化合物饮料可以改善患者的状态，减少脱水，以及降低大手术中的胰岛素抵抗。给予等张的碳水化合物饮料非常重要，否则可能导致胃排空损伤。

麻醉的实施

目前没有证据表明特殊的全身麻醉技术具有优势，但是应选用具有后遗效应的现代短效药物。氧化亚氮对肠道有影响，且引发恶心、呕吐的风险较高，应避免使用。瑞芬太尼和短效阿片类药物，如有需要可以使用。

胃肠道手术期间避免使用鼻胃管

不仅患者厌恶鼻胃管，鼻胃管还可影响肠道功能的恢复，增加术后发热、肺不张和肺炎的发生风险。对于低位胃肠道手术，只有患者发生胃扩张时才应使用鼻胃管（手术结束时应取出），或者是在外科医师要求时（通常为广泛粘连性疾病）。

抗生素预防

抗生素预防已经证实可以减少术中发生感染性并发症的风险[9]。由于耐药性的变异，抗生素的使用应遵循当地医院的政策。结直肠手术中使用抗生素的最佳时期为皮肤切开前1h。如果手术持续1h以上，应另外给予抗生素[9]。

尿管引流

目的是在手术次日早上拔除尿管，尽管镇痛剂此时仍有一定影响。腹膜返折以上结肠切除术后24h发生尿潴留的风险较低，即使是使用低浓度剂量硬膜外麻醉[10]。由于手术或其他生理问题导致排尿困难时，应留置尿管。近期的一项meta分析表明，膀胱穿刺导尿更容易为患者所接受，且用于盆腔手术时患者发病率较低[11]。

避免围术期低体温

为防止低体温的发生，进行体温监测是必要的。应使用暖风机，静脉注射液体也应加温，直至术后[12]。低体温会增加创口感染和出血/凝血障碍的风险，并导致输液需求增多[13-14]，但是可能会降低发生心脏事件的风险[15]。

预防术后恶心呕吐

PONV对患者康复有较大影响，可引起患者的消极情绪，延迟肠道功能的恢复，影响患者活动与代谢。所有患者均应预防性使用抗生素（如$5HT_3$拮抗剂或塞克利嗪）。使用评分系统确定PONV高危患者对其预防有所帮助，可以作为病房 PONV 早期处理的一项规范步骤[16]。女性、不吸烟、晕动病史以及术后使用阿片类药物均为重要的危险因素[17]。3 项或 3 项以上危险因素预示 PONV 风险较高，可能需要采取其他措施，如靶控输注丙泊酚维持麻醉或联合单剂量地塞米松。目前关于地塞米松在大手术中影响应激和代谢的机制尚不明确，但是如果使用地塞米松，应采取最低有效剂量。若术后使用吗啡止痛，可合用 0.0625～1.25 mg 氟哌利多，效果较好[17]。

术中监护与血管通路

应对心电图、脉搏血氧饱和度、血压、呼气末 CO_2 分压、吸入麻醉气体以及血氧浓度进行标准监测。动脉导管容易放置，常用于大手术。中心静脉导管仍常用于大型开放性手术。插入导管时使用消毒技术并用超声对颈内静脉进行定位，可以减少并发症的发生。然而，使用流量导向技术（如食管多普勒）优化液体治疗已经证实比记录中心静脉压更具优势，因为记录常常会产生不具代表性的数值，尤其是在腹腔镜操作期间。

个体化目标导向液体治疗

围术期液体治疗是麻醉师可以控制的能够影响手术预后的最重要因素之一。麻醉师在麻醉期间用以测量心输出量的方法越来越多。食管多普勒监测是唯一一项经随机对照研究证实有效的技术。Mythen 和 Webb[18] 首次提出了液体优化的方法。几项研究已经证实，在大手术期间采用食管多普勒监测使每搏输出量达最佳时手术预后亦随之改善[19-20]，尤其是结直肠手术[21-24]。液体量的改变可迅速反应于每搏输出量，持续补液至补液后每搏输出量不得高于 10%。图 47.1 示补液步骤。

大手术期间应使用哪种类型的液体仍存在争议。目前并没有证据支持胶体液或晶体液的使用。然而，使用食管多普勒优化每搏输出量的研究均使用胶体液来达到每搏输出量的目标，而在术后使用晶体液。《英国成人手术患者静脉液体治疗指南》推荐使用平衡盐溶液而非生理盐水[25]。术后在避免血容量不足的同时应使静脉输液维持在最低限度。鼓励早期进食，目的是尽快实现口服摄入以取代静脉输液。

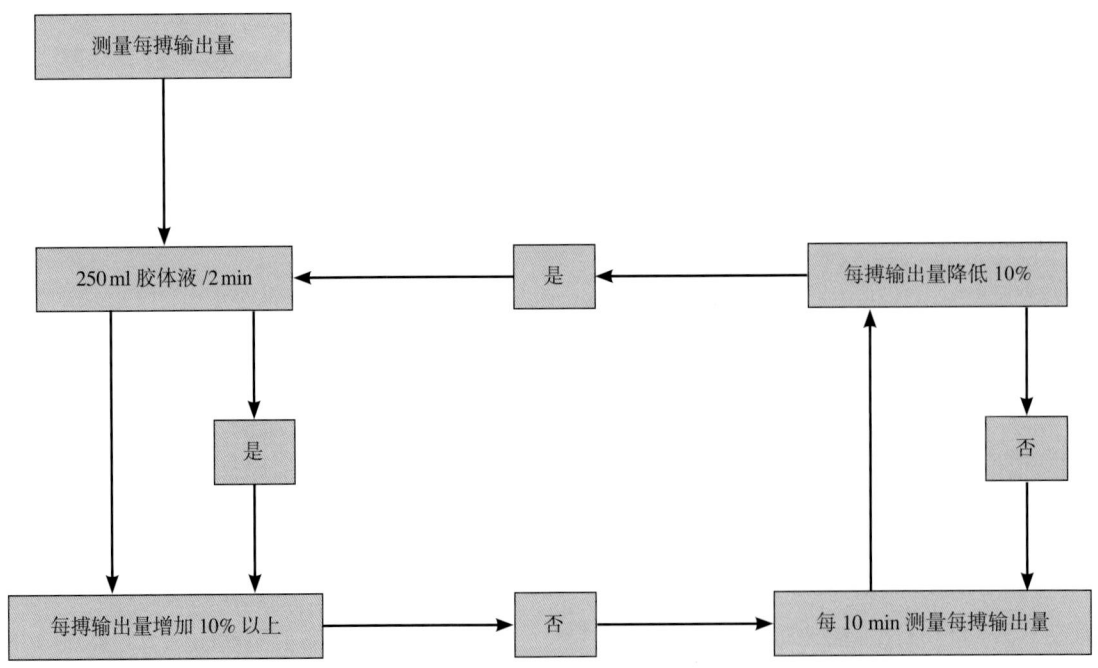

图 47.1　Mythen 使用胶体液优化每搏输出量的方法经随机对照实验证实，可以改善大手术预后

镇痛方法

镇痛剂对手术预后有重要影响，止痛方案应对患者有效，且能使患者实现早期活动。应避免使用长效阿片类药物。若无禁忌证，可给予对乙酰氨基酚和非甾体抗炎药。区域阻滞剂可以帮助调节患者对手术的应激反应并促进开放性手术后肠功能的恢复[10]。硬膜外麻醉仍广泛用于开放性手术，但可引起术后高血压、无法活动以及术后静脉液体负荷增加。局部麻醉导管技术如切口输液器和经腹平面阻滞已经得到越来越多的应用。在腹腔镜手术中，使用硬膜外麻醉已经证实会延长住院时间，局部麻醉似乎效果更佳，因为术后12～24h内的止痛通常可由口服镇痛药满足。

应激反应的调节

手术应激反应较为复杂，且具有多种通路。尽管传统观念侧重减少应激反应，但是显然人类应激反应的存在有其必要性。因此，我们要讨论的是应激反应的调节而不是缓解，因为一些应激反应的形式如愈合反应，由于局部炎症反应的存在是必需的，且不可避免的。ER中能够帮助调节应激反应的因素可以分成几组，但是对患者早期康复和身体状况具有重要意义的是这些因素的总和。重要因素包括：

- 目标导向液体治疗
- 最佳止痛方式
- 早期术后营养，避免饥饿

麻醉师的术中注意事项

在腹腔镜切除术中，进行骨盆手术的患者通常采取头低脚高位。由于患者可能会长时间保持某种姿势，因此仔细调整体位、包裹手臂，以及在可能受压的地方放置胶垫非常重要。Yellofin镫形座（Allen Medical Systems，美国马萨诸塞州，阿克顿）可以通过支托双腿而提高患者体位的稳定性，同时避免了小腿受压。用于移动患者的滑动片应予以移除，肩部支撑可以防止患者滑离手术台。图47.2所示的头低脚高位对患者的生理状况有显著影响，尤其是联合腹腔注气时。

后负荷的增长会导致每搏输出量降低。Levy等[8, 26]的研究表明，在液体优化的患者中，后负荷

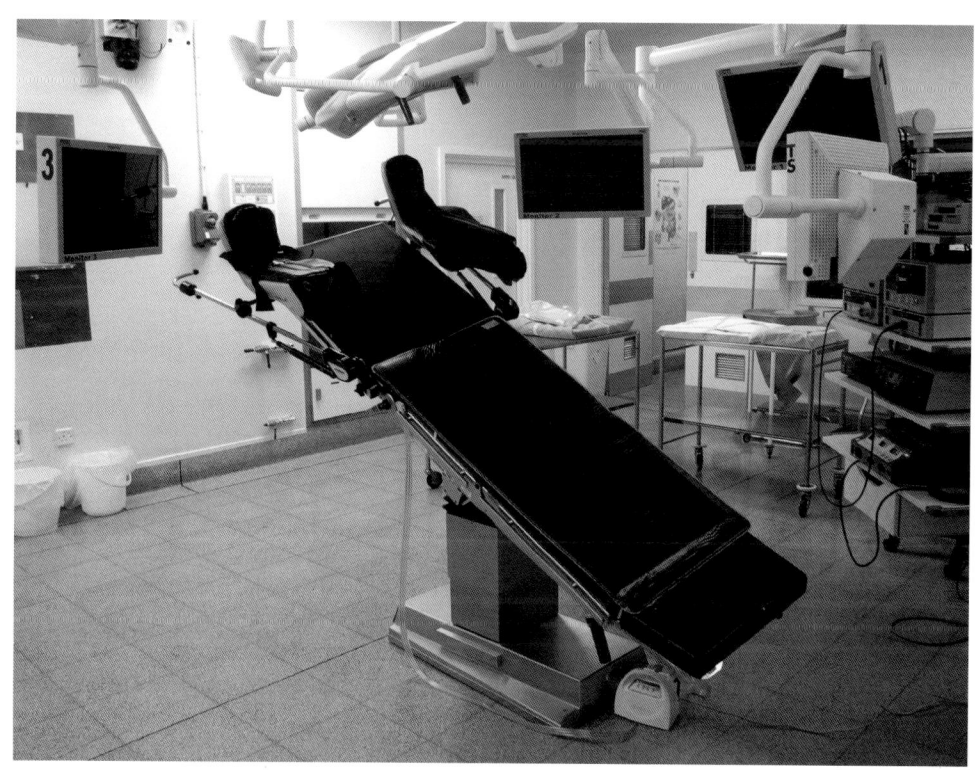

图47.2 腹腔镜直肠手术所采用的头低脚高位（Trendelenburg体位）

的增长持续约 20～25 min，无论患者是否行区域阻滞，后负荷的增长方式均相似。此后，体循环血管阻力将向正常水平恢复。左右心室充盈压均有所增长，肺循环压力及血管阻力也有所上升[26]。呼吸机参数的改变和呼气末正压的增长使平均气道压力升高，可能导致右心室负荷大幅上升。右心室负荷的增长已经通过经食管超声心动图得到证实，其原因在于呼吸机的使用和 CO_2 气腹[27-28]。在头低脚高位时，若要改变呼吸机参数以提高胸内平均气道压力，则需加强护理，因为这会导致右心室负荷增加。

CO_2 气腹使腹壁顺应性增强，且由于向膈肌施压而使肺容积下降。膈肌运动受限会影响呼吸，因此应该增加通气压力以维持与腹膜注气之前相同的潮气量。此外，头低脚高位的长时间（超过 4 h）腹腔镜手术会引起开放性手术之外的问题已经得到越来越多的认可。头低脚高位和人工气腹由于减少静脉回流会导致头部静脉怒张。同时动脉血 CO_2 升高以及脑血流增加可使问题进一步加重[29]。这可能导致意识模糊以及患者术后意识的改变，术后脑水肿继发颅内高压需呼吸机辅助通气的病例已有报道。

术后护理

大多数患者可从恢复区回到病房。特殊患者群体需要考虑术后监护，包括流量导向评估和针对性供氧 12 h。这些患者如下：

- 术前确定存在心肺储备受限或无氧阈值下降的患者（术前心肺试验测得无氧阈值 <10 的患者）；
- 术中优化每搏输出量之后供氧量意外降低的患者。

术后 12 h 对于细胞的损伤反应和愈合反应非常重要，该时段采取密切监护可以降低并发症的发生率。Pearse 等[30]的研究显示，术后 12 h 内进行液体治疗（有必要时可使用多培沙明）及针对性输氧可以减少术后并发症。该方法对于液体优化后无低氧状况的择期手术患者是否有效，目前仍不确切。

预防并发症

有效的止痛方法、最佳的体位以及早期活动可以改善术后肺功能。Levy 等[24]的研究表明，腹腔镜手术患者中采用或未采用区域阻滞者只有微小的肺功能(最大呼气流速和第 1 秒用力呼气容积)差异，各组患者均有肺功能下降。在开放性手术中，硬膜外麻醉可以改善肺功能。增加活动和早期步行是改善肺功能的最有效方式。围术期发生静脉血栓栓塞的风险可持续几周，甚至患者出院之后[31-33]。手术前应评估每位患者的个体风险，分数越高预示风险越高，深静脉血栓和肺栓塞的独立危险因素包括深静脉血栓史、癌症、年龄 60 岁以上以及术后长时间不活动[34]。小腿压力袜、术中小腿压迫装置以及低分子量肝素（参考当地医院治疗指南）的使用均可降低风险。早期活动亦非常重要。

结 论

麻醉相关问题对于结直肠手术患者的预后非常重要。ER 可以加快患者术后恢复正常功能。目标导向液体治疗、有效的镇痛以及早期进食是实现最佳预后的关键。优化每搏输出量的目标导向液体治疗可以实现最佳总体氧供，手术后避免开放性输入大量含盐液体可以减少肠麻痹的发生，促进肠功能的恢复以及早期进食。手术期间进行区域阻滞可以调节患者的应激反应，减少肠麻痹。早期进食可以降低患者对手术的分解代谢反应，促进愈合。结直肠手术后的早期活动和恢复稳态可以缩短住院时间，降低并发症的发生率，在再次手术、重建手术和长时间腹腔镜手术中具有同样的重要性[35-37]。今后可通过进一步的 ER 对照试验来研究其对手术相关再入院及患者随访的长期利益及影响[38]。

参考文献

1. Khuri SF, Henderson WG, DePalma RG, Mosca C, Healey NA, Kumbhani DJ. Determinants of long-term survival after major surgery and the adverse effect of postoperative complications. Ann Surg. 2005;242:326–43.
2. Lee TH, Marcantonio ER, Mangione CM, Thomas EJ, Polanczyk CA, Cook EF, et al. Derivation and prospective validation of a simple index for prediction of cardiac risk of major noncardiac surgery. Circulation. 1999;100:1043–9.
3. Older P, Hall A, Hader R. Cardiopulmonary exercise testing as a screening test for perioperative management of major surgery in the elderly. Chest. 1999;116:355–62.
4. Older P, Smith R, Hall A, French C. Preoperative cardiopulmonary risk assessment by cardiopulmonary exercise testing. Crit Care Resusc. 2000;2:198–208.
5. Snowden CP, Prentis JM, Anderson HL, Roberts DR, Randles D, Renton M, et al. Submaximal cardiopulmonary exercise testing predicts complications and hospital length of stay in patients undergoing major elective surgery. Ann Surg. 2010;251:535–41.

6. Fleisher LA, Beckman JA, Brown KA, Calkins H, Chaikof E, Fleischmann KE, et al. ACC/AHA 2007 Guidelines on Perioperative Cardiovascular Evaluation and Care for Noncardiac Surgery: Executive Summary: A Report of the American College of Cardiology/American Heart Association Task Force on Practice Guidelines (Writing Committee to Revise the 2002 Guidelines on Perioperative Cardiovascular Evaluation for Noncardiac Surgery): Developed in Collaboration with the American Society of Echocardiography, American Society of Nuclear Cardiology, Heart Rhythm Society, Society of Cardiovascular Anesthesiologists, Society for Cardiovascular Angiography and Interventions, Society for Vascular Medicine and Biology, and Society for Vascular Surgery. Circulation. 2007;116:1971–96.
7. Lassen K, Soop M, Nygren J, Cox PB, Hendry PO, Spies C, et al. Consensus review of optimal perioperative care in colorectal surgery: Enhanced Recovery After Surgery (ERAS) Group recommendations. Arch Surg. 2009;144(10):961–9.
8. Levy BF, Scott MJ, Fawcett WJ, Rockall TA. 23-hour-stay laparoscopic colectomy. Dis Colon Rectum. 2009;52:1239–43.
9. Song F, Glenny AM. Antimicrobial prophylaxis in colorectal surgery: a systematic review of randomized controlled trials. Br J Surg. 1998;85:1232–41.
10. Basse L, Madsen JL, Kehlet H. Normal gastrointestinal transit after colonic resection using epidural analgesia, enforced oral nutrition and laxative. Br J Surg. 2001;88:1498–500.
11. McPhail MJ, Abu-Hilal M, Johnson CD. A meta-analysis comparing suprapubic and transurethral catheterization for bladder drainage after abdominal surgery. Br J Surg. 2006;93:1038–44.
12. Wong PF, Kumar S, Bohra A, Whetter D, Leaper DJ. Randomized clinical trial of perioperative systemic warming in major elective abdominal surgery. Br J Surg. 2007;94:421–6.
13. Kurz A, Sessler DI, Lenhardt R. Perioperative normothermia to reduce the incidence of surgical-wound infection and shorten hospitalization. Study of Wound Infection and Temperature Group. N Engl J Med. 1996;334:1209–15.
14. Scott EM, Buckland R. A systematic review of intraoperative warming to prevent postoperative complications. AORN J. 2006;83:1090–104, 1107–1113.
15. Frank SM, Fleisher LA, Breslow MJ, Higgins MS, Olson KF, Kelly S, et al. Perioperative maintenance of normothermia reduces the incidence of morbid cardiac events. A randomized clinical trial. JAMA. 1997;277:1127–34.
16. Apfel CC, Kranke P, Eberhart LH, Roos A, Roewer N. Comparison of predictive models for postoperative nausea and vomiting. Br J Anaesth. 2002;88:234–40.
17. Carlisle JB, Stevenson CA. Drugs for preventing postoperative nausea and vomiting. Cochrane Database Syst Rev. 2006;(3):CD004125.
18. Mythen MG, Webb AR. Perioperative plasma volume expansion reduces the incidence of gut mucosal hypoperfusion during cardiac surgery. Arch Surg. 1995;130:423–9.
19. Gan TJ, Soppitt A, Maroof M, el-Moalem H, Robertson KM, Moretti E, et al. Goal-directed intraoperative fluid administration reduces length of hospital stay after major surgery. Anesthesiology. 2002;97:820–6.
20. Wakeling HG, McFall MR, Jenkins CS, Woods WG, Miles WF, Barclay GR, et al. Intraoperative oesophageal Doppler guided fluid management shortens postoperative hospital stay after major bowel surgery. Br J Anaesth. 2005;95:634–42.
21. Conway DH, Mayall R, Abdul-Latif MS, Gilligan S, Tackaberry C. Randomised controlled trial investigating the influence of intravenous fluid titration using oesophageal Doppler monitoring during bowel surgery. Anaesthesia. 2002;57:845–9.
22. Noblett SE, Snowden CP, Shenton BK, Horgan AF. Randomized clinical trial assessing the effect of Doppler-optimized fluid management on outcome after elective colorectal resection. Br J Surg. 2006;93:1069–76.
23. Kumar CM, Corbett WA, Wilson RG. Spinal anesthesia with a micro-catheter in high-risk patients undergoing colorectal cancer and other major abdominal surgery. Surg Oncol. 2008;17:73–9.
24. Levy BF, Tilney HS, Dowson HM, Rockall TA. A systematic review of postoperative analgesia following laparoscopic colorectal surgery. Colorectal Dis. 2010;12:5–15.
25. Soni N. British Consensus Guidelines on Intravenous Fluid Therapy for Adult Surgical Patients (GIFTASUP): Cassandra's view. Anesthesia. 2009;64:235–8.
26. Levy B, Scott M, Stoneham J, Fawcett W, Zuleika M, Rockall T. The effect of analgesic regime on post-operative lung function following laparoscopic colorectal surgery. Br J Surg. 2008;95(S3):57.
27. Galizia G, Prizio G, Lieto E, Castellano P, Pelosio L, Imperatore V, et al. Hemodynamic and pulmonary changes during open, carbon dioxide pneumoperitoneum and abdominal wall-lifting cholecystectomy. A prospective, randomized study. Surg Endosc. 2001;15:477–83.
28. Alfonsi P, Vieillard-Baron A, Coggia M, Guignard B, Goeau-Brissonniere O, Jardin F, et al. Cardiac function during intraperitoneal CO_2 insufflation for aortic surgery: a transesophageal echocardiographic study. Anesth Analg. 2006;102:1304–10.
29. Park EY, Koo BN, Min KT, Nam SH. The effect of pneumoperitoneum in the steep Trendelenburg position on cerebral oxygenation. Acta Anaesthesiol Scand. 2009;53:895–9.
30. Pearse R, Dawson D, Fawcett J, Rhodes A, Grounds RM, Bennett ED. Early goal-directed therapy after major surgery reduces complications and duration of hospital stay. A randomised controlled trial [ISRCTN38797445]. Crit Care. 2005;9:R687–93.
31. Catheline JM, Capelluto E, Gaillard JL, Turner R, Champault G. Thromboembolism prophylaxis and incidence of thromboembolic complications after laparoscopic surgery. Int J Surg Investig. 2000;2:41–7.
32. Huo MH, Muntz J. Extended thromboprophylaxis with low-molecular-weight heparins after hospital discharge in high-risk surgical and medical patients: a review. Clin Ther. 2009;31:1129–41.
33. Rasmussen MS, Jørgensen LN, Wille-Jørgensen P. Prolonged thromboprophylaxis with low molecular weight heparin for abdominal or pelvic surgery. Cochrane Database Syst Rev. 2009;(1):CD004318.
34. Spyropoulos AC, Anderson FA Jr, Fitzgerald G, Decousus H, Pini M, Chong BH, et al.; for the IMPROVE (International Medical Prevention Registry on Venous Thromboembolism) Investigators. Predictive and associative models to identify hospitalized medical patients at risk for venous thromboembolism. Chest. 2011;140(3):706–14. Epub 2011 Mar 24.
35. Wind J, Polle SW, Fung Kon Jin PH, Dejong CH, von Meyenfeldt MF, Ubbink DT, et al.; Laparoscopy and/or Fast Track Multimodal Management Versus Standard Care (LAFA) Study Group; Enhanced Recovery after Surgery (ERAS) Group. Systematic review of enhanced recovery programmes in colonic surgery. Br J Surg. 2006;93:800–9.
36. Delaney CP, Fazio VW, Senagore AJ, Robinson B, Halverson AL, Remzi FH. 'Fast track' postoperative management protocol for patients with high co-morbidity undergoing complex abdominal and pelvic colorectal surgery. Br J Surg. 2001;88:1533–8.
37. Gouvas N, Tan E, Windsor A, Xynos E, Tekkis PP. Fast-track vs standard care in colorectal surgery: a meta-analysis update. Int J Colorectal Dis. 2009;24:1119–31.
38. Nygren J, Hausel J, Kehlet H, Revhaug A, Lassen K, Dejong C, et al. A comparison in five European Centres of case mix, clinical management and outcomes following either conventional or fast-track perioperative care in colorectal surgery. Clin Nutr. 2006;24:455–61.

第 48 章 憩室病并发症的再手术治疗

Patricia L. Roberts

徐 靖译 王西墨 审校

摘 要

本章主要讨论 Hartmann 重建手术在憩室病并发症中的应用，以及憩室病复发后的手术治疗。在复发的憩室病患者出现严重急性憩室炎时手术可能性有多大，以及肠道功能和生活质量是否得到改善，我们知之甚少。但随着腔镜适应证放宽，传统的肠切除和肠道重建方法正在发生变化。本章讨论了在择期手术的憩室病患者中出现吻合口瘘和憩室病并发瘘管、脓肿或狭窄时再次手术的作用，以及解剖因素、手术时机、术前准备、术式和预后。

关键词

憩室病；再次手术；Hartmann 手术；造口；一期吻合；吻合口漏；瘘管；脓肿；狭窄；解剖因素；时机；术前准备；预后

引 言

复杂憩室病再手术的原因主要有两个：① Hartmann 的肠切除，近端造口远端封闭手术破坏了肠道的连续性，为恢复其连续性而行的计划性再次手术；②首次肠切除一期吻合后出现并发症或其他意外事件而行的非计划再次手术。后者的发生主要归因于吻合口瘘，但也可能是吻合后出现瘘管、脓肿或狭窄的结果。本章讨论了再次手术之前应该注意的一些因素，包括解剖因素、手术时机、术前准备、术式及预后。

Hartmann 肠切除术后的再次手术

Hartmann 手术首次由 Henri Hartmann[1] 描述，用来治疗直肠癌，在 2 例肠梗阻的患者中，他成功切除了肿瘤，并在没有破坏骨盆底的情况下关闭了直肠上端，使其留在腹腔里。该术式很快在 20 世纪下半叶成为大部分憩室炎合并穿孔患者急诊手术的首选术式，替代了由 Lockhart-Mummery[2] 和 Smithwick[3] 提倡的三阶段手术方式，即一期结肠造口，二期肠切除，三期造口还纳。虽然有研究者认为那些急诊手术的患者可以耐受一期肠切除肠吻合术而不需要肠道改道，但是一份系统回顾报道收集了从 1998—2005 年 267 000 例急性憩室炎患者，表明做一期吻合的患者并不多[4]。更重要的是，Hartmann 认为不应该尝试 Hartmann 还纳手术。当前，Hartmann 还纳手术仍然有很高的并发症发生率和死亡率，以及很低的还纳率。这个问题已经在第 45 章讨论过。出于这方面的考虑，高达 35% 的患者没有行造口还纳术[5]。报道显示吻合口瘘发生率是 2%～30%，死亡率是 0～10%，伤口感染率是 12%～50%[6-7]，再次回到手术室重新造口的风险同样很高。下面节段概述了术前、术中的注意事项，以及一些手术技巧可以最大限度降低 Hartmann 还纳手术带来的风险，使患者受益。

手术时机

慢性炎症性肠病患者在行肠切除术前已经知道自己患病多年，而急性憩室炎的患者从来没有生病过，也没想过在行肠切除术后要带着造口离开医院，所以这些患者更希望在首次做完 Hartmann 手术后能尽快行 Hartmann 还纳手术。Hartmann 还纳手术可以进行的早些（距离初次手术小于 3 个月）或晚些（距离初次手术大于 3 个月）。两种方法都有其支持者[8-12]。进行还纳手术太接近初次手术时间会有几点不利，主要是术后的粘连和急性炎症反应会造成解剖困难、意外切开肠道以及难以辨认直肠残端等问题。虽然等待大概 3 个月可以让患者有充足的时间得到恢复以及容易辨认直肠残端，但是等待的时间过长会由于直肠残端继发纤维化和收缩以至于更加难以辨认。这两种方法没有在随机实验中做过比较。我们通常会等到第 3 个月时再行 Hartmann 还纳手术。这个时间是考虑到炎症过程以及行粘连松解术的困难程度而确定的。

术前准备

患者术前应该做评估，保证营养状况要达到一个最佳状态，心肺疾病应该及早诊断并做相应评估。盆腔的再次手术有很高风险合并血栓性并发症，患者术前应做好预防。虽然越来越多的证据表明机械性肠道准备并不是必须的，但是在再次手术中是非常必要的，它可以降低手术区域肠道内容物的溢出率[13]。已经有术前静脉预防给予抗生素的疗法，但没有证据可以支持这一疗法。

术前影像学

之前没有做结肠评估的年龄大于 50 岁的患者，应该行纤维结肠镜检查或钡灌肠检查。在行 Hartmann 造口还纳之前，我们更喜欢通过造口做钡灌肠检查和通过直肠作泛影葡胺灌肠检查。泛影葡胺灌肠尤其有用，因为它可以显示直肠段的长度和结构，同时也可以发现任何残余的乙状结肠或憩室（图 48.1 a, b）。在初次手术中，由于某些原因，有很多患者在行肠切除术时适当地保留了一段乙状结

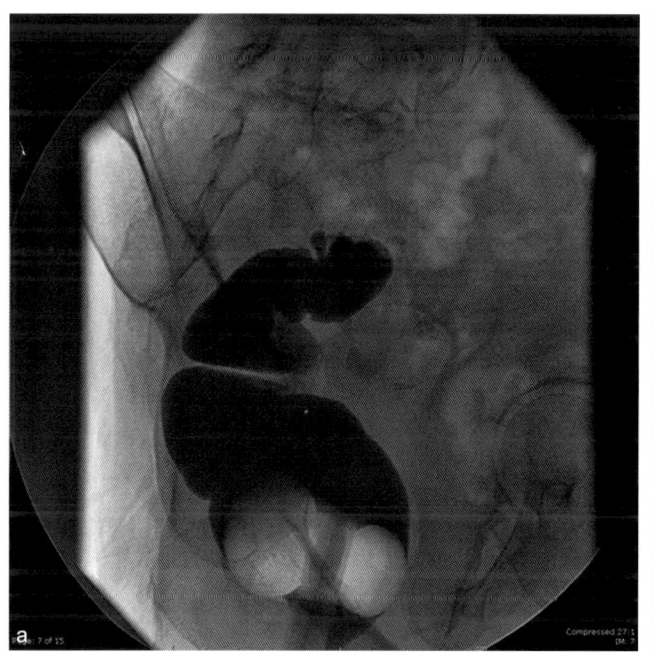
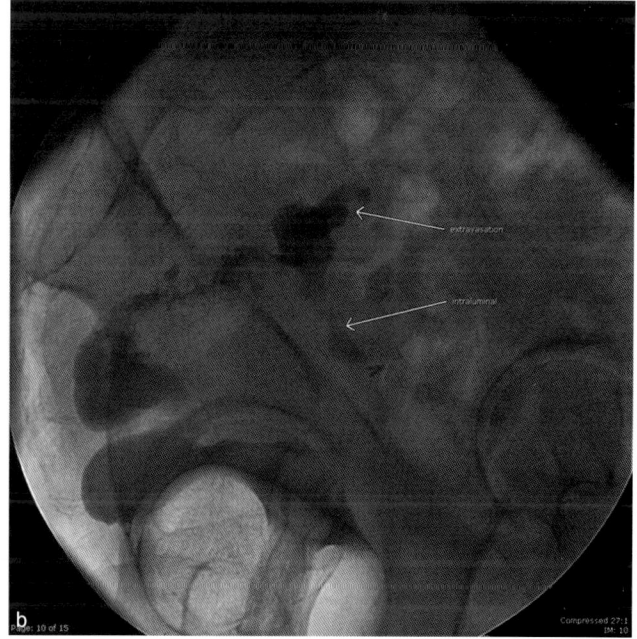

图 48.1 （a）泛影葡胺灌肠显示残留的乙状结肠和憩室；（b）泛影葡胺灌肠显示末端直肠顶部有造影剂外渗，部分造影剂进入小肠

肠。虽然两种方法都可以实现，但通过显影剂明确解剖结构要优于结肠镜检查。这些检查方法同时也可以帮助清除残余的粪渣。在初次做完 Hartmann 手术后残余直肠里会残留有排泄物，在还纳手术时应该清除掉这些排泄物或对末端直肠作冲洗以利于放置管腔探头和随后的端端吻合器。

术中注意事项

患者体位

如果预测手术时间较长，可以在患者骨突出的位置放置棉垫以防长时间受压。患者体位应为截石位或 Allen 脚蹬位，注意减缓压力防止腓神经受压和骶部皮肤破损。整个体位要保证髋关节伸展对称、膝关节弯曲和大腿外展。如果自动牵引器持续牵引超过了伸展的极限，当髋关节伸展超过 60° 时会导致大腿神经麻痹。会阴部略超出床板边缘以便留出空间放置端端吻合器。若需要可以对直肠进行清洗和放置蘑菇头导管，以便识别末端直肠袋。直肠镜和管腔探头同样可以在术中来识别末端直肠袋，阴道同样也要进行准备。我们常用的另外一种体位是患者仰卧在手术台上，两腿分开而不需要架起，这种体位避免了长时间截石位引起的一些不良反应，包括神经损伤和筋膜室综合征。再有，这种体位要保证臀部超出手术台足够的空间可以方便端端吻合器进入肛门。用约束带将患者上臂固定在两侧，这样可以防止身体向头侧滑行，尤其是在坡度较大的 Trendelenburg 体位的时候更要固定好。

手术方式

手术方法可以采用腹腔镜或开腹手术，由于之前的手术或腹腔感染会造成腹腔粘连，这不利于进行腹腔镜手术。腹腔粘连的程度和范围是很难预料的，有时腹腔的粘连程度并没有我们想象中的那么严重，手术可以很快地将粘连松解开。另外，如果是广泛的腹腔粘连，在我们进入腹膜腔的时候很有可能损伤肠道。有效的解决办法是在腹壁做一个小切口，通过这个小切口来评价腹腔的粘连程度[14]。一次性的腹腔镜器械像套管针可以在确定腹腔镜手术确实可行的情况下启封从而避免浪费。另外，这个小的切口也可以放置在远离第一次手术切口的地方来评估腹腔粘连程度和腹腔镜手术的可行性。

手术视野的暴露和照明

再次手术过程中手术视野的暴露和照明非常重要，如果是开腹手术，手术切口要延伸到耻骨联合，如果要游离结肠脾曲，中线切口可向头侧延伸。在患者两腿之间操作提供了对脾曲的最佳视角。

充足的手术室光源、头灯、带有光源的盆腔拉钩都是很有用的，一种带有保护膀胱叶片的自动拉钩已经在使用，直型和 S 型拉钩也用于盆腔手术，但是前者更利于深部盆腔手术暴露，有时在暴露直肠袋上端时会使用到，必须小心不要将拉钩放置在手术巾上以免引起燃烧。

初始解剖

进入腹腔后应集中松解盆腔的小肠粘连以便找到 Hartmann 直肠袋，最后，在大多数情况下从屈氏韧带到回盲部的小肠粘连被松解开，这样近端结肠游离起来后可以下放到盆腔而没有张力。由于初次的 Hartmann 手术，患者再次手术时面临着严重的腹腔粘连以至于没有办法去区分解剖结构，明智的方法就是先松解小肠粘连，然后再去处理比较复杂的粘连。粘连比较严重的地方通常是在 Hartmann 直肠袋的上部，当发现吻合钉的时候提示已经接近末端直肠。如果粘连很严重，可以用水分离或生理盐水对粘连区进行浸润，这对粘连松解有一定帮助[15]。阑尾有时可能会被拉进盆腔靠近 Hartmann 直肠袋的位置，这会导致外科医生把它误以为是右侧的输尿管。经过之前的手术，输尿管会更多靠近中间的位置，尤其是左侧的卵巢和输卵管可能会与 Hartmann 直肠袋粘在一起。盆腔侧壁的出血多是损伤了输卵管或卵巢静脉的分支造成的。

结肠造口松动后，分离黏膜与皮肤的连接处，尽可能保留肠系膜。在黏膜与皮肤的连接处周围注射生理盐水有助于解剖分离。造口切除后，新的肠组织将用于和末端直肠吻合。一旦造口游离出来，外科医生要评估在保障没有张力的情况下肠组织是否有足够长度做吻合。如果肠组织长度不够，可以通过下列几种方法获得足够长的肠组织，包括打开近端结肠的肠系膜、游离结肠脾曲、在主动脉起始部分离肠系膜下动脉、在胰腺下缘分离肠系膜下静脉，也可以游离末端直肠后将直肠拉向近端结肠。一旦近端结肠游离和粘连松解完成后，小肠和结肠就可以被推入上腹部。

辨别和松动 Hartmann 直肠袋

一旦小肠被松解开，我们就可以看见 Hartmann 直肠袋，一些外科医生会用不可吸收缝线来标记直肠袋的顶部，以便于再次手术时可以辨认直肠袋位置，但我们并没有发现这样做有任何帮助。吻合口的钉子可以辨别出直肠袋的位置，即使直肠袋位于骨盆缘以下，但是直肠袋的长度通常要比预期的长。如果末端直肠吻合口与骶前筋膜粘在一起，那么通常从正中线向下解剖是比较安全的，避开了输尿管和髂血管。直肠上动脉在上次手术的时候被完整保留下来非常常见，用 Babcock 钳住直肠袋的顶部向头侧牵拉以暴露肠系膜和直肠。从中部到近端直肠，至少这是我们松解和解剖出直肠袋的常用方法。用器械将直肠拉直很有必要，一旦直肠袋被游离出来，从直肠放入一个小的管腔探头以确保它可以很容易通过预定的吻合口。如果患者有过脓肿或再次手术距第一次手术时间较长，那么有必要做进一步的松解手术。我们发现在女性患者中，由于中段直肠是弯曲的以及与子宫粘在一起，需要做进一步解剖。即使进一步游离组织，有些患者盆腔纤维化仍然很严重，直肠本质上是正常的，但是周围纤维化却很严重以至于管腔探头不能通过直肠，在这种情况下，用吻合器做端端吻合不可行，而用手缝的方法更可取。将预定做吻合区域上部切除与近端结肠做吻合，然后将生理盐水倒满盆腔，从直肠吹入空气以确定直肠的完整性。

一定要避免损伤输尿管，外科医生应该意识到，在初次手术之后，输尿管更多的会出现在居中的位置。对于有严重的盆腔纤维化或解剖模糊的患者，可于术前留置输尿管导管，导管并不能避免输尿管损伤，但它可以让我们及早发现这种损伤。对于阴道与直肠粘连者，将手指放入阴道可帮助我们在解剖时不伤及阴道。

吻合操作

Hartmann 手术后，为恢复肠道连续性，我们常用端端吻合器做吻合。手工或用荷包钳在近端肠管做荷包缝合，将钉砧置入其中固定，将吻合器器身由直肠缓慢推入到达直肠袋顶部。有时，吻合器很难通过肛门，Khoury 和 Opelka[16] 介绍可以先放置一种 Faensler 或 Chelsey-Eaton 肛门镜，随着肛门括约肌的不断扩张，再由肛门镜置入吻合器，吻合器到达直肠顶端后，穿刺器由直肠袋顶端穿出后与钉砧结合，然后激发吻合器，将吻合器缓慢退出直肠，检查吻合环的厚度和完整性。夹闭近端肠管，由直肠镜或乙状结肠镜打入空气来检测吻合口是否有瘘[17]。

其他术式

在做吻合的时候，并不是只能采用一种吻合方式，使用一些其他的吻合方式也是必要的。由于直肠的纤维化和挛缩，吻合器可能并不能够穿过直肠的顶端，尤其是那些带着造口很多年的患者，在这种情况下，可以选用其他的吻合方式，包括手工吻合，或者将吻合器的穿刺头由直肠前壁穿出，做一个结直肠的端侧吻合（图 48.2）[15]。还可以采用双荷包吻合技术，即在近端结肠和直肠末端各作一个荷包，吻合器仍然由肛门进入。最后一种方法是在末端直肠作荷包，然后吻合器由近端结肠侧壁穿出与直肠做吻合，结肠的末端用 TA 直线缝合器横断封闭。

关闭腹膜

肠道吻合结束后，要进行腹腔冲洗和关闭腹膜。全筋膜层缝合要优于分层缝合，连续全层缝合可以降低伤口裂开率。而且，6 项随机对照研究的 meta 分析发现，连续缝合要比间断缝合形成切口疝的风险更小（不考虑缝线的种类）[18]。在伤口裂开发生率上，可吸收线和不可吸收线并无区别，但是不可吸收线可能会导致长期的窦道和慢性伤口问题。所以首选的最佳缝合是用可吸收线全层连续缝合，间距 1cm，边距 1cm[19]。腹腔镜可以缩短切口的长度和减少伤口创伤，可以最大限度降低伤口并发症的出现。

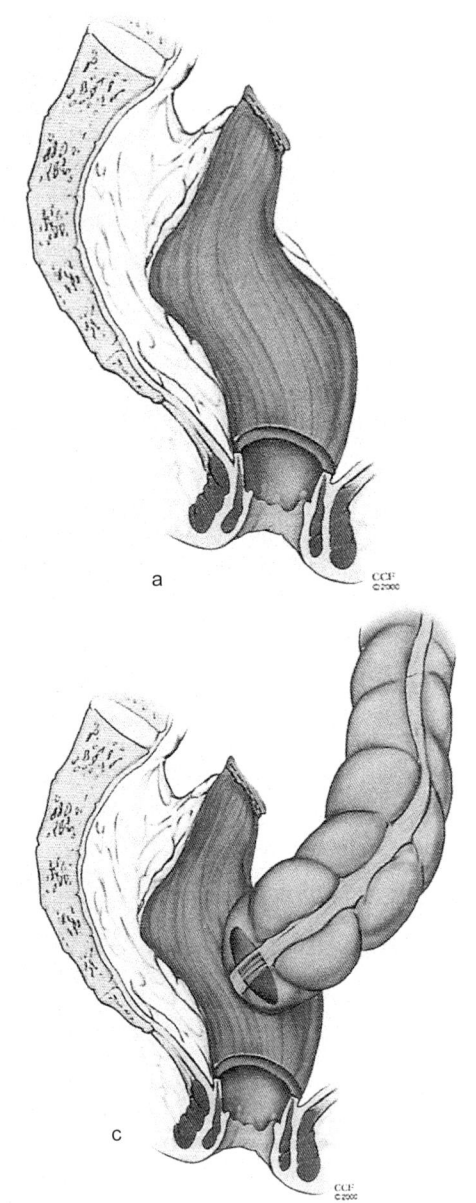
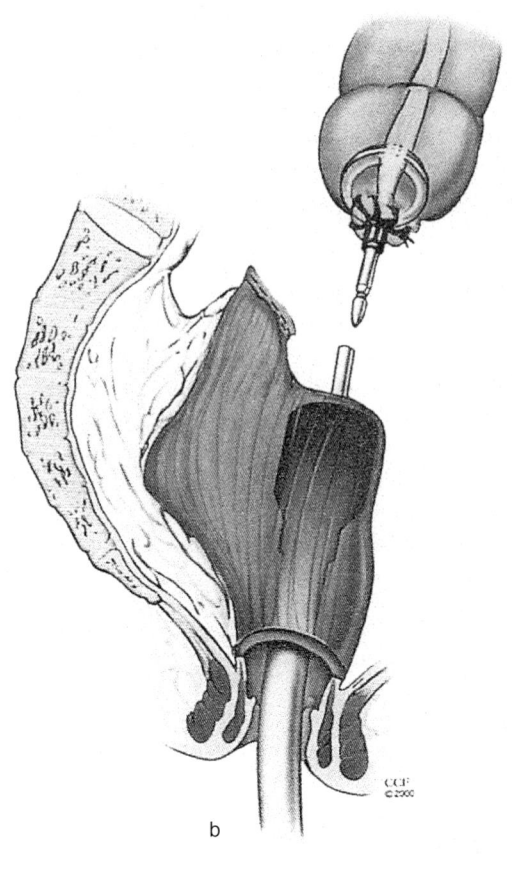

图48.2 直肠袋的松解比较困难，尤其是顶端瘢痕相对比较严重（a），在这种情况下，端端吻合器可以由直肠侧壁穿出（b），来完成结肠末端和直肠侧壁的吻合（c）（CCF 2000, reprinted with permission from the Cleveland Clinic Foundation）

还纳术后败血症和吻合口并发症的再次手术

造口还纳术后最严重的并发症之一就是吻合口瘘，对该并发症缺乏一个标准定义，使我们很难做出判断，我们甚至不清楚该并发症的准确发生率。我们使用了英国工作小组对消化道瘘做出的定义，该定义没有涉及由外科手术构建的吻合出现瘘的内容[20]。我们医院评估了998例左侧结直肠吻合术，吻合口瘘的发生率是4.8%[17]。在术中空气渗漏试验阳性者中，7.7%发生了临床吻合口瘘，而术中空气渗漏试验阴性组和未行空气渗漏试验组发生临床吻合口瘘的比例分别为3.8%和8.1%（$P<0.03$）。数据表明，在所有吻合术中都应该做空气渗漏实验，这样可以使外科医生能在第一时间发现和修补瘘口。

吻合口瘘的处理依赖于临床表现和患者的整体状况。吻合口裂开可以表现为腹膜炎、形成结肠与皮肤的瘘管或者形成脓肿，甚至可能没有症状。对于有弥漫性腹膜炎的患者，在抗感染、液体复苏之后要做急诊探查手术。理想的做法是术前标记造口的位置，患者的体位是截石位或劈腿位以便术中做乙状结肠镜。术中要考虑是保留吻合口然后近端作造瘘，还是切除吻合口，然后结肠造瘘。吻合口瘘的进一步处理细节将在第49章讨论。对于吻合口全层裂开的患者，最大的担心就是吻合口的生存能力，而将吻合口切除是明智的办法。远端直肠由直线缝合器或手工缝合关闭，近端结肠作造瘘，这些患者中大部分人不建议再做造口还纳术。

在一些相对稳定的患者中，如果只是出现了小的裂口，可以将吻合口保留下来，然后做改道手术，即做一个近端结肠造口术或回肠造口术。最近的一份 meta 分析表明回肠造口术较少出现造口并发症和腹壁疝[21]。有研究者担心这种方法会使残存的粪便由瘘口漏出而造成骨盆持续感染。对此，如果是做的回肠造口术，我们一般会对远端肠道作冲洗或在内镜下排空远端肠道。

慢性脓毒血症或者是吻合口瘘可以表现为结肠皮肤瘘，结肠皮肤瘘发展的一个主要风险因素就是保留了远端的乙状结肠，而与近端直肠无关[22]。虽然给予营养支持可以治愈瘘管，但是对于持续存在的瘘管，再次手术切除吻合口不可避免。

憩室病复发的再次手术

乙状结肠切除后憩室病复发的情况并不常见。憩室病肠切除后的患者出现腹痛，应排除是由其他疾病引起的腹痛，包括炎症性肠病、肠易激综合征、妇产科疾病、腹腔粘连疾病和来自初次肠切除引起的感染并发症。憩室病复发还应与肠切除术后缺乏特征的疼痛相鉴别，Munson 等[23]发现 27.2% 的憩室病患者在肠切除术后仍然会有疼痛，Parks 和 Connell[24] 注意到在分期手术的患者中有 1/4 会有持续存在的轻微症状。

憩室病复发常见的风险因素是由于保留了部分乙状结肠作为肠道末端，从而不能完成结直肠吻合。虽然只有一部分乙状结肠会发生憩室炎，但将整个乙状结肠及近端直肠切除是非常必要的。直肠没有结肠带，通常起自骶骨岬。近切缘有时很难掌握，虽然不需要切除所有近端憩室，但做吻合处的肠管要保证柔软易弯曲[25]。两项研究提到了吻合的位置和复发的风险因素，Bwnn 等[26]调查了 501 例由于憩室病经历乙状结肠手术的患者，吻合口在直肠和乙状结肠的复发率分别是 6.7% 和 12.5%。与此结果相似，Thaler 等[27] 的回顾性分析发现吻合口位置是预测复发的唯一因素，做结肠乙状结肠吻合复发的患者是做结直肠吻合的 4 倍。

在评价复发憩室炎患者时，获得之前的病案是非常有帮助的，包括病理报告和手术记录，以明确诊断和了解之前的手术细节。如果第一次手术就比较困难，伴随着解剖不清楚，或术后有盆腔感染以及吻合口并发症，那么术中应考虑使用输尿管支架。患者要有做临时造口的心理准备，尤其是吻合口较低的患者。充分的结肠松解是关键，尤其是脾曲的游离（见之前部分）。通过上诉方法仍然没有达到充分的活动度而无法保证无张力吻合时，可以将中结肠血管去除掉，残余结肠可以由右结肠和回结肠血管提供血供。还有就是可以将右结肠通过肠系膜或者进一步切除然后游离脾曲后将结肠拉下来与直肠吻合[28-29]。对于结肠长度不够的患者，两种方法可以用来确保与直肠的无张力吻合。一种方法就是在回结肠系膜打个窗口，横结肠由此穿过下降到直肠袋上部。还有就是进一步游离右结肠并结扎右结肠血管，然后再游离肝曲将其旋转到直肠上部。阑尾也应一并切除，因为解剖学上的改变将对阑尾炎的诊断造成困难。

先前的手术可能会使吻合口与骶前筋膜粘得比较严重，骶前筋膜是盆筋膜脏层凝结而成，到达正确的骶前筋膜层面非常重要；否则，损伤骶椎静脉会造成盆腔出血[30-31]。骶前大出血的处理不在这里具体讨论。盆腔交感神经向尾部走行并横跨骶前筋膜最后汇聚成盆腔丛，如果不能充分暴露这个层面会将其损伤。根据盆腔解剖难度和融合程度，做改道手术更可取。

结　论

再次手术是一个挑战，憩室病的再次手术也不例外。没有特别好的办法可以使用，外科医生必须有大量不同功能的医疗设备来确保患者可以得到更好的医治。在医院，急性憩室炎的发病率逐渐升高，患者呈现年轻化趋势[32]，最新的数据表明保守治疗急性疾病出院后，大部分人会由于出现并发症而再次入院治疗[33]。对于有结肠憩室病家族史的患者更会出现这种情况，多表现为腹膜后脓肿。不但外科治疗策略会影响到急诊手术和再次手术的发生率，疾病统计上的差异和初次手术治疗憩室病后的变化趋势，以及用腹腔镜手术，都会影响到急诊手术和再次手术的发生率。

参考文献

1. Hartmann H. Nouveau procede d'ablation des cancers de la partie terminale du colon pelvien. Congres Francais de Chirugia 1923;30:2241. Cited by: Corman ML. Classic articles in colonic and rectal surgery. Dis Colon Rectum. 1984;27:273.
2. Lockhart-Mummery JP. Late results in diverticulitis. Lancet. 1938;2:1401–2.
3. Smithwick RH. Experiences with surgical management of diverticulitis of sigmoid. Ann Surg. 1942;15:969–83.
4. Etzioni DA, Mack TM, Beart Jr RW, Kaiser AM. Diverticulitis in the United States: 1998–2005: changing patterns of disease and treatment. Ann Surg. 2009;249:210–7.
5. Maggard MA, Zingmoud D, O'Connell JB, Co CY. What proportion of patients with an ostomy for diverticulitis get reversed? Am Surg. 2004;70:9328–32.
6. Salem L, Flum DR. Primary anastomosis or Hartmann's procedures for patients with diverticular peritonitis? A systematic review. Dis Colon Rectum. 2004;47:1953–64.
7. Constantinides VA, Heriot A, Remzi F, Darzi A, Senapati A, Fazio VW, Tekkis PP. Operative strategies for diverticular peritonitis. Ann Surg. 2007;245:94–103.
8. Khan AL, Ah-See AK, Crofts TJ, Heys SD, Eremin O. Reversal of Hartmann's colostomy. J R Coll Surg Edinb. 1994;39:239–42.
9. Keck JO, Collopy BT, Ryan PJ, Fink R, Mackay JR, Woods RJ. Reversal of Hartmann's procedure: effect of timing and technique on ease and safety. Dis Colon Rectum. 1994;37:243–8.
10. Salem L, Anaya DA, Roberts KE, Flum DR. Hartmann's colectomy and reversal in diverticulitis: a population-level assessment. Dis Colon Rectum. 2005;48:988–95.
11. Fleming FJ, Gillen P. Reversal of Hartmann's procedure following acute diverticulitis: is timing everything? Int J Colorectal Dis. 2009;24:1219–25.
12. Albarran SA, Shimoens C, Van de Winkel N, Da Costa PM, Thill V. Restoration of digestive continuity after Hartmann's procedure: ASA score is a predictive factor for risk of postoperative complications. Acta Chir Belg. 2009;109:714–9.
13. Slim K, Vicaut E, Launay-Savary MV, Chipponi J. Updated systematic review and meta-analysis of randomized clinical trials on the role of mechanical bowel preparation before colorectal surgery. Ann Surg. 2009;249:203–9.
14. Read TE, Salgado J, Ferraro D, Fortunato R, Caushaj PF. "Peek port": a novel approach for avoiding conversion in laparoscopic colectomy. Surg Endosc. 2009;23:477–81.
15. Worsey MJ, Fazio VW. Reoperative pelvic surgery. In: Yeo CJ, Dempsey DT, Klein AS, Pemberton JH, Peters JH, editors. Shackelford's surgery of the alimentary tract. 6th ed. Philadelphia: Saunders/Elsevier; 2007. p. 2409–18.
16. Khoury DA, Opelka FG. Anoscopic-assisted insertion of end-to-end anastomosing staplers. Dis Colon Rectum. 1995;38:533–4.
17. Ricciardi R, Roberts PL, Marcello PW, Hall JF, Read TE, Schoetz DJ. Anastomotic leak testing after colorectal resection: what are the data? Arch Surg. 2009;144:407–12.
18. Hodgson NC. The search for an ideal method of abdominal fascial closure: a meta-analysis. Ann Surg. 2000;231:436–42.
19. Ceydeli A, Rucinski J, Wise L. Finding the best abdominal closure: an evidence-based review of the literature. Curr Surg. 2005;62:220–5.
20. Bruce J, Krukowski ZH, Al-Khairy G, Russell EM, Park KG. Systematic review of the definition and measurement of anastomotic leak after gastrointestinal surgery. Br J Surg. 2001;88:1157–68.
21. Tilney HS, Sains PS, Lovegrove RE, Reese GE, Heriot AG, Tekkis PP. Comparison of outcomes following ileostomy versus colostomy for defunctioning colorectal anastomoses. World J Surg. 2007;31:1141–5.
22. Fazio VW, Church JM, Jagelman DG. Colocutaneous fistulas complicated diverticulitis. Dis Colon Rectum. 1987;30:89–94.
23. Munson KD, Hensien MA, Jacob LN, Robinson AM, Liston WA. Diverticulitis – a comprehensive follow-up. Dis Colon Rectum. 1996;39:318–22.
24. Parks RG, Connell AM. The outcome of 455 patients admitted for treatment of diverticular disease of the colon. Br J Surg. 1970;57:775–8.
25. Rafferty J, Shellito P, Hyman NH, Buie WD, Standards Committee of American Society of Colon and Rectal Surgeons. Practice parameters for sigmoid diverticulitis. Dis Colon Rectum. 2006;49:939–44. 85–8.
26. Benn PL, Wolff BG, Ilstrup DM. Level of anastomosis and recurrent colonic diverticulitis. Am J Surg. 1986;151:269–71.
27. Thaler K, Baig MK, Berho M, Weiss EG, Nogueras JJ, Arnaud JP, et al. Determinants of recurrence after sigmoid resection for uncomplicated diverticulitis. Dis Colon Rectum. 2003;46:385–8.
28. Le TH, Gathright Jr JB. Reconstitution of intestinal continuity after extended left colectomy. Dis Colon Rectum. 1993;36:197–8.
29. Beck DE. Intraoperative anastomotic challenges. In: Whitlow CB, Beck DE, Margolin DA, Hicks TC, Timmcke AE, editors. Improved outcomes in colon and rectal surgery. London: Informa Healthcare; 2010. p. 33–55.
30. Wang QY, Shi WJ, Zhao YR, Zhou WQ, He ZR. New concepts in severe presacral hemorrhage during proctectomy. Arch Surg. 1985;120:1013–20.
31. Germanos S, Bolanis I, Saedon M, Baratsis S. Control of presacral venous bleeding during rectal surgery. Am J Surg. 2010;200:e33–5.
32. Jeyarajah S, Papagrigoriadis S. Diverticular disease increases and affects younger ages: an epidemiological study of 10-year trends. Int J Colorectal Dis. 2008;23:619–27.
33. Hall JF, Roberts PL, Ricciardi R, Read T, Scheirey C, Wald C, et al. Long-term follow-up after an initial episode of diverticulitis: what are the predictors of recurrence? Dis Colon Rectum. 2011;54:283–8.

第 49 章 肠吻合口瘘的外科问题

Yair Edden · Eric G. Weiss
李 民译 李 宁审校

摘 要

结直肠切除术后的肠吻合口瘘可以导致肠内容物经破裂的吻合口进入腹腔，不论对于患者还是外科医生，均是最严重的并发症之一。影像学技术的进步和肛门内真空负压引流装置在低位直肠吻合口瘘中的应用改善了部分肠吻合口瘘患者的预后。随着低位保肛手术和术前放射治疗的增加、近端肠管粪便转流手术实施率的变化，术后肠吻合口瘘的发生率也发生了改变。本章主要讨论肠吻合口瘘的危险因素和治疗原则。

关键词

吻合口瘘；吻合口；肠切除术；血液灌注；真空负压吸引；重建吻合口；回肠贮袋；结肠贮袋；放射线损伤的肠管

引 言

对于外科医生和患者而言，肠吻合口瘘是结直肠切除术后最严重的并发症之一，表现为肠内容物通过破裂的吻合口进入腹腔。切除病变结肠后行肠吻合术最初被认为很危险，在很多病例中失败并导致患者死亡。

20世纪初，William S Halsted[1]指出了黏膜下层（肠壁黏膜层和浆膜层中间组织）在成功的肠吻合术中的重要性。随着麻醉方法的进步、外科技术的改进和抗生素的使用，结合 William S Halsted 的经验，肠切除吻合术的应用越来越广泛，且越来越安全。然而，尽管腹部外科在过去几十年中发展迅猛，术后吻合口瘘仍然存在，且预后较差。

吻合口愈合的影响因素

获得完整和功能正常的吻合口需要几个步骤：①肠管的两个断端要以无张力的方式进行全层吻合；②吻合口重建（手工吻合或吻合器吻合）结束以后，局部组织的生长愈合非常重要。在吻合口完全愈合并有正常功能之前，创伤愈合过程中伴随的复杂炎症反应是必不可少的。创伤愈合需要几个重要因素，包括机体正常代谢状态、正常免疫能力和局部组织良好的血液灌注。其中任何一个因素出现异常均可影响吻合口愈合并最终导致吻合口瘘。吻合口愈合除了受创伤愈合过程中这些因素的影响以外，还与局部张力和细菌污染有关。最早出现的炎症反应过程是停滞期，期间胶原蛋白酶活性上调，胶原蛋白合成减少，导致吻合口抗张力能力降低，它出现在术后24h内，并可持续4天[2]。随后出现胶原组织增殖期，吻合口抗张力能力增加。吻合口重建后的几周出现塑型期，胶原组织的数量不再增加，但期间出现的胶原纤维交联进一步增加吻合口强度[3]。

局部组织中增高的溶胶原基质金属蛋白酶、MMP-2和MMP-9浓度可以增强浸润的中性粒细胞分泌的蛋白水解酶和胶原蛋白酶活性。吻合口周围组织的金属蛋白酶浓度与吻合口的抗张力能力相关[4]；研究表明，降低该酶的浓度可以在术后前3天内增强吻合口抗张力能力[5]。

代谢状态

伤口愈合的生理过程在肠吻合术中表现为肠管两个断端生长融合，进而封闭吻合口。受细胞因子调节的多个步骤依次发生，以形成具有一定强度的瘢痕。与其他瘢痕一样，吻合口瘢痕的形成和强度的增加同样依赖胶原蛋白，它是瘢痕的基本框架。胶原的形成依赖饮食中摄入的微量蛋白分子。该蛋白在体内的存储量非常少，因此，需要持续的营养摄入。在营养不良、代谢异常和术后呈分解代谢状态的患者中，腹壁切口和肠吻合口的愈合欠佳。因此，对于择期手术或条件允许的限期手术患者，术前应进行营养状态的评估。如患者白蛋白和前白蛋白水平降低，应考虑给患者进行术前静脉营养支持。对于老年患者或因长期慢性疾病（如炎性肠病）导致营养不良的患者，应重视患者营养状态。如果患者术前或术后长期不能正常进食，应考虑行营养支持，通常持续1周以上[6-7]。

免疫状态

如上所述，伤口愈合需要机体正常的免疫功能；细胞免疫和体液免疫在这一过程都起到非常重要的作用。通常情况下，伤口周围足量的活性白细胞和在不同阶段出现的具有调节功能的细胞因子是伤口愈合的重要因素。以下几种患者术后吻合口瘘的风险显著增加：存在可能导致免疫力低下的因素（如糖尿病、肥胖、高龄）；合并自身免疫性疾病；使用如类固醇类的免疫抑制剂；由于其他原因接受化学治疗。为了降低手术风险，术前应严格控制血糖、戒严和适当减肥；如果可能，择期手术前数周应停用免疫抑制剂。需要强调的是，对于使用类固醇激素的一些患者，应根据其之前使用的剂量给予适当的术前短效应激剂量[8]。多因素分析显示，服用类固醇激素患者需要输血，且慢性呼衰和其他围术期并发症的发生率显著增高[9]。

血液灌注

在伤口愈合的过程中，上述提到的所有因素（蛋白、细胞和体液免疫分子）均要到达局部组织方能发挥作用。虽然有些分子由局部组织分泌，白细胞在创伤后早期没有充分血液灌注的情况下也能够进入局部组织；但是，在没有良好血供的情况下，吻合口不可能充分愈合。在手术过程中，由于肠壁的正常血供被破坏，吻合口的血供相对较差。另外，由于存在个体差异，不可能预先判断离断血管后肠壁是否会出现血供不足。肠吻合之前确保肠管两个断端血供正常非常重要。对于合并血管疾病的患者，如血栓病史或其他能影响局部血供的疾病，更应特别注意吻合口血供情况。

手术操作

术前仔细的病情评估、术中精细操作都是减少吻合口瘘发生的重要方法。无论术者采用吻合器吻合还是手工吻合，肠吻合术的基本原则是使肠管两个断端的肠黏膜无张力靠拢并内翻吻合，确保吻合口良好愈合。由于黏膜下层是肠壁抗牵拉能力最强的一层，因此，吻合时应确保该层包含在缝线或吻合钉之内，确保吻合口能抵抗肠蠕动或其他原因产生的张力[10]。

如上所述，局部良好的血液灌注对于吻合口愈合非常重要；在进行肠吻合术之前，应注意检查肠管断端的血供情况。对于肠壁缺血，不论界限是否清除，应慎重考虑该段肠管是否适合进行肠吻合。肠壁断端没有活动性出血、局部肠系膜无可触及的或可视的动脉搏动都是血供不良的表现。一旦怀疑肠管血液灌注不佳，应切除局部肠管直至血供良好的部分[11]。确定肠壁血供良好以后，应保证肠管断端在无张力的情况下进行吻合，以确保吻合口正常愈合。局部张力可以引起缝线或吻合钉撕脱，还会导致敏感部位，尤其是肠壁断端血供不佳。如果肠管两个断端不能无张力靠拢，应继续松解两端肠管，确保无张力吻合。

吻合口瘘发生率

Kingham 和 Pachter[12] 统计分析了 15 篇研究共 12000 例患者，术后吻合口瘘的发生率是 2.4%~19%；对于有经验的结直肠外科医生，该发生率为 3%~6%。这一结果与其他报道基本相似，Ho 和 Ashour[10] 报道的吻合口瘘发生率是 1%~24%，Meade 和 Moran[13] 的研究结果为 3%~21%。不同类型的肠吻合，如小肠、小肠吻合与降结肠、远端直肠吻合，其吻合口瘘的发生率不同；被放射线照射过的肠管吻合与正常肠管间吻合的瘘的发生率不同；有基础疾病或长期口服药物的患者，其术后吻合口瘘的发生率显著高于其他患者。因此，没有一个准确的方法可以评价吻合口瘘的发生率。而且，国际上目前还没有吻合口瘘的诊断和治疗指南。

临床症状、影像学表现

肠吻合口瘘是指两端肠管连接处破裂，导致肠内容物进入腹腔。其临床表现的差异可以非常大：有的患者表现为严重的腹膜炎和脓毒症；有的患者则仅表现为心动过速或轻度体温升高，而很多术后原因都可以引起该症状；有些患者甚至没有任何腹腔感染的临床表现。吻合口瘘可以出现在术后 3~45 天内，术后 30 天以后的发生率最高达 12%[14]。由于吻合口瘘可能导致患者死亡，术后应进行密切随访并保持高度警觉。

临床上，当患者术后出现原因不明的心动过速、体温升高或血压变化时应高度警惕，因为这些症状可能与菌血症有关，预示着早期腹腔感染。当出现上述症状的时候，可以考虑行腹部 CT 检查以明确诊断。通常情况下，口服造影剂以后，应等待一段时间再行 CT 扫描，以确保造影剂通过吻合口，准确显示吻合口形态及是否有造影剂外漏（图 49.1）。当吻合口瘘存在时，由于病程长短不同，CT 可以显示出腹腔游离液体或脓肿。由于 CT 在大部分医院都可以进行，检查结果客观公正，可以提供结肠管腔以外的信息，是判断是否存在吻合口瘘的首选检查[15]。必须指出的是，约 1/3 的吻合口瘘患者 CT 检查仅表现为腹腔游离气体或液体，而不会有

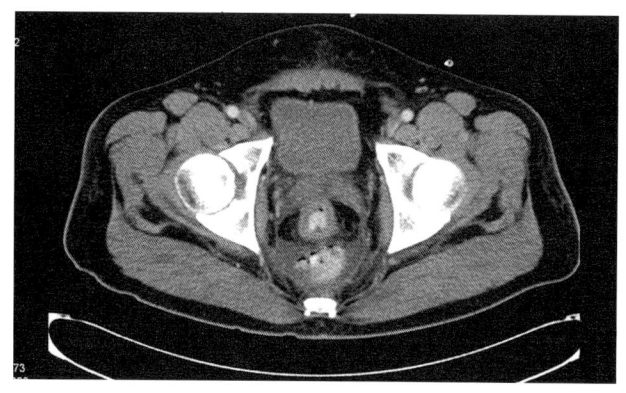

图 49.1　患者直肠低位前切除术后 7 天口服造影剂的盆腔 CT 成像。直肠后方可见造影剂和气体积聚

造影剂外漏的表现[16]。

另外一种目前很少使用的判断是否存在吻合口瘘的影像学检查方法是水溶性造影剂灌肠。通过灌肠使可视造影剂通过吻合口，以此判断是否存在破口。如果吻合口距齿状线较近，放置灌肠导管时应特别小心，以免损伤已经愈合的吻合口。这些先进的影像学方法不仅可以诊断，还可以治疗吻合口瘘。如果患者没有明显的弥漫型腹膜炎和休克症状，且腹腔脓肿局限包裹，可以进行 CT 引导下经皮穿刺引流[17]。对于一些患者，这种方法辅以营养支持和广谱抗感染治疗可以预防二次手术、治愈吻合口瘘。

近年来报道[18-19]一种特殊的负压引流装置（肛门内置海绵，产自德国 B. Braun Aesculap 公司）可以通过对骶前进行负压吸引治愈局限性的直肠吻合口瘘。平均更换 5 次内置海绵、引流 21 天以后，体温升高和菌血症可以得到控制。瘘口经影像学和内镜检查证实愈合通常需要两个月时间，该时间与患者年龄及瘘口周围脓腔大小有关：脓腔越大，愈合需要的时间越长；吻合口距肛门距离越近，瘘口愈合需要的时间越长。目前还不清楚治疗期间是否需要行预防性末端回肠袢式造口（图 49-2）。

二次手术

怀疑吻合口瘘的时候，应该根据临床经验和判断指导治疗。如果患者存在严重的弥漫性腹膜炎和败血症症状，应该在积极的复苏后行剖腹探查手术。如果患者的临床症状不明显，应行上述提到的影像学检查，根据检查结果制定下一步治疗方案。

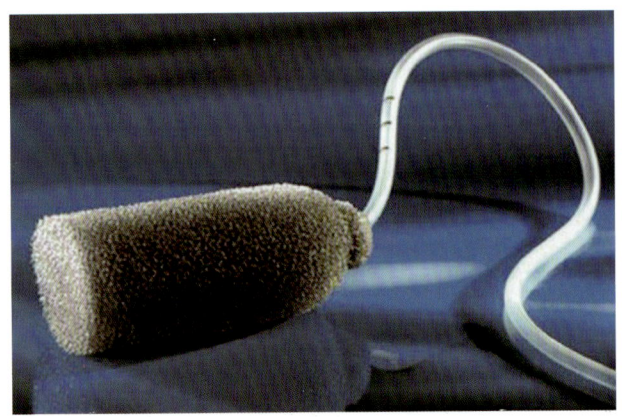

图 49.2　用于部分低位直肠吻合口瘘患者骶前吸引的真空海绵（一种单腔聚氨基甲酸乙酯海绵）（Reprinted with permission from Arezzo et al.[19]）

二次剖腹探查时，手术的基本原则包括：①尽量减少手术创伤；②尽量缩短手术时间；③充分的腹腔冲洗；④作好近端肠管粪便转流的准备。

二次剖腹探查的手术方式很多，但术者应该遵循几个原则。通俗地说，应该首先拯救患者生命，其次考虑患者的生活质量。术中也可以选择一些手术方式以减少后期干预，但是应该分清楚主次。在绝大部分情况，二次手术应选择经原切口进入腹腔。由于术后腹腔内瘢痕组织形成及腹腔感染，进腹时常碰到严重的腹腔粘连和脓肿，因此，进腹时应非常小心，以免造成新的损伤。缓慢、仔细地钝性分离可以避免不必要的损伤。术中应最大限度清除腹腔内的肠内容物，并行充分的腹腔冲洗，这样可以祛除病因、减少腹腔内细菌繁殖，降低败血症和腹腔脓肿形成的可能。

由于部分患者生命体征不稳定、严重腹腔感染和局部组织充血水肿、质地较脆，二次手术时修复吻合口是不提倡的。修复吻合口有时候看起来可行，但由于存在广泛腹腔感染，修复处通常难以愈合。因此，对于大部分患者而言，最安全、最省时的手术方式是腹腔冲洗引流、近端肠管粪便转流。对于生命体征稳定的患者，如果吻合口容易暴露、结肠相对健康且瘘口较小、不需要重新进行肠管吻合，可以考虑进行局部修补。即使修补了瘘口，为了帮助瘘口愈合，仍应进行近端肠管粪便转流。

再次吻合的转归

关于患者出现吻合口瘘后再次行肠吻合术预后的报道比较少。很多因为吻合口瘘接受腹腔探查、近端肠管粪便转流的患者不再接受确定性手术，而是永久保留肠造口[20-21]。由于死亡率不同，结肠瘘后永久保留肠造口的可能性大于直肠瘘[21]。Lefevre 等[22]近来报道了他们关于结肠-直肠吻合和直肠-肛管吻合失败后再次行肠吻合术的经验。这个研究中包括了多种需要二次行肠吻合的病例，而不是单纯的吻合口瘘。再次行肠吻合的失败率是15%（5例）。研究者指出，虽然再次行肠吻合是可行的，但是手术非常困难，且术后并发症发生率较高。

特殊情况

回肠贮袋

回肠贮袋手术常用于一些缺乏结肠存储能力的患者，这类患者是一个特殊的群体。这类患者术后如出现吻合口瘘，除了有上述提到的危险以外，还会有两方面远期影响。由于缺乏结肠吸收水分和粪便存储的功能，小肠的长度就显得尤为重要。二次手术时切除瘘的贮袋会导致小肠长度缩短、吻合口重建困难及生活质量降低。另一个远期影响就是盆腔纤维化和瘢痕化。盆腔组织对漏出的肠内容物的反应会减弱新贮袋的伸展和扩张的能力，从而降低新吻合口的顺应性。由于这些原因，很多外科医生在行回肠贮袋手术时会预防性地行近端肠管粪便转流[23-24]。关于回肠贮袋肛管吻合的二次手术问题在第 20 章叙述。

结肠贮袋

结肠 J 形贮袋（本书其他章节讨论）的目的是在术后 2~3 年内模仿直肠粪便存储功能。与回肠贮袋不同，接受结肠贮袋手术患者的结肠长度是足够的，一旦出现吻合口瘘行结肠造口术以后，患者的生活质量可以有保证。结肠贮袋手术经常行预防性近端肠管粪便转流，并能最终还纳造口肠管[25]。

放射线损伤的肠管

关于放射线损伤的肠管的讨论见第10章。与以前相比，越来越多的患者在肠管接受放射照射以后接受手术治疗。放射治疗目前是盆腔肿瘤术前新辅助治疗或综合治疗的重要方法，这导致该类患者在接受直肠或多脏器切除时是吻合口瘘的高危人群。放射线对肠管的损伤可以在照射后持续多年。放射线对血管的损伤主要是针对中、小血管，可以导致吻合口纤维化和直肠炎等远期并发症。在肠切除过程中，判断局部组织血供情况非常重要；肠吻合需要在未被照射的结肠和正常直肠间进行或行复杂的直肠成形术[26]。

结 论

在过去的30年里，虽然结肠-直肠吻合术的并发症显著减少，却没有完全消失。吻合口瘘的发生与否与吻合方式（手工吻合、吻合器吻合）无关[27-28]。由于其威胁生命、影响生活质量和近端粪便分流的肠管可能永远无法还纳，吻合口瘘是最严重的并发症。一旦出现吻合口瘘，应立即给予准确的处理措施；通常患者需要接受二次腹部探查手术：冲洗腹腔、切除破裂的吻合口、行临时或永久性近端肠管粪便转流。术前患者良好营养状态和正确的手术原则，如无张力吻合、肠管良好血供、内翻吻合，可以减少吻合失败的可能、减少住院费用和增加床位使用率[29-30]。高度的临床敏感性有助于早期诊断吻合口瘘。

参考文献

1. Halsted WS. Circular suture of the intestine: an experimental study. Am J Med Sci. 1887;94:436–61.
2. Thompson SK, Chang EY, Jobe BA. Healing in gastrointestinal anastomosis, part I. Microsurgery. 2006;26:131–6.
3. Martens MF, Hendricks T. Postoperative changes in collagen synthesis in intestinal anastomoses of the rat: differences between small and large bowel. Gut. 1991;32:1482–7.
4. De Hingh IH, de Man BM, Lomme RM, van Goor H, Hendriks T. Colonic anastomotic strength and matrix metalloproteinase activity in an experimental model of bacterial peritonitis. Br J Surg. 2003;90:981–8.
5. Syk I, Agren MS, Adawi D, Jepsson B. Inhibition of matrix metalloproteinases enhances breaking strength of colonic anastomoses in an experimental model. Br J Surg. 2001;88:228–34.
6. Schwenk W, Günther N, Haase O, Konschake U, Müller JM. Changes in perioperative treatment for elective colorectal resections in Germany 1991 and 2001/2002. Zentralbl Chir. 2003;128:1086–92.
7. Oguz M, Kerem M, Bedirli A, Mentes BB, Sakrak O, Salman B, et al. L-alanin-L-glutamine supplementation improves the outcome after colorectal surgery for cancer. Colorectal Dis. 2007;9:515–20.
8. Suding P, Jensen E, Abramson MA, Itani K, Wilson SE. Definitive risk factors for anastomotic leaks in elective open colorectal resection. Arch Surg. 2008;143:907–12.
9. Trésallet C, Royer B, Godiris-Petit G, Menegaux F. Effect of systemic corticosteroids on elective left-sided colorectal resection with colorectal anastomosis. Am J Surg. 2008;195:447–51.
10. Ho Y-H, Ashour MAT. Techniques for colorectal anastomosis. World J Gastroenterol. 2010;16:1610–21.
11. Holmes NJ, Cazi G, Reddell MT, Gorman JH, Fedorciw B, Semmlow JL, et al. Intraoperative assessment of bowel viability. J Invest Surg. 1993;6:211–21.
12. Kingham TP, Pachter HL. Colonic anastomotic leak: risk factors, diagnosis and treatment. J Am Coll Surg. 2009;208:269–78.
13. Meade B, Moran B. Reducing the incidence and managing the consequences of anastomotic leakage after rectal resection. Acta Chir Iugosl. 2004;51:19–23.
14. Hyman N, Manchester TL, Osler T, Burns B, Cataldo PA. Anastomotic leaks after intestinal anastomosis: it's later than you think. Ann Surg. 2007;245:254–8.
15. Doeksen A, Tanis PJ, Wüst AF, Vrouenraets BC, van Lanschot JJ, van Tets WF. Radiological evaluation of colorectal anastomoses. Int J Colorectal Dis. 2008;23:863–8.
16. Nicksa GA, Dring RV, Johnson KH, Sardella WV, Vignati PV, Cohen JL. Anastomotic leaks: what is the best diagnostic imaging study? Dis Colon Rectum. 2007;50:197–203.
17. Khurrum Baig M, Hua Zhao R, Batista O, Uriburu JP, Singh JJ. Percutaneous postoperative intra-abdominal abscess drainage after elective colorectal surgery. Tech Coloproctol. 2002;6:159–64.
18. Glitsch A, von Bernstorff W, Seltrecht U, Partecke I, Paul H, Heidecke CD. Endoscopic transanal vacuum-assisted rectal drainage (ETVARD): an optimized therapy for major leaks from extraperitoneal rectal anastomoses. Endoscopy. 2008;40:192–9.
19. Arezzo A, Miegge A, Garbarini A, Morino M. Endoluminal vacuum therapy for anastomotic leaks after rectal surgery. Tech Coloproctol. 2010;14:279–81.
20. Iancu C, Mocan LC, Todea-Iancu D, Mocan T, Acalovschi I, Ionescu D, et al. Host-related predictive factors for anastomotic leakage following large bowel resections for colorectal cancer. J Gastrointestin Liver Dis. 2008;17:299–303.
21. Thornton M, Joshi H, Vimalachandran C, Heath R, Carter P, Gur U, et al. Management and outcome of colorectal anastomotic leaks. Int J Colorectal Dis. 2011;26:313–20.
22. Lefevre JH, Bretagnol F, Maggiori L, Ferron M, Alves A, Panis Y. Redo surgery for failed colorectal or coloanal anastomosis: A valuable surgical challenge. Surgery. 2011;149:65–71.
23. Schoetz Jr DJ, Coller JA, Veidenheimer MC. Can the pouch be saved? Dis Colon Rectum. 1988;31:671–5.
24. Remzi FH, Fazio VW, Kirat HT, Wu JS, Lavery IC, Kiran RP. Repeat pouch surgery by the abdominal approach safely salvages failed ileal pelvic pouch. Dis Colon Rectum. 2009;52:198–204.
25. Jeyarajah S, Sutton C, Miller A, Hemingway D. Leicester Colorectal Specialist Group. Colo-anal pouches: lessons from a prospective audit. Colorectal Dis. 2008;10:599–604.
26. Steichen FM, Barber HK, Loubeau JM, Iraci JC. Bricker-Johnston sigmoid colon graft for repair of postradiation rectovaginal fistula and stricture performed with mechanical sutures. Dis Colon Rectum. 1992;35:599–603.
27. Khan AA, Wheeler JM, Cunningham C, George B, Kettlewell M, Mortensen NJ. The management and outcome of anastomotic leaks in colorectal surgery. Colorectal Dis. 2008;10:587–92.
28. Lustosa SAS, Matos D, Atallah AN, Castro AA. Stapled versus hand sewn methods for colorectal anastomosis surgery. Cochrane Database Syst Rev. 2001;3:CD003144.

29. Martínez JL, Luque-de-León E, Andrade P. Factors related to anastomotic dehiscence and mortality after terminal stomal closure in the management of patients with severe secondary peritonitis. J Gastrointest Surg. 2008;12:2110–8.

30. Frye J, Bokey EL, Chapuis PH, Sinclair G, Dent OF. Anastomotic leakage after resection of colorectal cancer generates prodigious use of hospital resources. Colorectal Dis. 2009;11:917–20.

第 50 章 直肠后肿瘤

Ursula M. Szmulowicz · Tracy L. Hull
张巨东 译　李国逊 审校

摘　要

直肠后（骶前）肿瘤相对比较少见。本章将阐述骶前的解剖及与这类特殊肿瘤分类有关的筋膜界限。手术方式取决于推测的病理结果和能够确定肿块水平的影像学检查。我们将讨论不同外科手术入路的优劣势。

关键词

直肠后肿瘤；骶前；胚胎学；发病率；病理学；症状学；囊肿；畸胎瘤

引　言

直肠后肿瘤在成人中相当少见。这类肿瘤的发病率在 0.0025%～0.015% 之间[1]。早期的有关直肠后肿瘤的文献普遍将这些病变称作 Middeldorpf 肿瘤。最早的 Middeldorpf 肿瘤类似于直肠重复畸形或者畸胎瘤，是在 1885 年利用 Kraske 方法从一名 1 岁小女孩身上切除的[2-4]。经典的直肠后肿瘤的描述出现在 1885 年，然而法国产科医师 Ph. Peu 在 17 世纪就已经记载了类似的肿物[4]。虽然这类肿瘤生长在同一部位，但是它们的病理学和病因学却存在着多样性。

本章将讲述骶前的解剖、直肠后肿瘤的胚胎学、发病率、病理学、症状学及如何诊断这类肿物，并将详细介绍直肠后肿瘤的不同手术入路及其预后。

解剖和胚胎学

直肠后/骶前间隙是一个存在于直肠上 2/3 和骶骨间潜在的凹陷[5]。其位于覆盖在直肠及直肠系膜上的固有筋膜和骶前筋膜之间，致密的结缔组织紧密附着于骶骨和尾骨（图 50.1）[7-8]。骶前间隙的上界为腹膜反折（位于 S_2～S_3 水平），下界为直肠骶骨筋膜[5,8,9]。Hannon 等[10] 把肛提肌和尾骨肌称为直肠后间隙的下界，尽管它们实际上是位于肛提肌上间隙的基底部。直肠骶骨筋膜是骶前筋膜的延续，它起自 S_3～S_4 椎体，止于直肠固有筋膜的后壁（大约在齿状线上方 3～5cm）[8]。在 Sato 和 Sato[11] 的尸检中，直肠骶骨筋膜 97.2% 起自 S_2～C_1，大部分（94.4%）还是起自 S_3～S_4；5 例尸体中有 2 例是双层直肠骶骨筋膜。这个筋膜间偶尔会有血管存在，如果不被发现会导致不可控制的出血[11]。直肠后间隙的外侧界为直肠侧韧带和梨状肌筋膜[7]。一些学者把输尿管、髂肌和髂血管也包括在内[8,10,12]。腹下神经从这个间隙中的疏松结缔组织和脂肪组织中穿过[7,13]。骶正中动脉、直肠上动脉、直肠中动脉、淋巴系统以及骶神经根也起源于直肠后间隙[8,10,14]。尽管直肠上动脉位于腹膜反折以上，但是这个部位正好是直肠固有筋膜和骶前筋膜的交界处[8]。直肠

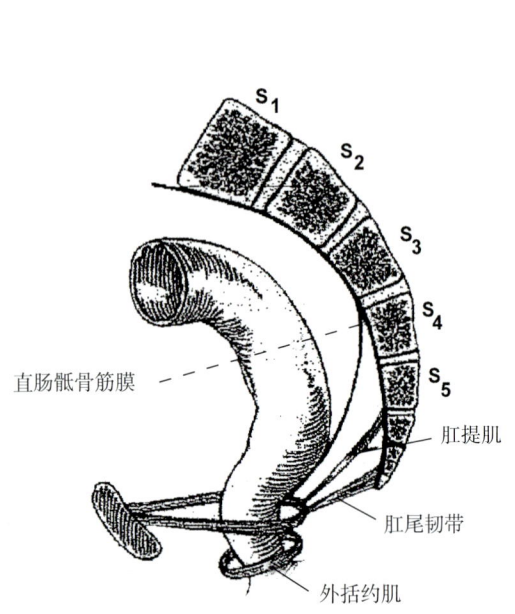

图 50.1 骶骨前间隙的解剖（Reprinted with permission from Dunn[6]）

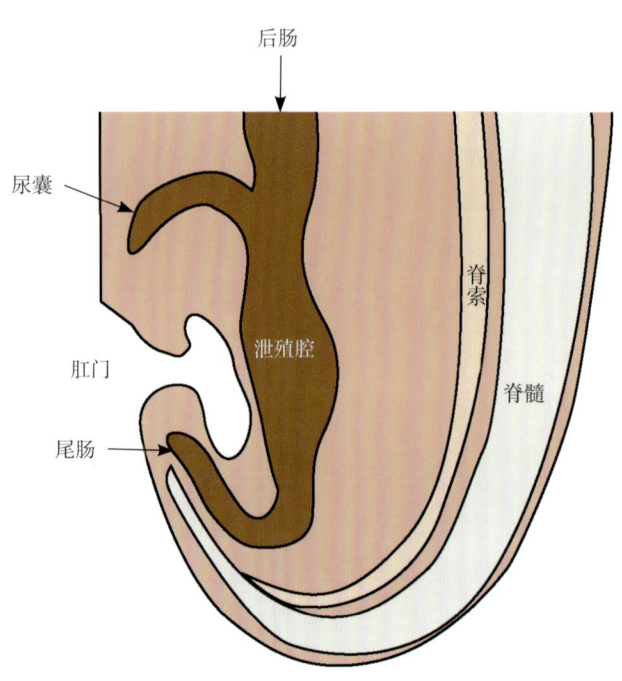

图 50.2 胚胎的肛后肠。妊娠 35 天，尾肠从尾部延伸到泄殖腔。肛后肠的残留会产生尾肠囊肿

后肿瘤的后面是骶前筋膜后的无血管区，避免了损伤细微的骶前静脉，它是位于直肠中动脉旁的一个主要出血静脉[7,15]。直肠后肿瘤的血运来源于从骶正中动脉和髂内动脉发出的滋养血管[10]。周围小的血管也会为肿瘤提供血运[10]。

了解直肠后间隙的胚胎学起源对于处理先天性直肠后肿瘤十分必要。大部分这类肿瘤是因为发育畸形产生：残留的胚胎残余、中线融合的缺陷和胚胎隔离[16]。

原始的内脏是由卵黄囊的内胚层发育而来，在怀孕第 4 周时分化为 3 个独立的部分——前肠、中肠和后肠[17-19]。后肠最后发育成远端 1/3 的横结肠至齿状线以上的肠管。在耻骨尾骨连线水平，后肠和前侧的尿囊产生泄殖腔，它是一个盲端[18]。在胚胎早期，后肠持续的超过泄殖腔形成尾肠或者肛后肠，妊娠 35 天是最好的界定时间（长 8mm）（图 50.2）[10,20]。在怀孕的第 4～6 周之间，尿直肠膈向下延伸至泄殖腔膜（内外胚层的交界），将泄殖腔分为前面的尿生殖窦和后面的肛门直肠[21]。泄殖腔膜是未来肛门的节点，它经历程序性细胞死亡后与羊水进行沟通[21-22]。同样，在怀孕 56 天时位于未来肛门尾部的尾肠完全分裂（长约 35mm）[10,20,22]。肛后肠生成尾肠囊肿。因为与出现在直肠后间隙的类癌和尾肠囊肿关系密切，因此 Ghosh 等[23]认为这两种病变可能存在相同的后肠的起源。

直肠后畸胎瘤的病因存在争议。骶前畸胎瘤被认为起源于直肠周围组织的多功能胚胎造血干细胞[10,24,25]。Hannon 等[10]认为这个组织起源于 Hensen 节。Larsen[26-27]以及 Coco 等[26-27]指出，这些原始生殖细胞在怀孕第 4～6 周期间不按正常途径，从卵黄囊沿着体壁的背侧到达生殖腺。

产生直肠重复畸形的胚胎缺陷是一个争辩的话题。虽然一些理论十分先进，但是没有一种能够系统的解释各种重复畸形[28]。这些病变代表了在胚胎形成的第 8 或第 9 周时短暂的肠道支囊的延续[29-30]。后来的研究者指出这些胚芽位于小肠系膜游离部表面，只包含黏膜和浆膜，但不会使它们成为重复畸形。这些胚胎支囊不是大肠的特征[31]。在怀孕第 6 周时，闭塞肠管再通的异常是形成两个肠腔的病因[29-32]。此外，Veeneklaas[33]认为胚胎脊索从内胚层分离时的缺陷可能会导致在背侧分出了一部分原始肠道，它进化成独立的胃肠道。Edwards[34]提出所有后肠衍生出的重复畸形都发生在原始消化道形成之前。

表皮样囊肿被认为起源于外胚层关闭缺陷[35]。不同的研究者将表皮样囊肿归咎于移位的外胚层残留部分[36-37]。皮样囊肿起源于外胚层残留的尾部[27]。Hannon 等[10]认为这些囊肿因为外胚层融合误差而产生，导致这个地方胚胎组织残留。泌尿生殖器"装置"的延续被当做皮样囊肿的起源[38]。同样，皮样囊肿由于椎管尾骨的退化障碍而形成[39]。脊索瘤从原始脊索演变而来[10]。中胚层脊索通常在怀孕3周时发育，但是最后退化形成软骨和椎体[10]。

分类

下面讲述直肠后肿瘤的各种分类方法。虽然它们有共同的发病空间，但是这些肿瘤有不同的病理学表现和起源。Lovelady 和 Dockerty[40] 在 1949 年提出了经典的分类体系的原型，将这些肿瘤分成为先天性、炎性、神经源性、骨性、软组织性和混合性。Uhlig 和 Johnson[2] 将软组织肿瘤归为混合性肿瘤来简化这个分类方法（表 50.1）。Wolpert 等[9] 更倾向于删除炎性肿瘤。一个更简单的分类方法由 Lev-Chelouche 等[41] 提出，这种分类方法包括良性先天性、恶性先天性、良性后天性、恶性后天性。这些研究者指出同一类型的肿瘤虽然有不同的病理类型，但是它们有类似的表现、治疗和预后。这种分类方法没有改变肿瘤的治疗，但有助于患者更好地了解这类疾病。Chêne 和 Voitellier[24] 更加简化了分类方法，将其分为发育性囊肿、畸胎瘤、脊索瘤和非胚胎肿瘤。

发病率

直肠后肿瘤在成年人群的发病率很低。这类肿瘤的观察结果大部分来源于个案病例报道和小宗的病例分析。总发病率在 0.0025%～0.015% 之间[1]。来自三级治疗中心的大宗病例分析认为每 40 000～63 000 例住院患者中只有 1 例被诊断为直肠后肿瘤（表 50.2）[45, 55, 56]。Spencer 和 Jackman[57] 证实在过去1年的时间里直肠后病变只占他们常规乙状结肠镜检查、治疗的 0.02%，其中 20 851 例患者中只检查出 3 例直肠后肿瘤。各种报道指出，美国每年的新增病例是 1.4～6.5 例[27]。这些数字只反映了转诊中心的水平，所以这类肿瘤的发病率可能比实际报道的要高[58]。Uhlig 和 Johnson[2] 预测在一个大都市里每年大约有 2 例直肠后肿瘤的患者被诊断出来。在极少的病例中，同时存在两种骶前肿瘤。Krivokapic 等[59] 曾描述了一名 37 岁女性同时合并有肠囊肿和骶前脑脊膜膨出。其他的直肠后肿物被发现同时可能合并有畸胎瘤、表皮样囊肿、脂肪瘤、

表 50.1　直肠后肿瘤的分类

先天性肿瘤
　进展性肿瘤
　　尾肠囊肿（囊性黏蛋白错构瘤）
　　畸胎瘤
　　畸胎癌
　　直肠重复畸形
　　表皮样囊肿
　　皮样囊肿
　骶前脊膜膨出
　脊索瘤
神经源性肿瘤
　室管膜瘤
　节细胞神经母细胞瘤
　节细胞神经瘤
　恶性施万细胞瘤
　神经母细胞瘤
　神经纤维瘤
　神经纤维肉瘤
　神经鞘瘤
　施万细胞瘤
骨肿瘤
　动脉瘤样骨囊肿
　软骨瘤
　软骨黏液肉瘤
　尤因肉瘤
　骨巨细胞瘤
　骨软骨瘤
　骨肉瘤
　骨瘤
单纯性骨囊肿
混杂性肿瘤
　动静脉畸形
　类癌
　腹外硬纤维瘤
　纤维瘤
　纤维肉瘤
　血管内皮瘤
　血管瘤
　血管外皮细胞瘤
　平滑肌瘤
　脂肪瘤
　淋巴瘤
　转移性肿瘤（如乳腺癌和前列腺癌）
　髓脂瘤

表 50.1 续

- 多发性骨髓瘤
- 软组织肉瘤
- 炎性肿瘤
  - 脓肿（直肠周、骨盆）
  - 复杂的憩室炎
  - 克罗恩病
  - 异物
  - 异物性肉芽肿（如矿物油、钡剂）
  - 内瘘

畸胎癌[45, 59]。成年人群中被确诊的直肠后肿瘤大多发生在中年（表 50.2）。不同的文献记录了这类肿瘤的手术年龄在 29～60 岁之间，大部分患者是在 40 岁左右[2]。直肠后肿瘤在女性中的发病率比男性高 2～15 倍[35, 45, 60]。来自 Uhlig 和 Johnson 的文章指出直肠后肿瘤 75% 是女性[2]。Aslan[35] 指出每个外科医生在他的职业生涯中将诊断出 1 例直肠后肿瘤，而且这个患者很有可能是女性。这类肿瘤常发生在女性的育龄期，尤其是围产期，这和可能与频繁进行常规盆腔检查有关，而不是性别差异[4, 61]。3%～30% 的直肠后肿瘤在产妇中确诊[4]。在 Uhlig 和 Johnson 的调查中，24 例育龄女性患者中有 7 例是在怀孕期间和产后被确诊的。

先天性肿瘤占直肠后肿瘤的 55%～81%[2, 27, 41, 45, 48]。而 Lev-Chelouche 等[41] 认为各种类型的直肠后肿瘤发病率相同。先天性肿瘤最常见的是发育性囊肿，另外 60% 包括尾肠囊肿、畸胎瘤、畸胎癌、直肠重复畸形、皮样囊肿和表皮样囊肿[8, 36]。Jao 等的文章[45]中指出平均诊断时间为 33 岁。发育性囊肿常见于中年妇女，尤其是在 30～50 岁之间[2, 23, 62]。各种的研究表明发育性囊肿男女发病率比为 1:3，而 Jao 等认为有更大的差距（1:15）[20, 62]。大多文献指出直肠后先天性囊肿在女性的发病率能达到 85%[2, 48]。

表 50.2 直肠后肿瘤的统计报告

研究者	持续时间（年）	病例数	平均年龄（岁）	女性	恶性	恶性（男性）
Freier 等[42](1971)	35	21	NR	12（57%）	12（57%）	NR
Uhlig and Johnson[2](1975)	30	63	NR	46（73%）	26（42%）	NR
Localio 等[43](1979)	15	20	45	10（50%）	12（60%）	9（75%）
Cody 等[44](1981)	28	39	NR	21（53.8%）	39（100%）	18（46%）
Jao 等[45](1985)	19	120（100 成人）	43	74（61.6%）	51（43%）	33（65%）
Hjermstad and Helwig[20](1987)	35	53	35	41（77%）	1（2%）	NR
Lee and Symmonds[46](1988)	15	70	NR	70（100%）	21（30%）	0（0%）
Böhm 等[1](1993)	12	24	29（DC）51（C）	19（79%）	4（17%）	2（50%）
Wang 等[47](1995)	14	45	41.1	25（25.5%）	22（48%）	20（91%）
Pidala 等[48](1999)	20	14	44	12（85.7%）	1（7%）	NR
Lev-Chelouche 等[41](2003)	10	42	40.6	28（67%）	21（50%）	11（52%）
Smith 等[49](2004)	23	43	49	26（60%）	9（39%）	NR
Glasgow 等[50](2005)	22	34	48	21（62%）	7（21%）	6（86%）
Buchs 等[51](2007)	9	16	37	13（81%）	0（0%）	0（0%）
Woodfield 等[16](2007)	8	27	30（B）60（M）	17（63%）	7（26%）	4（57%）
Grandjean 等[52](2008)	15	30	43	23（58%）	1（3%）	NR
Pappalardo 等[53](2009)	14	34	42	19（56%）	14（41%）	NR
Mathis 等[54](2008)	23	31	52	28（90%）	4（13%）	0（0%）

缩写：NR 未报道，DC 进展性囊肿，C 脊索瘤，B 良性，M 恶性

大约50%的发育性囊肿是尾肠囊肿，如囊性错构瘤、黏液分泌性囊肿（表50.3）[56]。Uhlig和Johnson[2]报道在他们研究的63例良性发育性囊肿患者中有16例是尾肠囊肿，其中93.7%是女性。来自于Hjermstad和Helwig的统计，大部分尾肠囊肿（77%）出现在女性中[20]。然而，Hannon等[10]发现尾肠囊肿常见于男性。Hjermstad和Helwig记录了平均年龄在35～53岁的尾肠囊肿患者，尽管女性患者的年龄分布符合贝尔曲线，研究者证实3例男性患者并没有类似的年龄分布区间。

畸胎瘤在成年人群中很罕见。大宗病例报道指出其发病率在0～37.5%之间（表50.3）。这类肿瘤常见于婴儿和儿童，30 000～43 000名婴儿中能发现1名[23, 62]。在成年人中，合并其他发育性囊肿的畸胎瘤主要在中年妇女中被确诊[6, 62]。Uhlig和Johnson[2]报道在过去30年被诊治的63例直肠后肿瘤患者中只有2例为畸胎瘤。Jao等的病例回顾报道了在成年患者中有7例畸胎瘤（7%）和1例畸胎癌（1%）[45]。

直肠重复畸形在成年人中极少见。这种畸形经常是在12岁之前的儿童中被确诊[25, 30]。Pappalardo等[53]研究了34例直肠后肿瘤的患者，其中仅有2例是直肠重复畸形（占5.8%）。这类肿瘤更常见于女性。大多数肠道重复畸形位于直肠外。截止到1951年，文献报道的315例肠道重复畸形中只有10例（3.2%）位于直肠[28, 63, 64]。直肠重复畸形占所有消化道重复畸形的1%～8%[25, 32, 62, 65]。

接近15%的直肠后肿瘤是表皮样囊肿[35, 45, 50]。在Jao等报道[45]中有12.5%被确诊为表皮样囊肿。直肠后皮样囊肿占所有皮样囊肿的很少一部分[25]。大量文献报道皮样囊肿占直肠后肿瘤的0～5%[43, 45, 53]。

骶前脑脊膜膨出是一种罕见的先天性囊性肿瘤。自从在1837年首次发现此病到2007年间，文献仅报道了240例[59, 66, 67]，其中女性患者占85%[45, 59]。Jao等[45]在120例直肠后肿瘤的患者中发现2例骶前脑脊膜膨出，这2例都是女性。部分骶前脑脊膜膨出被证实是常染色体显性遗传，是Currarino综合征的一部分[45, 62]。这种病变与Marfan综合征关系密切[66]。这类肿块与脊柱裂、脊髓栓系、脊柱闭合不全、双角子宫、直肠、子宫、卵巢重复畸形、肛管狭窄或肛管闭锁等有关[8, 59, 62]。

炎性肿瘤大约占直肠后肿瘤的5%[2]。然而，Hannon等[10]认为炎性肿瘤是最常见的直肠后肿瘤。直肠后炎性肿瘤可有不同的病理来源[68]。Uhlig和Johnson[2]描述了由于用苯酚或者矿物油硬化注射痔和隐匿憩室炎穿孔引起的这类肿块，其中1例是由于

表50.3 直肠后肿瘤的病理

	Localio等[43]	Jao等[45]	Lee and Symmonds[46]	Böhm等[1]	Lev-Chelouche等[41]	Glasgow等[50]	Pappalardo等[53]
尾肠囊肿	0	16	0	6	12	2	3
表皮样囊肿	0	15	5	5	0	5[a]	3
皮样囊肿	1	0	0	0	0	—	1
畸胎瘤	3	15	24	9	0	8	2
畸胎癌	0	3	4	0	0	1	1
直肠重复畸形	0	0	0	0	0	0	2
骶前脊膜膨出	0	2	1	0	0	0	3
脊索瘤	8	30	0	4	9	3	5
神经源性肿瘤	1	14	16	0	4	6	1
骨肿瘤	3	13	10	0	3	2	3
炎性肿瘤	0	0	0	0	0	0	3
混杂性肿瘤	2	14	10	0	14	7	7
总计	20	120	70	24	42	34	34

[a] 联合表皮样囊肿和皮样囊肿

溃疡性结肠炎行结肠次全切除术后脓肿所致。神经源性和骨性分别占直肠后肿瘤的10%和5%～10%[58]。混合性占直肠后肿瘤的10%～25%[8,58]。

恶性直肠后肿瘤

恶性直肠后肿瘤占直肠后肿瘤的一小部分。总体来说，1/3的直肠后肿瘤被确诊为恶性肿瘤[2]。Guillem等认为30%～50%的直肠后肿瘤为恶性肿瘤（表50.2）[60]。Uhlig和Johnson[2]发现在他们研究的63例直肠后肿瘤的患者中，恶性肿瘤的发病率为42%。然而，Spencer和Jackman[57]证实在他们研究的病例中恶性肿瘤占87%。平均年龄为60岁的老年人比平均年龄为30岁的年轻人更容易患恶性直肠后肿瘤[16]。Glasgow等[50]描述了直肠后肿瘤在63岁和43岁时其良恶性存在重要的偏差。来自于Jao等的报道：恶性肿瘤常见于男性，占所有恶性直肠后肿瘤的64.7%[45]。Glasgow等统计发现性别差异更明显（表50.2），86%的恶性直肠后肿瘤患者是男性。然而，Singer等[61]认为恶性瘤的发病率和性别无关。肿瘤的大小和肿瘤的良恶性无关联[10]，但是Wang等[47]记录了良恶性肿瘤的平均大小存在明显差异：恶性肿瘤的平均大小为16.5cm（5～40cm之间），良性肿瘤的平均大小为6.3cm（1.5～20cm之间）。

最常见的直肠后恶性肿瘤是脊索瘤[10,44,61]。Cody等[44]治疗的39例恶性直肠后肿瘤中大部分是脊索瘤（38%）。但是Uhlig和Johnson指出，在他们的研究中，这类肿瘤只有6例（占9.5%）。Freier等[8,42]统计脊索瘤的平均发病年龄为60～70岁，其中30岁之前被确诊的很少[8]。总体来说，脊索瘤中男性的发病率比女性高（2:1～5:1）。这和Uhlig及Johnson的报道[2]形成了对比，在他们的报道中有5例女性患者而没男性患者[10,45,48]。脊索瘤发生转移的概率高达20%[16]。当转移时，肿瘤能扩散至淋巴结、骨骼、肝、肺[1]。在Jao等[45]的统计中，17%的脊索瘤患者出现了转移；其中肺转移2例；肝转移1例；肋骨、股骨和腰椎转移1例；胸椎转移1例。

恶性囊性直肠后肿瘤十分罕见。实性肿瘤比囊性肿瘤更容易出现转移（分别为60%和10%）[23,58]。大量文献报道直肠后囊性肿瘤恶变的概率在10%～60%之间[61]。Chêne和Voitellier[24]认为恶性囊性直肠后肿瘤常出现在男性患者中。

尾肠囊肿很少出现恶变[20]。文献报道尾肠囊肿出现恶变的概率为2%[20,54]。Mathis等[54]确诊了4例恶性尾肠囊肿的女性患者，其中3例为腺癌，1例为类癌，她们的年龄在31～79岁。他们认为恶性肿瘤和年龄、临床症状、肿瘤大小没有关联[54]。在尾肠囊肿患者中类癌、腺癌、肉瘤、腺鳞癌均有报道[54,69-73]。Krivokapic等[74]报道了1例47岁尾肠囊肿合并腺鳞癌的女性患者。这个肿瘤最初是在子宫切除术后11年被发现。尾肠囊肿切除术后病理为高分化的黏液腺癌[75]。Yamaguchi等记载了1例32岁直肠癌经肛瘘侵犯尾肠囊肿的男性患者[76]。

畸胎癌在成年人中比较少见。畸胎瘤出现恶变的概率约1%～10%[2,25,29,58]。Jao等[45]报道他们的成年畸胎瘤患者中有12.5%为恶性肿瘤，儿童患者恶性肿瘤的发生率比成年人常见，但是在20岁以后开始下降[10,27,58]。成年人发生恶变与低分化的畸胎瘤密切相关。畸胎癌比良性肿瘤大，其主要是实性成分而不是囊性成分[10]。Uhlig和Johnson[2]报道了2例畸胎癌，1例为70岁女性，1例为49岁女性。前者合并有甲状腺滤泡癌，后者合并有呼吸道上皮起源的胚胎癌。这类恶性肿瘤大部分为腺癌和窦状瘤[10]。

恶性肿瘤在直肠重复畸形中很少见[30]。18%的直肠重复畸形为恶性肿瘤。这样的腺癌患者发现于在30岁以后的成年人[3]。Orr和Edwards[78]证实了一个囊性直肠重复畸形的患者为腺癌，术后8个月死亡。Yang等[37]认为表皮样囊肿恶变是囊壁的慢性炎症所致。在皮肤、肝、脑也有类似的恶性表皮样囊肿的报道[37]。脑部的表皮样囊肿恶变一般发生在良性病变被确诊后的3个月～33年（平均年龄为8.4±11.3岁）[37]。Yang等报道了1例63岁以急性尿潴留为临床表现的鳞状细胞癌性表皮样囊肿的女性患者。Thway等[25]报道了1例64岁男性皮样囊肿的患者，乳腺外Paget病引起了他的汗腺炎症。Roy等[79]描述了1例合并乳腺外Paget病的45岁男性皮样囊肿患者。

病理学

直肠后肿瘤包含多种不同的病理类型。其中囊性病变占了这类肿瘤的 40.8%[68]。而且，实性肿块和炎性肿块会发生囊变，这也增加了诊断的困难[55]。下面将讲述直肠后肿瘤的常见病理类型，包括尾肠囊肿、畸胎瘤、畸胎癌、直肠重复畸形、皮样和表皮样囊肿、骶前脑脊膜膨出、脊索瘤和神经鞘瘤。

尾肠囊肿常为多腔。来自 Hjermstad 和 Helwig[20] 的报道：一半的尾肠囊肿为单腔，但在显微镜下 81% 为多腔。这种病变由 1~2 个"母囊"和多个"子囊"组成[2]。它的上皮由鳞状上皮细胞、柱状上皮细胞和纤毛柱状上皮细胞演变而来[2,10]。Hjermstad 和 Helwig 认为鳞状上皮最常见。尽管在囊壁中发现了杂乱的平滑肌纤维，但是它不像直肠重复畸形有完整的肌层、肌间神经和浆膜[10,20]。这种病变不像皮样囊肿含有真皮组织，也不像直肠重复畸形含有肠上皮，也不像畸胎瘤起源于三胚层[61]。这些薄壁囊肿包含黄色清亮的浆液或者淡绿色的黏液[2,20,80]。虽然这些囊肿可能十分紧密的黏附于直肠后壁，但是除了医源性因素外，它和直肠没有交通[20]。Hjermstad 和 Helwig 统计：接近 50% 的囊肿和炎症（感染）有关，它好像产生了这些附属物。由于肿瘤局限在直肠后间隙，很少向直肠上、直肠两侧及直肠前扩散[20]，很少有直肠前囊肿的报道[81]。

重复畸形是一种可以出现于消化道任何部位（从食管到肛门）的发育畸形。大部分（94%）重复畸形是中空的囊状结构，也就是肠道囊肿或者肠源性囊肿[28-29]。管状重复畸形重复了或长或短的肠段，常合并尿道重复或骶骨畸形[28,64]。然而，大部分滋养重复畸形（80%）的不是管状结构，巨大的憩室起到了沟通的作用[28,31,32]。1969 年一篇文献报道了 70 例直肠重复畸形，54.3% 为管状畸形，45.7% 为囊肿畸形[29,31]。滋养型重复畸形附着于消化道的一部分，它们位于肠系膜表面，并且有同样的血供[25,29,30]。消化道重复畸形的特征是遵循了一段肠道的结构，有完整的平滑肌层，黏膜层由消化道的细胞类型组成[3,28,30,32]。然而，一些消化道重复畸形所含有的黏膜细胞并不在邻近的肠道中出现；La Quaglia 等[3,28,30,32,80] 证实 11 例直肠重复畸形中含有胃、结肠、移形、鳞状和尿道上皮细胞[28,30,32,80]。这种病变中很少能发现纤毛上皮[32]。不同类型的上皮细胞可能会共同存在于一种病变中[29]。在一些病例中可能会发现异位的胃、胰腺及尿道上皮细胞[62]。滋养型重复畸形和消化道一样由 3 层组成，即黏膜层、肌层和浆膜层[30]。很少有患者会有两种重复畸形[32]。如果邻近重复畸形的小囊肿不被发现和切除，会导致复发[29]。Alavanja 等[30] 描述了 1 例 60 岁直肠重复畸形的女性患者，病变的内层是类似黏膜的纤维组织，显微镜下证实为尿道上皮细胞、炎性的黏膜下层和骨骼肌。Monek 等[32] 治疗了 1 例 39 岁直肠重复畸形女患者，病理证实为：含有黏蛋白分泌细胞的异位柱状纤毛上皮、结缔组织和骨骼肌。与成对的后肠形成对比，孤立的直肠重复畸形和泌尿生殖畸形无关联[29]。

表皮样囊肿非常坚固，且是一种富有弹性、包膜完整的病变[82]。Ueda 等[82] 证实表皮样囊肿是一种缺乏血供病变。薄壁单室的表皮样囊肿是由一层含有透明角质蛋白的鳞状上皮组成[36,62,82]。囊液通常由水、角蛋白、胆固醇及脱落的上皮组成[36]。Sasaki 等[56] 发现了一种"干酪样物质"。虽然表皮样囊肿内也含有一层鳞状上皮，但是它还包含有毛囊、汗腺、钙化物（也就是牙蕾）等附件（图 50.3）[4,62]。这种多腔病变常含有角蛋白或皮脂液，但一部分[27,62,80] 是"混浊液"。有报道称这些病变中脂肪物质占 67%~75%，钙占 31%[62,80]。

骶前脑脊膜膨出是由于脊髓的蛛网膜和硬网膜通过一个缺损疝入骶骨腹侧所致[59]。这种单发的囊性病变内部是清亮的脑脊液[59]。脊索瘤从原始的脊索衍变而来，由胶冻样物质组成（图 50.4）[10]。这种分叶、生长缓慢的肿瘤常发生局部的浸润和破坏，很少远处转移[10,58]。尽管脊索瘤会出现在脊柱的任何部位，但骶尾部（30%~50%）是最常见的发病部位[6]。神经鞘瘤是最常见的神经源性肿瘤[23]。这种

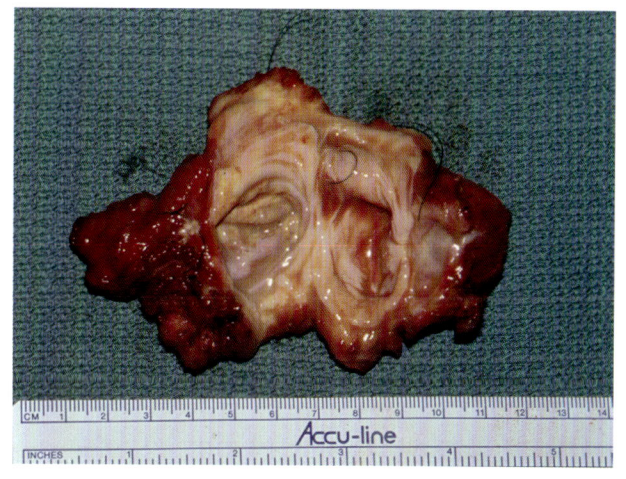

图 50.3 骶前表皮样囊肿。这个复发的囊肿是通过 Kraske 方法从一例 39 岁女性患者体内切除的

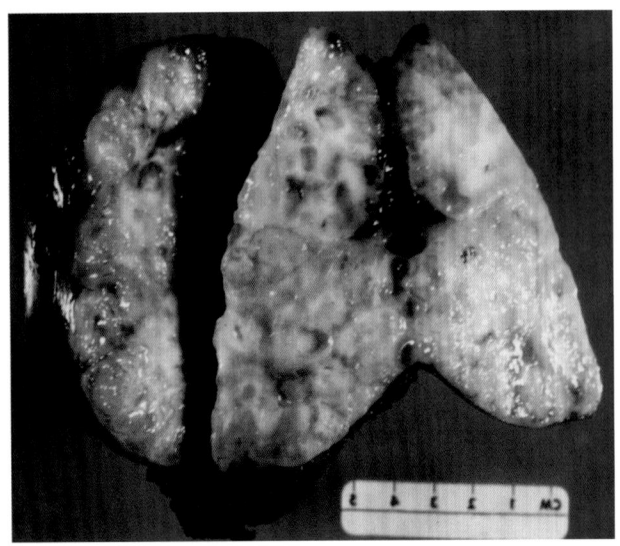

图 50.4　骶前脊索瘤。这个复发的脊索瘤是通过经骶入路从一例 35 岁男性患者体内切除的

肿瘤由成束的梭状细胞组成，表面有坚实的外膜[23]，经常发生明显的纤维化、钙化、出血和囊性变等退行性病变[23]。

症　状

大部分直肠后肿瘤无症状。Pidala[48] 报道了 14 例肿瘤患者中 57%（8 个）没有临床症状。Lev-Chelouche 等[41] 报道 26% 的患者没有临床症状。由于这些生长缓慢的病变引起的症状没有特征性，给诊断带来了困难。Singer 等[61] 报道此类疾病的症状平均持续 4.9 年才会被确诊，被诊断的时间范围在 1～11 年。同样，在 Uhlig and Johnson[2] 的文章中指出这种疾病症状的平均持续时间是 3.7 年。急性表现很少见[20]。患者的主诉通常与肿瘤的大小和位置有关[4,9,82]。症状常常与肿瘤的感染、坏死及恶性程度密切相关。Pidala 等[2,48,61,82] 发现 50% 有症状的患者是由直肠后囊肿感染所致，其他观察组也记录了这些症状[2,61,82]。侵犯周围组织也会引起相应的症状，尤其是侵犯神经[79]。侵犯神经根会引起疼痛、大小便失禁和运动感觉减退[43]。患者表现出的症状常为直肠、肛门及会阴部疼痛和坠胀；排便不畅、排便困难、排便疼痛和大便变细[27,30,43,59,61,83]。

疼痛（最常见的症状）常常为钝痛且定位不清[48,61]。来自 Hjermstad 和 Helwig[20] 的病例回顾，82% 有症状的尾肠囊肿患者表现为直肠和腰部疼痛，这些患者中有 7 例（39%）会因为排便而使疼痛加重[20]。脊索瘤除了持续的直肠疼痛外，还尤其会引起排便疼痛[10,84]。在一些患者中，直肠疼痛坐位时会加重，MacLeod 和 Purves[31] 曾报道了 1 例 39 岁的直肠重复畸形女性患者，她同时感觉到尾骨肿块。有些患者行走时会出现腰痛[61]。Localio 等[43] 报道了 18 例（90%）患者出现腰痛和骶骨疼痛，中位持续时间为 12 个月（从 2 天～8 年）。脊索瘤引起的腰痛与体位有关，坐位时会加重[45,61]。当侵犯骶神经丛时，神经性疼痛表现为腰痛、臀部疼痛以及下肢放射痛[10,61]。Chen 等[36] 认为腹痛可能由囊肿自发性破裂引起，他报道了 1 例 62 岁巨大直肠后表皮样囊肿患者，表现为右下 1/4 象限的钝痛。

有些患者回忆在确诊直肠后肿瘤之前尾骨受过外伤[2]。Cody 等[44] 的病例分析中 15% 的恶性直肠后肿瘤以及 Jao 等[45] 的病例回顾中 11% 的直肠后肿物所产生的症状都是在尾骨外伤后出现的。尽管外伤可能会使我们对之前无症状的肿瘤产生重视，但是 Sasaki 等[56] 认为外伤会直接导致表皮样囊肿和皮样囊肿等病变。Hjermstad 和 Helwig[20] 认为外伤后囊肿破裂会促进炎症反应，从而产生症状帮助诊断直肠后肿瘤。

直肠后肿瘤患者常常有肠道症状。在 Lee 和 Symmonds[46] 的研究中，31% 的女性患者有这样的症状；在 Wang 等[47] 的病例回顾中也有 44% 的患者有类似的症状。直肠角度的改变或挤压直肠管腔，或两种情况同时发生，都会引起排便习惯改变[58]。大便失禁可能是由于神经受累所导致[61]。

直肠后肿瘤有时会引起泌尿系统症状。Lee 和 Symmonds[46] 把泌尿系症状及肠道症状归咎于肿瘤的大小而不是肿瘤的病理基础。神经受累同样会导致泌尿系症状[61]。Lee 和 Symmonds 研究中的 10% 的患者以及 Wang 等[46,47] 病例回顾中的 13% 的患者都有尿潴留、尿失禁及尿急的症状。而且，尿频也与直肠后肿瘤有关[20,26,43]。Thway 等[25] 描述了 1 例 64 岁女性患者，患表皮样囊肿合并乳房外的 Paget 病，仅表现为多尿。Chen 等[36] 详细描述了患者因直肠后肿瘤而发展为尿路梗阻导致右侧肾盂和输尿管积水。同样，Yang 等[36] 报道了 1 例 64 岁女性患者，因为一个 17cm×11cm×10cm 的直肠后囊性肿瘤压迫膀胱、子宫及直肠，从而导致急性尿潴留和耻骨联合上方疼痛。

无痛性血便可能继发于直肠后肿瘤。在

Grandjean 等[20, 52]的病例回顾中，1 例患者因为直肠出血而输血，2 例患者为慢性失血。在 Wang 等[47]的研究中，4 例发育性囊肿患者有直肠出血或黏液便。大部分直肠重复畸形患者在年轻时就出现症状。1 例囊性直肠重复畸形患者因为黏膜扩张导致腹痛[30, 64]。异位黏膜会导致出血，有人报道 1 名 4 岁女孩因为异位胃黏膜在直肠巨大憩室内引发直肠溃疡而出血[28, 30]。扩大的重复畸形压迫直肠导致坏死也会引起出血[64, 78]。直肠重复畸形患者也可以出现肠梗阻，因为直肠容量大，所以肠梗阻在直肠重复畸形中出现的概率比其他部位的重复畸形中要少[3, 31]。此外，在很少一部分病例中直肠重复畸形会引发直肠脱垂[3]。La Quaglia 等[3]认为直肠重复畸形常常伴有感染。但这些患者首先表现为肛周脓肿，可能导致细菌进入无菌的直肠后肿物[3]。在手术前，1 个患有囊性病变的 39 岁女性行切开引流，放出大量的脓液；结果在切开部位形成了窦道，最后这个囊性病被确诊为直肠重复畸形[31]。直肠重复畸形合并有通向后正中线的窦道，会通过此窦道排黏液或脓性物质[3]。

直肠后肿瘤会引起妇科症状。1 名 27 岁的女性被报道有阴道口红肿和排便困难，伴有阴道后壁脱垂，开始认为和Ⅲ度直肠脱垂有关，但最后证实是由直肠后表皮样囊肿引起[35]。患者可能自诉有月经不调和性交疼痛[10, 61]。直肠后肿瘤也会导致妊娠困难。自 1996 年起，只有 15 例合并有此种并发症的妊娠病例报道[40]。在 Lovelady 和 Dockerty[4]的研究中，7.8% 的直肠后肿瘤患者（127 例）出现了产科并发症。盆腔性难产是由于分娩过程中阴道受到压迫引起[4, 27]。小的直肠后肿瘤患者可以顺产[59]。Uhlig 和 Johnson[2]描述了 3 例合并有小的直肠后肿瘤的女性患者，顺产后因为感染而出现了症状；大的直肠后肿瘤患者通常需要剖宫产。Krivokapic 等[59]描述了 1 例 37 岁女性患者因为骶前脑脊膜膨出和肠囊肿进行了剖宫产，这些病变是在产前检查时发现的。但是，有时大的直肠后肿瘤会影响剖宫产手术。Sobrado 等[59]报道了 1 例合并有巨大骶前肿瘤的 25 岁女性患者因为胎盘剥离导致出血而紧急行剖宫产术，最终胎儿死亡。在怀孕期间可以试图切除肿瘤，1 例患者因为星形胶质细胞瘤在怀孕 4 个月时行肿瘤切除[2, 4]。在怀孕晚期，盆腔血流速度的增加会加大肿瘤切除的风险[85]。

骶前脑脊膜膨出患者有 1/3 会出现头痛[59]。这种头痛伴有恶心，会由于咳嗽、拉伸、排便、下蹲及性交而引发[45, 59]。囊肿的颈部被压迫后脑脊液不能进入脑脊膜膨出，这导致了颅内压的升高[59]。当颅内压升高到一定水平后会刺激痛觉感受器引发头痛。脑膜炎的出现可能与直肠后肿瘤有关。反复发作的脑膜炎常常提示骶前脑脊膜膨出[9, 58]。一个自发的微小穿孔可能会引起脑膜炎，死亡率可达 30%[59]。由于活检造成的医源性穿孔也会导致脑膜炎，这种患者的死亡率几乎为 100%[59]。在骶前脑脊膜膨出患者中直肠鞘瘘是脑膜炎的一个病因，1 例 48 岁男性脑膜炎患者就归因于粪石性穿孔[86-87]。也有表皮样囊肿破裂进入蛛网膜下腔而引发脑膜炎的报道[10]。

直肠后肿瘤很容易和其他疾病混淆。Singer 等[61]报道，他们的 7 例患者在诊断为直肠后肿瘤前表现为其他疾病，如直肠周围脓肿、外伤性、精神性及产后疼痛、藏毛窦、骶前脓肿和肛瘘。他们的患者在做出正确诊断前平均经历 4.7 个诊断和治疗流程。反复发作的肛周脓肿或肛瘘均提示有可能患直肠后肿瘤[9]。1 例 39 岁患者开始表现为慢性的腹膜后脓肿，合并有左侧输尿管重复畸形，最后诊断为直肠重复畸形[32]。Localio 等[43]遇到过 1 例直肠后肿瘤感染却被诊断为盆腔脓肿的患者。反复地切开引流会引起炎性反应，这将给直肠后肿瘤的切除带来困难[10]。尾骨远端的藏毛窦可能是直肠后肿瘤的一个信号[10]。此外，反复发作和不能治愈的藏毛窦可能提示潜在的直肠后肿瘤。Satyadas 等[88]报道了 1 例和尾肠囊肿密切相关的藏毛窦，反复发作，在臀沟皮肤有 2 处不规则小孔。内科医师通过 B 超检查可能会把直肠后囊性肿瘤误认为卵巢囊肿或者其他腹腔内的病变，如果不进行腹腔镜检查或者开腹手术很容易做出错误的诊断[89-91]。同样，Localio 等报道了 1 例肿瘤破裂的患者仅表现为反复的发热和不适。

恶性直肠后肿瘤没有特征性的临床表现[10]。这些肿瘤都是被偶然发现的。在 Cody 等[44]的研究中，有 2 例无症状的恶性直肠后肿瘤（5%）是在常规检查后确诊。大部分恶性肿瘤患者有临床症状。Jao 等[45]认为有症状的直肠后病变是恶性肿瘤的可能性更大。Glasgow 等[50]也有同样的发现，他们认为良性肿瘤无症状的患者比恶性肿瘤无症状的患者多（良恶性肿瘤无症状的百分比分别为 14% 和 56%；$P = 0.09$）。尽管良性肿瘤也会引起同样的症状，但是恶性肿瘤常有先兆，如下肢感觉异常或者减弱[27]。Cody 等报道了 37 例恶性肿瘤患者中 95% 的患者有临床症状。恶性肿瘤常常表现为疼痛，包括骶尾部疼痛、臀部疼痛、后背部疼痛、直肠疼痛及神经痛。在 Cody 等的研究中：67% 有症状的患者有这些表现[36,44]。Glasgow 等的病例回顾中，恶性肿瘤常常表现为骶尾部疼痛（83%）。他们认为只有坐骨神经痛和骨盆疼痛与恶性肿瘤有密切的关系（$P=0.02$）。Jao 等统计，有 88% 的恶性肿瘤患者有疼痛症状，相反良性肿瘤只有 39%。Localio 等[43]报道，12 例恶性肿瘤中有 50% 的患者有神经根疼痛，他们认为大小便失禁与恶性肿瘤有关：2 例大小便失禁的患者被确诊为高分化的恶性肿瘤[9]。在 Cody 等[44]的报道中很少有肠道和膀胱并发症的表现。Wang 等[47]统计发现，良恶性肿瘤确诊的时间为 6.1~18.8 个月，两者之间没有统计学差异（$P=0.148$）。

感 染

直肠后囊性病变因为合并感染而被频繁报道。感染可首发或者继发出现[10]。Abel 等[61,85]认为 1/3 的直肠后囊性肿瘤都会继发感染。在 Spencer 和 Jackman[44,57]的研究中，手术的患者中有 31.6% 发现肿瘤合并有感染。Dahan 等[62]报道发育性囊肿（尤其是表皮样囊肿和肠囊肿）的感染率为 30%~50%。Verazin 等[92]认为直肠后肿瘤出现感染与直肠后间隙血运差、肿瘤紧邻直肠以及其对外伤和活检比较敏感有关。他们进一步证实：梭状芽孢杆菌在坏死及高分化的肿瘤中比较常见[92]。患者由于感染会出现间歇热、盗汗或者骨盆疼痛[61,62,85]。

Currarino 综合征

直肠后肿瘤的遗传基础是由 Currarino 在 1981 年首次以综合征的形式描述[93]。这种常染色体显性基因突变被证实为染色体 7q36 的 HLXB9 基因[94-95]。50% 的病例有家族性，其他的都是散发出现[93-94]。这种综合征的胚胎学基础不太清楚。在 Currarino 建立的"脊索裂"模型的胚胎早期，内外胚层的融合会引起这种综合征的特征性表现[93,94,96]。这种常染色体显性基因突变包括直肠后肿瘤、直肠肛门畸形（直肠肛门狭窄和低位肛门闭锁）和骶骨发育畸形[62]。包括骶前脑脊膜膨出、肠囊肿、尾肠囊肿、皮样囊肿以及畸胎瘤在内的大量直肠后肿瘤都涉及这种综合征[25,62]。这种综合征中最常见的直肠后肿瘤是骶前脑膜膨出和畸胎瘤[96]。也可能有多种直肠后肿瘤共同存在[62]。有报道：3 名 2 岁的儿童和 4 名成年人出现肿瘤的恶变，包括：5 例畸胎瘤、1 例平滑肌肉瘤和 1 例神经内分泌肿瘤[94]。典型的直肠后肿瘤、直肠肛门畸形和骶骨发育畸形三联征很少同时出现[93]。截止到 1984 年，只有 40 例典型的 Currarino 三联征患者被报道[93]。在 80% 的病例中，完整的 Currarino 三联征患者到 10 岁时才被诊断；那些不具备完整的 Currarino 三联征患者通常到成年时才被发现[96]。这种综合征通常都有骶骨畸形[97]，也可以合并有肾、输尿管、卵巢、子宫、输卵管的畸形[25,62]。在 Crétolle 等[94]的病例回顾中有 17 例患者（58.6%）被发现有脊髓栓系。尽管 33% 的患者无症状[24,94,98]，但最常见的症状还是便秘[62]。患者可能会出现肠梗阻、肛周脓肿和脑膜炎[95]。家庭成员可以通过骶骨 X 片和遗传咨询来进行筛查[93]。

诊 断

直肠后肿瘤正确诊断的前提是开始时就怀疑这个病变存在。这些肿瘤的鉴别首先依赖于体格检查。主要的影像学检查包括：ERUS、CT 和 MRI。如果临床需要，可以使用内镜、钡灌肠、血管造影及脊髓造影等其他检查。

尾小凹代表了直肠后囊性病变和肛周皮肤有关联。尾小凹和囊肿间的通路不恒定[2]。锥形的外口出现在臀沟处，越过肛周皮肤可能在末端肛管内[3-4]。尾小凹和肛瘘的区别在于它在齿状线没有内口[23]。然而，Grandjean 等[52]报道了 1 例尾小凹符合肛瘘表现，他们治疗了 2 例同时存在尾小凹和括约肌间瘘的患者。20% 囊性直肠重复畸形患者会出现尾小凹[29]。在一项有 11 例儿童患者的研究中，La Quaglia 等[52]证实有 5 例患者（45%）有小凹征。2%~34% 的先天性病变（如尾肠囊肿和表皮样囊肿）可出现尾小凹症状[1,48,61]。在 Uhlig 和 Johnson[2,50]的研究中，34.6% 的直肠后囊肿发现有尾小凹，但是在 Glasgow 等[50]的研究中只有 5.8%。Singer 等[2,50]描述了 1 例 18 岁女性患者，她有一个高分化上皮覆盖的外口通向直肠后囊肿（尾肠囊肿），伴有血水或脓液溢出。尾小凹的起源不太清楚。Hjermstad

和 Helwig[20] 认为尾小凹是由于胎儿发育过程中肛周皮肤被终丝牵引所致。

在成年人中很少遇到外部肿块。在新生儿中这些肿块（通常为畸胎瘤）会向盆腔内延伸[6, 9]。Coco 等[27] 描述了 1 例 40 岁女性患者，自幼就发现盆腔肿块，伴有骨盆疼痛和右臀肿物，最后确诊为畸胎瘤。他们还描述了 1 例 50 岁男性患者，他在有临床表现之前已经发现盆腔肿块 25 年，伴有右臀部明显的肿物，最后确诊为皮样囊肿。类似的报道还有 1 例 39 岁直肠重复畸形女患者表现为左臀部肿物[32]。在体格检查中可能发现尾骨畸形。Uhlig 和 Johnson[2] 报道了 6 例（9.5%）直肠后肿瘤合并尾骨畸形的患者。

大部分直肠后病变都能通过直肠指诊发现。针对无症状的患者，这些评估经常是在常规体格检查和产前检查期间进行的[80]。Jao 等[45] 指出 97% 的直肠后肿瘤患者是通过直肠指诊发现。然而，Glasgow 等[50] 统计发现：只有 35% 的直肠后肿瘤能通过直肠指诊触及。示指一般能在中线（偶尔在中线的左边或右边）区分是固定的肿物还是骶前的饱满[10]。在 Bellotti 等[99] 的研究中，有 3 例直肠后肿瘤位于骶前间隙的后外侧。因为大部分肿瘤（尤其是囊性病变）是柔软、可压缩的，所以常常被忽视。不同的研究者[2, 27, 61] 均强调指诊可以了解直肠后空间。1 例表皮样囊肿[68, 82] 在直肠指诊时表现为坚硬、有弹性、无痛的肿块。1 例骶前脑脊膜膨出表现为柔软的、有波动感的肿块[59]。当患者完成 Valsalva 动作时，骶前脑脊膜膨出在直肠指诊过程中会增大[45]。直肠后间隙饱满、固定的肿块常意味着它是感染的囊肿[10]。由于肿瘤的存在，直肠及肛门的移位和管腔的狭窄会比较明显[30, 65]。骶神经的侵犯表现为肛门扩张和会阴部感觉减退[61]。瘘管在检查时会被发现：在 Mathis 等[54] 的研究中有 4 例直肠后肿瘤患者在直肠指诊时发现直肠瘘。直肠指诊未必能区分出肿瘤的良恶性。Localio 等[43] 发现原发的恶性肿瘤的特征是比较固定，但是有 5 例良性肿瘤也符合这种表现。Yang 等[37] 描述了 1 例在直肠指诊时"橡胶感"的直肠后肿瘤，最后确诊为含有鳞状细胞癌的表皮样囊肿。在 Localio 等的研究中 8 例肿瘤患者有 2 例为分叶状肿瘤，但脊索瘤一般表现为光滑、无痛、坚韧的肿块[10, 43, 45]。相反，Lev-Chelouche 等[41] 指出他的脊索瘤患者为固定于尾骨的实性肿块。当肿瘤侵犯尾骨时，尾骨在直肠触诊期间比较柔和[41]。

特殊的肿瘤标记物能提高一些直肠后肿瘤的诊断。Coco 等[27] 报道了 1 例 CA125 高达 109ng/mL 的畸胎瘤患者，他的 CA15-3、CA19-9、AFP、HCT 水平在正常范围。畸胎瘤中癌胚抗原和甲胎蛋白升高的患者分别占 82% 和 53%[45]。Chêne 和 Voitellier[24] 认为癌胚抗原单独升高可能提示为表皮样囊肿。一例 CA-125 升高至 103.4 U/mL（正常 <35 U/mL）的 62 岁女性患者开始考虑为卵巢癌，最终被确诊为表皮样囊肿[36]。一例直肠后尾肠囊肿患者的 CA19-9 升高，术后 1 个月时降至正常水平[100]。当某一肿瘤标记物很高时可能提示为恶性肿瘤。Rogers 等[71] 描述了 1 例 54 岁恶性肿瘤复发的女性患者，起初表现为 CEA 升高的良性囊肿。血清甲胎蛋白升高与畸胎癌有关[24, 45]。这些肿瘤标记物对术后患者复发的评估价值不确定。1 例含有低分化腺癌的尾肠囊肿复发患者经过手术及放疗后，CEA 和 CA19-9 较治疗前升高（其治疗前 CEA 和 CA19-9 就明显升高）。

纤维内镜和硬式直肠镜能除外直肠黏膜病变。这些检查能显示正常的直肠黏膜，可能会发现直肠后壁压迹[68]。Palanivelu 等[65] 发现巨大表皮样囊肿患者在行乙状结肠镜检查时会有外在的压迫。Alavanja 等[30] 报道了 1 例直肠后病变在行结肠镜时表现为"凸出的肿块"，最终被确诊为直肠重复畸形。Abel 等[85] 认为黏膜的点状红斑和直肠后肿瘤引起的直肠后壁饱满有关。20% 的直肠重复畸形和直肠有交通，内镜检查可能发现这种交通。直肠后肿瘤侵犯直肠时内镜检查也不太明显[1]。Glasgow 等[50] 发现单独直肠镜检查诊断直肠后肿瘤的敏感率为 52%。

普通的骨盆 X 片对直肠后肿瘤的评估价值有限。在 Grandjean 等的研究中[52] 85% 的普通腹部 X 片都是正常的。Wolpert 等[9] 认为有价值的表现（甚至是骶骨畸形）经常被重叠的肠管及周围的软组织掩盖。X 片能显示骶尾骨的破坏、移位、软组织肿块或者钙化灶[9, 61]。骶前脑脊膜膨出表现为病理性半月征、尾骨缺失，有 50% 的病例这两种征象共存；这个发现和肿瘤引起的异常骨发育形成的肿块有关[59, 62]。类似的骶骨畸形在尾肠囊肿中很少见。Hjermstad 和 Helwig[10, 20] 在他们尾肠囊肿的患者中遇到了 4 例脊柱裂、1 例尾骨骨折、1 例前屈尾骨、1 例骶骨畸形伴有尾骨缺失；他们认为骶尾部畸形是由肛后肠缺陷所导致[10]。尽管皮样囊肿也可以因为齿胚显示钙化，但是钙化灶首先是在成熟的畸胎瘤中发现的[27]。尾肠囊肿里的钙化可能提示为恶性肿瘤[20]。骶骨破坏和恶性肿瘤密切相关[9,45]。Localio 等[43]证实 11 例（92%）恶性肿瘤有骶骨破坏，尤其是全部 8 例脊索瘤；良性肿瘤均没有骶骨破坏。在 Jao 等[45]的经历中，79% 有骶骨破坏的肿瘤为恶性肿瘤；有 9 例良性肿瘤也有类似的骨破坏，他们把这种情况归咎于巨大的肿块压迫所致。脊索瘤 X 片表现为骨膨胀、骨小梁形成、骨质疏松、外周钙化和"幽灵外表"[1,10,45,84]，但是在 Jao 等的研究病例中有 1/3 没有这些表现。骶骨 X 片可作为鉴别诊断的一种方法，鉴别骨样骨瘤、骨囊肿和骨肉瘤[23]。

在 CT 及 MRI 还没有引进之前，直肠后肿瘤靠钡灌肠来诊断。他能显示黏膜外直肠后肿块对直肠的挤压[43,82]。从侧面观直肠后空间比正面尺寸宽2cm[10,62,83]。Hannon 等[10]报道钡剂成功识别了 6 例直肠后病变中的 4 例。然而，小的或低位直肠后病变可能会在这种检查中被漏诊[10]。通过尾小凹的窦道造影能够进一步识别囊性直肠后病变的解剖[61-62]。

已经主张使用直肠内超声来评价直肠后肿瘤。Glasgow 等[50]认为联合直肠镜检查，直肠内超声对直肠后肿瘤诊断的敏感度为 100%。这种技术能够很好地区分囊实性肿瘤，并且能够识别直肠后病变的层次关系（图 50.5）[23,50]。它同样能发现淋巴结的情况[50]。良性囊肿内部没有回声[10]。表皮样囊肿为不均匀的低回声和后方极小的增强[36,68]。

评估直肠后肿瘤最好的技术是盆腔 CT 和盆腔MRI。Glasgow 等[50]认为这两种技术对直肠后肿块的诊断敏感率为 100%。这些影像学技术能够区分肿瘤的囊实性[61]。这两种检查在测量肿瘤大小方面有很高的敏感性和特异性，这对外科手术方案的设计很重要[27]。此外，这些影像学检查能够准确地显示邻近组织是否受到肿瘤的侵犯[61]。Pappalardo 等[53]遇到了 1 例畸胎瘤患者，骶前的侵犯在外科手术前的 CT 或 MRI 上没有任何表现；而且，这两种检查对病理学诊断都不能做出预判[27]。MRI 比 CT 对直肠后肿瘤类别的诊断正确率高（28% vs 18%）[50]。Pappalardo 等也发现 MRI 在识别肿瘤（直肠后的、骶前的、直肠的）的起源和评价邻近器官是否受到侵犯比 CT 更可靠。

CT 在直肠后肿瘤的诊断中扮演重要的角色（图 50.6 和图 50.7）。这些肿瘤可能在 CT 检查其他病

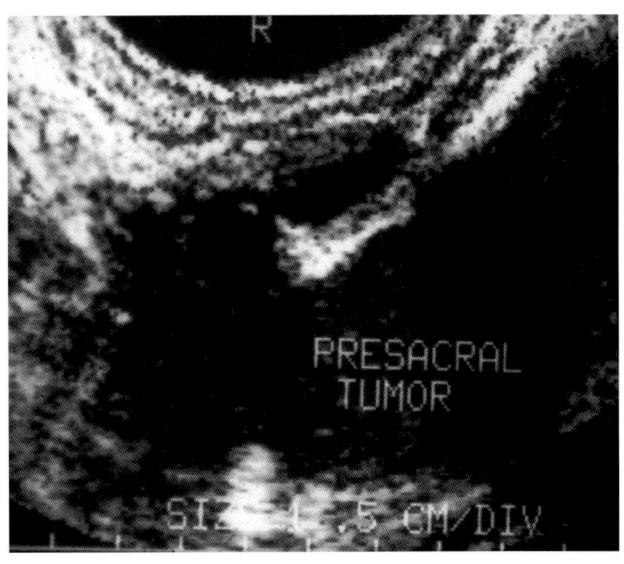

图 50.5 一个骶前肿物的直肠内超声。直肠内超声证实这是一个囊性肿瘤，最终结果是一个皮样囊肿

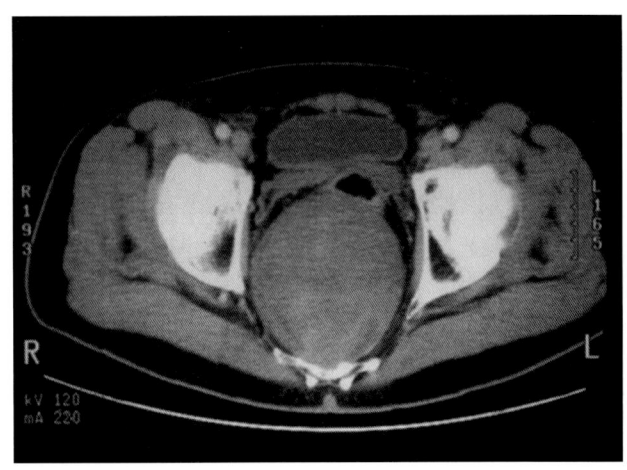

图 50.6 骶前肿物的轴向 CT 图像

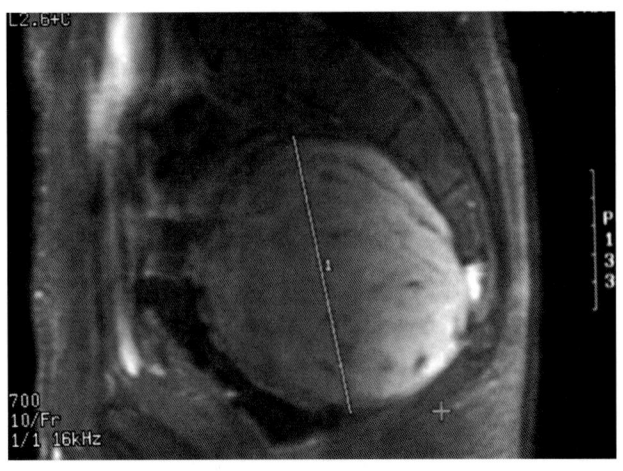

图 50.7 骶前肿物的 CT 矢状位重建图像

变而被无意发现的，就有这样 1 例 67 岁表皮样囊肿女性患者[30, 55]。在 Singer 等的研究中，盆腔 CT 联合体格检查正确诊断出了所有的直肠后囊肿[61]。CT 能够显示肿瘤的大小、区分邻近器官，这对治疗方案有很大帮助。有 1 例 20cm×15cm×12cm 多房的直肠后表皮样囊肿在 CT 上被误认为右侧卵巢恶性肿瘤，因此直肠后肿瘤应该与巨大的腹部肿瘤进行鉴别[36]。Localio 等[43] 认为直肠后肿瘤的骨转移在 CT 上可能会被误判。表皮样囊肿在 CT 上表现为薄壁、水样密度；由于角蛋白的沉积一般密度均匀，偶尔密度不均匀[37, 68]。像表皮样囊肿一样，皮样囊肿也表现为薄壁、低密度、不强化，而且常常为多房[83]。皮样囊肿的特征为：一般囊性肿块中有脂肪密度（衰减少）颗粒或钙化灶，或者两者同时存在[25, 80, 83]。瘤体内脂肪的发现能够确切的区分皮样囊肿和尾肠囊肿[80]。Yang 等[37] 报道了 1 例含有鳞状细胞癌的表皮样囊肿，他认为恶性囊性肿瘤的特征为：灶状的和不规则的囊壁增厚。在 1 例反复溢液的 18 岁女性窦道患者，通过尾小凹的窦道造影 CT 检查更好地描绘出囊性病变的相应轮廓[61]。

直肠后肿瘤在 MRI 上有特殊的形态，因此 MRI 比 CT 更有优势。与 CT 相比，MRI 在多个平面上提高了软组织的分辨率，尤其能更好地显示骶前筋膜是否受侵犯[9, 23, 58]。MRI 在脊髓成像方面更有优势，同时能够识别像蛛网膜囊肿、脊柱闭合不全这样的畸形[9]。表皮样囊肿在 T1 加权表现为不均匀的低信号，而在 T2 加权表现为高信号[37, 68]。储存在表皮样囊肿里的角蛋白在 T2 加权表现为多发细小的低信号[37, 68]。皮样囊肿表现为薄壁、内部无分隔，由于含有脂肪成分在 T2 加权为高信号[80, 83]。化学位移成像用来显示皮样囊肿里的脂肪[80]。Nishie 等[80] 认为皮样囊肿由于其内含有的角蛋白成分能在弥散 MRI 中显影而最终被确诊。畸胎瘤是一种不均质肿瘤，它的囊实成分比例不恒定[62]。肿瘤含有不规则或增厚的边缘被认为是恶性肿瘤，尽管 1 例复发的良性肿瘤有同样的特征[16, 62]。Yang 等[37] 描述了 1 例含有不规则软组织肿块（鳞状细胞癌）的囊性病变在 T1 和 T2 加权均为低信号，但是注射钆喷酸葡胺后有不同的强化。脊索瘤的特征是注射钆后，其边缘出现模糊的强化、瘤内有钙化灶、T2 加权为高信号[16, 102]。这些恶性肿瘤在 MRI 上有多种表现，在 T1 加权上与骨骼肌的信号相等[84]。

在一些直肠后肿瘤中，脊髓造影常常被用来评估中枢神经是否受侵犯。如果 MRI 或 CT 不能识别可疑的骶前脑脊膜膨出的颈部，那么可以行脊髓造影得到这个结果。这种技术可以显示不透明的对比剂从尾囊转移至骶前囊肿[45]。脊髓造影同样对评价骨侵犯有很大帮助。Cody 等[44] 建议用脊髓造影来帮助诊断侵犯骶骨的巨大肿瘤以及神经根性疼痛。

血管造影在直肠后肿瘤的诊断中很少使用。在 Localio 等[43] 的研究中，通过髂内血管造影，1 例含有血管外皮细胞瘤的血运丰富的肿瘤显影。1981 年，Cody 等推荐血管造影作为剖腹手术计划的一部分，尽管这一点没有成为公认或被推荐的指南。

活检的作用

活检在直肠后肿块的作用存在争议。由于骶骨的屏障作用，接近这些直肠后病变很困难[9]。术前活检有不同的方法，包括经直肠、经骶骨背侧、经骶骨旁、经尾骨前和经臀肌的入路（经过较大的坐骨孔）[9, 103]。Rapport 和 Ferguson[103] 描述了经骶骨背侧入路的活检方法，用螺旋钻在骶骨上钻孔，经过此孔对直肠后肿块取活检。Localio 等[43] 推荐切取活检。活检可以经腹部进行，其中通过剖腹手术或经 CT 引导活检可以二选一[103]。Ghosh 等[23] 推荐经腹部活检，此方法适用于膀胱上方、膀胱前方和膀胱侧方的肿瘤。在大部分病例中，CT 矢状位引导能够通过适当的途径到达肿瘤[9]。Singer 等[61] 推荐 CT 引导下的骶骨前入路。低位直肠后肿瘤通过直肠腔内超声引导可以经直肠取活检[9, 103]。一些活检的方法，细针在到达肿瘤前需要通过一层脂肪组织，在肥胖患者中会阻碍标本的收集[9]。细针穿刺活检很少能提供有用的标本[23]。Alavanja 等[30] 经直肠细针穿刺活检从在 1 例直肠重复畸形患者中获取了非诊断性组织，它包含有坏死的和变形的细胞碎片。术前活检增加了肛门尾骨韧带、交感神经节或坐骨神经损伤的风险，这将导致神经痛或活检后疼痛[9]。骶正中动脉或臀部血管损伤会导致大出血[90]。Ghosh 等指出经腹部活检有损伤肠管的风险[22]。在 Cody 等的研究中，有 39 例恶性肿瘤在术前进行了经骶骨或经腹的开放活检以及经骶骨或经直肠的细针活检，没有任何并发症[44]。

活检会增加直肠后无菌肿瘤的感染风险。在 Smith 等[49] 的研究中，有 23% 的病例行术前活检后导致肿瘤感染。尤其是经直肠活检细菌可能会进入无菌的囊性病变[9, 26]。Verazin 等报道了 1 例 55 岁直肠后肿块男性患者，肿块为侵犯了髂血管和直肠的非骨性 Ewing 肉瘤，经直肠细针活检后患者出现了感染性休克，最终死于产气梭状芽孢杆菌和大肠杆菌引起的感染。研究者认为操作前预防使用抗生素会阻止这种结果的发生，尤其是经直肠活检[92]。他们进一步申明：他们的患者如果术前证实为坏死性肿瘤均避免经直肠活检。Kraft[29] 描述了 1 例 34 岁直肠重复畸形女性患者，通过肛门后开放切口取活检，导致了需切开引流的感染；这个患者随后反复出现了经肛门后两个窦道流脓的症状。Jao 等报道了 2 例术前活检后直肠脓肿和 1 例术前活检后粪瘘[45]，但是在 Glasgow 等研究的 12 例术前活检的病例无任何并发症[50]。骶前脑脊膜膨出是活检的禁忌证，因为活检后脑膜炎和死亡的风险很高，几乎是 100% 的死亡率[9, 45, 59, 61]。

直肠后肿瘤的活检也会增加细针穿刺管腔内种植的风险[26, 61]。术前进行活检的肿瘤在手术切除时需连同活检管腔，一并完整切除；尤其是恶性肿瘤。脊索瘤的术前活检会增加局部复发的风险[16, 45]。Jao 等发现 9 例术前经直肠或经骶前活检的脊索瘤患者，虽然进行了有效的"外科切除"，但是仍有 6 例（67%）局部复发或远处转移。与此相比，7 例没有进行活检的患者中 6（85.7%）例出现了复发或远处转移。Bergh 等提出术前活检能够确诊脊索瘤[102]。

术前活检仅仅在特殊的情况下可取。大部分研究者认为术前活检对不能手术的肿瘤患者或术后很差的患者的放化疗有重要意义[9]。如果怀疑术前放化疗对肿瘤有效果，活检也是可以接受的，如 Ewing 肉瘤、硬纤维瘤、成骨细胞肉瘤、神经纤维瘤[8]。活检在先前其他部位有恶性肿瘤的患者中可以用来排除直肠后恶性肿瘤[6]。Guillem 等[60] 强调活检由于存在抽样误差，阴性时不能完全排除恶性肿瘤。与经直肠活检相比 Glasgow 等降低了经骶骨活检感染的风险[50]。尽量避免经腹膜、腹膜后及阴道入路的活检方法[8]。一个可切除的直肠后肿瘤（尤其是囊性病变）不应该活检[8, 61]。Ueda 等认为最好的活检是完整地去除肿瘤或者至少术中冰冻[82]。

治 疗

手术切除是大多数直肠后肿瘤的最佳治疗，甚至对于无症状的、怀疑是良性的肿瘤也推荐进行手术切除。这是因为即使通过高级的影像学检查及组织活检都很难达到充分的术前诊断，可能无法发现恶变的肿瘤[45, 82]，而且良性病变也可能会发生恶变[45, 82]。直肠后囊性肿瘤容易发生感染，导致手术切除变得很困难，会增加发生术后并发症和肿瘤复发的风险[45, 58, 82]。对于骶前脑脊膜膨出患者，如果不予治疗，死亡率高达 30%，但这个数据可能是错误的，因为只包括得到诊疗的患者[45, 67]。与大多数研究者[44, 66, 104] 不同，Ashley 和 Wright[46, 66, 104] 建议只有当影像学提示肿瘤体积逐渐增大，或是症状逐渐明显时才需行手术治疗，除了处于育龄期的女性患者。对于怀孕的女性，肿瘤可能会引起阴道梗阻，可能引起致命性难产，因此我们应切除所有的直肠后肿瘤[27]。肿瘤还可能会发生瘤内出血[60]。尤其对于直肠重复畸形的患者，异位的胃黏膜可能会导致出血[31]。只有对于淋巴瘤和直肠后转移肿瘤，才推荐使用化学治疗联合或不联合放射治疗，而不首选手术治疗[41]。

术前计划是一个成功的直肠后肿瘤切除术的开始。应通过各种影像学检查来明确肿瘤的范围（肿瘤的大小、上下界限、毗邻及侵犯的器官），从而制定最好的手术路径[9, 10, 60]。Woodfield 等[16] 指出 4 项有助于术前计划的肿瘤特征，包括肿瘤与骶椎的位置关系、肿瘤的大小、形态学表现及是否侵犯周围结构，如骶骨、骨盆侧壁、盆腔脏器等。Pappalardo 等的综述指出在 94.1% 的病例中，术前影像学检查指导了手术的选择[53]。肿瘤是原发还是复发也影响手术方式的选择[9]。当肿瘤较大并侵犯骶骨或膀胱时，可能需要更多外科专家的参与，包括骨科医师、神经外科医师、泌尿外科医师和整形外科医师[9]。尽管我们已经制定了手术计划，但我们应考虑到有联合切除骶骨和尾骨的可能[27]。

我们应该考虑到将直肠后肿瘤与直肠分离可能会很困难，所以术前我们应做好充分的肠道准备，以防发生直肠损伤或意料之外的直肠切除[9, 60, 61, 105]。囊性病变尤其会引起明显的异物反应，通常会发生感染或囊肿破裂，可能是自发性或是医源性，这造成手术更困难[36]。一部分结肠壁可能需要随着囊肿一并切除[7]。此外，直肠壁的肌肉可能与肛提肌无法区分，导致医院性损伤[58]。直肠损伤大部分可以修复，而不需行直肠切除术。Pidala 等[48] 缝合了由于分离囊肿导致的直肠撕裂，并没有发生后遗症。在直肠后壁固有肌层的会聚处完全切除直肠重复畸形，会导致直肠缺陷[64]。MacLeod 和 Purves[31] 在通过后入路切除囊性直肠重复畸形后，将直肠摺叠，在直肠后间隙留出一个引流。但是完全直肠切除术对于完全切除肿瘤有时也很必要，尤其是对于恶性直肠后肿瘤的患者[61]。在 Glasgow 等的研究中，34 例患者里共有 5 例行直肠切除术[50]。恶性直肠重复畸形应行完全直肠切除术，因为病变和直肠共用一段肠壁[32]。在对良性病变或复发率低的恶性肿瘤进行全直肠切除术后，我们应使用或不使用转流性肠造口来重建直肠的连续性[8]。Lev-Chelouche 等在 3 例脊索瘤的患者中进行了直肠后壁的部分切除，并行一期缝合和转流性结肠造瘘[41]。损伤直肠会增加发生术后肠瘘的风险[58]。对于术中可能损伤直肠或可能行直肠切除术的患者，推荐术前进行吻合口标记和告知患者[1]。在 Böhm 等的病例中，有 3 例患者因为直肠损伤进行了临时性结肠造口术[1]。Hassan 和 Wietfeldt[7] 进一步建议对于行骶骨切除而分离两侧 S_3 神经根的患者，应行乙状结肠造口术，这是因为这些患者可能会发生大便失禁。

手术过程中可能会发生严重的出血，尤其是对于大的直肠后肿瘤。严重出血的危险因素包括术前放疗、血管瘤或合并骶骨切除[8]。而且黏附于骶前筋膜的肿瘤尤其倾向于发生大量出血，由于可能损伤骶前静脉丛[23]。在 Lee 和 Symmonds[46] 的综述中，患者有 7% 需要输血，输血量从 1～17 单位浓缩红细胞。提前分离骶中血管和髂内血管可能会减少出血的程度[8]，McCune[55] 建议这样的结扎，还能预防肿瘤细胞的扩散。Hassan 和 Wietfeldt[7] 还指出保护骶前动脉前支能预防会阴部坏死。术前的血管造影和肿瘤血管栓塞对富血运肿瘤的切除有帮助。Dozois 等[106] 为了减少一个 13cm×15cm 的直肠后脂肪瘤样血管外皮细胞瘤的术中出血，对其供应动脉进行了弹簧圈栓塞（髂前动脉前支的分支和臀下动脉）；两天后，动脉造影提示肿瘤的动脉灌注减少了 90%～95%。他们指出术前血管栓塞可能会引起周围同样接受髂内动脉供应的器官缺血，这限制了它的使用[106]。尽管术前进行了栓塞，术中出血也达到了 3900ml，主要由于肿瘤上覆的静脉出血[106]。同样，Yang 等[107] 术前对 30 例骶脊索瘤患者进行肿瘤主要供应血管的栓塞，使术中平均出血量为 1200ml，术后平均需要输血 1080ml，术后没有发生盆腔坏死的患者。Yang 等指出术前经导管动脉栓塞术能使完全切除脊索瘤成为可能，此手术的出血量从 2000～24 200ml，若不进行动脉栓塞，我们只能采取效果略差但出血较少的局部切除术。

术中应能进行冰冻切片检查。若术中意外发现肿瘤恶变，可能会改变手术方式，需要进行广泛的完全切除术或变为经腹、骶入路进行手术[9]。切除直肠后肿瘤时有损伤输尿管的风险，Glasgow 等的一例患者就因术中横断输尿管而变得复杂[50]。对于那些肿瘤较大或经过术前放疗的患者，放置输尿管支架可能对预防输尿管损伤有帮助[8]。在骶骨切除术前，可以游离并保护输尿管[8]。如果肿瘤导致输尿管梗阻从而引发肾盂积水，应经皮放置肾造瘘管来缓解泌尿系统梗阻[36]。不管何种手术方式都应在直肠后间隙放置闭式引流[43, 60, 61]。Guillem 等[60] 推荐，尤其在损伤直肠或术中不慎损伤肿瘤后，应采用骶前引流和抗生素治疗。

根治性切除的最佳机会是在初次手术时，良性肿瘤比恶性肿瘤更容易达到完整切除。LevChelouche 等[41] 报道的良性肿瘤完整切除率达到 100%，而恶性肿瘤只有 71%。如果切除后的良性肿瘤包膜完整，那么就认为是完整切除[16]。Palanivelu 等[65] 警告若原位保留一部分囊肿壁，可能会提高肿瘤的复发率。完全切除恶性肿瘤并达到切缘阴性要优于将瘤体切除得支离破碎，这很容易残留病变[16, 44]。局灶切除只适用于组织面扭曲的患者，为了保证手术安全和缓解患者症状，而不为了达到肿瘤学上的根治[46, 106]。对于恶性肿瘤的完整切除，应包括预先的活检和引流部位[8]。不管是良性还是恶性肿瘤，切除不完全都会导致术后肿瘤的复发[9]。Sciubba 等[84] 指出，是否彻底切除肿瘤是决定无病生存率的首要因素。经后入路对肿瘤多次复发的反复治疗会增加大便失禁的风险[9]。

直肠后肿瘤的主要手术方式会在下面讨论，包括前入路（腹部）、腹骶联合入路、腹腔镜和后入路（表 50.4）；也介绍了几种比较少见的后入路方式的变型，包括经阴道/阴道旁、经直肠、经括约肌间和经肛内镜显微手术。还描述了适用于直肠后囊性肿物、骶前脑脊膜突出和直肠重复畸形等特定病理类型肿瘤的手术方式。

前入路/经腹入路

经腹入路最适合用于位于第 4 骶骨以上的直肠后肿瘤[27, 57, 61]，Woodfield 等[16] 将分界点定在第 3

骶骨。Guillem 等[60] 推荐这种方法最适用于直肠后上间隙的小肿瘤或是位于骶骨岬水平的大肿瘤。畸胎瘤和子宫内膜异位症的最佳治疗方法是开腹手术[53]。要使手术成功，必须术前保证骶骨不受累及[8, 58]。在最近的回顾性分析中，使用此方式的比例在 0～42.9% 之间（表 50.4）[41, 51]。此种方式能对盆腔结构，包括骶中动脉、骶前静脉和神经进行充分的评估[9, 26]。Woodfield 等支持在切除肿瘤之前，早期控制瘤蒂的血管，主要是骶中动脉；如果有必要，还包括髂内血管。但 Guillem 等指出在他们的病例中，没有发现肿瘤真正的血管蒂，而这些肿瘤的血供来自于髂内动脉和直肠上动脉放射状的小动脉[9, 60]。Jao 等[45] 的临床回顾中报道了 21 例经腹入路治疗的患者。Guillem 等[60] 使用经腹入路治疗了 6 例直肠后肿瘤的女性患者，肿瘤大小从 5cm～9cm，更多使用普凡嫩施蒂尔切口（n=5），而不是正中脐下切口（n=1）。在骶骨岬水平切开腹膜，并评估直肠后间隙，然后将直肠与肿物分离（图 50.8）[60, 108]，最后将肿物从骶前筋膜上分离下来[58]。Guillem 等指出，即使肿瘤位于直肠后间隙的下部，也是可以触及的；但是其他研究者指出，单独经腹部入路无法达到肿瘤的最远端[9]。Guillem 等为其

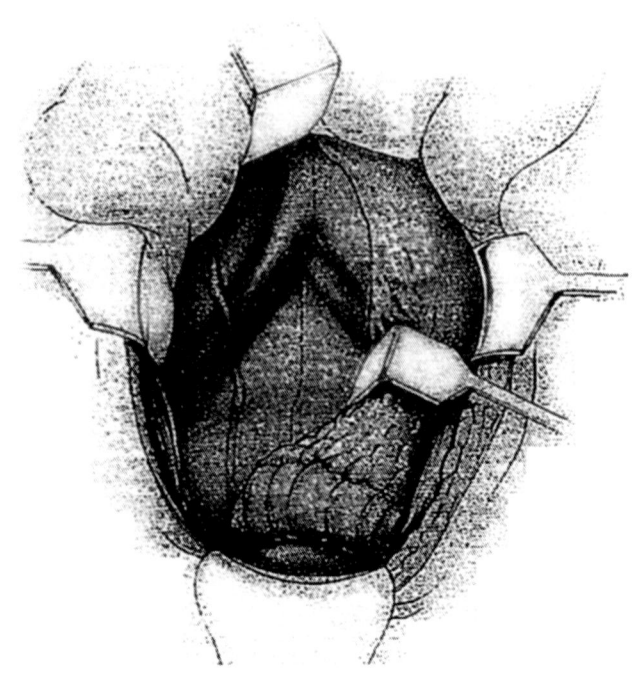

图 50.8 通过前入路 / 经腹入路到达骶前间隙的通路，通过游离直肠和乙状结肠进入直肠后间隙（Reprinted with permission from Grundfest-Broniatowski et al.[108, 159-160]）

表 50.4 手术方式的类型

研究者	病例数	前入路	联合入路	后入路	其他	尾骨切除术 / 骶骨切除术
Freier 等[42](1971)	21	2	0	15TS	4NS	NR
Localio 等[43](1979)	20	3	13	4TS		NR
Cody 等[44](1981)	39	8	10	8TS	1 盆腔清除术	NR
Jao 等[45](1985)	102	21	2	79	18 活检	12/31
Hjermstad and Helwig[20](1987)	53	22	0	9TA	1APR 2 造袋 22NS	NR
Lee and Symmonds[46](1988)	70	39	6	20TS 5TP		0/0
Wang 等[47](1995)	45	24	6	13TS	2 活检	0/0
Pidala 等[48](1999)	14	0	0	11TR 3PR		0/0
Lev-Chelouche 等[41](2003)	42	18	3	21		NR
Glasgow 等[50](2005)	34	14	9	11		11[a]
Buchs 等[51](2007)	16	0	0	16		NR
Woodfield 等[16](2007)	27	11	4	12		NR
Grandjean 等[52](2008)	30	2	2	23		15/0
Mathis 等[54](2009)	31	9	2	20		7/1

APR：腹会阴联合切除术；NR：未报道；NS：未详细说明；TS：经骶骨；TA：经肛门；TR：经直肠；TP：经会阴；PS：骶骨旁
[a] 每个的例数未详细说明

所有的病例都切除了肿瘤，并且没有发生重大的出血、术后并发症和术后复发。Bellotti 等[99]对大多数直肠后肿瘤也采用经腹入路，从而避免了采用后入路的并发症。

腹骶联合入路

腹骶联合入路适用于大的肿瘤，一般超过 3~4cm，超过了第 4 骶椎的上下界，但 Hassan 和 Wietfeldt 使用第 3 骶椎作为分界点[7]。尤其是侵犯周围结构（如骶骨）的恶性肿瘤，通过此种方法更容易达到完全切除[16, 26, 41, 48, 68, 92]。Ueda 等[82]建议如果在开腹手术中发现直肠后肿瘤恶变，那么应该改为经腹骶联合入路。此外较大和感染的直肠后肿瘤，经常与周围器官粘连紧密，最适用于此种入路[10, 58]。在治疗直肠后肿瘤的手术中，腹骶联合入路约占 2%~65%，但近期的回顾性分析中，此种方式占所有病例的 6.4%~26.4%（表 50.4）[43, 45, 50, 54]。此种联合手术方式能很好地暴露肿瘤及周围结构，尤其是神经，并能达到更好的血流控制[61]。Singer 等[61]推荐初始行开腹手术，随后采用俯卧折刀位，这是标准技术。在 Monek 等的个案报道中[32]，一例 39 岁的女性患者，通过腹部入路对一个巨大的多囊的直肠后重复畸形进行了部分切除，并在 21 天后采用后矢状入路进行了完全切除。Localio 等[8, 43, 58]建议两个手术应同时进行，患者采取"sloppy lateral"卧位[8, 58]。虽然 Cody 等[44]指出侧卧位时通过双手触诊能清楚地识别完全骶骨切除的平面，但此种姿势不利于分离坐骨神经和骶骨旁结构。Hannon 等[10]提出患者在手术中可以一直采用截石位。

大多数研究者都支持使用脐下正中切口[8]。对于侧卧位，Localio 等[43]则描述了一种腹部斜切口，从右髂嵴到左肋缘，平行于腹股沟韧带。在游离乙状结肠和直肠后，在骶骨岬水平进入骶前间隙[8, 43]。止血带环绕髂血管放置，使其能被阻断，以防发生大出血[43]。Cody 等[44]不仅结扎骶中动静脉，还会结扎两侧的髂内动脉。术中还应识别输尿管，放置输尿管支架会有帮助[10]。从直肠到肛提肌的水平将肿瘤分离出来，剩下的过程就采用后入路完成[43]。

腹腔镜技术

腹腔镜技术对于直肠后肿瘤的诊断和治疗是一个更新的选择。它能更好地显示直肠后肿瘤的病理和狭小盆腔里邻近的结构[65]。Bax 和 van der Zee[109]描述了 1 例经腹腔镜结扎骶正中动脉（它可能是大出血的原因）的案例。腹腔镜技术瘢痕小、疼痛轻、恢复快[65, 110]。一些研究者提议腹腔镜技术只能应用于未怀疑恶变的囊性病变，而实性病变则需开放手术[65]。然而，在儿科中的实性直肠后畸胎瘤中，通过腹腔镜切除可获得良好的效果[109, 111]。

用腹腔镜技术治疗成人直肠后肿瘤只有散在的个案报道[77, 89, 112, 113]。Witherspoon 等[112]建议患者保持仰卧位。然而，Bax 等[109]建议在操作过程中取肛门截石位。Salameh 等[77]认为改良的截石位效果更好。手术孔的位置及数量在不同的报道中存在差异。Witherspoon 等通过 5 孔法切除了 1 例 10cm×7cm×7cm 的直肠后神经鞘瘤，包括 1 个 10mm 放置腹腔镜的 trochar、3 个 12mm 的 trochar 和 1 个 5mm 的 trochar[112]。Chen 等[110]利用 4 孔法（1 个 10mm 的脐部 trochar、2 个位于双侧髂前上棘内侧 3cm 的 5mm 的 trochar 和 1 个位于左侧锁骨中线脐上 2cm 的 10mm 的 trochar）切除了 1 例 10cm×8.5cm×8.5cm 的直肠后畸胎瘤。Konstantinidis 等[113]除了 1 个脐下 10mm 放置腹腔镜的孔，还分别于左、右髂窝及耻骨上插入了 3 个 5mm 的 trochar。二氧化碳气腹应该维持在 10~12mmHg[89, 112, 114]。在开放手术中，输尿管、髂血管及下腹神经的识别至关重要[110]。切开腹膜从直肠的左侧或右侧进入直肠后间隙，在骶骨岬从肿瘤的上方和侧方牵拉直肠来进行手术[110, 112]。经腹缝合时子宫被向前牵拉[77]。Witherspoon 等认为一个手助装置或经尾骨的对口切开有利于解剖巨大直肠后神经鞘瘤的下极，困难在于肿瘤的"赤道"、最大直径的位置、肿瘤的"南极点"和近尾部的范围。在 Salameh 等的经验中，术中吸出囊性肿瘤和直肠重复畸形的内容物，能改善直肠间隙下极的视野。Yang 等[114]进行了良性直肠后神经鞘瘤的摘除，这有利于肿瘤囊壁的切除。相反，Witherspoo 等强烈建议尽量减少肿瘤的触碰，避免囊壁的损伤和术后的复发。将肿瘤从骶前筋膜分离至直肠骶骨筋膜水平，避免损伤骶前静脉丛[77, 110]。Chen 等认为：电外科器械能更好地控制肿瘤的供应血管。然而 Konstantinidis 等却使用血管夹。应尽量避免经肛门镜下疏忽地直肠切开。Salameh 等在行肿瘤切除时同时用硬式乙状结肠镜检查直肠，这样可以保证直肠回缩，并与肿瘤分离[110]。这些研究者进一步建议应经肛滴注美兰来评估直肠有无损伤。Witherspoon等将切除的神经鞘瘤最后通过放置切口保器的Pfannenstiel切口取出，然而Yang等更愿意在左髂窝使用爱惜康的Lap-Disc。在Chen等的报道中，在切除1个畸胎瘤时进行减压，并通过标本袋从1cm的trochar取出。Gunkova等[89]报道了1例在切除9.3cm×5.8cm×6.4cm的尾肠囊肿后关闭盆底，并于道格拉斯窝放置引流管。这些病例术后没有并发症[77, 89, 109, 110, 112, 114, 115]。绝大数研究者并没有报道腹腔镜的远期疗效。Yang等记录了1例神经鞘瘤患者，术后6个月都没有复发。同样，Konstantinidis等描述了2例患者分别于术后25个月和32个月都没任何症状。Sharma等[83]发现尽管腹腔镜手术时损伤了表皮样囊肿的囊壁，但术后12个月也没有复发。

腹腔镜技术作为联合方法的一部分来解决延伸至骶4上极和下极水平的巨大肿瘤。Palanivelu等[65]描述了他们切除巨大"哑铃状"表皮样囊肿的手术方法，通过腹腔镜处理16cm×10cm的盆腔病变，通过后入路处理9cm×6cm的会阴部的组成部分。共刺入了4个trochar：1个10mm的脐上孔，2个锁骨中线的腰部孔，1个10mm的上腹部孔。显示器放于手术台的下方，助手站在患者的头部控制腹腔镜，主刀从右侧操作。囊肿先通过减压，释放出脓性液体。开始游离囊肿时，利用超声刀打开囊肿侧方的腹膜；囊肿壁从直肠后组织分离至肛提肌；发现了与囊肿会阴部组成部分的连接点。Palanivelu等指出：曾有患者由于供应囊壁小的血管破裂引起直肠后间隙持续性渗血，导致出血360ml而输注1个单位浓缩红细胞[65]。盆腔的死腔用网膜填充并放置引流管。囊肿壁利用标本袋从脐下3.5cm的横切口取出。囊肿会阴部的组成部分通过后入路处理。外科医生报道：尽管解剖过程"冗长"，但整个操作只持续了174min。患者术后第4天出院。随访26个月没有复发。

后入路

后入路是切除直肠后病变最常用的方法，包括经括约肌、经骶骨、经直肠和经骶尾部入路[2, 8, 60]。在一些报道中，有高达80%的直肠后肿瘤，平均直径在4cm，通过后入路来治疗[23, 45, 48, 68]。在Hjermstad和Helwig[20]的报道中，有71%的尾肠囊肿病例通过后入路解决。绝大多数研究者建议后入路用于直径小于4cm和低于S_3水平的直肠后肿瘤[8, 16, 48, 51, 105]，直肠指诊时示指可触及这些肿瘤的最下极[61]。其他研究者认为如果切除尾骨和骶骨下端（S_4~S_5）时，直径在8cm~10cm的良性肿瘤能被游离[16, 43]。Woodfield等[16]指出要保证手术的成功，术前应该排除内脏、骨盆和骶骨受累。相反，Ghosh等[23]主张：这种入路适用于所有骶骨受累的肿瘤。Lev-Chelouche等[41]建议只有小于1cm的脊索瘤或累及骶尾骨最下方10cm的良性肿瘤才适用于这种方法。一些研究者主张除了脊索瘤以外的恶性肿瘤不应用此方法，因为它有发生不可控大出血的可能[41, 44]。Pappalardo等[16]推荐经骶骨旁或经会阴部入路治疗感染的直肠后囊肿，因为经腹入路增加了腹腔感染的机会，经骶骨入路会导致骨髓炎[61]。由于这种入路能很好地显露神经，所以Hobson等[16]认为它是治疗神经性肿瘤或肿瘤累及神经的理想方法。

后入路很少有并发症[51]。Glasgow等[16]认为，后入路（尤其是与经会阴入路和经骶骨入路比较）与经腹入路或经腹骶联合入路相比，能减少术中的出血和术中用血（330mL vs 1260mL）[85, 105]。尽管Guillem等[60]指出这种方法会损伤到髂血管，但是Ghosh等[23]指出他们经腹膜外的方法会保护血管。在Pappalardo等[53]经骶骨旁治疗皮样囊肿的报道中就遇到不可控制的大出血，开腹进行止血[16, 54, 85]。在Mathis等[16, 54, 85]的治疗经历中，经后入路比经腹或经腹骶联合入路术后恢复时间短[16, 54, 85]，平均住院时间为2.6天 vs 6.9天（$P = 0.002$）。而在Woodfield等[16]的报道中经后入路的住院时间和开腹的住院时间差不多，为7天 vs 7.5天。在Mathis等的统计中，后入路的并发症比前路或联合入路要少（$P = 0.007$）。而Guillem等[60]指出经后入路发生术后坐位慢性疼痛的概率可能会增加。此外，Bellotti等[99]认为经后入路手术会出现骨炎、直肠破裂、肛门功能紊乱、粪瘘的风险。

后入路有若干体位。大部分研究者把患者摆放成俯卧折刀位，用带子将臀部回缩[8, 61, 64]。然而，Localio等[43]将患者摆放成侧卧位，通过经骶骨入路切除了4例良性直肠后肿块。同样，Hannon等认为可以把患者摆成截石位进行手术[46]。不同的切口均可到达肿瘤，包括经骶尾旁切口、正中切口、弧形切口、倒V字切口、水平切口（横切口）[61, 109]。

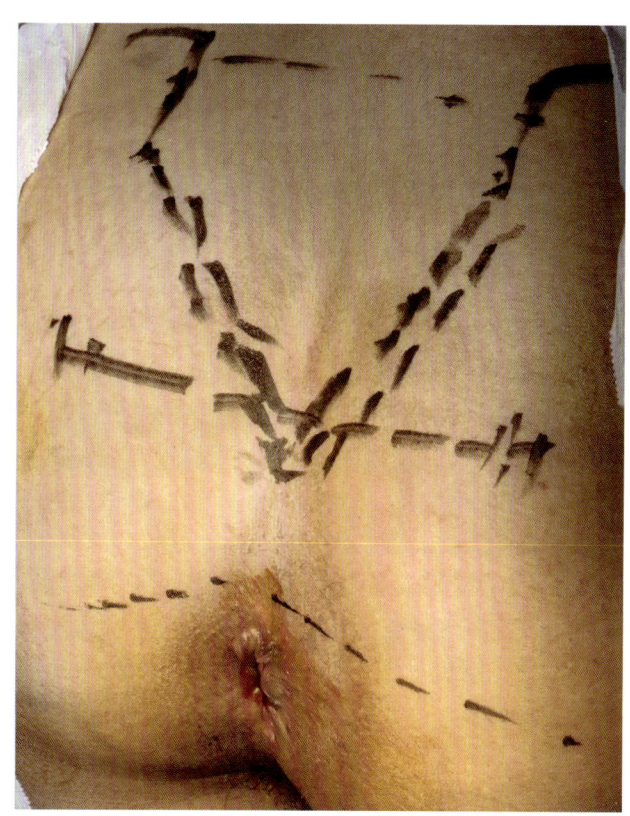

图 50.9 经骶尾的横切口。一例 36 岁女性患者，做经骶的横切口，通过后入路切除 12cm 的直肠后血管黏液瘤

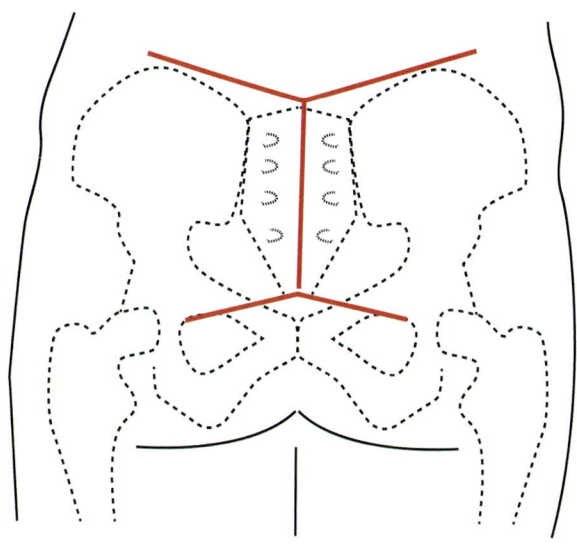

图 50.10 Yang 的 I 形方法，做一个 I 形切口来切除脊索瘤

横切口应越过骶尾关节（图 50.9）[10]。经骶尾旁切口可以从左侧或右侧到达骶骨[41, 85]。在中线经骶骨切口通过第 5 骶椎到达外括约肌，避免损伤括约肌[116]。Yang 等[107]更喜欢 I 形切口来切除脊索瘤（图 50.10）。在截石位，做一弧形切口从阴道后部到肛门后部[46]。大多数研究者采用横切口或垂直中线的骶骨切口来切除尾骨，但是 Böhm 等[107]喜欢采用越过 S_2~S_3 的倒"V"形切口，来避免损伤骶神经[8]。切开皮下脂肪，分离肛门尾骨韧带和肛提肌，到达肿瘤（图 50.11）[58, 61]。横断臀肌、骶棘和骶结节韧带以便更好地显露手术视野[44]。通过尾骨或部分骶骨（S_4~S_5）切除，更好地到达直肠后间隙[9, 23, 105]。Hannon 等建议戴双层手套的示指在直肠内进行指引，能避免直肠壁后方切开时直肠损伤，尤其在致密粘连的感染囊肿（图 50.12）[9, 16]。Sciaudone 等[105]描述了通过"双重"入路从术者示指周围切除了 1 例 5cm×5cm 的直肠后囊肿，另一只手的示指在直肠内做指引。与肛后隐窝相通的囊性直肠后肿瘤，Singer 等[61]推荐从外口插入 Foley

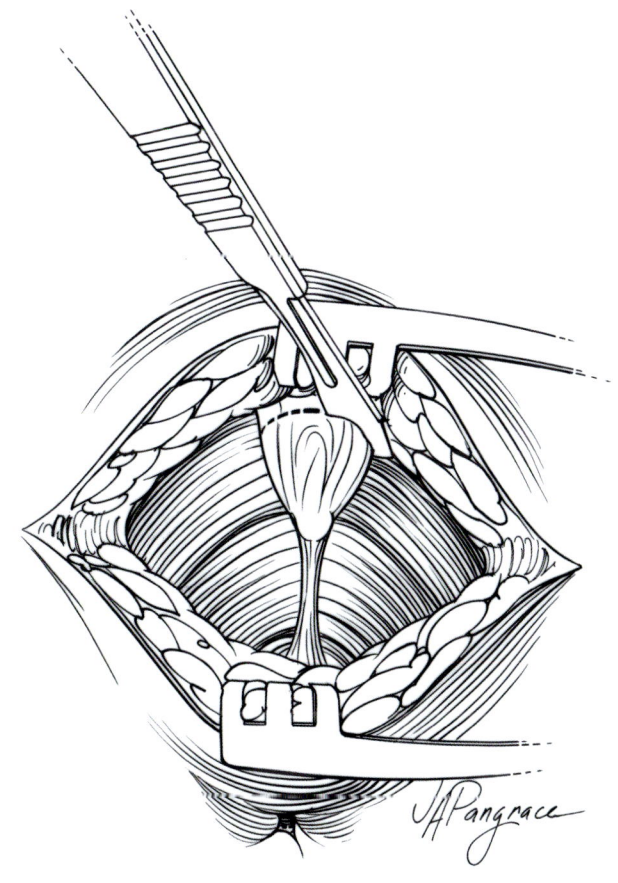

图 50.11 分离肛尾韧带进入直肠后间隙（Reprinted with permission from Böhm et al.[1]）

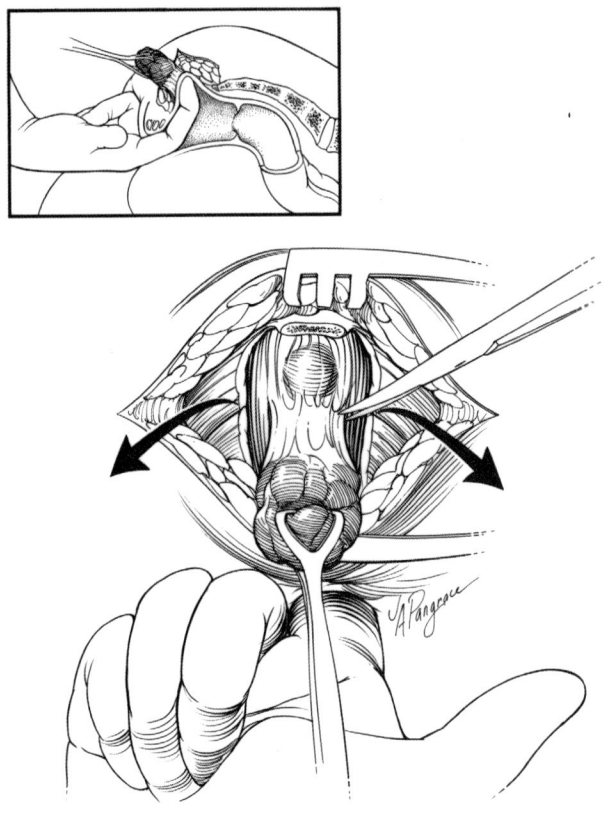

图50.12 在分离肿瘤的过程中,将示指放在直肠中可以避免损伤肠道(Reprinted with permission from Böhm et al.[1])

尿管以便更好地区分这类肿块的界限,研究者通过这种方法经骶尾旁切口成功切除了1例表皮样囊肿。尾小凹不一定要连同标本完整切除[52]。术前切开引流或活检部位必须连同肿瘤一并切除,以防止肿瘤的复发,尤其是针对恶性肿瘤[10]。

经肛门切除

经直肠或经肛门入路在直肠后肿瘤中很少使用。Hjermstad和Helwig的报道中:有29%的尾肠囊肿患者经肛门入路手术[20]。大多当代研究者只通过这种入路来切除小的感染囊肿(这些病变有窦道与直肠相通或自发破裂)的窦道[9-10]。这种有争议的入路的适应证包括低位、未定位、小的囊性病变和侵及直肠后壁浆膜或固有肌层的良性肿瘤[9, 23, 48, 68]。Hannon等[10]认为小的表皮样囊肿或皮样囊肿也可以采用这种入路。Pidala等[48]指出只有不含实性物质的单纯囊肿才能通过这种入路治疗,他们14例1~4cm的囊性直肠后肿瘤患者中有11例进行了经肛门入路手术[20, 48]。在截石位,使用贯穿直肠后壁全层的横切口(大约邻近齿状线2~3cm)[48],而Hannon等建议采用纵切口,分两层关闭直肠切口,经切口放置引流,而一些研究者则建议敞开伤口[10, 48]。Pidala等报道了11例囊性患者中有10例完整切除,没有切除的1例囊肿是因为术前活检而感染,最后只取病理、放引流。有1例患者最后发展成骶前脓肿而经直肠引流。完整切除囊肿的患者没有复发的病例,而只进行引流的囊肿患者在5年后复发。Hjermstad和Helwig[20]有类似的报道,9例经肛门入路切除的患者都获得了良好的疗效。然而,在Hannon等的报道中2例患者中有1例复发,他们把这归咎于暴露不充分。直肠后间隙的暴露不好会遗漏部分病变,尤其是多囊性病变[20, 51]。暴露不充分会增加出血的风险[51]。虽然没有具体的报道,但是这种入路有可能损伤括约肌导致大便失禁。

经内镜的微创手术是经肛门入路一个新的变化。只有Zoller等[117]报道使用这种技术治疗了3例尾肠囊肿。他们认为经内镜的微创手术的最大优势是立体放大的图像能够很好地显露手术视野[117]。Zoller等还指出这种技术比经骶骨入路的损伤更小。这种方法的细节和疗效没有被报道过,在1个病例中囊肿无意中被刺破,流出大量的灰色液体[117]。

经括约肌间入路

Buchs等[51]报道使用经括约肌间入路治疗低位的良性直肠后肿瘤,患者可采用俯卧折刀位或截石位[8]。在肛门后做一V形或放射状切口,并经此到达括约肌间层。对括约肌间的无血管区进行钝性分离,到达耻骨直肠肌水平[8, 51]。Buchs等指出在分离直肠骶骨筋膜时可能需要改善手术视野。值得注意的是,由于直肠骶骨筋膜是直肠后间隙最下方的界限,必须切断这个筋膜带才能触及一个真正的直肠后肿瘤。在Buchs等的系列研究中,有8例患者经括约肌间入路切除了2~7cm的良性直肠后肿瘤。在24~120个月的随访中,没有一例患者发生复发。由于这种技术并发症发生率低,他们更情愿使用此种技术,并宣称能维持括约肌功能,但Wolpert等[9]指出可能会导致括约肌损伤的并发症。Buchs等进一步指出此方法能防止损伤骶神经,从而避免了术后泌尿系统后遗症[9, 23]。

经阴道或阴道旁入路

经阴道入路治疗直肠后肿瘤只有 2 例个案报道。Madanes 等[118]建议经阴道的手术用来治疗低位直肠后肿瘤女性患者，列举了经腹、经骶骨和经后入路手术存在损伤腹腔脏器、骶神经和直肠的风险。位于中线的直肠后肿瘤是这个方法的唯一指征[9, 51]。Madanes 等描述了经阴道手术来治疗 1 例 28 岁女性患者，在中线右侧有一个光滑的、坚实的大小约 5cm×6cm 的直肠后肿块（畸胎瘤）。患者取截石位，行右侧阴道旁切口：从后穹窿的右下方 3cm 处切开，沿着阴道的右侧后外侧壁，到达距后正中线约 3cm 的右侧后联合。从右侧后联合，行弧形切口到达坐骨结节，距肛门 3cm。而 Aslan[35]用长约 8cm 的右侧阴道旁正中纵切口治疗了 1 例患有右后外侧直肠后肿瘤（表皮样囊肿）的 27 岁女性患者。分离会阴浅横肌和耻骨直肠肌，游离直肠壁，到达肿瘤。切除病变后逐层关闭伤口，并放置引流管。在这两篇报道中，患者排便后也没有任何围术期的并发症[35, 118]。Madanes 等认为 Schuchardt 切口（这个切口最早在 1893 年是用来进行阴式子宫切除术）如果离后正中线太近会损伤直肠，如果太靠外侧会损伤到球海绵体肌[118]。研究者认为耻骨直肠肌的局部切除"应该不会"导致大便失禁[118]。手术后泌尿系统的并发症是由于骶神经受到损伤而导致的[9]。对于低位直肠后肿瘤，Aslan 指出经阴道入路的优势在于视野清楚、手术时间短、出血少。然而，这两个患者的远期效果都不好[35, 118]。

囊性肿瘤

薄壁囊性直肠后肿瘤对手术切除通常是个挑战。从邻近组织解剖囊肿的过程中，不小心就进入囊肿，导致囊内容物流出。在大部分病例中，如果囊内容物无感染，溢出不会引起不良后果。Sharma 等[83]经腹腔镜切除了 1 例 8cm×7cm 的直肠后表皮样囊肿，在操作过程中"混浊"的液体溢出增加了手术难度，但是这个病例在 12 个月后随访时没有复发。在日本文献中，Ueda 等[82]报道了 1 例手术过程中囊肿破裂的案例，此后 2 年的随访中没有复发。术后脓肿是由于损伤感染性囊肿导致。一些研究者报道，常规进行囊壁的切开和囊内容物的吸引[10, 85]。在 Ueda 等的报道中，通过缩小表皮样囊肿的大小能够使肿物的切除更容易。Bax 等[109]主张巨大囊性肿瘤的经腹减压有利于腹腔镜下肿物的切除。巨大囊肿减压后有机会经后路切除，否则需经腹入路切除[20]。在日本文献中，15 例表皮样囊肿手术切除前进行了 3 次囊肿吸引，其中 2 例经骶骨入路，1 例经腹入路，术后 5 个月～2 年间没有任何并发症和复发迹象[82]。1 例感染性囊肿在正式切除之前进行了引流[61]。Ghosh 等[23]建议感染性囊肿可以通过不同入路经皮细针穿刺引流。非确定性肿物切除的切开引流会增加复发的风险。

骶前脑脊膜膨出

骶前脑脊膜膨出需要与直肠后囊性肿瘤鉴别。在 1960 年之前，大约 40% 骶前脑脊膜膨出死亡病例与手术有关，这些病例术前诊断错误，从而进行了错误的手术[45]。这些囊性病变需要多学科参与，尤其是神经外科医生。切除这些囊肿的手术关键是要把疝出的硬脑膜和蛛网膜的颈部结扎牢靠，来避免脑脊液漏和由此导致的脑膜炎[58, 59]。Ashley 和 Wright[66]认为仅结扎囊肿颈部而不手术切除，可能会引起囊肿自身退化。他们建议骶前脑脊膜膨出最好通过经腹入路来处理[9, 66]。巨大的脑脊膜膨出或与此相关的直肠后肿块最适合这种入路[67]。神经外科医生采用腹腔镜技术治疗骶前脑脊膜膨出。Jeon 等[104]描述了 1 例腹腔镜操作的过程：硬式腹腔镜通过经脐 3cm 的横切口插入一个 10cm×10cm×12cm 的骶前脑脊膜膨出中，通过植入来源于腹部的脂肪移植物来阻断硬膜囊和脑脊膜膨出间的通路。这个病例 1 年后复查 MRI 没有复发。Trapp 等[67]在 5 例患者中经腹腔镜利用 2 个塑料夹子夹闭了囊肿颈部，有 4 例患者术后 3～4 个月症状减轻，但是有 1 例患者术后 2 个月症状反复。神经外科医生习惯通过切除骶骨椎板来治疗这些肿瘤，尤其是囊肿颈部位置比较低时[59, 66, 67, 104]。在 1938 年，Adson[59, 119]描述了 19 例骶骨椎板切除后结扎囊肿颈的患者，没有 1 例死亡[59]。经后入路被用于治疗合并有脊椎畸形的患者，比如脊髓栓系[67]。Hobson 等[9, 58]建议经腹骶联合入路，通过后入路寻找囊肿颈部，通过前入路进行结扎[9]。Krivokapic 等[59]通过这种联合入路治疗了 1 例 8.5cm×8.9cm×14cm 骶前脑脊膜膨出患者。

直肠重复畸形

很多方法均可以治疗直肠重复畸形（图 50.13）。手术切除首为推荐[29]。尤其是恶性直肠重复畸形需通过低位前切或经腹会阴联合完整切除直肠[4,77]。直肠重复畸形复发是由于原位残留了卫星灶[4,31,120]。此外，由于直肠重复畸形和直肠有共同的血供，手术很少因为直肠的缺血而变得复杂[30,120]。还有一种较保守的方法是切除直肠重复畸形的黏膜[30]。扩肛后通过直肠黏膜的横切口进入直肠重复畸形，剥离它的黏膜，把病变留在原位[4]。这项技术遗留了肿瘤恶变的风险，但同时阻止了黏液的分泌，去除了引起临床症状的源头[4,30]。Stockman 等[9,64]建议可以打开直肠重复畸形与直肠间的壁，形成一个独立的巨大腔隙来治疗直肠重复畸形，但通过这种方法没有去除肿瘤恶变的可能。感染的直肠重复畸形在确定性手术前先要进行引流和造瘘[4]。

尾骨切除术

是否常规进行尾骨切除存在争议。尾骨切除的最大优势是能够充分暴露手术视野，尤其是经后路治疗巨大直肠后肿瘤时[20,50]。切口越过骶尾联合，避免损伤侧面的盆神经[9]。分离肛门尾骨韧带前切断骶尾关节[9]。尾骨切除和某些直肠后肿瘤复发的关联存在争议。一些研究者认为尾骨是癌细胞潜在的定植地，规范的尾骨切除（尤其是巨大的直肠后良性肿瘤）能够保证直肠后肿瘤的完整切除，从而防止肿瘤的复发[9,20,26,44,50]。Hjermstad 和 Helwig[20]建议应该切除尾骨，来清除尾肠囊肿的残留细胞。有类似的报道：表皮样囊肿和皮样囊肿也采用尾骨切除术[50]。尾骨留在原位会增加畸胎瘤复发的可能[50,58]。Glasgow 等[50]发现尾骨切除（有 11 例患者）和肿瘤的复发没有关联。其他研究者提倡只有良性囊肿或恶性肿瘤明显侵犯尾骨时才进行尾骨切除[27,50,54]。Lev-Chelouche 等[41]通过后入路连同脊索瘤、下端骶骨及尾骨的整块切除治疗了 7 例患者。

骶骨切除术

骶骨切除术是某些直肠后肿瘤的外科治疗手段。手术通常需要矫形外科医生、神经外科医生、整形外科医生和结直肠外科医生的共同参与。临床很少应用这个手术，但是部分切除远端骶骨（通常 $S_4 \sim S_5$ 椎体）的后入路术式，可以有效提高直肠后间隙的视野。Mathis 等[54]完成了一个尾肠囊肿患者远端骶骨的切除手术；然而，部分或全部的骶骨切除术更多应用于像脊索瘤这样局部浸润的直肠后肿瘤，手术患者通常健康、有活力[45,50,54]。Tomita 和 Tsuchiya[50,58,102,121,122]指出经腹部和腹骶联合入路是常见的手术方法，而后入路术式是最常见的手术方式[50,58,102,122]。腹骶联合手术是肿瘤半体切除术、完整骶骨切除术、某些高位的骶骨肿瘤切除和当肿瘤侵犯腹膜后结构时的最佳手术方式[102]。在骶骨切除术中，应游离骶结节、骶棘、下肢骶髂韧带、臀肌和梨状肌，暴露坐骨神经[43,108]。在适当的水平面上进行骶尾骨切除术及截骨术，关闭硬膜囊，截断神经根（图 50.14）[43,102,108]。Sciubba 等们[43,84]建议，为获得切缘阴性，应切除肿瘤以上至少一个骶段[43]。第 1 和第 2 骶椎骨对于载荷传递和生理起重要作用，因此对于 S_3 椎骨水平以上的骶骨切除术，必须分离骶髂关节，以排除腰椎骨盆的失调[58,84,102]。对于涉及超过 50% 以上的骶髂关节的骶骨切除术，稳定腰椎骨盆必须使用骨移植（如胫骨或腓骨）、回肠骶螺丝和固定装置进行固定（图 50.15）[58,84,102]。肿瘤累及 S_1 椎体的骶骨切除术，术后会发生明显的术后并发症，如神经源性膀胱、大便失禁和结构不稳[58]。总体而言，不建议行涉及 $S_1 \sim S_2$ 椎间盘间隙的骶骨切除术[9]。诸如脊索瘤这样的肿瘤，虽然他们不侵犯骶神经根，而是完全围绕着骶神经根生长，但是仍不能保留这些肿瘤[102]。同双侧分离骶神经

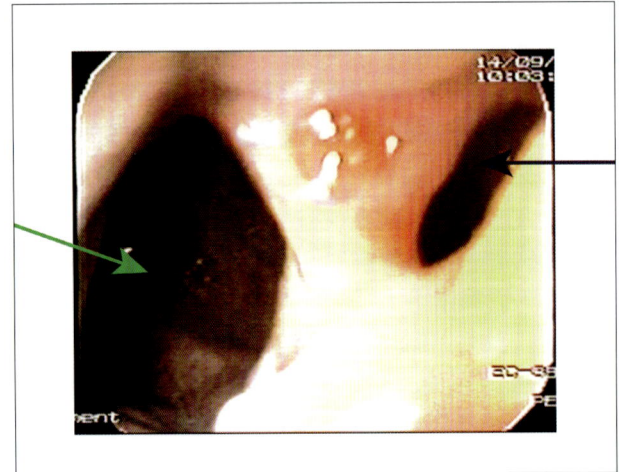

图 50.13　直肠重复畸形囊肿的内镜表现。重复畸形（左侧箭头）和原始管腔（右侧箭头）

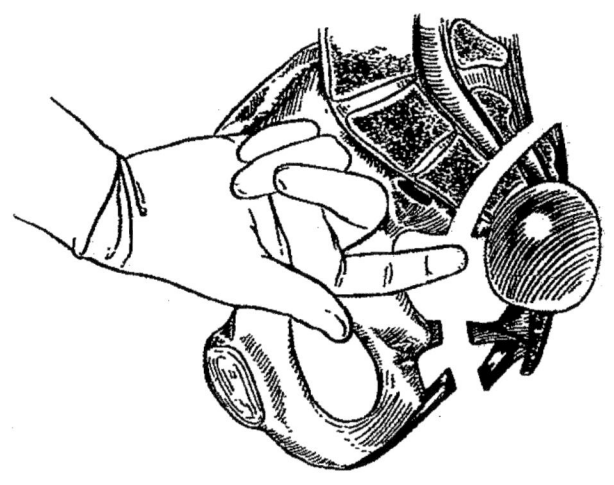

图 50.14 作为骶骨切除的一部分，将骶棘韧带和骶结节韧带横向分离。行骶骨椎板切除术，并切断神经根，关闭鞘膜。在完成椎板切除术后，对骶骨行骨切除术，并切除肿瘤（Reprinted with permission from Grundfest-Broniatowski et al.[108], 159-160）

相比，单侧分离骶神经能够更好的维持尿便功能[58]。近端 S_3 神经根切除后出现尿便失禁和阳痿（表 50.5）[50, 84, 123]。如要保留尿便功能应至少保存一侧 S_2 神经根[16, 50, 58, 84]。如果骶骨切除术没有损害第 5 腰椎神经，患者通常可以下地行走[102]。骶骨半切手术虽然不引起排泄障碍，但会造成单侧运动及感觉障碍[84]。如果骶神经的保留妨碍了根治性手术，那就应当将骶神经切除[1]。但是健侧的骶神经根应当保留[44]。臀部的缺损往往需要肌皮瓣进行闭合，尤其是接受术前放射治疗的患者[7, 102]。

表 50.5 骶骨切除术后的预期并发症

骶骨切除水平	涉及的神经根	缺　　陷
高位	$S_1 \sim S_5$	运动功能减弱
		便/尿失禁
		感觉麻木（鞍状）
		性功能障碍
中位	$S_2 \sim S_5$	很少出现运动功能减弱
		括约肌功能障碍
		感觉麻木（鞍状）
		性功能障碍
低位	$S_4 \sim S_5$	可变的性功能障碍
		感觉麻木（会阴部）

Adapted from Refs[84, 102]

辅助治疗

目前，辅助治疗对于直肠后肿瘤的治疗意义不大，术后患者最佳的辅助治疗方案存在很大争议。对于某些特定的恶性肿瘤，冷冻治疗已经成为一种手术切除的辅助治疗手段。Schwab 等描述的关于骶尾部肿瘤的治疗方法涉及了 3 种冷冻及解冻方式[124]。Lev-Chelouche 等[41]将冰冻治疗加入到 3 例脊索瘤患者的手术切除治疗中。Cody 等[44]报道应用液氮治疗 5 例不完全切除后切缘阳性或局部复发的患者。这项技术被认为对于治疗侵犯骶骨的肿瘤复发，尤其是部分骶骨切除术的患者是有帮助的[44]。Cody 等指出原发肿瘤因为太大无法完全冰冻，固冷冻治疗不能作为其主要的治疗手段。

包括畸胎癌、腺癌、肉瘤、脊索瘤等在内的某些直肠后肿瘤可能会通过术后的化学治疗及放射治疗获益[45]。患有畸胎瘤的儿童，经放射治疗及化学治疗（长春新碱、放线菌素 D、环磷酰胺）治疗后，

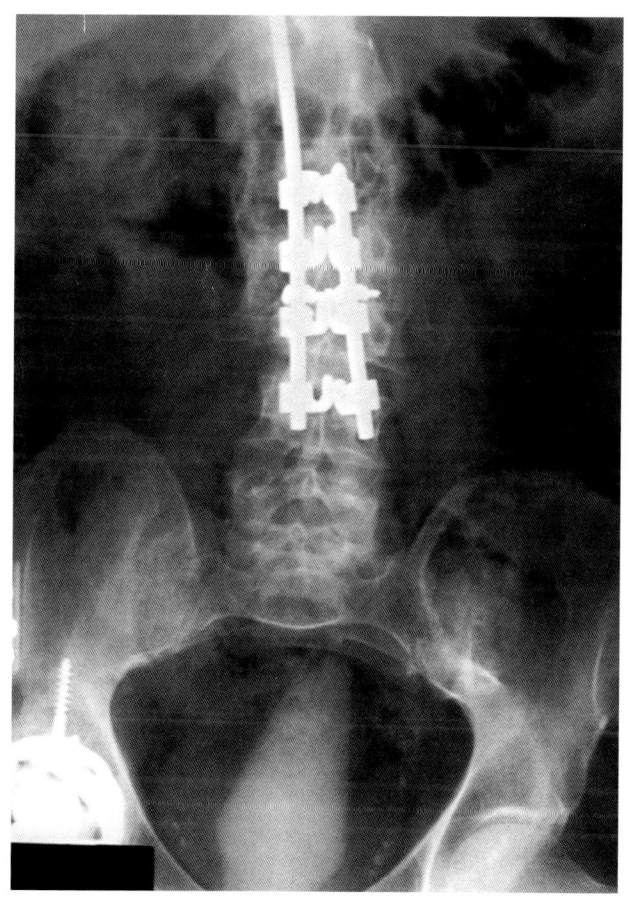

图 50.15 广泛骶骨切除术后的腰椎骨盆稳定，脊索瘤手术后放置固定装置的 X 片

取得了比单纯手术更好的结果[1]。Pidala 等[48]指出，一例患有尾肠囊肿包含侵袭性腺癌的患者接受放射治疗，1年后未发现肿瘤学证据。Lev-Chelouche 等[41]对两例盆腔肉瘤切除术后切缘阳性的患者进行术后放射治疗，两例患者术后复发时间为 12 个月和 18 个月。以前认为脊索瘤对放射治疗不敏感，但是近期短疗程，高剂量照射（40～80 GYS 超过 4～8 周）已经产生了良好的治疗效果[1]。脊索瘤手术切除联合术后辅助放射治疗的患者与单纯手术相比，其无病生存期已延长（甚至两倍）[50, 84]。然而，上述显著的治疗效果只针对原发和非复发的脊索瘤[84]。脊索瘤次全切除术后辅助放疗的患者无病间隔也显著延长[107]。Baratti 等[122]指出，病灶切除术后切缘阳性联合辅助放疗的患者同切缘阴性完全切除的患者相比，其局部复发率相近[102]。经皮瘤内注射无水酒精对脊索瘤已获得良好的治疗效果，而传统的化学治疗对脊索瘤治疗无效[7, 125]。

对脊索瘤的治疗正制定新的治疗方式。晚期脊索瘤已经对多种生物治疗疗法表现出良好的反应，这其中包括血小板衍生生长因子 β- 受体抑制剂伊马替尼，其正处于Ⅱ期研究[7, 125, 126]。对于脊索瘤接受伊马替尼治疗过程中进展的患者可加用西罗莫司（mTOR）。从 Stacchiotti 等[125]的 10 例患者的研究中可以得知上述治疗获益率为 89%，其中 7 例患者 PET 阳性。这些研究者断定，雷帕霉素可能会增强伊马替尼的效果。结合低剂量顺铂与伊马替尼可获得类似的结果[102]。此外，当脊索瘤局部复发和出现肺转移表现超过 9 个月时，应用表皮生长因子受体抑制剂西妥昔单抗和吉非替尼治疗的患者可部分缓解[126-127]。

并发症

许多研究指出直肠后肿瘤术后并发症率较低。在各种大系列直肠后肿瘤的研究中，术后并发症发生率的记录则高达 31%～36%（表 50.6）[46, 47, 52]。Glasgow 等[50]报道称，恶性直肠后肿瘤同良性直肠后肿瘤相比，更容易发生并发症，无论短期或长期并发症，而且他们发现手术方法和这些并发症的发病率之间的无相关性。

直肠瘘是直肠后病变术后少见的并发症。这些肿瘤许多紧密附着在直肠上，造成肿物分离困难，

表 50.6 整理后的直肠后肿瘤的术后并发症发生率（手术方式不同）

研究者	病例数	死亡率	并发症发生率	感染	肠/膀胱	性功能	神经性
Localio 等[43](1979)	20	1 (5%)	8 (40%)	0	5UR 1UI	0	2 LE 缺陷
Cody 等[44](1981)	39	1 (2.5%)	8 (21%)	0	3UR	0	1 足下垂
Jao 等[45](1985)	102	0	48 (47%)	11 创面 3 脓肿 1 瘘	15UR 7FI	0	7 缺陷
Lee and Symmonds[46](1988)	70	0	22 (31%)	4 创面 2 脓肿	4UR 2FI	0	0
Böhm 等[1](1993)	24	0	8 (33%)	3 创面	1UI	0	1 "外周缺陷"
Wang 等[47](1995)	45	0	16 (36%)	2 脓肿 1 瘘	7UR 4FI	0	2 缺陷
Pidala 等[48](1999)	14	0	2 (14%)	1 脓肿	0	0	0
Lev-Chelouche 等[41](2003)	42	0	15 (36%)	5 创面 2 脓肿	2UR	0	1 LE 缺陷
Glasgow 等[50](2005)	34	0	5 (15%)	0	0	0	0
Buchs 等[51](2007)	16	0	1 (6%)	0	0	0	0
Woodfield 等[16](2007)	27	0	4 (15%)	3 创面	0	0	0
Grandjean 等[52](2008)	30	0	6 (20%)	3 创面 2 漏	0	0	0
Mathis 等[54](2008)	31	0	8 (26%)	0	0	1	0

UR：尿潴留/神经源性膀胱；UI：尿失禁；FI：大便失禁；LE：下肢

并伴有实质损伤的风险。据报道，接近 1%～3% 的患者术后发生瘘[27, 44, 45, 47]。直肠后肿瘤经治疗后可能并发脓肿及伤口感染，术后感染的发生率为 1%～11%[45, 58]。Woodfield 等[16] 报道称在调查的 27 例术后患者中，有 11% 发生了伤口感染。Hobson 等[58] 称这些术后感染是由先前肿瘤感染而促进其发生的。脓肿的治疗需经皮穿刺引流和抗生素治疗，而伤口感染需要清创和二次缝合。部分骶骨切除术还有着后部伤口裂开的风险，Glasgow 等[50] 调查的 3 例这类患者中，2 例患者需盆底网状重建及臀肌推进皮瓣。

直肠后肿瘤术后泌尿系统症状可能加重，多达 15%～27% 的患者术后膀胱功能受损[84, 110, 123]。骶神经损伤是造成排尿功能障碍的原因，可能由于骶神经切除或术中意外损伤。在 Wang 等[47] 的研究中，神经源性膀胱是最常见的并发症（15.5%）。Localio 等[43] 报道了 5 例（25%）术后尿潴留患者，其中两例需要经尿道行前列腺切除术，而有 1 例患者术后尿失禁。Cody 等[44] 的研究中有 3 例患者进行 $S_1 \sim S_2$ 水平的骶骨切除术，术后出现神经源性膀胱，需要自行导尿。大便失禁也可能受到直肠后肿瘤手术的影响；这种并发症占手术治疗的患者的 7%[110]。大便失禁可能是由于外科手术损伤括约肌复合体，主要是后路手术。由于分离骶神经根的缘故，部分骶骨切除术（如脊索瘤）的大便失禁发生率高达 70%[84, 123]。两例尾肠囊肿患者经后路手术后出现的盆底功能障碍，Mathis 等[54] 使用生物反馈方法将其成功治愈。性功能障碍在直肠后肿瘤切除术后很少报道。Woodfield 等[16] 发现了双侧 S_2 神经根分离后发生的性功能障碍。

某些直肠后肿瘤的手术治疗可并发术后神经系统后遗症。骶脊膜膨出术后可能出现脑膜炎。Krivokapic 等[59] 指出，1 例 37 岁女性患者在脊膜膨出和肠道囊肿切除后第 10 天出现脑膜炎，即使长期使用抗生素后，仍存在难以下床活动、畏光、头痛等症状。骶前脑脊膜膨出手术的其他并发症包括伴随截瘫的蛛网膜炎及脑脊液瘘 / 泄漏[59]。脊索瘤切除术过程中硬膜损伤也可能导致脑膜炎，特别是在 $S_2 \sim S_3$ 水平[1]。

直肠后肿瘤切除术的其他神经源性并发症也已被报道。7% 的患者出现触觉迟钝[110]。低例神经根受损的患者可能出现会阴部感觉丧失[43]。下肢运动功能受损可能主要出现在骶神经根分离后。Bergh 等的回顾性研究[123]中指出，1 例患者在单侧切除 L_5/S_1 神经根（作为骶骨切除术的一部分）后出现一只脚瘫痪。

这些手术的术后死亡率低。在大规模的直肠后肿瘤的研究中，死亡率为 0～5%[43, 44]。Localio 等[43] 报道，1 例骶骨脊索瘤患者在术后 18 天死于"严重的泌尿系和创面脓毒症"。Cody 等报道一例 74 岁女性患者，对已侵犯直肠、膀胱、子宫的肿瘤进行松解，术后出现大出血导致围术期死亡[44]。表 50.6 显示了一系列直肠后肿物切除术后的并发症及死亡率。

术后随访

目前术后随访没有统一的方案。总之，观察的方法和持续时间是依赖于病理学结果和切除是否充分。Grandjean 等[52] 建议良性囊性肿瘤术后 1 年行 ERUS 或 MRI 检查。Mathis 等[54] 建议对于尾肠囊肿患者要每年进行直肠指诊，术后 1 年和 5 年进行 CT 扫描。应在术前评估如 CA19-9 和 CEA 等肿瘤标志物水平，并在术后对其水平进行复查，评估肿瘤有无复发。观察期应该是长期的，因为有报道良性和恶性肿瘤术后复发时间可长达 5～30 年。

预　后

由于这些直肠后肿瘤的异质性，它们作为一个单一实体的预后无法评估。总之，良性肿瘤比恶心肿瘤有更好的结局[27]。有病例报道提示，完全切除肿物能改善预后[47]。大多数报道指出，良性肿瘤外科手术治疗后生存率可达 100%[8, 58]。然而，直肠后肿物的复发率高，从 0～22.4%（表 50.7）[41, 46]。在平均随访时间为 9.6 年的时间里，Jao 等[45] 发现 66 例良性肿瘤（6 例先天性囊肿及 4 例巨细胞瘤）中有 10 例复发（15.1%）。其中有 3 例患者开始时出现感染性囊肿，因此研究者认为复发率高[45]。相反，Glasgow 等[50] 的综述指出，平均 22 个月的平均随访时间后，未出现良性肿瘤的复发。有未成熟组织的畸胎瘤比含有成熟组织的畸胎瘤更容易复发[10]，在部分病例中，对复发的良性肿瘤进行再次切除是可能的。Jao 等报道 4 例直肠后囊性肿瘤患者中 3 例行再次手术切除成功。Hannon 等[10] 发现尾肠囊肿经肛门切除术后 1 年复发的患者，经骶尾部切除治愈。

Uhlig 和 Johnson[2] 评价说恶性直肠后肿瘤的预

表 50.7 良性直肠肿瘤切除术后复发率

研究者	平均随访时间（年）	病例数	复发率
Jao 等[45](1985)	9.6（3~23）	66	10（15.1%）
Hjermstad and Helwig[20](1987)	10.7（0.5~26）	53	4（7.5%）
Lee and Symmonds[46](1988)	NR	49	11（22.4%）
Böhm 等[1](1993)	1.75（0.5~7.6）	20	3（15%）
Wang 等[47](1995)	4.9（0.8~14.9）	23	5（21.7%）
Pidala 等[48](1999)	3.25	13	1（7.7%）
Lev-Chelouche 等[41](2003)	4.5（0.17~7.8）a	21	0a（0%）
	2.25b		0b（0%）
Glasgow 等[50](2005)	1.8	27	0（0%）
Woodfield 等[16](2007)	4.1（0.17~6）	20	1（5%）
Grandjean 等[52](2008)	3.2（0.5~15）	29	2（6.9%）
Mathis 等[54](2008)	2（1~22.6）	27	1（3.7%）

a 先天性良性肿瘤
b 获得性良性肿瘤

后对于男性和女性来说都很差。他们发现患有恶性直肠后肿瘤的人群中，77%的男性和64%的女性均死于该病[2]。在一些文章中，患者被诊断出恶性直肠后肿瘤后的5年生存率总体低至17%[45, 58]。而在 Cody 等的回顾性分析中，患有恶性直肠后肿瘤的患者经手术治疗后的5、10、15年生存率分别为85%、56%、42%[44]。然而在 Wang 等[47]在一项有22例患者的报告中提出其5年生存率为40.7%。在 Glasgow 等的文章中[50]指出总体疾病相关生存期的中位数为61个月（37~108个月）。来自 Cody 等的数据显示，4例患有畸胎瘤的患者中有3例在术后1年内死亡[44]。Wang 等[47]指出完整切除能明显提高患者的生存率（$P=0.034$）。然而 Cody 认为，外科治疗对其生存期的延长并无效果，恶性肿瘤经常会在局部或者全身复发[27]。在 Cody 等的综述中显示，27例经外科治疗的恶性直肠后肿瘤患者，约48%在局部出现了肿瘤复发[44]。Pindala 等[48]指出含有侵袭性腺癌的尾肠囊肿会导致更早的局部复发及远处转移。同样，尽管采用了经腹会阴联合切除术，1例尾肠囊肿中含有腺癌的患者在手术后8个月死于该病[20]。在出现局部复发后，在某些特定的情况下再次切除是有可能的，Cody 等谈到，在他们出现局部复发的13例患者中，其中4例患者又进行了最多3次的再次切除[44]。

最常见的直肠后恶性肿瘤——脊索瘤，已经得到充分的研究。在 Jao 等的文章[45]中，在16例采用根治性手术切除和8例采用姑息性手术切除的患者中，5年生存率达到了75%（表50.8）。Bergh 等[123]记录的5年和10年的生存率估计为84%和64%，并且大约有40%的局部复发率和30%的全身复发率。在更大宗的回顾性研究中，总体10年生存率为9%~35%不等[6]。在脊索瘤手术后经常会发生局部复发，常见的部位是骶骨周围、直肠周围、肛周、臀部软组织和骶部残端[122]。众多回顾性分析报道的局部复发率在40%~93%之间[122]。在一项中位随访期为26个月的随访中，Woodfield 等的记录显示有2例脊索瘤的患者发生了复发（28.5%）[16]。切缘阳性对于局部复发是最有意义的标志，在所有的病例中约有70%的复发率[8]。病灶内的切除增加了局部复发的风险[124]。这种高复发率也有可能是因为手术中凝胶样薄壁肿瘤的泄漏[1]。术后发生局部复发和全身复发的时间分别为1.4~12.7年和0.2~13.3年[123]。Varga 等的经验中，有患者经过全骶骨切除后达到广泛的阴性切缘，但在术后的15~52个月诊断了臀部和骶骨的局部复发[102]。其中影响预后的不良因素包括局部复发、Ki-67细胞免疫组化染色超过5%的细胞、镜下肿瘤坏死、手术切缘阳性、肿瘤体积大[123]。局部复发是全身复发和疾病相关性死亡的一个重要前兆[123]。来自 Baratti 等的数据显示，局部复发后的中位生存期为27个月[122]。在 Lev-Chelouche 的回顾性分析[41]中，4例脊索瘤患者（44%）中发现了局部复发，其中有2例进行了边缘性切除，复发是在他们手术后的18~36个月发生的。Böhm 等[1]发现在这些复发中有局部疼

表 50.8 脊索瘤切除术后存活率及复发率

研究者	5 年生存率（%）	10 年生存率（%）	局部复发率（%）
Cody 等 [44] (1981)	69	50	93
Jao 等 [45] (1985)	75	35	67
Bergh 等 [123] (2000)	84	64	44
Baratti 等 [122] (2002)	87.8	48.9	53.5
Schwab 等 [124] (2009)	59	35	40

痛和神经干扰信号。对这些局部侵犯、复发的肿瘤，Cody 等 [44] 建议进行完全再切除，如果完全再切除不可行，可以进行部分切除、刮除术、冷冻疗法来达到缓解的目的。他们提出外科切除术只能推迟而不能阻止复发的发生和疾病相关的死亡。而且多种外科手术由于可能导致术后功能的丧失而受限 [58]。在 Lev-Chelouche 的文章中，所有的 4 例脊索瘤复发患者进行了再次切除，其中有 1 例患者尽管进行了多达 7 次手术包括 1 次半骨盆切除术，但仍在最初发病后的 118 个月后死亡 [41]。经过 2 年的随访，Lev-Chelouche 断定剩余的 3 例患者中，2 例没有疾病的迹象，而 1 例发生了转移 [41]。复发的脊索瘤患者也可用外照射治疗，如同在 Böhm 的文章中提到的 2 例应用成功的患者。Localio 展示了 1 例脊索瘤患者，在术后 5 年发生复发，尽管企图行再次切除失败，但对姑息性放射治疗反应良好，结果增加了 14 年的寿命 [43]。在极罕见的转移病例中可能会行转移肿瘤切除术 [58]。在 Bergh 的回顾性分析中，虽然报道 2 例肺和骨转移患者分别存活 10 年和 7.5 年，但是诊断远处转移后的生存期平均为 0.2 年 [123]。来自 Baratti 的数据提示患者的中位生存期为 11 个月。

结　论

在成人中，直肠后间隙不是原发肿瘤的常见位点。这些直肠后病变在病因和病理上多种多样。进展性囊肿代表大多数直肠后肿瘤。虽然直肠后肿瘤大部分是良性，但恶性并非少见，在更大的研究中其发生率从 0～60% 不等。大多数直肠后肿瘤是在常规查体中偶然发现。因为与这些肿瘤相关的症状很不典型，对该疾病的高度怀疑需要进行正确的病理诊断。除了数字直肠检查，先进的成像系统、CT、MRI 可在外科手术计划前作为必要的检查，极少推荐术前组织活检，而手术对于良恶性直肠后肿瘤均获得推荐。直肠后间隙可经多种途径到达，主要有经腹骶联合入路及后入路。腹腔镜是近来治疗肿瘤的外科手术方式。尾骨切除不常规应用。良性肿瘤提示高生存率及低复发率，而恶性肿块总体预后很差。非手术治疗作为脊索瘤的辅助治疗仍在继续发展。

参考文献

1. Böhm B, Milsom JW, Fazio VW, Lavery IC, Church JM, Oakley JR. Our approach to the management of congenital presacral tumors in adults. Int J Colorectal Dis. 1993;8:134–8.
2. Uhlig BE, Johnson RL. Presacral tumors and cysts in adults. Dis Colon Rectum. 1975;18:581–96.
3. La Quaglia MP, Feins N, Fraklis A, Hendren WH. Rectal duplications. J Pediatr Surg. 1990;25:980–4.
4. Sobrado CW, Mester M, Simonsen OS, Justo CR, de Abreu JN, Habr-Gama A. Retrorectal tumors complicating pregnancy: report of two cases. Dis Colon Rectum. 1996;39:1176–9.
5. Nivatvongs S, Gordon PH. Surgical anatomy. In: Gordon PH, Nivatvongs S, editors. Principles and practice of surgery for the colon, rectum, and anus. 2nd ed. St. Louis: Quality Medical Publishing, Inc.; 1999. p. 3–39.
6. Dunn KB. Retrorectal tumors. Surg Clin North Am. 2010;90:163–71.
7. Hassan I, Wietfeldt ED. Presacral tumors: diagnosis and management. Clin Colon Rectal Surg. 2009;22:84–93.
8. Church JM, Raudkivi PJ, Hill GL. The surgical anatomy of the rectum – a review with particular relevance to the hazards of rectal mobilisation. Int J Colorectal Dis. 1987;2:158–66.
9. Wolpert A, Beer-Gabel M, Lifschitz O, Zbar AP. The management of presacral masses in the adult. Tech Coloproctol. 2002;6:43–9.
10. Hannon J, Subramony C, Scott-Conner CEH. Benign retrorectal tumors in adults: the choice of operative approach. Am Surg. 1994;60:267–72.
11. Sato K, Sato T. The vascular and neuronal composition of the lateral ligament of the rectum and the rectosacral fascia. Surg Radiol Anat. 1991;13:17–22.
12. Gordon PH. Retrorectal tumors. In: Gordon PH, Nivatvongs S, editors. Principles and practices of surgery for the colon, rectum, and anus. 2nd ed. St. Louis. Quality Medical Publishing, Inc.; 1999. p. 428–45.
13. Chapuis P, Bokey L, Fahrer M, Sinclair G, Bogduk N. Mobilization of the rectum: anatomic concepts and the bookshelf revisited. Dis Colon Rectum. 2002;45:1–9.
14. Dozois EJ, Jacofsky DJ, Dozois RR. Presacral tumors. In: Wolff BG, Fleshman JW, Beck DE, Pemberton JH, Wexner SD, editors. The ASCRS textbook of colon and rectal surgery. New York:

Springer; 2007. p. 501–14.
15. Garcia-Armengol J, Garcia-Botello S, Martinez-Soriano F, Roig JV, Lledo S. Review of the anatomic concepts in relation to the retrorectal space and endopelvic fascia: Waldeyer's fascia and the rectosacral fascia. Colorectal Dis. 2008;10:298–302.
16. Woodfield JC, Chalmers AG, Phillips N, Sagar PM. Algorithms for the surgical management of retrorectal tumors. Br J Surg. 2007;95:214–21.
17. Larsen WJ. Development of the gastrointestinal tract. In: Human embryology. New York: Churchill Livingstone; 1993. p. 205–34.
18. Moore K, Persaud T. The developing human: clinically oriented embryology. 7th ed. Philadelphia: Saunders; 2003.
19. Sadler T. Langman's medical embryology. 10th ed. Philadelphia: Lippincott Williams & Wilkins; 2006.
20. Hjermstad BM, Helwig EB. Tailgut cysts: report of 53 cases. Am J Clin Pathol. 1988;89:139–47.
21. Penington EC, Hutson JM. The cloacal plate: the missing link in anorectal and urogenital development. BJU Int. 2002;89:726–32.
22. Akita K, Yamaguchi K, Sasaki C, Sato T. An embryological study of the anorectal system in mice. J Anat. 2002;201:417–34.
23. Ghosh J, Eglinton T, Frizelle FA, Watson AJM. Presacral tumours in adults. Surgeon. 2007;5:31–8.
24. Chene G, Voitellier M. Teratome benin mature pre-sacre et formations kystiques vestigiales retro-rectales chez l'adulte. J Chir. 2006;143:310–3.
25. Thway K, Polson A, Pope R, Thomas JM, Fisher C. Extramammary paget disease in a retrorectal dermoid cyst: report of a unique case. Am J Surg Pathol. 2008;32:635–9.
26. Larsen WJ. Human embryology. 1st ed. New York: Churchill Livingstone; 1993.
27. Coco C, Manno A, Mattana C, Verbo A, Sermoneta D, Franceschini G, et al. Congenital tumors of the retrorectal space in the adult: report of two cases and review of the literature. Tumori. 2008;94:602–7.
28. Stockman JM, Young VT, Jenkins AL. Duplication of the rectum containing gastric mucosa. JAMA. 1960;173:1223–5.
29. Kraft RO. Duplication anomalies of the rectum. Ann Surg. 1962;155:230–2.
30. Alavanja G, Kaderabek DJ, Habegger ED. Rectal duplication in an adult. Am Surg. 1995;61:997–1000.
31. MacLeod JH, Purves JKB. Duplications of the rectum. Dis Colon Rectum. 1970;13:133–7.
32. Monek O, Martin L, Heyd B, Mantion G. Rectal duplication in an adult: unusual cause of a buttock mass. Dis Colon Rectum. 1999;42:816–8.
33. Veeneklaas G. Pathogenesis of intrathoracic gastrogenic cysts. Am J Dis Child. 1952;83:500–7.
34. Edwards H. Congenital diverticula of the intestine: with the report of a case exhibiting heterotopia. Br J Surg. 1929;17:7–21.
35. Aslan E. Transvaginal excision of a retrorectal tumor presenting as rectocele. Int Urogynecol J. 2008;19:1715–7.
36. Chen M-L, Su J-M, Cheng Y-M, Chou C-Y, Kuo P-L. Presacral epidermoid cyst with right hydronephrosis. Taiwan J Obstet Gynecol. 2006;45:155–8.
37. Yang DM, Kim HC, Lee HL, Lee SH, Kim GY. Squamous cell carcinoma arising from a presacral epidermoid cyst: CT and MR findings. Abdom Imaging. 2007;33:498–500.
38. Sharpe LA, Van Oppen DJA. Laparoscopic removal of a benign pelvic retroperitoneal dermoid cyst. J Am Assoc Gynecol Laparosc. 1995;2:223–6.
39. Wagner M, Zastrow R, Reasa DA. Presacral tumors: case report, review of the literature. Clin Anat. 1995;8:227–30.
40. Lovelady S, Dockerty M. Extragenital pelvic tumors in women. Am J Obstet Gynecol. 1949;58:215–34.
41. Lev-Chelouche D, Gutman M, Goldman G, Even-Sapir E, Meller I, Issakov J, et al. Presacral tumors: a practical classification and treatment of a unique and heterogenous group of diseases. Surgery. 2003;133:473–8.
42. Freier DT, Stanley JC, Thompson NW. Retrorectal tumors in adults. Surg Gynecol Obstet. 1971;132:681–6.
43. Localio SA, Eng K, Ranson JHC. Abdominosacral approach for retrorectal tumors. Ann Surg. 1980;191:555–9.
44. Cody HS, Marcove RC, Quan SH. Malignant retrorectal tumors: 28 years' experience at Memorial Sloan-Kettering Cancer Center. Dis Colon Rectum. 1981;24:501–6.
45. Jao S-W, Beart RW, Spencer RJ, Reiman HM, Ilstrup DM. Retrorectal tumors: mayo clinic experience, 1960–1979. Dis Colon Rectum. 1985;28:644–52.
46. Lee RA, Symmonds RE. Presacral tumors in the female: clinical presentation, surgical management, and results. Obstet Gynecol. 1988;71:216–21.
47. Wang JY, Hsu CH, Changchien CR, Chen JS, Hsu KC, You YT, et al. Presacral tumor: a review of forty-five cases. Am Surg. 1995;61:310–5.
48. Pidala MJ, Eisenstat TE, Rubin RJ, Salvati EP. Presacral cysts: transrectal excision in select patients. Am Surg. 1999;65:112–5.
49. Smith JJ, Tekkis PP, Heriot AG, Tarioni D, Talbot IC, Northover JMA. Retrorectal tumours: tertiary unit experience and management. Colorectal Dis. 2004;6(1):84.
50. Glasgow SC, Birnbaum EH, Lowney JK, Fleshman JW, Kodner IJ, Mutch DG, et al. Retrorectal tumors: a diagnostic and therapeutic challenge. Dis Colon Rectum. 2005;48:1581–7.
51. Buchs N, Taylor S, Roche B. The posterior approach for low retrorectal tumors in adults. Int J Colorectal Dis. 2007;22:381–5.
52. Grandjean J-P, Mantion G-A, Guinier D, Henry L, Cherki S, Passebois L, et al. Tumeurs cystiques vestigiales retrorectales de l'adulte: une serie de 30 cas. [Vestigial cystic retrorectal tumours in adults: a series of 30 cases]. Gastroenterol Clin Biol. 2008;32:769–78.
53. Pappalardo G, Frattaroli FM, Casciani E, Moles N, Mascagni D, Spoletini D, et al. Retrorectal tumors: the choice of surgical approach based on a new classification. Am Surg. 2009;75:240–8.
54. Mathis KL, Dozois EJ, Grewal MS, Metzger P, Larson DW, Devine RM. Malignant risk and surgical outcomes of presacral tailgut cysts. Br J Surg. 2010;97:575–9.
55. McCune WS. Management of sacrococcygeal tumors. Ann Surg. 1964;159:911–8.
56. Sasaki A, Sugita S, Horimi K, Yasuda K, Inomata M. Retrorectal epidermoid cyst in an elderly woman: report of a case. Surg Today. 2008;38:761–4.
57. Spencer J, Jackman RJ. Surgical management of precoccygeal cysts. Surg Gynecol Obstet. 1962;115:449–52.
58. Hobson KG, Ghaemmaghami V, Roe JP, Goodnight JE, Khatri VP. Tumors of the retrorectal space. Dis Colon Rectum. 2005;48:1964–74.
59. Krivokapic Z, Grubor N, Micev M, Colovic R. Anterior sacral meningocele with presacral cysts: report of a case. Dis Colon Rectum. 2004;47:1965–9.
60. Guillem P, Ernst O, Herjean M, Triboulet JP. Tumeurs retrorectales: interet de la voie abdominale isolee. Ann Chir. 2001;126:138–42.
61. Singer MA, Cintron JR, Martz JE, Schoetz DJ, Abcarian H. Retrorectal cyst: a rare tumor frequently misdiagnosed. J Am Coll Surg. 2003;196:880–6.
62. Dahan H, Arrive L, Wendum D, Ducou le Pointe H, Djouhri H, Tubiana J-M. Retrorectal developmental cysts in adults: clinical and radiographic-histopathologic review, differential diagnosis and treatment. Radiographics. 2001;21:575–84.
63. Dohn K, Povlsen O. Enterocystomas: report of six cases. Acta Chir Scand. 1951;102:21.
64. Stockman JM, Young VT, Sholes DM. Duplication of the rectum. Dis Colon Rectum. 1960;13:223–9.
65. Palanivelu C, Rangarajan M, Senthilkumar R, Madankumar MV, Annapoorni S. Laparoscopic and perineal excision of an infected "dumb-bell" shaped retrorectal epidermoid cyst. J Laparoendosc Adv Surg Tech A. 2008;18:88–92.
66. Ashley WW, Wright NM. Resection of a giant anterior sacral meningocele via an anterior approach: case report and review of literature. Surg Neurol. 2006;66:89–93.
67. Trapp C, Farage L, Clatterbuck RE, Romero FR, Rais-Bahrami S, Long DM, Kavoussi LR. Laparoscopic treatment of anterior sacral meningocele. Surg Neurol. 2007;68:443–8.

68. Negro F, Mercuri M, Ricciardi V, Massari M, Destito C, Mafucci S, et al. Presacral epidermoid cyst. A case report. Ann Ital Chir. 2005;77:75–7.
69. Lin S-L, Yang A-H, Liu H-C. Tailgut cyst with carcinoid: a case report. Chin Med J (Taipei). 1992;49:57–60.
70. Lim K-E, Hsu W-C, Wang C-R. Tailgut cyst with malignancy: MR imaging findings. AJR Am J Roentgenol. 1997;170:1488–90.
71. Rogers A, Simpson E, Atherstone A. Adenocarcinoma in a retrorectal cystic hamartoma. S Afr J Surg. 2007;45:148–50.
72. Tampi C, Lotwala V, Lakdawala M, Coelho K. Retrorectal cyst hamartoma (tailgut cyst) with malignant transformation. Gynecol Oncol. 2007;105:266–8.
73. Jarboui S, Jarraya H, Ben Mihoub M, Abdesselem MM, Zaouche A. Retrorectal cystic hamartoma associated with malignant disease. Can J Surg. 2008;51:E115–6.
74. Krivokapic Z, Dimitrijevic I, Barisic G, Markovic V, Krstic M. Adenosquamous carcinoma arising within a retrorectal tailgut cyst: report of a case. World J Gastroenterol. 2005;11:6225–7.
75. Zappa L, Godwin TA, Sugarbaker PH. Tailgut cyst, an ususual cause of pseudomyxoma peritonei. Tumori. 2009;95:514–7.
76. Yamaguchi K, Okushiba S, Katoh H, Shimizu M, Taneichi H. Tailgut cyst invaded by rectal cancer through an anal fistua: report of a case. Dis Colon Rectum. 2001;44:447.
77. Salameh JR, Votanopoulos KI, Hilal RE, Essien FA, Williams MD, Barroso AO, Sweeney JF, Brunicardi FC. Rectal duplication cyst in an adult: the laparoscopic approach. J Laparoendosc Adv Surg Tech A. 2002;12:453–6.
78. Orr MM, Edwards AJ. Neoplastic change in duplications of the alimentary tract. Br J Surg. 1975;62:269–74.
79. Roy J, Mirnezami A, Gatt M, Sasapu KK, Scott N, Sagar PM. A rare case of Paget's disease in a retrorectal dermoid cyst. Colorectal Dis. 2010;12:944–7.
80. Nishie A, Yoshimitsu K, Honda H, Irie H, Aibe H, Shinozaki K, et al. Presacral dermoid cyst with scanty fat component: usefulness of chemical shift and diffusion-weighted MR imaging. Comput Med Imaging Graph. 2003;27:293–6.
81. Jang S-H, Jang K-S, Song Y-S, Min KW, Han HX, Lee KG, et al. Unusual prerectal location of a tailgut cyst: a case report. World J Gastroenterol. 2006;12:5081–3.
82. Ueda K, Tsunoda A, Nakamura A, Kobayashi H, Shimizu Y, Kusano M, et al. Presacral epidermoid cyst: report of a case. Jpn J Surg. 1998;28:665–8.
83. Sharma D, Nandini R, Goel D, Ghosh A, Shukla RC, Shukla VK. Retrorectal dermoid cyst in an adult. ANZ J Surg. 2008;78:408.
84. Sciubba DM, Petteys RJ, Garces-Ambrossi GL, Noggle JC, McGirt MJ, Wolinsky JP, et al. Diagnosis and management of sacral tumors: a review. J Neurosurg Spine. 2009;10:244–56.
85. Abel ME, Nelson R, Prasad L, Pearl RK, Orsay CP, Abcarian H. Parasacrococcygeal approach for the resection of retrorectal developmental cysts. Dis Colon Rectum. 1985;28:855–8.
86. Sanchez AA, Iglesias CD, López CD, Cecilia DM, Gómez JA, Barbadillo JG, et al. Rectothecal fistula secondary to an anterior sacral meningocele. J Neurosurg Spine. 2008;8:487–9.
87. Phillips JT, Brown SR, Mitchell P, Shorthouse AJ. Anaerobic meningitis secondary to a rectothecal fistula arising from an anterior sacral meningocele: report of a case and review of the literature. Dis Colon Rectum. 2006;49:1633–5.
88. Satyadas T, Davies M, Nasir N, Halligan S, Akle CA. Tailgut cyst associated with a pilonidal sinus: an unusual case and a review. Colorectal Dis. 2002;4:201–4.
89. Gunkova P, Martinek L, Dostalik J, Gunka I, Vavra P, Mazur M. Laparoscopic approach to retrorectal cyst. World J Gastroenterol. 2008;14:6581 3.
90. Piura B, Rabinovich A, Sinelnikov I, Delgado B. Tailgut cyst initially misdiagnosed as ovarian tumor. Arch Gynecol Obstet. 2005;272:301–3.
91. Menassa-Moussa L, Kanso H, Checrallah A, Abboud J, Ghossain M. CT and MR findings of a retrorectal cystic hamartoma confused with an adnexal mass on ultrasound. Eur Radiol. 2005;15:263–6.
92. Verazin G, Rosen L, Khubchandani IT, Sheets JA, Stasik JJ, Riether R. Retrorectal tumor: is biopsy risky? South Med J. 1986;79:1437–9.
93. O'Riordain DS, O'Connell PR, Kirwan WO. Hereditary sacral agenesis with presacral mass and anorectal stenosis: the Currarino triad. Br J Surg. 1991;78:536–8.
94. Crétolle C, Zérah M, Jaubert F, Sarnacki S, Révillon Y, Lyonnet S, et al. New clinical and therapeutic perspectives in Currarino syndrome (study of 29 cases). J Pediatr Surg. 2006;41:126–31.
95. Arora P, Purai N, Rajpurkar M, Kamat D. A missed case of currarino syndrome. Clin Pediatr. 2010;49:183–5.
96. Kochling J, Pistor G, Brands SM, Nasir R, Lanksch WR. The currarino syndrome – hereditary transmitted syndrome of anorectal, sacral and presacral anomalies. Case report and review of the literature. Eur J Pediatr Surg. 1996;6:114–9.
97. Emans PJ, Kootstra G, Marcelis CLM, Beuls EAM, van Heurn LWE. The Currarino triad: the variable expression. J Pediatr Surg. 2005;40:1238–42.
98. Lynch SA, Wang Y, Strachan T. Autosomal dominant sacral agenesis: Currarino syndrome. J Med Genet. 2000;37:561–6.
99. Bellotti C, Montori J, Capponi MG, Cancrini G, Cancrini A. The management of retrorectal congenital tumors. Hepatogastroenterology. 2002;49:687–90.
100. Garcia-Donas J, Rodriguez N, Jara C, Urioste M, Nevado M, Cañamero M, et al. Retrorectal cystic hamartoma as benign cause of CA 19-9 elevation. J Clin Oncol. 2007;25:4012–4.
101. Cho BC, Kim NK, Lim BJ, Kang SO, Sohn JH, Roh JK, et al. A Carcinoembryonic antigen-secreting adenocarcinoma arising in tailgut cyst: clinical implications of Carcinoembryonic antigen. Yonsei Med J. 2005;46:555–61.
102. Varga PP, Bors I, Lazary A. Sacral tumors and management. Orthop Clin North Am. 2009;40:105–23.
103. Rapport RL, Ferguson GS. Dorsal approach to presacral biopsy: technical case report. Neurosurgery. 1997;40:1087–8.
104. Jeon B, Kim D, Kwon K. Anterior endoscopic treatment of a huge anterior sacral meningocele: technical case report. Neurosurgery. 2003;52:1231–3.
105. Sciaudone G, Di Stazio C, Guadagni I, Pellino G, De Rosa M, Selvaggi F. Retrorectal epidermoid cyst – a rare entity: the effectiveness of a transperineal posterior approach. Acta Chir Belg. 2009;109:392–5.
106. Dozois EJ, Malireddy KK, Bower TC, Stanson AW, Sim FH. Management of a retrorectal lipomatous hemangiopericytoma by preoperative vascular embolization and a multidisciplinary surgical team: report of a case. Dis Colon Rectum. 2009;52:1017–20.
107. Yang H, Zhu L, Ebraheim NA, Liu J, Shapiro A, Castillo S, et al. Surgical treatment of sacral chordomas combined with transcatheter arterial embolization. J Spinal Disord Tech. 2010;23:47–52.
108. Grundfest-Broniatowski S, Marks K, Fazio VW. Diagnosis and management of sacral and retrorectal tumors. In: Fazio VW, Church JM, Delaney CP, editors. Current therapy in colon and rectal surgery. 2nd ed. Philadelphia: Elsevier Mosby; 1990. p. 153–60.
109. Bax NMA, van der Zee DC. The laparoscopic approach to sacrococcygeal teratomas. Surg Endosc. 2003;18:128–30.
110. Chen Y, Xu H, Li Y, Li J, Wang D, Yuan J, et al. Laparoscopic resection of presacral teratomas. J Minim Invasive Gynecol. 2008;15:649–51.
111. Lee KH, Tam YH, Chan KW, Cheung ST, Sihoe J, Yeung CK. Laparoscopic-assisted excision of sacrococcygeal teratoma in children. J Laparoendoscand Adv Surg Tech A. 2008;18:296–301.
112. Witherspoon P, Armitage J, Gatt M, Sagar PM. Laparoscopic excision of retrorectal schwannoma. Dis Colon Rectum. 2010;53:101–3.
113. Konstantinidis K, Theodoropoulos GE, Sambalis G, Georgiou M, Vorias M, Anastassakou K, et al. Laparoscopic resection of presacral schwannomas. Surg Laparosc Endosc Percutan Tech. 2005;15:302–4.
114. Yang C-C, Chen H-C, Chen C-M. Endoscopic resection of a presacral schwannoma: case report. J Neurosurg Spine. 2007;7:86–9.
115. Melvin WS. Laparoscopic resection of a pelvic schwannoma. Surg Laparosc Endosc. 1996;6:489–91.
116. Kanemitsu T, Kojima T, Yamamoto S, Koike A, Takeshige K,

Naruse T. The transsphincteric and transsacral approaches for the surgical excision of rectal and presacral lesions. Jpn J Surg. 1993;23:860–6.
117. Zoller S, Joos A, Dinter D, Back W, Horisberger K, Post S, et al. Retrorectal tumors: excision by transanal endoscopic microsurgery. Rev Esp Enferm Dig. 2007;99:547–50.
118. Madanes AE, Kennison RD, Mitchell GW. Removal of a presacral tumor via a Schuchardt incision. Obstet Gynecol. 1981;57:94S–6.
119. Adson AW. Spina bifida cystica of the pelvis: diagnosis and surgical treatment. Minn Med. 1938;21:468–75.
120. Mousseau L, Konno T. Duplication of the rectum. Can J Surg. 1963;6:438–44.
121. Tomita K, Tsuchiya H. Total sacrectomy and reconstruction for huge sacral tumors. Spine. 1980;15:1223–7.
122. Baratti D, Gronchi A, Pennacchioli E, Lozza L, Colecchia M, Fiore M, et al. Chordoma: natural history and results in 28 patients treated at a single institution. Ann Surg Oncol. 2002;10:291–6.
123. Bergh P, Kindblom L-G, Gunterberg B, Remotti F, Ryd W, Meis-Kindblom JM. Prognostic factors in chordoma of the sacrum and mobile spine: a study of 39 patients. Cancer. 2000;88:2122–34.
124. Schwab JH, Healey JH, Rose P, Casas-Ganem J, Boland PJ. The surgical management of sacral chordomas. Spine. 2009;34:2700–4.
125. Stacchiotti S, Marrari A, Tamborini E, Palassini E, Virdis E, Messina A, et al. Response to imatinib plus sirolimus in advanced chordoma. Ann Oncol. 2009;20:1886–94.
126. Stacchiotti S, Ferrari S, Ferraresi V. Imatinib mesylate in advanced chordoma: a multicenter phase II study. J Clin Oncol. 2007;25(18):10003.
127. Hof H, Welzel T, Debus J. Effectiveness of cetuximab/gefitinib in the therapy of a sacral chordoma. Onkologie. 2006;29:572–4.

第 51 章 直肠脱垂手术失败后的治疗方法

David J. Maron · Juan J. Nogueras
杨 东 译 王荫龙 审校

摘 要

本章介绍了佛罗里达州克利夫兰医学中心治疗复发性直肠脱垂的方法。目前对于初发完全性直肠脱垂患者的治疗方法还存在争议，而对于复发型则更是如此。但是对于原本不太适合开腹手术的患者，现在越来越倾向于选择腹腔镜及机器人辅助手术。在这种背景下，会阴部手术也在逐渐改变，对于复发性直肠脱垂合并大便失禁患者，肛镜下直肠切除术的作用目前还不清楚，需要有一个专家共识。

关键词

直肠脱垂；完全性直肠脱垂；Ripstein 术；Ivalon 海绵植入术；经腹直肠固定术；经腹直肠固定 + 乙状结肠切除术；经会阴直肠乙状结肠切除术；Delorme 术；Thiersch 术

引 言

直肠脱垂是指直肠全层通过肛门括约肌向外突出。直肠全层脱垂产生并进展的因素除了解剖缺陷，如肛提肌分离、肛门括约肌松弛、直肠前凸、乙状结肠冗长、由于附着于骶骨及盆壁的组织疏松导致的直肠水平位置的改变等，还有很多其他因素。直肠脱垂在女性中更常见，并且往往合并有慢性便秘及精神疾病。

尽管直肠脱垂早在公元前 1500 年即被人们认识，但迄今为止一直没有一种完美的手术修补方法。直肠脱垂的手术方式有很多，包括直肠固定术、直肠固定联合直肠切除术、经会阴直肠乙状结肠切除术、黏膜袖状切除术、Thiersch 术等，手术方式的选择主要受到手术死亡率及复发率的影响，所以，对于老年人及高风险患者通常避免经腹修补。另外，对于完全性直肠脱垂的男性患者，经腹修补术后可能存在的性功能改变也是需要考虑的一个因素。

由于修补方式的不同（表 51.1），文献报道的术后复发率也不一样。一般来说，经腹手术要比经会阴手术复发率低，后者复发率可高达 50%。Ripstein 术是用补片包绕直肠并将其固定于骶前筋膜。Tjandra 等[1]报道了 142 例经腹直肠前悬吊术病例，术后便秘更普遍，术后复发 11 例，占 8%。

治疗直肠脱垂更常采用的经腹方法为直肠固定术及直肠固定联合冗长乙状结肠切除术，后者通常适用于有慢性便秘病史的患者。Husa 等[2]报道了 48 例直肠固定联合乙状结肠切除术患者，对他们随访平均 4.3 年（1~10 年），复发率为 9%。尽管理论上由于有吻合口与骶前组织间纤维化形成，直肠

表 51.1 不同手术方法的复发率

研究者（年代）	患者数量	复发率（%）
Ripstein procedure		
Ripstein (1972)[13]	289	0
Biehl 等 (1978)[14]	22	10
Gordon and Hoexter (1978)[15]	1111	2.3
Eisenstat 等 (1979)[16]	30	0
Failes et 等 (1979)[17]	53	5.7
Romero-Torres (1979)[18]	24	0
Morgan (1980)[19]	64	1.6
Roberts 等 (1988)[20]	135	9.6
Leenen and Kuijpers (1989)[21]	64	0
Tjandra 等 (1993)[1]	134	8
Winde 等 (1993)[22]	35	0
Schultz 等 (2000)[23]	105	2
Ivalon sponge procedure		
Morgan 等 (1972)[24]	150	3.2
Penfold and Hawley (1972)[25]	101	3
Stewar (1972)[26]	41	7.3
Boutsis and Ellis (1974)[27]	26	11.5
Anderson 等 (1984)[28]	42	2.4
Atkinson and Taylor (1984)[29]	40	10
Boulous 等 (1984)[30]	32	15.6
Kuijpers and de Morree (1988)[31]	30	0
Arndt and Pircher (1988)[32]	62	6.4
Yoshioka 等 (1989)[33]	165	1.5
Sayfan 等 (1990)[34]	16	0
Luukkonen 等 (1992)[35]	15	0
Novell 等 (1994)[36]	31	3.2
Abdominal rectopexy		
Loygue 等 (1971)[37]	140	3.6
Blatchford 等 (1989)[38]	42	2
Solomon and Eyers (1996)[39]	45	0
Boccasanta 等 (1999)[40]	23	13
Solomon 等 (2002)[41]	39	2.5
Byrne 等 (2008)[42]	321	4
Abdominal rectopexy and sigmoid resection		
Watts 等 (1985)[43]	102	1.9
Husa 等 (1985)[2]	48	9
Sayfan 等 (1990)[34]	13	0
Mckee 等 (1990)[44]	9	0
Luukkonen 等 (1992)[35]	15	0
Huber 等 (1995)[45]	39	0
Xynos 等 (1999)[46]	18	0
Perineal rectosigmoidectomy		
Altemeier 等 (1971)[47]	106	3

表 51.1 续

研究者（年代）	患者数量	复发率（%）
Gopal 等 (1984)[48]	18	6
Finlay and Aitchison (1991)[49]	17	6
Williams 等 (1992)[50]	114	11
Johansen 等 (1993)[51]	20	0
Agachan 等 (1997)[52]	32	13
Kim (1999)[53]	183	16
Azimuddin 等 (2001)[54]	36	16
Kimmins (2001)[55]	63	16
Schutz (2001)[56]	31	0
Zbar 等 (2002)[57]	80	4
Delorme procedure		
Uhlig and Sullivan (1979)[58]	44	7
Monson 等 (1986)[59]	27	7
Graf 等 (1992)[60]	14	21
Senapati 等 (1994)[61]	32	13
Oliver 等 (1994)[62]	41	22
Tobin and Scott (1994)[63]	43	26
Liberman 等 (2000)[64]	34	0
Watts 等 (2000)[65]	101	27
Watkins 等 (2000)[66]	52	10
Thiersch procedure		
Jackaman 等 (1980)[67]	52	33
Labow 等 (1980)[68]	9	0
Hunt 等 (1985)[69]	41	44
Poole 等 (1985)[70]	15	33
Vongsangnak 等 (1985)[71]	25	39
Earnshaw and Hopkinson (1987)[72]	21	33
Khanduja 等 (1988)[73]	16	0

固定联合乙状结肠切除术具有优势，但实际上联合乙状结肠切除术与单纯直肠固定术相比术后复发率并没有显著不同。用腹腔镜实施上述两种手术方式具有相似的成功率[3-7]。

而最常采用的经会阴部手术方式为 Delorme 术及经会阴直肠乙状结肠切除术。Thiersch 术是指用人造合成补片包绕肛管一周，以此来缩窄肛门并提供机械支撑，但它并没有根治直肠脱垂，仅仅是阻止脱垂肠管的进一步下降，由于复发率高达 44%，这种手术方式已逐渐被淘汰。

Delorme 术指切除脱垂肠管的黏膜及黏膜下层并将肠壁肌肉折叠缝合，这种手术方式的复发率为

0～27%。经会阴直肠乙状结肠切除术指切除直肠及脱垂的乙状结肠，这种手术方式的复发率也可高达16%，但跟前者相比，其复发率要低。

虽然文献上有很多关于初发完全性直肠脱垂的报道，但对于复发性病例则相对报道较少。Hool等[8]报道了克利夫兰医学中心24例复发性直肠脱垂病例，其中9例患者第1次接受的是经会阴手术，而15例患者第1次手术则是经腹完成，后者有10例行Ripstein术。对这些复发病例，采用了25例次的经腹手术以及4例次的经会阴手术，其中有1例再次复发患者经历了3次经腹手术。而复发的原因仅仅在其中12例患者中找到，主要是Ripstein术后补片失去作用。初次复发时间平均为2年，34%的患者术后7个月内即复发。

Fengler等[9]报道了14例复发型直肠脱垂病例，这些患者第1次手术主要采用的是经会阴术式。其中10例采用经会阴直肠切除及肛提肌成形术，2例采用Thiersch术，1例采用Delorme术，1例采用前切除术，其平均复发时间为14个月。10例经会阴直肠切除术的患者中再次手术时5例采用了同样的经会阴直肠切除术，4例采用直肠固定术（其中1例联合直肠切除术），1例采用Thiersch术。直肠前切除术后复发的患者则采用了Delorme术，而Delorme术后复发的患者采用了经会阴直肠切除术，术后平均随访50个月，无再次复发病例。

Pikarsky等[10]比较了两组27对原发性及复发性直肠脱垂病例。对照组原发直肠脱垂病例中7例采用直肠固定术，7例采用Delorme术，7例采用经会阴直肠乙状结肠切除术，4例采用Thiersch术，2例采用直肠切除固定术。而复发病例中14例采用经会阴直肠乙状结肠切除术，8例采用直肠切除固定术，2例采用直肠固定术，2例采用Thiersch术，1例采用Delorme术。原发直肠脱垂组复发率为11.1%，而复发组再次复发率为14.8%，两组复发率无明显差异。研究者得出结论：两组病例在术式选择及术后效果方面无明显差别。

明尼苏达大学的Steele等[11]报道了78例复发性直肠脱垂病例，这也是文献中能找到的最大宗病例报道。该78例病例中61例第一次手术采用经会阴术式，第1次平均复发时间为33个月，29%的复发病例在术后7个月内发生。78例复发病例中，51例二次手术时采用经会阴术式，27例采用经腹术式，术后平均随访9个月，再次复发23例，占29%。二次手术后再次复发率明显升高，经会阴手术组再次复发19例，占全部51例的37.3%，经腹手术组再次复发4例，占全部27例的14.8%。经会阴部手术后再次复发的19例病例中，有6例接受了再一次的经会阴部手术，其中2例再一次复发，占6例再次手术的33%，有11例接受经腹手术，第3次复发率为9.1%。研究者把前后3次手术的复发率一并统计，结果发现经腹入路手术复发率为13%，经会阴入路手术复发率为39%，前者复发率明显低于后者。

经腹腔镜治疗复发性直肠脱垂也有报道。Tsugawa等[12]报道了2例经腹腔镜治疗复发性直肠脱垂病例，该2例病例先前均接受了Gant-Miwa手术，这一术式在日本广为流行，即结扎脱垂肠管的黏膜并联合肛管缩窄术。研究者于腹腔镜下行直肠缝合固定，术后2例患者随访2年，均未复发。

复发性直肠脱垂患者的便秘、大便失禁以及其他盆底异常情况有必要重新评估。排粪造影和直肠测压有利于检测直肠肛管的生理性疾病，而内镜检查有利于排除病理性疾病。年龄及一般健康状况的评估对于选择最佳治疗方式也很重要。了解第一次手术记录也非常必要。无论初发型还是复发型直肠脱垂患者，都没有一个快速可靠的评估方法。对儿童，我们采用超声或者磁共振的方法去确诊合并有巨结肠的罕见病例，治疗上考虑到术后便秘问题，多比较保守[74]。对于那些准备再次行经会阴直肠乙状结肠切除术的患者，似乎（尽管未经证实）术前行肛管直肠测压有一定的价值，只有在排除诱导肛管直肠反射失败或肛管静息压低或两者均排除后，我们才把经会阴直肠乙状结肠切除作为再次手术的一部分[57,75,76]。我们对直肠脱垂术后的复杂生理了解的还不多，也许会有附近直肠顺应性的改变以及其他改变，如提高直肠黏膜的敏感性、继发于脱垂本身的括约肌的破坏、直肠内括约肌舒张功能的改变、直肠肛管向前蠕动协调能力的提高等，术前我们也经常发现直肠蠕动波消失[57,77]。没有证据表明存在直肠脱垂修补术后依然会遗留大便失禁的决定因素[78]。手术治愈直肠脱垂的同时也使80%术前合并大便失禁的患者得到改善[79]。尽管应用术前超声内镜去评估括约肌形态看似合乎逻辑，但没有客观实验证据表明肌肉折叠术会改善原发或继发性直肠脱垂的预后[80]。

复发性直肠脱垂的修补方式主要决定于脱垂本

身以及第一次手术。那些再次手术患者残余结直肠的血供将明显减少，患者可能会遭遇两吻合口之间肠段缺血的情况，这也是我们应该避免的。这个问题既可发生在经会阴直肠乙状结肠切除后再行乙状结肠切除的患者身上，也可发生在先行乙状结肠切除，再行经会阴直肠乙状结肠切除的患者身上，除非术者将吻合口也一并切除，尤其是对于后者。当我们将第一次手术的吻合口一并切除时，经会阴行二次直肠乙状结肠切除术是安全的[111]。Delorme 术是行肠管部分切除术后复发直肠脱垂患者的另一个选择。之前行经会阴直肠乙状结肠切除术的患者再次手术时，如果仅行直肠固定而不切除部分肠管，将非常困难。因为没有足够的周围组织用来固定于骶前。另外，应用腹腔镜技术去治疗经腹直肠固定术后失败的直肠脱垂患者也极具挑战性，即使是对于那些用腹腔镜行直肠骶前固定术很有经验的医生而言也是如此[41]。应用补片行经腹直肠固定术（现在几乎不再采用）后有几乎一半的复发病例主要是跟补片相关技术有关，有的是因为补片自直肠分离或自骶骨分离，有的是因为补片太松弛，有的是因为固定于直肠壁的位置太低[8]。对于儿童的原发和复发性直肠脱垂的治疗在本章范围之外，但是有一些未在成人中采纳的方法可应用于儿童，如经骶骨直肠固定术（Ekehorn 术）[81-82]以及后矢状切口肛门直肠成形术[83]。在这组患者中，直肠脱垂通常见于 4 岁以下儿童，在 1 岁内发病率最高[84]。许多治疗很保守，大部分的儿童复发主要发生在该年龄段之外，通常脱垂更严重，也更需要手术治疗，并且应该考虑采用成人手术方法。完全性直肠脱垂的治疗原则见图 51.1。

完全性直肠脱垂术后复发非常普遍，尤其是经会阴手术，再次复发率也很高，这说明当前治疗手段并没有完全消除其病理基础。尽管如此，再手术对于复发性直肠脱垂患者也是有效的，尤其是经腹部修补[85]。虽然从直观上我们看到对于术后持续大便失禁的患者重要括约肌的损伤可能在后面一段时间内需要处理，但术前成像及生理检测的作用仍不明确。腹腔镜技术和一些新技术（包括便秘患者保留神经的经腹直肠固定术及大便失禁患者的经阴道骶前直肠固定术）[86-89]使得在决定采用标准经肛会阴手术时更困难；最小创伤入路可能会使一些虚弱患者更容易地实施经腹手术[90]。就这一点而言，我们需要做前瞻性对照试验，但考虑到不同年龄以及不同患者并发症的不同，随机起来很困难[91]。

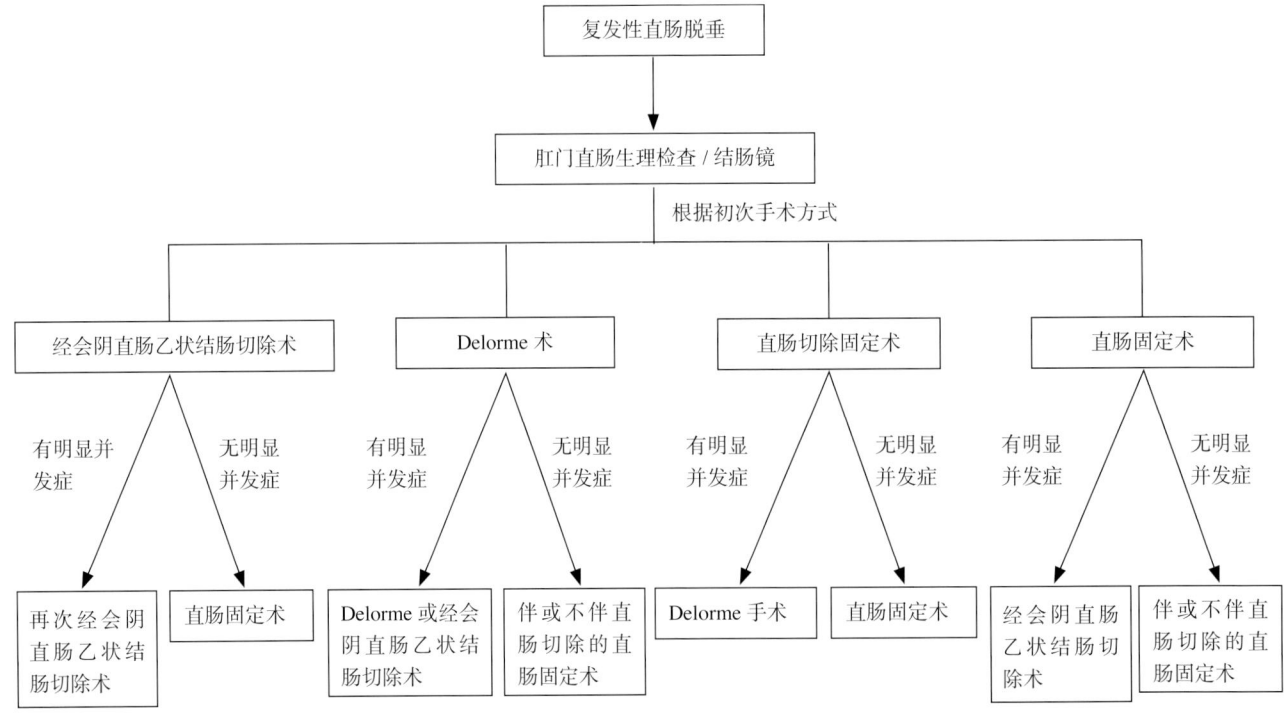

图 51.1　完全性直肠脱垂的治疗原则

讨 论

个体化评估每个患者是非常重要的，因为为每个患者选择最佳治疗方案需要高度地个体化考虑。结直肠吻合术在决定应用于复杂状况之前，如慢性便秘、大便失禁、多盆腔器官脱垂，以及了解它们在原发或复发性直肠脱垂中各自独立的作用之前，有待于了解使用新技术进行纵向、独立研究所得长期随访的复发率。在这些病例中，只有在复发病例中取得足够的成功才能提高生活质量[92]。在这些情况下，提出一种系统的治疗方法有一定难度，这需要术前灵活应用排粪造影、经会阴超声以及核磁共振直肠排粪造影，以明确其他盆腔脏器及软组织是否异常。对于部分这样的患者，需要采取灵活的手术方式[93-95]。

参考文献

1. Tjandra JJ, Fazio VW, Church JM, Milsom JW, Oakley JR, Lavery IC. Ripstein procedure is an effective treatment for rectal prolapse without constipation. Dis Colon Rectum. 1993;36:501–7.
2. Husa A, Sainio P, von Smitten K. Abdominal rectopexy and sigmoid resection (Frykman-Goldberg operation) for rectal prolapse. Acta Chir Scand. 1988;154:221–4.
3. Ashari LH, Lumley JW, Stevenson AR, Stitz RW. Laparoscopically-assisted resection rectopexy for rectal prolapse: ten years' experience. Dis Colon Rectum. 2005;48:982–7.
4. Baker R, Senagore AJ, Luchtefeld MA. Laparoscopic-assisted vs. open resection. Rectopexy offers excellent results. Dis Colon Rectum. 1995;38:199–201.
5. Heah SM, Hartley JE, Hurley J, Duthie GS, Monson JR. Laparoscopic suture rectopexy without resection is effective treatment for full-thickness rectal prolapse. Dis Colon Rectum. 2000;43:638–43.
6. Kairaluoma MV, Viljakka MT, Kellokumpu IH. Open vs. laparoscopic surgery for rectal prolapse: a case-controlled study assessing short-term outcome. Dis Colon Rectum. 2003;46:353–60.
7. Stevenson AR, Stitz RW, Lumley JW. Laparoscopic-assisted resection-rectopexy for rectal prolapse: early and medium follow-up. Dis Colon Rectum. 1998;41:46–54.
8. Hool GR, Hull TL, Fazio VW. Surgical treatment of recurrent complete rectal prolapse: a thirty-year experience. Dis Colon Rectum. 1997;40:270–2.
9. Fengler SA, Pearl RK, Prasad ML, Orsay CP, Cintron JR, Hambrick E, Abcarian H. Management of recurrent rectal prolapse. Dis Colon Rectum. 1997;40:832–4.
10. Pikarsky AJ, Joo JS, Wexner SD, Weiss EG, Nogueras JJ, Agachan F, Iroatulam A. Recurrent rectal prolapse: what is the next good option? Dis Colon Rectum. 2000;43:1273–6.
11. Steele SR, Goetz LH, Minami S, Madoff RD, Mellgren AF, Parker SC. Management of recurrent rectal prolapse: surgical approach influences outcome. Dis Colon Rectum. 2006;49:440–5.
12. Tsugawa K, Sue K, Koyanagi N, Hashizume M, Wada H, Tomikawa M, et al. Laparoscopic rectopexy for recurrent rectal prolapse: a safe and simple procedure without a mesh prosthesis. Hepatogastroenterology. 2002;49:1549–51.
13. Ripstein CB. Procidentia: definitive corrective surgery. Dis Colon Rectum. 1972;15:334–6.
14. Biehl AG, Ray JE, Gathright Jr JB. Repair of rectal prolapse: experience with the Ripstein sling. South Med J. 1978;71:923–5.
15. Gordon PH, Hoexter B. Complications of the Ripstein procedure. Dis Colon Rectum. 1978;21:277–80.
16. Eisenstat TE, Rubin RJ, Salvati EP. Surgical treatment of complete rectal prolapse. Dis Colon Rectum. 1979;22:522–3.
17. Failes D, Killingback M, Stuart M, De Luca C. Rectal prolapse. Aust N Z J Surg. 1979;49:72–5.
18. Romero-Torres R. Sacrofixation with Marlex in massive prolapse of the rectum. Surg Gynecol Obstet. 1979;22:522–3.
19. Morgan B. The teflon sling operation for repair of complete rectal prolapse. Aust N Z J Surg. 1980;50:121–3.
20. Roberts PL, Schoetz Jr DJ, Coller JA, Veidenheimer MC. Ripstein procedure. Lahey Clinic experience: 1963-1985. Arch Surg. 1988;123:554–7.
21. Leenen LP, Kuijpers JH. Treatment of complete rectal prolapse with foreign material. Neth J Surg. 1989;41:129–31.
22. Winde G, Reers B, Nottberg H, Berns T, Meyer J, Bunte H. Clinical and functional results of abdominal rectopexy with absorbable mesh-graft for treatment of complete rectal prolapse. Eur J Surg. 1993;159(5):301–5.
23. Schultz I, Mellgren A, Dolk A, Johansson C, Holmström B. Long-term results and functional outcome after Ripstein rectopexy. Dis Colon Rectum. 2000;43:35–43.
24. Morgan CN, Porter NH, Klugman DJ. Ivalon (polyvinyl alcohol) sponge in the repair of complete rectal prolapse. Br J Surg. 1972;59:841–6.
25. Penfold JC, Hawley PR. Experiences of Ivalon-sponge implant for complete rectal prolapse at St. Mark's Hospital, 1960-70. Br J Surg. 1972;59:846–8.
26. Stewart R. Long-term results of Ivalon wrap operation for complete rectal prolapse. Proc R Soc Med. 1972;65:777–8.
27. Boutsis C, Ellis H. The Ivalon-sponge-wrap operation for rectal prolapse: an experience with 26 patients. Dis Colon Rectum. 1974;17:21–37.
28. Anderson JR, Wilson BG, Parks TG. Complete rectal prolapse–the results of Ivalon sponge rectopexy. Postgrad Med J. 1984;60:411–4.
29. Atkinson KG, Taylor DC. Wells procedure for complete rectal prolapse. A ten-year experience. Dis Colon Rectum. 1984;27:96–8.
30. Boulos PB, Stryker SJ, Nicholls RJ. The long-term results of polyvinyl alcohol (Ivalon) sponge for rectal prolapse in young patients. Br J Surg. 1984;71:213–4.
31. Kuijpers JH, de Morree H. Toward a selection of the most appropriate procedure in the treatment of complete rectal prolapse. Dis Colon Rectum. 1988;31:355–7.
32. Arndt M, Pircher W. Absorbable mesh in the treatment of rectal prolapse. Int J Colorectal Dis. 1988;3:141–3.
33. Yoshioka K, Heyen F, Keighley MR. Functional results after posterior abdominal rectopexy for rectal prolapse. Dis Colon Rectum. 1989;32:835–8.
34. Sayfan J, Pinho M, Alexander-Williams J, Keighley MR. Sutured posterior abdominal rectopexy with sigmoidectomy compared with Marlex rectopexy for rectal prolapse. Br J Surg. 1990;77:143–5.
35. Luukkonen P, Mikkonen U, Jarvinen H. Abdominal rectopexy with sigmoidectomy vs. rectopexy alone for rectal prolapse: a prospective, randomized study. Int J Colorectal Dis. 1992;7:219–22.
36. Novell JR, Osborne MJ, Winslet MC, Lewis AA. Prospective randomized trial of Ivalon sponge versus sutured rectopexy for full-thickness rectal prolapse. Br J Surg. 1994;81:904–6.
37. Loygue J, Huguier M, Malafosse M, Biotois H. Complete prolapse of the rectum. A report on 140 cases treated by rectopexy. Br J Surg. 1971;58.847–8.
38. Blatchford GJ, Perry RE, Thorson AG, Christensen MA. Rectopexy without resection for rectal prolapse. Am J Surg. 1989;158:574–6.
39. Solomon MJ, Eyers AA. Laparoscopic rectopexy using mesh fixation with a spiked chromium staple. Dis Colon Rectum. 1996;39:279–84.

40. Boccasanta P, Venturi M, Reitano MC, Salamina G, Rosati R, Montorsi M. Laparotomic vs. laparoscopic rectopexy in complete rectal prolapse. Dig Surg. 1999;16:415–9.
41. Solomon MJ, Young CJ, Eyers AA, Roberts RA. Randomized clinical trial of laparoscopic versus open abdominal rectopexy for rectal prolapse. Br J Surg. 2002;89:35–9.
42. Byrne CM, Smith SR, Solomon MJ, Young JM, Eyers AA, Young CJ. Long-term functional outcomes after laparoscopic and open rectopexy for the treatment of rectal prolapse. Dis Colon Rectum. 2008;51:1597–604.
43. Watts JD, Rothenberger DA, Buls JG, Goldberg SM, Nivatvongs S. The management of procidentia. 30 years' experience. Dis Colon Rectum. 1985;28:96–102.
44. McKee RF, Lauder JC, Poon FW, Aitchison MA, Finlay IG. A prospective randomized study of abdominal rectopexy with and without sigmoidectomy in rectal prolapse. Surg Gynecol Obstet. 1992;174:145–8.
45. Huber FT, Stein H, Siewert JR. Functional results after treatment of rectal prolapse with rectopexy and sigmoid resection. World J Surg. 1995;19:138–43.
46. Xynos E, Chrysos E, Tsiaoussis J, Epanomeritakis E, Vassilakis JS. Resection rectopexy for rectal prolapse. The laparoscopic approach. Surg Endosc. 1999;13:862–4.
47. Altemeier WA, Culbertson WR, Schowengerdt C, Hunt J. Nineteen years' experience with the one-stage perineal repair of rectal prolapse. Ann Surg. 1971;173:993–1006.
48. Gopal KA, Amshel AL, Shonberg IL, Eftaiha M. Rectal procidentia in elderly and debilitated patients. Experience with the Altemeier procedure. Dis Colon Rectum. 1984;27:376–81.
49. Finlay IG, Aitchison M. Perineal excision of the rectum for prolapse in the elderly. Br J Surg. 1991;78:687–9.
50. Williams JG, Rothenberger DA, Madoff RD, Goldberg SM. Treatment of rectal prolapse in the elderly by perineal rectosigmoidectomy. Dis Colon Rectum. 1992;35:830–4.
51. Johansen OB, Wexner SD, Daniel N, Nogueras JJ, Jagelman DG. Perineal rectosigmoidectomy in the elderly. Dis Colon Rectum. 1993;36:767–72.
52. Agachan F, Reissman P, Pfeifer J, Weiss EG, Nogueras JJ, Wexner SD. Comparison of three perineal procedures for the treatment of rectal prolapse. South Med J. 1997;90:925–32.
53. Kim DS, Tsang CB, Wong WD, Lowry AC, Goldberg SM, Madoff RD. Complete rectal prolapse: evolution of management and results. Dis Colon Rectum. 1999;42:460–9.
54. Azimuddin K, Khubchandani IT, Rosen L, Stasik JJ, Riether RD, Reed JF. Rectal prolapse: a search for the "best" operation. Am Surg. 2001;67:622–7.
55. Kimmins MH, Evetts BK, Isler J, Billingham R. The Altemeier repair: outpatient treatment of rectal prolapse. Dis Colon Rectum. 2001;44:565–70.
56. Schutz G. Extracorporal resection of the rectum in the treatment of complete rectal prolapse using a circular stapling device. Dig Surg. 2001;18:274–8.
57. Zbar AP, Takashima S, Hasegawa T, Kitabayashi K. Perineal rectosigmoidectomy (Altemeier's procedure): a review of physiology, technique and outcome. Tech Coloproctol. 2002;6:109–16.
58. Uhlig BE, Sullivan ES. The modified Delorme operation: its place in surgical treatment for massive rectal prolapse. Dis Colon Rectum. 1979;22:513–21.
59. Monson JR, Jones NA, Vowden P, Brennan TG. Delorme's operation: the first choice in complete rectal prolapse? Ann R Coll Surg Engl. 1986;68:143–6.
60. Graf W, Ejerblad S, Krog M, Påhlman L, Gerdin B. Delorme's operation for rectal prolapse in elderly or unfit patients. Eur J Surg. 1992;158:555–7.
61. Senapati A, Nicholls RJ, Thomson JP, Phillips RK. Results of Delorme's procedure for rectal prolapse. Dis Colon Rectum. 1994;37:456–60.
62. Oliver GC, Vachon D, Eisenstat TE, Rubin RJ, Salvati EP. Delorme's procedure for complete rectal prolapse in severely debilitated patients. An analysis of 41 cases. Dis Colon Rectum. 1994;37:461–7.
63. Tobin SA, Scott IH. Delorme operation for rectal prolapse. Br J Surg. 1994;81:1681–4.
64. Liberman H, Hughes C, Dippolito A. Evaluation and outcome of the delorme procedure in the treatment of rectal outlet obstruction. Dis Colon Rectum. 2000;43:188–92.
65. Watts AM, Thompson MR. Evaluation of Delorme's procedure as a treatment for full-thickness rectal prolapse. Br J Surg. 2000;87:218–22.
66. Watkins BP, Landercasper J, Belzer GE, Rechner P, Knudson R, Bintz M, et al. Long-term follow-up of the modified Delorme procedure for rectal prolapse. Arch Surg. 2003;138:498–503.
67. Jackaman FR, Francis JN, Hopkinson BR. Silicone rubber band treatment of rectal prolapse. Ann R Coll Surg Engl. 1980;62:386–7.
68. Labow S, Rubin RJ, Hoexter B, Salvati EP. Perineal repair of rectal procidentia with an elastic fabric sling. Dis Colon Rectum. 1980;23:467–9.
69. Hunt TM, Fraser IA, Maybury NK. Treatment of rectal prolapse by sphincteric support using silastic rods. Br J Surg. 1985;72:491–2.
70. Poole Jr GV, Pennell TC, Myers RT, Hightower F. Modified Thiersch operation for rectal prolapse. Technique and results. Am Surg. 1985;51:226–9.
71. Vongsangnak V, Varma JS, Smith AN. Reappraisal of Thiersch's operation for complete rectal prolapse. J R Coll Surg Edinb. 1985;30:185–7.
72. Earnshaw JJ, Hopkinson BR. Late results of silicone rubber perianal suture for rectal prolapse. Dis Colon Rectum. 1987;30:86–8.
73. Khanduja KS, Hardy Jr TG, Aguilar PS, Plasencia G, Hartmann RF, Bowers F, et al. A new silicone-prosthesis in the modified Thiersch operation. Dis Colon Rectum. 1988;31:380–3.
74. Hutson JM, McNamara J, Gibb S, Shin YM. Slow transit constipation in children. J Paediatr Child Health. 2001;37(5):426–30.
75. Glasgow SC, Birnbaum EH, Kodner IJ, Fleshman JW, Dietz DW. Preoperative anal manometry predicts continence after perineal proctectomy for rectal prolapsed. Dis Colon Rectum. 2006;49:1052–8.
76. Zbar AP, Nguyen H. Management guidlines for full-thickness rectal prolapsed, Ch. 26. In: Altomare D, Pucciani F, editors. Rectal Prolapse: Diagnosis and Clinical Management. Italy: Springer Verlag; 2008. p. 201–7.
77. Plusa SM, Charig JA, Balaji V, Watts A, Thompson MR. Physiological changes after Delorme's procedure for full-thickness rectal prolapse. Br J Surg. 1995;82:1475–8.
78. Schultz L, Mellgren A, Nilsson BA, Dolk A, Homström B. Preoperative electrophysiologic assessment cannot predict continence after rectopexy. Dis Colon Rectum. 1998;41:1392–8.
79. Bondurri A, Zbar AP, Tapia H, Boffi F, Pescatori M. The relationship between etiology, symptom severity and indications of surgery in cases of anal incontinence: a 25-year analysis of 1046 patients at a tertiary coloproctology practice. Techn Coloproctol. 2011;15(2):159–64.
80. Chun SW, Pikarsky AJ, You SY, Gervaz P, Efron J, Weiss E, et al. Perineal recotsigmoidectomy for rectal prolapse: role of levatorplasty. Techn Coloproctol. 2004;8:3–9.
81. Chino ES, Thomas CG. Transsacral approach to repair of rectal prolapse in children. Am Surg. 1984;50:70–5.
82. Schepens MA, Verhelst AA. Reappraisal of Ekehorn's rectopexy in the management of rectal prolapse in children. J Pediatr Surg. 1993;28:1494–7.
83. Pearl RH, Ein SH, Churchill B. Posterior sagittal anorectoplasty for pediatric recurrent rectal prolapse. J Pediatr Surg. 1989;24:1100–2.
84. Flum AS, Golladay ES, Teitelbaum DH. Recurrent rectal prolapse following primary surgical treatment. Pediatr Surg Int. 2010;26:427–31.
85. Riansuwan W, Hull TL, Bast J, Hammel JP, Church JM. Comparison of perineal operations with abdominal operations for full-thickness rectal prolapse. World J Surg. 2010;34:1116–22.
86. Boons P, Collinson R, Cunningham C, Lindsey I. Laparoscopic ventral rectopexy for external rectal prolapse improves constipation and avoids de novo constipation. Colorectal Dis. 2010;12:526–32.
87. Laubert T, Kleemann M, Schorcht A, Czymek R, Junbluth T, Bader

FG, et al. Laparoscopic resection rectopexy for rectal prolapse: a single-center study during 16 years. Surg Endosc. 2010;24:2401–6.
88. Gurland B, Garrett KA, Firoozi F, Goldman HB. Transvaginal sacrospinous rectopexy: initial clinical experience. Tech Coloproctol. 2010;14:169–73.
89. Lee SH, Lakhtaria P, Canedo J, Lee YS, Wexner SD. Outcome of laparoscopic rectopexy versus perineal rectosigmoidectomy for full-thickness rectal prolapse in elderly patients. Surg Endosc. 2011;25(8):2699–702.
90. Wijffels N, Cunningham C, Dixon A, Greenslade G, Lindsey I. Laparoscopic ventral rectopexy for external rectal prolapse is safe and effective in the elderly. Does this make perineal procedures obsolete? Colorectal Dis. 2011;13:561–6.
91. Phillips RKS. Rectal prolapse – update on the PROSPER trial. Royal Australasian College of Surgeons Annual Scientific Congress 2004; CR 33
92. Kim M, Reibetanz J, Boenicke L, Germer CT, Jayne D, Isbert C. Quality of life after transperineal rectosigmoidectomy. Br J Surg. 2010;97:269–72.
93. Holley RL, Vamer RE, Gleason BP, Apffel LA, Scott S. Recurrent pelvic support defects after sacrospinous ligament fixation for vaginal vault prolapse. J Am Coll Surg. 1995;180:444–8.
94. Tou S, Brown SR, Malik AI, Nelson RL. Surgery for complete rectal prolapse in adults. Cochrane Database Syst Rev 2008: CD001758
95. Huebner M, Krzonkalla M, Tunn R. Abdominal sacrocolpopexy – standardized surgical technique, perioperative management and outcome in women with posthysterectomy vaginal vault prolapse. Gynakol Geburtschilifliche Rundsch. 2009;29:308–14.

第 52 章　藏毛窦疾病复发的治疗

Asha Senapati

曹　磊 译　王荫龙 审校

摘　要

本章概述了对于藏毛窦疾病复发的专科处理。很多更简单的术式正在逐步取代偏离中线皮瓣闭合术对于预后改善的作用。目前有上百种藏毛窦的治疗方法，但这也从另一个角度说明对于藏毛窦的复发，目前仍没有完全有效的治疗方法。

治疗失败往往比原发病更严重，并且在治疗失败后，患者可能出现多年经久不愈的伤口。症状轻微或单个急性脓肿引流的藏毛窦疾病患者，有可能不需要任何干预及随诊。藏毛窦疾病的非外科治疗，如注射苯酚及单独去毛并注意臀沟卫生可能有效，但长期效果未知。简单的疾病需要简单的手术。Pit-picking 术使用 Bascom 技术，具有良好的效果，这种使用环锯去除中心凹陷的技术可以重复应用。改良瓣手术可用于治疗复杂或复发未愈合的中线伤口。

关键词

藏毛窦疾病复发；藏毛窦；不对称切除皮内缝合术（Karydakis 术式）；Bascom 的挑坑术；广泛切除；暴露；皮瓣

引　言

藏毛窦疾病最早在 19 世纪被描述[1]，是一种较常见的疾病[2]，并且在大多数患者中都是很小的问题。目前已经提出 100 多种治疗此病的方法，这更清楚地表明没有一种治疗完全有效，因此治疗失败和疾病复发是不可避免的。然而，由于藏毛窦大多没有症状，应采取失败率和复发率较小的治疗方法，避免采用会导致患者出现严重并发症的治疗方法。

治疗失败往往比原发病更严重，并且在治疗失败后，患者可能出现多年经久不愈的伤口。复发性藏毛窦疾病包括在初始治疗后一段时间内已治愈又再次复发、初始治疗没有成功以及留有进展的后遗症的患者。虽然一旦涉及研究结果的发表，上述分类应具体区分开，但是其治疗方案均相似。为进一步治疗，每种患者的治疗应该一并讨论。在这方面，许多文献刊物不分开讨论这些问题，使得很难从其中获得确切的结论。然而，研究者试图总结已发表的结果[3-5]。

并发症的问题应包括对藏毛窦治疗中平均住院日过长的关注，因为藏毛窦疾病的手术治疗只有极少需要住院。尽管如此，英格兰和威尔士在 2001 年有 11 534 例患者入院治疗，平均住院日为 4.3 天(共 49 596 床日)[6]。自 20 世纪 80 年代以来，40 000 名藏毛窦疾病患者在美国的住院日为 208 000 天，在这方面，估计如果避免过度住院治疗，全美国每年可以节省多达 4 亿美元[7]。

多家中心仍采取完整广泛切除进行治疗[4-5]，

尽管在过去70年中，人们越来越认识到这种治疗方法产生严重并发症的风险很高，现在许多外科医生避免采取广泛切除治疗[8]。手术并发症可能导致患者长时间无法上学或工作，住院治疗一年，伤口填充15个月[9]，伤口不愈长达37年[10-11]，多次（最多13次）手术[10]，中厚皮瓣移植[12]，使用肌肉瓣重建甚至采取放疗[9, 11, 13]。虽然治疗方法已得到改进[4-5]，对某些患者来说，术后并发症仍然比原发病更加严重[14-15]。

藏毛窦疾病的病因学

从复发性疾病病因学开始研究才能够做到对于疾病真正的防止，了解疾病的病因学很有必要。现在人们认识到这是一种获得性、自限性、多发生在青春期的疾病[16]。藏毛窦疾病的危险因素包括年龄在18～30岁之间[2, 17, 18]（很少出现年轻或年长的患者[11, 17, 19, 20]）、男性[2, 18, 21]、多毛症[2, 18, 21]、肥胖和较深的臀沟[17, 21, 22]，以及恶劣的卫生条件（曾被称为"吉普座位"或军事疾病）[2, 9, 17, 21]。此病多见于地中海沿岸国家，东亚、大洋洲和非洲撒哈拉以南地区较罕见。

毛囊[7]或皮肤隐窝的扩大可能是由于束带和皮肤中线拉伸时受力不均[2, 7, 23, 24]、皮肤炎症以及与痤疮类似的毛囊堵塞。Karydakis[25]、Bascom和Bascom[11]发现，在"推移皮瓣"手术术后，"新臀沟"的皮肤，而非别的部位，可能出现毛囊扩张，增加了发展为藏毛窦疾病的可能。然而，在上述过程后，往往是病情反复发作，这是由于在皮瓣下出现慢性感染，而不是新的病灶。高达50%的藏毛窦疾病患者在窦内或脓肿内可能没有毛发[23]，或者毛发并不来自患者自身[26-27]，因此毛发可能是重要的次要因素，而不是原发性原因[7, 28]。

藏毛窦疾病的治疗结果

治疗藏毛窦疾病的方案有很多种，这也反映了没有一种治疗方法是完全安全的，均存在治疗失败及复发的事实。不同治疗方法的成功也证明有不同治疗方案均可供选择。

非外科治疗

对于无症状的患者可以定期观察。活动期患者的非手术治疗包括注意肛周卫生及单独去毛，此法是因为在二战时期由于手术治疗导致长期残疾，在1947年推出[29]。其他3项研究[8, 30, 31]证实超过170例保守治疗的患者的后续手术率较低。去除毛发是重要的治疗之一，最近使用多种不同的脱毛方法[31-32]。自从首次报道藏毛窦疾病，就开始使用注射硬化剂的治疗方法。无需手术切除脓肿，苯酚注射治愈率达到70%以上[33-39]。

非广泛切除脓肿的简单手术

第一次出现急性脓肿的患者超过50%可通过使用单纯引流治疗治愈[40]，即在未来的5年中，没有进一步的问题出现。McLaren的一项研究[41]表明，许多表现为急性脓肿的患者通过非切除手术可以治愈。藏毛窦脓肿应该是通过一个尽量小的切口直接引流。这使得后续手术的计划和实行不会因为过度初始治疗而受到阻碍。

一项近期的大型研究显示[45]，单纯的切开脓肿和藏毛窦以及切口袋形缝合术[42-44]，可以取得良好的疗效，在441例随访1～10年的患者中复发率为1%～6%。进一步研究表示，使用相同治疗但不做袋形缝合术的815例患者也有相似结果，即5%的复发率[46-49]。虽然简单切开有很好的疗效，但是存在开放切口，在某些患者中可能较深，导致修复手术不能达到满意效果。此外，选择偏移由于其主要用于较轻患者而产生。

20世纪60年代，Lord和Millar[28]简化了非切除手术，使用尼龙毛刷清洗藏毛窦，无需切开并第一次正式通过微小的中线切口切除皮肤坑。Bascom[22]强调切除皮肤的重要性，但同时应通过远离中线的外侧切口清洗脓肿（图52.1），这能达到

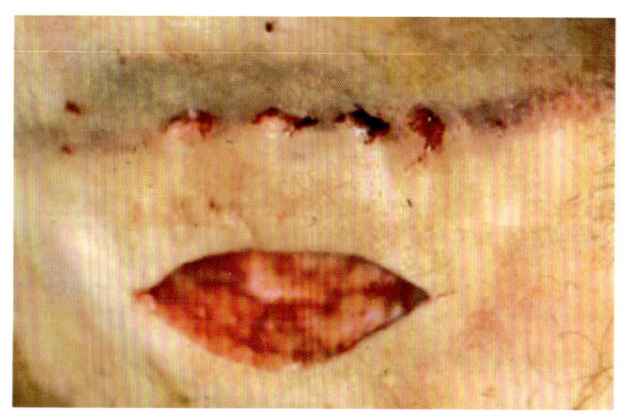

图52.1 侧面切口切开4个皮凹引流

近100%的一期愈合率和10%的复发率。每个坑去除组织量应不大于"一粒米粒"[50]。此过程的总体目标是简单地通过小型中线切口"挑坑"和"留出沟"[51-52]即臀沟。其他患者用此法取得令人满意的预后[52]。

在最近的一项涉及1435例患者的研究表示，使用植皮环钻可简单使中线坑和继发开口达到空心，通过环钻清理脓肿，并不用进行缝合。平均随访近7年后有16.2%的复发率[53]。

单纯切除皮肤坑后的复发率相对较高[22, 28, 52-55]，此治疗可多次重复，这意味着虽然此方法第1次治疗只有不到85%的治愈率，第2次的治愈率则可超过95%。开放性伤口是此治疗方案的另一个缺点。然而，Bascom法治疗后的侧切口，50%在3周时愈合，99%在3个月可愈合，4个月时所有伤口可完全愈合[52]。由于患者可以自理，一个开放的侧切伤口不会推迟其返回正常活动的时间[22,53]。

广泛切除脓肿伴（或不伴）中线皮肤缝合

广泛切除脓肿将导致手术并发症，包括中线切口不愈合[10, 56-58]。目前很少有资料涉及其发生率，但可能高达2%～7%[59-60]。在这方面，因为不愈的伤口大多发生在中线，且藏毛窦疾病是由臀沟环境所造成的，所以在广泛切除术后，无论是缝合或非缝合的中线切口，都有较高风险出现并发症或复发。手术是伤口经久不愈和术后并发症的一个主要原因。然而，应当指出，在臀沟无手术史的患者中也可能出现自发不愈合的伤口。

关于广泛切除治疗的多项非随机研究的系统综述[4-5]指出，虽然完全愈合的时间在中线封闭后可能会缩短，复发率仍可高达22%～41%[14, 15]，而单纯切开非切除治疗的复发率仅约6%[42-46, 48, 61]。

偏离中线皮肤缝合伴（或不伴）广泛脓肿切除

两篇系统综述[4-5]分析了6项随机对照试验（RCTs）[4]后得出的结论是，在切除脓肿后，标准的缝合方法应该是偏离中线皮肤缝合，而不是中线的皮肤缝合[62]。Karydakis偏离中线皮瓣法（图52.2），指一个椭圆形的不对称广泛切除皮肤、脓肿、藏毛窦，游离靠近中线的皮肤边缘从而产生厚的皮瓣，然后将其缝合到远离中线的一侧。皮瓣深面固定于骶尾筋膜[21]。在一项包括从1966—1990年7471病例的研究中，95%的患者随访达到2～20年，Karydakis[25]研究发现，平均住院日为1～3天。大多数迅速愈合，平均休假为9天，55例患者（1%）复发。

Kitchen[62-63]和Bascom[10, 11, 56]改进了Karydakis术式，他们使用较薄的皮瓣及Bascom的"挑坑"术（图52.3、图52.4和图52.5），避免任何的脓肿切除或二次开口。如果脓肿壁较硬，呈立方状，而更容易塌陷。远离中线的脓肿壁的二次切口不需要被包括在切除的伤口中。如果因为引流而扩大开口或者残留的毛发及碎屑形成了窦道，将原来的中线皮坑切除后，切口将愈合。最初的Karydakis术式是在全身麻醉下进行的，改良术已经逐渐能在局部

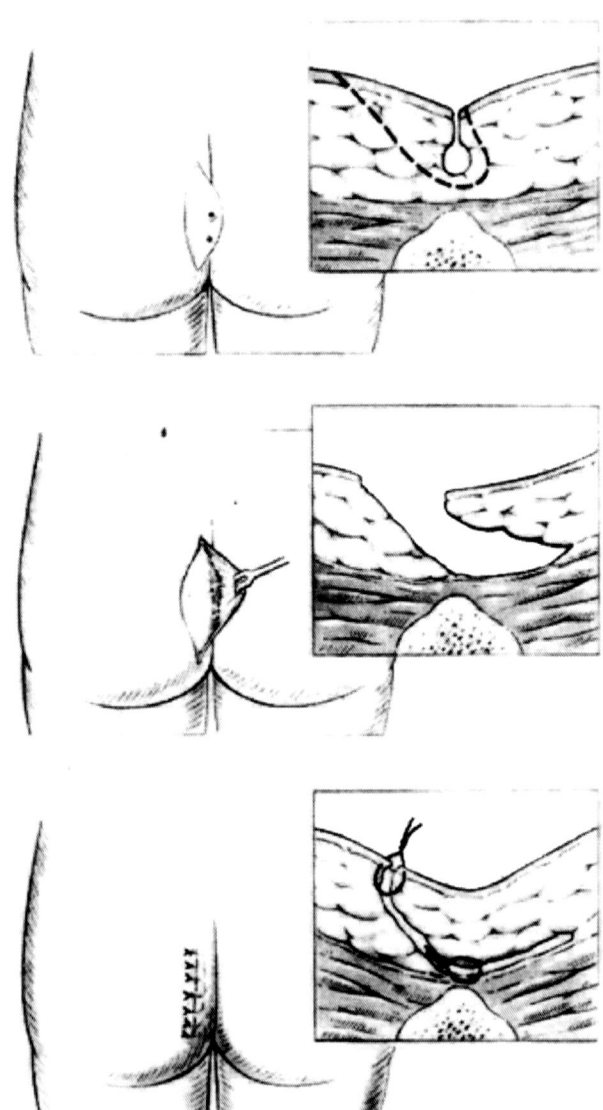

图52.2 图示Karydakis术式。与皮肤一起切除藏毛窦和脓肿（上）和从臀沟的一侧（中）至偏离中线的皮肤缝合（下）

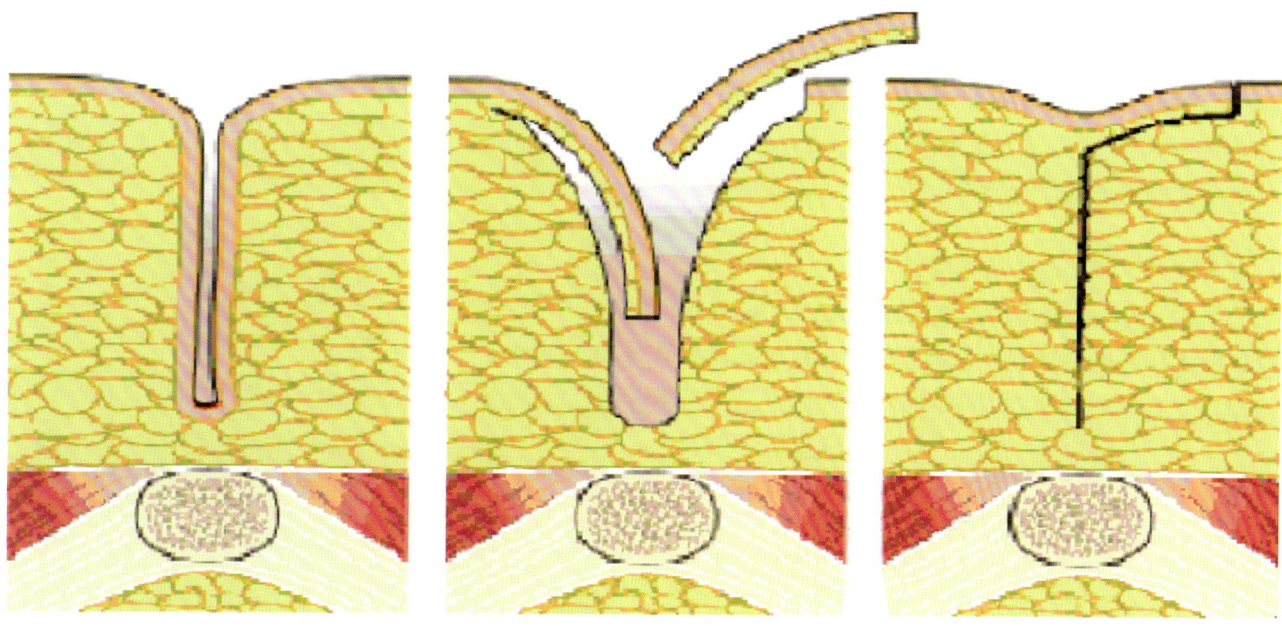

图 52.3　图解 Bascom 挑坑术，从臀沟的一个侧面切除皮肤（左，中），封闭裂口，缝合皮肤至中线的一侧（右）

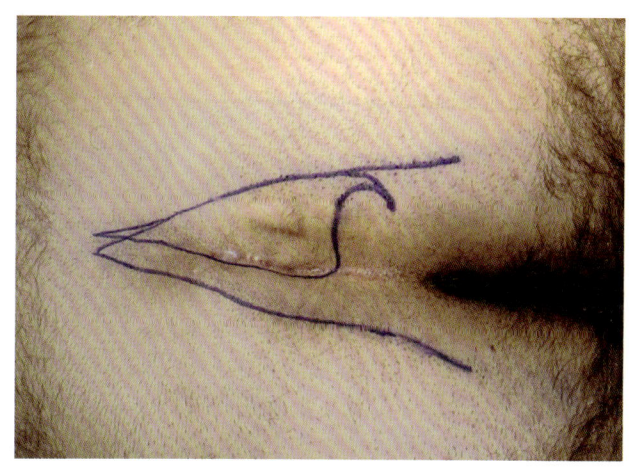

图 52.4　Bascom 挑坑术后的皮肤外观，包括中线皮肤凹坑和臀沟患侧皮肤。将标记的皮肤划线，当患者站起来时，边缘显得自然

麻醉下进行[11,62,63]。

过去的几年中，对 Karydakis 术式的研究[64-74]显示其日益普及，大多数研究得出较好结果，除了一项随机对照试验[75]显示与 Limberg 皮瓣相比，本术具有较高的伤口感染率（26% 和 8%）。虽然有 4%~26% 的患者有切口并发症，包括皮肤坏死、感染、血清肿、血肿、伤口裂开，这些大多可以通过门诊得到治疗。在 60%~70% 的患者伤口在 1 周内完全愈合，在 1~4 周内患者需要极少的社区照顾，

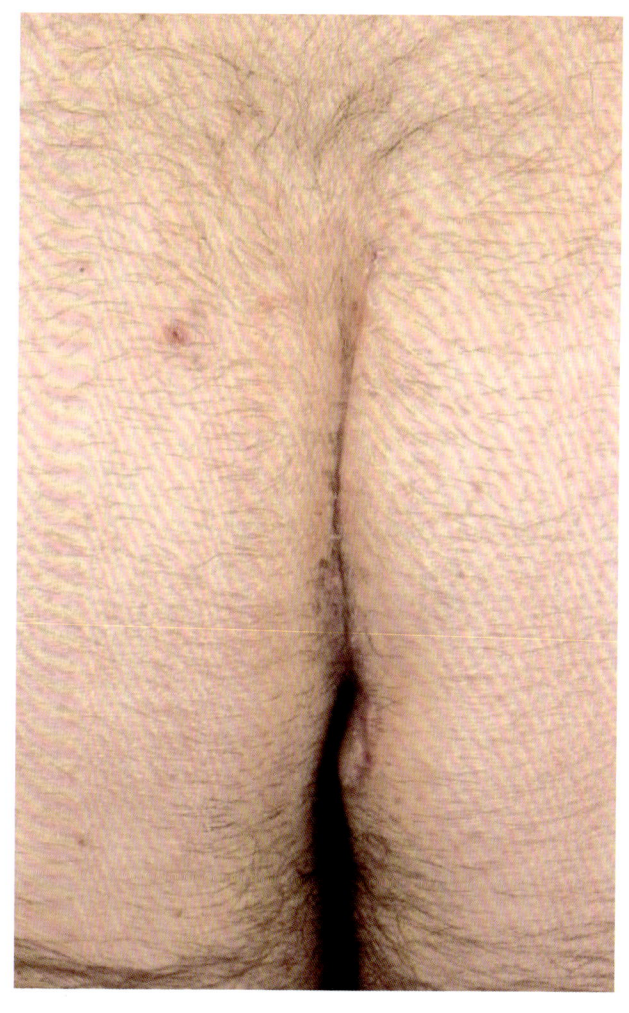

图 52.5　单侧伤口愈合后的中线皮肤

并能重返工作岗位。严重的手术并发症尚未见报道。

一项随机对照试验显示治疗原发藏毛窦疾病，Bascom 术相比单纯切开术具有较好效果[76]。Bascom 的挑坑术对于具有较深的臀沟和多个坑的多毛患者可能是最好的操作[76-80]。

广泛切除手术后更复杂的皮瓣术

虽然 Z/V-Y 成形术和菱形/Limberg 皮瓣术已经取得了良好的疗效[81-92]，但是两项随机对照试验显示：V-Y 和 Limberg 皮瓣术的疗效不优于基本的闭合术[93]或切开袋形缝合术[94]。这些更复杂的皮瓣术包括切除脓肿，并要求全身麻醉和更长的住院天数，偶尔也会发生需要进一步住院手术的并发症。总的来说，与改良 Karydakis 术相比，它提供很少或根本没有额外的好处[80]。

失败和复发

在文献报道中，往往很难区分失败和复发，而事实上，一旦手术失败已经持续很多个月，外科医生和患者均认为是复发。这类患者的治疗也是治疗藏毛窦疾病的一部分。最严重的是中线伤口不愈合。

术后中线伤口未愈

虽然中线伤口不愈合可能比较少见（图 52.6），但它是藏毛窦手术和复发性疾病的"眼中钉"，手术后伤口并发症的数量，开放或裂开的缝合伤口的愈合时间，是比较不同的治疗方式需要考察的因素。很少有研究记录所有这些参数[4]，特别是中线伤口不愈的频率及为实现完全愈合所需要的手术数量。这些参数的精确测量需要大量患者的长期随访。在较小的短期随访研究，有存在漏报最明显和最严重的藏毛窦疾病的术后并发症的风险[14]。如果没有这些数据，我们很难通过对比不同的外科治疗方式来得到一个确切的结论，而随机化实验中经常缺乏这些信息[4-5]。

失败和复发的治疗

非手术治疗

有些很轻微的复发很少困扰患者。间断换药和抗生素可能比手术更可取。剃毛可能保留一些肛周

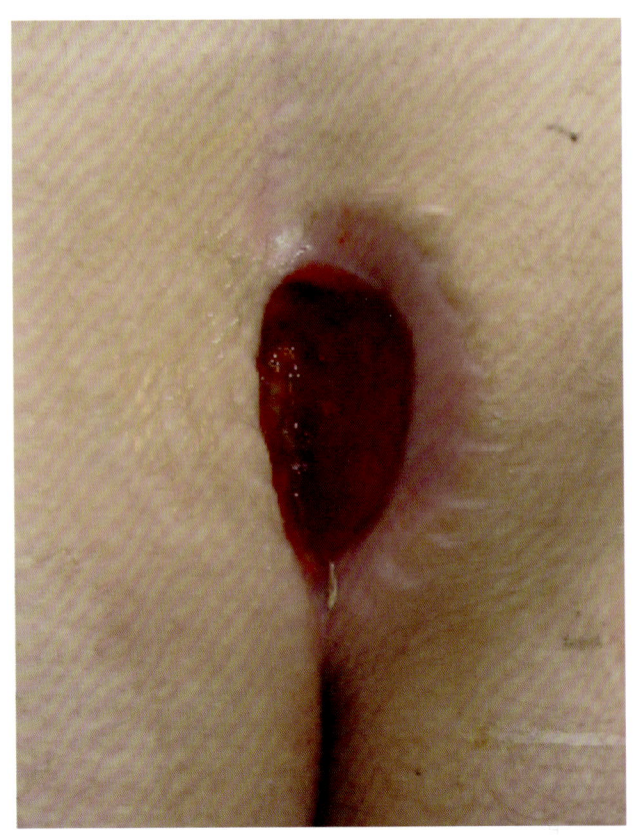

图 52.6　广泛切除后中线伤口不愈

症状。当其他治疗的手术范围更大并有治疗失败的风险时，应采取此种方法。

单纯切开术

袋形缝合术可解决一部分轻微情况。这是许多外科医生经常采取的治疗，可能未予报道。手术可在门诊进行。

广泛切除伴（或不伴）一期缝合

广泛切除术不应该被采用，因为许多失败发生于广泛切除术后，且中线伤口不愈合是一种严重的并发症。目前，当证明偏离中线缝合效果更好的情况下，广泛切除术存在如此高的切口不愈合的风险是不能接受的[4-5]。此术失败的风险与原发手术的失败风险相类似。

偏离中线皮肤缝合

Karydakis 术用于疾病复发或失败。此术治疗复发或失败患者的成功率与治疗原发病类似，是一个不错的选择。然而，它手术范围相当大，已逐渐被

改良术式取代。Bascom 的挑坑术也具有了类似的疗效。它完全适用于中线伤口不愈合，可快速痊愈。150 例患者接受 Bascom 的挑坑术，其中复发或中线伤口不愈的患者占 63%，成功愈合率为 96%[80]。没有患者出现重大并发症，只有 5% 复发患者需要进一步手术治疗。

更复杂的皮瓣术

这些术式也用于治疗失败和复发性疾病。它们更适合这种情况，而不是治疗原发疾病，除非原发性疾病的病变范围十分广泛。更复杂的皮瓣术更适于 Karydakis 术失败后。

结 论

症状轻微或那些进行引流的单发急性脓肿的藏毛窦患者，可能不需要任何干预，只需定期复查。非手术治疗如苯酚注射剂和单独去毛，并注意臀沟卫生，可能有效，但其长期结果尚不清楚。治疗的并发症很可能可以避免，但复发率可能会很高。

较轻的病情需要简单的手术。Pit-picking 采用 Bascom 术，具有很好的疗效。也可以使用环钻取芯，并能重复使用。更复杂或复发性疾病可以使用改良 Karydakis 术成功地治疗，如 Bascom 的挑坑术，从而避免了广泛脓肿切除。如今越来越多地在局部麻醉下进行，具有良好的长期预后和良好的美容效果。Z 和 V-Y 皮瓣术，以及广泛脓肿切除后的 Limberg 皮瓣已经取得成功，但需要全身麻醉，很难用于门诊手术，手术失败可能更难纠正。它们的美容效果也可能不尽如人意。在挑坑术失败和广泛疾病复发的情况下最好不要使用。

非切除手术的成功和中线皮肤坑是藏毛窦疾病的原因理论，显示目前没有对藏毛窦疾病行脓肿切除术合理的依据。然而，这种简单方法的主要好处是避免过长地缝合或臀裂中线不愈合的伤口，从而避免了偶然发生的严重手术并发症。目前，许多藏毛窦疾病治疗的并发症可以预防。患者应了解这些情况，并选择合适的治疗方法。对这种情况没有足够研究的外科医生，应该避免治疗这些患者，因为治疗失败的后果可能非常严重。大多数的手术失败和并发症可以有良好预后。因此，不应允许患者存在持续未愈合的伤口和因感染而导致不良的预后。

参考文献

1. Hodges RM. Pilonidal sinus. Boston Med Surg J. 1880;103:485–6.
2. Brearley R. Pilonidal sinus. A new theory of origin. Br J Surg. 1955;43:62–8.
3. Allen-Mersh TG. Pilonidal sinus: finding the right track for treatment. Br J Surg. 1990;77:123–32.
4. Petersen S, Koch R, Stelzner S, Wendlandt TP, Ludwig K. Primary closure techniques in chronic pilonidal sinus: a survey of the results of different surgical approaches. Dis Colon Rectum. 2002;45:1458–67.
5. McCallum IJ, King PM, Bruce J. Healing by primary closure versus open healing after surgery for pilonidal sinus: systematic review and meta-analysis. BMJ. 2008;336(7649):868–71.
6. No Authors Listed. Pilonidal sinus: is surgery alone enough? Colorectal Dis. 2003; 5:205.
7. Miller RJ. Pilonidal disease. A logical approach. Postgrad Med. 1967;41:382–5.
8. Armstrong JH, Barcia PJ. Pilonidal sinus disease. The conservative approach. Arch Surg. 1994;129:914–7.
9. Kronborg O, Christensen K, Zimmermann-Nielsen C. Chronic pilonidal disease: a randomized trial with a complete 3-year follow-up. Br J Surg. 1985;72:303–4.
10. Bascom JU. Repeat pilonidal operations. Am J Surg. 1987;154:118–22.
11. Bascom J, Bascom T. Failed pilonidal surgery: new paradigm and new operation leading to cures. Arch Surg. 2002;137:1146–50.
12. Guyuron B, Dinner MI, Dowden RV. Excision and grafting in treatment of recurrent pilonidal sinus disease. Surg Gynecol Obstet. 1983;156:201–4.
13. Hodgson WJ, Greenstein RJ. A comparative study between Z-plasty and incision and drainage or excision with marsupialization for pilonidal sinuses. Surg Gynecol Obstet. 1981;153:842–4.
14. Doll D, Krueger CM, Schrank S, Dettmann H, Petersen S, Duesel W. Timeline of recurrence after primary and secondary pilonidal sinus surgery. Dis Colon Rectum. 2007;50:1928–34.
15. Rabie ME, Al Refeidi AA, Al HA, Hilal S, Al AH, Al Amri AA. Sacrococcygeal pilonidal disease: sinotomy versus excisional surgery, a retrospective study. ANZ J Surg. 2007;77:177–80.
16. Patey DH. A reappraisal of the acquired theory of sacrococcygeal pilonidal sinus and an assessment of its influence on surgical practice. Br J Surg. 1969;56:463–6.
17. Clothier PR, Haywood IR. The natural history of the post anal (pilonidal) sinus. Ann R Coll Surg Engl. 1984;66:201–3.
18. Bascom JU. Pilonidal sinus. Curr Pract Surg. 1994;6:175–80.
19. Hopping RA. Pilonidal disease; review of the literature with comments on the etiology, differential diagnosis and treatment of the disease. Am J Surg. 1954;88:780–8.
20. Corman ML. Classic articles in colonic and rectal surgery, Pilonidal Sinus. Dis Colon Rectum. 1981;24:324–6.
21. Karydakis GE. New approach to the problem of pilonidal sinus. Lancet. 1973;2(7843):1414–5.
22. Bascom J. Pilonidal disease: long-term results of follicle removal. Dis Colon Rectum. 1983;26:800–7.
23. Millar DM. Etiology of post-anal pilonidal disease. Proc R Soc Med. 1970;63:1263–4.
24. Lord PH. Anorectal problems: etiology of pilonidal sinus. Dis Colon Rectum. 1975;18:661–4.
25. Karydakis GE. Easy and successful treatment of pilonidal sinus after explanation of its causative process. Aust N Z J Surg. 1992;62:385–9.
26. Lord PH. Unusual case of pilonidal sinus. Proc R Soc Med. 1970; 63:967–8.
27. Elliot D, Quyyumi S. A "pennanidal" sinus. J R Soc Med. 1981; 74:847–8.

28. Lord PH, Millar DM. Pilonidal sinus: a simple treatment. Br J Surg. 1965;52:298–300.
29. Klass AA. The so-called pilo-nidal sinus. Can Med Assoc J. 1956;75:737–42.
30. Hardaway RM. Polonidal cyst; neither pilonidal nor cyst. AMA Arch Surg. 1958;76:143–7.
31. Raffman RA. A re-evaluation of the pathogenesis of pilonidal sinus. Ann Surg. 1959;150:895–903.
32. Odili J, Gault D. Laser depilation of the natal cleft–an aid to healing the pilonidal sinus. Ann R Coll Surg Engl. 2002;84:29–32.
33. Maurice BA, Greenwood RK. A conservative treatment of pilonidal sinus. Br J Surg. 1964;51:510–2.
34. Stephens FO, Sloane DR. Conservative management of pilonidal sinus. Surg Gynecol Obstet. 1969;129:786–8.
35. Shorey BA. Pilonidal sinus treated by phenol injection. Br J Surg. 1975;62:407–8.
36. Blumberg NA. Pilonidal sinus treated by conservative surgery and the local application of phenol. S Afr J Surg. 1978;16:245–7.
37. Kelly SB, Graham WJ. Treatment of pilonidal sinus by phenol injection. Ulster Med J. 1989;58:56–9.
38. Stansby G, Greatorex R. Phenol treatment of pilonidal sinuses of the natal cleft. Br J Surg. 1989;76:729–30.
39. Dogru O, Camci C, Aygen E, Girgin M, Topuz O. Pilonidal sinus treated with crystallized phenol: an eight-year experience. Dis Colon Rectum. 2004;47:1934–8.
40. Jensen SL, Harling H. Prognosis after simple incision and drainage for a first-episode acute pilonidal abscess. Br J Surg. 1988;75:60–1.
41. McLaren CA. Partial closure and other techniques in pilonidal surgery: an assessment of 157 cases. Br J Surg. 1984;71:561–2.
42. Abramson DJ. Outpatient management of pilonidal sinuses: excision and semiprimary closure technic. Mil Med. 1978;143:753–7.
43. Meban S, Hunter E. Outpatient treatment of pilonidal disease. Can Med Assoc J. 1982;126:941.
44. Spivak H, Brooks VL, Nussbaum M, Friedman I. Treatment of chronic pilonidal disease. Dis Colon Rectum. 1996;39:1136–9.
45. Solla JA, Rothenberger DA. Chronic pilonidal disease. An assessment of 150 cases. Dis Colon Rectum. 1990;33:758–61.
46. Bissett IP, Isbister WH. The management of patients with pilonidal disease–a comparative study. Aust N Z J Surg. 1987;57:939–42.
47. Dwight RW, Maloy JK. Pilonidal sinus; experience with 449 cases. N Engl J Med. 1953;249:926–30.
48. Rickles JA. Ambulatory surgical management of pilonidal sinus. Am Surg. 1974;40:237–40.
49. Broadrick GL, Ehrlich FE, Kramer SG. Simplified treatment of pilonidal disease on an outpatient basis. Surgery. 1971;70:635–7.
50. Bascom J. Pilonidal disease: origin from follicles of hairs and results of follicle removal as treatment. Surgery. 1980;87:567–72.
51. Bascom J. Surgical treatment of pilonidal disease. BMJ. 2008;336(7649):842–3.
52. Senapati A, Cripps NP, Thompson MR. Bascom's operation in the day-surgical management of symptomatic pilonidal sinus. Br J Surg. 2000;87:1067–70.
53. Gips M, Melki Y, Salem L, Weil R, Sulkes J. Minimal surgery for pilonidal disease using trephines: description of a new technique and long-term outcomes in 1,358 patients. Dis Colon Rectum. 2008;51:1656–62.
54. Edwards MH. Pilonidal sinus: a 5-year appraisal of the Millar-Lord treatment. Br J Surg. 1977;64:867–8.
55. Mosquera DA, Quayle JB. Bascom's operation for pilonidal sinus. J R Soc Med. 1995;88:45P–6.
56. Bascom J. Pilonidal sinus: experience with the Karydakis flap. Br J Surg. 1998;85:874.
57. de Hyppolito Silva J. Pilonidal cyst. Cause and treatment. Dis Colon Rectum. 2000;43:1146–56.
58. Bascom J, Bascom T. Utility of the cleft lift procedure in refractory pilonidal disease. Am J Surg. 2007;193:606–9.
59. Rainsbury RM, Southam JA. Radical surgery for pilonidal sinus. Ann R Coll Surg Engl. 1982;64:339–41.
60. Testini M, Piccinni G, Miniello S, Di VB, Lissidini G, Nicolardi V, et al. Treatment of chronic pilonidal sinus with local anaesthesia: a randomized trial of closed compared with open technique. Colorectal Dis. 2001;3:427–30.
61. Notaras MJ. A review of three popular methods of treatment of postanal (pilonidal) sinus disease. Br J Surg. 1970;57:886–90.
62. Kitchen PR. Pilonidal sinus: excision and primary closure with a lateralised wound – the Karydakis operation. Aust N Z J Surg. 1982;52:302–5.
63. Kitchen PR. Pilonidal sinus: experience with the Karydakis flap. Br J Surg. 1996;83:1452–5.
64. Mann CV, Springall R. 'D' Excision for sacrococcygeal pilonidal sinus disease. J R Soc Med. 1987;80:292–5.
65. Anyanwu AC, Hossain S, Williams A, Montgomery AC. Karydakis operation for sacrococcygeal pilonidal sinus disease: experience in a district general hospital. Ann R Coll Surg Engl. 1998;80:197–9.
66. Patel H, Lee M, Bloom I, Allen-Mersh TG. Prolongued delay in healing after surgical treatment of pilonidal sinus is avoidable. Colorectal Dis. 1999;1:107–10.
67. Akinci OF, Coskun A, Uzunkoy A. Simple and effective surgical treatment of pilonidal sinus: asymmetric excision and primary closure using suction drain and subcuticular skin closure. Dis Colon Rectum. 2000;43:701–6.
68. Sakr M, El-Hammadi H, Moussa M, Arafa S, Rasheed M. The effect of obesity on the results of Karydakis technique for the management of chronic pilonidal sinus. Int J Colorectal Dis. 2003;18:36–9.
69. Gurer A, Gomceli I, Ozdogan M, Ozlem N, Sozen S, Aydin R. Is routine cavity drainage necessary in Karydakis flap operation? A prospective, randomized trial. Dis Colon Rectum. 2005;48:1797–9.
70. Morden P, Drongowski RA, Geiger JD, Hirschl RB, Teitelbaum DH. Comparison of Karydakis versus midline excision for treatment of pilonidal sinus disease. Pediatr Surg Int. 2005;21:793–6.
71. Abdul-Ghani AK, Abdul-Ghani AN, Ingham Clark CL. Day-care surgery for pilonidal sinus. Ann R Coll Surg Engl. 2006;88:656–8.
72. Kulacoglu H, Dener C, Tumer H, Aktimur R. Total subcutaneous fistulectomy combined with Karydakis flap for sacrococcygeal pilonidal disease with secondary perianal opening. Colorectal Dis. 2006;8:120–3.
73. Keshava A, Young CJ, Rickard MJ, Sinclair G. Karydakis flap repair for sacrococcygeal pilonidal sinus disease: how important is technique? ANZ J Surg. 2007;77:181–3.
74. Anderson JH, Yip CO, Nagabhushan JS, Connelly SJ. Day-case Karydakis flap for pilonidal sinus. Dis Colon Rectum. 2008;51:134–8.
75. Ersoy E, Devay AO, Aktimur R, Doganay B, Ozdogan M, Gundogdu RH. Comparison of the short-term results after Limberg and Karydakis procedures for pilonidal disease: randomized prospective analysis of 100 patients. Colorectal Dis. 2009;11:705–10.
76. Nordon IM, Senapati A, Cripps NP. A prospective randomized controlled trial of simple Bascom's technique versus Bascom's cleft closure for the treatment of chronic pilonidal disease. Am J Surg. 2009;197:189–92.
77. Bessa SS. Results of the lateral advancing flap operation (modified Karydakis procedure) for the management of pilonidal sinus disease. Dis Colon Rectum. 2007;50:1935–40.
78. Abdelrazeq AS, Rahman M, Botterill ID, Alexander DJ. Short-term and long-term outcomes of the cleft lift procedure in the management of nonacute pilonidal disorders. Dis Colon Rectum. 2008;51:1100–6.
79. Rushfeldt C, Bernstein A, Norderval S, Revhaug A. Introducing an asymmetric cleft lift technique as a uniform procedure for pilonidal sinus surgery. Scand J Surg. 2008;97:77–81.
80. Senapati A, Cripps NPJ, Flashman K, Thompson MR. Cleft closure for the treament of pilonidal sinus disease. Colorectal Dis. 2011;13:333–6.
81. Mansoory A, Dickson D. Z-plasty for treatment of disease of the pilonidal sinus. Surg Gynecol Obstet. 1982;155:409–11.

82. Azab AS, Kamal MS, Saad RA. Radical cure of pilonidal sinus by a transposition rhomboid flap. Br J Surg. 1984;71:154–5.
83. Morrison PD. Is Z-plasty closure reasonable in pilonidal disease? Ir J Med Sci. 1985;154:110–2.
84. Toubanakis G. Treatment of pilonidal sinus disease with the Z-plasty procedure (modified). Am Surg. 1986;52:611–2.
85. Jimenez RC, Alcalde M, Martin F, Pulido A, Rico P. Treatment of pilonidal sinus by excision and rhomboid flap. Int J Colorectal Dis. 1990;5:200–2.
86. Khatri VP, Espinosa MH, Amin AK. Management of recurrent pilonidal sinus by simple V-Y fasciocutaneous flap. Dis Colon Rectum. 1994;37:1232–5.
87. Schoeller T, Wechselberger G, Otto A, Papp C. Definite surgical treatment of complicated recurrent pilonidal disease with a modified fasciocutaneous V-Y advancement flap. Surgery. 1997;121:258–63.
88. Dylek ON, Bekereciodlu M. Role of simple V-Y advancement flap in the treatment of complicated pilonidal sinus. Eur J Surg. 1998;164:961–4.
89. Milito G, Cortese F, Casciani CU. Rhomboid flap procedure for pilonidal sinus: results from 67 cases. Int J Colorectal Dis. 1998;13:113–5.
90. Bozkurt MK, Tezel E. Management of pilonidal sinus with the Limberg flap. Dis Colon Rectum. 1998;41(6):775–7.
91. Tekin A. A simple modification with the Limberg flap for chronic pilonidal disease. Surgery. 2005;138:951–3.
92. Jamal A, Shamim M, Hashmi F, Qureshi MI. Open excision with secondary healing versus rhomboid excision with Limberg transposition flap in the management of sacrococcygeal pilonidal disease. J Pak Med Assoc. 2009;59:157–60.
93. Nursal TZ, Ezer A, Caliskan K, Torer N, Belli S, Moray G. Prospective randomized controlled trial comparing V-Y advancement flap with primary suture methods in pilonidal disease. Am J Surg. 2010;199:170–7.
94. Karakayali F, Karagulle E, Karabulut Z, Oksuz E, Moray G, Haberal M. Unroofing and marsupialization vs. Rhomboid excision and Limberg flap in pilonidal disease: a prospective, randomized, clinical trial. Dis Colon Rectum. 2009;52:496–502.

第 53 章 结直肠子宫内膜异位症的外科治疗

Adam Janusz Dziki · Łukasz Adam Dziki · Przemysław Galbfach

崔志刚 译　王西墨 审校

摘　要

本章讨论结直肠子宫内膜异位症这一临床难题的病因、检查和治疗。腹腔镜辅助技术在该领域的应用越来越多，但关于这种方法对远期受孕能力的影响还存在争议。对直肠子宫内膜异位症要根据不同患者及病情进展程度进行个体化治疗，对于梗阻、出血、穿孔和少数的恶性变等并发症，需要多学科协作的外科治疗方法。本章描述了疑难病例的手术技巧。

关键词

结直肠子宫内膜异位症；子宫内膜异位种植；子宫内膜腺体；子宫内膜间质；含铁血黄素色素沉着；吞噬含铁血黄素的巨噬细胞浸润；恶性变；腹腔镜切除术；性激素治疗；经腹子宫全切术；双侧输卵管卵巢切除术

引　言

子宫内膜异位症是妇产科医疗工作中经常遇到的疾病。根据不同文献，有4%～8%的育龄女性会发生这种疾病，而最常见年龄段是30～40岁[1-3]。子宫内膜异位症这一概念可以理解为，子宫内膜异位种植于子宫内膜层以外的组织器官[4]。子宫内膜异位症的异位病灶可能发生在远离子宫腔的位置，使得该病有时与浸润性和转移性肿瘤类似。但组织病理学检查通常会认定其为良性组织。局限于盆腔的，有3%～37%的患者消化道受累及[2,5,6]。消化道子宫内膜异位症分为肠型和肠外型。

病因学和发病机理

确诊子宫内膜异位症需要具备以下3项组织学典型特征中的两项，即存在子宫内膜腺体、存在子宫内膜基质和出血史的组织学证据，如含铁血黄素沉着或含铁血黄素巨噬细胞浸润[4]。由于子宫内膜异位症最常见于育龄女性，卵巢激素控制下的腺体上皮增殖和分泌周期性变化，也会发生在异位的子宫黏膜，包括月经前期水肿、黏膜脱落及伴随的出血。相反，绝经后女性的子宫内膜异位症有着不同的发病机制，根据诊断标准，有2%～5%的女性可以确诊。进入绝经后年龄，由于缺乏雌激素的刺激，异位的子宫内膜组织通常会发生退化；但情况也并不总是这样。如果在绝经后继续应用雌激素，就会导致有此病史女性的子宫内膜异位病灶持续存在。绝经后继续应用雌激素可能会导致两种情况：外源性性激素供给（雌激素替代疗法）或者肾上腺雌烯二酮经过外周转化形成雌激素（大部分发生在脂肪组织）。脂肪组织比较多的患者，经过肾上腺雌烯二酮外周转化形成的雌激素就占明显高的比例；已经发现绝经后肥胖女性雌激素水平明显高于正常体重的女性，而她们绝经后子宫内膜异位症的发病率较高[7,8,10]。子宫内膜异位的病灶组织含有雌激素受体和芳香化酶，这种酶能够催化雄激素向雌激素转化，这提示了局部生成的雌激素在刺激病灶进展方面起重要作用。在子宫内膜异位病灶的标本中，雌激素和孕酮的表达与正常子宫内膜是不一样的。已经认为 ER-a 基因和编码芳香化酶的 CYP19 基因的多态性与子宫内膜异位症的高风险有关[11]。

子宫内膜异位症的确切发病机制还不清楚。相关学说有很多，而最常被引用的有两个。第一个是体腔上皮化生学说，即壁层腹膜是一种多潜能组织，异位子宫内膜病灶是通过上皮衍化形成的，而这一过程又是在起源于原始体腔内苗勒氏管或肾内上皮组织的影响下进行的。被普遍认可的是另外一个理论，即经血逆流学说，意思是经血通过输卵管反流或逆流至腹膜腔，从而导致子宫内膜细胞的种植[12]。异位种植的子宫内膜组织与腔内浆膜上皮的黏合是很快的，这个过程仅需要约 1h。随后的上皮内浸润在 18~24h 内发生。机体对这一过程有一个防御机制，即透明质酸酶，能抑制子宫内膜细胞黏附于腹膜[13]。有证据表明，诸多因素使经血逆流的女性容易出现子宫内膜细胞的异位种植，包括免疫应答的变化、基因转导的变化，以及环境因素的影响。这种倾向性可能还与腹膜自洁、破坏外来细胞和子宫内膜碎片的功能降低有关。在正常情况下，女性腹腔内的液体能够阻止子宫内膜组织的侵入。该功能下降或消失会导致子宫内膜种植的形成。在那些局部有炎症反应的部位，这一过程与巨噬细胞活化和分泌各种生长因子、细胞因子以诱导腹膜细胞的转化有关[14-16]。另外还有一些关于子宫内膜症发病机制及其扩散的理论没有得到广泛认同，如局部淋巴管种植学说，脐部等子宫内膜异位症的部位对此学说有支持意义[17-18]。血行播散学说也被提出过，可以用来解释肺部子宫内膜异位症等少见病例[19]，还有就是直接种植机制，即子宫内膜脱落至皮肤，可以解释剖宫产或子宫切除术后的皮肤内子宫内膜异位种植，包括手术瘢痕内的种植[20-22]。

消化道子宫内膜异位症分为肠型和肠外型。肠型子宫内膜异位症更为多见，病灶通常位于乙状结肠和直肠。在一项大宗病例回顾性研究中，子宫内膜异位症患者 7000 多例，其中 12% 的病例有肠道受累[23]。在这项研究中，病灶最常见于直肠和乙状结肠（占 72%），其次是阴道直肠膈（14%）、盲肠（4%）及阑尾（3%）。直肠子宫陷凹区域的直肠前壁是最典型和常见的位置[24-25]。肠外型子宫内膜异位症少见得多，尽管曾有肝[26-28]和胰腺[29-30]子宫内膜异位症的个案报告。

消化道子宫内膜异位症最典型的表现是肠道内"肿瘤样"的实性肿块，导致由于外在压迫而形成不对称狭窄，或者是环形浸润引起小段肠管的瘢痕挛缩狭窄。也有肠腔内息肉样肿块增殖，但并不常见[24]。子宫内膜异位症并发溃疡或消化道内出血的病例也很少见[31]。在消化道，子宫内膜异位症最常见的部位是直肠。种植通常发生在与子宫直肠陷凹毗连的直肠前壁[24-25]。子宫内膜异位症病灶一般位于浆膜层内，肌层和黏膜下层相对很少，同样很少浸润到直肠黏膜[24,25,32]，其病理过程通常是从累及肠管浆膜面开始，再向腔内发展。子宫内膜异位病灶周围常常有明显的炎症反应，继发形成周围组织粘连。其结果是导致在直肠和子宫后壁、阴道、甚至骶骨骨膜之间形成紧密坚韧的粘连。直肠和周围组织的紧密粘连在手术中通过肉眼观察即可看到，使得切除的难度增加。纤维组织环状突向直肠肠腔，通常会累及环周的肠壁，使肠腔变窄。这种病灶有时会被误诊为癌症或 Leśniowski-Crohn 病[32-33]。病灶广泛时，通过直肠阴道检查可触及到与直肠壁毗连的子宫直肠陷凹内的肿块。

子宫内膜异位症的恶性病变

如前所述，子宫内膜异位症病灶的表现可能像盆腔恶性肿瘤。而且需要强调的是，子宫内膜异位症病灶也会发生恶性病变，尽管很少。根据目前的文献，子宫内膜异位症病灶恶性病变发生于 0.7%~1.0% 的病例[34-40]。在这些病例中，有不少通过结肠镜活检甚至冰冻切片组织学检查的术中切除活检都可能做不出明确诊断。癌症通常只能通过随后的手术标本蜡块组织病理学检查得到诊断[10,32,41]。1925 年由 Sampson[34] 首次对子宫内膜异位症病灶恶性病变进行了报道。在生殖器官以外的异位子宫内膜组织癌变的诊断标准（所谓 Sampson 标准）即由此研究者制订，目前仍在使用。这个标准包括：①包含子宫内膜形态的基质及腺体的病灶存在；②在同一位置并存癌组织和异位子宫内膜组织；③没有其他部位来源的癌组织转移的征象（尤其是子宫内膜/子宫体、卵巢或输卵管）。癌变病灶大部分是来源于异位子宫内膜腺体上皮的腺癌[10,35-38,42,43]。透明细胞癌比较少见[40,44]，起源于子宫内膜间质的肉瘤则更不多见[45-46]。目前认为这些肿瘤的形成，在很大程度上与围绝经期和绝经后年龄女性应用雌激素替代疗法有关。已确诊的消化道异位子宫内膜病灶癌变的患者中，接近50%曾用过绝经后激素疗法[42-43]。Magtibay等[10]的报道中，最详细地描述并且最清晰地呈现了子宫内膜异位症病灶癌变的病例。该报道精确地描述了组织学进展过程，包括从异位子宫内膜病灶到伴有细胞异型性的完整增生，再到直肠异位子宫内膜病灶来源的腺癌最终形成。其中所记录的患者最早是因为可疑子宫内膜癌而进行的手术。组织病理学检查发现仅仅是囊性增生和异位子宫内膜，没有典型的癌组织成分。20年后，该患者因为持续发作的周期性腹泻和直肠出鲜血住进另一家医院；临床检查提示盆腔肿物。对该患者再次进行手术，并在紧邻直肠前壁处发现肿瘤。与肿瘤毗邻的阴道上部被切除，肿瘤后缘也从直肠前壁上分离下来。切除病灶组织学检查显示子宫内膜腺体和间质明显纤维化，伴有子宫内膜增生和不典型增生的细胞学表现。当时没有发现明显特征性的癌组织成分。26个月后，该患者在随访期间又发现了第二个盆腔肿瘤。因肿瘤位于直肠，再次手术行直肠前切除术，组织细胞学检查显示肿块为腺癌。这个病例清晰地显示了子宫内膜异位症潜在进展的不同类型[10]，并验证了Kurman等[47]以前所提出的建议，即异位子宫内膜病灶伴有细胞异型性的组织增生提示其恶变的高度风险。

症 状

子宫内膜异位症的症状没有特异性，但这些症状可以对诊断性检查起重要的提示作用。大多数患者的症状特点是周期性发作并与月经周期密切相关，有时会直接表示以前确诊过盆腔子宫内膜异位症[32]。直肠子宫内膜异位症最常见症状是腹部、盆腔或直肠疼痛，通常在月经来潮前加重或在月经期出现疼痛。月经期前出现的疼痛与病灶处水肿有关，而月经期出现的疼痛则是在局限的间隙内血液积聚的结果。此期间，异位子宫内膜病灶肿胀并压迫周围组织。育龄女性常常会同时出现典型的妇科症状，包括痛经、月经过多和性交疼痛。直肠子宫内膜异位症其他可能的症状包括便秘、腹泻、伴有疼痛的里急后重、直肠出血，以及细如铅笔样的大便[32,48]。这些症状（排除结直肠癌后）常常让人怀疑为肠炎或者可能会将其归咎于肠道激惹综合征[49]。需要强调的是，以直肠溃疡和出血为主要表现的病例相对少见[31]。然而，有一定比例的患者没有明显症状，不孕症可能是该疾病的唯一表现[50]。症状的轻重与病灶的大小或范围没有直接关系。小的异位子宫内膜病灶可能会引起严重的症状，而大的腺肌症病灶引起的症状也可能较轻微。通常最有意义的症状，尤其是从外科角度来看，是大肠的梗阻[25,32,51,52]或肿瘤样病灶/肿块的存在[41,48]，这些都需要尽快手术。在直肠子宫内膜异位症的病程中出现肠穿孔的格外少见，有报道的不足20例。出现这种情况时，症状比较特殊，在左髂窝有明显的腹膜刺激征，并可触及肿瘤样包块。刚开始时常常被诊断为憩室炎[53]。极少情况下，在怀孕期间会出现子宫内膜异位症的直肠穿孔[54]。

诊 断

对直肠和直乙交界区有症状的子宫内膜异位症患者做出诊断并不容易。需要着重强调的是，精确、详细并且完整的病史尤其重要，有助于医生考虑到该病的诊断。上面列出的症状虽然没有特异性，但同时出现时则提示本病。在一些情况下，所有检查的诊断价值都有限，只能起到补充的作用。基本检查包括结肠（或直肠）钡灌肠双重对比检查、直肠镜和结肠镜等内镜检查、CT检查、磁共振成像，以及经直肠或阴道超声检查。诊断性腹腔镜探查能够对生殖器官子宫内膜异位病灶进行确切判定，但对于消化道子宫内膜异位症尤其是直肠病灶的诊断却不能同样有效。结肠钡灌肠双重对比检查通常会发现直肠腔外肿瘤样异位子宫内膜病灶。这种"肿瘤"与直肠黏膜一般没有关系，也没有典型癌肿浸润的征象。但有时，由于肠壁增厚或者甚至是小段肠管的瘢痕挛缩而表现为直肠肠腔狭窄。这主要是由于异位子宫内膜浸润到肠壁黏膜层引起。显而易见的是，没有哪个单独病例具有特异性表现。类似的影像结果也可见于其他几种疾病，包括癌症、脓肿、Leśniowski-Crohn病或憩室炎[31,55]。用结肠钡灌肠双重对比来检查直肠子宫内膜异位症是一种廉价的方法，并且由于其敏感性高而被推荐为术前评估的检查方法[56-58]。在一些对照研究中，该检查方法的特异性优于磁共振成像[58]。

第 53 章 结直肠子宫内膜异位症的外科治疗

腹部和盆腔 CT 检查能够发现增厚的直肠壁、实性肿瘤或者复杂的囊肿样肿块。但这些同样是没有特异性的影像检查，不能快速与癌肿或脓肿鉴别。磁共振成像是一种敏感性和特异性均较高的影像技术，能够发现所检查病灶内的出血情况，也能对子宫内膜异位症和癌肿加以鉴别[58-59]。阴道或直肠内加入对比介质特别有助于评价直肠的子宫内膜异位病灶。这种方法使得盆腔内各种结构之间的分界更加清晰，能够清楚显示它们的位置与其他异位子宫内膜病灶的关系。近来有研究者指出磁共振弥散加权成像技术能够区别癌肿与深层浸润的子宫内膜异位症：癌肿表现为高信号强度，而子宫内膜异位症表现为低信号强度[60-61]。磁共振结肠成像技术中将水灌注入结肠（多层螺旋 CT 小肠造影），显示异位子宫内膜病灶的部位及范围，其结果与腹腔镜探查高度一致，但这项技术有赖于影像学专家；当经验少的影像学医生应用磁共振技术时，其敏感性、特异性和阳性预测值均会大打折扣[62, 63]。

更加精确地确定异位子宫内膜的病灶局部范围，能够更好地对病灶进行术前评估，自然也就能制定更好的手术方案。经直肠超声被认为是目前最精准的检查技术，在诊断方面有高敏感性和特异性[64-67]。这种方法能精细检查直肠壁各层，并能追踪直肠周围间隙。该检查能够对"肿瘤"做出精密诊断，确定其与直肠壁各层特别是黏膜层的关系。在检查过程中，异位子宫内膜病灶表现为低回声、不均匀、多囊并含有液体的肿块[65]。经直肠超声检查的重要一点在于其实时性，因此该检查可以显示直肠阴道间隙内的异位子宫内膜及其对直肠壁的浸润[68]。为了举例说明，图 53.1a-d 中展示了与癌肿相似的直肠异位子宫内膜团块在 CT、经直肠超声、经阴道超声和矢状面经会阴超声图像上的不同结果。

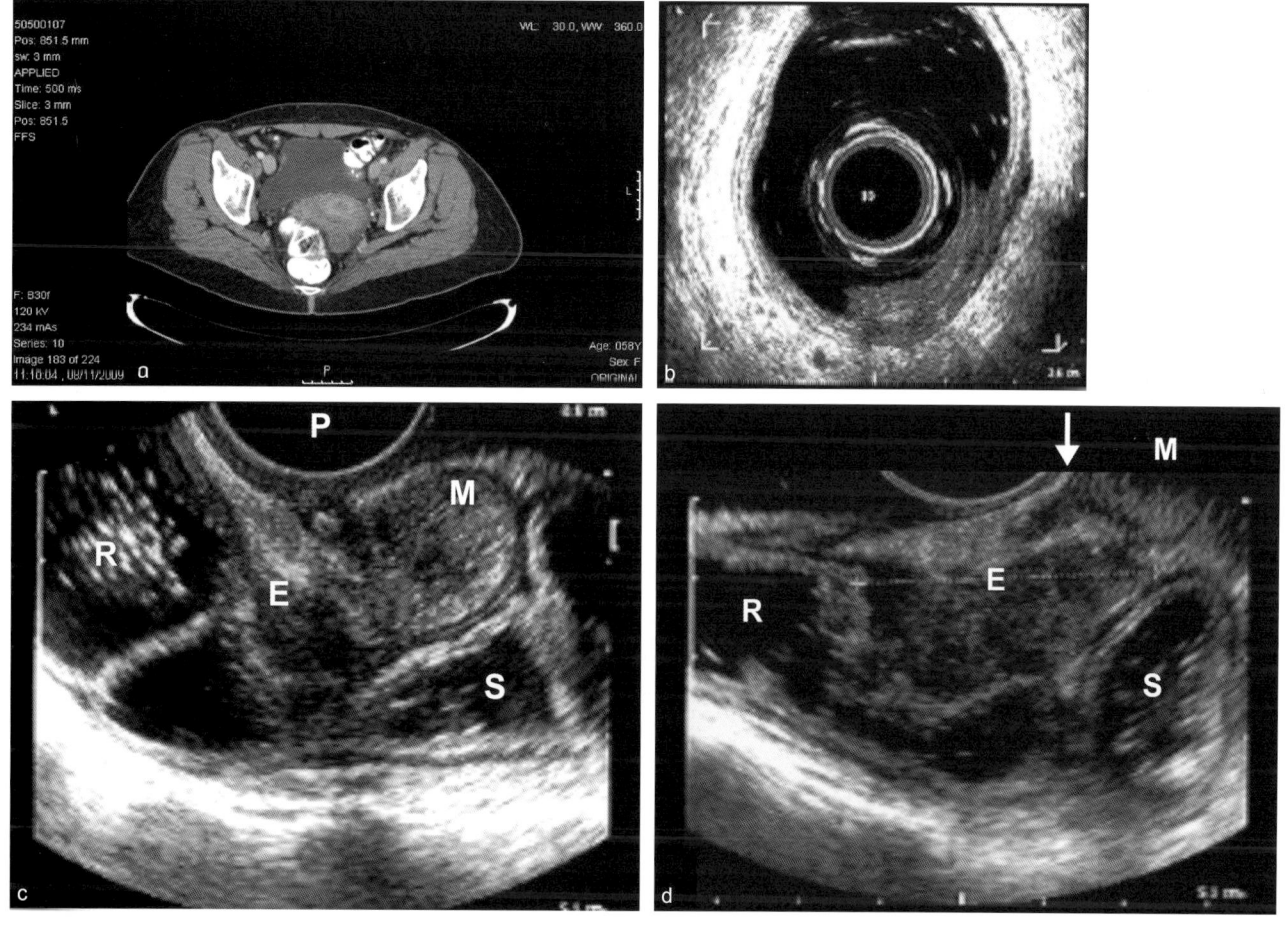

图 53.1 （a）腹部 CT 显示恶性表现肿块累及乙状结肠；（b）经直肠超声显示低回声团块浸润近端直肠壁各层；（c）经阴道超声，矢状面。探头位于阴道穹窿（P）后壁，左侧，直肠（R）被水充盈，右侧，乙状结肠（S）同样显示。异位子宫内膜结节（E）具有典型的低回声并位于直肠乙状结肠前壁；（d）经直肠超声，矢状面，显示异位子宫内膜团块浸润远端乙状结肠的黏膜固有层和黏膜下层

结肠镜通常只能发现直肠或乙状结肠狭窄，而黏膜没什么异常，有时也会合并有肠道激惹和轻度水肿表现，尤其在月经期二者会同时存在，或者肠道不蠕动，造成肠壁僵直而难于注入气体。需要提醒的是，有的子宫内膜异位症患者行结肠镜检查操作困难而不能完成。这是因为纤维化和粘连造成肠管游离度差，或形成锐角使镜身不能通过[25]。结肠镜活检常没什么用处，因为病灶很少累及黏膜[32]。这在一项研究中得到验证，26例经结肠镜活检诊断为慢性结肠炎的患者，肠切除后的最终组织病理学检查显示为其他良性疾病，包括2例子宫内膜异位症[69]。不过在某些病例，结肠镜检查仍是必要的，因为在排除尤其是结直肠癌等其他直肠出血疾病方面，其价值还是不容置疑的[25]。在最近韩国Kim等[70]关于结肠镜对子宫内膜异位症诊断的重要性报道中，检出80%病例有异常肠壁增厚，18%患者有息肉样病灶，78%患者有表面结节病变。结肠镜对结节样病灶有较高的组织学确诊率，但也为数不多，需要由外科医生/内镜医师对高度可疑的病灶直接进行活组织检查。

尽管对子宫内膜异位症的诊断方法有其局限性，而且组织学检查常常假阴性，但对于排除结直肠没有黏膜浸润的肿瘤性疾病有帮助，无论是癌肿还是间质来源的肿瘤（包括胃肠间质瘤）。需要强调的是，正确诊断子宫内膜异位症的关键是全面而详细的病史[71]。最近已应用氟脱氧葡萄糖正电子发射断层扫描（PET）在腹腔镜检查前对卵泡期患者进行检查，尽管其结果与腹腔镜探查结果相符，但使用时并不具备特殊的高代谢敏感性[72]。在影像方法和腹腔镜探查之间，根据美国生育学会关于子宫内膜异位症分期的指南进行了比较，该分期对怀孕有预测性[73-74]。该分级系统共4期，结直肠受累时则划为重型。

Ⅰ期（微型）

检查结果仅限于表浅病灶，可能有少数紧密粘连；

Ⅱ期（轻型）

Ⅰ期表现和子宫直肠窝的深在病灶；

Ⅲ期（中型）

Ⅰ期和Ⅱ期表现，加上卵巢子宫内膜异位症及粘连加重

Ⅳ期（重型）

Ⅰ～Ⅲ期表现，加上大的异位子宫内膜瘤、广泛粘连及消化道受累。

目前认为，在腹腔镜探查评估腹膜粘连和子宫内膜异位症方面，存在相当大的主观差异，但对于卵巢异位子宫内膜瘤并不至于此[75]。

治 疗

对直肠子宫内膜异位症要根据不同患者及病情进展程度进行个体化治疗。这需要一个由外科医生和妇产科医生组成的团队协作。通常是在出现并发症时，才对子宫内膜异位症做出诊断并开始治疗，这是更常见的情况，包括梗阻、出血、穿孔，或者异位子宫内膜病灶恶变。对于没有并发症和症状的子宫内膜异位症，要根据病灶大小、患者年龄及其有无怀孕要求进行治疗[33,48]。存在疼痛、直肠出血、直肠结构改变、肠梗阻迹象及怀疑恶性变，尤其是不能排除时，要考虑手术治疗。

对于有子宫内膜异位症症状并有生育要求的年轻女性，以及病灶局限的患者，可以考虑腹腔镜下切除，继以性激素治疗。曾经有几年，许多研究者提出，切除直肠和乙状结肠子宫内膜异位症病灶的同时切除受累的肠段，效果很好[76-82]。据报道，术后并发症仅为8%～16%[79,80,82]，中转开腹率为3.2%～3.9%[79,80]。术后复发的患者占2%～3.4%[80,83]，而开腹手术后复发率高达13.2%（平均约8%）[79]。然而，腹腔镜技术还未被广泛掌握，只能作为直肠子宫内膜异位症病灶治疗方法的一种选择。选择合适患者及术者经验很重要。腹腔镜对于大块及粘连紧密的病灶切除困难，并且根据我们的经验，这种情况还很多。腹腔镜技术在分离直肠和阴道之间的粘连时没有直接的手感，容易导致直肠阴道瘘这种可怕的结果，据报道有3.2%的患者会出现这种情况[80]。应用腹腔镜技术时，有必要对病灶进行直接、快速的组织病理学检查。不能排除恶性变的病灶，必须开腹对肿瘤及其周围组织进行广泛的整块切除。

道格拉斯窝封闭是腹腔镜下盆腔子宫内膜异位症的特征[84]。尽管腹腔镜下切除结直肠子宫内膜异位病灶是可行的，但在技术上仍是个挑战，只用于经过筛选的病例[85]。希望手术切除子宫内膜异位病灶后能够怀孕的女性应该知道，大约40%的不孕患者在腹腔镜手术后能够受孕，但腹腔镜术后患者自然妊娠率仅仅略高于开腹手术的患者。如果施行的是开腹结直肠切除术（与不行切除的简单腹

腔镜治疗相反），以及如果同时存在子宫腺肌症，那么随着时间推移，成功怀孕的可能性就会降低，所以患者群之间并没有严格的可比性[86]。如果是腹腔镜切除结直肠病灶结节而不是结直肠切除，则子宫和肠道很少发生功能障碍，但这类患者不能准确分组[87]。

治疗子宫内膜异位症的基本手术操作包括直肠前切除并一期吻合，或前切除后行乙状结肠造口或其他部位结肠造口术。少数情况下行直肠前壁的局部切除后继以性激素治疗，这用于以后想生育的女性或不愿接受直肠全切除的患者[33,48]。直肠前切除并一期吻合的方法最常用。很多研究者都证明术后长期效果良好[25,48,83]。就像在该区域施行其他结直肠手术那样进行结肠准备，然后手术开始。手术之中需要牢记的是，要将一个组织区域内种植的异位子宫内膜全部切除。在直肠阴道隔进行剥离相当困难，因为存在不断进展的瘢痕、紧密的粘连和炎性浸润。在手术同时用妇产科检查的方法对阴道后壁施压，可能会对该区域的剥离有帮助。直肠前壁可以用经典的方法切除，沿着阴道后壁直至远端经触诊证实的柔软没有变化的组织[48]，这种方法在开腹的复杂病例中有独特的优势。

对于将来要生孩子的年轻女性，手术后要应用性激素治疗来清除肉眼不能发现的残留病灶以防止复发[33,48,88]。该治疗包括联合应用雌激素和孕激素，也可以单独使用孕激素或达那唑。使用性激素类似物会导致黄体生成素的释放，而芳香化酶抑制剂也被推荐使用，据报道可以缓解痛经或非经期疼痛以及排便困难[89]。虽然激素治疗会很成功，并被推荐用来缩小异位子宫内膜组织，但应该知道陈旧、纤维化、形成瘢痕的及无活性病灶对激素刺激不会有反应[90]。激素治疗本身即可将子宫内膜转化成纤维组织，造成直肠狭窄和肠道症状加重[32]。对于围绝经期和绝经后的女性要考虑手术范围，应该行开腹子宫全切术和双侧输卵管－卵巢切除术。该术式可以清除子宫内膜异位症的来源及其播散途径。直肠子宫内膜切除术联合子宫全切术/双侧输卵管－卵巢切除术这么大范围的治疗，使其94%的患者收到了长期无复发的良好疗效，相比之下，保留卵巢的病例没有复发的仅占77%[91]。

虽然直肠子宫内膜异位症与整个消化道子宫内膜异位症相似，但并不常见。与这类病例相关的最适合的治疗方案，包括明确的手术适应证、推荐的手术方式及切除的范围等，还没有统一。尽管如此，还是建议手术治疗子宫内膜异位症时要彻底切除病理上有改变的肠管，因为这些病灶有恶变的可能[10,46]。总之，选择治疗方法时要考虑到症状明显缓解、生育能力和受孕率，并且在多数病例还要考虑生活质量参数的改善[92]。

参考文献

1. Gray L. Endometriosis. Clin Obstet Gynecol. 1960;3:472–9.
2. Ranny B. Etiology, prevention, and inhibition of endometriosis. Clin Obstet Gynecol. 1980;23:875–83.
3. Zwas FR, Lyon DT. Endometriosis: an important condition in clinical gastroenterology. Dig Dis Sci. 1991;36:353–64.
4. Czernobilsky B. Endometriosis. In: Fox H, Wells M, editors. Haines and Taylor's obstetrical and gynaecological pathology. 4th ed. Edinburgh: Churchill Livingstone; 1995. p. 1043–62.
5. Farinon AM, Stroppa I, Chiarelli C. Therapy of colorectal endometriosis. Colo Proctology. 1992;14:230–4.
6. Panebianco V, Poli A, Blandino R, Pistritto A, Puzzo L, Grasso A, et al. Low anterior resection of the rectum using mechanical anastomosis in intestinal endometriosis. Minerva Chir. 1994;49:215–7.
7. Ranny B. Endometriosis III: complete operations: reasons, sequelae, treatment. Am J Obstet Gynecol. 1971;109:1137–44.
8. Punuonem R, Klemi PJ, Nikkanen V. Postmenopausal endometriosis. Eur J Obstet Gynecol Reprod Biol. 1980;11:195–200.
9. Deval B, Rafii A, Felce-Dachez M, Kermanash R, Levardon M. Sigmoid endometriosis in a postmenopausal woman. Am J Obstet Gynecol. 2002;187:1723–5.
10. Magtibay PM, Heppel J, Leslie KO. Endometriosis-associated invasive adenocarcinoma involving the rectum in a postmenopausal female: report of a case. Dis Colon Rectum. 2001;44:1530–3.
11. Kitawaki J, Kado N, Ishihara H, Koshiba H, Kitaoka Y, Honjo H. Endometriosis: the pathophysiology as an estrogen – dependent disease. J Steroid Biochem Mol Biol. 2002;83:149–55.
12. Sampson JA. The development of the implantation theory for the origin of peritoneal endometriosis. Am J Obstet Gynecol. 1942;40:549–62.
13. Witz CA, Allsup KT, Montoya-Rodriguez IA, Vaughan SL, Centonze VE, Schenken RS. Pathogenesis of endometriosis – current research. Hum Fertil (Camb). 2003;6:34–40.
14. Vinatier D, Orazi G, Cossou M, Dufour P. Theories of endometriosis. Eur J Obstet Gynecol Reprod Biol. 2001;96:21–34.
15. Gazvani R, Templeton A. New considerations for the pathogenesis of endometriosis. Int J Gynaecol Obstet. 2002;76:117–26.
16. Witz CA. Pathogenesis of endometriosis. Gynecol Obstet Invest. 2002;53 Suppl 1:52–62.
17. Boufettal H, Zekri H, Majdi F, Noun M, Hermas S, Samouh N. Primary umbilical endometriosis. Ann Dermatol Venereol. 2009;136:941–3.
18. Fukuda H, Mukai H. Cutaneous endometriosis in the umbilical region: the usefulness of CD10 in indentifying the interstitium of ectopic endometriosis. J Dermatol. 2010;37:545–9.
19. Kiyan E, Kilicaslan Z, Caglar E, Yilmazbayhan D, Tabak L, Gürgan M. An unusual radiographic finding in pulmonary parenchymal endometriosis. Acta Radiol. 2002;43:164–6.
20. Zhu Z, Al-Beiti MA, Tang L, Liu X, Lu X. Clinical characteristic analysis of 32 patients with abdominal incision endometriosis. J Obstet Gynaecol. 2008;28:742–5.
21. Shelat VG, Low CH. Scar endometriosis. ANZ J Surg. 2009;79:311–2.
22. Brown AS, Malone JC, Brown TS, Callen JP. Cutaneous incisional

endometriosis. Arch Dermatol. 2009;145:605–6.
23. MacAfee CHG, Greer HLH. Intestinal endometriosis: a report of 29 cases and a survey of the literature. J Obstet Gynaecol Br Emp. 1960;67:539–55.
24. Graham B, Mazier WP. Diagnosis and management of endometriosis of the colon and rectum. Dis Colon Rectum. 1988;31:952–6.
25. Collin GR, Russell JC. Endometriosis of the colon: its diagnosis and management. Am Surg. 1990;56:275–9.
26. Bohra AK, Diamond T. Endometrioma of the liver. Int J Clin Pract. 2001;55:286–7.
27. Huang WT, Chen WJ, Chen CL, Cheng YF, Wang JH, Eng HL. Endometrial cyst of the liver: a case report and review of the literature. J Clin Pathol. 2002;55:715–7.
28. Goldsmith PJ, Ahmad N, Dasgupta D, Campbell J, Guthrie JA, Lodge JP. Case hepatic endometriosis: a continuing diagnostic dilemma. HPB Surg. 2009;2009:407206.
29. Marchevsky AM, Zimmerman MJ, Aufses Jr AH, Weiss H. Endometrial cyst of the pancreas. Gastroenterology. 1984;86:1589–91.
30. Lee DS, Back JT, Ahn BM, Lee EH, Han SW, Chung IS, et al. A case of pancreatic endometrial cyst. Korean J Intern Med. 2002;17:266–9.
31. Szucs RA, Turner MA. Gastrointestinal tract involvement by gynecologic diseases. Radiographics. 1996;16:1251–70.
32. Midorikawa Y, Kubota K, Kubota K, Kawai K, Mori M, Kajiura N. Endometriosis of the rectum causing bowel obstruction: a case report. Hepatogastroenterology. 1997;44:706–9.
33. Schröder J, Löhner M, Doniec J, Dohrmann P. Endoluminal ultrasound diagnosis and operative management of rectal endometriosis. Dis Colon Rectum. 1997;40:614–7.
34. Sampson JA. Endometrial carcinoma of the ovary, arising in endometrial tissue in that organ. Arch Surg. 1925;10:1–72.
35. Lott JV, Rubin RJ, Salvati EP, Salazar GH. Endometrioid carcinoma of the rectum arising in endometriosis: report of a case. Dis Colon Rectum. 1978;21:56–60.
36. Amano S, Yamada N. Endometrioid carcinoma arising from endometriosis of the sigmoid colon: a case report. Hum Pathol. 1981;12:845–8.
37. Duun S, Roed-Petersen K, Michelsen JW. Endometrioid carcinoma arising from endometriosis of the sigmoid colon during estrogenic treatment. Acta Obstet Gynecol Scand. 1993;72:676–8.
38. Han AC, Hovenden S, Rosenblum NG, Salazar H. Adenocarcinoma arising in extragonadal endometriosis: an immunohistochemical study. Cancer. 1998;83:1163–9.
39. Yantis RK, Clement PB, Young RH. Neoplastic and pre-neoplastic changes in gastrointestinal endometriosis: a study of 17 cases. Am J Surg Pathol. 2000;24:513–24.
40. McCluggage WG, Desai V, Toner PG, Calvert CH. Clear cell adenocarcinoma of the colon arising in endometriosis: a rare variant of primary colonic adenocarcinoma. J Clin Pathol. 2001;54:76–7.
41. Kim JS, Hur H, Min BS, Kim H, Sohn SK, Cho CH, et al. Intestinal endometriosis mimicking carcinoma of rectum and sigmoid colon: a report of five cases. Yonsei Med J. 2009;50:732–5.
42. Jones KD, Owen E, Berresford A, Sutton C. Endometrial adenocarcinoma arising from endometriosis of the rectosigmoid colon. Gynecol Oncol. 2002;86:220–2.
43. Petersen VC, Underwood JC, Wells M, Shepherd NA. Primary endometrioid adenocarcinoma of the large intestine arising in colorectal endometriosis. Histopathology. 2002;40:171–6.
44. Pokieser W, Schmerker R, Kisser M, Peters-Engl C, Mühlbauer H, Ulrich W. Clear cell carcinoma arising in endometriosis of rectum following progestin therapy. Pathol Res Pract. 2002;198:121–4.
45. Baiocchi G, Kavanagh JJ, Wharton JT. Endometrioid stromal sarcomas arising from ovarian and extraovarian endometriosis: report of two cases and review of the literature. Gynecol Oncol. 1990;36:147–51.
46. Bosincu L, Massarelli G, Cossu Rocca P, Isaac MA, Nogales FF. Rectal endometrial stromal sarcoma arising in endometriosis: report of a case. Dis Colon Rectum. 2001;44:890–2.
47. Kurman RJ, Kamiński PF, Norris HJ. The behavior of endometrial hyperplasia. A long-term study of "untreated" hyperplasia in 170 patients. Cancer. 1985;56:403–12.
48. Urbach DR, Reedijk M, Richard CS, Lie KI, Ross TM. Bowel resection for intestinal endometriosis. Dis Colon Rectum. 1998;41:1158–64.
49. Kumar D. Irritable bowel syndrome, chronic pelvic inflammatory disease and endometriosis. Eur J Gastroenterol Hepatol. 2004;16:1251–2.
50. Yantis RK, Clement PB, Young RH. Endomeriosis of the intestinal tract: a study of 44 cases of a disease that may cause diverse challenges in clinical and pathologic evaluation. Am J Surg Pathol. 2001;25:445–54.
51. Varras M, Kostopangiotou E, Katis K, Farantos C, Angelidou-Manika Z, Antoniou S. Endometriosis causing extensive intestinal obstruction simulating carcinoma of the sigmoid colon: a case report and review of the literature. Eur J Gynaecol Oncol. 2002;23:353–7.
52. Takai N, Ueda T, Nishida M, Nasu K, Narahara H. Bowel obstruction due to endometriosis in the rectovaginal septum. Clin Exp Obstet Gynecol. 2008;35:295–6.
53. Garg NK, Baul NB, Doughan S, Rowe PH. Intestinal endometriosis – a rare cause of colonic perforation. World J Gastroenterol. 2009;15:612–4.
54. Pisanu A, Deplano D, Angioni S, Ambu R, Uccheddu A. Rectal perforation from endometriosis in pregnancy: case report and literature review. World J Gastroenterol. 2010;16:648–51.
55. Gordon RL, Evers K, Kressel HY, Laufer I, Herlinger H, Thompson JJ. Double-contrast enema in pelvic endometriosis. Am J Roentgenol. 1982;138:549–52.
56. Ribeiro HS, Ribeiro PA, Rossini PA, Rossini L, Rodrigues FC, Donadio N, et al. Double-contrast barium enema and transrectal endoscopic ultrasonography in diagnosis of intestinal deeply infiltrating endometriosis. J Minim Invasive Gynecol. 2008;15:315–20.
57. Faccioli N, Manfredi R, Mainardi P, Dalla Chiara E, Spoto E, Minelli L. Barium enema evaluation of colonic involvement in endometriosis. AJR. 2008;190:1050–4.
58. Faccioli N, Manfredi R, Mainardi P, Spoto E, Ruffo G, Minelli L. Evaluation of colonic involvement in endometriosis: double-contrast barium enema vs. magnetic resonance imaging. Abdom Imaging. 2010;35(4):414–21.
59. Tagashi K, Nishimura K, Kimura I, Tsuda Y, Yamashita K, Shibata T, et al. Endometrial cysts: diagnosis with MR imaging. Radiology. 1991;180:73–8.
60. Busard MP, Pieters-van den Bos IC, Mijatovic V, Van Kuijk C, Bleeker MC, van Waesberghe JH. Evaluation of MR diffusion-weighted imaging in differentiating endometriosis infiltrating the bowel from colorectal carcinoma. Eur J Radiol. 2011;81(6):1376–80.
61. Marcal L, Nothaft MA, Coelho F, Choi H. Deep pelvic endometriosis: MR imaging. Abdom Imaging. 2010;35(6):708–15.
62. Biscaldi E, Ferrero S, Fulcheri E, Ragni N, Remorgida V, Rollandi GA. Multislice CT enteroclysis in the diagnosis of bowel endometriosis. Eur Radiol. 2007;17:211–9.
63. Scardapane A, Bettocchi S, Lorusso F, Stabile Ianora AA, Vimercati A, Ceci O. Diagnosis of colorectal endometriosis: contribution of contrast enhanced MR-colonography. Eur Radiol. 2011;21(7):1553–63.
64. Delpy R, Barthet M, Gasmi M, Berdah S, Shojai R, Desjeux A, et al. Value of endorectal ultrasonography for diagnosing rectovaginal septal endometriosis infiltrating the rectum. Endoscopy. 2005;37:357–61.
65. Pishvaian AC, Ahlawet SK, Garvin D, Haddad NG. Role of EUS and EUS-guided FNA in the diagnosis of symptomatic rectosigmoid endometriosis. Gastrointest Endosc. 2006;63:331–5.
66. Ribeiro HS, Ribeiro PA, Rossini L, Rodrigues FC, Donadio N, Aoki T. Double-contrast barium enema and transrectal endoscopic ultrasonography in the diagnosis of intestinal deeply infiltrating endometriosis. J Minim Invasive Gynecol. 2008;15:315–20.
67. Huang XF, Han CN, Lin KQ, Zhang J, Xu H, Zhang XM. Meta-analysis of ultrasonography in diagnosis of deeply infiltrating endometriosis. Zhonghua Fu Chan Ke Za Zhi. 2010;45:269–72.
68. Pascual MA, Guerriero S, Hereter L, Barri-Soldevila P, Ajossa S,

Graupera B, et al. Diagnosis of endometriosis of the rectovaginal septum using introital three-dimensional ultrasonography. Fertil Steril. 2010;94:2761–5.
69. Gupta J, Shepherd NA. Colorectal mass lesions masquerading as chronic inflammatory bowel disease on mucosal biopsy. Histopathology. 2003;42:476–81.
70. Kim KJ, Jung SS, Yang SK, Yoon SM, Yang DH, Ye BD, et al. Colonoscopic Findings and Histologic Diagnostic Yield of Colorectal Endometriosis. J Clin Gastroenterol. 2011;45(6):536–41.
71. Roman H, Vassilieff M, Gourcerol G, Savoye G, Leroi AM, Marpeau L, et al. Surgical management of deep infiltrating endometriosis of the rectum: pleading for a symptom-guided approach. Hum Reprod. 2011;26:274–81.
72. Fastrez M, Nogarède C, Tondeur M, Sirtaine N, Rozenberg S. Evaluation of 18FDG PET-CT in the diagnosis of endometriosis: a prospective study. Reprod Sci. 2011;18(6):540–4.
73. Buttram Jr VC. Evolution of the revised American fertility society classification of endometriosis. Fertil Steril. 1985;43:347–50.
74. Adamson GD, Pasta DJ. Endometriosis fertility index: the new, validated endometriosis staging system. Fertil Steril. 2009;94(5):1609–15.
75. Weijenborg PT, ter Kuile MM, Jansen FW. Intraobserver and interobserver reliability of videotaped laparoscopy evaluations for endometriosis and adhesions. Fertil Steril. 2007;87:373–80.
76. Sharpe DR, Redwine DS. Laparoscopic segmental resection of the sigmoid and rectosigmoid colon for endometriosis. Surg Laparosc Endosc. 1992;2:120–4.
77. Nezhat C, Nezhat F, Pennington E, Ambroze W. Laparoscopic disc excision and primary repair of the anterior rectal wall for the treatment of full-thickness bowel endometriosis. Surg Endosc. 1994;8:682–5.
78. Nezhat F. Laparoscopic segmental resection for infiltrating endometriosis of rectosigmoid colon: a preliminary report. Surg Laparosc Endosc. 2001;11:67–8.
79. Minelli L, Fanfani F, Fagotti A, Ruffo G, Ceccaroni M, Mereu L, et al. Laparoscopic colorectal resection for bowel endometriosis: feasibility, complicationa, and clinical outcome. Arch Surg. 2009;144:234–9.
80. Ruffo G, Scopelliti F, Scioscia M, Ceccaroni M, Mainardi P, Minelli L. Laparoscopic colorectal resection for deep infiltrating endometriosis: analysis of 436 cases. Surg Endosc. 2010;24:63–7.
81. Juhasz-Böss I, Lattrich C, Fürst A, Malik E, Ortmann O. Severe endometriosis: laparoscopic rectum resection. Arch Gynecol Obstet. 2010;281:657–62.
82. Dousset B, Leconte M, Borghese B, Millischer AE, Roseau G, Arkwright S, et al. Complete surgery for low rectal endometriosis: long-term results of a 100-case prospective study. Ann Surg. 2010;251:887–95.
83. Meyers W, Kelvin F, Jones R. Diagnosis and surgical treatment of colonic endometriosis. Arch Surg. 1979;114:169–75.
84. Khong SY, Bignardi T, Luscombe G, Lam A. Is pouch of Douglas obliteration a marker of bowel endometriosis? J Minim Invasive Gynecol. 2011;18:333–7.
85. Daraï E, Dubernard G, Coutant C, Frey C, Rouzier R, Ballester M. Randomized trial of laparoscopically assisted versus open colorectal resection for endometriosis: morbidity, symptoms, quality of life, and fertility. Ann Surg. 2010;251:1018–23.
86. Daraï E, Lesieur B, Dubernard G, Rouzier R, Bazot M, Ballester M. Fertility after colorectal resection for endometriosis: results of a prospective study comparing laparoscopy with open surgery. Fertil Steril. 2011;95:1903–8.
87. Roman H, Rozsnayi F, Puscasiu L, Resch B, Belhiba H, Lefebure B, et al. Complications associated with two laparoscopic procedures used in the management of rectal endometriosis. JSLS. 2010;14:169–77.
88. Kilgus M, Schöb O, Largiadèr F. Rectal endometriosis: transanal endoscopic microsurgery or laparoscopic resection? Eur J Surg. 1998;164:231–2.
89. Ferrero S, Camerini G, Ragni N, Venturini PL, Biscaldi E, Seracchioli R, et al. Letrozole and norethisterone acetate in colorectal endometriosis. Eur J Obstet Gynecol Reprod Biol. 2010;150:199–202.
90. Coronado C, Franklin RR, Lotze FC, Bailey HR, Valdés CT. Surgical treatment of symptomatic colorectal endometriosis. Fertil Steril. 1990;53:411–6.
91. Bailey HR, Ott MT, Hartendorp P. Aggressive surgical management for advanced colorectal endometriosis. Dis Colon Rectum. 1994;37:747–53.
92. Meuleman C, Tomassetti C, D'Hoore A, Van Cleynenbreugel B, Penninckx F, Vergote I, et al. Surgical treatment of deeply infiltrating endometriosis with colorectal involvement. Hum Reprod Update. 2011:17:311–26.

第 54 章 结直肠肛门外科再手术的医疗法律问题

David C.C. Bartolo

邵 伟 译　王西墨 审校

摘　要

本章为结直肠科的执业医师概述了涉及医疗法律风险的若干问题。对于重建手术和再次手术尤其值得注意，因为这些手术更容易发生伴随和预期的并发症。专科情况包括吻合口瘘、肛门内括约肌切开术后发生令人烦恼的大便失禁的潜在可能、因功能性盆底紊乱行手术治疗的潜伏危险等。本文还探讨了投诉的方法，必须有客观详尽的证明文件。如果出现并发症而治疗未能达到最高标准，并不构成过失。我们所需要做的是我们的行为符合职责要求，与其他理性医生所做的一样。避免医学法律诉讼是成功实践的关键环节之一，而法律诉讼常与三级肛肠科转诊基地有关。在那里，直肠、肛门和会阴部重建手术的患者占转诊患者的很大一部分。新技术的利用导致了医学法律投诉新领域的出现；新技术涉及的适应证、禁忌证、技术培训问题，还涉及没有经过试验的操作等，由于这些情况，医学技术衍生出了它自身的医学法律附属专业。

关键词

医学法律；肛肠科；医疗责任；英国 *Bolam* 测试；苏格兰 *Hunter* 诉 *Hanley* 测试标准；*Bolitho* 测试；吻合口瘘；产科损伤；失禁；肛门内括约肌切开术；盆底疾病

引　言

医疗实践最重要的一个方面是知情同意的过程。这里并不是指要患者签署文书，而是向他们详细地解释治疗所涉及的各个方面以及相关的风险。在我个人的实践中，我愿意解释如果事情朝着不幸的方向发展，最糟糕的病例情况可能会怎样。如直肠重建手术后，可能会发生吻合口瘘并且需要造口，甚至在极个别情况下，造口需要永久保留。又如术后有可能发生直肠阴道瘘，那么，造口就会显得尤为必要。有时，患者会认为我是在试图阻止他们接受手术。在作决断的时候，彻底地想清楚最糟糕的病情变化十分重要。同样，为患者提出一些重要的问题，让他们自己回答，也是一项重要的工作。这些问题可以包括"我的情况是否十分严重，以至于值得冒险；即使风险很小，是否有可能继发严重的并发症？"。

与处理癌症患者或那些伴有梗阻和严重炎性肠病的重症患者相比，在处理良性病变时，认同过程要复杂得多。在紧急情况下，认同成为生死攸关的事情。显然，如果腹膜炎患者或严重梗阻的患者不接受治疗性手术，那么一定要告知他们结局很可能是致命的。在可选择的情况下或处理良性疾病时，认同过程就变得更为重要，因为患者可以选择带病生活。如一例患者患失禁，或者直肠脱垂，或者严重便秘，虽然可以继续生活，但他正在寻求一种更高质量的生活，所以可能寻求重建手术来改善生活质量。甚至很多轻微的病症如痔疮，有时可以在手术后变得更加糟糕，所以临床医生有责任既解释预期效果，还要告知各种罕见的和意想不到的可能，即使给予最好的治疗，也有偶尔发生的可能性。

医疗责任

因为我在英国行医，所以我将论述英格兰和苏格兰的相关法律。在世界上的大部分地区，法律的基本原则会有许多相似之处。本文可能无法涵盖不同国家在法律上所存在的细微差别，因此我将重点论述我对英国法律的理解，因为它涉及了结肠肛门外科的医疗实践。

医生有治疗患者的责任。这与关心患者的职责不尽相同。医疗责任要求医生在治疗期间必须采取合理的措施而不能伤害患者。要履行这一职责，医生一定不要忽视正规医疗机构所要求的标准。医疗责任以民法为基础，而不是刑法。如果由于医生的医疗行为未能达到正规医疗机构所认可的最低标准从而使患者遭受伤害或损失，那么这项法律可以保证患者得到补偿（伤害赔偿）。履行医疗职责时，我们应该保证良好的治疗效果，既不要伤害患者，也不要因此种伤害承担法律赔偿责任。如果符合以下几条将追究其责任：①从业者的行为低于行业认可的标准；②患者因此遭受伤害。许多的医学法律实践是以以下两项测试为基础：英格兰的 *Bolam* 测试和苏格兰的 *Hunter v. Hanley* 测试。

英国法律

在英国的法律规则中，确定一个医生是否存在疏忽的测试被称为 *Bolam* 测试标准。就实用性来说，英格兰的 *Bolam* 测试和苏格兰的 *Hunter v. Hanley* 测试之间并没有多少差别。甚至，*Bolam* 测试基于（并专门引用了）苏格兰的 *Hunter v. Hanley* 测试，因为在 *Bolam* 决议提出前两年，苏格兰的法院就已经表述了 *Hunter v. Hanley* 测试的理念。*Bolam* 测试提出的背景是 1957 年 *Bolam* 诉 Friern 医院管理委员会一案。*Bolam* 测试主要表述的是："从医学观点出发，如果一名医生达到了正规医疗机构所认可的标准，他就不应负过失责任。" *Bolam* 先生是一名行动自如的精神病院住院患者，精神病院由 Friern 医院管理委员会管理运行。*Bolam* 先生同意接受电休克疗法。他没有被给予任何放松药物，他的身体也没有被限制。治疗期间，他由于剧烈挣扎而受伤，其中包括髋臼骨折。他起诉了医院委员会，并认为院方存在过失，因为他们未使用放松药物，也没有限制他的身体，更没有警告他治疗所涉及的风险。医院委员会提出医疗观点不赞成使用放松药物，而且人工限制有时会增加骨折的风险。此外，在当时，如果治疗的风险很小，医疗行业的惯例是不向患者提出风险警告（除非他们询问）。法官认为行业惯例与医疗必须达到的标准高度相关。

Bolam 先生认为，"如果一个人的医疗行为未能达到适当的标准，他们就存在过失，特别是如果他们未能符合一个合格人员在当时条件下应有的行为。" 法官希望医生有一个更高的治疗标准，但是他认为如果 "医生按照某种规范行事，而该专业领域里的资深专家团队认可其行为，他就不应负过失责任。" 他接着说："换句话讲，如果医生按照这样的一种规范行事，那么他就没有过失，并且不能仅仅因为存在相反的观点而认定他有过失。与此同时，这并不意味着一位医疗人员可以固执和愚蠢地去坚守一些旧的做法，如果这些做法被证明明显地有悖于最新的医学观点"，他继续说："否则，今天你可能会听到某位医生说我不相信麻醉学。我不相信抗感染治疗。我打算采用 18 世纪的术式来做手术，这显然是错误的。" 在 *Bolam* 案件中，由于陪审团接受了电休克治疗实践中所认可的主要医学观点，所以其判决有利于被起诉的医院。他们的结论是医院实施治疗的方式没有过失。在过去的 50 年中，这条原则成为认定专业过失的基础。

苏格兰法律

在苏格兰，确定一个医生是否存在疏忽的测试被称为 *Hunter v. Hanley* 测试标准。这一测试标准源于已故的克莱德勋爵在 1955 年所表述的一段著名的文字，他当时是（苏格兰）最高民事法庭庭长，这段话这样写道：

若要成功地对医生或其他人做出是否存在过失

的判定，那么建立一种失职的标准是十分必要的，这也是法律所需要的，当然构成过失的懈怠程度一定会因情况的不同而划分。但是就医生或其他的专业人士工作的环境而言，情况就不会像正常案例一样，那么的精确和清楚。在诊断和治疗领域，存在许多真诚的不同意见，很明显，一个人不能仅因为他的结论与其他专业人士有异就认定其存在过失，也不能因为他所展示的技能和知识逊于其他人就认定其存在过失。在诊断和治疗领域认定医生过失的真正的测试标准是，是否能够证明他应对其行为承担责任，与此同时，一个具有通常技能的医生如果谨慎行事是不会承担责任的。

克莱德勋爵的进一步阐述指出了到底是什么常被称为第三方测试：

如果有什么地方与常规存在偏离，那么有三个事实需要确立。首先必须证明存在一个常规标准；其次，必须证明被告没有采用这种常规做法；第三（这一点至关重要），必须证明具有通常技能的专业人士，如果谨慎行事，是不会采用被告医生的治疗方式的。

患者抱怨时会发生什么？

患者可能会决定按照国家卫生服务内部投诉程序去投诉。对于患者所提出的问题，如果能提供令人满意的回应和详尽的解释，许多针对医生的投诉和指控可以得到处理，当然解释的内容应涉及手术时到底发生了什么，使得事情没有按照计划发展，以及为何会出现并发症。如果患者对给出的应答不满意，那么他可能会去找申诉专员，进而寻求医院的赔偿。在苏格兰，无论是国家卫生服务投诉程序还是申诉专员，均不能对补偿的问题做出处理。

除了国家卫生服务投诉程序，患者还可以选择向律师咨询，他将提供一些法律意见。律师将会指派一位独立的专家准备案例报告。有一点很重要，那就是这位专家一定是同一医学领域的从业人员；例如，如果指控针对的是一位全科医生，那么人们会希望由一位全科医生提供报告。如果投诉一位结直肠外科的专科医生，那么应该由另一位结直肠外科的医生提供报告。如果患者的律师指派的专家证实存在过失，那么代表患者利益的索赔将被提出。一旦索赔被提出，被告也会需要一个对等的专家来出具一份关于他们行为的报告。在英格兰，报告通常可以相互交换，但在苏格兰却不是这样。有时，对被告而言，事实也许很明确，他们未能妥善行事，接下来可以进行讨论以达成和解。如果没有达成协议，下一步，专家们可以决定是否同意对方观点或者求同存异。此后，此案例可能提交至法院。而苏格兰尚未采纳专家会议的形式。

专业过失的测试设置了一个很高的门槛。实际上，必须证明在这一专业领域，即使是普通的医生也不会犯案例中的错误。未遵循最佳治疗实践不能作为裁定的依据，甚至未实施常规的治疗也不能作为依据，而后一条是广泛适用的法律测试标准，主要针对非专业领域涉及过失的案例（例如交通事故或工伤事故）。判定专业过失的依据是没有提供最低限度的被认可的规范治疗。实际上，独立的医疗专家常常会说："我是不会这样做的，但是我也不能说本专业的合格医生不会采用这种做法。"如果专家这么说，那么没有通过专业过失的测试。

差错的后果

当确定差错如何严重（即到底有多么疏忽）时（也许只是轻微的失误，或者是严重的错误），通常其后果并不被考虑在内。最好的比喻是驾驶。粗心驾驶就是粗心驾驶，不管是否有人在事故中丧生或者是否只构成轻伤。两者粗心的程度是相同的。在确定一个司机是否粗心大意时，法庭感兴趣的只是驾驶行为本身的"恶劣"，而不是"后果的恶劣程度。"于是，患者可能由于医疗差错遭受重大的损失，但这一切与必须提出的首要问题并无关联，这个问题就是"给予患者的治疗是否存在失误，而合格的结直肠外科的医生是否应该采用这样的方式"？

原 因

对于任何一个医疗事故中，突破两种障碍是十分重要的。首先要证明存在过失，而且要证明合格的医生不会采用这一方案。其次要证明因果关系，有必要证明是差错导致了严重后果。通常的法律测试是基于"如果没有"的测试。一般情况下，肯定要问到的问题是"如果没有"差错，可能的结果会是什么？

在这里，举例说明一下，一名年轻的患者可能因腹痛到外科就诊，外科医生没有经过详查就诊断为肠易激综合征，并将其打发回家。如果两周后她因肠穿孔再次就诊且需要急症手术，病因是之前未能确诊的肠癌，她可能会认为治疗存在差错，因为在门诊就诊时并没有经过详查，她就被打发回家。然而，如果一个人着眼于事实，他就有可能发现两者之间不一定存在因果关系。因此，如果专科医生要求钡灌肠或结肠镜检查，而且考虑最可能的诊断是肠易激综合征，那么检查要求将被视为例行公事，有可能直到就诊后的 2~3 个月才进行检查。照此推断，作出诊断的时间有可能是在患者发生肠穿孔之后很久的时候了，因此这其中并不存在因果关系。有人可能会认为医生未能实施合适的治疗，但因果关系不会被证明，因为即使他的行为是合适的，也不会使最终结果有丝毫的改变。参照可能性平衡的原则，"如果没有"疏忽，结果仍将是现在这样。另一方面，如果患者因肛周脓肿就诊而医生未能及时处理，导致病变继续发展直至出现福耳尼埃氏坏疽，那么医生存在差错，理应为后果负责。这是因为合格的从业者通过适当引流，不应该治疗不了这样的脓肿。也许福耳尼埃氏坏疽无论怎样都会发生，但是参照可能性平衡的原则，司法界会认为它不会发生，所以医疗差错和坏疽的发生之间存在因果关系。

需要患者证明的唯一的一件事是如果没有发生差错，那么，基于可能性平衡的原则，脓肿会被引流，坏疽的发生是有可能避免的。患者只需要证明不发生坏疽的可能性有 51% 或者更大。因此，如果可能性是 51% 而不是 49%，那么法院会裁决支持当事人。

Bolitho 案例

一名医生被指控存在过失，专家的观点支持医生所采取的专业措施，并且专家表述一大群医疗观点相同的合格医生均会采用这种治疗方法，那么，根据 *Bolam* 测试标准，医生不存在医疗过失，因而无罪。作为结果，这个案子会被驳回。然而，*Bolam* 测试标准有诸多限制。对于被告来说，仅仅表述其专业领域的其他医生也会以相同方式治疗患者还不足以脱罪。他必须证明，这种采用相同方式的"别人"，其行为有理由充分、合乎逻辑的基础。

什么是 *Bolitho* 测试，它的适用范围是什么，最好的解释见于 2006 年 Lord Hodge 对于 *Honisz* 诉 *Lothian* 医疗委员会的裁决。在 Lord Hodge 的判定中，他说了下面的话：

首先，一般情况下，判断某一特定医疗行为是否恰当，在负责任的医疗从业人员相关群体中往往存在两种彼此对立的流派，法院所扮演的角色绝不倾向某一种流派的选择而压制另一派（*Maynard* 诉 *West Midlands Regional Health Authority*，Scarman 法官 见于 p.639F-G）。其次，法院不能完全听从相关专业人士的意见，以至于一旦辩护者提出证据证明相关执业医师群体中其他负责任的专业人员也会采用与受指责的医师相同的做法时，法官无论如何都会判定不存在过失。这是因为，第三，在特殊情况下，法院可以判定负责任的执业医师所坚持的某一做法经不起理性分析（*Bolitho* 诉 *City and Hackney Health Authority*，Browne-Wilkinson 法官，见于 p.241G-242F，243A-E）。法官充分了解了辩护者所依赖的主流专业意见，但他判定这些意见并不合理或可靠，或许会认为执业医师有医疗过错，尽管主流意见认可其行为。这种情况很少发生，因为评估和平衡医疗的风险与益处是临床判断的问题。因此做出这一裁定，通常需要由令人信服的专家提供证据，证明涉案的医学专家所持的观点不被其他专家认可，当然前提是这些专家认真分析了实践基础。根据 *Hunter* 诉 *Hanley* 一案，当专家经过深思熟虑，对某一做法的风险和益处进行评估并做出了经得起推敲的结论后，法庭没有理由去否定它，也就不能支持原告，做出存在医疗差错的判决……正如 Browne-Wilkinson 法官在 Bolitho 一案（见于 p.243D-E）中说的，'如果法官认为主流专家意见逻辑上缺乏基础，那么这些意见就不能成为评估被告行为的基准。

一个罕见的案例是 *Hucks* 诉 *Cole* [1993] 4, Med L R 393，Browne-Wilkinson 法官采用 Bolitho 测试来讨论案情。在那个病例中，产科病房的一位女士出现了脓点，而一位全科医生并未给其开出青霉素，最终这位女士发展成暴发性败血症。被告很聪明地承认其诊断存在风险，他考虑女士可能是产褥热，因为这种疾病的风险小，同时他的决定得到了知名专家证人的支持。不过，法官认为他是有过失的，而且上诉法院支持法官的决定，Sachs LJ 认为其专业行为中存在空白，而被告故意承担了一个容易避免的风险，仅通过初步培养就可以使其避免风险。因此，在法庭的判决书中，没给青霉素并没有一个合理的原因，对于执业医师来说，使患者暴露于风险之中是不合理的。

有关 Bolitho 测试的案例于 1997 年 11 月 13 日被提交至英国上议院。在这一案例中，一个 2 岁的儿童似乎时不时出现呼吸困难。一名资深护士呼叫了资深专业医师，但是她没有到场，在第二次出现呼吸急症情况时，儿童出现了心跳停搏，继而遭受到了严重的脑部损害，最终死亡。医生因未到场行使职责而被起诉，但是要证实因果关系却相当复杂。5 名著名的专家证人认为医生应到场，并且应实施气管插管，这样就可以防止出现这样的结果。但另一方面，医生说即使到场，也不会采取插管措施。之前这个儿童有好几次发作，每次脸色都会变得青紫，但之后每次都完全恢复，并且开始在周围玩耍，甚至在一次发作以后，还吃了很多饭。她不会采取插管措施的观点得到了另外 3 名知名专家的支持，他们引用了与不适当插管相关的发病率和死亡率作为风险的说明。这也就意味着法官必须面对不同的意见，而这些意见均由同样知名的专家支持。在英国上议院，Browne Wilkinson 法官提到了 1984 年 5 月 Scarman 法官在 Maynard 诉 West Midlands Regional Health Authority 一案中的意见，他是这样表述的：

……我必须指出，如果同时存在两种知名的专业意见，而法官却偏好其中一种主流意见，那么其判定从业人员存在过失的依据就不充分，而该人员的行为恰恰被那种未得到法官垂青的意见所认可，当然，这种意见也是真实公正的。如果个人喜好成为该法官进行裁决的真实原因，那么他的法律工作就走上了歧途，即使在其他地方他所做的法律裁决是正确的。在诊断和治疗领域，不能因为偏好某种受追捧的主流意见而不看好另一种来判定是否存在过失。医生（如果他是某相关专业的专科医生）未能实施基本的技能是判定存在过失所必须的。

在 Bolitho 一案中，法官几乎被两名最知名专家的意见所说服，而这两人的意见是不同的，尽管截然相反，但均代表了一种负责任的主流的专业意见，这些主流意见均由杰出和诚实的专家支持。法官认为如果医生到场诊查患者，并决定不实施插管，那么实际上她已达到技术和能力的适度水平（即，这一标准是由支持专家的观点所描述的）。因此，法官认为不能证明是由已被认可的医生的某些失职造成了灾难的发生，导致孩子不治。这个案例被提交至上诉法院，被驳回后又上诉至上议院。Browne Wilkinson 法官进一步引用了 McNair 法官在 Bolam 诉 Friern 医院管理委员会一案中对陪审团的陈述，具体如下：

我本人更愿意这样表达，如果他按照一个做法行事，而该种做法被熟知那种特定技能的一群负责任的医疗人员接受为适当，他就不应负过失责任……换句话讲，如果一个人按照这种做法行事，不能仅因为存在一种相反的意见就认定他有过失。

在这一案例中，关于因果关系，法官必须要确定如下问题：

1. 如果这名医生到场对孩子进行了诊查，那么她会做什么，或者批准做什么？
2. 如果她没有行气管插管，那她是否有过失？

Bolam 测试被认为与第一个问题没有关联，但对于第二个问题却极为重要。最终，上诉法院的法官和上议院认为，假如这名儿童很快从前两次的严重呼吸危机中恢复，那么为防止再一次的呼吸衰竭所带来的预知的风险而实施插管，插管将是有创的，而且并非没有风险。因此，法官驳回了上诉。对于原告指控存在过失，Bolam 案例和 Hunter 诉 Hanley 案都设置了相当高的门槛。二者的基础都是"一名合理的和负责任的医生会做什么"。而且，Bolitho 案例严重依赖 Bolam 测试，但尽管如此，最终还是要由法官在两种彼此冲突却同样权威的医学观点中做出决定。按照我的理解，上述案例提供了医疗诉讼的背景。现在，我将举例说明，这些例子涉及首次结直肠手术和结直肠重建手术，而我均作为一名顾问参与其中。

吻合口瘘

我非常感谢圣马克医院的 Robin Phillips 教授，正是他建议把吻合口瘘作为阐明 Bolitho 测试的一个方面。我们都知道吻合口瘘会使直肠癌手术变得复杂，而且新辅助放化疗有可能增加瘘的风险。一些研究者提出应强制性实施环状回肠造口术，它可以保护患者避免发生吻合口瘘的结果[1]，特别是老年病患，他们还将致死性的后果的瘘的发生率作为佐证。在 Matthiessen 等所做的随机试验[1]显示 defunctioning 的环状回肠造口术可以大大降低吻合口瘘的发生率。而后，涉及术前肠道准备的问题被提了出来。一项大型 Meta 分析得出的结论是：肠道准备不会影响瘘的发生率和死亡率[2]。这一结论连同由 Henrik KehletKehlet 倡导的强制恢复计划所获得的证据，导致结肠手术的肠道准备被大规模地摒弃，直肠手术的肠道准备在某种程度上也被舍弃了。最近，法国[3]进行了一项卓越的研究，此研究将接受直肠吻合术的患者随机分为行肠道准备组和非肠道准备组。未行肠道准备的患者，其瘘的发生率为19%，而那些行肠道准备的患者的瘘的发生率为10%。这还未具备统计学的显著性（$P=0.09$），但也高度提示了两者的差别。

接下来的问题是，当一名医生为一个化学治疗的患者实施了吻合手术，一切事情进展得几近完美时，还有什么是必须要做的？吻合口没有张力，断端有丰富的血供，充气试验为阴性，患者情况稳定，只有极少量的失血。（我们都知道这一状况，因为我们希望实施的每个吻合手术都能达到这一目标。）我们没有进行肠道准备，而且我们没有实施回肠造口术。很不幸，患者发生了瘘，患者和医生都崩溃了。当尽了最大努力，尽管尽可能提供最好的治疗仍无法弥补，事情依旧变得糟糕时，前者就会起诉，后者会接受其选择医学专业所带来的残酷性。T. Oresland在瑞典哥德堡工作，其指出功能不全的结肠会自行关闭，因此肠道准备并不重要，但是其他人认为，由于存在粪便，即使加做了环状回肠造口术，也不能预防瘘的发生。因此，Phillips辩称，在这种情况下，他不会批评外科医生未行造口。显然，依照Bolitho测试标准，会有许多不同意见，我希望这个讨论有助于解决专业的争论，并为通过法律处理类似案例提供手段。

必须提醒大家，吻合口瘘及其后果是常见的投诉，但是要想通过仔细分析病例记录中的各种因素来鉴定十分困难，尽管这些因素可能会暗示外科医生存在医疗过失。显然，如果吻合时的张力低于公认的张力，吻合处的肠管看上去颜色暗淡或苍白缺血，或吻合不能令人满意，那么除非医生采取适当的措施来处理手术时的缺陷，否则他们就没有尽到医疗的责任，也就应该为各种后果负责。另外，我们都认识到，吻合时即使没有张力、血液供应良好、兼顾了种种注意事项，一些患者仍然会随着病情的发展出现吻合口并发症，进而需要造口，而这个造口有时可能是永久性的。评论这些事件是很困难的。在大多数情况下，无论如何也未能发现存在过失，这种结局仅仅是不走运的后果。

是否要建立预防性造口一直是一个存在争议的话题。一例男性患者因低位直肠癌接受了放化疗，此次医生为其实施了恢复性吻合手术，在大多数情况下，人们可能会认为造口术是明智的选择。可是，如果手术完美而术后问题接踵而至，能否认为外科医生没有尽到治疗职责？很明显，高龄患者的死亡风险实际上比吻合口开裂所导致的死亡风险更大，在这种情况下，大多数医生宁可谨慎小心而选择造口术。如理性的外科医生进行了一台十分理想的手术，手术不是过分地困难，如果医生决定不行环形造口而结束手术，术后患者出现问题，我不确定是否能证明医生无须承担医疗过失之责。外科手术总会有风险平衡的考虑，毫无疑问有很多风险与造口的建立及闭合有关。这些情况本身可能有十分重大的意义，所以没有被轻易地忽略，因为有时候，患者恰恰死于造口相关并发症，此外还有相当比例的患者因造口出现严重的并发症，更不用说造口对于术后生活质量的影响。

产科损伤

经阴道分娩的产妇中，有1%~9%的人会发生产后括约肌损伤。在宾夕法尼亚州的费城，一项大型研究表明7.3%的患者存在三度或四度撕裂[4]。修复通常由产科医生实施，效果立竿见影，绝大多数女性恢复顺利，可以达到合理的控制，但有时会出现一些尿急或不能控制的排气，但大多数可以恢复正常的控制。这主要是由于括约肌这一结构有相当大的储备，可以允许伤害某种程度的损伤而不影响控制能力。控制能力恶化的原因有很多种：如女性的年龄，尤其是更年期前后；多次经阴道分娩，尤其是如果在分娩的第二阶段有延迟或需借助医疗干预，特别是使用了产钳；如果婴儿出生时体重超标（大于4kg）或头围特别大；或者是在下一次的阴道分娩时又发生了撕裂。最近的研究表明多达30%的女性在头胎分娩时经历了肛门括约肌损伤；这一损伤被称为"隐性损伤。"在一项由Sultan等[5]所做的研究中，研究者认为由技术熟练的产科医生做出的专家评估，会确定大多数的这类撕裂，而助产士和初级产科医生漏掉这类损伤的概率较高。另一项研究表明，三度或四度撕裂发生之后即由产科医生进行最初的修复，这以后的一段时期借助超声影像评估肛门括约肌时，可以发现超过90%的患者存在持续性的功能缺陷[6]。此外，经随访，这些缺陷通常变得更大[7]。

事实表明，产科损伤是常见的，大部分妇女似乎能够应付得当。目前尚不清楚究竟有多少人会恶化，尤其是更年期左右的妇女。产科的观点认为，如果三度的撕裂被修复，绝大多数的女性会达到可接受的控便效果。因此，当产科损伤被漏诊或处理得不尽完美，或者继发伤口感染和自制能力恶化时，许多产科专家认为，临床医生没有尽到他们的医疗职责，二者存在因果关系，因为如果处理得当，患者的控便能力会很好。换句话说，由于治疗中的感知失败，患者会出现大便失禁。

我经常被要求检视这样的病例并提供涉及因果关系的报告，同时涵盖病情和预后。许多患病女性的病情会进展，根据不同的病情，结直肠科的专家会为其进行择期修复手术，这一天往往被称为"cool light of day"。有些患者会恢复得很好，但是其他患者就不一定会这样。对于那些恢复糟糕的患者来说，这就深化了因果关系，加重了创伤，因此她们会因产科损伤的漏诊而寻求赔偿。此外，大多数修复肛门括约肌的结直肠专家认为，在绝大多数情况下，不能修复肛门内括约肌，而妇产科专家则认为可以；因此，这是专业的妇产科证据引证因果关系的另一个方面。Vaizey 和 Philips 在 Clinical Risk 中讨论道，妇产科医师在产房内的评估难免出现错误，因为在创伤分娩后，面对血淋淋、瘀紫和水肿的组织时，评估损伤程度存在很大困难。因此，看似全层的损伤实际上可能是不全层的，如我们认为已离断的内括约肌的一部分可能是完整的[8]。此外，他们认为即使采用了不恰当的修复，许多妇女也会恢复，但是因损伤需要正规修复而就诊于结直肠专家的患者毫无疑问是最严重的病例。从某种意义上说，因为存在严重的大便失禁，他们自己已经进行了选择，而许多的类似情况往往不会就诊，因为他们有残留的括约肌功能，在很大程度上是可以控制的。

George 等[9] 在给《journal Colorectal Disease》杂志的信中以"比较不能比较的：早期和延迟的括约肌成形术的比较"为标题，认为早期修复由产科医生现场进行。参与修复的医生并不知道正在修复的损伤是否有任何功能上的意义，且通常情况下妇产科医生往往并不精通对肛门括约肌的评估[8-9]。因此，不能确定确切的损伤程度。George 等质疑，损伤是涉及部分还是整个肛门外括约肌，同样，肛门内括约肌是否真正受损。另一方面，延迟修复通常由专业的结直肠外科医师在全面评估后进行，包括肛门超声检查，且只能在有显著功能缺陷的女性中进行。George 等做出了如下评论："在对待存在争议的病例时，这种比较的固有缺陷也是很重要的。"

有争议的是，与训练有素的产科医生相比，由有经验的专业结直肠外科医生修复肛门括约肌的预后可能会更好。事实上，Sultan 在一篇文章中报道，许多产科医师和高级学员在面对产科损伤时会感觉到训练得不充分，而难以做到令人满意的修复。我发现，这些案例经常会以原告胜诉而告终，而产科专家往往受到责难。虽然我们可以看到，在这些案例几乎都是患者自己做主进行选择的，而且事实上即使不能诊断出产科损伤，也不一定有因果关系。这是一个持续存在的争论。我们也确实知道，许多女性的产科损伤经超声扫描评估后会真实地存在严重损伤，但其中只有少数会出现二便失禁。另一方面，二便失禁的患者可能会认为他们的整体治疗是不理想的。而正是这些患者提起了诉讼。鉴于常见的血泪史，可以相对容易的证实，患者一旦确诊，适当的修复会发挥作用，女性患者会保留有二便的控制功能。其他未考虑的缓解因素包括持续存在的便溏或伴发的肠易激综合征。

当建议患者在产科损伤后进行延迟修复时，对于医师来说，现实中最重要的是为双方可能的期望值提供令人满意的证据。例如，如果患者的主诉是排气失禁，这是不太可能纠正的。同样如果他们的主诉是泻下急迫，虽然可以改善，但是患者很可能会持续存在这种令人烦恼的症状。如果他们的主诉是轻微失禁，通常是由于内括约肌功能缺陷所致。我们认识到，在试图修复肛门内括约肌时，我们的结果总是很差，因此失禁症状可能会持续存在，只有当出现可控性固体粪便，括约肌修复的结果才是满意的，而且会随着时间而持续。在我的实践中，告诉患者我不能使其恢复到正常，但是我希望做的是提高他们的控制力。此外，重要的是要告诫患者，其控制力可能会恶化，特别是如果存在并发症时。虽然轻微的创伤性脓毒症比较常见，但严重脓毒症很罕见。它可能导致可怕的后果，并可使患者出现直肠阴道瘘，在极少数情况下，需要预防性造口术。

因此，在患者开始手术前，了解获益与风险的平衡，适当的信息可以使其做出合理的判断。

肛门括约肌切开术

肛裂的括约肌切开术对于粗心的医生是一个潜在的雷区。对于不能采用保守方法治愈的、适当筛选的合适的年轻肛裂患者，限制性横向内括约肌切开术具有良好的预后，且导致粪便失禁的可能性很小。另外，具有肛裂的产后女性患者可能已经出现外括约肌的产科损伤，进行括约肌切开术可能会危及其控制力。此外，值得注意的是，女性括约肌切开术的范围通常比外科医师看到的大，而且如果切开全部内括约肌会有不良的预后。因此，在评估过程中需要非常谨慎。此外，肛裂的诊断必须准确。裂缝有时不是一个真正的肛裂。典型的慢性肛裂通常在中线，暴露内括约肌，且经常伴有前哨皮赘和肥大的肛乳头。失禁的患者由于损伤的原因可能会产生肛裂。根据定义，这些患者具有薄弱的括约肌，且遗憾的是，患有典型肛裂的患者很少能够诊断，且接受括约肌弱化程序完全不合适。

我已提出了一个经典的方案。一般患者四五十岁，且已经采用一氧化氮供体和钙通道阻滞剂治疗不成功，继续使用肉毒杆菌毒素注射，还是没有成功或愈合，最终采用内括约肌切开术，使其遗留有受损的控制力。这里的问题是，不通过括约肌切开术也可恰当地治疗典型的高压肛裂。同样，在产科损伤病例中，括约肌经常被婴儿的头部削弱或损伤，因而括约肌切开术不合适。我可以想象在法庭上形成与Bolitho相似的争论，有专家支持使用括约肌切开术而其他专家则反对。除外法律方面的原因，在病情方面，表象未必反映本质时，我会强调仔细临床评估和准确诊断的重要性。如果评估准确，且患者表现为典型的高压肛裂时，Brown等[10]和其他研究者已经证实，括约肌切开术的结果是理想的，且事实上控制力恶化的可能性极小。许多人可能已经存在大便失禁，令人惊讶的是部分医师在这类患者中不谨慎地开展括约肌切开术。我一直相信病史至关重要。当患者因为疼痛害怕排便时，这与肛裂一致。另一方面，疼痛在排便过程中不发生，而是在其后发生，这更符合肛门区域损伤后肛瘘和肛门刺激征，也就是更符合肛门区域损伤的泄漏和刺激。唯一的体征可能是薄线性裂纹样"裂隙"或溃疡。

这是肛瘘和失禁所致，当然不需要进行括约肌弱化程序。

横向与中线括约肌切开术

医疗证据表明，与中线括约肌切开术相比，侧向内括约肌切开术与手术后失禁的相关性可能更小。因此可以认为不应该再进行中线括约肌切开术。而且，因为中后位括约肌切开术的医学观念实践的合理性，在正中入路手术后，很难认为患者出现节制机制或大便失禁的术后损伤是不能接受的。这同样适用于开放与封闭的括约肌切开术。没有任何证据表明一个是比另一个更好或更安全。

再次手术：事情出问题时或当无过错而情况还没有得到解决时

一名外科医生有责任决定他们是否是进行其所计划进行手术的最佳人选。术后有可能会出现并发症，抑或是问题可能没有得到纠正。后者常见的例子是肛瘘和骶尾窦。前者的例子是进行贮袋后的脓毒症性并发症。外科医生需要首先确定他们是否有修复的必要技能，并试图寻求解决方案，或者是否应该将患者转诊给另一名更有经验的临床医生。寻求另一种观点听起来总是法律医师的做法，将有助于Hunter V. Hanley或Bolam的检验履行法律的字面意思。在一个多学科团队会议上，另一种策略将会讨论这种情况，使得其可越来越多地被应用到各种专业领域。我所看到的情况是，如果一名外科医生反复治疗肛瘘没有成功，最终外科医师会因为没能愈合病情而被患者责难。事实上，当节制力恶化时，这也可能阻碍外科医师的脚步。令人遗憾的是，节制力一定程度上的损伤可能是治愈肠瘘所付出的代价。另外，适当的劝告，详细的解释，同时为患者提供另一个选择的机会，可以使外科医生处于一个舒服的位置，他的患者充分知情，并能决定是否寻求其他意见。

在外科实践中，在有成功希望时，重复一个手术可能是恰当的。但此后外科医生必须认识到在反复失败的情况下，这种程序明显是不恰当的。手术可能会失败，因为外科医生仍未能提供恰当的标准，由于不能胜任，或更多的是因为存在一种并发症。前一种情况下是防不胜防的，但后者则是可以预防的，且再次手术可能是适当的。然而，如果再次手术失败了，那么我的观点是第三次手术是错误的，因为很明确，很多因素正在背向成功。

虽然我曾在不同场合下提出建议，但是最简单的例子就是肛瘘和骶尾窦。对于肛瘘，在很大程度上是一个技术问题。外科医生必须引流主要窦道和次要窦道，并确定主瘘。如果他们能够准确地做到这一点，并解决这一问题，患者将被治愈。如果保持开放是唯一可用的手术，那么提供建议会是容易的。目前的选择包括纤维蛋白胶，有或没有成纤维细胞和胶水的不同来源的胶原蛋白栓，推进皮瓣，有或没有挂线的开放方式。正如所有的所谓的手术中的新黎明，早期成功并不一定能够对抗时间的力量。纤维蛋白胶整体上是令人失望的，且栓子的结果并不像首次报道的一样好。皮瓣相对较少能够获得部分极佳的报道的结果。因此外科医生应该怎么办？在理想的情况下，他们应该对文献有一个很好的掌握，但不是每一名外科医生都可以实现这一目标。他们有责任出席会议，以继续其教育，且不断更新，使他们能够为患者提供适当的建议。期望必须是现实的，且必须评估这些技术失败的可能性。这样一来，患者的治疗会符合规则。另外，我确实相信反复进行同样的手术是不能接受的，在反复失败时，是时候寻求具备已证实技能的人，以治疗此类患者。

骶尾窦是沿着这些线路进行讨论的另一个领域。有研究者可能会保持开放、切除、切除与闭合、切除瘢痕、裂痕封闭与切除、并旋转皮瓣。该主题将会在第52章中进行详细讨论。哪个程序是最好的。对于每个患者来说，并不总是显而易见的。在我的实践中，我认识到多毛肌肉发达的男性的潜在难度，其骶尾窦位于臀部形成的深沟之下的较深位置。在大多数情况下，我会向已成为裂隙闭合专家的同事请教。以前对于我接手的复发病例，我会使用皮瓣，但显然裂隙闭合更简单。一名具有平坦新生裂隙的女性可以简单地通过单纯的保持开放和瘘管造口术治疗，并能很快治愈。

关于医学法律方面，我相信当外科医生简单地一遍又一遍地重复相同的手术时，问题即会出现。我曾经被问及一个患者的情况，该患者反复进行广泛的局部切除，然后再进行数月的敷药，伴随伤口慢慢变得粗糙，最后只有骶尾窦复发。这种情况持续了很多年都没有成功。最后，患者寻求另一种观念，且有了成功的皮瓣技术。对于外科医生来说，应该很清楚原来的程序不会发挥作用。一个假设就是外科医生不知道对于骶尾窦如何作别的东西。显然，当主要程序和重复手术失败时，他们应该考虑别的东西。如果医生缺乏专业知识，那么我相信他们有责任询问别人，以得到建议，并取得成功的预后。三级外科医生在寻求解决方法的时候，也可能有困难，但是这就是手术，在适当的治疗和知情时，失败也不存在过错。

另一个区域以并发症的治疗为中心，如恢复性直肠结肠切除术（即回肠粪袋手术）。是不是每个对结直肠手术有兴趣的外科医师应该进行粪袋手术？这可能会导致一般的外科医生会一年作一例或两例这样的手术。他们从来不会积累多少经验，且虽然有些人可能会取得极好的结果，但毫无疑问的是，这种困难手术的经验和熟练度会产生更好的预后。不可避免的是，这将是一个持续的争论，除非患者实际上在接受手术前既已质疑外科医师的经验。据我所知，没有任何法规、法律或其他，可以提示外科医生在将这种手术作为其经验的一部分之前应该有一定水平的经验。事实上，新任命的外科医生如何开始实践？显然他们在任命前既已接受了培训，但真正的"培训"和经验应遵循一个明确的实质性任命。

当事情出现错误时，我确实相信这种情况可能会不同，且对于并发症的治疗，采取有经验的外科医生的意见可能是一个明智之举。例如，外科医师可能不能充分处理正在发生的脓毒症，可能被视为在其治疗职责上已经失败，对于错误希望试图保留粪袋的患者，当脓毒症再次发作时，可能将这些患者置于危险当中，且损害健康，甚至偶尔会死亡。如果功能较差的患者使用磁共振成像扫描或其他症状证实盆腔存在脓毒症特征，然后外科医生有责任去处理这一切，如果他们没有信心或不能做到这样的话，建议请教另一名专家，因为不采取措施就会被解释为违反职责。即使外科医生认为他们知道如何处理这一个问题，从其他专家那里听取意见不是一个坏主意，然后返回到患者的讨论预后。这在知识上给患者安全感，他们正在沿着正确的道路前进。

当脓毒症使粪袋复杂化时，有明确的某些先决条件。这种问题不能遗留，如果外科医生不知道如何纠正这种情况，那么他们有责任向有相关经验的人需求帮助。不这样做将招致合理的批评，因为这不仅是外科医生治疗责任的失败，而且他们将对后果负责，且存在因果关系。

任何外科医生和"团队工作"

我所关心问题是，在英国医院内通常有越来越多的等候名单。有争论的是，在一个机构中所有的外科医生应该具有相似的能力，所以无所谓谁做手术。如在疝气手术中，一旦患者安排进行手术以修复腹股沟疝，谁进行手术不重要，只要如最初讨论的那样执行操作。这可能是我没有认识到疝气手术的复杂性，但我相信结直肠病的知情过程更为复杂。为了说明这一点，我举一个曾进行了2次痔切除术患者的例子，患者就诊于专家进行吻合器痔切除术，就诊的外科医生告之这种操作具有相对较小的痛苦。专家同意且安排患者进行吻合器手术。在能进行手术之前，外科医生离开，患者被安排在来自海外的代理医师的手术单中。该外科医生从来没有做过这种手术，所以进行了传统的结扎切除的痔切除术。术后患者非常不高兴，因为他出现了痛苦的肛裂，对此需要推进皮瓣进行医治。此外，术前患者抱怨的大小便失禁没有得到解决。

显然，在这里讨论的问题有很多。失禁方面，在恰当使用了3种手术中的任何一种后都没有得到解决，显然应该被进一步讨论。在这方面，患者有抱怨的理由，在进行任何手术前，应该详细研究。事实上，值得强调的是，患者不应该因为痔疮进行任何第三次手术。不幸的是，在现实生活中，这些决定是很容易的，二便失禁方面的专家很容易受到责难；我知道许多外科医生在面对明显脱垂的痔疮时，可能会做出类似的决定。因此如果征求我医学法律方面的意见，我想说作为一个专家，我不会同意手术的决定，但我会相信很多人会进行手术，所以我不会批判，并奉劝法院这一决策是正当医师采取的一个可以接受的决定。

接下来的问题围绕临时代理医生做了什么，应该已经做了什么。患者进行手术时承受了相当大的压力，患者可能有等待，有期望。外科医生可能会处于压力之下，特别是如果他或她相对缺乏经验，或是一个代理医师。在上述的情况下，代理外科医生进行了手术，这不是患者期待的。知情书中说"痔切除术"，所以缺乏详细说明。该案件解决了，并没有去法院，但我听到的意见是，在本案中做了"错误"的手术被认为是一个缺陷，因为这并不是所期待的。在一个理想的世界中，手术医师应该探望其所医治的每一例患者，在手术之前应该进行适当讨论，但目前的事实并非如此。

我们目前面临，从常规等候名单中收入院的患者，患有所谓的轻微的肛门直肠疾病，包括痔疮和肛瘘。不同的医生有不同的方法，差别可能很小，但已经形成了知情同意的一部分。如出现在一般肛瘘名单中的患者可能会出现持续的脓毒症问题。安排的外科医生可能从来没有讨论过影响控制力的因素，仅仅在手术前才是深入讨论危险因素的正确时间吗？我相信不是，但我们越来越多地被放置在这个位置上，除了这样做，没有别的选择。如果患者有每天定期排便的习惯，且控制力较好，没有腹泻，那么采用开放手术治疗时，控制力显著恶化的可能性较小。尽管如此，仍然需要讨论风险，且患者可能会被延期，或如前面讨论过的那样害怕新的外科医生。肛瘘保持开放，而不是持续使用引流，可能发挥最佳的作用，但这可能不是患者所期望的。而且，这涉及知情同意的问题。

结 论

我已经开始学习关于初次和再次结肠直肠肛门手术的医学法规方面的法律。正如我所说的一样，要求我们对患者尽职尽责，且大多数医师会尽其所能做到这一点。如果出现并发症而未能达到最高标准，也不构成玩忽职守。现在需要我们行为得当，且做到其他正规医师所做到的。当出现困难时，来自同事的讨论和建议是明智的，我相信团队法可以使患者得到保障。现在，在英国医院内，这是许多治疗的标准做法。可悲的是，失误一定会发生，患者和外科医生都不得不面对相应的后果。如果正规的外科医生不会以特殊的方式行事，那么患者或其亲属将没有理由申诉。另一方面，如果竭尽了所有努力，预后仍然是不成功的，那么医生将不承担任何责任。

致 谢

感谢 Andrew Pollock 高级律师、Peacock Johnston 律师及 Glasgow 的仔细阅读，并检查我对法律解释的准确性。感谢 Lord Hodge 总结列入文中的法律知识，感谢他非常有帮助的建议；同样感谢他指导我在苏格兰建议并研究非常有意义的案例。

参考文献

1. Matthiessen P, Hallbook O, Rutegard J, Simert G, Sjodahl R. Defunctioning stoma reduces symptomatic anastomoticleakage after low anterior resection of the rectum for cancer: a randomized multicenter trial. Ann Surg. 2007;246:207–14.
2. Slim K, Vicaut E, Launay-Savary MV, Contant C, Chipponi J. Updated systematic review and meta-analysis of randomized clinical trials on the role of mechanical bowel preparation before colorectal surgery. Ann Surg. 2009;249:203–9.
3. Bretagnol F, Panis Y, Rullier E, Rouanet P, Berdah S, Dousset B. Rectal cancer surgery with or without bowel preparation. The French Greccar III Multicenter Single-Blinded Randomized Trial. Ann Surg. 2010;252:863–8.
4. Dandolu V, Gaughan JP, Chatwani AJ, Harmanli O, Mabine B, Hernandez E. Risk of recurrence of anal sphincter lacerations. Obstet Gynecol. 2005;105:831–5.
5. Andrews V, Sultan AH, Thakar R, Jones PW. Occult anal sphincter injuries–myth or reality? Br J Obstet Gynaecol. 2006;113:195–200.
6. Starck M, Bohe M, Valentin L. Results of endosonographic imaging of the anal sphincter 2–7 days after primary repair of third- or fourth-degree obstetric sphincter tears. Ultrasound Obstet Gynecol. 2003;22:609–15.
7. Starck M, Bohe M, Valentin L. The extent of endosonographic anal sphincter defects after primary repair of obstetric sphincter tears increases over time and is related to anal incontinence. Ultrasound Obstet Gynecol. 2006;27:188–97.
8. Vaizey CJ, Phillips RKS. A twisted tale. Clin Risk. 2005;11:53–6.
9. George AT, Vaizey CJ, Phillips RKS. Comparing the incomparable: a comparison between primary and delayed sphincteroplasty. Colorectal Dis. 2009;11:656–7.
10. Brown CJ, Dubreuil D, Santoro L, Liu M, O'Connor BI, McLeod RS. Lateral internal sphincterotomy is superior to topical nitroglycerin for healing chronic anal fissure and does not compromise long-term fecal continence: Six-year follow-up of a multicenter, randomized, controlled trial. Dis Colon Rectum. 2007;50:442–8.